£ 22·50

D1363086

'A

7

Strength and Power in Sport

VOLUME III OF THE ENCYCLOPAEDIA OF SPORTS MEDICINE

AN IOC MEDICAL COMMISSION PUBLICATION

IN COLLABORATION WITH THE

INTERNATIONAL FEDERATION OF SPORTS MEDICINE

EDITED BY

PAAVO V. KOMI

**Blackwell
Science**

© 1992 International Olympic Committee

Published by
Blackwell Science Ltd
Editorial Offices:
Osney Mead, Oxford OX2 0EL
25 John Street, London WC1N 2BL
23 Ainslie Place, Edinburgh EH3 6AJ
238 Main Street, Cambridge
  Massachusetts 02142, USA
54 University Street, Carlton
  Victoria 3053, Australia

Other Editorial Offices:
Arnette Blackwell SA
  1, rue de Lille, 75007 Paris
  France

Blackwell Wissenschafts-Verlag GmbH
  Kurfürstendamm 57
  10707 Berlin, Germany

  Zehetnergasse 6, A-1140 Wien
  Austria

First published 1991
Reissue in paperback 1993
Reprinted 1994, 1996

Set by Excel Typesetters, Hong Kong
Printed and bound in Great Britain by
Butler & Tanner Ltd, Frome and London

DISTRIBUTORS

Marston Book Services Ltd
  PO Box 87
  Oxford OX2 0DT
  (*Orders:* Tel: 01865 791155
       Fax: 01865 791927
       Telex: 837515)

North America
  Blackwell Science, Inc.
  238 Main Street
  Cambridge, MA 02142
  (*Orders:* Tel: 800 215-1000
       617 876-7000
       Fax: 617 492–5263)

Australia
  Blackwell Science Pty Ltd
  54 University Street
  Carlton, Victoria 3053
  (*Orders:* Tel: 03 9347-0300
       Fax: 03 9349-3016)

British Library
Cataloguing in Publication Data

Strength and power in sport.
  1. Sports. Physical fitness
  I. Komi, Paavo V.   II. Series
  613.71

  ISBN 0-632-03031-3 (hbk)
  ISBN 0-632-03806-3 (pbk)

Library of Congress
Cataloging-in-Publication Data

Strength and power in sport/edited by Paavo V. Komi
       p.   cm.—(The Encyclopaedia of sports medicine)
  ISBN 0-632-03031-3 (hbk)
  ISBN 0-632-03806-3 (pbk)
  1. Sports—Physiological aspects.   2. Muscle strength.
  3. Athletic training.   I. Komi, Paavo V.   II. Series.
  RC 1235.S76   1992
  612'.044—dc20

Part title illustrations by Grahame Baker

Contents

v

List of Contributors

R. BILLETER PhD, *Department of Anatomy, University of Bern, CH-3000 Bern 9, Switzerland*

G.A. DUDLEY PhD, *Biomedical Operations and Research Office, National Aeronautics and Space Administration, Kennedy Space Center, Florida 32899, USA*

V.R. EDGERTON Prof PhD, *Brain Research Institute and Department of Kinesiology, University of California at Los Angeles, Los Angeles, CA 90024-1761, USA*

K.A.P. EDMAN Prof MD, *Department of Pharmacology, University of Lund, S-223 62 Lund, Sweden*

S.J. FLECK PhD, *Sport Science Division, US Olympic Commitee, Colorado Springs, Colorado 80909, USA*

J. GARHAMMER Prof PhD, *Biomechanics Laboratory, Department of Physical Education, California State University, Long Beach, CA 90840, USA*

G. GOLDSPINK Prof PhD, *Department of Veterinary Basic Sciences, Royal Veterinary College, University of London, London NW1, UK*

G. GRIMBY Prof MD, *Department of Rehabilitation Medicine, University of Göteborg, Sahlgren's Hospital, S-413 45 Göteborg, Sweden*

R.T. HARRIS, MS, *Department of Zoological and Biomedical Sciences, Ohio University, Athens, Ohio 45701, USA*

J.G. HAY Prof PhD, *Department of Exercise Science, University of Iowa, Iowa City, IA 52242, USA*

H. HOPPELER Prof MD, *Department of Anatomy, University of Bern, CH-3000 Bern 9, Switzerland*

P.A. HUIJING PhD, *Faculteit Bewegingswetenschappen, Vrije Universiteit, Amsterdam, NL 1081 BT, The Netherlands*

R.S. HUTTON* Prof PhD, *formerly of Department of Psychology, University of Washington, Seattle, WA 98195, USA*

S. ISRAEL Prof MD, *Faculty of Sport Science, University of Leipzig, D-7010 Leipzig, Germany*

H.G. KNUTTGEN Prof PhD, *Center for Sports Medicine, Pennsylvania State University, University Park, PA 16802, USA*

P.V. KOMI Prof PhD, *Department of Biology of Physical Activity, University of Jyväskylä, 40100 Jyväskylä, Finland*

W.J. KRAEMER PhD, *Center for Sports Medicine, Pennsylvania State University, University Park, PA 16802, USA*

B.J. LOITZ PhD, *Department of Kinesiology, University of California at Los Angeles, Los Angeles, CA 90024-1568, USA*

*Dr R.S. Hutton unfortunately died during publication of this volume.

J.D. MacDOUGALL Prof PhD,
*Department of Physical Education and Department of
Medicine, McMaster University, Hamilton L8S 4K1,
Ontario, Canada*

T. MORITANI PhD, *Laboratory of Applied
Physiology, College of Liberal Arts and Sciences, Kyoto
University, Kyoto 606, Japan*

J. NOTH Prof MD, *Neurological Clinic with
Clinical Neurophysiology, Alfried Krupp Hospital,
D-4300 Essen 1, Germany*

R.R. ROY PhD, *Brain Research Institute,
University of California at Los Angeles, Los Angeles,
CA 90024-1761, USA*

D.G. SALE Prof PhD, *Department of Physical
Education, McMaster University, Hamilton L8S 4K1,
Ontario, Canada*

D. SCHMIDTBLEICHER Prof PhD,
*Institut für Sportwissenschaften, Johann Wolfgang
Goethe Universität Frankfurt/Main, D-6000
Frankfurt/Main 90, Germany*

M.H. STONE Prof PhD, *Health, Leisure and
Exercise Science, Appalachian State University, Boone,
NC 28608, USA*

B. TAKANO *United States Weightlifting
Federation, Biology Faculty, Van Nuys Math/Science
Magnet School, Van Nuys, CA 91411, USA*

P.A. TESCH PhD, *Department of Physiology,
Karolinska Institutet, S-104 01 Stockholm, Sweden*

K. TITTEL Prof MD, *Faculty of Sport Sciences,
University of Leipzig, D-7010 Leipzig, Germany*

H. WUTSCHERK Prof PhD, *Faculty of Sport
Sciences, University of Leipzig, D-7010 Leipzig,
Germany*

R.F. ZERNICKE Prof PhD, *Department of
Surgery, University of Calgary, Calgary, Alberta T2N
4N1, Canada*

Preface

It was an honour to receive an invitation to serve as editor of the volume *Strength and Power in Sport*. This volume is the third one in the series of publications entitled *Encyclopaedia of Sports Medicine*, which presents state-of-the art information about current topics of clinical and scientific importance. The initial volume, *The Olympic Book of Sports Medicine*, resulted from extensive collaboration between the Medical Commission of the International Olympic Committee (IOC) and the Scientific Commission of the International Federation of Sports Medicine (FIMS). The success of this publication resulted in the establishment of the IOC Publications Advisory Committee, which was formed for the purpose of planning and producing succeeding volumes of the *Encyclopaedia of Sports Medicine*. The second volume in this series *Endurance in Sport* was published only a few weeks prior to the current volume *Strength and Power in Sport*.

Acceptance of the editorial leadership for the present volume placed me in a very demanding but challenging situation. The first stages of the editorial work required formation of the outline of the content of the volume. It was a rewarding and motivating experience to receive full support for the intended content from the IOC Publications Advisory Committee. Selection of the potential contributors for the various chapters is naturally a difficult task, but I was fortunate to receive acceptance from all the scientists contacted. The recruited team of 29 contributing authors represents the most prominent scientists and clinicians, all of whom have interest in the various problems related to strength and power training. But, more importantly, they have all established themselves as world leaders in their particular research or applied area.

Several books have been published related to strength and power which have advanced our understanding of the subject area. In the present volume we have made an effort to take a slightly different approach to the problem. While it is very easy to demonstrate improvement of muscle strength with almost any method—if sufficiently intensive—the present volume, *Strength and Power in Sport*, examines the basic mechanisms and reasons for beneficial strength exercises. In order to give state-of-the-art information—as is the purpose of the *Encyclopaedia of Sports Medicine*—a great portion of the book is devoted to the basics of strength and power and their adaptation. The material is divided into five sections.

1 Definition of fundamental terms and concepts.

2 A comprehensive coverage of the biological basis for strength and power including the structural, hormonal, neural and mechanical aspects.

3 A detailed examination of the reasons (mechanisms) leading to the adaptations of the organism when subjected to various strength and power exercises. This section covers eight different topics ranging from cellular and neural adaptation to endocrine and cardiovascular responses.

4 Special problems of strength and power training including age-related changes, the potential use of electrical stimulation, and clinical aspects.
5 The volume finishes with a more applied and solely sports-orientated section where three chapters cover the current knowledge of the practical strength and power training principles, as based on available scientific knowledge.

The way the material has been presented varies slightly between chapters. In some cases, considerable depth and detail were necessary; on the other hand, a few chapters have been written in a more readable and overview-type format. Whatever the writing style has been, the material should be accessible to readers with a background in biological aspects of sport sciences. Because of the wide coverage of basic mechanismic features of strength and power training, it is expected that this volume will become required reading for many graduate programmes in medicine and the science of sport. The study of strength and power is one of the major components of sports science, and understanding of the relationships between neural, hormonal, muscular and mechanical factors is central to athletic performance as well as to strength and power needs of other human populations.

Paavo V. Komi, *Jyväskylä, Finland*

Units of Measurement and Terminology*

Units for quantifying human exercise

Mass	kilogram (kg)
Distance	metre (m)
Time	second (s)
Force	newton (N)
Work	joule (J)
Power	watt (W)
Velocity	metres per second $(m \cdot s^{-1})$
Torque	newton-metre (N·m)
Acceleration	metres per second^2 $(m \cdot s^{-2})$
Angle	radian (rad)
Angular velocity	radians per second $(rad \cdot s^{-1})$
Amount of substance	mole (mol)
Volume	litre (l)

Terminology

Muscle action: The state of activity of muscle.
   Concentric action: One in which the ends of the muscle are drawn closer together.
   Isometric action: One in which the ends of the muscle are prevented from drawing closer together, with no change in length.
   Eccentric action: One in which a force external to the muscle overcomes the muscle force and the ends of the muscle are drawn further apart.

*Compiled by the Publications Advisory Committee, IOC Medical Commission.

Force: That which changes or tends to change the state of rest or motion in matter. A muscle generates force in a muscle action. (SI unit: newton.)

Work: Force expressed through a displacement but with no limitation on time. (SI unit: joule; note: 1 newton × 1 metre = 1 joule.)

Power: The rate of performing work; the product of force and velocity. The rate of transformation of metabolic potential energy to work or heat. (SI unit: watt.)

Energy: The capability of producing force, performing work, or generating heat. (SI unit: joule.)

Exercise: Any and all activity involving generation of force by the activated muscle(s). Exercise can be quantified mechanically as force, torque, work, power, or velocity of progression.

Exercise intensity: A specific level of muscular activity that can be quantified in terms of power (energy expenditure or work performed per unit of time), the opposing force (e.g. by free weight or weight stack) isometric force sustained, or velocity of progression.

Endurance: The time limit of a person's ability to maintain either an isometric force or a power level involving combinations of concentric and/or eccentric muscle actions. (SI unit: second.)

Mass: The quantity of matter of an object which is reflected in its inertia. (SI unit: kilogram.)

Weight: The force exerted by gravity on an object. (SI unit: newton; traditional unit: kilogram of weight.) (Note: mass = weight/acceleration due to gravity.)

Free weight: An object of known mass, not attached to a supporting or guiding structure, which is used for physical conditioning and competitive lifting.

Torque: The effectiveness of a force to overcome the rotational inertia of an object. The product of force and the perpendicular distance from the line of action of the force to the axis of rotation. (SI unit: newton-metre.)

Strength: The maximal force or torque a muscle or muscle group can generate at a specified or determined velocity.

PART 1

DEFINITIONS

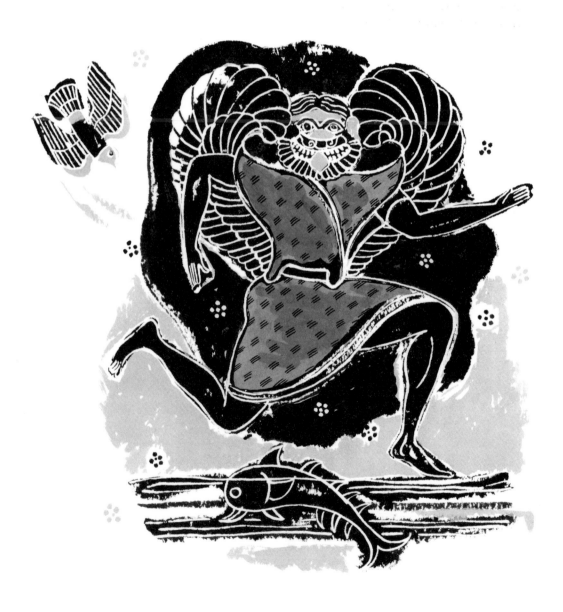

Chapter 1

Basic Definitions for Exercise

HOWARD G. KNUTTGEN AND PAAVO V. KOMI

Physical exercise and sport performance are made possible by means of forces developed by the voluntary muscles of the body acting through the lever systems of the skeleton. Unfortunately, the description and measurement of human performance of exercise and sport have been plagued through the years by the use of a variety of terms and measurement systems. Frequently, terms have been misused and units of measurement inappropriately applied. For these reasons, communication among scientists, physicians, coaches, and athletes has been hampered.

When the threshold of excitation of a muscle cell (fibre) is attained, the elements of the cell's sarcomeres act to shorten the cell along its longitudinal axis. Even when the cell is prevented from shortening, the term that has been traditionally applied to this event is *contraction* as, without restraint, a diminishment in the length of the muscle cell would occur. The microstructures that make up the sarcomeres of a muscle cell are routinely referred to as the contractile elements.

During the performance of sport skills, the recruitment of motor units for the purpose of developing force between the attachments of muscles to bones may or may not result in shortening the muscle and drawing the attachments closer together. The basic objective of muscle cell activation is to cause filament sliding as a result of the crossbridge attachments from myosin to actin filaments so that the Z-discs of an active sarcomere are drawn closer together. Depending on the ratio between the total activation (neural signal input) and any opposing force acting on the attachments of a muscle, the sarcomere movement may be either shortening or lengthening or there may be no change in the total muscle length. In forceful lengthening of the muscle, the muscle activation may not be capable of causing shortening but, instead, it resists the stretch while muscle is lengthening.

Another objective of the muscle activation, especially in submaximal force development, is to recruit selectively an appropriate pool of motor units so that the movement is controlled and may result in shortening of the muscle, the maintenance of a particular length (as in the stabilization of body parts), or a controlled lengthening of muscle length as the distance between bony attachments increases.

To describe the state of activity of muscle as a 'contraction' when the muscle may be shortening, maintaining the same length, or being increased in length seems inappropriate. Therefore, the term *muscle action* has been proposed (Cavanagh, 1988) to describe the result of skeletal muscle force development interacting with the external forces that affect the body parts of an organism which, in the context of this volume, is the exercising human.

Muscle actions

The interaction of muscle force development and the external forces will result in actions that

Table 1.1 Classification of exercise and muscle action types

Exercise	Muscle action	Muscle length
Dynamic	Concentric	Decreases
	Eccentric	Increases
Static	Isometric	No change

produce static exercise (no movement about the related joints) or in dynamic exercise (involving either an increase or decrease in joint angles). Static exercise of activated muscle is traditionally referred to as *isometric*. Force is developed but, as there is no movement, no work is performed. All other muscle actions involve movement and are termed *dynamic*. The term *concentric* is traditionally used to identify a shortening action and the term *eccentric* is used to identify a lengthening action (see Table 1.1).

Isometric and dynamic actions can be assessed at any particular length of the muscle and/or positioning of the related body parts in terms of: directly measured force from the muscle or its tendon; force at a particular point on the related body parts; or torque about the axis of rotation. A dynamic action must be further described in terms of directionality (shortening or lengthening) and the velocity of muscle length change or body part movement.

Because of variation in mechanical advantages as a joint angle is changed as well as differences in maximal force capability of a muscle through its range of length, no dynamic action of a muscle in exercise and sport performance involves constant force development. Therefore, the term 'isotonic,' implying uniform force throughout a dynamic muscle action, is inappropriate for the description of human exercise performance and should not be employed.

Furthermore, a variation in linear movement occurs with muscles in both sport skill performance and exercise on mechanical devices. For this reason, the term 'isokinetic' to denote constant velocity should not be employed

to describe a muscle action. Although the controlled movement of an exercise machine or ergometer may be at constant velocity and described as being isokinetic, this provides no guarantee that the muscles that are providing force in the movement are acting at constant velocity.

Human locomotion seldom involves pure forms of isolated concentric, eccentric, or isometric actions. This is because the body segments are periodically subjected to impact forces, as in running or jumping, or because some external force such as gravity causes the muscle to lengthen. In many situations, the muscles first act eccentrically with a concentric action following immediately. The combination of eccentric and concentric action forms a natural type of muscle function called a *stretch–shortening cycle* or SSC (Norman & Komi, 1979; Komi, 1984). The SSC is an economical way to cause movement and, consequently, the performance of the muscle can be enhanced. A chapter in this volume has been especially devoted to muscle performance in SSC.

Quantification of exercise performance

If *exercise* can be defined as any and all activity involving force generation by activated skeletal muscles (Knuttgen & Kraemer, 1987), the resultant performance can be assessed in terms of the physical concepts of force, torque, work, power, and velocity. *Force* is that which changes or tends to change the state of rest or motion in matter (SI unit of force: newton (N)). *Torque* is the effectiveness of a force to produce rotation of an object about an axis and is measured as the product of the force and the perpendicular distance from the line of action of the force to the axis of rotation (SI unit of torque: newton metre (N · m)). *Work* is equivalent to a force expressed through a displacement with no limitation on time (SI unit of work: joule (J)). *Power* is the rate of performing work or the rate of transformation of metabolic potential energy to work and/or heat (SI unit of power: watt (W)). It should be noted that the force of 1 N expressed through the displacement of 1 m results in 1 J of work. The transformation of 1 J of metabolic potential energy to work or heat in 1 s results in 1 W of power. The basic unit of measurement for *velocity* is metre per second.

The *exercise intensity* can, therefore, be quantified in various situations as: the opposing force in dynamic exercise, e.g. provided by a free weight, exercise machine, or ergometer; isometric force sustained; power (energy expenditure or work performed per second); or velocity of progression, e.g. running, cycling, rowing. *Endurance* is the time limit of a person's ability to maintain either an isometric force or a power level of dynamic exercise (basic SI unit of time: second (s)).

Strength and power

The ability to exert maximal force is commonly referred to as the *strength* of the muscles that control particular body movements. However, the muscles may perform maximal effort as either isometric, concentric, or eccentric actions and the two dynamic actions may be performed at a wide range of velocities. An infinite number of values for the strength of muscle(s) may be obtained either for an isolated muscle preparation or for a human movement as related to the type of action, the velocity of the action, and the length of the muscle(s).

Therefore, strength is not the result of an assessment performed under a single set of conditions. Because of the number of variables or conditions involved, strength of a muscle or muscle group must be defined as the maximal force generated at a specified or determined velocity (Knuttgen & Kraemer, 1987).

For comparative purposes, the force and/or torque measurements must be performed when the muscle or muscle groups are at similar lengths or as the peak force obtained during a dynamic action. The measurements may be obtained directly from the muscle or its tendons, from a particular point on one of the body

parts, or as torque developed on a testing device. Regardless of the measurement technique, the assessment must precisely identify the muscle action, the velocity of the action, and the muscle length (alternatively, the joint angle).

Power can be determined for a single body movement, a series of movements, or, as in the case of aerobic exercise, for a large number of repetitive movements. Power can be determined instantaneously at any point in a movement or averaged for any portion of a movement or bout of exercise.

For the simple movement of lifting and/or lowering a free weight, the force (N) necessary to oppose the force of gravity (N) acting on the free weight mass (kg) operates through a displacement (change in altitude in metres) during a determined time (s)*. Force (N) multiplied by the displacement (m) determines the work (J) which, divided per unit of time (s), yields the power (W). The same determinations can be accomplished for any mechanical device where a weight stack is employed to provide the force opposing the body movement being performed.

An alternative system developed for exercise programmes in rehabilitation medicine (De Lorme, 1945) has been adopted in many situations in which strength assessment and strength development is carried out. While the testing methodology does not readily yield precise information about force and/or torque development at specific muscle lengths and joint angles, the system offers the advantage of ease of test administration. Either free weights or an exercise machine can be employed.

The basic test consists of determining the number of repetitions a person can perform to exhaustion in lifting a certain mass. The mass (kg) is then described in terms of a 'repetition maximum' or RM. For example, a person lifts

*It should be noted that the work done in lifting a weight should not be calculated using a force value equal to force of gravity (weight). The definition must consider the fact that the lifting force depends on both the weight and its acceleration.

a mass of 72 kg 10 times before exhaustion; therefore, 72 kg is identified as the person's 10 RM for the particular body movement and conditions of the test (e.g. free weight vs. machine, free cadence vs. controlled cadence). If the largest mass the person can lift without repetition is 98 kg, this mass is identified as the 1 RM, the person's strength score for the movement according to this procedure. Performance assessment and exercise prescription can then be accomplished in terms of the mass of a specific RM or percentages of the mass of the 1 RM. Determination of a 1 RM in this manner for each body movement constitutes one approach for assessing the strength of the muscles in performing the movement.

Summary

Accurate and reproducible determinations of strength and power can be accomplished through careful control of testing procedures and adherence to an internationally accepted system of measurement. Such practice guarantees confidence in the evaluation of changes occurring in individual athletes and the comparison of results among athletes. Appropriate use of standardized terminology in scientific and lay publications enhances meaningful communication among all concerned.

References

Cavanagh, P.R. (1988) On 'muscle action' vs. 'muscle contraction'. *Journal of Biomechanics*, **22**, 69.

De Lorme, T.L. (1945) Restoration of muscle power by heavy resistance exercises. *Journal of Bone and Joint Surgery*, **27**, 645–67.

Knuttgen, H.G. & Kraemer, W.J. (1987) Terminology and measurement in exercise performance. *Journal of Applied Sports Science Research*, **1**, 1–10.

Komi, P.V. (1984) Physiological and biomechanical correlates of muscle function: effects of muscle structure and stretch–shortening cycle on force and speed. In R.L. Terjung (ed.) *Exercise and Sport Sciences Reviews*, Vol. 12, pp. 81–121. The Collamore Press, Lexington, Mass.

Norman, R.W. & Komi, P.V. (1979) Electromechanical delay in skeletal muscle under normal movement conditions. *Acta Physiologica Scandinavica*, **106**, 241–8.

PART 2

BIOLOGICAL BASIS FOR STRENGTH
AND POWER

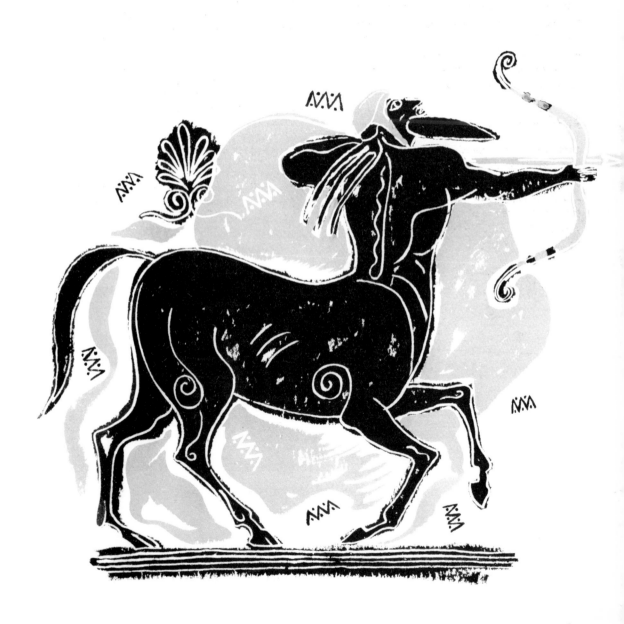

Chapter 2A

Cortical and Peripheral Control

JOHANNES NOTH

Our motor system must cope with a great diversity of internal and external demands and constraints. These include the regulation of upright posture and locomotion, goal-directed movements of the arms, manipulative finger movements, the oculomotor system and even our repertoire of gestures. The sensorimotor control of these various systems while showing some common features, also differs in fundamental aspects. Extraocular eye muscles, for instance, lack a direct feedback system via muscle spindle afferents. No external load can influence the movement of the eyeballs, thus making a load-compensating feedback loop impossible. The main task of the oculomotor system is to keep the fovea precisely on target. This is achieved by control systems in the brain stem and the cerebellum utilizing information from the visual and vestibular system. The arm and leg muscles, on the other hand, deal with varying loads that are not predictable. They require information from skin and deep receptors, which is fed back via different spinal and supraspinal pathways in order to assist in the central control of movements and posture. In addition, cues about the spatial coordinates of objects in the environment of the body are relayed to the central motor system via exteroceptors. This information is necessary for the accurate planning of goal-directed movements, for locomotor tasks, and for postural adjustments.

As it is impossible to describe the specific control features of the various motor systems in isolation, an attempt will be made to delineate the basic principles of motor control, with special reference to the skeletomotor system, which plays the major role in the control of strength and power in sports. This approach will be guided by the functional anatomy of the main motor components and by their interactions, in so far as they are known.

Hierarchical structure of central motor systems

The central motor system is organized in a hierarchical fashion (Fig. 2.1). Motor programming takes place in the premotor cortex (PMC), the supplementary motor area (SMA) and other association areas of the cortex. Inputs from these areas, from the cerebellum and, to some extent, from the basal ganglia converge to the primary motor cortex (MI, area 4 according to Brodmann) and finally excite or inhibit the corticobulbar and corticospinal neurones of MI. These output neurones of MI have a powerful influence on interneurones and motoneurones of the brain stem and of the spinal cord. In primates, a monosynaptic link exists between the corticospinal tract and alpha-motoneurones, providing direct cortical control of muscle activity. The influence of descending motor systems from the brain stem on the spinal cord has become less important in primates, especially in the case of the rubrospinal tract. Thus, the primary motor cortex can influence the spinal cord directly via the pyramidal tract

9

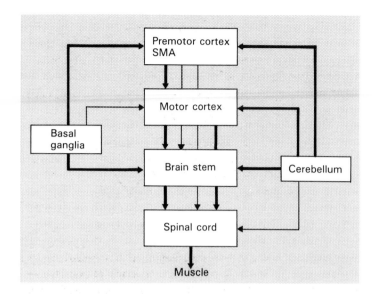

Fig. 2.1 Diagram of hierarchical organization of central motor systems. Thickness of lines indicates importance of connections.

and, indirectly, by modulating the activity of the descending brain stem systems (mainly the vestibulospinal and the reticulospinal tracts). The alpha-motoneurone is the final point of summation for all the descending and reflex input, and the net membrane current of this motoneurone determines the firing pattern of the motor unit and thus the muscle activity. Sherrington recognized the unique task of these neurones by characterizing them as the 'final common pathway'.

The motor cortex

Premotor areas

In humans, the PMC has reached a considerable size and is about six times larger than the primary motor cortex (Bonin, 1949). The corresponding ratio in the monkey is 1:1, which indicates the importance of this cortical area in human motor control. Together with the SMA (Fig. 2.2), these premotor cortices constitute an important relay for information from other cortical areas and subcortical nuclei (basal ganglia and cerebellum via the thalamus) to the primary motor cortex. In addition, the PMC

projects to the brain stem and to the spinal cord via the cortico-reticulospinal tract, and this route is thought to be responsible for the control of the muscles of the trunk and the proximal limb. The functional role of the PMC, as derived from clinical observations (Foerster, 1909; Freund & Hummelsheim, 1985) and from single cell studies in monkeys (Weinrich *et al.*, 1984) includes the preparation of movements, the postural control, the visual guidance of movements, and rapid corrections of ongoing movements in response to novel sensory cues.

The SMA is located medial to the PMC (Fig. 2.2). Its motor function is not, as yet, fully understood. A dominant afferent input comes from the motor loop of the basal ganglia, via the thalamus. This loop is involved in the initiation of movements that are generated by internal motivation. Wise and Strick (1984) have therefore speculated that 'perhaps those aspects of movement that depend on internal guidance are particularly the province of the supplementary motor cortex, whereas those aspects that depend upon an interaction of both exteroceptive and internal guidance are the province of the non-primary motor cortex as a whole'.

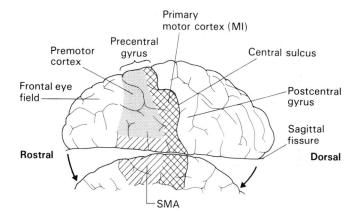

Fig. 2.2 Scheme of the motor cortex of the right hemisphere. Primary motor cortex extends deep into the central sulcus. The lateral border reaches the Sylvian fissure (not shown). The medial aspect of the right hemisphere is turned up in order to show the medial border of MI and of SMA.

The primary motor cortex

The MI lies in the precentral gyrus and extends deep into the rostral bank of the central sulcus (Fig. 2.2). The main output is the corticospinal tract, which originates from large (Betz cells), medium-sized and small neurones of layer 5 of MI. Betz cells only amount to 3% of the over 1 million corticospinal fibres passing the medullary pyramid. This number compares well with the 2% of thick myelinated axons of the corticospinal tract. Thus, only a small number of the corticospinal tract fibres carry information at high speed (about $65\,\mathrm{m}\cdot\mathrm{s}^{-1}$), whereas the majority of fibres are involved in processing information at a slower speed. Corticospinal fibres terminate on motoneurones and interneurones (Phillips, 1969). Monosynaptic control dominates in distal arm and leg muscles and subserves the independent control of these muscles. More proximal limb muscles are mainly linked via polysynaptic interconnections with the corticospinal tract. Proximal limb muscles and, as mentioned above, still more so the axial muscles receive, in addition, input via the premotor area and the reticulospinal system.

There exists a long-standing debate about the organization of the motor cortex, i.e. whether functional connections with muscles are represented in single spots within MI or whether there are multiple representations. Sherrington raised this question by asking whether the motor cortex thinks in terms of muscles or movements. Recent experiments performed in monkeys by using the microstimulation technique have clearly shown that action of distal arm muscles can be elicited by stimulation of multiple, well separated foci within MI (Strick & Preston, 1982; Sato & Tanji, 1989). This observation is in line with the notion that the motor cortex is organized in such a way as to optimize the selection of muscle synergies and not for the selection of a single muscle. Thus, to answer Sherrington's question, the motor cortex thinks in terms of movements and not of muscles.

Coding of dynamic and kinematic parameters of movements

In recent years, experiments have been performed to elucidate the coding of motor parameters by neurones of the primate motor cortex. The first studies were focused on the relationship between the activity of identified pyramidal tract neurones and the magnitude of the force generated by arm muscles (Cheney & Fetz, 1980; Fromm, 1983). Task-related neurones exhibited a positive relation between discharge rate and force and showed a steady-state activity, which was consistent with the length–tension relation of the muscle, i.e. force production at a smaller muscle length was associated with higher discharge rate, and vice versa. In addition, force was graded by the activation of higher threshold neurones, similarly to the recruitment of alpha-motoneurones at increasing muscle force (Fromm, 1983). Unlike the behaviour of motoneurones, however, low discharge rates of pyramidal tract neurones were observed during tasks requiring maximal actions of synergistic muscles, i.e. during execution of the power grip of the hand, whereas finely graduated finger movements were associated with much higher discharge rates (Muir & Lemon, 1983).

The coding of neurones during arm movements of monkeys in three-dimensional space was recently investigated by Georgopoulos and coworkers. The activity of task-related cells varied in an orderly fashion with the direction of movement, i.e. the discharge rate was highest with movements in the preferred direction (Schwartz et al., 1988). The vector sum of the contribution of the neuronal population determined the direction of the arm movement in space well before the movement began (Georgopoulos et al., 1988). It could further be shown that different classes of neurones with phasic and tonic action subserve these dynamic and kinematic aspects of motor planning (Kalaska et al., 1989). Which parts of the motor programme are delegated to subcortical centres such as the basal ganglia and the cerebellum will be discussed in a later section.

Stimulation of the motor cortex in man

Non-invasive tools are today available to assess the normal and disturbed function of the corticospinal tract in humans. Single shocks, which are delivered by specially designed electric or magnetic stimulators and which are applied to the scalp over the motor cortex, can evoke muscle twitches in skeletal muscles. The activation of the muscle can be quantified by electromyography (EMG). This method has provided some interesting new insights into the function of the corticospinal tract. Firstly, cortical stimulation elicits larger EMG responses in distal hand muscles than in more proximal arm muscles. Secondly, in slightly preactivated muscles, the amplitude of the EMG response to cortical stimulation may exceed that evoked by maximal stimulation of the corresponding muscle nerve. Thirdly, the central conduction speed, calculated from the difference in latency between cortical and cervical stimulation, has been found to be around $65 \, \text{m} \cdot \text{s}^{-1}$ (Day et al., 1987; Hess et al., 1987; Rothwell et al., 1987).

These results show that the corticospinal tract has a powerful action on human arm muscles. The excitation reaches the target muscles via the central and peripheral pathway with a fast conduction velocity of $65 \, \text{m} \cdot \text{s}^{-1}$. A single cortical shock can elicit multiple excitatory potentials, which, in turn, can induce repetitive discharges in alpha-motoneurones. However, these results only reflect the function of the fast component of the corticospinal tract. Much less is known about the role of the vast majority of slowly conducting corticospinal fibres.

The oculomotor system

The principles of the central and peripheral control mechanisms of the oculomotor systems are better understood than those of the skeletomotor system. This is mainly due to the fact that the design of the oculomotor system is more easily comprehended. The eyes can be rotated around three imaginary axes that intersect in the centre of the eyeball, and each rotation (horizontal, vertical, torsional) is controlled by a pair of antagonistic muscles. Rotations outside these principal directions are controlled by the vector contribution of muscles operating in synergy. In most situations both eyes move together. These conjugate eye movements, when performed around one of the principal axes, are induced by pairs of synergistic muscles. For example, horizontal gaze to the left side is caused by activation of the left lateral rectus and the right medial rectus muscles.

This uniform principle of organization persists in the vestibular nuclei of the brain stem and in the semicircular canal system of the labyrinth. This means that two corresponding semicircular canals, which measure the rotation of the head around a principal axis, control a pair of vestibular nuclei on either side of the brain stem, and these nuclei, in turn, govern the bilateral pair of eye muscles via the motor nuclei (Büttner-Ennever, 1981). By this device, head rotations lead to opposite rotations of the eyes, in order to stabilize the image on the retina during active and passive head movements. This automatic compensation is called the vestibulo-oculomotor reflex (VOR).

When the surrounding visual field is moved and the head is kept in a stable position in space, an optokinetic nystagmus is induced. This type of eye movement is characterized by a tracking movement of the eyes followed by a fast saccade bringing the eyes back to a neutral position. During active and passive head movements, both the VOR and the optokinetic system act together to stabilize the eyes in space.

The smooth pursuit system is concerned with tracking or fixation of a small target once it has been located. The aim of this system is to keep the image on the fovea (the centre of the visual field with the highest visual acuity). The three systems described so far and the vergence system are controlled by neurones in the brain stem and in the cerebellum. The most voluntary system, the saccadic eye system, is, in addition, controlled by the prefrontal eye field (Fig. 2.2). This cortical area can initiate eye movements to any target of interest in the visual space. In man, voluntary saccades can reach angular velocities of $8-10$ rad $\cdot$ s^{-1}, which is much faster than any active or passive limb movements under normal conditions. In order to achieve these high angular velocities, the motoneurones of the eye muscles can fire at rates of about 500 impulses $\cdot$ s^{-1}. Spinal motoneurones, in contrast, discharge at the onset of fast movements at maximal rates of about 200 impulses $\cdot$ s^{-1} for two or three initial

spikes. Discharge rates then quickly drop to 40 impulses $\cdot$ s^{-1} or less. Thus, the oculomotor system is the fastest movement system in the body.

The oculomotor system has to operate with high precision. Even the smallest misalignments of the eyes can cause double vision, which grossly disturbs visual accuracy. Factors that can produce misalignment are the growth of the body, changes in refraction of the eyes, wearing of glasses, deterioration of the gain of the VOR due to lesions of the semicircular canals, as well as many other causes. Therefore, the gain of these control systems requires a continuous readjustment, which is the task of the cerebellum.

Cerebellum as an adaptive control system

General function of the cerebellum

The cerebellum is a neuronal network that contains half of all the neurones in the brain. In contrast to the cerebrum, the neuronal matrix of the cerebellum is entirely uniform, which indicates that the internal functioning of all areas of the cerebellum is similar. The huge number of cellular compartments is needed for parallel processing and storage of information. The cerebellum is, in fact, involved in the learning and execution of all motor programmes in the body, from the most voluntary commands to the least voluntary reflexes.

A scheme of the neuronal organization of the cerebellum is shown in Fig. 2.3. Two excitatory input systems reach the cerebellum, the mossy fibre system and the climbing fibre system. Both provide collaterals to the deep cerebellar nuclei, which contain the output cells of the cerebellum. Mossy fibres synapse on the granule cells, which send their axons via the parallel fibres to the dendritic trees of the Purkinje cells. These parallel fibres make excitatory contact with a large number of Purkinje cells. The climbing fibres, on the other hand, ascend directly to the dendrites of the

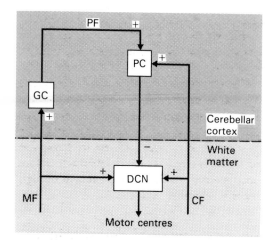

Fig. 2.3 Simplified scheme of input and output systems of the cerebellum. Inhibitory neuronal circuits within the cerebellar cortex are neglected. CF, climbing fibres; DCN, deep cerebellar nucleus; GC, granule cells; MF, mossy fibres; PC, Purkinje cells; PF, parallel fibres.

action potential of a climbing fibre elicits one 'complex spike' in the Purkinje cell. This is an action potential followed by a number of smaller spikes. Mossy fibres only evoke 'simple spike' activity. Due to the low discharge rate, climbing fibre activity is not directly related to the ongoing control of motor activity. It is believed that the occurrence of complex spikes, which depends on the firing of climbing fibres, modifies the gain of the excitatory pathway from mossy fibres to Purkinje cells. This change in gain is stored and becomes manifest in subsequent executions of the same motor programme. According to this concept, the cerebellar cortex has an important task in motor learning. It is not the part of the brain in which motor programmes are stored, but rather is the site where the main adaptive control of all motor systems resides.

In order to fulfil the function sketched out above, the cerebellum requires information about the intended motor plan and the actual performance of the movement. The two input systems to the cerebellum, the mossy fibres and the climbing fibres, provides this information by connecting all relevant sensory systems and integrative motor centres with the cerebellar cortex. The nature of the specific information carried in the two afferent systems is one of the current questions in cerebellar research.

Purkinje cells. One climbing fibre excites only a single Purkinje cell. The Purkinje cell is the sole output neurone of the cerebellar cortex, with all of them making inhibitory synaptic contacts with the deep cerebellar nuclei.

The firing pattern of the mossy and climbing fibres differs markedly. The former have high discharge rates (50–100 impulses · s^{-1}) and provide the excitatory background for the Purkinje cells. The climbing fibres discharge at low rates, but due to their tight coupling with the dendrites of the Purkinje cells, a single

Of the various cerebellar subsystems, the control of the VOR is the best described system, and this will be selected in order to exemplify the fundamental working mechanisms of the cerebellum.

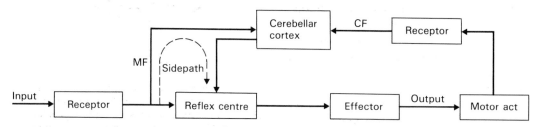

Fig. 2.4 Cerebellar sidepath model. A copy of the input signal reaches the cerebellar cortex via the mossy fibre system (MF) and is transmitted via the Purkinje cells to the reflex centre. The gain of this loop is modified by a feedback signal from the climbing fibre system (CF), which acts as an error detector.

Cerebellar control of the vestibulo-ocular reflex

The VOR has already been introduced as a feedforward device to stabilize the image on the retina during active and passive head movements. A pure feedforward system has the disadvantage that changes in gain are not detectable and that they therefore cause misalignments between the desired and the actually achieved eye position in space. The network sketched in Fig. 2.4 demonstrates how the cerebellum compensates for this default. The mossy fibre system adds a sidepath to this feedforward system. These fibres transmit a copy of the output of the vestibular receptors to the Purkinje cells, which, in turn, have direct synaptic connections with the vestibular nuclei. The climbing fibres, on the other hand, signal the performance of the motor act, i.e. shifts of the visual image on the retina during the head movements, to Purkinje cells. This feedback signal is thought to adjust the gain in the side-path of the VOR by modulating the mossy fibre–Purkinje cell pathway.

The validity of this concept is supported by lesioning experiments, which have shown that a disruption of the cerebellar sidepath abolishes the adaptation of the VOR (for review see Ito, 1984). According to this model, the efference copy of the motor command is transmitted via the mossy fibre system and the Purkinje cells to the reflex centre, whereas the climbing fibre system relays the error between the intended and the accomplished motor act to the Purkinje cells. Error signals reaching the Purkinje cells modify the gain of the mossy fibre pathway, until the error is minimized. Whether this concept can be generally applied to cerebellar control systems is an open question, but it is a useful working hypothesis with a sound experimental background.

The cerebellum is also involved in most voluntary motor acts. A powerful cerebro-cerebellar loop exists, which relays information from the sensorimotor cortex back to the pre-motor and the primary motor cortex. The func-tion of this loop is not known, but it may be speculated that it adjusts the output of the motor cortex in a similar way to the mechanism demonstrated for the VOR. A lesion of the cerebellum never causes a paresis of skeletal muscles, which shows that the maximum force output is not dependent on an intact cerebellar function. The cerebellum is responsible for the adaptation of any motor act to changes of internal or external restraints, and it is therefore most relevant for the accomplishment of high motor precision.

Motor functions of the basal ganglia

The basal ganglia consists of five major nuclei, the caudatum, the putamen, the globus pallidus, the nucleus subthalamicus, and the substantia nigra (Fig. 2.5). Two of these nuclei, the globus pallidus and the substantia nigra,

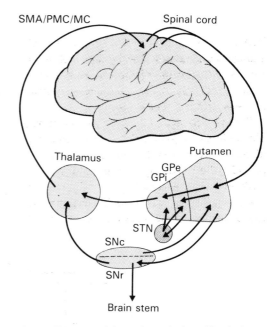

Fig. 2.5 Diagram of the main extrinsic and intrinsic connections of the motor loop of the basal ganglia. GPe, globus pallidus externus; GPi, globus pallidus internus; MC, primary motor cortex; PMC, premotor cortex; SMA, supplementary motor area; SNc, substantia nigra pars compacta; SNr, substantia nigra pars reticulata; STN, subthalamic nucleus.

can be further subdivided into functionally separate subunits. The main receiving nuclei are the caudatum and the putamen, which obtain information from almost all cortical areas. In contrast to the cerebellum, the basal ganglia are not directly fed with signals from receptor systems, and the specific nature of the information sent to these receiving nuclei of the basal ganglia is, up until now, obscure. Recordings from single neurones within the putamen and the caudatum and the effects of microstimulations suggest that both nuclei are embedded in two functionally different loops, the motor loop and the cognitive loop (DeLong et al., 1984). Within the motor loop, the putamen receives input from the premotor cortices, the MI and the somatosensory cortex. The internal segment of the globus pallidus and the pars reticulata of the substantia nigra are the output nuclei. They project to some brain stem nuclei and via a powerful thalamo-cortical pathway to the SMA and the PMC, and, according to new data, to a lesser degree also to the MI. The pathway to the brain stem is mainly involved in the control of eye movements, whereas the cortical projection is concerned with the control of the skeletomotor system.

The processing of information within the basal ganglia is currently one of the most extensively studied topics in motor control. It is beyond the scope of this introduction to cover this new field, which is excellently reviewed by Alexander and Crutcher (1990). Instead, some ideas about the putative function of the basal ganglia in motor control will be developed. The first notion that the basal ganglia might be concerned with the release of motor programmes following external or internal stimuli came from animal experiments, in which lesions of the basal ganglia produced neglect, i.e. an inability of the animal to respond to familiar stimuli. This concept found support in clinical observations. Parkinsonian patients, who are afflicted with a deficiency of a major neurotransmitter in the striatum, dopamine,

are severely impaired in the initiation of movements and especially in the release of internally released motor programmes (for recent review see Marsden, 1989).

Modern neurophysiological methods allow the analysis of the response pattern of neurones within the basal ganglia in the behaving monkey. The results obtained in these studies support the view that this system deals with the selection and sequencing of motor programmes. In the striatum, functionally different classes of neurones have been found. A number of cells responded in close relation to a sensory stimuli; the firing of others were related to the execution of the behavioural response, and a third class was involved in the recognition of behaviourally important stimuli; they quickly adapted when the stimulus was given without a behavioural context (Rolls, 1984; Hikosaka et al., 1989a,b; Kimura, 1990). Functionally similar neurones have been identified in the main cortical projection areas of the basal ganglia, the SMA and the PMC. From this and neuroanatomical findings it can be concluded that the basal ganglia are involved in the preparation of axial and proximal limb muscles for the execution of goal-directed movements. The preparation for and the execution of a movement requires exact timing, and it is likely that the elaboration of these commands is an important task of the basal ganglia. They select those internal and external cues that are behaviourally relevant, and initiate the preparation and execution of movements by sending the appropriate commands to the premotor centres in the cortex and the brain stem.

Spinal cord and the principles of peripheral motor control

The spinal cord is the lowest level in the hierarchical structure of the central motor system. Together with the brain stem, it is the site where all motoneurones are located. A major function of the spinal cord is the integration of

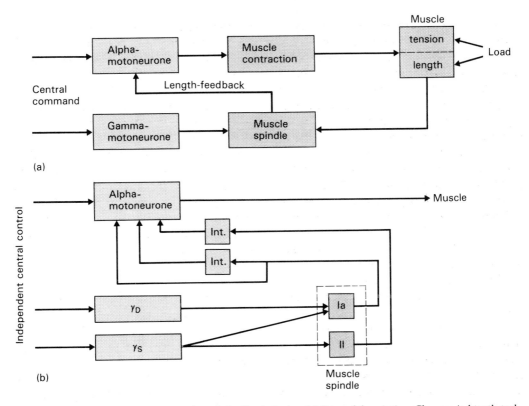

Fig. 2.6 Muscle spindle loop acting as a length-feedback device. (a) General description. Changes in length and tension of the muscle depend on the degree of muscle activation and on the load force. (b) Diagram to illustrate operation of dynamic (γ_D) and static gamma-motoneurones (γ_S). γ_D regulates velocity sensitivity of Ia afferents. γ_S determines the position sensitivity of both types of afferents. Ia afferents make monosynaptic and polysynaptic contacts with alpha-motoneurones via spinal interneurones (Int.), whereas monosynaptic contacts of group II muscle spindle afferents are scanty.

descending commands with peripheral inputs. In addition, interneurones in the spinal cord are capable of generating rhythmic activity, and they modulate the output of motoneurones and the gain of spinal reflexes. Another important function of the spinal cord in motor control is the processing of afferent information and the transmission of this information to supraspinal centres. Most important in this context are the ventral and dorsal spinocerebellar tracts in the lateral funiculus, and the dorsal columns. The latter relay cutaneous and proprioceptive information to the somatosensory cortex.

The understanding of the function of the local neuronal networks and of the descending and ascending pathways in the spinal cord is rapidly growing, and the reader is referred to the survey of Baldissera *et al.* (1980). In the following section, current concepts about the functional role of the stretch reflex and of its fusimotor control are presented.

The spinal stretch reflex

A simplified scheme of the muscle spindle loop is depicted in Fig. 2.6. Changes in muscle length are sensed by muscle spindle endings, which make monosynaptic and polysynaptic contacts with alpha-motoneurones innervating their own and synergistic muscles. An increase in load acting on the muscle evokes an increment in muscle length, and, via the excitation of muscle spindle endings, an extra-depolarization of the alpha-motoneurones, which counteracts the change in length (Fig. 2.6a). Thus, the muscle spindle loop functions as a feedback system, which stabilizes the muscle length. The sensitivity of muscle spindle endings can be regulated by virtue of gamma-motoneurones, which innervate the intrafusal muscle fibres. The sensory region of the muscle spindle can thus be viewed as a comparator, which signals differences between the length of extrafusal and intrafusal muscle fibres to the alpha-motoneurones.

In such a system, activation of gamma-motoneurones can induce length changes of the extrafusal muscle via the feedback loop. In engineering terms, such an operation is called a follow-up servo-loop mechanism, and, for a long time, at least slow movements were thought to be caused by an independent central drive of gamma-motoneurones.

This concept has been disproved by Vallbo (1971), who managed to record the firing of primary muscle spindle endings (Ia afferents) of human arm muscles during voluntary movements. There was no evidence for Ia excitation preceding the onset of muscle activation, which would be a prerequisite for servo action. This observation called for a reformulation of the servo-loop hypothesis, and today it is believed that the muscle spindle loop operates, under certain conditions, in a 'servo-assistance' manner. This means that the inevitable unloading of the muscle spindle during self-induced shortening actions of a muscle is counteracted by a concomitant shortening of the intrafusal muscle fibres. This is accomplished by a central command exciting both the alpha-motoneurones and the gamma-motoneurones. Under functional considerations, this model has some apparent advantages. Firstly, a quick onset of the contraction due to a direct feedforward command utilizing the high conduction velocity of alpha-fibres. Secondly, a resetting of the length-feedback system, which would otherwise counteract the shortening action.

Fusimotor control of muscle spindle endings

However, this model does not take into account that the muscle spindle loop is equipped with two types of gamma-motoneurones (Fig. 2.6b). The two types can be distinguished by their specific influence on the sensitivity of primary muscle spindle endings (Ia) to ramp and hold stretches: dynamic gamma-motoneurones (γ_D) enhance the velocity sensitivity of Ia fibres, whereas static gamma-motoneurones (γ_S) increase the position sensitivity of Ia fibres and reduce their velocity sensitivity. Secondary muscle spindle endings are exclusively innervated by γ_S. The two types of gamma-motoneurones have similar conduction velocities, which are about one-third of that of the alpha-fibres. A similar ratio of $3:1$ holds true for the conduction velocities of primary (Ia) and secondary (II) muscle spindle endings.

It has long been debated whether or not γ_D and γ_S can be independently controlled during various motor tasks. Stimulation of distinct centres in the brain can elicit fusimotor effects in restricted animal preparations, which makes separate fusimotor control likely. More recently, Ia firing recorded in freely moving cats has been simulated by different modes of fusimotor stimulation in anaesthetized cats (Hulliger et al., 1985). Although the simulation technique has been criticized for disregarding the effect of muscle contraction on the Ia firing, some principal findings emerged from this study.

1 There is evidence for an independent control of alpha- and gamma-motoneurones, and of γ_D and γ_S, respectively.

2 Under many conditions, fusimotor activity is steady and provides a certain set of velocity or position sensitivity of Ia fibres, which can change with the type of movement selected.

3 A linkage between alpha and gamma activity

can occur during powerful muscle actions. In this situation, the concomitant gamma-drive may prevent the unloading of muscle spindles as mentioned above.

Functional considerations

Regarding the functional meaning of the stretch reflex, an attractive hypothesis has been put forward by Nichols and Houk (1976). They suggest that an important role of the spinal stretch reflex is the control of muscle stiffness. A muscle deprived of its reflex control only reacts insufficiently to a sudden increase in load. After a short steep increase in tension (short-range elastic stiffness), the muscle tension gives way, in spite of ongoing muscle lengthening. With intact reflex loop, the stretch reflex comes into play during this 'yielding' phase and leads to an extension of the high stiffness range. These experiments have been performed in cats, but human data suggest that in man, too, the stretch reflex can compensate for the yielding of muscles exposed to forcible stretches during forward falls onto the outstretched arms (Dietz et al., 1981). During running and jumping, the Ia-mediated stretch reflex can even be utilized for the active shortening of a muscle following a stretch (Dietz et al., 1979; for review see Komi, 1984). Although not yet proven, it is reasonable to assume that under these conditions γ_D activity provides a high 'dynamic' gain around the muscle spindle loop.

In contrast, during standing and walking these fast, Ia-mediated spinal reflexes are suppressed, as experiments with treadmill perturbation have shown (Dietz et al., 1985). Under these conditions, compensatory reflexes are dominant that have longer latencies and which are resistant to ischaemic blocking of Ia-fibres. These polysynaptic reflexes do not obey the synergistic pattern of the monosynaptic spinal reflex, but are bilaterally expressed, even during unilateral displacement of a leg (Berger et al., 1984). From these and other observations it has been concluded that these polysynaptic compensatory reflexes are mainly mediated via secondary muscle spindle endings (group II), which have access to spinal interneuronal circuits (for review see Dietz, 1987).

These are only a few examples demonstrating how the spinal stretch reflex and its gain can be adjusted to cope with the functional demands of the various motor tasks. Two principal mechanisms can be distinguished: (i) switching from one motor programme to another, with a profound change in reflex control; and (ii) gain adjustment during the execution of a motor programme according to internal and external restraints. For the latter, the cerebellum plays an important role by selecting the appropriate gain during repeated executions of the same motor programme.

References

Alexander, G.E. & Crutcher, M.D. (1990) Functional architecture of basal ganglia circuits: neural substrates of parallel processing. *Trends in Neurosciences*, **13**, 266–76.

Baldissera, F., Hultborn, H. & Illert, M. (1980) Integration in spinal neuronal systems. In V.B. Brooks (ed.) *Handbook of Physiology. Section 1. The Nervous System. Vol. 2, Motor control*, pp. 509–95. Williams & Wilkins, Baltimore.

Berger, W., Dietz, V. & Quintern, J. (1984) Corrective reactions to stumbling in man: neuronal coordination of bilateral leg muscle activity during gait. *Journal of Physiology*, **357**, 109–25.

Bonin, G. von (1949) Architecture of the precentral motor cortex and some adjacent areas. In P.C. Bucy (ed.) *The Precentral Motor Cortex*, pp. 7–82. University of Illinois Press, Urbana.

Büttner-Ennever, J.A. (1981) Vestibular–oculomotor organization. In A.F. Fuchs & W. Becker (eds) *Progress in Oculomotor Research*, pp. 361–70. Elsevier, Amsterdam.

Cheney, P.D. & Fetz, E.E. (1980) Functional classes of primate corticomotoneuronal cells and their relation to active force. *Journal of Neurophysiology*, **44**, 773–91.

Day, B.L., Rothwell, J.C., Thompson, P.D., Dick, J.P.R., Cowan, J.M.A., Berardelli, A. & Marsden, C.D. (1987) Motor cortex stimulation in intact man. 2. Multiple descending volleys. *Brain*, **110**, 1191–209.

DeLong, M.R., Alexander, G.E., Georgopoulos, A.P., Crutcher, M.D., Mitchell, S.J. & Richardson, R.T. (1984) Role of basal ganglia in limb movements. *Human Neurobiology*, **2**, 235–44.

Dietz, V. (1987) Role of peripheral afferents and spinal reflexes in normal and impaired human locomotion. *Revue Neurologique*, **143**, 241–54.

Dietz, V., Noth, J. & Schmidtbleicher, D. (1981) Interaction between pre-activity and stretch reflex in human triceps brachii during landing from forward falls. *Journal of Physiology*, **311**, 113–25.

Dietz, V., Quintern, J. & Berger, W. (1985) Afferent control of human stance and gait: evidence for blocking of group I afferents during gait. *Experimental Brain Research*, **61**, 153–63.

Dietz, V., Schmidtbleicher, D. & Noth, J. (1979) Neuronal mechanisms of human locomotion. *Journal of Neurophysiology*, **42**, 1212–22.

Foerster, O. (1909) Der Lähmungstypus bei corticalen Hirnherden. *Deutsche Zeitschrift für Nervenheilkunde*, **37**, 349–414.

Freund, H.-J. & Hummelsheim, H. (1985) Lesions of premotor cortex in man. *Brain*, **108**, 697–733.

Fromm, C. (1983) Changes of steady state activity in motor cortex consistent with the length–tension relation of muscle. *Pflügers Archiv*, **398**, 318–23.

Georgopoulos, A.P., Kettner R.E. & Schwartz, A.B. (1988) Primate motor cortex and free arm movements to visual targets in three-dimensional space. II. Coding of the direction of movement by a neuronal population. *Journal of Neuroscience*, **8**, 2928–37.

Hess, C.W., Mills, K.R. & Murray, N.M.F. (1987) Responses in small hand muscles from magnetic stimulation of the human brain. *Journal of Physiology*, **388**, 397–419.

Hikosaka, O., Sakamoto, M. & Usui, S. (1989a) Functional properties of monkey caudate neurons. I. Activities related to saccadic eye movements. *Journal of Neurophysiology*, **61**, 780–98.

Hikosaka, O., Sakamoto, M. & Usui, S. (1989b) Functional properties of monkey caudate neurons. III. Activities related to expectation of target and reward. *Journal of Neurophysiology*, **61**, 814–32.

Hulliger, M., Zangger, P., Prochazka, A. & Appenteng, K. (1985) Simulations reveal large variations in fusimotor action in normal cats: 'fusimotor set'. In J.A. Boyd & M.H. Gladden (eds) *The Muscle Spindle*, pp. 311–15. Stockton Press, New York.

Ito, M. (1984) *The Cerebellum and Neural Control*. Raven Press, New York.

Kalaska, J.F., Cohen, D.A.D., Hyde, M.L. & Prud'homme, M. (1989) A comparison of movement direction-related versus load direction-related activity in primate motor cortex, using a two-dimensional reaching task. *Journal of Neuroscience*, **9**, 2080–102.

Kimura, M. (1990) Behaviorally contingent property of movement-related activity of the primate putamen. *Journal of Neurophysiology*, **63**, 1277–96.

Komi, P.V. (1984) Physiological and biomechanical correlates of muscle function: effects of muscle structure and stretch–shortening cycle on force and speed. In R.L. Terjung (ed.) *Exercise and Sport Sciences Review, Vol. 12*, pp. 81–121. The Collamore Press, Lexington, Mass.

Marsden, C.D. (1989) Slowness of movement in Parkinson's disease. *Movement Disorders*, **4** (suppl. 1), S26–S37.

Muir, R.B. & Lemon, R.N. (1983) Corticospinal neurons with a special role in precision grip. *Brain Research*, **216**, 312–16.

Nichols, T.R. & Houk, J.C. (1976) Improvement in linearity and regulation of stiffness that results from actions of stretch reflex. *Journal of Neurophysiology*, **39**, 119–42.

Phillips, C.G. (1969) Motor apparatus of the baboon's hand. *Proceedings of the Royal Society of London B*, **173**, 141–74.

Rolls, E.T. (1984) Response of neurons in different regions of the striatum of the behaving monkey. In J.S. McKenzie, R.E. Kemm & L.N. Wilcock (eds) *The Basal Ganglia. Structure and Function*, pp. 467–93. Plenum Press, New York.

Rothwell, J.C., Thompson, P.D., Day, B.L., Dick, J.P.R., Kachi, T., Cowan, J.M.A. & Marsden, C.D. (1987) Motor cortex stimulation in intact man. 1. General characteristics of EMG responses in different muscles. *Brain*, **110**, 1173–90.

Sato, K.C. & Tanji, J. (1989) Digit-muscle responses evoked from multiple intracortical foci in monkey precentral motor cortex. *Journal of Neurophysiology*, **62**, 959–70.

Schwartz, A.B., Kettner, R.E. & Georgopoulos, A.P. (1988) Primate motor cortex and free arm movements to visual targets in three-dimensional space. I. Relations between single cell discharge and direction of movement. *Journal of Neuroscience*, **8**, 2913–27.

Strick, P.L. & Preston, J.B. (1982) Two representations of the hand in area 4 of a primate. I. Motor output organization. *Journal of Neurophysiology*, **48**, 139–49.

Vallbo, A.B. (1971) Muscle spindle response at the onset of isometric voluntary contractions in man. Time difference between fusimotor and skeletomotor effects. *Journal of Physiology*, **318**, 405–31.

Weinrich, J., Wise, S.P. & Mauritz, K.-H. (1984) A neurophysiological study of the premotor cortex in the rhesus monkey. *Brain*, **197**, 385–414.

Wise, S.P. & Strick, P.L. (1984) Anatomical and physiological organization of the non-primary motor cortex. *Trends in Neurosciences*, **7**, 442–6.

Chapter 2B

Motor Units

JOHANNES NOTH

Basic structure and function

Sherrington was the first to recognize that muscle contractions are induced by the excitation of the motoneurones of the spinal cord. He introduced the term 'motor unit' for the structural entity consisting of the motoneurone, its motor axon, and the muscle fibres supplied by the motoneurone (Fig. 2.7). The number of muscle fibres belonging to a single motor unit can vary from 5–10 to more than 100. As a general rule, small muscles with precision tasks, such as the intrinsic hand muscles, are composed of motor units with few muscle fibres, whereas trunk and proximal limb muscles contain motor units with a large number of muscle fibres. The muscle fibres of a single motor unit occupy varying amounts of the transverse section of a muscle. In the human biceps brachii muscle, the territory of a single motor unit has a diameter of about 5–10 mm (Fig. 2.7). Muscle fibres from different motor units are intermingled. Besides its physical benefits, this overlap has implications for the energy supply of a tonic muscle during long-lasting, submaximal contractions, because it improves the ratio between active muscle fibres and capillaries for a given cross-section of a muscle.

The excitation of a single motoneurone causes the contraction of all muscle fibres belonging to its motor unit. This occurs in several steps. The action potential of the motoneurone travels along the myelinated axon to the muscle in an 'all-or-nothing' manner. At the end plate (the synapse between axon terminals and muscle fibres), the action potential causes the release of acetylcholine (ACh) from the presynaptic terminals. Acetylcholine binds to specific receptors of the subsynaptic membrane of the muscle fibre. This reaction depolarizes the muscle fibre membrane. As the end plate region lies in the middle part of the muscle fibre, the action potential then travels out in both directions to the polar regions of the muscle fibre, with a conduction velocity of around $2-5\,\mathrm{m \cdot s^{-1}}$. The transmission of excitation from the axon to the muscle occurs with a high security factor. The events occurring between the excitation of the muscle fibre and the resulting contraction are termed excitation–contraction coupling. This term includes, in brief, the invasion of the depolarization into the muscle fibre via the transverse tubular system, the release of calcium into the myoplasma, and the subsequently induced sliding of the myofilaments, actin and myosin, which finally causes the muscle action (for details see Chapter 3).

Types of motor unit

The tension developed by a motor unit in response to a single action potential invading the axon terminals is called a twitch. Twitch tension is normally measured under isometric conditions. When the firing frequency increases, overlap of twitches begins to appear

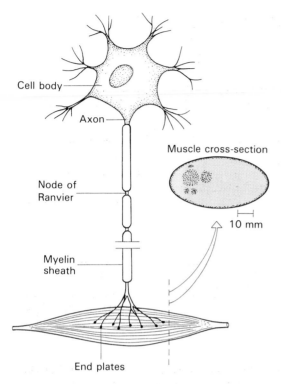

Fig. 2.7 Main features of a motor unit. The cell body is located in the brain stem or in the spinal cord. The axon travels along the peripheral nerves to the muscle of destination. The unmyelinated axon terminals make contacts with the muscle fibres via the end plates in a one-to-one fashion. The transmitter released at the end plate is acetylcholine. Muscle fibres belonging to one motor unit occupy a certain amount of the cross-section of a muscle, exemplified for the human biceps brachii on the right; each dot represents one motor fibre.

between 7 and 10 impulses $\cdot$ s^{-1}. With further increase in firing rate, tension becomes more and more fused, and at a certain frequency, the tension output is completely fused (Fig. 2.8). Measurement of these contraction parameters reveals that marked differences exist between motor units, even for motor units belonging to the same muscle. Muscle fibres of the same motor unit, on the other hand, exhibit similar physical, biochemical and ultrastructural properties, which indicates the importance of the motoneurone in controlling these parameters. As long as 60 years ago, Denny-Brown (1929) had realized that motoneurones with low reflex thresholds innervate motor units in slowly contracting, fatigue-resistant 'red' muscles, while those with high thresholds innervate muscle units in the fast contracting, fatiguable 'white' muscles. Since then, physiological properties such as speed of shortening, force development and endurance have been studied in many different muscles and species, in order to classify motor units. Today, the classification of Burke (1981) is widely accepted among physiologists (Kernell, 1986). According to this classification, developed from animal models and based on contractile speed and sensitivity to fatigue during a fused tetanus, three types of motor units can be distinguished: (i) fast-twitch, fatigue-sensitive (FF); (ii) fast-twitch, fatigue-resistant (FR); and (iii) slow-twitch (S), which are most resistant to fatigue. Motor units of the FF-type are predominantly found in pale

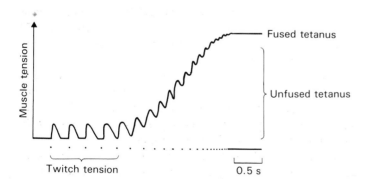

Fig. 2.8 Rate coding of muscle force. Isometric force development of a motor fibre during electrical stimulation at progressively increasing rate. At low rates of stimulation, single twitches are evoked. Unfused tetanus starts to develop at rates between 7 and 10 Hz and becomes a fused tetanus at rates between 20 and 30 Hz, depending on the type of motor unit. (From Buchthal, 1942.)

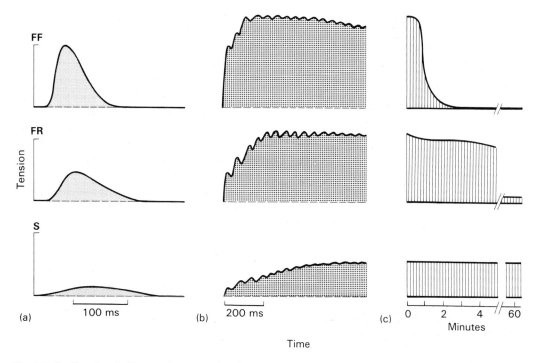

Fig. 2.9 Graphs of typical isometric tension development of the three types of motor unit (FF, FR, S) as found in the cat gastrocnemius muscle. (a) Twitch tension; (b) unfused tetanus evoked by stimulus train of $20 s^{-1}$; (c) curve of isometric maxima obtained by train of stimulation at $40 s^{-1}$, lasting 330 ms and repeated every 1 s. Note large twitch force in the FF unit, slow build-up of tetanic force in the S unit and rapid decline in tension within 2 mm in the FF unit. The FR unit behaves in an intermediate fashion. (From Burke *et al.*, 1971.)

muscles, while red muscles such as the soleus are exclusively composed of type S motor units. The gastrocnemius muscle of the cat contains all three types of motor unit, and the typical characteristics of force production of these motor units are depicted in Fig. 2.9.

Types of human muscle fibre

In human muscles, a characterization of motor units based on their physical properties is difficult to achieve, and in most studies a classification based on histochemical criteria has been used: type I muscle fibres, which have high levels of ATPase activity (stained at pH 9.4) and low levels of succinic dehydrogenase (SDH), and type II fibres, which show the reverse pattern of enzyme activity. In normally exercised

human muscles, there is a clear cut division in ATPase staining, which makes the classification unambiguous. Type I fibres correspond to the type S units (classification of Burke), while type II fibres are found in fast, fatigue-sensitive muscles and are therefore innervated by type FF units.

When slices of human muscles are preincubated in acid, ATPase staining reveals further subgroups of fast-twitch (type II) muscle fibres. The following classification can be made:

Type I: slow-twitch fibres; fatigue-resistant; low glycogen content; high mitochondrial content. Used for long-lasting, low level force production; energy supply via dense capillarization in red muscles.

Type IIA: fast-twitch fibres, fatigue-resistant. High glycolytic and oxidative enzyme content.

Suitable for prolonged and relatively high force output.

Type IIB: fast-twitch fibres, fatigue-sensitive. High glycogen and low mitochondrial content. Short-term energy supply via glycolysis. Suited for intermittent, high-force production, i.e. during fast sprinting.

Type IIC: intermediary fibres, between types I and II. Histochemically they react both with fast-twitch and slow-twitch antimyosins.

It should be emphasized, however, that the correlation between histochemical and contractile parameters is largely indirect, due to the small number of experiments performed on single motor units in man that are directly comparable with those performed in animals (see, for instance, Garnett *et al.*, 1979). The results of these experiments are not conclusive. It is also noteworthy that a large interindividual variation exists in histochemical properties of the muscle fibres of non-trained human subjects (cf. Lexell *et al.*, 1983), and that fibre composition and metabolic properties differ between males and females (Komi & Karlsson, 1978; Henriksson-Larsén, 1985). Any discussion of the effects of exercise on muscle fibre parameters must take these variations into account.

Neuronal influences on properties of motor units

Mammalian skeletal muscle differentiates during the postnatal period into red (slow), pale (fast) or mixed muscles. This differentiation is based on a complex trophic and neurophysiological interaction between motoneurones and muscle fibres. The classical experiment demonstrating the importance of the motoneurones for the expression of the contractile properties of a muscle was performed by Buller *et al.* (1960). In the cat hindlimb, cross-reinnervation of the nerve supply to the slow soleus muscle and to the fast flexor digitorum longus muscle altered the contractile properties of the re-innervated muscles: the fast muscle acquired

properties of the former slow muscle and vice versa. Numerous later studies have confirmed and expanded these early findings (see, for instance, Dubowitz, 1967). It is now well established that not only the biomechanical properties are changed, but also that many of the histochemical, mitochondrial and structural differences between fast and slow muscles are under neuronal control. As a rule, transformation from a fast to a slow muscle is much easier to obtain following cross-reinnervation than the reverse (Dum *et al.*, 1985).

Kinesiological investigations have shown that the motoneurone activation pattern during unrestrained movements remains qualitatively unaltered when motor axons reinnervate foreign muscles (O'Donovan *et al.*, 1985). Transformation can therefore be caused by trophic factors and/or by the specific activity pattern of the motoneurones. This question has been addressed through chronic stimulation of muscle nerves, which has convincingly demonstrated the powerful effect of the patterns of use of motor units on the physiological, enzymatic and ultrastructural properties of muscle fibres and even on their gene transcription (for reviews see Salmons & Henriksson, 1981; Pette & Vrbová, 1985; Brownson *et al.*, 1988). The 'state of the art' regarding the influence of the amount and the activity pattern of chronic nerve stimulation on the contractile and histochemical properties of the cat peroneus longus muscle has been recently summarized by Kernell (1990). The main points are the following.

1 Chronic stimulation transforms the fibre composition of a mixed hindlimb muscle, which becomes a slow muscle with homogeneous myosin ATPase staining (type I) of its muscle fibres. This was achieved even with burst rates of 100 Hz. Effects were apparent even with a stimulation pattern covering only 0.5% of a 24-hour cycle.

2 The speed of an isometric twitch action is markedly slowed, independent of the activity pattern applied (cf. Fig. 2.10).

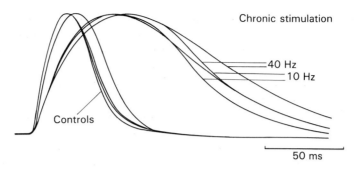

Fig. 2.10 Time course of isometric twitch tension of four normal peroneus longus muscles (left) and four peroneus longus muscles subjected to chronic nerve stimulation in the cat (right). The pattern of stimulation consisted of 1-s bursts of 10 Hz or 40 Hz as indicated, interrupted by 1-s pauses, covering 50% of the total time. Stimulation was applied 24 hours per day over the 8-week period, before the test contractions were elicited. Note the lack of influence of stimulation rate on time course of twitch tension. (From Eerbeek *et al.*, 1984.)

3 Maximum tetanic force decreases following extreme amounts of daily activation. This is partly due to shrinkage in fibre diameter. For the maintenance of maximum force and fibre size, high-frequency stimulation is necessary.
4 Resistance to fatigue improves. Chronic stimulation also counteracts EMG depression as measured during a fatigue test. These effects are not strongly correlated with each other.

Kernell (1990) concluded that non-neuronal factors during ontogeny set '. . . the adaptive range within which the adult muscle properties may become further adjusted by means of long-term effects of usage'. For the training of muscle in various sport disciplines, these experimental findings have two major implications. Firstly, the transformation of a slow muscle into a fast muscle by training programmes involving short periods of maximal muscle actions is probably impeded by normal daily use of these muscles in postural activity. Secondly, the transformation of a fast muscle into a muscle with slow contractile properties must involve maximal actions, because motor units with fast-contracting properties (FF units) are also those with the highest threshold. The experimental finding of a decline in maximal force output with large amounts of daily usage is an important factor in this context.

Motor unit recruitment

The size principle

Force gradation within a muscle can occur in two different ways. When the discharge rate of a motor unit increases, the forces generated by each impulse summate (unfused tetanus). Thus, force output is positively related to the discharge rate of a motor unit in the frequency range of the unfused tetanus. Additionally, the force output may be graded by the recruitment of higher threshold motor units. The recruitment follows a certain rule, which was first discovered by Henneman and colleagues, and which has turned out to be one of the most reliable laws in neurobiology: the 'size principle' (Henneman *et al.*, 1965). This states that during reflex activation of motoneurones, those with the smallest spikes (and thus with the smallest cell bodies) have the lowest threshold, and the largest cells have the highest threshold. Motoneurones with small spikes, as a rule, innervate motor units with little force output, while motoneurones with large spikes generate high amounts of tension. Thus, the Hennemann principle also predicts a positive correlation between recruitment threshold and twitch tension. This has been shown to be valid

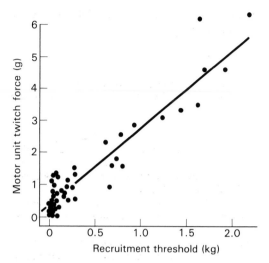

Fig. 2.11 Relationship between motor unit twitch force and recruitment threshold of the first dorsal interosseus muscle during slowly increasing isometric abduction of the index finger. The twitch force of each motor unit is obtained by spike triggered averaging, using the motor unit potential as trigger for the force measurement. The correlation is highly linear (correlation coefficient >0.9). (From Desmedt, 1981.)

in both animal and human muscle. An example of this relation is given in Fig. 2.11 for the human first dorsal interosseus muscle.

It has been shown that the soma size of a motoneurone is positively correlated with many other parameters, such as the diameter and the conduction velocity of its axon and the resting input conductance of the neurone (Kernell, 1983). Large motoneurones innervate muscle fibres that are fatigue-sensitive, whereas small neurones innervate fatigue-resistant muscle fibres (for reviews see Buchthal & Schmalbruch, 1980; Freund, 1983; Kernell, 1986). It is well established, furthermore, that the size principle also holds for many other types of muscle actions. A fixed recruitment order of motoneurones has been observed during locomotor movements in the cat (Hoffer *et al.*, 1987) and during ballistic arm movements in man (Desmedt & Godaux, 1978).

Much emphasis has been placed on exceptions from the size principle. These have however, in most instances turned out to contain no real contradiction. After EMG recordings with small needles had been introduced to record from single motor units in human muscles during sustained voluntary contractions, drop-out of tonically active motor units and recruitment of fresh units could be observed. This 'rotation' occurred only between units with similar force threshold. This phenomenon is therefore due to adaptation of motor units that discharge over unduly long periods. In order to keep the force level on target after a drop-out of such a unit, the motor unit with the next higher force threshold will come into play.

Another misleading situation is the investigation of fast reflex or voluntary muscle actions, during which a reversal of the orderly recruitment order can occur. It is, however, evident that a strong excitatory drive is able to discharge a whole motoneurone pool within a few milliseconds. Given the long peripheral pathway of human limb nerves, these small differences may be overridden by the difference in conduction delay between small and large motoneurones, the excitation of large motoneurones reaching the muscle first. The size principle, however, predicts the timing of the central excitation of a motor unit and not the peripheral excitation. In spite of this peripheral counteraction, the normal rank order is mostly preserved, even during fast ballistic contractions in man (Desmedt & Godaux, 1978).

Finally, the size principle is only valid when the motoneurone pool is functionally homogeneous. Even in seemingly uniform muscles, such as the cat sartorius muscle and the human first dorsal interosseus, task-related subgroups of motoneurones exist, which differ in their central and peripheral synaptic weighting. It is not surprising that a shift in the central or peripheral command from one to the other subgroup can mimic a reversal of the recruitment order.

Exceptions from the size principle

There are, nevertheless, a few true exceptions to the size principle. During very rapid stereotyped movements, such as paw shaking, high-threshold units can be activated without firing of small low-threshold units (Smith *et al.*, 1980). Another observation of recruitment reversal is the response of motor units to electrical stimulation of cutaneous nerves (Kanda *et al.*, 1977; Garnett & Stephens, 1981). It is likely that under these conditions synaptic connections are active which are preferentially made with higher threshold motoneurones. A so far unexplained finding is the observation of Nardone *et al.* (1989) that high-threshold motoneurones of the triceps surae muscle are recruited during voluntary eccentric muscle actions in man, when lower threshold units cease firing. The authors emphasize that the control of the eccentric muscle action is a rather skilled task, and they speculate that fast relaxing motoneurones are selectively brought into action via a central command.

Another example of a change in excitability of motor units during ongoing muscle actions has been recently detected in behaving monkeys. In accordance with earlier findings in man (Dietz *et al.*, 1979, 1981), motor units begin to fire during the preparation for a movement. When a monkey was trained to perform a rapid forearm flexion movement triggered by a light after a preparatory period, the firing of low-threshold motor units was completely suppressed at the time when higher threshold motor units were recruited (Mellah *et al.*, 1990).

Apart from these exceptions, the size principle has been proved to be valid in most reflex and voluntary motor acts in man (for a recent review, see Thomas *et al.*, 1987). It is not possible, within the limits of this introduction, to discuss the membrane and synaptic properties of motoneurones, which are nevertheless important for the rate- and recruitment-gradation of muscle force: the interested reader is referred, therefore, to recent articles concerned with these questions (Kernell, 1986; Kernell & Hultborn, 1990).

References

Brownson, C., Isenberg, H., Brown, W., Salmons, S. & Edwards, Y. (1988) Changes in skeletal muscle gene transcription induced by chronic stimulation. *Muscle and Nerve*, **11**, 1183–9.

Buchthal, F. (1942) The mechanical properties of the single striated muscle fibre at rest and during contraction and their structural interpretation. *Det Kongelige Danske Videnskabernes Selskab Biologiske Meddelelser*, **17**, 1–138.

Buchthal, R. & Schmalbruch, H. (1980) Motor unit of mammalian muscle. *Physiological Reviews*, **60**, 90–142.

Buller, A.J., Eccles, J.C. & Eccles, R.M. (1960) Interactions between motoneurones and muscles in respect of the characteristic speeds of their responses. *Journal of Physiology*, **150**, 417–39.

Burke, R.E. (1981) Motor units: anatomy, physiology, and functional organization. In V.B. Brooks (ed.) *Handbook of Physiology. Section I, The Nervous System II*, pp. 345–422. American Physiological Society, Washington.

Burke, R.E., Levine, D.N. & Zajac, F.E. (1971) Mammalian motor units: physiological–histochemical correlation in three types in cat gastrocnemius. *Science*, **174**, 709–12.

Denny-Brown, D.E. (1929) On the nature of the postural reflexes. *Proceedings Royal Society London Series B*, **104**, 252–301.

Desmedt, J.E. (1981) The size principle of motoneuron recruitment in ballistic or ramp-voluntary contractions in man. In J.E. Desmedt (ed.) *Progress in Clinical Neurophysiology, Vol. 9, Motor Unit Types, Recruitment and Plasticity in Health and Disease*, pp. 250–304. Karger, Basel.

Desmedt, J.E. & Godaux, E. (1978) Ballistic contractions in fast or slow human muscles: discharge patterns of single motor units. *Journal of Physiology*, **285**, 185–96.

Dietz, V., Noth, J., & Schmidtbleicher, D. (1981) Interaction between pre-activity and stretch reflex in human triceps brachii during landing from forward falls. *Journal of Physiology*, **311**, 113–25.

Dietz, V., Schmidtbleicher, D. & Noth, J. (1979) Neuronal mechanisms of human locomotion. *Journal of Neurophysiology*, **42**, 1212–22.

Dubowitz, V. (1967) Cross-innervated mammalian skeletal muscle: histochemical, physiological and biochemical observations. *Journal of Physiology*, **193**, 481–96.

Dum, R.P., O'Donovan, M.J., Toop, J., Tsairis, P., Pinter, M.J. & Burke, R.E. (1985) Cross-reinnervated motor units in cat muscle. II. Soleus muscle reinnervated by flexor digitorum longus motoneurons. *Journal of Neurophysiology*, **54**, 837–51.

Eerbeek, O., Kernell, D. & Verhey, B.A. (1984) Effects of fast and slow patterns of tonic long-term stimulation on contractile properties of fast muscle in the cat. *Journal of Physiology*, **352**, 73–90.

Freund, H.-J. (1983) Motor unit and muscle activity in voluntary motor control. *Physiological Reviews*, **63**, 387–436.

Garnett, R., O'Donovan, M.J., Stephens, J.A. & Taylor, A. (1979) Motor unit organization of human medial gastrocnemius. *Journal of Physiology*, **287**, 33–43.

Garnett, R. & Stephens, J.A. (1981) Changes in the recruitment threshold of motor units produced by cutaneous stimulation in man. *Journal of Physiology*, **311**, 463–73.

Henneman, E., Somjen, G. & Carpenter, D.O. (1965) Functional significance of cell size in spinal motoneurones. *Journal of Neurophysiology*, **28**, 560–80.

Henriksson-Larsén, K. (1985) Distribution, number and size of different types of fibres in whole cross-sections of female m. tibialis anterior. An enzyme histochemical study. *Acta Physiologica Scandinavica*, **123**, 229–35.

Hoffer, J.A. Loeb, G.E., Marks, W.B., O'Donovan, M.J., Pratt, C.A. & Sugano, N. (1987) Cat hindlimb motoneurons during locomotion. I. Destination, axonal conduction velocity and recruitment threshold. *Journal of Neurophysiology*, **57**, 510–73.

Kanda, K., Burke, R.E. & Walmsley, B. (1977) Differential control of fast and slow twitch motor units in the decerebrate cat. *Experimental Brain Research*, **29**, 57–74.

Kernell, D. (1983) Functional properties of spinal motoneurons and gradation of muscle force. In J.E. Desmedt (ed.) *Motor Control Mechanisms in Health and Disease*, pp. 213–26. Raven Press, New York.

Kernell, D. (1986) Organization and properties of spinal motoneurones and motor units. In H.-J. Freund, U. Büttner, B. Cohen & J. Noth (eds) *Progress in Brain Research, Vol. 64*, pp. 21–30. Elsevier Science Publishers, Amsterdam.

Kernell, D. (1990) Spinal motoneurones and their muscle fibers: mechanisms and long-term consequences of common activation patterns. In M.D. Binder & L.M. Mendell (eds) *The Segmental Motor System*, pp. 36–57. Oxford University Press, New York, Oxford.

Kernell, D. & Hultborn, H. (1990) Synaptic effects on recruitment gain: a mechanism of importance for the input–output relations of motoneurone pools? *Brain Research*, **507**, 176–9.

Komi, P.V. & Karlsson, J. (1978) Skeletal muscle fibre types, enzyme activities and physical performance in young males and females. *Acta Physiologica Scandinavica*, **103**, 210–18.

Lexell, J., Henriksson-Larsén, K. & Sjöström, M. (1983) Distribution of different fibre types in human skeletal muscles. 2. A study of cross-sections of whole m. vastus lateralis. *Acta Physiologica Scandinavica*, **117**, 115–22.

Mellah, S., Rispal-Padel, L. & Riviere, G. (1990) Changes in excitability of motor units during preparation for movement. *Experimental Brain Research*, **82**, 178–86.

Nardone, A., Romanò, C. & Schieppati, M. (1989) Selective recruitment of high-threshold human motor units during voluntary isotonic lengthening of active muscles. *Journal of Physiology*, **409**, 451–71.

O'Donovan, M.J., Pinter, M.J., Dum, R.P. & Burke, R.E. (1985) Kinesiological studies of self- and cross-reinnervated FDL and soleus muscles in freely moving cats. *Journal of Neurophysiology*, **54**, 852–66.

Pette, D. & Vrbová G. (1985) Neural control of phenotypic expression in mammalian muscle fibres. *Muscle and Nerve*, **8**, 676–89.

Salmons, S. & Henriksson, J. (1981) The adaptive response of skeletal muscle to increased use. *Muscle and Nerve*, **4**, 94–105.

Smith, J.L., Betts, B., Edgerton, V.R. & Zernicke, R.F. (1980) Rapid ankle extension during paw shakes: selective recruitment of fast ankle extensors. *Journal of Neurophysiology*, **43**, 612–20.

Thomas, C.K., Ross, B.H. & Calancie, B. (1987) Human motor-unit recruitment during isometric contractions and repeated dynamic movements. *Journal of Neurophysiology*, **57**, 311–24.

Chapter 2C

Neuromuscular Basis of Stretching Exercises

ROBERT S. HUTTON

Few topics have received greater attention in the rehabilitation and exercise science literature than the study of joint mobility and the maintenance of a fully functional range of motion (ROM) to meet the demands of daily, recreational, or sports activities. However, there have been very few studies that have addressed the problem from a mechanistic level *vis-à-vis* the testing of stretching techniques that putatively produce the best results. Therefore, this chapter will assess flexibility training techniques from a mechanistic view-point and derive implications for future clinical applications.

In evaluating the effectiveness of a stretching technique, there are two levels of concern: (i) acute changes in ROM; and (ii) chronic changes in ROM. The research literature primarily addresses the latter problem without concern for causal mechanisms associated with improved flexibility. Basically, any form of sustained or repetitive stretch that places joints toward their maximum ROM will produce an enhancement in their ROM capacity over time. The outward limitations will be dictated by the articulation of the joint(s) under investigation. Since the initial stage of flexibility training must address acute adaptations, mechanisms associated with these changes will be considered first.

Mechanisms underlying acute adaptive changes in ROM

Resistance to any movement, either passive or active (involving muscle activation), can be broken down to the following mechanistic constraints.

1 Neurogenic constraints, i.e. voluntary and reflex control over the muscle group undergoing stretch.

2 Myogenic constraints, the passive and active resistive properties of whole muscle undergoing stretch. If the condition is active, then the neurogenic and myogenic constraints are interactive.

3 Joint constraints. These resistive forces comprise the articular tissues, which involve the physical structures of the articulation of bones, the joint capsule structure, and the related ligamentous attachments.

4 Skin, subcutaneous connective tissue, and frictional constraints.

Stretching techniques

Of the four mechanistic groupings, only groups 1 and 2 can be subjected to voluntary control in an acute setting. Most emphasis on stretching exercises used in rehabilitation medicine and athletic training has been placed on the neurogenic component by employing stretching techniques that are presumed to promote the level of inhibition to the muscles undergoing stretch. Sherringtonian concepts (Sherrington, 1906) of reflex control based on animal studies formed the major rationale for the use of these stretching procedures. Typically, the stretch techniques considered are the following.

Ballistic stretch

The stretch torque is applied by a dynamic and fast movement into the extreme ROM limits of the joints of concern.

Static stretch (SS)

The joints are first placed in the outer limits of their present ROM and then subjected to a stretch torque. The stretch torque is either passively induced by the pull of gravity on the anatomical segment(s) involved in the stretch, by passively applied manual manipulation, or through the application of weights to increase the amount of the stretch torque normally induced by the anatomical segmental weight(s).

Proprioceptive neuromuscular facilitation (PNF) stretch

These stretch procedures usually involve a maximum precontraction of the muscle groups about to undergo elongation. The most commonly used in clinical settings are shown below.

Contract or hold relax (CR or HR). The muscles to be stretched are first maximally contracted and then stretched in the manner of the SS technique. The neurological basis for this procedure is usually attributed to Sherrington's observation of 'successive induction' (Sherrington, 1906). However, the procedure bears little resemblance to the original description of successive induction, wherein the agonists (e.g. flexors when the direction of stretch is into flexion) were successively excited to induce less reflex activity from the antagonists (extensors or the muscles to undergo stretch). The basis for this confusion in the literature remains a mystery. Others have claimed that the prior contraction of the muscle to be stretched will evoke more inhibitory activity from Golgi tendon organs (Etnyre & Abraham, 1986). There is no research evidence to support this conclusion, but there is experimental evidence to the contrary, which will be discussed later.

Contract (hold) relax, agonist contract (CRAC or HRAC). This procedure begins with the CR technique but differs in that the subject is asked to assist the stretch with contraction of the agonists. In either the CR or CRAC procedure, the stretch torque is usually increased by assistance from the therapist, trainer, or co-athlete. The rationale for an agonist contraction to assist the stretch torque on the muscles undergoing elongation is well founded in the research literature (Hultborn, 1972; Shindo *et al.*, 1984) and has been described as 'alpha–gamma-linkage in reciprocal inhibition'. The neural circuitry for this response is illustrated in Fig. 2.12. The evidence suggests that through alpha–gamma coactivation, not only is the gamma-loop involved but supraspinal pathways have direct access to the Ia reciprocal inhibitory interneurones engaged with the motor command. The inhibitory response is not obligatory, however, since the Renshaw cell feedback loop can override the reciprocal inhibitory input to antagonists (Haase *et al.*, 1975; Malmgren, 1988). The possibility of mutual inhibition between antagonistic pairs of Ia reciprocal inhibitory interneurones (Fig. 2.12) has also been shown (Hultborn *et al.*, 1974; Baldissera *et al.*, 1981).

Acute adaptive changes in neuromuscular tissue undergoing elongation

As stated before, in an acute setting one can only exert control over the neurogenic and myogenic constraints of joint ROM. The controlled variable is 'muscle stiffness', which is defined as the ratio of a change in muscle force divided by a change in muscle length, e.g. a small change in muscle length that gives rise to a large increment in muscle force would indicate a stiffer muscle response and one that would be contraindicated during the course of a flexibility exercise. Since muscle stiffness cannot be directly measured without the use of invasive techniques, the control of 'joint stiffness', or a change in joint angle divided by

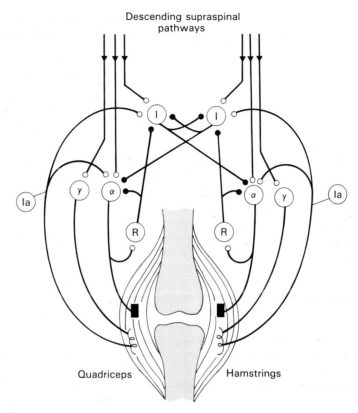

Fig. 2.12 The proposed stretch reflex neural circuitry and neural–mechanical coupling between antagonistic pairs of limb musculature. Neuromusculature interactions for each muscle group (quadriceps or hamstrings) occurs through alpha (α) motoneuronal innervation of extrafusal muscle fibres (black rectangles), Renshaw cell (R) recurrent inhibition, gamma (γ) motoneuronal innervation of intrafusal muscle fibres (tail of circular ring), Ia afferent fibres (Ia), and the Ia reciprocal inhibitory interneurone (I). Interactions between the two muscle groups occur through mechanical coupling via the bony–articular system and neural coupling through the Ia reciprocal inhibitory interneurone and less direct routes (not shown). Descending supraspinal inputs to the alpha- and gamma-motoneurones and the Ia reciprocal inhibitory interneurones are shown (corticospinal and subcorticospinal pathways). Open synaptic terminals are excitatory and closed synaptic terminals are inhibitory. See text for further explanation. (From Moore & Hutton, 1980.)

a change in joint torque or moment, would be the typical variable monitored. However, joint stiffness also includes resistances offered by joint structures, skin, subcutaneous connective tissue, or in other words, those mechanistic constraints identified in groups 3 and 4 (p. 29). Perhaps for these reasons, joint stiffness tends not to be the typical dependent variable used in flexibility studies on humans.

The prevailing focus in the clinical literature has been on the neurogenic constraint as the major factor in limiting the effectiveness of a stretch technique. It would seem intuitively obvious that a muscle that is in some state of neural activation, as evidenced by elevated electromyographic (EMG) activity, would be more resistive to stretch. Consequently, the stretching techniques identified earlier, excluding ballistic stretch, are putatively designed to minimize EMG activity in the muscle(s) to be stretched. As it turns out, the issue of stretch effectiveness and muscle relaxation is far more

complicated than previously realized as revealed in the following review.

In recent years, a great deal of attention
has been placed on the use of PNF stretching
techniques on the assumption that they are the
'most' effective methods for increasing ROM
(Holt *et al.*, 1970; Tanigawa, 1972; Markos, 1979;
Sady *et al.*, 1982; Wallin *et al.*, 1985; Etnyre &
Abraham, 1986; Etnyre & Lee, 1988); however,
several published reports have shown no significant differences in ROM achieved between
PNF techniques and static stretching procedures (Medeiros *et al.*, 1977; Hartley-O'Brien,
1980; Moore & Hutton, 1980; Lucas & Koslow,
1984; Condon & Hutton, 1987). Part of the
disparity in findings may be associated with
whether the study cited was acute or chronic
in design, and whether the stretch torque was
held relatively constant across the stretch techniques employed. Nevertheless, it is generally assumed that a maximum action prior to
stretch, as is done in the PNF procedure, promotes muscle relaxation through mechanisms
previously discussed (see above) and therefore
greater ROM is achieved. Ironically, this
assumption prior to 1980 (see Moore & Hutton,
1980) was never systematically tested nor was
an association drawn between the 'short term
activation history' of muscle and its subsequent
tonic and/or dynamic level of EMG excitability,
even though an abundant amount of basic
research literature existed on the subject.

Contrary to the general assumption of
contraction-induced muscle relaxation prior to
stretch, moderate to intense actions of skeletal
muscle increase the excitability of the activated
neuromuscular pathway for several seconds.
The sites of these changes in post-contraction
excitability are both neurogenic and myogenic
in origin (see Hutton, 1984 for a review). Of
critical importance is the observation that the
gamma-motoneurone and the stretch reflex
pathway (Fig. 2.12) are both tonically and
dynamically facilitated leading to an enhanced
response to subsequent stretch. This appears
to be due to two adaptive mechanisms in the
so-called gamma-loop: (i) an afterdischarge of

gamma-motoneurones to the previous activation, and (ii) a postcontraction persistence
of binding between some intrafusal actin and
myosin filaments leading to a stiffening of these
muscle fibres in the polar region of the muscle
spindle. As a consequence, a positive 'bias' of
stretch is placed on the spindle receptors. This
being the case, application of a PNF procedure
should promote muscle activation, not alleviate
it. This assumption can be directly tested by
recording EMG activity as well as changes in
ROM during the application of a stretching
technique.

Moore and Hutton (1980) tested the above
assumption by recording EMG activity from
the hamstrings (Hs) and quadriceps (Q) while
subjects performed in random order a series of
S, CR and CRAC stretches of the Hs musculature. Range of motion was monitored by an
electrogoniometer and a constant stretch torque
was applied to the ankle with the subject in a
supine position. The knee joint was braced in
full extension. The experimental condition is
shown in Fig. 2.13. The stretching techniques
utilized are explained in the caption (see also
the section on stretching techniques).

The most common finding in EMG magnitude (ordered least to most) during stretch was
S < CR < CRAC (*n* = 11 of 21 subjects), with
CR < S < CRAC (*n* = 7) the second most
common trend. Statistical significance at the *P*
< 0.05 level was reached in 9 and 3 subjects in
these groupings, respectively. For changes
in ROM, there was no significant difference
between the S and CRAC condition, but the
CRAC stretch produced a greater increase in
ROM than the CR condition. The findings that,
overall, the PNF procedures produced greater
EMG activity in stretched muscle have been
replicated in subsequent studies (Condon &
Hutton, 1987; Osternig *et al.*, 1987; Osternig
et al., 1990).

Since the CRAC technique involves voluntary assistance through agonist action in
combination with the stretch torque, the question arises whether alpha–gamma linkage
in reciprocal inhibition is occurring with Q

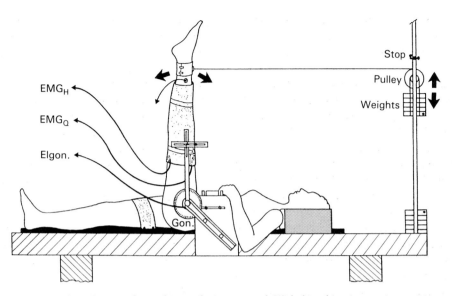

Fig. 2.13 Experimental condition and stretching techniques tested. With the subject in a supine position, surface electromyographic activity (EMG) was recorded from the hamstring (H) and the quadriceps (Q) muscles. An electrogoniometer (Elgon.) and calibration goniometer (Gon.) monitored hip angle. The lower extremity was held in full knee extension by a brace and attached at the ankle to a pulley system and weights (8.54 kg). Within the range of hip angles observed, the rise and fall of the weights (with changes in hip angle) allowed a constant angle of pull on the leg thereby providing a constant stretch torque. A 'stop' on the pulley assembly allowed isometric actions against the stabilized weights. Static stretch was achieved by the subject relaxing the hamstring muscles. For a contract–relax stretch, the subject performed a 5 s maximum isometric action of the hamstring muscles followed by the static stretch procedure. In the contract–relax, agonist contract condition, the subject maximally contracted the hamstring muscles for 5 s and then assisted the stretch torque of the weights by a submaximal quadriceps action. The EMG data can be used to check that the techniques are correctly performed. (From Moore & Hutton, 1980.)

contraction, i.e. reciprocal inhibition of the Hs muscles during stretch. To test for this Condon and Hutton (1987) employed the Hoffmann (H) reflex as a probe of neural excitation during stretch of plantar flexors undergoing different stretching procedures. Since the H-reflex tests the excitability of the alpha-motoneuronal pool by electrical stimulation of the muscle spindle Ia afferent fibres, changes in the evoked response in the soleus muscle would be an indirect assessment of whether the reciprocal Ia inhibitory pathway was operative during voluntary dorsiflexion. It was found that despite the greater EMG tonic activity observed in the CRAC stretch (and additionally in this study, in an agonist contraction (AC) without a conditioning contraction) the H-reflex ampli-

tude was significantly lower in the CRAC (and AC) condition than in the CR or S procedure. This suggests that reciprocal inhibition was operative but 'masked' by other sources of excitatory current to the soleus motoneuronal pool. These H-reflex findings have been supported and extended by Guissard et al. (1988) to include tendon reflexes. Nevertheless, the observation remains that the PNF procedure employing a precontraction and, in particular, agonist assistance to the stretch torque gives rise to *greater* EMG activity not *less*.

Since in most studies, S and CRAC stretch techniques yield similar acute improvements in ROM, one is left with the paradoxical observation that the effectiveness of a particular stretching procedure is independent of the level of EMG activity at the time of muscle displacement. This appears counter intuitive until one probes deeper into the mechanisms that may oppose muscle stretch.

It appears that myogenic constraints in determining ROM have long been underestimated and the role of connective tissue, as the major resistance to stretch, overestimated. The notion that actin and myosin filaments are totally detached when in a resting state, thus allowing them to move passively past each other during muscle stretch, has been seriously challanged and, in fact, is no longer valid as initially demonstrated by Hill (1968). Hill demonstrated in frog muscle that a 'short range stiffness' exists in relaxed muscle, which is caused by the presence of bonds between actin and myosin. More recently, Magid and Law (1985) reported muscle stiffness ratios in whole frog sartorius muscle, intact single fibres, and in skinned single fibres (fibres with the sarcolemma dissolved thus eliminating contributions from the membrane protein elastin) to be essentially identical. When the rise in force was expressed relative to the change in sarcomere length, it was calculated that in whole muscle significant contributions from muscle connective tissue did not occur until the degree of actin–myosin filament overlap was minimal, indicating that contributions from connective tissue play a major role at considerably longer muscle lengths than previously suspected. These observations suggest that much of what has been attributed to resistive properties of connective tissue in the attainment of maximum ROM may actually be due to intrinsic molecular properties of the muscle fibre.

Evidence for the existence of similar intrinsic resistive properties in human muscle has been reported recently by Hagbarth et al. (1985) and Lakie and Robson (1988). Hagbarth and coworkers measured inherent muscle and reflex stiffness of human finger flexor muscles combined with EMG and microneurographic recordings (axonal recordings from the peripheral nerve). Inherent muscle stiffness (tested under passive conditions) in response to manually applied movement was found to be enhanced following a brief finger flexion and reduced after a brief finger extension. Following a conditioning concentric action, finger flexion muscle stiffness was enhanced as was the multiunit afferent discharge, attributed to muscle spindle stretch receptors, transmitted through the median nerve. A decrease in muscle stiffness was found when the conditioning muscle action was performed isometrically or eccentrically. Since passive or active disturbance of a muscle appears to alter intrinsic properties of a muscle and its subsequent stiffness response to stretch, muscle fibres are said to show *thixotropic* behaviour, a rheologic term used to describe a change in viscosity of a gel and resistance to molecular deformation when it is shaken or stirred.

Lakie and Robson (1988) studied the stiffness of relaxed forearm extensor muscles acting across the metacarpophalangeal joint. In a resting state and over the course of several minutes, the stiffness of these muscles increased twofold (Fig. 2.14). Repetitive eccentric actions or passive oscillations of the muscles (so-called 'stirring'), prior to the application of a flexor torque to measure stiffness, lowered the initial stiffness, whereas (in contrast to the findings of Hagbarth et al., 1985 and earlier reports by Hutton & Suzuki, 1979 and Suzuki & Hutton, 1976), isometric actions increased the initial stiffness response to applied torques (Fig. 2.14).

It therefore appears that certain active or passive movements conducted prior to the application of a stretch torque may either loosen or increase thixotropic bonds (presumably between actin and myosin filaments) in both extrafusal and intrafusal muscle fibres. Pre-stretch conditions that tend to loosen these bonds are passive oscillations or active repetitive eccentric actions of the muscles to be stretched. The effectiveness of this 'stirring' is mostly determined by the amplitude of the movement(s) with duration playing a secondary role. The CRAC PNF procedure most likely involves a small eccentric action component,

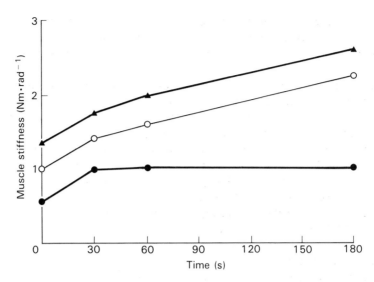

Fig. 2.14 Muscle stiffness responses in extensor forearm muscles are shown as a function of time and a pre-stretch conditioning contraction stimulus. Open circles denote a gradual rise in muscle stiffness as a function of time in undisturbed relaxed muscle. If prior to each stiffness measurement at the designated times (0, 30, 60 and 180 s) the muscle is 'stirred' (see text) by repetitive concentric or isometric actions, the initial stiffness level sampled at each time period is higher (▲). In contrast, repetitive eccentric actions or passive oscillatory stretches lowers the initial stiffness levels (●) across all time periods sampled relative to the other pre-stretch conditioning stimuli. (From Lakie & Robson, 1988.)

particularly as the technique is usually performed with the aid of an assistant. This may account for the effectiveness of this stretching technique in spite of its lingering effects on ongoing tonic EMG activity, which may amount to only a small portion of the total muscle mass remaining electrically active.

Interestingly, based upon analyses at the mechanistic level, it follows that repetitive smaller movements of passive oscillations of the muscle group(s) about to be stretched to the limits of their ROM, may respond with lower intrinsic resistance to deformation than when stretched from an initial static state of relaxation. Since intrafusal muscle fibres also exhibit this thixotropic property, it follows that any pre-stretch conditioning stimulus that increases or decreases their level of stiffness likewise causes a parallel change in the amplitude of the stretch reflex responses mediated over the group Ia and II receptors (Hutton, 1984; Hagbarth *et al.*, 1985). It remains to be resolved,

however, why Hagbarth and his colleagues' findings differed from those of Lakie and Robson when the conditioning pre-stretch stimulus was an isometric action. However, the muscles tested and the manner in which muscle stiffness was assessed differed between the two experiments and this may have accounted for the discrepancy between their findings.

Mechanisms underlying chronic adaptive changes in ROM

As previously mentioned, most studies on flexibility training have focused on long-term (chronic) gains in ROM as a function of the stretching techniques employed. Historically, the results have been rather mixed, but the CRAC PNF procedure has often been shown to produce the greatest 'absolute' gains in ROM over other PNF procedures, static stretch, or ballistic stretch, although the results reported or emphasized are sometimes not statistically significant. Studies of this nature were recently reviewed by Etynre and Lee (1987). None of these investigations, however, shed any light on the adaptive mechanisms involved in accounting for these improvements in ROM. The underlying assumption is that a permanent deformation in connective tissue and, perhaps, tendons has occurred due to repeated exposure to stress and strain. Such yield characteristics can be demonstrated even under acute conditions providing that a load of sufficient magnitude and duration is applied (Warren et al., 1976; Butler et al., 1978).

Based on observations initially associated with developmental growth of skeletal muscle from birth through full maturation, it has been shown that skeletal muscle fibres adapt to growth by an increase in muscle length through the addition of new sarcomeres added in-series to the fibre as well as an increase in fibre girth (Williams & Goldspink, 1971). These findings led to the use of immobilization experiments (e.g. by plaster casting) to determine if prolonged stretch or shortening of muscles would lead to similar adaptations in sarcomere numbers resulting from induction of protein synthesis of contractile proteins and other cell structures of muscle fibres. A consistent finding has been that immobilization of limb joints in either an extended or shortened position results in the number of sarcomeres along the fibre (in-series) to increase or decrease in numbers, respectively, when compared to contralateral control muscle (Williams & Goldspink, 1971; Tabary et al., 1972). Further experimentation has shown that this new induced functional length of the muscle is not under direct neuronal control since denervated muscles show similar adaptations under immobilized conditions (Goldspink et al., 1974). To determine the role of muscle length vis-à-vis muscle tension in determining the nature of sarcomere adaptation, Huet de la Tour et al. (1979) replicated the immobilization experiments with conditions wherein some experi-

mental groups were subjected to permanent muscle contraction (elicited by tetanus toxin) during an imposed length change, while others were subjected to length changes with either the tendon cut or the nerve innervation compromised in addition to tenotomy. The results implicated muscle length, and not tension, as the major determining factor in sarcomere number regulation.

It should be noted that when muscles are immobilized in the shortened position muscle stiffness is increased (Tabary et al., 1972). This may be due to an increase in connective tissue as observed by Williams et al. (1988). To determine if increases in muscle stiffness were primarily due to a decrease in sarcomere numbers in-series, a decrease in contractile activity, or to the proliferation of connective tissue, Williams et al. (1988) determined whether contractile activity, through electrical stimulation, would prevent connective tissue accumulation in rabbit soleus muscle immobilized in a shortened position. They found that connective tissue proliferation could be prevented by contractile activity during the immobilized period.

Interestingly, no similar accumulation of connective tissue occurs when the muscle is immobilized in the lengthened position suggesting that passive stretch alone may also prevent increases in connective tissue. Reversals in sarcomere numbers after immobilization (e.g. after the cast is removed) takes about 4 weeks to return to control levels (Tabary et al., 1972). While one can only speculate as to the implications these findings have to chronic flexibility training, it would appear that, once again, the plasticity of the myogenic component plays a major role in determining the muscle stiffness as long as the muscle remains active or is passively stretched.

While these extreme cases from the animal research literature clearly imply that a myogenic factor is involved in chronic regulation of muscle length and thereby resistance to maximum ROM, it remains to be determined how important this myogenic component might be in chronic adaptations to long-term involvement in flexibility training such as that seen in gymnasts, ballet dancers and other various sport and art forms. The current research literature would suggest that in both acute and chronic adaptations to flexibility training, myogenic constraints to ROM appear to have been underestimated. Neural constraints appear to set rather than dictate the myogenic response to extreme changes in ROM, i.e. intrinsic myogenic mechanisms (e.g. through the type of pre-stretch contraction or tonic activity induced) may represent the major determinant of resistance to muscle deformation rather than neural activation *per se*. Likewise, adaptive responses in sarcomere number and in-series length may represent a major chronic factor in allowing full joint ROM with eventual attendant stress on connective tissue and joint structures. The latter constraints, though long held as the major adaptive components to improved ROM, are in great need of further experimental investigation to determine at what range of ROM do they play a major role in limiting joint flexibility.

References

Baldissera, F., Hultborn, H. & Illert, M. (1981) Integration in spinal neuronal systems. In V.B. Brooks (ed.) *Handbook of Physiology Section 1, Vol. 1, Motor Control.* pp. 509–96. American Physiological Society, Bethesda.

Butler, D.L., Grood, E.S. & Noyes, F.R. (1978) Biomechanics of ligaments and tendons. *Exercise and Sport Sciences Reviews*, **6**, 125–81.

Condon, S.M. & Hutton, R.S. (1987) Soleus muscle electromyographic activity and ankle dorsiflexion range of motion during four stretching procedures. *Journal of American Physical Therapy Association*, **67**, 24–30.

Etnyre, B.R. & Abraham, L.D. (1986) H-reflex changes during static stretching and two variations of proprioceptive neuromuscular facilitation techniques. *Electroencephalography and Clinical Neurophysiology*, **63**, 174–9.

Etnyre, B.R. & Lee, E.J. (1987) Comments on proprioceptive neuromuscular facilitation stretching techniques. *Research Quarterly for Exercise and Sport*, **58**, 184–8.

Etnyre, B.R. & Lee, E.J. (1988) Chronic and acute flexibility of men and women using three different stretching techniques. *Research Quarterly for Exercise and Sport*, **59**, 222–8.

Goldspink, G., Tabary, C., Tabary, J.C., Tardieu, C. & Tardieu, G. (1974) Effect of denervation on the adaptation of sarcomere number and muscle extensibility to the functional length of the muscle. *Journal of Physiology*, **236**, 733–42.

Guissard, N., Duchateau, J. & Hainaut, K. (1988) Muscle stretching and motoneuron excitability. *European Journal of Applied Physiology*, **58**, 47–52.

Haase, J., Cleveland, S. & Ross, H.-G. (1975) Problems of postsynaptic autogenous and recurrent inhibition in the mammalian spinal cord. *Review of Physiology, Biochemistry and Pharmacology*, **73**, 73–129.

Hagbarth, K.-E., Hagglund, J.V., Nordin, M. & Wallin, E.U. (1985) Thixotropic behaviour of human finger flexor muscles with accompanying changes in spindle and reflex responses to stretch. *Journal of Physiology*, **368**, 323–42.

Hartley-O'Brien, S.J. (1980) Six mobilization exercises for active range of hip flexion. *Research Quarterly for Exercise and Sport*, **51**, 625–35.

Hill, D.K. (1968) Tension due to interaction between the sliding filaments in rested striated muscle. *Journal of Physiology*, **199**, 637–84.

Holt, L.E., Travis, T.M. & Okita, T. (1970) Comparative study of three stretching techniques. *Perceptual and Motor Skills*, **31**, 611–16.

Huet de la Tour, E., Tabary, J.C., Tabary, C. & Tardieu, C. (1979) The respective roles of muscle length and muscle tension in sarcomere number adaption of guinea-pig soleus muscle. *Journal of Physiology (Paris)*, **75**, 589–92.

Hultborn, H. (1972) Convergence on interneurones in the reciprocal Ia inhibitory pathway to motoneurons. *Acta Physiologica Scandinavica*, **85** (suppl. 375), 5–42.

Hultborn, H., Illert, M. & Santini, M. (1974) Disynaptic Ia inhibition of the interneurones mediating the reciprocal Ia inhibition of motoneurones. *Acta Physiologica Scandinavica*, **91**, 14–15A.

Hutton, R.S. (1984) Acute plasticity in spinal segmental pathways with use: implications for training. In M. Kumamoto (ed.) *Neural and Mechanical Control of Movement*, pp. 90–112. Yamaguchi Shoten, Kyoto.

Hutton, R.S. & Suzuki, S. (1979) Postcontraction discharge of motor neurons in spinal animals. *Experimental Neurology*, **64**, 567–78.

Lakie, M. & Robson, L.G. (1988) Thixotropic changes in human muscle stiffness and the effects of fatigue. *Quarterly Journal of Experimental Physiology*, **73**, 487–500.

Lucas, R.C. & Koslow, R. (1984) Comparative study

of static, dynamic, and proprioceptive neuro-muscular facilitation stretching techniques on flexibility. *Perceptual and Motor Skills*, **58**, 615–18.

Magid, A. & Law, D.J. (1985) Myofibrils bear most of the resting tension in frog skeletal muscle. *Science*, **230**, 1280–2.

Malmgren, K. (1988) On premotoneuronal integration in cat and man. *Acta Physiologica Scandinavica*, **134** (suppl. 576), 7–53.

Markos, P.D. (1979) Ipsilateral and contralateral effects of proprioceptive neuromuscular facilitation techniques on hip motion and electromyographic activity. *Physical Therapy*, **59**, 1366–73.

Medeiros, J.M., Smidt, G.L., Burmeister, L.F. & Soderberg, G.L. (1977) The influence of isometric exercise and passive stretch on hip joint motion. *Physical Therapy*, **57**, 518–23.

Moore, M.A. & Hutton, R.S. (1980) Electromyographic investigation of muscle stretching techniques. *Medicine and Science in Sports and Exercise*, **12**, 322–9.

Osternig, L.R., Robertson, R., Troxel, R. & Hansen, P. (1987) Muscle activation during proprioceptive neuromuscular facilitation (PNF) stretching techniques. *American Journal of Physical Medicine*, **66**, 298–307.

Osternig, L.R., Robertson, R.H., Troxel, R.K. & Hansen, P. (1990) Differential responses to proprioceptive neuromuscular facilitation (PNF) stretch techniques. *Medicine and Science in Sports and Exercise*, **22**, 106–11.

Sady, S.P., Wortman, M. & Blanke, D. (1982) Flexibility training: ballistic, static or proprioceptive neuromuscular facilitation? *Archives of Physical Medicine and Rehabilitation*, **63**, 261–3.

Sherrington, C.S. (1906) *The Integrative Action of the Nervous System*. Yale University, New Haven.

Shindo, M., Harayama, H., Kondo, K., Yanagisawa, N. & Tanaka, R. (1984) Changes in reciprocal Ia inhibition during voluntary contraction in man. *Experimental Brain Research*, **53**, 400–8.

Suzuki, S. & Hutton, R.S. (1976) Postcontractile motoneuronal discharge produced by muscle afferent activation. *Medicine and Science in Sports and Exercise*, **8**, 258–64.

Tabary, J.C., Tabary, C., Tardieu, C., Tardieu, G. & Goldspink, G. (1972) Physiological and structural changes in the cat's soleus muscle due to immobilization at different lengths by plaster casts. *Journal of Physiology*, **224**, 231–44.

Tanigawa, M.C. (1972) Comparison of the hold–relax procedure and passive mobilization on increasing muscle length. *Physical Therapy*, **52**, 725–35.

Wallin, D., Ekblom, B., Grahn, R. & Nordenborg, T. (1985) Improvement of muscle flexibility. A comparison between two techniques. *American Journal of Sports Medicine*, **13**, 263–8.

Warren, C.G., Lehmann, J.F. & Koblanski, J.N. (1976) Heat and stretch procedures: an evaluation using rat tail tendon. *Archives of Physical Medicine and Rehabilitation*, **57**, 122–6.

Williams, P.E., Catanese, T., Lucey, E.G. & Goldspink, G. (1988) The importance of stretch and contractile activity in the prevention of connective tissue accumulation in muscle. *Journal of Anatomy*, **158**, 109–14.

Williams, P.E. & Goldspink, G. (1971) Longitudinal growth of striated muscle fibres. *Journal of Cell Science*, **9**, 751–67.

Chapter 3

Muscular Basis of Strength

RUDOLF BILLETER AND HANS HOPPELER

Contractile machinery of skeletal muscle fibre types

The sarcomere

Muscle fibres, the cells of skeletal muscles, have but one function: to generate force. They are large single cells about 50 µm wide and up to 10 cm long with thousands of nuclei, and filled to 80% by cylindrical contractile organelles, the myofibrils. These myofibrils are 1–2 µm in diameter and often extend the whole length of a muscle fibre. They are built of a series of sarcomeres, the contractile units, which consist of longitudinal thick and thin filaments precisely arranged between the so-called Z-discs that are spaced about 2.5 µm apart (Fig. 3.1). Upon the addition of calcium to isolated myofibrils in a test tube, the sarcomeres contract by sliding the thick and thin filaments against each other, pulling their Z-discs closer together, as shown in the electron micrographs of Fig. 3.2. This is the basis of muscle contraction. The availability of calcium ions in the space around the myofibrils decides if the thick and thin filaments can slide against each other. The simultaneous sliding of tens of thousands of sarcomeres in series generates considerable length changes and force development in this cell.

A consequence of the 'sliding filament' model is that the forces generated between actin and myosin are unidirectional in the sense that they tend to shorten the sarcomere.

Extension while the muscle is activated (eccentric contraction) or while the muscle is inactive (relaxation) has to be accomplished by an outside force. Every muscle in our body is therefore matched by another muscle that can counteract its action, a so-called antagonist. Skeletal muscles work on the agonist–antagonist principle. For some muscles, gravity can take the function of the antagonist.

The filament: myosin

The principal protein of the thick filament is myosin. A single myosin molecule consists of two heavy chains with long intertwined tails connected to pear-shaped heads to which a total of four light chains are bound (Fig. 3.3). Isolated myosin molecules can spontaneously form filaments because their tails have a tendency to aggregate alongside each other. In the skeletal muscle sarcomeres, such interactions are thought to be controlled by various accessory proteins, leading to thick filaments with a bipolar structure, composed of about 250 myosins with a bare zone in the middle of the filament where the tails are packed in an antiparallel fashion such that no heads are found in this region (Fig. 3.4). The myosin heads are the force generating sites in muscle. The energy for contraction is derived from the hydrolysis of adenosine triphosphate (ATP) to adenosine diphosphate (ADP) (see below). The ATP cleaving site, the ATPase activity, is located in the myosin head. This

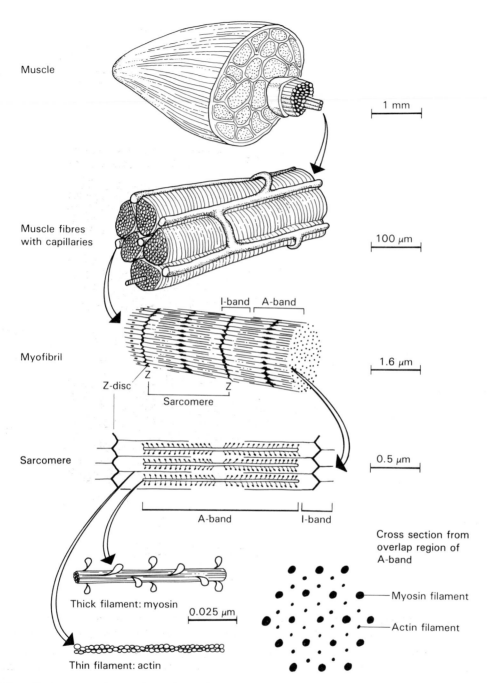

Fig. 3.1 Diagrammatic representation of the structural composition of skeletal muscle tissue. (From di Prampero, 1985.)

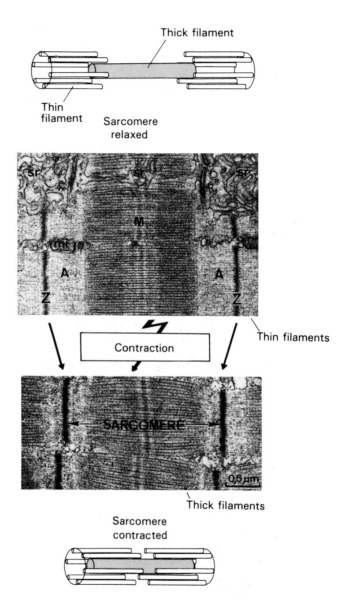

Fig. 3.2 Illustration of the 'sliding filament' theory of muscle contraction. In the relaxed extended state, the Z-lines are spaced about 2.5 μm apart. The thick and thin filaments overlap only partially. In the shortened state, the Z-lines have moved closer, and the thin and thick filaments overlap over most of their lengths. (From Alberts *et al.*, 1989.) A, A-band; M, M-line; mi, mitochondria; sr, sarcoplasmic reticulum; Z, Z-line.

ATPase is activated several hundred fold when the myosin head (with the light chains bound to it) interacts with an actin molecule of the thin filament, as will be described below.

The filament: actin with troponin and tropomyosin

The thin filaments (Fig. 3.5) consist of two intertwined strings of adjoining actin molecules (also called actin monomeres or G-actin). Both actin strands are flanked by a continuous string of tropomyosin molecules, long rod-shaped proteins spanning a length of seven actin residues each. Every tropomyosin molecule carries a troponin complex, consisting of the globular-shaped proteins troponin C and troponin I as well as the elongated troponin T. Troponin C can bind calcium ions (the triggers of contraction), which leads to a conformational

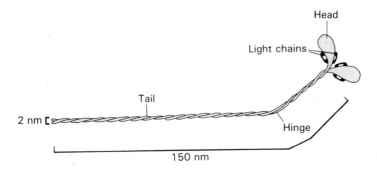

Fig. 3.3 A myosin molecule: myosin consists of six protein chains, two intertwined heavy chains and four light chains. The ATPase activity is located in the heads. (From Alberts *et al.*, 1989.)

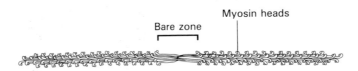

Fig. 3.4 Drawing of a thick filament, consisting of aligned myosin molecules. The myosins are aggregated with their tails, with the heads sticking out of the filament. The bare zone in the middle, where the myosin molecules change their orientation relative to the filament, is composed of tails. Its middle binds the M-line proteins. (From Alberts *et al.*, 1989.)

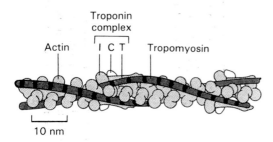

Fig. 3.5 Model of a section of a thin filament, indicating the positions of actin, tropomyosin and the troponin subunits. Each tropomyosin has seven evenly spaced regions of considerable homology, each of which are thought to bind to a single actin residue. Since every tropomyosin has one troponin complex bound (consisting of one molecule each of troponin I, C and T), there is one troponin complex per seven actin residues. One tropomyosin molecule in combination with the troponin complex forms a so-called regulatory unit. (From Alberts *et al.*, 1989.)

Since tropomyosin interacts with every actin monomer along its length, the actin molecules also are 'bent' slightly into a state that lets them activate the myosin ATPase (Fig. 3.6). One tropomyosin unit with its adjoining troponin complex forms a so-called 'regulatory unit'. A thin filament of 1 µm length has 52 regulatory units and therefore consists of about 360 actin molecules.

The cross-bridge cycle: myosin 'walks' along actin

In a muscle, force is generated by the concerted action of billions of myosin heads interacting with actin, moving, detaching, interacting with another actin and so on. This repeated actin–myosin interaction (linked to the breakdown of ATP) is called the cross-bridge cycle (Fig. 3.6). The cross-bridge cycle involves four different states of myosin. In state 1, the myosin head is not interacting with actin (in fact has just been released) and has ATP bound in the 'pocket' of the ATPase enzyme site in the head. The ATP is

change; the molecule is 'bent' differently. This different shape of the troponin C in turn leads to conformational changes in troponin I and troponin T and also tropomyosin.

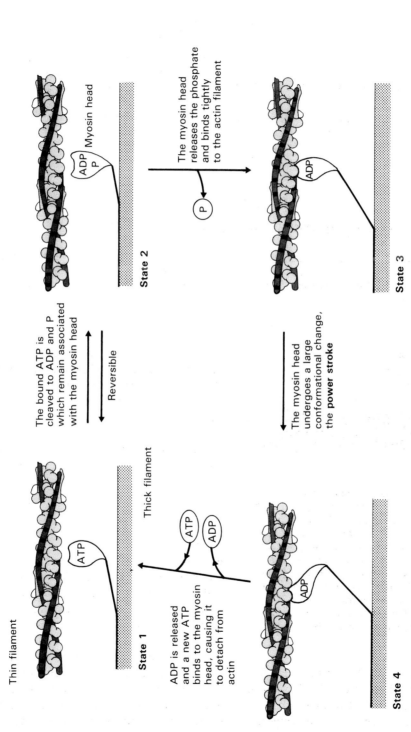

Fig. 3.6 Model of the cross-bridge cycle. Myosin binds ATP upon detachment from actin, splits it into ADP and phosphate (P) but retains both molecules in the ATPase site until it attaches to actin, upon which the phosphate is released and the head undergoes a conformational change, the 'power stroke', which shifts the actin filament and generates force. The head is then detached from the actin, whereby it releases ADP and binds a new ATP in order to start another cycle. The different states (1–4) correspond to different conformations of the myosin head. Only the transition between states 1 and 2 is reversible, the others are not. (From Alberts *et al.*, 1989.)

then cleaved to ADP plus phosphate (Pi) but the products are not released, they stay bound tightly at the ATPase site. The myosin head does not yet interact with actin. This is named state 2. The reaction between state 1 and state 2 is reversible. The myosin head, still in a free swinging state, then binds to an actin residue on the thin filament, upon which the phosphate of the previous ATP is released (state 3). This somehow makes that head bend and move in such a way that the bound actin (and therefore the whole filament) is shifted towards the middle of the sarcomere (state 4). This is called the 'power stroke' of myosin. The step from state 2 (head away from myosin, ADP and phosphate bound) to state 3 (phosphate released, head interacts with actin) is the main regulatory step in this cycle: actin in its 'bent' state, caused by the conformational changes of the regulatory units due to calcium binding on troponin C, allows the transition from state 2 to state 3 to go much more rapidly than actin in the 'off' state (no calcium bound to troponin C). It should be noted in this context that recent evidence argues against the classic 'steric hindrance' model of regulation of the step between states 2 and 3. According to this model, tropomyosin alters its position on the actin filament as a consequence of calcium binding to troponin C and this allows the myosin head to gain access to actin at a site that was previously obstructed by the tropomyosin.

After the myosin head has performed its 'power stroke', it detaches from the actin only after binding an ATP molecule. This brings the myosin back to state 1, but with the thin filament shifted by the distance of the power stroke. With each thick filament having about 500 heads and each head going through the cycle from step 1 through step 4 a few hundred times every second in the course of a rapid shortening, thick and thin filaments can slide past each other at rates of up to $15\,\mu m \cdot s^{-1}$.

It should also be noted that the ATP-requiring step, namely the detachment of the myosin head from the actin filament after the power stroke (state 4 to state 1), is not the regulatory step of the cross-bridge cycle. Calcium regulation affects the step from state 2 to state 3. A muscle that is completely depleted of its ATP gets very stiff because the heads cannot be released from the actin filament, as is the case in the muscles of a dead animal, which fall into rigor mortis.

The sarcomere is built of many more proteins

While actin and myosin are clearly the most abundant proteins in the sarcomere, many more are necessary for its build-up, maintenance and function. Figure 3.7 locates most of these better known 'auxiliary' proteins on the sarcomere. Table 3.1 indicates their function. There are still more proteins in the structure of the sarcomere. Some of them have been isolated by biochemists, but their function and locations are not well known.

Titin is the largest protein so far isolated. It is loosely bound alongside the myosin molecules of the thick filament. It also strongly binds to M-protein in the M-line. One titin molecule stretches from the M-line to the Z-line and is thought to form an elastic filament. These elastic filaments keep the thick filaments centred exactly in the middle between the two Z-lines. Without them, they could pull themselves very close to one end and away from the other Z-line. They also keep the sarcomere together when it is stretched beyond the point of overlap between thick and thin filaments (Fig. 3.8).

Excitation–contraction coupling

The large skeletal muscles in our body consist of up to a million fibres. The exact coordination of the contraction of all these fibres and muscles is achieved by a subdivision of this huge population of fibres into functional units, the motor units.

The motor unit

Motor units consist of a motor nerve, which in the case of the limb muscles has its nerve body

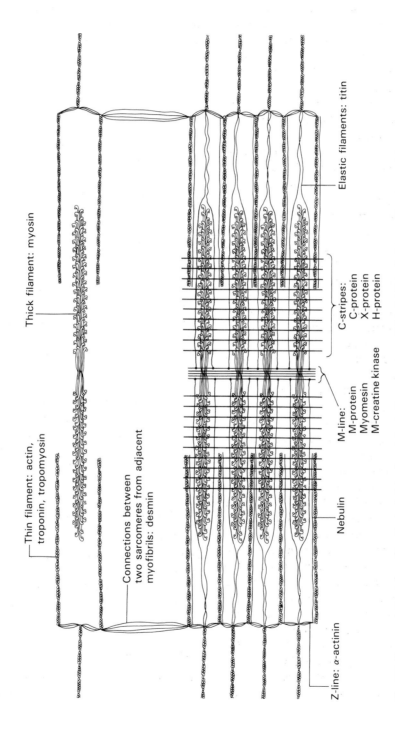

Thick filament: myosin

Thin filament: actin, troponin, tropomyosin

Connections between two sarcomeres from adjacent myofibrils: desmin

Nebulin

Z-line: α-actinin

Elastic filaments: titin

C-stripes:
C-protein
X-protein
H-protein

M-line:
M-protein
Myomesin
M-creatine kinase

Fig. 3.7 Representation of auxiliary (cytoskeleton) proteins in the sarcomere. Table 3.1 lists the known functions of the proteins indicated in this figure.

Table 3.1 Sarcomere proteins and their function

Element	Protein	Function
Z-line	α-actinin	Holds thin filaments in place and in register. Z-lines of slow fibres have more α-actinin than fast ones
	Desmin	Forms the connection between adjacent Z-lines from different myofibrils. This keeps their sarcomeres in register. Desmin is thus responsible for the regular striated appearance of muscle fibres
Thin filament	Actin	Interacts with myosin Forms the core of the thin filament
	Tropomyosin	Transduces the conformational change of the troponin complex to actin
	Troponin	Binds calcium, changes upon binding and affects tropomyosin Represents 'switch' that transforms the calcium signal into molecular signals inducing cross-bridge cycling
	Nebulin	Alongside thin filaments Thought to control the number of actin monomers joined to each other in a thin filament
Thick filament	Myosin	Spilts ATP Responsible for 'power stroke' of the head
C-stripes	C-protein	Thought to hold the thick filaments in a regular array Speculated to hold H-protein of neighbouring thick filaments at even distance during force generation; also thought to control the number of myosin molecules in the thick filament
M-line	M-protein	Holds thick filaments in a regular array
	Myomesin	Forms strong anchoring point for titin
	M-CK	Provides ATP from creatine phosphate; located close to the myosin heads
Elastic filament	Titin	Keeps the thick filament in the middle between the two Z-lines during contraction; also thought to control the number of myosin molecules contained in the thick filament

and nucleus located in the grey matter of the spinal cord and forms a long axon going all the way down the limb to the muscle, where it branches out and innervates several fibres (up to 1000 in large 'fast' motor units) through one single synapse located in the middle of the muscle fibre (Fig. 3.9).

When a motor unit is activated, impulses travel down the axon at a speed of several metres per second and are simultaneously distributed to all the fibres in the motor unit. The excitation of the nerve is transferred by the synapse to the muscle fibre's membrane. The depolarization of the muscle cell membrane travels via the T-tubular system into the muscle fibre, where calcium is released from the sarcoplasmic reticulum stores. These calcium ions activate the troponin complex, which in turn 'switches' the contractile machinery on. The whole activation process takes only a few milliseconds. Since all the fibres in a motor unit are contracting simultaneously, they are of the same histochemical fibre type, and moreover have very similar metabolic and physiological properties.

The synapse

The site of signal transduction of the electrical impulses from the motor nerve's membrane to the muscle fibre's membrane is the synapse (Fig. 3.10), the 'blob'-like end of the axon, which is separated from the muscle membrane by a cleft of 0.05 μm. This is called the 'neuro-

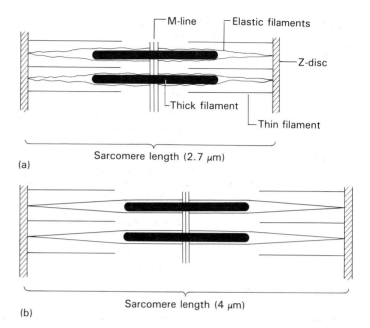

Fig. 3.8 Illustration of elastic filament function. (a) Elastic filaments, composed of titin molecules, link the M-lines of the thick filaments to the Z-discs and keep the thick filaments centred at rest. (b) An overstretched sarcomere is still kept together despite the loss of overlap between thin and thick filaments. (From Horowitz & Podolsky, 1987.)

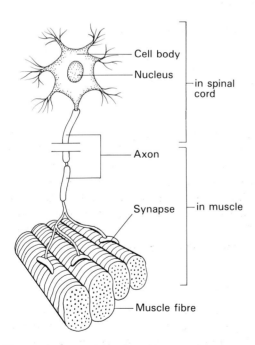

Fig. 3.9 A motor unit consists of its motor nerve, which branches out to form connections to many muscle fibres through synapses, called motor end plates. (From Brooks & Fahey, 1985.)

muscular junction'. When an electrical impulse arrives at the synapse, acetylcholine, a small molecule, is released by the nerve terminal and diffuses rapidly through the small cleft to the muscle membrane. There it is bound to an acetylcholine receptor, which in turn opens sodium ion channels giving rise to an electrical impulse travelling down the muscle cell membrane. The acetylcholine is rapidly cleaved (and thus rendered non-functional) and taken back up by the nerve terminal. From the neuromuscular junction, the electrical impulse not only travels up and down the muscle fibre's membrane (at a speed exceeding $1 \text{ m} \cdot \text{s}^{-1}$), it also reaches the inside of the muscle fibre by way of the membranes of the T-tubular system (Fig. 3.11).

The sarcoplasmic reticulum regulates intracellular calcium

The T-tubules inside the fibre are connected by knob-like structures to the sarcoplasmic reticulum, a sheet of anastamosing flattened

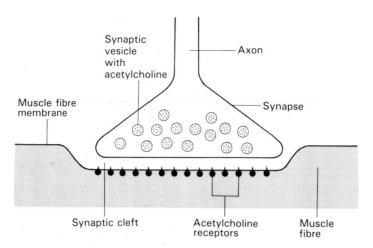

Fig. 3.10 The synapse is a broadened nerve terminal, separated from the target cell (in this case a muscle fibre) by a very small space, the synaptic cleft. A motor end plate uses acetylcholine as transmitter substance. It is stored in the synapse in the synaptic vesicles. When an electrical impulse from the axon reaches the synapse, acetylcholine is released into the synaptic cleft and taken up by acetylcholine receptors located on the muscle side of the cleft in the membrane. The acetylcholine receptors then generate an electrical impulse travelling down the muscle fibre membrane. (From Brooks & Fahey, 1985.)

vesicles that surround each myofibril like a net stocking (Fig. 3.11). The sarcoplasmic reticulum is a calcium store. Inside it, the calcium ion concentration is about 10 000-fold higher than in the sarcoplasm of the muscle fibre. The knob-like structures connecting T-tubules and sarcoplasmic reticulum are called 'junctional feet' (Fig. 3.12). It has been hypothesized that the junctional feet undergo conformational changes upon the arrival of an electrical impulse on the T-tubule. The conformational change of the feet proteins lead to a change in calcium channel proteins, which are located right next to the junctional feet. These channel proteins are normally in a closed state. With the change of the junctional feet complex they open for a short moment and release a small quantity of calcium ions, enough to permit the calcium concentration inside the muscle fibre to rise about 100-fold. The calcium release is driven by the large concentration difference between the sarcoplasmic reticulum and the muscle fibre's sarcoplasm.

If no other impulse comes along the T-tubules, the calcium ions are quickly pumped back by the calcium pumps of the sarcoplasmic reticulum membranes. These pumps are assumed to be situated further away from the junctional feet than the channels. After a single impulse, the calcium concentration in the cytosol is restored to resting levels typically within 30 ms. The calcium pumps derive their energy to bring the ions back into the sarcoplasmic reticulum through splitting of ATP. Up to 30% of a muscle fibre's ATP used during contraction is accounted for by the sarcoplasmic reticulum calcium pumps. Inside the sarcoplasmic reticulum, excess calcium ions are bound to calsequestrin, a special calcium-binding protein.

When a muscle fibre is activated during a normal contraction it generally does not receive just a single impulse, but rather a volley of several impulses. The calcium ions cannot be pumped back fast enough between these impulses. Calcium can thus accumulate to higher levels in the fibre's interior. More regulatory units are activated and higher forces can be developed during such 'tetanic bursts' compared to a single stimulus. The rise in

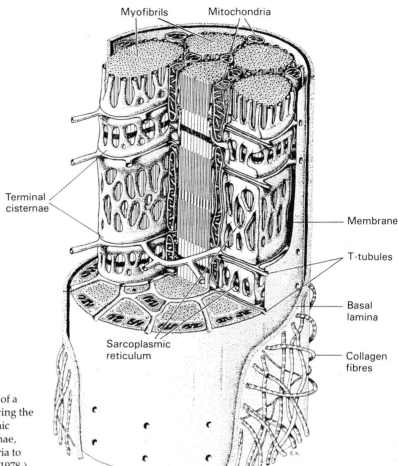

Myofibrils   Mitochondria

Terminal
cisternae

Membrane

T-tubules

Basal
lamina

Sarcoplasmic
reticulum

Collagen
fibres

Fig. 3.11 Drawing of part of a skeletal muscle fibre showing the relationship of sarcoplasmic reticulum, terminal cisternae, T-tubules and mitochondria to myofibrils. (From Krstić, 1978.)

intracellular calcium concentration also has a stimulating effect on the mitochondrial metabolism; thus ATP generation is enhanced at the same time that ATP use by the myofibrils is activated.

Muscle fibre types

Isoforms of myofibrillar proteins

Nearly all the proteins that build up the sarcomere and the sarcoplasmic reticulum exist in different molecular forms, so-called isoforms. Isoforms are different 'editions' of the same protein, differing only slightly in their structure. Functional differences between isoforms include different reaction speeds, tighter binding to target proteins, etc.

The isoforms of myosin are the basis of the nomenclature of muscle fibre types. These myosin isoforms differ in the rate at which the ATPase operates. Heads of the faster myosins split ATP about 600 times per second, slower myosins at about half this rate. The different ATPase reaction rates relate well to the contractile properties of the muscle fibres containing the particular myosin: the contraction time for 'fast' fibres is 40–90 ms, and for slow fibres 90–140 ms. Since fibres with fast myosins have

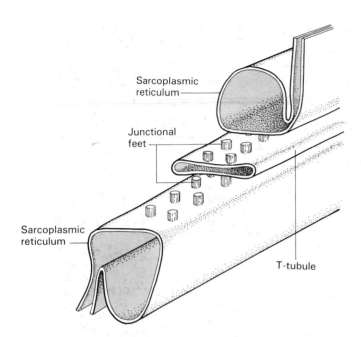

Sarcoplasmic
reticulum

Junctional
feet

Sarcoplasmic
reticulum

T-tubule

Fig. 3.12 Connection between T-tubules and the sarcoplasmic reticulum. The two structures are connected by large protein complexes, called 'junctional feet', which are thought to transfer the impulse signal from the T-tubules to the parts of the sarcoplasmic reticulum adjacent to it. (From Eisenberg, 1983.)

a faster cross-bridge cycle, they are optimally used in quick movements. Fibres with slow myosins, which have a slower cross-bridge cycle, are best suited for static (tonic) work and in the relatively slow everyday movements. It is thought that at a given moment during a contraction, more myosin heads are attached to actin in slow compared to fast fibres, since their heads detach more slowly. At their optimal speed of contraction, slow fibres use less ATP per unit force generated than fast fibres, whose heads have to go through more cross-bridge cycles to generate that same power. Slow fibres therefore have a higher efficiency of contraction than fast fibres. The price is a slower contraction.

The exact number of different myosin isoforms in skeletal muscle is still a matter of controversy. Molecular biologists have found at least five different forms in human limb muscle on the basis of slight differences in the amino acid sequences of their tails; it would not be surprising, however, if biochemists find many more skeletal muscle myosin isoforms in the wake of the ever-growing sophistication of analytical techniques.

Muscle fibre typing is based on myofibrillar ATPase histochemistry

The classic histochemical way of fibre typing relies on the recognition of the three distinct myosin isoforms, which can be distinguished on the basis of the sensitivity of their ATPase activity to acid and alkali solutions (Fig. 3.13). When a muscle cryostat section (from a needle biopsy, for example) is incubated in a solution of pH 10.6 before the myosin ATPase reaction is performed, only fibres with predominantly fast myosin show the coloured reaction product and therefore ATPase reactivity. Such fibres are called fast, fast twitch or type II fibres. When a muscle cryostat section is incubated at pH 4.3 before the ATPase reaction, only the fibres with the slow myosin show the product and thus ATPase activity. These fibres are called slow, slow twitch or type I fibres. Preincubation at pH 4.6 reveals that the myosin ATPase of some of the type II fibres shows some resistance against this pH, the myosin of others does not. Fibres staining slightly after incubation at pH 4.6 are called type IIB, the blank fibres are type IIA. As indicated by the differences in

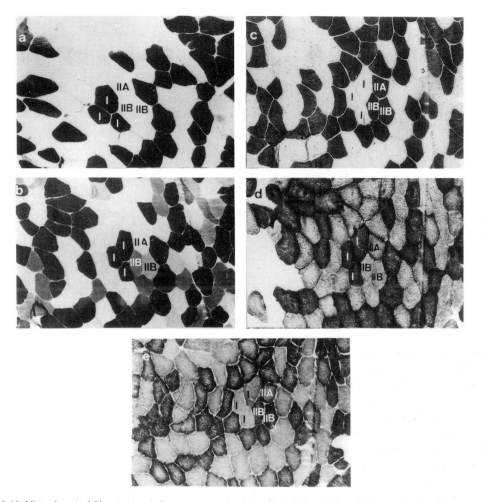

Fig. 3.13 Histochemical fibre typing in human m. vastus lateralis. (a) Myofibrillar ATPase reaction of a 10-μm cryostat section after preincubation at pH 4.3. The ATPase of type I fibres is still active, type II fibre ATPase is destroyed. (b) Myofibrillar ATPase reaction after preincubation at pH 4.6. The ATPase of type I fibres is active, type IIB fibre ATPase is moderately affected, type IIA fibre ATPase is destroyed. (c) Myofibrillar ATPase reaction after preincubation at pH 10.6. The ATPase of type II fibres is activated, type I fibre ATPase is destroyed. (d) Succinate dehydrogenase reaction, indicating the oxidative capacities of the muscle fibres. Note the slightly higher activity of the IIA fibre compared to IIB. (e) α-glycerophosphate dehydrogenase reaction, indicating the glycolytic (lactate forming) capacities of the fibres. Note the variability in type I fibres and slightly lower reaction in some type IIA fibres compared to IIB.

acid sensitivity of their ATPase reactions, the myosin isoforms of type IIA and IIB fibres are different.

Figure 3.13 also shows that these muscle fibre types have quite different metabolic capacities. Type I (slow twitch) fibres stain stronger for succinate dehydrogenase than type II (fast twitch) fibres. They therefore have higher oxidative capacities, i.e. more mitochondria with more enzymes of the pathways of lipid and glucose oxidation. They generate their ATP mainly through the oxidation of glucose units and fatty acids (see below). Only when producing very high power output do they form lactate. They can also use lactate as an energy source. This is done by taking up lactate from the bloodstream or from the interstitial tissue between the fibres, turning it into pyruvate and oxidizing it in the mitochondria. As already mentioned, slow fibres have lower contraction velocities than fast fibres. Due to their oxidative metabolism and their higher efficiency, they show a much greater resistance to fatigue.

Type II (fast twitch) fibres stain weaker for succinate dehydrogenase than type I, but they stain stronger for α-glycerophosphate dehydrogenase. The α-glycerophosphate dehydrogenase staining intensity indicates the glycolytic capacity of a muscle fibre. This is the ability to form lactate from the glycogen stores in the fibre. Type II fibres generate the ATP for force production mainly through anaerobic glycolysis, which results in the production of lactate. They have smaller amounts of mitochondria, and their power output during repetitive activation could not be achieved through ATP produced in their mitochondria. They tend to fatigue quickly because they accumulate lactate (up to 30-fold the concentration in resting muscle). The low pH associated with this lactate accumulation as well as the corresponding rise in free phosphate inhibits the myosin ATPase, slowing contraction speed or stopping active contraction entirely. Type IIA fibres are intermediate to type I and type IIB fibres in contractile and metabolic characteristics.

As previously mentioned type II fibres exhibit greater shortening velocities than type I fibres. Within each fibre type, however, one finds relatively large variations in physiological parameters, such as contraction velocity, relaxation time or fatiguability. The distribution of these parameters among the fibres of a particular muscle looks more like a continuum than clearly distinct, narrowly defined fibre type groups. Careful analysis of the myofibrillar protein isoform composition of a large number of muscle fibres has shown that many different combinations of isoforms of troponin, tropomyosin, C-protein, myomesin and other proteins occur in fibres of the same ATPase type. People have speculated that different combinations of these protein forms are a way of 'fine-tuning' the contractile properties of a given fibre to the exact pattern of use. This is probably because the rate of operation of ATPase of the myosin head cannot be modulated to a large degree. Fibres belonging to the same motor unit, however, have all essentially the same contractile properties and should therefore also have the same myofibrillar isoprotein combination.

Motor unit recruitment

In most voluntary everyday contractions, slow (type I) motor units are the first to be recruited. With increasing power output, more and more fast (type II) units are activated. Trained people can activate all the motor units in a large limb muscle during a static, maximal, voluntary contraction, whereas this is not possible for untrained people. The 'fastest' (type IIB) motor units are preferentially activated in fast corrective movements and reflexes. Explosive maximal contractions are thought to activate fast and slow motor units simultaneously. Slow motor units generally contain only few fibres; fast motor units are larger and may contain up to 1000 fibres. For other details of motor unit recruitment see Chapter 2B.

Strength is related to fibre diameter, not fibre type

While the different fibre types show clear differences in contraction speed, the force developed in a maximal static action is independent of the fibre type, but related to the cross-sectional diameter. Since type I (slow) fibres tend to have smaller diameters than type II (fast) fibres, a high percentage of type I fibres is believed to be associated with a smaller muscle diameter.

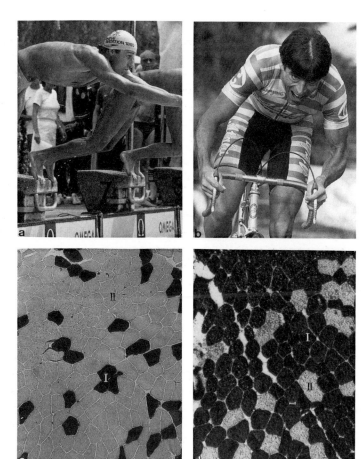

Fig. 3.14 Fibre type composition of two selected top athletes. (a) A swimmer whose speciality is the 50-m crawl sprint. (b) A professional cyclist of world-class 'roller' type. (c–d) Cryostat sections of the swimmer and cyclist's m. vastus lateralis stained for myofibrillar ATPase after preincubation at pH 4.3. Type I fibres stain dark, type II fibres remain unstained. (c) The vast majority of the swimmer's fibres are type II (fast twitch). (d) The vast majority of the cyclist's fibres are type I (slow twitch).

Athletes may have extreme fibre type distributions

It has been known for several decades that top athletes in sports requiring either high speed or very good endurance have very different fibre type compositions in their muscles. Figure 3.14 illustrates this fact with a muscle sample from a swimmer whose speciality was the 50 m crawl sprint; it is compared to a muscle sample from a professional cyclist. The swimmer has about 80% type II (fast twitch) fibres in his m. vastus lateralis, the cyclist about 80% type I (slow twitch) fibres. It is still a matter of debate to what extent such extreme fibre type compositions are genetically predetermined or caused by the hard training the athletes perform. Both factors certainly play some role. Endurance training over periods of several months has been shown to induce fibre type conversions from type IIB to IIA in most type IIB fibres and from type IIA to I in a few percent of the type IIA fibres. However, training periods of several years, typical for most top athletes, have not been analysed so far.

Energy supply systems

The contractile machinery of muscle tissue previously discussed occupies some 80% of the muscle fibre volume and thus represents about one-third of our body mass. The intricately

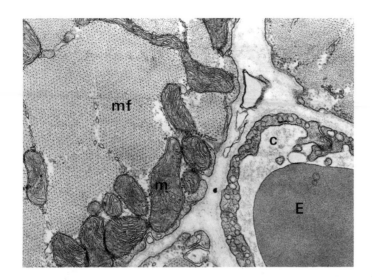

Fig. 3.15 Electron micrograph of cross-sections of portions of skeletal muscle fibres. The capillary (C) contains an erythrocyte (E). In the muscle fibre thin actin and thick myosin filaments (mf) and mitochondria (m) can be distinguished.

interwoven network of tubules and cisternae that regulates the interaction of actin and myosin is relatively compact and occupies only some 5% of the volume of a muscle fibre. However, both the processes of muscle contraction as well as the maintenance of the necessary ion gradients within and around the muscle cells are critically dependent on the energy status of the muscle cell. This section explores the various pathways by which energy is channelled into muscle contraction.

Aerobic metabolism

When a muscle cell is not supplying external mechanical energy but is simply ticking over, the little energy it consumes is derived through cell respiration or 'oxidative phosphorylation'. In this process foodstuff, mainly sugars and lipids, are being broken down in a cellular furnace located in specific submicroscopic organelles called mitochondria (Fig. 3.15). These processes allow the capture of some 50% of the energy stored in the chemical bonds of these foodstuffs. If we take the example of sucrose or fructose that we may ingest when we eat an apple this energy essentially represents solar energy that served to bind atmospheric CO_2 at the time the fruit was

growing on its tree. Respiration can thus be considered to be a form of cellular combustion, which allows for liberation of energy in a form that can be reused for the energy-requiring processes of the cell. The unused or waste energy is lost as heat and serves to maintain our body temperature.

It has been demonstrated that the processes of cellular combustion are occurring at rather fixed efficiencies. As a consequence, we find that the quantity of oxygen consumed during respiration is directly proportional to the power yield of this process to the organism. The production of 1 W of metabolic power requires the consumption of $3\,ml \cdot min^{-1}$ of oxygen. At rest a human consumes some $300\,ml \cdot min^{-1}$ of oxygen and is thus producing metabolic energy at a rate of approximately 100 W. At rest the main oxygen consumers are the brain, heart, kidneys and the intestinal organs, while despite its large size the musculature consumes less than 20% of the total energy. This is different during work. With increasing workloads, such as when doing an aerobic performance test on a bicycle ergometer, it is noted that the oxygen consumption increases in proportion to the external load (Fig. 3.16). Eventually the oxygen consumption levels off and further energy for

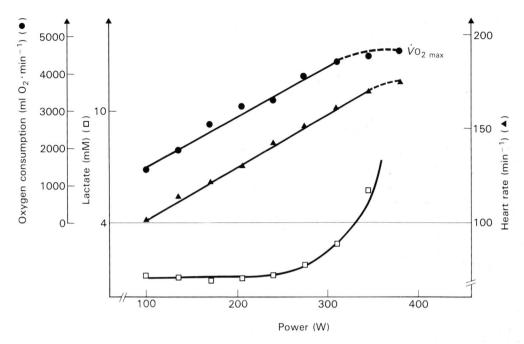

Fig. 3.16 Evolution of oxygen consumption (●), heart rate (▲) and plasma lactate concentration (□) during a typical bicycle ergometer performance test. The power was increased by 35 W every second minute until the subject was exhausted.

muscle contraction must be supplied by anaerobic glycolysis. As a consequence we observe a rapid rise in plasma lactate levels at these power settings. We will further explore the process of glycolysis below.

Provided we carry out the performance test with a large enough muscle mass, we observe a plateau of oxygen consumption beyond which oxygen consumption cannot be increased. We call this plateau *maximal oxygen consumption* or $\dot{V}_{O_{2max}}$. At $\dot{V}_{O_{2max}}$ it has been shown that over 90% of the oxygen taken up by the lungs goes to skeletal muscle mitochondria (Åstrand & Rodahl, 1986). There is thus a large dynamic range of functional regulation of cellular respiration in skeletal muscles, which outstrips by far the regulatory capacity of other organs. It has been hotly debated in the past which of all the transfer steps from lungs to skeletal muscle mitochondria might be the limiting step, responsible for setting the pace of aerobic energy flow in humans. There is growing evi-

dence that all transfer steps add some resistance to oxygen flow into the periphery (Fig. 3.17). However, during work with a large muscle mass in humans in normoxia the major resistance (some 80%) resides in cardiovascular oxygen transport (di Prampero, 1985). In that sense cardiovascular oxygen transport can be considered to be the most 'important' step of oxygen transfer during heavy exercise.

In order to maintain the largest possible power output for a prolonged period of time (i.e. over 30 min; Fig. 3.18) muscle cell respiration must be near maximal. It can be observed that an untrained young man may be capable of maintaining a power output of 200 W by consuming just over $3 \, l \cdot min^{-1}$ of oxygen. A highly trained professional bicyclist may be capable of a power output of just over 400 W with a corresponding oxygen uptake close to 6 $l \cdot min^{-1}$. As previously discussed, the limit for aerobic mechanical power production does not reside in the contractile machinery of the

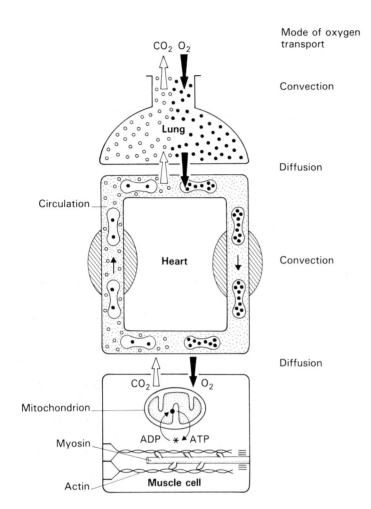

Fig. 3.17 Model of gas exchange in the human respiratory system.

muscles but rather in the characteristics of the entire respiratory system. We will now address the problem of how energy is stored in muscle and how it is moved around in muscle cells.

Energy storage and energy transfer

We have seen that, during aerobic muscular exercise, oxygen must be supplied constantly to muscle fibres such that the oxygen flow rate essentially represents energy flux at the level of the active muscle cells. This is because only small quantities of oxygen can be stored in muscle tissue in humans. Thus the oxygen supply must continuously be renewed. This is not the case for the substrates of cellular

combustion. Glucose in its storage form of glycogen as well as lipids are stored intra-cellularly in muscle cells. It has been demonstrated that continuous athletic activity, such as running 100 km, leads to an almost complete depletion of these stores (Kayar et al., 1986; Fig. 3.19). Nutrient supply through the capillaries can, except during very low intensity exercise, always only account for a fraction of the total cellular substrate needs. It is believed that active transport across the cell membrane is a bottleneck for the entry of both glucose and free fatty acids into the muscle cell. The breakdown of amino acids plays a very minor role for the energy budget of the working muscle cell in well-nourished people. However, certain

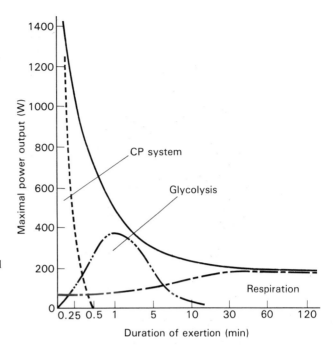

Fig. 3.18 Decrease of maximal mechanical power output on a bicycle ergometer as a function of duration of the exercise. The approximate contribution of the different systems of cellular energy supply is indicated under the curve.

amino acids or their degradation products have been hypothesized to play a role in fatigue-related phenomena (Åstrand & Rodahl, 1986).

If substrates are degraded through the Krebs cycle in muscle mitochondria and terminally oxidized to H_2O and CO_2, both of these compounds are innocuous and rapidly leave the muscle cells to be carried away by the capillary bloodstream (Fig. 3.20). Likewise the excess metabolic heat is dissipated and may, if heavy exercise is carried out in a hot environment, represent a serious hazard for the exercising subject. The 'useful' energy is captured in a highly specialized chemical substance, ATP, which is composed of the purine base adenine and the sugar ribose to which three phosphate residues are reversibly bound (Fig. 3.21). The enzymatic cleavage of these phosphate residues yields energy that can directly be used in all energy-requiring processes of the muscle cell such as contraction, ion pumping, biosynthesis, etc. The largest quantity of chemical energy is made available by splitting off the terminal phosphate from ATP liberating one ADP and one free phosphate. As we will see below, the

remaining two phosphates of the ADP can also be split off. However, the energy gain per bond is smaller and different enzymatic systems must be involved. Mitochondria maintain the energy charge of the muscle cell essentially by rephosphorylating ADP from ATP keeping ATP at a relatively constant and high level.

The creatine phosphate shuttle system

In many mammalian cells there is a close apposition of mitochondria to those structures that are the major energy consumers. Cells that need to transfer energy from mitochondria to some distant consumer (i.e. to myofilaments in muscle cells) have developed an energy shuttle system. In this system a specialized enzyme in the mitochondrial intermembrane space transfers the 'high energy' phosphate from ATP to a creatine molecule (Fig. 3.21). Creatine phosphate (CP) is a much smaller molecule than ATP and is thus more easily diffusible in the muscle cell. An additional advantage of this system resides in the fact that only those structures that have an enzyme capable of

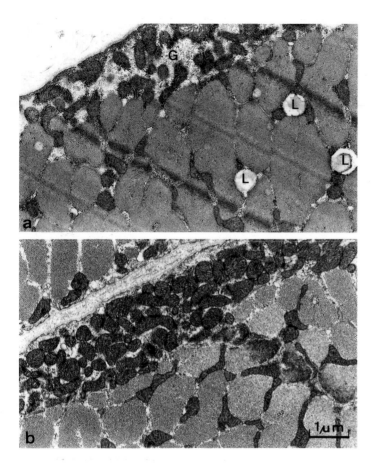

Fig. 3.19 Cross-sections of muscle fibres (a) before and (b) after running 100 km in 7 hours. It is evident that the cellular substrate stores of glycogen (G) and lipid (L) have almost completely disappeared.

retransferring the energy from CP to ADP can utilize this energy (Fig. 3.20). In muscle cells only the myofilaments can access the creatine phosphate pool. This allows for accumulation of CP in relatively large concentrations in muscle cells. Creatine phosphate thus represents an intracellular energy buffer that can be degraded at an extremely high rate for the myosin ATPase if need arises. During intensive exercise, such as sprinting, the CP pool only lasts some 10 s (Fig. 3.18).

With the new technology of magnetic resonance spectroscopy (MR spectroscopy) muscle physiologists have obtained a tool by which the different phosphate pools, as well as the intracellular pH, in muscle cells can be monitored non-invasively (Fig. 3.22). It has thus become possible to evaluate the energy

status of muscle cells while they work. A major limitation of this technique is that to date measurements can only be obtained from relatively large 'volumes' of muscle tissue comprising hundreds of muscle fibres. The MR spectroscopy data therefore represent an average over many muscle fibres, which may be in different states of activation and fatigue.

Glycolysis

So far we have considered respiration capable of furnishing a relatively low power output over a very long time period as well as the associated creatine phosphate system, which can be used for short bursts of very intense exercise (Fig. 3.18). Glycolysis represents an additional system of energy supply that may

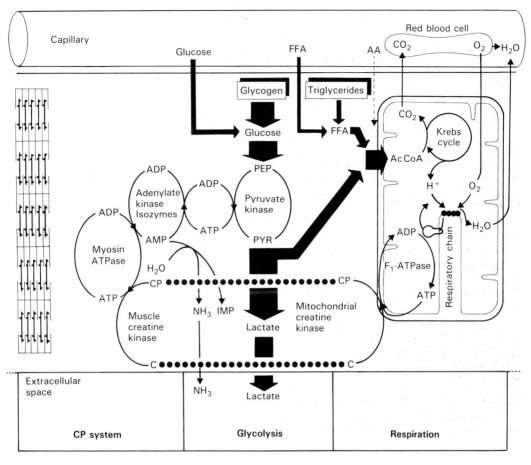

Fig. 3.20 Integrated schematic view of pathways of energy supply to myofibrils. Thickness of arrows approximate the relative importance of some of the substrate fluxes. AA, amino acids; AcCoA, acetyl coenzyme A; CP, creatine phosphate; FFA, free fatty acids; IMP, inosine monophosphate; PEP, phosphoenolpyruvate; PYR, pyruvate.

produce intermediate levels of power output for intermediate periods of time. Furthermore, glycolysis produces the metabolite pyruvate, which is a major fuel for mitochondrial oxidative phosphorylation (Fig. 3.20). During aerobic work glycolysis furnishes pyruvate, which is transferred to mitochondria where its carbon skeleton is entirely degraded to CO_2. This process of full oxidation of glucose in mitochondria yields 36 ATP for each glucose molecule degraded. Glycolysis of glucose to pyruvate only yields 2 ATP.

Why then does the muscle cell bother about glycolysis? The reason is that glycolysis can proceed at a very high rate, indicated in Fig. 3.20 by the different thickness of the arrows. If glycolysis occurs at a rate exceeding the uptake capacity of mitochondria for pyruvate, there is a build-up of lactic acid in the muscle cells. Lactic acid lowers the intracellular pH, thus interfering with muscle contractile activity as previously mentioned. Lactic acid has to be removed from the muscle cell if contractile activity is to proceed. Lactate removal is a relatively slow process, again indicated by the thickness of the arrow in Fig. 3.20.

Adenosine triphosphate (ATP)

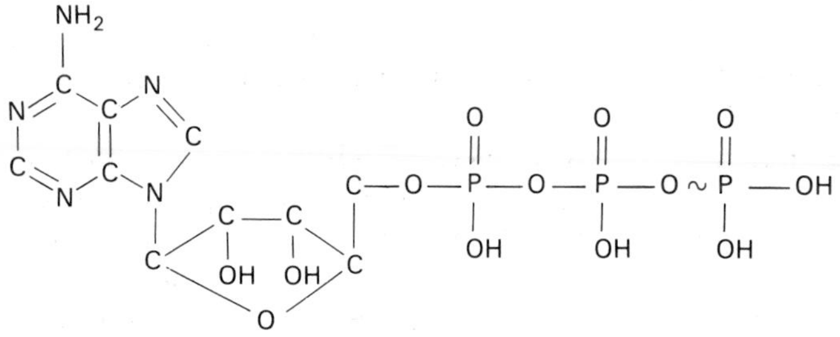

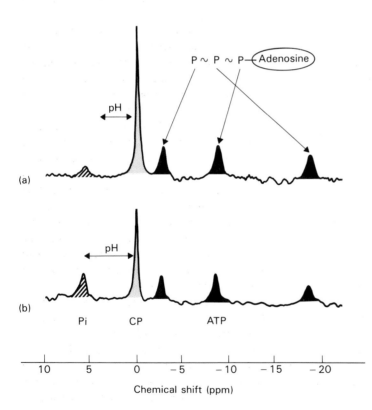

Creatine phosphate (CP)

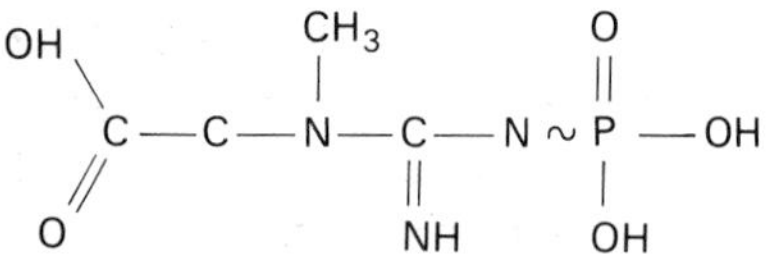

Fig. 3.21 Molecular composition of ATP and CP. Note the much larger size of the ATP molecule.

Fig. 3.22 Representative ^{31}P magnetic resonance spectra obtained (a) at rest and (b) during 2-Hz stimulation in rat muscle tissue. Area under peaks represent metabolite concentration. Note that the separation of the CP and Pi peak is an indicator of intracellular pH. (From Kushmerick, 1986.)

There are some interesting particularities of ATP turnover in glycolysis only recently uncovered and still somewhat controversial (Bessmann & Carpenter, 1985; Zeleznikar *et al.*, 1990). Glycolysis may not participate to a large extent in the CP-shuttle system. In turn, it probably acts through a special tandem isozyme adenylate kinase system. In the proposed metabolic scheme (Fig. 3.20) two ADP, produced by the action of the myosin ATPase as well as by the adenylate kinase, are converted into one ATP and one AMP (adenosine monophosphate). The ATP can be re-utilized by the myosin ATPase. The AMP is rephosphorylated to ADP by ATP produced in glycolysis and then takes part in another cycle of ADP transphosphorylation. The formation of AMP in muscle cells may give rise to the production of IMP catalysed by the enzyme AMP deaminase. In this process ammonia is produced, which is liberated to the bloodstream. Heavy muscle exercise with the activation of glycolysis is thus characterized by the appearance of lactate and ammonia in the bloodstream (Fig. 3.20).

Interdependence of muscle energetics and substrate choice

The different metabolic pathways are activated depending on the intensity and the duration of exercise (Fig. 3.18). It is quite evident that the CP system can be switched on immediately because the energy is available in a directly degradable form. Glycolysis can also be turned on rather rapidly; however, it takes a few minutes before oxidative phosphorylation is in full swing. The metabolites and substrates for the CP system and for glycolysis can be considered to be on-board the muscle cell. In contrast, stimulating respiration involves activating many processes throughout the entire body. Muscle microcirculation must be increased in the working muscles, cardiac output must be stepped up by increasing the heart rate, and ventilation in the lung must be augmented so that a larger blood flow can be

oxygenated. This takes some time. All these regulatory steps are mainly mediated by the nervous system; however, there are local metabolic and hormonal influences that are also involved.

If we go for a full-out sprinting activity for 10 s, we are capable of lowering the CP levels to extremely low values, without much glycolysis occurring, i.e. we are incurring an alactic oxygen (energy) debt. If we then wait for a few minutes for respiration to reload the CP system the same power output as before can be obtained. This is not the case when we run very hard for 800–1000 m. Glycolysis will be fully activated and plasma lactate levels may rise to very high levels (over 20 mmol · l^{-1} in trained athletes). This will seriously disturb acid–base balance and plasma pH may drop well below 6.9 (normal 7.4). More importantly, because of the relatively slow lactate removal from muscle cells, intracellular homeostasis is even more disturbed than what is apparent from the plasma concentrations of the relevant metabolites. When we stop such an exercise it will take not minutes but hours before the muscle cell has regained its equilibrium. It must also be considered that the CP system uses nucleotides that are shuttled around in the muscle cell but that are not 'used up' in the process. This is different for glycolysis. If glycolysis was not switched off quickly by the accumulation of lactic acid in the muscle cell, it would be capable of breaking down all the available glycogen in only a few minutes. To reload the glycogen stores from external (nutritional) sources takes at least a full day under optimal conditions of substrate supply.

If we engage in an aerobic exercise that we know will last for a prolonged period of time we know to pace ourselves so that we do not accumulate excess lactate levels at the beginning of the exercise. Despite that, glycolysis will have to energetically cover the time period until respiration is fully activated. If we thus start to run at a pace of say 75% of our maximal aerobic capcity we will see an initial rise of lactate in the plasma, which later subsides when the muscle cells turn to oxidative phosphorylation.

The maximal rate at which we can work aerobically with a particular muscle or muscle group is essentially given by the quantity of mitochondria it contains provided the capillary supply and cardiovascular oxygen delivery match mitochondrial oxidative capacity. It is likely that aerobic exercise training not only augments all of these factors but also serves to fine-tune all of the energy transfer systems. In most mammals it looks as if cell respiration could proceed at rates higher than the maximal transport capacities of substrates (glucose and free fatty acids, FFA) across the cell membrane. High intensity aerobic work thus necessarily leads to a gradual depletion of the intracellular substrate stores. Once these are used up, respiration continues maximally at the rate of the membrane transport of the substrates. This is believed to be around 50% of the maximal possible rate of respiration. From this it can be seen that in short-time work mitochondrial oxidative capacity limits aerobic work, while the longer the exercise lasts the more important substrate supply becomes.

Structural basis of muscle training

Under given neuronal activation conditions muscle force is proportional to the total number of cross-bridges that can be formed, as mentioned previously. As each myofilament contains the same number of ATPase heads, muscle force is proportional to the total number of myofilaments on the muscle cross-section or roughly to the muscle cross-sectional area. There is to our knowledge no experimental evidence indicating that the intrinsic force of the actin–myosin interaction could be modulated *in vivo*. On the structural level, strength training acts through an increase of muscle cross-sectional area. Likewise, there is no indication that the CP pool of a muscle cell could be increased sizeably. If this were possible it would improve the 'sprint' capacity of an individual. Glycolysis may be improved

with high intensity or interval type of training, although probably only to a limited degree. Additionally, an individual seems to be able to train for tolerance to acidosis and high levels of lactic acid both on a muscle cell level and on a systemic level. Respiration may be the most readily malleable part of the muscle energy supply system. Both muscle capillarity and mitochondrial content can rapidly and largely be increased with an appropriate training stimulus. Furthermore, the size of the heart and hence maximal cardiac output can also be increased under aerobic training conditions.

Perspective

The major challenge to basic muscle research is currently to uncover the mechanisms by which the precise molecular properties of the contractile, the regulatory and the energetic systems are controlled and if need arises modified. It is likely that the next few years will bring major breakthroughs in our understanding of muscle regulatory events. This will not only benefit athletes but all humans. This is because for all of us the quality of our lives is largely dependent on an intact and fully functional locomotor system. We will better understand what to do to keep our muscles optimally functional and how we can get them back to function once they should fail.

Acknowledgements

The excellent technical help of L. Tüscher, K. Babl and B. Krieger in preparing this manuscript is gratefully acknowledged. The work of both authors has been supported over many years by the Swiss National Science Foundation.

References and further reading

Alberts, B., Bray, D., Lewis, J., Raff, M., Roberts, K. & Watson, J.D. (1989) *Molecular Biology of the Cell*, 2nd edn. Garland Publishing, New York.
Åstrand, P.-O. & Rodahl, K. (1986) *Textbook of Work*

Physiology. Physiological Bases of Exercise, 3rd edn. McGraw-Hill International Editions, New York.

Bessmann, S.P. & Carpenter, C.L. (1985) The creatine–creatine phosphate energy shuttle. *Annual Review of Biochemistry*, **54**, 831–62.

Brooks, G.A. & Fahey, T.D. (1985) *Exercise Physiology: Human Bioenergetics and its Applications*. Macmillan, New York.

Cashwell, A.H. & Brandt, N.R. (1989) Does muscle activation occur by direct mechanical coupling of transverse tubules to sarcoplasmic reticulum? *Trends in Biochemical Sciences*, **14**, 161–5.

di Prampero, P.E. (1985) Metabolic and circulatory limitations to VO_{2max} at the whole animal level. *Journal of Experimental Biology*, **115**, 319–32.

Donaldson, S.K. (1989) Mechanisms of excitation–contraction coupling in skinned muscle fibers. *Medicine and Science in Sports and Exercise*, **21**, 411–17.

Eisenberg, B.R. (1983) Quantitative ultrastructure of mammalian skeletal muscle. In L.D. Peachy, R.H. Adrian & S.R. Geiger (eds) *Handbook of Physiology. Skeletal Muscle*, pp. 73–112. Williams & Wilkins, Baltimore.

Horowitz, R. & Podolsky, R. (1987) The positional stability of thick filaments in activated skeletal muscle depends on sarcomere length: Evidence for the role of titin filaments. *Journal of Cell Biology*, **105**, 2217–23.

Howald, H. (1982) Training-induced morphological and functional changes in skeletal muscle. *International Journal of Sports Medicine*, **3**, 1–12.

Kayar, S.R., Hoppeler, H., Howald, H., Claassen, H. & Oberholzer, F. (1986) Acute effects of endurance exercise on mitochondrial distribution and skeletal muscle morphology *European Journal of Applied Physiology*, **54**, 578–84.

Krstić, R.V. (1978) *Die Gewebe des Menschen und der Säugetiere*. Springer Verlag, Berlin.

Kushmerick, M.J. (1986) Spectroscopic applications of magnetic resonance to biomedical problems. *Cardiovascular and Interventional Radiology*, **8**, 382–9.

Payne, M.R. & Rudnick, S.E. (1989) Regulation of vertebrate striated muscle contraction. *Trends in Biochemical Sciences*, **14**, 357–60.

Warrick, H.M. & Spudich, J.A. (1987) Myosin structure and function in cell motility. *Annual Review of Cell Biology*, **3**, 379–421.

Zeleznikar, R.J., Heyman, R.A., Graeff, R.M., Walseth, T.F., Dawis, S.M., Butz, E.A. & Goldberg, N.D. (1990) Evidence for compartmentalized adenylate kinase catalysis serving a high energy phosphoryl transfer function in rat skeletal muscle. *Journal of Biological Chemistry*, **265**, 300–11.

Chapter 4

Hormonal Mechanisms Related to the Expression of Muscular Strength and Power

WILLIAM J. KRAEMER

Muscle fibres play an important role in the production of force and subsequent expression of strength and power. Hormonal mechanisms are part of a complex integrated system that helps mediate and influence the adaptive changes made in the muscle's metabolic and cellular remodelling process involved in the adaptation to resistance exercise training. The training adaptations that occur result in improved force production capabilities and increased size of the muscle cells. The hormonal mechanisms involved are dependent upon the configuration of the exercise stimulus and mediated via molecular mechanisms. The relationship between hormonal release and subsequent cellular interactions provides the theoretical paradigm for the adaptive influence of neuroendocrine factors.

The primary anabolic hormones involved with muscle tissue growth and remodelling are growth hormone, insulin, testosterone, and thyroid hormones (Florini, 1987). In addition, *in vitro* studies have demonstrated that insulin-like growth factors (IGF) also have dramatically potent effects on muscle cell growth (Florini, 1985, 1987). Thus, neuroendocrine factors span a wide variety of hormonal mechanisms affecting metabolism and cellular changes related to growth. Such mechanisms appear to be operational in response to a training stimulus provided by heavy resistance exercise. Still, the exact mechanisms that mediate such changes remain speculative. The purpose of this chapter will be to provide a basic overview

of some of the possible mechanisms where interactions between hormones and receptors may result in adaptive changes consequent to acute resistance exercise stress. Heavy resistance exercise has been classically shown to result in significant adaptive responses resulting in the enhanced size, strength, and power of trained musculature (Fleck & Kraemer, 1987). It might be hypothesized that hormonal increases observed consequent to the performance of heavy resistance exercise routines interact with or influence various cellular mechanisms and enhance the development of the muscle's protein contractile unit thereby providing for the improved force production capabilities observed.

Hypothalamic–pituitary axis

It has long been recognized that growth hormone (GH), a polypeptide hormone secreted from the anterior pituitary gland, is intimately involved with the growth process of skeletal muscle and other tissues in the body. Over the past 10 years, it has also become quite evident that GH actions are mediated to a certain extent by a secondary set of hormones called insulin-like growth factors (IGF), also referred to as somatomedins (Florini, 1987). The secretion of GH is regulated by a complex system of neuroendocrine feedback mechanisms. Various feedback mechanisms have been elucidated and these are presented in Fig. 4.1. For more in-depth examination of this topic, a

64

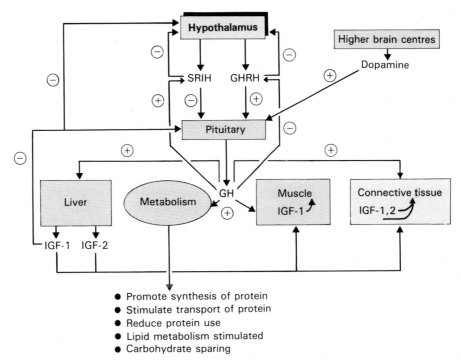

Fig. 4.1 A basic scheme for the cybernetic regulatory neuroendocrine control of growth hormone secretion. GHRH, growth hormone-releasing hormone; IGF, insulin-like growth factor; SRIH, somatotropin release-inhibiting hormone.

number of comprehensive reviews have been published (Clemmons *et al.*, 1989a; Rogol, 1989; Sonntag *et al.*, 1982).

Growth hormone stimulates the release of growth factors and the availability of amino acids for protein synthesis. Together such conditions promote recovery and tissue repair. The many reports of IGF being released from non-hepatic tissues, including muscle itself, really suggests that GH could also stimulate the intracellular increase in IGF synthesis (Florini, 1987; Han *et al.*, 1987; Daughaday & Rotwein, 1989). Growth hormone plays a crucial role in augmenting IGF release. Alone, IGF cannot manifest such a complex system of external signals (Florini, 1987). Thus, GH promotes IGF release from hepatic sources that interacts with the various cells. In addition, it stimulates synthesis and release of IGF from within the cell itself to influence growth promoting actions.

Growth hormone is secreted in a 'burst-like' or pulsatile fashion and has definite diurnal variations with the highest levels observed at night during sleep phases (Finkelstein *et al.*, 1972; Sonntag *et al.*, 1982). It has been hypothesized that such increases are involved with various tissue repair mechanisms. Thus, it is possible that such GH secretion and release may directly influence adaptations of the contractile unit of muscle and subsequent expression of strength and power. A typical diurnal response curve of GH is presented in Fig. 4.2. Various external factors such as sleep, nutrition, alcohol consumption, and exercise have all been shown to alter GH release patterns (Buckler, 1971; Okayama, 1972; Sonntag *et al.*, 1982; Chang *et al.*, 1985).

Growth hormone is released into the peripheral circulation where it attaches to specific binding proteins, which represent the extracellular domain of the GH receptor (Leung

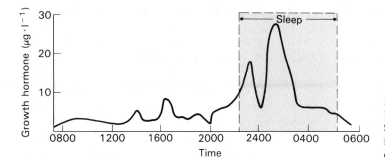

Fig. 4.2 A 24-hour growth hormone diurnal response curve. Sleep stimulates dramatic increases in the magnitude and duration of GH release.

et al., 1987). It acts by binding to plasma membrane-bound receptors on the target cells. Less is understood about the subsequent cellular effects and molecular events that mediate effector changes. A glycosylated single polypeptide appears to be important for GH binding. These binding proteins provide the basis for the biological actions of GH. It is still unclear how extracellular domain binding of the receptor leads to a signal transduction in the cytosolic domain via such a short trans-membrane sequence (Clemmons *et al.*, 1989a). Growth hormone binding may produce aggregates of receptors that traverse laterally in the fluid plasma membrane. Subsequently, the cell membrane-bound receptor also interacts and binds specifically with GH. Thus, the GH receptor interactions are operational within a number of different molecular domains where various binding and subsequent biological actions occur (Clemmons *et al.*, 1989a).

Growth hormone has many biological roles in metabolism and growth promoting actions in tissues (Sonntag *et al.*, 1982; Florini, 1987; Clemmons *et al.*, 1989a). Many of these biological actions are mediated via IGF mechanisms. Such effects as muscle tissue growth are mediated by a variety of cellular mechanisms, which promote such adaptations. Some of the basic physiological roles initiated by GH are shown in Table 4.1.

It appears that the role of GH in muscle tissue is related to events involving an immature muscle cell. This has been hypothesized as GH has few direct effects on embryonic muscle

Table 4.1 Basic direct and indirect physiological actions of growth hormone

Reduction of glucose utilization
Decreased glycogen synthesis
Increased amino acid transport across cell membrane
Increased protein synthesis
Increased utilization of fatty acids
Increased lipolysis
Metabolic sparing of glucose and amino acids
Collagen synthesis
Stimulation of cartilage growth
Increased uptake of chondroitin sulphate
Rentention of nitrogen, sodium, potassium and phosphorus
Increased renal plasma flow and glomerular filtration
Promotion of compensatory renal hypertrophy

tissue cultures (Florini, 1987). The enhancement of the contractile unit by such interactions would appear to contribute to the development of the intact muscle and subsequent force production characteristics. Still, further research is needed to clarify how it is involved with exercise-induced hypertrophy. Studies outlined by Rogol (1989) show that the GH treatment alone is not effective in causing strength increases and that the total motor unit involvement is probably necessary. Thus, any apparent ergogenic effect may be outweighed by a wide variety of secondary effects not related to strength changes in muscle tissue (Rogol, 1989). It seems plausible that the endogenous mechanisms that are related to the exercise stimulus have greater specificity and would be more effective in mediating the specific mechanisms related to strength and hypertrophy development. It now appears that exercise-induced hypertrophy is quite different from GH-stimulated hypertrophy. The muscle fibre's force production characteristics are superior consequent to exercise-induced size increases compared to GH-treated muscle (Goldberg & Goodman, 1969; Riss *et al.*, 1986; Rogol, 1989).

Insulin-like growth factors (somatomedins)

As previously discussed, many of the effects of GH are mediated through small polypeptides called insulin-like growth factors: IGF-I is a 70 amino acid polypeptide and IGF-II is a 67 amino acid polypeptide whose function is less clear. Typical of many polypeptide hormones, both growth factors are synthesized as a larger precursor peptide and undergo significant post-translational processing to the final end-products, IGF-I and IGF-II peptides. In muscle fibres, virtually all biological actions attributed to GH appear to be mediated by IGF (Florini, 1987; Fagin *et al.*, 1989). Growth hormone stimulated DNA synthesis of IGF typically takes 3–9 hours. Speculation of a non-GH-mediated release of IGF from intracellular release mechanisms remains a very distinct possibility but more definite evidence is needed (Allen *et al.*, 1979; Florini, 1987; Han *et al.*, 1987; Adem *et al.*, 1989; Hill *et al.*, 1989; Horikawa *et al.*, 1989). Over the past 10 years, there has been a virtual explosion in the number of investigations that have examined these polypeptides (i.e. IGF-I, IGF-II). Since providing a review of such a large amount of data is beyond the scope of this chapter, a number of reviews are available for more detailed study (Florini, 1987; Clemmons *et al.*, 1989a; Czech, 1989).

It now appears that IGF are important stimulators of a number of biological activities involving anabolic processes in skeletal muscle (Allen & Boxhorn, 1988; Turner *et al.*, 1988; Zorzano *et al.*, 1988). Various findings also suggest that IGF-I may be secreted locally in various tissues and stimulate growth prior to any release into the circulation. The hypothesized autocrine/paracrine mechanisms proposed are supported in theory by the fact that IGF receptors are found in most cell lines. The circulating transport binding and membrane binding are related to at least five distinct macromolecules. The various interactions between GH and IGF for cellular release and stimulation are shown in Fig. 4.3, while the various relationships between the different circulating and membrane-bound protein-binding interactions are depicted in Fig. 4.4.

Circulating IGF are apparently associated with binding proteins. At least two circulating binding proteins have been identified and regulate the amount of IGF that is available in the plasma and capable of initiating any signal transduction. Binding proteins are important factors in the transport and physiological mechanisms related to IGF (Forbes *et al.*, 1988; Clemmons *et al.*, 1989a,b). Insulin-like growth factors have been shown to stimulate the secretion of their own binding proteins from within the muscle cell itself thus modulating its responsiveness to IGF (McCusker *et al.*, 1989). The circulating IGF binding proteins play a major role in restricting access of the IGF peptides to receptors and are influenced by GH concentrations. The regulation of IGF concentration and availability is a function of many factors including hormonal regulation influenced by growth hormone secretion and insulin, while other factors such as nutritional status also have been shown to be an important signal mechanism for IGF release. The nutritional influence on IGF transport, production, and regulatory control is a dramatic variable affecting cellular interactions. Acute changes in nitrogen balance, protein intake, and nutritional status all affect a variety of mechanisms and have been previously reviewed (Clemmons *et al.*, 1989a; Maiter *et al.*, 1989; Rogol, 1989). It also appears that binding proteins act as a reservoir of IGF and, in a pulsatile manner, respond to the receptor

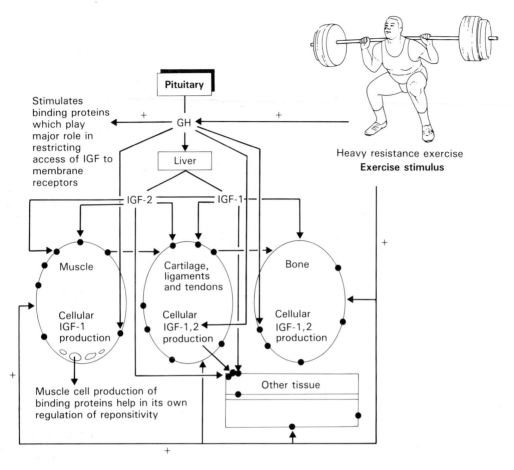

Fig. 4.3 Possible influences for IGF production. IGF is stimulated in both hepatic and extrahepatic tissues through both autocrine and paracrine mechanisms. GH, growth hormone; IGF, insulin-like growth factor; •, IGF receptors.

occupancy by releasing IGF when receptors are available (Blum *et al.*, 1989). This could theoretically reduce degradation and allow IGF to have more effective and longer response times as receptor interactions could be maintained for longer periods of time.

Type I and type II IGF receptors and IGF-II/mannose-6-phosphate receptors all interact with IGF in addition to insulin receptors, which have cross-reactivity but show a much lower affinity for IGF. The membrane-bound receptor's interactions and regulation are complex and just starting to be understood (Baxter & Martin, 1989; Baxter *et al.*, 1989;

Czech, 1989). For example, the type I IGF receptor complex presents exofacial ligand binding domains (alpha subunit) and intracellular tyrosine kinase domains (beta subunit). The receptor tyrosine kinase signal pathways are activated by insulin or IGF receptor binding and appear necessary for signal transmission (see Fig. 4.4).

In strength training it is easy to see that many of these mechanisms would be influenced by the exercise stress, acute hormonal responses, and the need for tissue remodelling (e.g. muscle, nerve, bone) at the cellular level (Skottner *et al.*, 1988; Hansson *et al.*, 1989; Ishii,

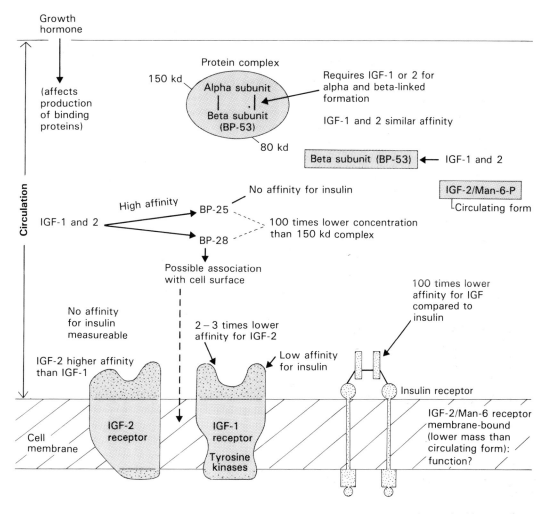

Fig. 4.4 Theoretical scheme for circulating and membrane-bound binding interactions for insulin-like growth factors (IGF-1 and IGF-2). BP, binding protein; Man-6-P, mannose-6-phosphate.

1989). The dramatic interactions of multiple hormones and receptors provide possible powerful adaptive mechanisms in the response to resistance exercise training and theoretically contribute to the subsequent changes in muscular strength and power.

Insulin

A vast amount of research has underscored the importance of insulin in energy metabolism and disease states such as diabetes. Insulin also plays an important role in protein metabolism and, therefore, in the subsequent development of the contractile unit via effects on protein metabolism. Insulin, similar to IGF, inhibits protein degradation and apparently offsets the catabolic effects of other hormones, especially cortisol. The net effects of greater receptor occupancy of insulin and IGF appear to antagonize or offset the catabolic actions promoted when greater net receptor occupancy

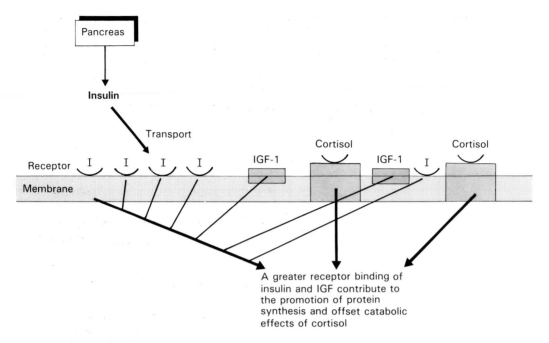

Fig. 4.5 A basic scheme showing the antagonistic relationship of insulin and insulin-like growth factors (IGF) in net binding effects versus cortisol in the development of a muscle fibre.

of glucocorticoids (i.e. cortisol) are observed. Anabolic actions of insulin are related to its nitrogen sparing effects and promotion of nitrogen retention. The interaction with insulin receptors and the cross-reactivity with IGF-I receptors help contribute to an overall anabolic status for protein metabolism and synthesis in muscle. Thus, insulin is critical for normal development of muscle tissue and contributes to the dramatic regulatory mechanisms that have been previously described in detail (Pruett, 1985; Florini, 1987). An overview of insulin's theoretical actions in skeletal muscle is depicted in Fig. 4.5.

Testosterone

The mechanism of action concerning testosterone's influence on skeletal muscle have been at times misinterpreted due to parallel research performed on sex-linked tissue such as the prostate, seminal vesicles, and levator ani, which respond quite differently from skeletal muscle and where testosterone is not the primary androgen (Rance & Max, 1984; Florini, 1985, 1987). Testosterone has been used as a physiological marker or contributor to various hormonal ratios to evaluate the 'anabolic status' of the body (Häkkinen et al., 1985; Kuoppasalmi & Adlercreutz, 1985). The direct effects of testosterone on skeletal muscle growth in culture are not as dramatic as other hormones, e.g. IGF, and it is possible that testosterone mechanisms involve a variety of direct and indirect actions (Florini, 1987; Young et al., 1989). Such observations reflect the augmentation role played by testosterone in the development of the protein contractile unit of muscle (Griggs et al., 1989).

Testosterone, not dihydrotestosterone, directly interacts and binds with the skeletal muscle receptors. Such actions include transport, a membrane-bound protein, a theoretical secondary messenger, and cytoplasmic receptor with subsequent migration to the nucleus where the potential interactions with nuclear

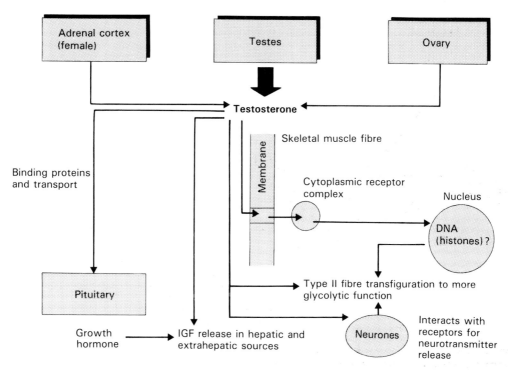

Fig. 4.6 A basic theoretical scheme for the primary influences of testosterone on factors in muscle cell development. Adrenal cortex is a significant source for females compared to males.

proteins exists (Michel & Baulieu, 1980; Sherman & Stevens, 1984; Florini, 1985; Griggs *et al.*, 1986; Vermeulen, 1988; Rosner, 1990). Such interactions with the nucleus may reflect the direct actions of testosterone on muscle cell development.

Examining the possible effects on strength expression, testosterone may play a more dramatic role by influencing neural factors and the possible muscle fibre transition of type II fibres to more glycolytic profiles (Bleisch *et al.*, 1984; Kelly *et al.*, 1985). In addition, enhanced stimulation of GH secretion by testosterone increases the production of IGF via GH-mediated mechanisms and may also help produce various anabolic properties typically attributed to testosterone in the whole animal (Florini, 1987). These potential interactions with other hormones demonstrate the highly interdependent nature of the neuroendocrine system in influencing the expression of a per-formance characteristic such as strength and power of the intact muscles. Thus, how testosterone influences such changes in muscle structure and function may be in large part due to the interaction of testosterone with many tissues (e.g. nervous tissue) and other hormones in the body (e.g. GH). The hormonal cybernetic controls of testosterone release have been previously overviewed in detail (Gharib *et al.*, 1990; Kraemer, 1988). An overview of the influence of testosterone on the contractile elements of muscle and subsequent strength and power expression are outlined in Fig. 4.6.

Thyroid hormones

The effects of thyroid hormones on metabolism are well known in the scientific and medical literature (Tapperman, 1980). Such data have shown that thyroid hormones have dramatic effects on tissue metabolism and hypertrophy

Table 4.2 Effects of thyroid hormones in skeletal muscle

Primary increase in concentration of fast isozymes independent of GH and innervation of muscle
Induced GH secretion
Higher content of fast myosin heavy chain mRNAs variable across types of muscles
Metabolic effects
Increased mitochondrial synthesis
Increased enzymatic concentration related to energy metabolism
Protein synthesis

in the human if not in normal concentrations, e.g. hyposecretion. Still, whether thyroid hormones influence skeletal muscle through indirect, i.e. other hormones (e.g. IGF) or direct effects is unclear (Florini, 1987; Ikeda *et al.*, 1989; Wolf *et al.*, 1989). The lack of evidence for changes related to tissue growth effects using *in vitro* culture experiments suggest that thyroid hormones affect skeletal muscle through secondary mechanisms in contrast with their other physiological interactions. Extensive interaction with binding proteins also influence physiological actions (Bartalena, 1990). Changes in muscle tissue attributed to thyroid hormones are shown in Table 4.2.

Glucocorticoids (cortisol)

In a classic sense, glucocorticoids and more specifically cortisol have been viewed as catabolic hormones in skeletal muscle (Kuoppasalmi & Adlercreutz, 1985; Florini, 1987). In situations of disease, joint immobilization, or injury, a nitrogen wasting effect is observed with a net loss of contractile protein and muscle atrophy with associated reductions in force production capabilities (MacDougall, 1986; Florini, 1987). Since the balance of anabolic and catabolic activities in the muscle affects the protein contractile unit, strength would be directly influenced. The search for markers of anabolic and catabolic states in the body have persuaded many investigators to examine cortisol responses in this light. Again, due to the multiplicity of roles played by each hormone, varying success has been realized with this approach (see Chapter 11). Still, cortisol acts

Table 4.3 Overview of catabolic functions related to cortisol actions in muscle

Conversion of amino acids to carbohydrates
Increase in proteolytic enzymes
Inhibition of protein synthesis
Increased protein degradation
Greater catabolic effects in fast-twitch muscle fibres

as one of the major catabolic influences at the molecular level in skeletal muscle fibres. Progesterone to a lesser degree is also associated with catabolic activities in muscle tissue. The major catabolic effects of cortisol in muscle are listed in Table 4.3.

While the cellular mechanisms and the molecular biology of catabolism remain to be completely elucidated, a number of possibilities exist. The catabolic activities appear to be mediated at the glucocorticoid receptor complex level (Konagaya *et al.*, 1986). As previously noted, antagonism with the receptor binding of insulin and IGF-I appears plausible. Also, glucocorticoids may influence mRNA mechanisms for production of proteolytic enzymes (Florini, 1987). Additionally, the acute increases in circulating cortisol following exercise also implicate acute inflammatory response mechanisms to be involved in the tissue remodelling processes. Various extensive reviews of receptor interactions with binding proteins and cytoplasmic receptors have been published (Housley *et al.*, 1989; Schmidt *et al.*, 1989; Rosner, 1990). A scheme of cortisol interaction and subsequent catabolic effects is depicted in Fig. 4.7.

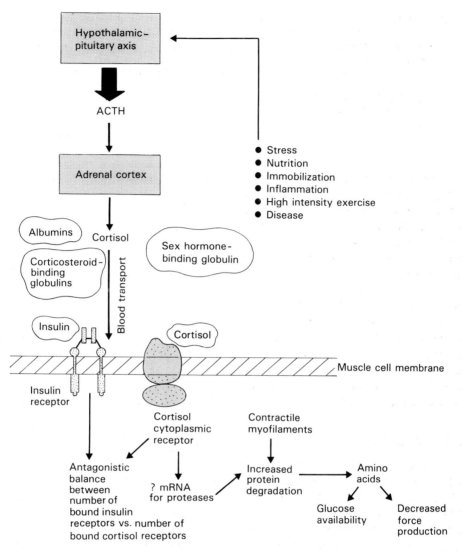

Fig. 4.7 A theoretical scheme for the interaction of cortisol with other hormones and cellular effects in muscle cells. ACTH, adrenocorticotrophic hormone.

Catecholamines

Catecholamines, i.e. adrenaline, noradrenaline and dopamine, are probably more important for the acute expression of strength than any other hormone. Their role in promoting growth of muscle tissue is less clear but may be important during certain stages of prenatal development to accelerate the growth process (Florini, 1985, 1987; Carmichael, 1986). The physiological functions in muscle of adrenaline and noradrenaline are overviewed in Table 4.4.

Summary

The hormonal regulation of strength and power expression is related to the various neuro-endocrine mechanisms involved with the

Table 4.4 Basic direct and indirect actions of catecholamines for muscle function

---

Increased force production
Increased contraction rate
Increased blood pressure
Increased energy availability
Augmentation of secretion rates of other hormones
 (e.g. testosterone)

---

growth and development of muscle tissue. This system presents a complex array of molecular mechanisms. A variety of neuroendocrine feedback and feedforward loops exist and external factors, e.g. behavioural activities, nutrition, can also dramatically influence the magnitude of the hormonal responses. The anabolic/ catabolic balance of the body are affected by the exercise stimulus, nutrition, overtraining, sleep, substance abuse (e.g. alcohol, drugs), and health status. The molecular mechanisms are now becoming elucidated with the improvement of cellular techniques in molecular biology and biochemistry. This multivariate paradigm is dependent on a variety of potential mechanisms, which all can interact and mediate strength and power expression. Understanding how various factors in strength training affect neuroendocrine mechanisms and muscle tissue responses will provide greater understanding of tissue adaptation, e.g. hypertrophy, and subsequent performance gains in strength and power.

References

Adem, A., Jossan, S.S., D'Argy, R., Gillberg, P.G., Nordberg, A., Windbald, B. & Sara, V. (1989) Insulin-like growth factor I (IGF-1) receptors in the human brain: Quantitative autoradiographic localization. *Brain Research*, **503**, 299–303.

Allen, R.E. & Boxhorn, L.K. (1988) Regulation of skeletal muscle satellite cell proliferation and differentiation by transforming growth factor-beta, insulin-like growth factor I, and fibroblast growth factor. *Journal of Cell Physiology*, **138**, 311–15.

Allen, R.E., Merkel, R.A. & Young, R.B. (1979) Cellular aspects of muscle growth: myogenic cell proliferation. *Journal of Animal Science*, **49**, 115–27.

Bartalena, L. (1990) Recent achievements in studies on thyroid hormone binding proteins. *Endocrine Reviews*, **11**, 47–64.

Baxter, R.C. & Martin, J.L. (1989) Structure of the M_r 140 000 growth hormone-dependent insulin-like growth factor binding protein complex: Determination by reconstitution affinity-labeling. *Proceedings of the National Academy of Sciences, USA*, **86**, 6898–902.

Baxter, R.C., Martin, J.L. & Beniac, V.A. (1989) High molecular weight insulin-like growth factor binding protein complex: Purification and properties of the acid-labile subunit from human serum. *Journal of Biological Chemistry*, **264**, 11843–8.

Bleisch, W., Lunie, V.N. & Nottebohm, F. (1984) Modification of synapses in androgen-sensitive muscle. Hormonal regulation of acteylcholine receptor number in the songbird syrinx. *Journal of Neuroscience*, **4**, 786–92.

Blum, W.F., Jenne, E.W., Reppin, F., Kietzmann, K., Ranke, M.B. & Bierich, J.R. (1989) Insulin-like growth factor I (IGF-I)-binding protein complex is a better mitogen than free IGF-I. *Endocrinology*, **125**, 766–72.

Buckler, J.M.H. (1971) The relationship between exercise, body temperature and plasma growth hormone levels in a human subject. *Journal of Physiology*, **214**, 25–6.

Carmichael, S.W. (1986) *The Adrenal Medulla, Vol. 4.* Cambridge University Press, Cambridge.

Chang, F., Dodds, W., Sullivan, M., Kim, M. & Malarkey, W. (1985) The acute effects of exercise on prolactin and growth hormone secretion: comparison between sedentary women and women runners with normal and abnormal menstrual cycles. *Journal of Clinical Endocrinology and Metabolism*, **62**, 551–6.

Clemmons, D.R., Busby, H.W. & Underwood, L.E. (1989a) Mediation of the growth promoting actions of growth hormone by somatomedin-C/insulin like growth factor I and its binding protein. In J.M. Tanner & M.A. Preece (eds) *The Physiology of Human Growth*, pp. 111–28. Cambridge University Press, Cambridge.

Clemmons, D.R., Thissen, J.P., Maes, M., Ketelslegers, J.M. & Underwood, L.E. (1989b) Insulin-like growth factor-I (IGF-I) infusion into hypophysectomized or protein-deprived rats induces specific IGF-binding proteins in serum. *Endocrinology*, **125**, 2967–72.

Czech, M.P. (1989) Signal transmission by the insulin-like growth factors. *Cell*, **59**, 235–8.

Daughaday, W.H. & Rotwein, P. (1989) Insulin-like growth factors I and II. Peptide, messenger ribonucleic acid and gene structures, serum and tissue concentrations. *Endocrine Reviews*, **10**, 68–91.

Fagin, J.A., Fernandez-Mejia, C. & Melmed, S. (1989)

Pituitary insulin-like growth factor-I gene expression: Regulation by triiodothyronine and growth hormone. *Endocrinology*, **125**, 2385–91.

Finkelstein, J.W., Roffwarg, H.P., Boyar, R.M., Kream, J. & Hellman, L. (1972) Age related change in the twenty-four hour spontaneous secretion of growth hormone. *Journal of Clinical Endocrinology and Metabolism*, **35**, 665–70.

Fleck, S.J. & Kraemer, W.J. (1987) *Designing Resistance Training Programmes*. Human Kinetics, Champaign, Illinois.

Florini, J.R. (1985) Hormonal control of muscle cell growth. *Journal of Animal Science*, **61**, 20–7.

Florini, J.R. (1987) Hormonal control of muscle growth. *Muscle and Nerve*, **10**, 577–98.

Forbes, B., Szabo, L., Baxter, R.C., Ballard, F.J. & Wallace, J.C. (1988) Classification of the insulin-like growth factor binding proteins into three distinct categories according to their binding specificities. *Biochemical and Biophysical Research Communications*, **157**, 196–202.

Gharib, S.D., Wioerman, M.E., Shupnik, M.A. & Chin, W.W. (1990) Molecular biology of the pituitary gonadotropins. *Endocrine Reviews*, **11**, 177–99.

Goldberg, A. & Goodman, H. (1969) Relationship between growth hormone and muscular work in determining muscle size. *Journal of Physiology*, **200**, 655–66.

Griggs, R.C., Halliday, D., Kingston, W. & Moxley R.T. III (1986) Effect of testosterone on muscle protein synthesis in myotonic dystrophy. *Annals of Neurology*, **20**, 590–6.

Griggs, R.C., Kingston, W., Jozefowicz, R.F., Herr, B.E., Forbes, G. & Halliday, D. (1989) Effect of testosterone on muscle mass and muscle protein synthesis. *Journal of Applied Physiology*, **66**, 498–503.

Häkkinen, K., Pakarinen, A., Alén, M. & Komi, P.V. (1985) Serum hormones during prolonged training of neuromuscular performance. *European Journal of Applied Physiology*, **53**, 287–93.

Han, V.K.M., D'Ercole, A.J. & Lund, P.K. (1987) Cellular localization of somatomedin (insulin-like growth factor) messenger RNA in the human fetus. *Science*, **236**, 193–6.

Hansson, H.A., Brandsten, C., Lossing, C. & Petruson, K. (1989) Transient expression of insulin-like growth factor I immunoreactivity by vascular cells during angiogenesis. *Experimental and Molecular Pathology*, **50**, 125–38.

Hill, D.J., Camacho-Hubner, C., Rashid P., Strain A.J. & Clemmons, D.R. (1989) Insulin-like growth factor (IGF)-binding protein release by human fetal fibroblasts: Dependency on cell density and IGF peptides. *Journal of Endocrinology*, **122**, 87–98.

Horikawa, R., Asakawa, K., Hizuka, N., Takano, K. & Shizume, K. (1989) Growth hormone and insulin-like growth factor I stimulate Leydig cell steroidogenesis. *European Journal of Pharmacology*, **166**, 87–94.

Housley, P.R., Sanchez, E.R. & Grippo, J.F. (1989) Phosphorylation and reduction of glucocorticoid components. In V.M. Moudgil (ed.) *Receptor Phosphorylation*, pp. 289–314. CRC Press, Boca Raton.

Ikeda, T., Fujiyama, K., Takeuchi, T., Honda, M., Mokuda, O., Tominaga, M. & Mashiba, H. (1989) Effect of thyroid hormone on somatomedin-C release from perfused rat liver. *Experientia*, **45**, 170–1.

Ishii, D.N. (1989) Relationship of insulin-like growth factor II gene expression in muscle to synaptogenesis. *Proceedings of the National Academy of Sciences, USA*, **86**, 2898–902.

Kelly, A., Lyongs, G., Gambki, B. & Robinstein, N. (1985) Influences of testosterone on contractile proteins of the guinea pig temporalis muscle. *Advances in Experimental Medicine and Biology*, **182**, 155–68.

Konagaya, M., Bernar, P.A. & Max, S.R. (1986) Biocade of glucocorticoid receptor binding and inhibition of dexamethasone-induced muscle atrophy in the rat by RU38486 a potent glucocorticoid antagonist. *Endocrinology*, **119**, 375–80.

Kraemer, W.J. (1988) Endocrine responses to resistance exercise. *Medicine and Science in Sports and Exercise*, **20**, (suppl.), S152–7.

Kuoppasalmi, K. & Adlercreutz, H. (1985) Interaction between catabolic and anabolic steroid hormones in muscular exercise. In K. Fotherby & S.B. Pal (eds) *Exercise Endocrinology*, pp. 65–98. Walter de Gruyter, Berlin.

Leung, D.W., Spencer, S.A., Cachianes, G., Hammonds, R.G., Collins, C., Henzel, W.J., Barnard, R., Waters, M.J., & Wood, W.I. (1987) Growth hormone receptor and serum binding protein: purification, cloning and expression. *Nature*, **330**, 537–43.

McCusker, R.H., Camacho-Hubner, C. & Clemmons, D.R. (1989) Identification of the types of insulin-like growth factor-binding proteins that are secreted by muscle cells *in vitro*. *Journal of Biological Chemistry*, **264**, 7795–800.

MacDougall, J. (1986) Morphological changes in human skeletal muscle following strength training and immobilization. In N.L. Jones, N. McCartney & A.J. McComas (eds) *Human Muscle Power*, pp. 269–84. Human Kinetics, Champaign, Illinois.

Maiter, D., Fliesen, T., Underwood, L.E., Maes, M., Gerard, G., Davenport, M.L. & Ketelslegers, J.M. (1989) Dietary protein restriction decreases insulin-like growth factor I independent of insulin and liver growth hormone binding. *Endocrinology*, **124**, 2604–11.

Michel, G. & Baulieu, E. (1980) Androgen receptor in rat skeletal muscle: Characterization and physiological variations. *Endocrinology*, **107**, 2088–97.

Okayama, T. (1972) Factors which regulate growth hormone secretion. *Medical Journal*, **17**, 13–19.

Pruett, E.D. (1985) Insulin and exercise in non-diabetic and diabetic man. In K. Fotherby & S.B. Pal (eds) *Exercise Endocrinology*, pp. 1–24. Walter de Gruyter, Berlin.

Rance, N.E. & Max, S.R. (1984) Modulation of the cytosolic androgen receptor in striated muscle by sex steroids. *Endocrinology*, **115**, 862–6.

Riss, T., Novakofski, J. & Bechtel, P. (1986) Skeletal muscle hypertrophy in rats having growth hormone-secreting tumor. *Journal of Applied Physiology*, **61**, 1732–5.

Rogol, A.D. (1989) Growth hormone: physiology, therapeutic use and potential for abuse. In K.B. Pandolf (ed.) *Exercise and Sport Sciences Reviews, Vol. 17*, pp. 353–77. Williams & Wilkins, Baltimore.

Rosner, W. (1990) The functions of corticosteroid-binding globulin and sex-hormone-binding globulin: Recent advances. *Endocrine Reviews*, **11**, 80–91.

Schmidt, T.J., Miller-Diener, A.S., Kirsch, T.M. & Litwack, G. (1989) Association of phosphorylation reactions with glucocorticoid receptor. In V.M. Moudgil (ed.) *Receptor Phosphorylation*, pp. 315–32. CRC Press, Boca Raton.

Sherman, M.R. & Stevens, J. (1984) Structure of mammalian steroid receptors: Evolving concepts and methodological developments. *Annual Review of Physiology*, **46**, 83–105.

Skottner, A., Kanie, M., Jennische, E., Sjögren, J. & Fryklund, L. (1988) Tissue repair and IGF-1. *Acta Paediatrica Scandinavica*, **347**, 110–12.

Sonntag, W.E., Forman, L.J., Miki, N. & Meiters, J. (1982) Growth hormone secretion and neuroendocrine regulation. In G.H. Gass & H.M. Kaplan (eds) *Handbook of Endocrinology*, pp. 35–9. CRC Press, Boca Raton.

Tapperman, J. (1980) *Metabolic and Endocrine Physiology*. Year Book Medical Publishers, Chicago.

Turner, J.D., Rotwein, P., Novakofski, J. & Bechtel, P.J. (1988) Induction of messenger RNA for IGF-I and -II during growth hormone-stimulated muscle hypertrophy. *American Journal of Physiology*, **255**, E513–17.

Vermeulen, A. (1988) Physiology of the testosterone-binding globulin in man. In R. Frairia, H.L. Bradlow & G. Gaidano (eds) *The New York Academy of Sciences*, pp. 103–11. The New York Academy of Sciences, New York.

Wolf, M., Ingbar, S.H. & Moses, A.C. (1989) Thyroid hormone and growth hormone interact to regulate insulin-like growth factor-I messenger RNA and circulating levels in the rat. *Endocrinology*, **125**, 2905–14.

Young, I.R., Mesiano, S., Hintz, R., Caddy, D.J., Ralph, M.M., Browne, C.A. & Thorburn, G.D. (1989) Growth hormone and testosterone can independently stimulate the growth of hypophysectomized prepubertal lambs without any alteration in circulating concentrations of insulin-like growth factors. *Journal of Endocrinology*, **121**, 563–70.

Zorzano, A., James, D.E., Ruderman, N.B. & Pilch, P.F. (1988) Insulin-like growth factor I binding and receptor kinase in red and white muscle. *FEBS Letters*, **234**, 257–62.

Chapter 5

Exercise-Related Adaptations in Connective Tissue

RONALD F. ZERNICKE AND BARBARA J. LOITZ

Fibrous and bony connective tissues provide the essential infrastructure that allows the human body to strive for the Olympic ideal— *citius, altius, fortius* (faster, higher, stronger). During movements, strong but pliant tendons transmit the forces generated by muscles to bones serving as effective levers, while ligaments and menisci maintain the intricate articulations of the skeletal levers. The adaptation ability of fibrous and bony connective tissues in response to training and exercise are discussed in this chapter. The dynamism and adaptive responses of a bone to its functional demands have been recognized for more than a century, but the responsiveness of fibrous connective tissues to exercise and conditioning has been appreciated only more recently. It is becoming more and more apparent that all fibrous and bony connective tissues are sensitive to mechanical loads. The quality and quantity of the loading to the tissue, however, can determine whether the outcome is positive or injurious.

There is a plethora of significant information about connective tissues, much more than could be covered in this chapter. Thus, we limit our discussion to major load-transmitting connective tissues (bone, tendon, ligament, and meniscus) and emphasize the adaptive and maladaptive changes that occur in these tissues as a consequence of exercise and conditioning after providing an overview of the structure of each tissue.

Bone

The dynamic nature of bone has long been recognized as Wolff, in 1892, stated that: 'every change in the . . . function of bone . . . is followed by certain definite changes in . . . internal architecture and external configuration in accordance with mathematical laws' (Carter, 1984, p. S19). To date, however, the mechanisms underlying bone's ability to translate loading events into cellular responses remain largely unexplained. Indeed, Cowin *et al.* (1984) list several questions that persist about bone remodelling dynamics, including: (i) How do mechanically derived stimuli compete with systemic stimuli? (ii) What is the nature of the mechanical stimuli that influence bone remodelling? (iii) What are the structural objectives of bone remodelling?

Structure

Bone matrix comprises three elements: organic, mineral, and fluid. Organic components account for 39% of bone's total volume, containing 95% type I collagen and 5% proteoglycans. Minerals include primarily calcium hydroxyapatite crystals and contribute 49% to bone's total volume. Fluid-filled vascular channels and cellular spaces constitute the remaining volume (Frost, 1987). Mineral components give bone its stiffness, while the organic matrix contributes to bone strength. Resistance to deformation under load may be

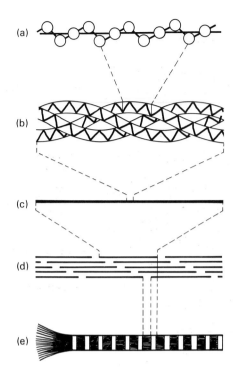

Fig. 5.1 Schematic diagram of a collagen fibril: (a) amino acids join to form an alpha chain; (b) three alpha chains coil to form the triple helix procollagen molecule; (c) procollagen bundles link to form tropocollagen, which packs in a staggered orientation (d) that gives the collagen fibril (e) a striated appearance. (From Prockop & Guzman, 1977; Nordin & Frankel, 1989.)

the most important physical property of bone (Albright & Skinner, 1987), and thus bone must be of adequate stiffness and strength not to break under dynamic or static loading (Currey, 1984). Bone mechanical characteristics reflect a balance between mineral and organic phases.

Collagen, the most abundant mammalian protein (Buckwalter & Cooper, 1987), provides a major structural support for connective tissues. Collagen constitutes perhaps one-third of the total protein in the body and, therefore, about 6% of body weight (White *et al.*, 1964). Collagen tensile strength results from polypeptides arranged in alpha chains (Fig. 5.1). Each alpha chain consists of amino acids, with

glycine, lysine, and proline being particularly important. Glycine, the smallest of the three, occupies every third position in the alpha chain and, in so doing, allows the chain to assume a helical shape. Hydroxyl groups attach to lysine and proline molecules in a completed alpha chain, and hydroxylation plays a critical role in determining collagen's stiffness. After hydroxylation and attachment of carbohydrates, the alpha chains coil around each other to form a triple helix called procollagen. Osteoblasts secrete procollagen into the surrounding matrix where cleavage of terminal peptides allows procollagen bundles to link together, forming tropocollagen molecules, the most fundamental molecular structure of collagenous tissues (White *et al.*, 1964; Ham, 1974). Strong crosslinks between procollagen's hydroxylysine molecules give tropocollagen its strength. Intramolecular crosslinks join tropocollagen molecules to form collagen fibrils. The extent of hydroxylysine crosslinking changes with age and between types of connective tissues; more crosslinks produce a stiffer tissue (Butler *et al.*, 1978).

Mineral content distinguishes bone from other connective tissues and gives bone its unique stiffness and a role in maintaining mineral homeostasis in the body. Skinner (1987) suggests that bone mineralization relies on a specific link between type I collagen and hydroxyapatite crystals in bone.

Although different in shape and size, all bones share certain structural features. Bone has two forms, woven and lamellar. Woven bone forms quickly and assumes an irregular pattern of collagen fibres and osteocytes. A sporadic mineral distribution also limits woven bone's ability to withstand mechanical loads (Albright & Skinner, 1987). Fracture callus, active endochondral ossification sites, and some pathological sites contain woven bone, but it is not typically found in the healthy, adult human skeleton. During skeletal maturation, lamellar bone systematically replaces woven bone, providing the adult skeleton with its functional stiffness (Frost, 1987).

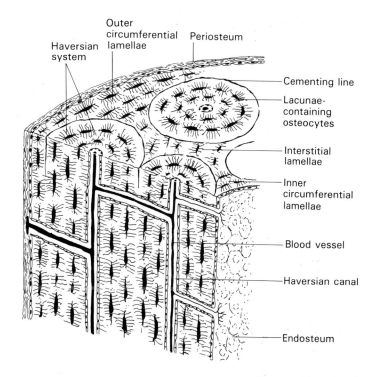

Fig. 5.2 Compact lamellar bone, with the transverse plane showing osteocytes arranged in Haversian systems and circumferential and interstitial lamellae. Vascular channels course longitudinally and transversely throughout the bone. (From Ham, 1974.)

Lamellar bone plays an important role in transmitting loads. Compact lamellar bone (Fig. 5.2) always surrounds cancellous lamellar bone, covering all external bony surfaces. Its relative thickness varies, from thin vertebral bodies to thick long bone diaphyses. Cancellous lamellar bone assumes a three-dimensional latticework continuous with the endosteal surface of cortical bone. Individual columns or plates of bone (trabeculae) orient parallel to the principal strain axes, providing maximal strength with minimum material (Clark *et al.*, 1975)

Remodelling

Electrical phenomena may alter remodelling and fracture repair, and electrical effects are a likely means of information transfer between mechanical deformation and cellular response. While the mechanisms producing electrical potentials remain questionable, Currey (1984) cites two possible sources of electrical phenomena: piezoelectricity and streaming potentials. Crystals having a lattice structure and no central symmetry develop a net separation of charge between anions and cations when deformation occurs. Charge separation causes a potential difference, the piezoelectric potential, to develop between opposite ends of the crystals. Wet collagen stiffened by minerals may react like a lattice crystal when deformed and may provide the piezoelectric potentials generated by bone strain (Eriksson, 1976). Piezoelectricity is highly directional, a noteworthy feature that may help to explain bone's differing sensitivity to compressive and tensile strains.

When a solid surface carrying a surface charge contacts a polar liquid, oppositely charged ions from the fluid migrate toward the surface. If the fluid flows, weakly bonded ions move, creating a current such that a potential difference (streaming potential) develops between upstream and downstream sites. When bone deforms, polarized extracellular fluid tends to move. The resulting streaming potentials may provide information concerning the strain stimulus.

Lanyon and Hartman (1977) demonstrated that during bending, the tensile surface of a wet bone sample developed a positive charge, the compressive side became negatively charged, and the peak difference depended both on the strain rate and magnitude. When bone experienced a static load, the potential decayed to zero within approximately 2 s (Cochran et al., 1968). Eriksson (1976) postulated that such strain-induced polarization resulted from streaming potentials generated by unidirectional flow of positively charged extracellular fluid in transversely oriented channels. Bending forced channel diameters to decrease on the concave surface and increase on the convex surface, moving fluid toward the convexity, thereby creating a strain-induced voltage. This theory supports bone's insensitivity to static load (Hert et al., 1971; Lanyon & Rubin, 1984) and sensitivity to variations in strain rate and magnitude (Rubin & Lanyon, 1985). When static loading is superimposed upon normal activity, however, new periosteal bone apposition results (Meade et al., 1984). Not unexpectedly, when intermittent bending loads are applied in physiological ranges, Liskova and Hert (1971) report that periosteal and endosteal bone is deposited. O'Connor et al. (1982) suggest that a principal determinant of new bone deposition in a weight-bearing bone is the rate of change of strain that closely approximates that developed during normal locomotion. Several investigators (Carter et al., 1981; Churches & Howlett, 1981) have reported a differential response to bending loads, indicating that more bone deposition occurs in areas of increased compressive strains as opposed to areas of tensile strains.

Skerry et al. (1988, 1990) proposed that load-related reorientation of proteoglycans may be a link between mechanical loading and remodelling. They measured collagen and proteoglycan reorientation following load applications, and collagen orientation showed no difference between loaded and control bones. Proteoglycans, however, showed a significant 36% difference in orientation between control and loaded bones. Forty-eight hours after the cessation of loading, no difference was found in control and loaded bones. Skerry et al. concluded that dynamic loading affected the proteoglycan orientation in a manner related to the load's magnitude and distribution, similar to previous descriptions relating strain and bone remodelling. Proteoglycan reorientation may, therefore, provide a strain-induced stimulus to the osteocyte that signals the bone's recent dynamic strain history.

Studies measuring prostaglandin (PG) concentrations in cultured osteoblasts led Yeh and Rodan (1984) and Binderman et al. (1984) to conclude that PGE_2 may act as a transducer between mechanical strain and osteoblasts. Yeh and Rodan compared PG synthesis between bone cells cultured on collagen ribbons left undisturbed and cells cultured on ribbons stretched eight times over a 2-hour period. Stretching increased PG synthesis 3.5-fold compared to the non-stretched ribbons, supporting PG's role in the translation of mechanical stimuli to cellular activity. Binderman et al. concluded, similarly, that the osteoblast's membrane may have a specific mechanoreceptor system capable of being stimulated by strains to increase PGE_2 synthesis.

Remodelling occurs when existing bone undergoes degradation and new bone forms in its place. Therefore, the first step in remodelling is activation of osteoclasts to resorb existing bone. A line of osteoclasts, the osteoclastic front, cuts a longitudinal cone through the bone by secreting acid phosphatase, collagenase, and other proteolytic enzymes (Buckwalter & Cooper, 1987). The cutting cone resorbs approximately three times its volume and, when completed, leaves a resorptive channel 1000–10 000 µm deep (Albright & Skinner, 1987).

Osteoblasts follow the resorptive front, first

laying mineralized matrix around the walls of the resorptive channel, forming a cement line. Cement lines contain 10–15% less mineral than surrounding bone, rendering the lines less stiff and providing paths for crack propagation. Osteoblasts then produce new matrix that fills the volume eroded by the osteoclasts. Refilling the cone requires three times longer than resorption, in spite of osteoblasts outnumbering osteoclasts by more than 200 to one (Jaworski, 1984). The distance between the osteoclasts and osteoblasts represents the time needed to reverse the resorptive process into one of formation. Generally, this latent period is about 1 week (Albright & Skinner, 1987). Osteoblasts deposit a non-mineralized matrix initially that calcifies 8–10 days later. Osteoblasts then become osteocytes as they trap themselves within the new matrix, changing their role from bone formation to bone maintenance.

Examination of a long bone cross-section reveals that remodelling occurs in three separate areas or envelopes. Though the sequence of osteoclast and osteoblast activity applies to all three envelopes, each surface exhibits unique behaviour to given stimuli and, therefore, needs to be considered independently when describing remodelling. The inner and outer bony surfaces are the endosteal and periosteal envelopes, and the cortical bone in between forms the intracortical envelope. Measurement of changes in periosteal and endosteal diameters and cortical density, therefore, is important in studying skeletal diseases and effects of disuse or exercise on bone.

Functional adaptation and exercise-related changes

Lanyon (1987) described remodelling as an 'interpretation and purposeful reaction' to a bone's strain state, allowing for adaptation to both increased and decreased strains. 'Functional strains are both the objective and the stimulus for the processes of adaptive modelling and remodeling' (Lanyon, 1987, p. 1084). Similarly, Rubin and Lanyon (1985) hypo-

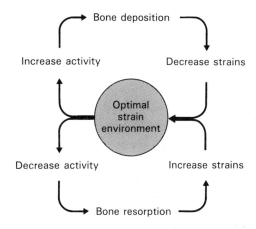

Fig. 5.3 Hypothesized relationship among activity level, bone strain and remodelling response. The bone resorption and deposition balance appears to maintain an optimal strain environment. (From Rubin & Lanyon, 1987.)

thesized that if functional strains were too high, the incidence of damage and probability of failure increased. If strains were too low, the bone was unnecessarily active, and energy was wasted in the synthesis and maintenance of its matrix. Thus, functional strain appears to be the most relevant parameter to control (Fig. 5.3).

During the past 20 years, experimental data have emerged to describe, quantitatively, the relationship between structure and function in bone. Numerous studies have been conducted to correlate known loading events with changes in bone geometry and strength. Among the approaches that have been used are functional overload, artificial loading, and *in vivo* strains.

Functional overload

Skeletal adaptation to overload has been documented in dogs (Chamay & Tschantz, 1972; Carter *et al.*, 1980; Meade *et al.*, 1984), sheep (Radin *et al.*, 1982), swine (Goodship *et al.*, 1979; Woo *et al.*, 1981), rats (Smith, 1977; Gordon *et al.*, 1989), mice (Saville & Whyte, 1969; Kiiskinen & Heikkinen, 1973; Kiiskinen, 1977), and humans (Jones *et al.*, 1977; Krolner et al., 1983; Smith et al., 1984; Simkin et al., 1987). Chamay and Tschantz (1972) performed unilateral radial excisions on dogs, placing the entire forelimb load-bearing responsibility on the ulna. Within 9 months, ulnar cortical thickness increased twofold. Following ulnar excision in swine, Goodship et al. (1979) reported rapid bone deposition, and after 3 months the area of the remodelled radius equalled that of the contralateral radius and ulna together. Surface strains were approximately equal in the radius before ulnar removal and after remodelling, despite dramatic changes in bone geometry. These overload studies support a hypothesis that mechanical loads stimulate bone remodelling and that remodelling continues until strains achieve a predetermined, site-specific level.

Artificial loading

Artificial load application through cortical pins facilitates precise measurement of loads experienced by bone and allows correlations between loads and remodelling changes. Applied loads may produce strains less than, equal to, or greater than those applied during normal activities. In this way, effects of both diminished and excessive loads can be quantified. Rubin and Lanyon (1985) deprived turkey ulnae of normal loads by performing metaphyseal osteotomies, then applied known loads through diaphyseal pins. A dose:response relationship ($r = 0.83$) was found, with loads producing strain less than 1000 µstrain resulting in bone loss, strains between 1000 and 2000 µstrain maintaining bone mass, and strains exceeding 2000 µstrain stimulating osteogenesis. Using a similar experimental design, Lanyon and Rubin (1984) also reported the remodelling effects of dynamic vs. static loads. Ulnae deprived of all loads and those that experienced static loads displayed increased endosteal diameters and intracortical porosity, resulting in a 13% decreased cortical cross-section. Ulnae exposed to cyclical loading of 1 Hz for $100 \, \text{s} \cdot \text{day}^{-1}$ showed a 24% increased cortical cross-section,

with new bone deposited primarily on the periosteal surface. Rubin (1984) reported maintained bone mass in rooster ulnae with only four bending cycles per day. Strain magnitudes generated by loads in each of these experiments did not exceed strains measured during wing flapping. From their numerous studies, Lanyon and Rubin conclude that bone appears to be sensitive to magnitude and distribution of dynamic strains and that the insensitivity to static experimental strain reflects the skeleton's natural insensitivity to adapt to static loading situations.

In vivo strains

Evans (1953) reported the first use of a strain gauge to measure bone strains of a dog's tibia during walking. Single element strain gauges have been used to measure strains in canine (Cochran, 1972, 1974), sheep (Lanyon & Smith, 1969, 1970), and horse (Turner et al. 1975; Rybicki et al., 1977) long bones during locomotion and sheep vertebrae (Lanyon, 1971, 1972) during walking and respiration. Use of single element gauges limits a study's impact because data reflect strains engendered only along the bones' longitudinal axes, but Lanyon (1973) rectified this when he placed rosette (three-element) gauges on sheep calcanei and calculated compressive, tensile, and shear strains during walking.

Carter et al. (1980) recorded strains from rosette gauges placed on various sites of canine radii and ulnae. Following full surgical recovery, strains were measured during normal walking. Results indicated, not surprisingly, that tensile strains developed along the bones' longitudinal convex cortices and compressive strains developed along the bones' longitudinal concave cortices. Shear and transverse tensile and compressive strains were more difficult to interpret but suggested that the bone experienced significant torsional loads during stance. Biewener et al. (1986) and Keller and Spengler (1989) used strain gauges to characterize growth-related changes in immature chickens and rats. Both studies noted similar strain magnitudes and distributions throughout growth in spite of threefold increases in bone length (chicken) and animal mass (rat). They suggested that strain state strongly influenced growth-related changes in bone mass and geometry.

Exercise effects

Disuse-related changes in bone resulting from immobilization (e.g. Uhthoff & Jaworski, 1978), spaceflight (e.g. Morey & Baylink, 1978; Jee et al., 1983; Shaw et al., 1988), and hind-limb suspension (Shaw et al., 1987) support a hypothesis that bone requires load-bearing strains to maintain its mass. Similarly, studies quantifying exercise-related changes in bone reiterate bone's dynamic nature by demonstrating increased cortical thickness (Jones et al., 1977; Woo et al., 1981) and bone mineral content (Krolner et al., 1983) following exercise regimes. Variations among exercise protocols and measurement techniques, however, limit the generalizability of results and conclusions about precise effects of exercise on bone.

Woo et al. (1981) studied the effects of long-term exercise on cortical bones. Five immature swine ran approximately $40 \, km \cdot week^{-1}$ at 65–80% maximum heart rate for 12 months. After the animals were killed, 4-mm wide strips of cortical bone taken from the anterior, posterior, medial, and lateral femoral diaphysis were loaded in four-point bending tests to failure. Biochemical components of cortical samples were also measured. The authors reported exercise-related increases in bone strength resulting from changes in bone geometry, with exercised animals developing a 17% increased cortical thickness and 23% increased cortical cross-sectional area. Analyses of bone composition showed similar biochemical constituents and bone density between exercise and control animals. Woo et al. concluded that exercise-induced internal stresses stimulated remodelling changes without altering bone's composition. No attempt was made, however,

to differentiate between growth- and exercise-related influences. Matsuda et al. (1986) studied exercise effects on growing chicks and found that moderate exercise increased cortical cross-sectional area but decreased the bone's strength. From the findings of Matsuda et al., it is conceivable that the bones may have initially laid down poorly mineralized matrix in response to the early exercise-related stresses. Given the duration of the Woo et al. exercise protocol, remodelling may have improved the quality of the immature bone so that after a year the resulting bone would be no different than that of the control bones. A relationship that appears to exist between remodelling and duration of an exercise protocol may account for the disparity between data from these studies.

Defining exactly how 'exercise or conditioning' affects the skeletal system is a profoundly complex problem. Exercise intensity, skeletal maturity, type of bones (trabecular or cortical), and anatomical location (axial or extremity bones) all can influence the specific response of a bone to exercise. Regular, prolonged exercise can increase the skeletal mass of adults and athletes (Dalen & Olsson, 1974; Pirnay et al., 1987), but particularly strenuous training, in the immature skeleton, can delay collagen crosslink maturation in joint connective tissues (Pedrini-Mille et al., 1988), slow the rate of long bone growth (Kiiskinen & Heikkinen, 1973; Kiiskinen, 1977; Matsuda et al., 1986), or deleteriously affect bone mechanical characteristics (Matsda et al., 1986). Rapidly growing bone appears to be more affected by mechanical loading environment than mature bone (Steinberg & Trueta, 1981; Carter, 1984), and trabecular bone, with its rapid turnover (Bhasin et al., 1988), may be even more sensitive to remodelling stimuli than is cortical bone (Rambaut & Johnson, 1979). McDonald et al. (1986) reported age-related differences in rat bone mineralization patterns after exercise, with axial bones being less mineralized than weight-bearing bones. In response to a programme of strenuous running, Hou et al. (1991)

have recently shown the differential effects that strenuous exercise may have on the mechanical properties of immature trabecular bone in the rat femoral neck as opposed to the lumbar vertebrae. In response to the 10 weeks of strenuous exercise, the structural and material properties of the weight-bearing femoral neck were significantly and adversely affected, but the lumbar vertebrae did not change significantly. It is not clear that a more moderate training programme would have the same effect on bone and its mechanical properties. Careful and well-controlled studies need to be conducted to characterize the dose–response relationship of exercise training to bone geometry and mechanical properties. On the plus side, Silbermann *et al.* (1990) examined the effects of long-term, moderate physical exercise on trabecular bone volume and composition. They showed that if the physical activity started at an early age (prior to middle age) and was extended until old age, the exercise positively influenced trabecular bone mass and mineralization. They did not find the same benefits if the training programme was initiated after middle age. Silbermann *et al.* suggested that while young animals (mice) responded favourably to moderate physical exercise, older animals lost this ability to adapt.

Exercise–growth interaction

Exercise-related changes in growing bones have been examined by Keller and Spengler (1989), Biewener *et al.* (1986), and Matsuda *et al.* (1986). Interest in the exercise–growth interaction stems from the lack of quantitative descriptions of whether all growing bones react similarly to exercise and whether such reactions are site-specific within the same bone.

Keller and Spengler (1989) implanted *in vivo* strain gauges on femora of 6–30-week-old rats. One treatment group walked on a wire-mesh wheel for $2 \min \cdot day^{-1}$, while the other exercised $45 \min \cdot day^{-1}$ at the same rate $(0.2 m \cdot s^{-1})$ and intensity (25% maximum effort). No statistically significant differences

were found for any *in vivo* stress or strain parameters between the activity groups. Compared with sedentary age-matched controls, the exercise animals also showed no significant differences. Keller and Spengler concluded that the loading threshold for positive bone change may have been greater than that elicited by the estimated 25% effort. Biewener *et al.* (1986) performed a similar study with 3-week-old chicks trained to run on a treadmill at 35% maximum speed $15 \min \cdot day^{-1}$. The exercise regime continued until animals reached 4–17 weeks of age. *In vivo* strain measurements were made on the tibiotarsus of animals 4, 8, 12 and 17 weeks old. Their data closely paralleled those reported by Keller and Spengler, with strain magnitudes, orientations, and distributions remaining consistent despite growth- and exercise-related stimuli. Biewener and colleagues postulated a genetically predefined strain environment directing bone remodelling. A conclusion similar to that made by Keller and Spengler relative to exercise intensity must also be considered.

Matsuda *et al.* (1986) addressed the limitations of the previous studies by exercising growing chicks at a moderate intensity (70–80% of maximum aerobic capacity). Animals ran on a treadmill for $35–45 \min \cdot day^{-1}$, 5 days a week for 5 or 9 weeks. Muscle fumerase activity of the lateral gastrocnemius demonstrated significantly increased aerobic capacity in the exercised animals. Significant differences were found in the geometry and structural properties of the tarsometatarsus bones between runners and controls. The runners' average flexural rigidity was 40% less than those of controls after 5 weeks of exercise and 52% less than those of controls after 9 weeks of exercise. Runners had greater cortical cross-sectional areas after both 5- and 9-week exercise bouts. The cortical cross-sectional area results support the hypothesis that exercise stimulates surface bone remodelling in growing animals. Data, however, also suggest that high intensity exercise produces a decrease in material strength. The authors theorized that high

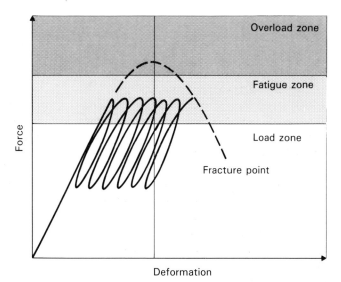

Fig. 5.4 Force–deformation curve illustrating fatigue that may result from repetitive loading (solid line) or fracture from a single load application (dashed line). Cyclic forces in the fatigue zone can lead eventually to fatigue failure. Fracture may result from a single application of load with magnitude within the overload zone. (From Chamay & Tschantz, 1972.)

intensity exercise undertaken during rapid growth may have altered calcification of the newly deposited matrix, making the bone less stiff despite an increased cortical area.

These data suggest that exercise below a certain threshold intensity does not alter a predetermined (perhaps genetic) strain state that bone attempts to maintain during modelling/remodelling. Exercise above a threshold intensity, however, elicits a local or systemic response that modifies bone's predisposition toward a given strain state.

Fatigue

'Fatigue in compact bone is the process of gradual mechanical failure caused by repetitive loading at stresses or strains far lower than those required to fracture bone in a single application of force' (Schaffler *et al.*, 1989, p. 207) (Fig. 5.4). Multiple loading of a bone may eventually lead to fatigue processes that are intimated in normal and pathological physiology of bone. Fatigue-related microdamage during exercise may stimulate bone remodelling. But if the loading is too extensive and the microdamage excessive, fatigue fractures may develop (Lafferty & Raju, 1979;

Carter & Caler, 1985). As compact bone fatigues, it progressively loses its stiffness and strength, leading to a fatigue failure (Carter & Caler, 1985). The exact characteristics of the multiple loading episodes—the number, magnitude, and strain rate—remain to be quantified. Vigorous exercise undoubtedly generates high strain rates as well as high strain magnitudes. Because bone is viscoelastic—exhibits strain rate dependency—the loading at higher strain rates may increase bone stiffness (Currey, 1988; Schaffler & Burr, 1988), which may increase the fatigue resistance in compact bone. The fatigue behaviour of compact bone is like that in composite materials that exhibit a progressive loss of stiffness and strength (Hahn & Kim, 1976). Nevertheless, the details of how exercise-related strain rates and magnitudes relate to bone fatigue properties remain to be quantified.

Tendons and ligaments

Without tendons and ligaments, normal motion of the human skeleton could not occur. But while important information has already been determined about the properties of tendons and ligaments (for reviews, see Booth

& Gould, 1975; Tipton *et al.*, 1975; Butler *et al.*, 1978; Akeson *et al.*, 1985; Buckwalter *et al.*, 1987; Zernicke & Loitz, 1990), significant gaps exist in our explanation of the effects of training and conditioning on these important dense fibrous connective tissues. Part of the lack of information related to training can be linked to earlier suggestions that tendons and ligaments were virtually inert (Butler *et al.*, 1978). In the past decade, however, it has become clear that these dense fibrous tissues exhibit a viable metabolism and are adaptable (e.g. Vailas *et al.*, 1981).

Structure

The principal fibre in tendons and ligaments is collagen. As described earlier, the tropocollagen molecule (Viidik, 1973) provides the fundamental molecular structure in tendons and ligaments. Generally, five parallel tropocollagen molecules are staggered to form a microfibril (Viidik, 1973; Kastelic *et al.*, 1978). Sequentially, microfibrils are organized into

fibrils and into collagen fibres (Viidik, 1973) (Fig. 5.5). A primary fibre bundle is a group of fibres enclosed in an endotenon. A group of these primary bundles is called a fascicle (Kastelic *et al.*, 1978) and is surrounded by an epitenon sheath. The eventual tendon or ligament is a group of collagen fascicles enclosed within a sheath called a paratenon (Butler *et al.*, 1978). The arrangement and organization of the fascicles within a tendon or ligament is thought to relate to the direction of pull in the collagen fibres (Elliott, 1965). Tendons are usually thick, white collagenous bands that connect muscle to bone and transmit tensile forces. The collagen content of tendon is roughly 70% of its dry mass (Harkness, 1968). The fascicles within a tendon are usually parallel to each other (Viidik, 1973), but the insertion of tendon into bone involves a gradual transition from tendon to fibrocartilage, to mineralized fibrocartilage, to lamellar bone (Cooper & Misol, 1970). Collagenous Sharpey's fibres connect the tendon to the underlying subchondral bone and blend with the col-

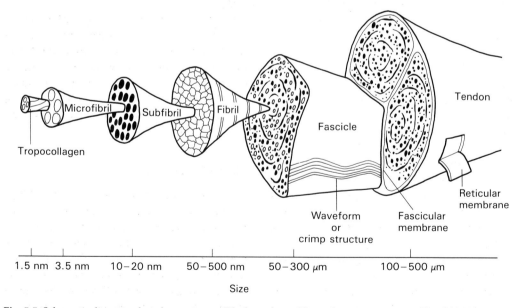

Fig. 5.5 Schematic diagram of tendon structure. Fibrils are bound by endotenons; epitenons bind fibril bundles together to form a fascicle; and these are bundled together by paratenons to form the tendon. (From Kastelic *et al.*, 1978.)

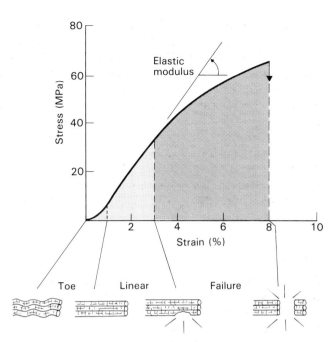

Fig. 5.6 Exemplar stress–strain curve for collagen. Each area of the curve reflects collagen's behaviour during tensile loading. (From Butler *et al.*, 1978.)

lagenous fibres of the periosteum. On the other end, tendon attaches to the muscle via the myotendinous junction. In the specialized region of the myotendinous junction, intracellular myofibrils join to extracellular collagen fibres. Recent studies have revealed the relatively complex multi-layered interface that is found at the connection of the actin filament of the terminal sarcomere to the tendon collagen fibres (Trotter *et al.*, 1983; Ovalle, 1987). The membranous foldings in the myotendinous junction enhance the surface area and thus reduce the stress on the junction. Recent work by Tidball (1983, 1984) reveals that the strength of the adhesive junction between the muscle and tendon depends both on the properties of the adjoining tissues and on the orientation of the forces that cross the junction. Junctions loaded in shear are stronger than junctions that have a large tensile component which is perpendicular to the membrane.

Under a light microscope, tendon appears crimped and wave-like because of the buckling phenomena created by the intercellular matrix impinging on collagen fibres (Butler *et al.*,

1978). In the intercellular matrix, besides collagen, tendon contains small amounts of mucopolysaccharides and elastin (Hooley *et al.*, 1980).

Ligaments join together adjacent bones at their ends and may support organs (Butler *et al.*, 1978). Ligaments can be internal or external to the joint capsule or they may blend with the capsule. The colour of collagenous ligaments is a dull white due to the greater percentage of elastic and reticular fibres between the collagen fibre bundles.

Mechanical properties

Collagenous tissues, such as tendons and ligaments, provide resistance to tensile loads. During a typical force elongation test, the initial load applied to the tissue results in a concave portion of the curve, termed the 'toe' region (Elliott, 1965; Viidik, 1973) (Fig. 5.6). The relative elongation of the tissue at the end of this region has been reported to be between 1.5 and 4% (Viidik, 1973; Butler *et al.*, 1978). Following the toe region is a relatively linear response. The fibres in the tissue become more parallel and lose their wavy appearance (Viidik, 1973; Butler et al., 1978). If collagen fibres are tested alone, the strain limit of the linear region may be from 2 to 5% (Elliott, 1965). Microfailure occurs at the end of the linear loading region; and once maximum load is attained, complete failure occurs rapidly, and the load-supporting ability of the ligament is lost (Butler et al., 1978). As with bone, fibrous connective tissues are viscoelastic and display a sensitivity to different strain rates (Fung, 1967, 1972; Butler et al., 1978). Noyes et al. (1974a) demonstrated that strain rate has a significant effect on the maximum loads that a ligament can withstand.

The myotendinous junction is also viscoelastic, and its mechanical behaviour depends on the duration, frequency, and magnitude of the applied loads (Tidball & Daniel, 1986). Tidball and Daniel (1986) suggest that the duration of loading helps establish the degree of myotendinous membranous folding that occurs at the junction. They have reported that slow twitch muscle cells have a greater junctional surface area than fast twitch muscle cells. Presumably, the greater surface area prevents muscle cell lysis under conditions of prolonged loading because of the reduction in stress at the membrane.

Exercise effects

Dense fibrous tissues have been shown to be sensitive to both disuse and training (Booth & Gould, 1975; Buckwalter et al., 1987). The underlying mechanisms responsible for these adaptive changes, however, are not clearly understood. Most of the information on the response of dense fibrous tissues to exercise is related to ligaments. Little quantitative information exists about exercise-related adaptations of tendon (Woo et al., 1982; Michna, 1984). Tipton et al. and Viidik et al. have provided some of the most systematic and extensive investigations of the influences of training and physical activity on ligaments (Viidik, 1973; Tipton et al., 1975). Generally, it has been

shown that with immobilization or significant disuse, noteworthy changes will occur in the substance of ligaments (Akeson et al., 1967; Woo et al., 1975) (Fig. 5.7). Immobilization decreases the glycosaminoglycan and water content of ligamentous and tendinous tissues, increases the non-uniform orientation of the collagen fibrils, and increases collagen cross-linking. The collagen synthesis and degradation rates increase with immobilization so that the proportion of new collagen to old increases in unloaded ligaments (Amiel et al., 1982). Total collagen mass (Amiel et al., 1982) and the stiffness of the ligament may also decrease (Noyes et al., 1974b; Tipton et al., 1974). Tipton and colleagues (1975) concluded that the strength of the junction between the bone and ligament was closely related to the type of exercise regimen and not due only to the duration of the exercise. Most researchers investigating exercise effects on ligaments report an increase in the ultimate strength of the maximum load at separation—junction strength (Adams, 1966; Tipton et al., 1967, 1970, 1974, 1975; Zuckerman

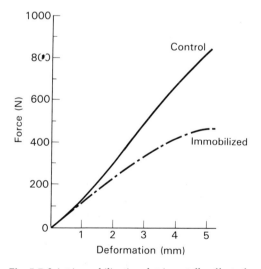

Fig. 5.7 Joint immobilization detrimentally affects the structural properties of the femur–anterior cruciate ligament–tibia unit. Immobilized tissues are less stiff and withstand less load at maximum and failure points. (From Butler et al., 1978.)

& Stull, 1969, 1973; Laros *et al.*, 1971). Single exercise bouts or sprint training, however, does not appear to result in significant increases in junction strength although the sprint training produced marked increases in ligament mass (Tipton *et al.*, 1967, 1974). Tipton and co-workers have also shown that although tendons and ligaments can be influenced by hormones (Dougherty & Berliner, 1968), chronic endurance training can increase the knee ligament junction strengths of thyroidectomized and hypophysectomized rats (Tipton *et al.*, 1971; Vailas *et al.*, 1978).

Of the few studies available that specifically quantify tendon's response to changes in load environment, Michna (1984), Woo *et al.* (1980), and Curwin *et al.* (1988) have provided details of the changes that occur with exercise. Mice that were exercised 1 week on a treadmill showed increased numbers and size of the collagen fibrils and larger cross-sectional areas in digital flexor tendons than did sedentary controls (Michna, 1984). After 7 weeks of continued training, the average fibril diameter was less than the control group, and it appeared that fibrils were splitting. By the end of the 10 weeks, the flexor tendon cross-sectional areas were comparable for both groups. Woo and colleagues (1980) exercised immature swine for 1 year and examined the adaptations in the extensor tendons. After this period of moderate exercise, there were no differences in the mechanical properties or cross-sectional area between the control and exercised swine. Currently, there is no quantitative information about how weight-bearing, mature extensor tendons adapt to exercise, but Curwin *et al.* (1988) have shown marked biochemical changes in immature tendon after a regimen of strenuous exercise. Collagen synthesis increased dramatically, but the Achilles tendon dry weight and collagen concentration did not change, suggesting that synthesis matched degradation.

Using a compensatory overload model, Zamora and Marini (1988) reported marked changes in plantaris tendon morphology. They reported a substantial increase in a number of active fibroblasts in the tendon. The fibroblast cytoplasm contained many vacuoles, indicating active protein synthesis. Zamora and Marini further described the changes in the myotendinous junction after an overload regimen. The adaptive changes to the overloading consisted of enhanced collagen synthesis, with intensive membrane renewal and recycling. Barfred (1973) summarized an extensive set of literature related to human tendons, indicating that physical activity and training apparently maintain tendon strength and integrity and reduce the probability of tendon rupture with age.

Meniscus

Menisci are fibrocartilage structures that bear loads and enhance rotation in synovial joints (Slocum & Larson, 1968; Shrive, 1974; Krause *et al.*, 1976), and the absence of knee menisci, for example, can result in increased joint laxity and a propensity for articular cartilage degeneration (Slocum & Larson, 1968; Lufti & Sudan, 1975). After meniscectomy, articular cartilage has been shown to degenerate morphologically and biochemically (Cox *et al.*, 1975; Krause *et al.* 1976).

While it is apparent that menisci must transmit a variety of mechanical loads (Shrive, 1974; Walker & Erkman, 1975; Krause *et al.*, 1976; Uezaki *et al.*, 1979; Jaspers *et al.*, 1980), little information is available about the adaptability of the important meniscal fibrocartilage in response to exercise. Some *in vitro* experiments involving chondrocytes obtained from fibrocartilage indicate that cyclic compression enhances the synthesis of collagen, proteoglycans, and deoxyribonucleic acid (Veldhuijzen *et al.*, 1979; De Witt *et al.*, 1984). In addition, a recent study by Vailas *et al.* (1986) suggests the meniscal fibrocartilage also is sensitive to exercise-related loading. After detailing the distinct regional characteristics of the rat knee meniscus composition, morphology and biomechanical properties (Vailas *et al.*, 1985;

Zernicke *et al.*, 1986), Vailas and co-workers trained rats to run on a motor-driven treadmill, 5 days a week for 12 weeks. There was a significant training effect that occurred, as evidenced by the 65% increase in gastrocnemius succinate dehydrogenase. In addition, in the region of the meniscus (posterior lateral horn) that most likely received the principal compressive cyclic loading, there was a significant increase in collagen, proteoglycan, and calcium concentrations.

Egner (1982) indicated that the longitudinal fibres of collagen ensure tension resistance in the meniscus while the transverse fibre bundles bind the longitudinal fibres to retain the shape of the meniscus. The increase in collagen and proteoglycan concentration in the meniscus as a result of exercise-induced loading should enhance the tissue's ability to accommodate mechanical loading (Mow *et al.*, 1984). Although researchers have doubted the capacity of meniscal fibrocartilage for adaptation—because of its low metabolic activity and poor blood supply (Videman *et al.*, 1979; Danzig *et al.*, 1983; Amiel *et al.*, 1985)—data indicate that the amount of nutrient delivery to the tissue is strongly related to the degree of tissue surface exposure to synovial fluid (Amiel *et al.*, 1985). During exercise, cyclic loading and unloading may improve the effectiveness of nutrient delivery to the matrix.

Concluding comments

In the past two decades, significant research has emerged in the area of the response of connective tissues to exercise and training. It is readily apparent from available data that fibrous and bony connective tissues are adaptive and very sensitive to the type of mechanical loads that are transmitted. Nevertheless, many of the relationships between the biochemical, morphological and biomechanical properties of bony and fibrous connective tissues and the quantity and quality of physical activity remain to be established. The search for the underlying mechanisms of remodelling and adaptation in

these tissues remains as a prime challenge for future research.

References

Adams, A. (1966) Effect of exercise upon ligament strength. *Research Quarterly for Exercise and Sport*, **37**, 163–7.

Akeson, W.H., Amiel, D. & La Violette, D. (1967) The connective-tissue response to immobility. *Clinical Orthopaedics and Related Research*, **51**, 183–97.

Akeson, W.H., Frank, C.B., Amiel, D. & Woo, S.L-Y. (1985) Ligament biology and biomechanics. In G.A.M. Finerman (ed.) *Symposium on Sports Medicine: The Knee*, pp. 111–51. C.V. Mosby, St Louis.

Albright, J.A. & Skinner, H.C. (1987) Bone: Structural organization and remodeling dynamics. In J.A. Albright & R.A. Brand (eds) *The Scientific Basis of Orthopaedics*, 2nd edn, pp. 161–98. Appleton-Lange, Connecticut.

Amiel, D., Abel, M.F. & Akeson, W.H. (1985) Nutrient delivery in the diarthrial joint: An analysis of synovial fluid transport in the rabbit knee (Abstract). *Transactions of the Orthopaedic Research Society*, **10**, 196.

Amiel, D., Woo, S.L., Harwood, F.L. & Akeson, W.H. (1982) The effect of immobilization on collagen turnover in connective tissue. *Acta Orthopaedica Scandinavica*, **53**, 325–32.

Barfred, T. (1973) Achilles tendon rupture: aetiology and pathogenesis of subcutaneous rupture assessed on the basis of the literature and rupture experiments on rats. *Acta Orthopaedica Scandinavica*, suppl. 152.

Bhasin, S., Sartoris, D.J., Fellingham, L., Zlatkin, M.B., Andre, M. & Resnick, D. (1988) Three dimensional quantitative CT of the proximal femur: Relationship to vertebral trabecular bone density in postmenopausal women. *Radiology*, **167**, 145–9.

Biewener, A.A., Swartz, S.M. & Bertram, J.E. (1986) Bone modelling during growth: Dynamic strain equilibrium in the chick tibiotarsus. *Calcified Tissue International*, **39**, 390–5.

Binderman, I., Shimshoni, Z. & Somjen, D. (1984) Biochemical pathways involved in the translation of physical stimulus into biological message. *Calcified Tissue International*, **36**, S82–S85.

Booth, F.W. & Gould, E.W. (1975) Effects of training and disuse on connective tissue. *Exercise and Sport Sciences Reviews*, **3**, 83–112.

Buckwalter, J.A. & Cooper, R.R. (1987) The cells and matrices of skeletal connective tissue. In J.A. Albright & R.A. Brand (eds) *The Scientific Basis of*

Orthopaedics, 2nd edn, pp. 1–30. Appleton-Lange, Connecticut.

Buckwalter, J.A., Maynard, J.A. & Vailas, A.C. (1987) Skeletal fibrous tissues: Tendon, joint capsule, and ligament. In J.A. Albright & R.A. Brand (eds) *The Scientific Basis of Orthopaedics*, 2nd edn, pp. 387–405. Appleton-Lange, Connecticut.

Butler, D.L., Grood, E.S., Noyes, F.R. & Zernicke, R.F. (1978) Biomechanics of ligaments and tendons. *Exercise and Sport Sciences Reviews*, **6**, 125–81.

Carter, D.R. (1984) Mechanical loading histories and cortical bone remodelling. *Calcified Tissue International*, **36**, S19–S24.

Carter, D.R. & Caler, W.E. (1985) A cumulative damage model for bone fracture. *Journal of Orthopaedic Research*, **3**, 84–90.

Carter, D.R., Caler, W.E., Spengler, D.M. & Frankel, V.H. (1981) Fatigue behavior of adult cortical bone: The influence of mean strain and strain range. *Acta Orthopaedica Scandinavica*, **52**, 481–90.

Carter, D.R., Smith, D.J., Spengler, D.M., Daly, C.H. & Frankel, V.H. (1980) Measurement and analysis of *in vivo* bone strains on the canine radius and ulna. *Journal of Biomechanics* **13**, 27–38.

Chamay, A. & Tschantz, P. (1972) Mechanical influences in bone remodelling. Experimental research on Wolff's law. *Journal of Biomechanics*, **5**, 173–80.

Churches, A.E. & Howlett, C.R. (1981) The response of mature cortical bone to controlled time-varying loading. In S.C. Cowin (ed.) *Mechanical Properties of Bone, Vol. 45*, pp. 69–80. American Society of Mechanical Engineers, New York.

Clark, E.A., Goodship, A.E. & Lanyon, L.E. (1975) Locomotor bone strain as the stimulus for bone's mechanical adaptability. *Journal of Physiology*, **245**, 57P.

Cochran, G.V. (1972) Implantation of strain gauges on bone *in vivo*. *Journal of Biomechanics*, **5**, 119–23.

Cochran, G.V. (1974) A method for direct recording of electromechanical data from skeletal bone in living animals. *Journal of Biomechanics*, **7**, 563–5.

Cochran, G.V., Pawluk, R.J. & Bassett, C.A. (1968) Electromechanical characteristics of bone under physiologic moisture conditions. *Clinical Orthopaedics and Related Research*, **58**, 249–70.

Cooper, R.R. & Misol, S. (1970) Tendon and ligament insertion. *Journal of Bone and Joint Surgery*, **52A**, 1–21.

Cowin, S.C., Lanyon, L.E. & Rodan, G. (1984) The Kroc Foundation conference on functional adaptation in bone tissue. *Calcified Tissue International*, **36**, S1–S6.

Cox, J.S., Nye, C.E., Schaefer, W.W. & Woodstein, I.J. (1975) The degenerative effects of partial and total resection of the medial meniscus in dogs'

knees. *Clinical Orthopaedics and Related Research*, **109**, 178–83.

Currey, J.D. (1984) *The Mechanical Adaptations of Bones*. Princeton University Press, New Jersey.

Currey, J.D. (1988) Strain rate and mineral content in fracture models of bone. *Journal of Orthopaedic Research*, **6**, 32–8.

Curwin, S.L., Vailas, A.C. & Wood, J. (1988) Immature tendon adaptation to strenuous exercise. *Journal of Applied Physiology*, **65**, 2297–301.

Dalen, N. & Olsson, K.E. (1974) Bone mineral content and physical activity. *Acta Orthopaedica Scandinavica*, **45**, 170–4.

Danzig, L., Resnick, D., Gonsalves, M. & Akeson, W.H. (1983) Blood supply to the normal and abnormal menisci of the human knee. *Clinical Orthopaedics and Related Research*, **172**, 271–6.

De Witt, M.T., Handley, C.J., Oakes, B.W. & Lowther, D.A. (1984) *In vitro* response of chondrocytes to mechanical loading. The effect of short-term mechanical tension. *Connective Tissue Research*, **12**, 97–109.

Dougherty, T.F. & Berliner, D.L. (1968) The effects of hormones on connective tissue cells. In B.S. Gould (ed.) *Treatise on Collagen. Vol. 2, Biology of Collagen, Part A*, Chapter 9. Academic Press, London.

Egner, E. (1982) Knee joint meniscal degeneration as it relates to tissue fibre structure and mechanical resistance. *Pathology, Research and Practice*, **173**, 310–24.

Elliott, D.H. (1965) Structure and function of mammalian tendon. *Biological Reviews*, **40**, 392–421.

Eriksson, C. (1976) Electrical properties of bone. In G.H. Bourne (ed.) *The Biochemistry and Physiology of Bone. Vol. IV, Calcification and Physiology*, 2nd edn, pp. 329–84. Academic Press, New York.

Evans, F.G. (1953) Methods of studying the biomechanical significance of bone form. *American Journal of Physical Anthropology*, **11**, 413–36.

Frost, H.M. (1987) Mechanical determinants of skeletal architecture. In J.A. Albright & R.A. Brand (eds) *The Scientific Basis of Orthopaedics*, 2nd edn, pp. 241–65. Appleton-Lange, Connecticut.

Fung, Y.C.B. (1967) Elasticity of soft tissues in simple elongation. *American Journal of Physiology*, **213**, 1532–44.

Fung, Y.C.B. (1972) Stress–strain relations of soft tissues in simple elongation. In Y.C.B. Fung, N. Perrone & M. Anliker (eds) *Biomechanics: Its Foundations and Objectives*, pp. 181–209. Prentice-Hall, Englewood Cliffs.

Goodship, A.E., Lanyon, L.E. & MacFie, H. (1979) Functional adaptation of bone to increased stress. *Journal of Bone and Joint Surgery*, **61A**, 539–46.

Gordon, K.R., Perl, M. & Levy, C. (1989) Structural

alterations and breaking strength of mouse femora exposed to three activity regimens. *Bone*, **10**, 303–12.

Hahn, H.T. & Kim, R.V. (1980) Fatigue behavior of composite laminates. *Journal of Composite Materials*, **10**, 156–80.

Ham, A.W. (1974) *Histology*. J.B. Lippincott, Philadelphia.

Harkness, R.D. (1968) Mechanical properties of collagenous tissues. In B.S. Gould (ed.) *Treatise on Collagen, Vol. 2, Biology of Collagen, Part A*, Chapter 6. Academic Press, London.

Hert, J., Liskova, M. & Landa, J. (1971) Reaction of bone to mechanical stimuli. Part 1. Continuous and intermittent loading of tibia in rabbit. *Folia Morphologica*, **19**, 290–300.

Hooley, C.J., McCrum, N. & Cohen, R.E. (1980) The viscoelastic deformation of tendon. *Journal of Biomechanics*, **13**, 521–8.

Hou, J. C-H., Salem, G.J., Zernicke, R.F. & Barnard, R.J. (1991) Structural and mechanical adaptations of immature trabecular bone to strenuous exercise. *Journal of Applied Physiology*, **69**, 1309–14.

Jaspers, P., Lange, A., Huiskes, R. & Van Reus, T.G. (1980) The mechanical function of the meniscus, experiments on cadaveric pig knee joints. *Acta Orthopaedica Belgica*, **46**, 663–8.

Jaworski, Z.F.G. (1984) Lamellar bone turnover system and its effector organs. *Calcified Tissue International*, 36, S46–S55.

Jee, W.S., Wronski, E.R., Morey, E.R. & Kimmel, D.B. (1983) Effects of spaceflight on trabecular bone in rats. *American Journal of Physiology*, **244**, R310–14.

Jones, H.H., Priest, J.B., Hayes, W.C., Tichenor, C.C. & Nagel, A. (1977) Humeral hypertrophy in response to exercise. *Journal of Bone and Joint Surgery*, **59A**, 204–8.

Kastelic, J., Galeski, A. & Baer, E. (1978) The multicomposite structure of tendon. *Connective Tissue Research*, **6**, 11–23.

Keller, T.S. & Spengler, D.M. (1989) Regulation of bone stress and strain in the immature and mature rat femur. *Journal of Biomechanics*, **22**, 1115–28.

Kiiskinen, A. (1977) Physical training and connective tissue in young mice—physical properties of Achilles tendon and long bone growth. *Growth*, **41**, 123–7.

Kiiskinen, A. & Heikkinen, E. (1973) Effects of physical training on development and strength of tendons and bones in growing mice. *Scandinavian Journal of Clinical and Laboratory Investigation*, **29** (suppl. 123), 60.

Krause, W.R., Pope, M.H., Johnson, R.J. & Wilder, D.G. (1976) Mechanical changes in the knee after meniscectomy. *Journal of Bone and Joint Surgery*, **58A**, 599–604.

Krolner, B., Toft, B., Nielson, S.P. & Tondevold, E. (1983) Physical exercise as prophylaxis against involutional vertebral bone loss: a controlled trial. *Clinical Science*, **64**, 541–6.

Lafferty, J.F. & Raju, P.V.V. (1979) The influence of stress frequency on the fatigue strength of cortical bone. *Journal of Biomechanical Engineering*, **101**, 112–13.

Lanyon, L.E. (1971) Strain in sheep lumbar vertebrae recorded during life. *Acta Orthopaedica Scandinavica*, **42**, 102–12.

Lanyon, L.E. (1972) *In vivo* bone strain recorded from thoracic vertebrae of sheep. *Journal of Biomechanics*, **5**, 277–81.

Lanyon, L.E. (1973) Analysis of surface bone strain in the calcaneus of sheep during normal locomotion. *Journal of Biomechanics*, **6**, 41–9.

Lanyon, L.E. (1987) Functional strain in bone tissue as an objective and controlling stimulus for adaptive bone remodelling *Journal of Biomechanics*, **20**, 1083–93.

Lanyon, L.E. & Hartman, W. (1977) Strain related electrical potentials recorded *in vitro* and *in vivo*. *Calcified Tissue Research*, **22**, 315–27.

Lanyon, L.E. & Rubin, C.T. (1984) Static vs. dynamic loads as an influence on bone remodelling. *Journal of Biomechanics*, **16**, 897–905.

Lanyon, L.E. & Smith, R.N. (1969) Measurement of bone strain in the walking animal. *Research in Veterinary Science*, **10**, 93–4.

Lanyon, L.E. & Smith, R.N. (1970) Bone strain in the tibia during normal quadrupedal locomotion. *Acta Orthopaedica Scandinavica*, **41**, 238–48.

Laros, G.S., Tipton, C.M. & Cooper, R.R. (1971) Influence of physical activity on ligament insertions in the knees of dogs. *Journal of Bone and Joint Surgery*, **53A**, 275–86.

Liskova, M. & Hert, J. (1971) Reaction of bone to mechanical stimuli. Part 2: Periosteal and endosteal reaction of tibial diaphyses in rabbit to intermittent loading. *Folia Morphologica*, **19**, 301.

Lufti, A.M. & Sudan, K. (1975) Morphological changes in the articular cartilage after meniscectomy: An experimental study in the monkey. *Journal of Bone and Joint Surgery*, **57B**, 525–7.

McDonald, R., Hegenauer, J. & Saltman, P. (1986) Age-related differences in the bone mineralization pattern of rats following exercise. *Journal of Gerontology*, **41**, 445–52.

Matsuda, J.J., Zernicke, R.F., Vailas, A.C., Pedrini, V.A., Pedrini-Mille, A. & Maynard, J.A. (1986) Structural and mechanical adaptation of immature bone to strenuous exercise. *Journal of Applied Physiology*, **60**, 2028–34.

Meade, J.B., Cowin, S.C., Klawitter, J.J., Van Buskirk, W.C. & Skinner, H.B. (1984) Bone remodeling to continuously applied loads. *Calcified Tissue International*, **36**, S25–S30.

Michna, H. (1984) Morphometric analysis of loading-induced changes in collagen-fibril populations in young tendons. *Cell and Tissue Research*, **236**, 465–70.

Morey, E.R. & Baylink, D.J. (1978) Inhibition of bone formation during space flight. *Science*, **201**, 1138–41.

Mow, V.C., Holmes, M.H. & Lai, W.M. (1984) Fluid transport and mechanical properties of articular cartilage: A review. *Journal of Biomechanics*, **17**, 377–94.

Nordin, M. & Frankel, V.H. (1989) *Basic Biomechanics of the Musculoskeletal System*, 2nd edn. Lea & Febiger, Philadelphia.

Noyes, F.R., De Lucas, J.L. & Torvik, P.J. (1974a) Biomechanics of anterior cruciate ligament failure: An analysis of strain-rate sensitivity and mechanisms of failure in primates. *Journal of Bone and Joint Surgery*, **56A**, 236–53.

Noyes, F.R., Torvik, P.J., Hyde, W.B. & De Lucas, J.L. (1974b) Biomechanics of ligament failure. *Journal of Bone and Joint Surgery*, **56A**, 1406–18.

O'Connor, J.A., Lanyon, L.E. & McFie, H. (1982) The influence of strain rate on adaptive bone remodeling. *Journal of Biomechanics*, **15**, 767–81.

Ovalle, W.K. (1987) The human muscle-tendon junction: A morphological study during normal growth and at maturity. *Anatomy and Embryology*, **176**, 281–94.

Pedrini-Mille, A., Pedrini, V.A., Maynard, J.A. & Vailas, A.C. (1988) Response of immature chicken meniscus to strenuous exercise: Biochemical studies of proteoglycan and collagen. *Journal of Orthopaedic Research*, **6**, 196–204.

Pirnay, F., Bodeux, M., Crielaard, J.M. & Franchimont, P. (1987) Bone mineral content and physical activity. *International Journal of Sports Medicine*, **8**, 331–5.

Prockop, D.J. & Guzman, N.A. (1977) Collagen diseases and the biosynthesis of collagen. *Hospital Practice*, **December**, 61–8.

Radin, E.L., Orr, R.B., Kelman, J.L., Paul, I.L. & Rose, M.R. (1982) Effect of prolonged walking on concrete on the knees of sheep. *Journal of Biomechanics*, **15**, 487–92.

Rambaut, P.C. & Johnson, R.S. (1979) Prolonged weightlessness and calcium loss in man. *Acta Astronautica*, **6**, 1113–22.

Rubin, C.T. (1984) Skeletal strain and the functional significance of bone architecture. *Calcified Tissue International*, **36**, S11–18.

Rubin, C.T. & Lanyon, L.E. (1985) Regulation of bone mass by mechanical strain magnitude. *Calcified Tissue International*, **37**, 411–17.

Rubin, C.T. & Lanyon, L.E. (1987) Osteoregulatory

nature of mechanical stimuli: Function as a determinant for adaptive remodeling in bone. *Journal of Orthopaedic Research*, **5**, 300–10.

Rybicki, E.F., Mills, E.J., Turner, A.S.D. & Simonen, F.A. (1977) In vivo and analytical studies of forces and moments in equine long bones. *Journal of Biomechanics*, **10**, 701–5.

Saville, P.D. & Whyte, M.P. (1969) Muscle and bone hypertrophy: Positive effect of running exercise in the rat. *Clinical Orthopaedics and Related Research*, **65**, 81–8.

Schaffler, M.B. & Burr, D.B. (1988) Stiffness of compact bone: The effects of porosity and density. *Journal of Biomechanics*, **21**, 13–16.

Schaffler, M.B., Radin, E.L. & Burr, D.B. (1989) Mechanical and morphological effects of strain rate on fatigue of compact bone. *Bone*, **10**, 207–14.

Shaw, S.R., Vailas, A.C., Grindeland, R.E. & Zernicke, R.F. (1988) Effects of one-week spaceflight on the morphological and mechanical properties of growing bone. *American Journal of Physiology*, **254**, R78–R83.

Shaw, S.R., Zernicke, R.F., Vailas, A.C., DeLuna, D., Thomason, D.B. & Baldwin, K.B. (1987) Mechanical, morphological and biochemical adaptations of bone and muscle to hindlimb suspension and exercise. *Journal of Biomechanics*, **20**, 225–34.

Shrive, N. (1974) The weight-bearing role of the menisci of the knee. *Journal of Bone and Joint Surgery*, **56B**, 381–7.

Silbermann, M., Bar-Shira-Maymon, B., Coleman, R., Reznick, A., Weisman, Y., Steinhagen-Thiessen, E., von der Mark, H. & von der Mark, K. (1990) Long-term physical exercise retards trabecular bone loss in lumbar vertebrae of aging female mice. *Calcified Tissue International*, **46**, 80–93.

Simkin, A., Ayalon, J. & Leichter, I. (1987) Increased trabecular bone density due to bone-loading exercises in postmenopausal osteoporotic women. *Calcified Tissue International*, **40**, 59–63.

Skerry, T.M., Bitensky, L., Chayen J. & Lanyon, L.E. (1988) Loading-related reorientation of bone proteoglycan in vivo. Strain memory in bone tissue? *Journal of Orthopaedic Research*, **6**, 547–51.

Skerry, T.M., Suswillo, R., El Haj, A.J., Ali, N.N., Dodds, R.A. & Lanyon, L.E. (1990) Load-induced proteoglycan orientation in bone tissue in vivo and in vitro. *Calcified Tissue International*, **46**, 318–26.

Skinner, H.C. (1987) Bone mineralization. In J.A. Albright & R.A. Brand (eds) *The Scientific Basis of Orthopaedics*, 2nd edn, pp. 199–212. Appleton-Lange, Connecticut.

Slocum, D.B. & Larson, R.L. (1968) Rotatory instability of the knee. *Journal of Bone and Joint Surgery*, **50A**, 211–25.

Smith, E.L., Smith, P.E., Ensign, C.J. & Shea, M.M. (1984) Bone involution decrease in exercising middle-aged women. *Calcified Tissue International*, **36**, 5129–38.

Smith, S.D. (1977) Femoral development in chronically centrifuged rats. *Aviation Space and Environmental Medicine*, **48**, 828–35.

Steinberg, M.E. & Trueta, J. (1981) Effects of activity on bone growth and development in the rat. *Clinical Orthopaedics and Related Research*, **156**, 52–60.

Tidball, J.G. (1983) The geometry of actin filament-membrane associations can modify adhesive strength of the myotendinous junction. *Cell Motility*, **3**, 439–47.

Tidball, J.G. (1984) Myotendinous junction: Morphological changes and mechanical failure associated with muscle cell atrophy. *Experimental and Molecular Pathology*, **40**, 1–12.

Tidball, J.G. & Daniel, T.L. (1986) Myotendinous junctions of tonic muscle cells: Structure and loading. *Cell and Tissue Research*, **245**, 315–22.

Tipton, C.M., James, S.L., Mergner, W. & Tcheng, T.K. (1970) Influence of exercise on strength of medial collateral knee ligaments of dogs. *American Journal of Physiology*, **218**, 894–902.

Tipton, C.M., Matthes, R.D., Maynard, J.A. & Carey, R.A. (1975) The influence of physical activity on tendons and ligaments. *Medicine and Science in Sports*, **7**, 165–75.

Tipton, C.M., Matthes, R.D. & Sandage, D.S. (1974) *In situ* measurements of junction strength and ligament elongation in rats. *Journal of Applied Physiology*, **37**, 758–61.

Tipton, C.M., Schild, R.J. & Tomanek, R.J. (1967) Influence of physical activity on the strength of knee ligaments in rats. *American Journal of Physiology*, **212**, 783–7.

Tipton, C.M., Tcheng, T.K. & Mergner, W. (1971) Influence of immobilization, training, exogenous hormones, and surgical repair on knee ligaments from hypophysectomized rats. *American Journal of Physiology*, **221**, 1144–50.

Trotter, J.A., Eberhard, S. & Samora, A. (1983) Structural connections of the muscle–tendon junction. *Cell Motility*, **3**, 431–8.

Turner, A.S., Mills E.J. & Gabel, A.A. (1975) *In vivo* measurement of bone strain in the horse. *American Journal of Veterinary Research*, **36**, 1573–9.

Uezaki, N., Kobayashi, A. & Matsushige, K. (1979) The viscoelastic properties of the human semilunar cartilage. *Journal of Biomechanics*, **12**, 65–73.

Uhthoff, H.K. & Jaworski, Z.F. (1978) Bone loss in response to long-term immobilization. *Journal of Bone and Joint Surgery*, **60B**, 420–9.

Vailas, A.C., Tipton, C.M., Laughlin, H.L., Tcheng, T.K. & Matthes, R.D. (1978) Physical activity and hypophysectomy on the aerobic capacity of ligaments and tendons. *American Journal of Physiology*, **44**, 542–6.

Vailas, A.C., Tipton, C.M., Matthes, R.D. & Gart, M. (1981) Physical activity and its influence on the repair process of medial collateral ligaments. *Connective Tissue Research*, **9**, 25–31.

Vailas, A.C., Zernicke, R.F., Matsuda, J., Curwin, S. & Durivage, J. (1986) Adaptation of rat knee meniscus to prolonged exercise. *Journal of Applied Physiology*, **60**, 1031–4.

Vailas, A.C., Zernicke, R.F., Matsuda, J. & Peller, D. (1985) Regional biochemical and morphological characteristics of rat knee meniscus. *Comparative Biochemistry and Physiology*, **82B**, 283–5.

Veldhuijzen, J.P., Bourret, L.A. & Rodan, G.A. (1979) *In vitro* studies of the effect of intermittent compressive forces on cartilage cell proliferation. *Journal of Cellular Physiology*, **98**, 299–306.

Videman, T., Eronen, I., Friman, C. & Langenskiold, A. (1979) Glycosaminoglycan metabolisms of the medial meniscus, the medial collateral ligaments and the hip joint capsule in experimental osteoarthritis caused by immobilization of the rabbit knee. *Acta Orthopaedica Scandinavica*, **50**, 465–70.

Viidik, A. (1973) Functional properties of collagenous tissues. *International Review of Connective Tissue Research*, **6**, 127–215.

Walker, P.S. & Erkman, M.J. (1975) The role of menisci in force transmission across the knee. *Clinical Orthopaedics and Related Research*, **109**, 184–91.

White, A., Handler, P. & Smith, E.L. (1964) *Principles of Biochemistry*. McGraw-Hill, New York.

Woo, S.L.-Y. Gomez, M.A., Woo, Y.K. & Akeson, W.H. (1982) Mechanical properties of tendons and ligaments: II. The relationships of immobilization and exercise on tissue remodeling. *Biorheology*, **19**, 397–408.

Woo, S.L.-Y., Kuei, S.C., Amiel, D., Gomez, M.A., Hayes, W.C., White F.C. & Akeson, W.H. (1981) The effect of physical training on the properties of long bone: A study of Wolff's law. *Journal of Bone and Joint Surgery*, **63A**, 780–7.

Woo, S.L.-Y., Matthews, J.V., Akeson, W.H., Amiel, D. & Convery, F.R. (1975) Connective tissue response to immobility. Correlative study of biochemical measurements of normal and immobilized rabbit knees. *Arthritis and Rheumatism*, **18**, 257–64.

Woo, S.L.-Y., Ritter, M.A., Amiel, D., Sanders, T.M., Gomez, M.A., Kuei, S.C., Garfin, S.R. & Akeson, W.H. (1980) The biomechanical and biochemical properties of swine tendons—long-term effects of exercise on the digital extensors. *Connective Tissue Research*, **7**, 177–83.

Yeh, C.K. & Rodan, G.A. (1984) Tensile forces enhance prostaglandin E synthesis in osteoblastic cells grown on collagen ribbons. *Calcified Tissue International*, **36**, S67–S71.

Zamora, A.J. & Marini, J.F. (1988) Tendon and myo-tendinous junction in an overloaded skeletal muscle of the rat. *Anatomy and Embryology*, **179**, 89–96.

Zernicke, R.F. & Loitz, B.J. (1990) Myotendinous adaptation to conditioning. In J. Buckwalter, S. Gordon & W. Leadbetter (eds) *Sports-Induced Inflammation*, pp. 687–98. American Academy Orthopaedic Surgeons, Illinois.

Zernicke, R.F., Vailas, A.C., Shaw, S.R., Bogey, R.S., Hart, T.J. & Matsuda, J. (1986) Heterogeneous mechanical response of rat knee menisci to thermomechanical stress. *American Journal of Physiology*, **250**, R65–R70.

Zuckerman, J. & Stull, G.A. (1969) Effects of exercise on knee ligament separation force in rats. *Journal of Applied Physiology*, **26**, 716.

Zuckerman, J. & Stull, G.A. (1973) Ligamentous separation force in rats as influenced by training, detraining and cage restriction. *Medicine and Science in Sports*, **5**, 41–9.

Chapter 6A

Contractile Performance of Skeletal Muscle Fibres

K.A. PAUL EDMAN

Skeletal muscle represents the largest organ of the body. It makes up approximately 40% of the total body weight and it is organized into hundreds of separate entities, or body muscles, each of which has been assigned a specific task to enable the great variety of movements that are essential to normal life. Each muscle is composed of a great number of subunits, muscle fibres, that are arranged in parallel and typically extend from one tendon to another. In order to understand the performance of muscle it is essential to know the mechanical properties of the individual fibres. With the laboratory techniques now available it is possible to study, in considerable detail, the contractile behaviour of intact single fibres that have been isolated from amphibian muscles and kept immersed in a physiological salt solution. Such fibres, if properly treated, are remarkably stable in their contractile behaviour, showing almost identical responses to electrical stimulation over a whole day of experimentation. In addition, the single fibre preparation offers the possibility to study the mechanical performance under strict control of sarcomere length. The latter aspect is of particular importance as the sarcomere length reflects the state of overlap between the two sets of interdigitating filaments that constitute the main functional elements of the contractile system. The following account will elucidate some basic contractile properties of the skeletal muscle fibre, and an attempt will be made to relate these properties to the structure of the contractile system.

Structure of the force generating system

The muscle fibre is a cable-like structure that is composed of tightly packed subunits, myofibrils, that fill up most of the fibre volume (Fig. 6.1). The myofibrils are approximately 1 μm wide and run the entire length of the fibre. They contain the contractile apparatus and are therefore the structures within the muscle that are responsible for force generation and active shortening. The myofibrils exhibit a characteristic band pattern of alternating dark and light segments when viewed in an ordinary light microscope. As the dark and light segments coincide in adjacent myofibrils the entire muscle fibre assumes a striped appearance in the microscope. Skeletal muscle is therefore often referred to as 'striated muscle'. As will become apparent from the following, the striated appearance is an expression of the remarkable regularity in which the contractile machinery is organized within the myofibril.

The principal elements in the myofibrillar structure are two sets of filaments of different thickness that show a highly ordered, segmental arrangement that corresponds to the striated appearance of the myofibril. The thicker filaments occupy the dark bands of the fibre (see above) and are made up of a fibrous protein, myosin (Hanson & Huxley, 1953; Hasselbach, 1953). It is the specific optical properties of these filaments in their ordered state in the muscle that make the segment

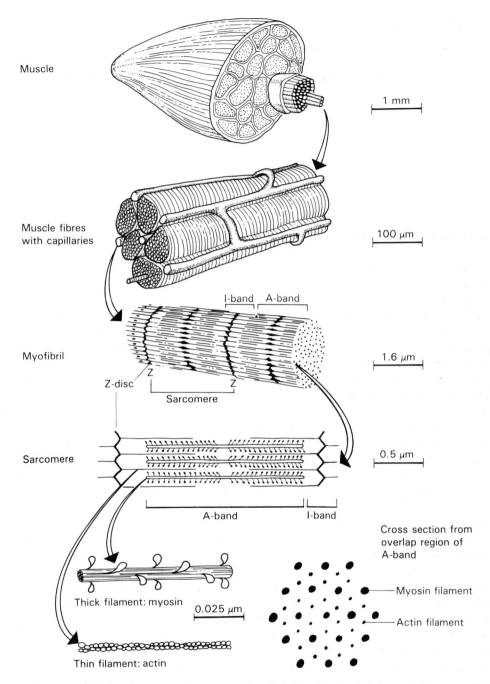

Muscle

1 mm

Muscle fibres
with capillaries

100 μm

I-band   A-band

Myofibril

Z-disc   Z   Z

Sarcomere

1.6 μm

Sarcomere

A-band   I-band

0.5 μm

Thick filament: myosin

0.025 μm

Thin filament: actin

Cross section from
overlap region of
A-band

Myosin filament

Actin filament

Fig. 6.1 Schematic illustration of muscle structure. For further explanation, see text. (From di Prampero, 1985.)

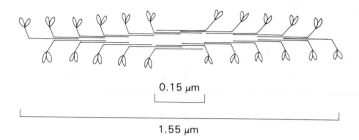

0.15 μm

1.55 μm

Fig. 6.2 Simplified drawing of the myosin filament (not drawn to scale) illustrating arrangement of myosin molecules. Note that the two halves of the filament are symmetrical and that a central zone, *c.* 0.15 μm wide, is free of myosin extensions (bridges). (After model presented by Huxley, 1963.)

appear dark in the microscope when the fibre is illuminated under standard conditions. Synonymous names of the filaments are: thick filaments, myosin filaments or, referring to their (anisotropic) optical properties, A-filaments.

The second set of filaments are mainly built up of a globular protein, actin. These filaments are anchored in the Z-disc that is located in the centre of the light band. They extend from either side of the Z-disc and reach into the adjacent A-band where they overlap to some degree with the thick filaments (Hanson & Huxley, 1953). The thin (actin) filaments have optical properties (isotropic) that differ from those of the thick filaments explaining the characteristic appearance of the segment they occupy. The thin filaments are often referred to as I-filaments, and the segments they fill up are generally named I-bands. A cross-sectional view of the myofibril makes clear that the two sets of filaments are arranged in a highly ordered fashion relative to one another (Fig. 6.1). Each A-filament is surrounded by six I-filaments in a hexagonal array. An individual A-filament is thus in a position to interact simultaneously with six adjacent I-filaments, and each I-filament is able to interact with three neighbouring A-filaments. This spatial arrangement of the myofilaments is of great functional significance as it lends stability to the contractile system during activity. The fact that any given filament is able to interact with several adjacent filaments simultaneously ensures that the individual filaments do not coalesce side to side but remain separated from one another during muscle contraction.

Myosin, which is the main constituent of the thick filament, is a large club-like structure composed of a long shaft with two globular heads at one end. The myosin molecules are packed together in such a way (Fig. 6.2) that the shafts form the backbone of the thick filament. However, a substantial portion of the myosin molecule, namely the two heads and a part of the shaft, extends from the rod-like structure to form side pieces (myosin cross-bridges) at regular intervals along the filament. The cross-bridges are spaced in such a way that every sixth bridge, going from the centre towards the tip of the filament, will face a given thin filament. The two halves of the filament are mirror images of one another (Fig. 6.2), and there is a central region, *c.* 0.15 μm in length, that is free of cross-bridges (the 'inert zone'). The total length of the thick filament is approximately 1.55 μm.

As is shown in Fig. 6.3 the actin monomer is the main building stone of the thin filament. The actin molecules are polymerized to form two helical strands that are wound together. Each actin molecule constitutes a site where an adjacent thick filament may interact to form a cross-bridge connection during muscle activity (see further below). Another important constituent of the thin filament is the protein system that regulates the degree of interaction between the thick and thin filaments. This system is located in the grooves between the two actin strands and is an integral part of the thin filament. It is formed by tropomyosin and troponin, whose functions are now quite well understood (Ebashi & Endo, 1968; Ebashi, 1980). The tropomyosin molecules are rod-

Fig. 6.3 Schematic drawing of a portion of the thin filament showing the two helical strands of actin molecules. The regulatory proteins, troponin and tropomyosin, are positioned in each of the two grooves between the actin strands. (From Ebashi, 1980.)

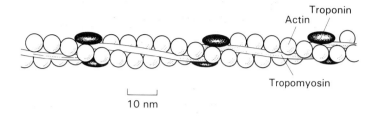

shaped. They are polymerized end to end to form a string that lies in each of the two grooves between the actin strands along the entire I-filament. Each tropomyosin molecule has a troponin entity attached to it as is shown in Fig. 6.3. Troponin, in reality a protein complex, has a high affinity for calcium. Binding of calcium to troponin causes a structural change of the troponin–tropomyosin complex that leads to contractile activation as is described subsequently.

For more information about the structure of the contractile system see monographs by Squire (1981) and Woledge *et al.* (1985).

Molecular events during contraction

Our knowledge about the structural organization of the contractile system in the form of two discrete sets of filaments, as outlined above, stems from the pioneering work of H.E. Huxley and J. Hanson in the early 1950s (Hanson & Huxley, 1953; Huxley, 1953; Huxley & Hanson, 1954). Their observation that the thick and thin filaments remain constant in length during muscle contraction, while the region of overlap between the two filaments changes with fibre length, led these authors to suggest that muscle contraction is based on a sliding motion of the two sets of interdigitating filaments. A similar conclusion was reached at the same time by A.F. Huxley & Niedergerke (1954). The latter authors were able to demonstrate that the length of the A-bands (occupied by the thick filaments) stays essentially constant as a muscle fibre shortens whereas the I-band spacing varies with the overall length

of the fibre. The idea that muscle contraction involves a sliding movement of the thick and thin filaments, with no significant change of their length, has now gained general acceptance. According to this view the driving force for the sliding motion is generated by the myosin cross-bridges within the region where the thick and thin filaments overlap. The experimental evidence suggests that the myosin bridges make repeated contacts with adjacent thin filaments and that each such contact makes a contribution to the force developed during contraction. However, the precise mechanism by which force is generated by the cross-bridge still remains to be established.

Figure 6.4 is a schematic illustration of the cross-bridge cycle according to current views. The process starts as the calcium concentration around the myofibrils is raised above a certain level. This occurs when the fibre is stimulated and calcium is released into the myoplasm from its storage site in the sarcoplasmic reticulum. Binding of calcium to troponin initiates a conformational change of the troponin–tropomyosin complex that leads to retraction of tropomyosin into the groove between the actin strands of the thin filament (Ebashi & Endo, 1968; Squire, 1981). In this way, the steric hindrance for interaction between the thick and thin filaments is eliminated, and myosin cross-bridges get the opportunity to attach to actin molecules that are within their reach on neighbouring thin filaments.

The following events are likely to occur during a cross-bridge cycle (Fig. 6.4a–d). A connection is formed between the globular head of the bridge and an actin site (b). This

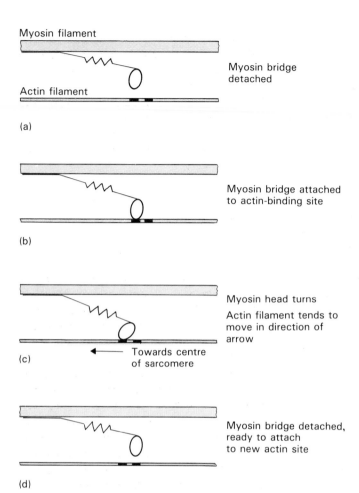

Myosin filament

Actin filament

Myosin bridge detached

(a)

Myosin bridge attached to actin-binding site

(b)

Myosin head turns

Actin filament tends to move in direction of arrow

Towards centre of sarcomere

(c)

Myosin bridge detached, ready to attach to new actin site

(d)

Fig. 6.4 Schematic illustration of the cross-bridge cycle. Two binding sites on the actin filament are marked to illustrate the sliding of the thin filament relative to the cross-bridge from (a) to (d).

leads to a conformational change within the bridge that alters the angle of the head relative to the thin filament in this way putting strain on the shaft of the bridge (c). The force so produced will tend to move the thin filament further into the array of thick filaments. After the 'power stroke' the cross-bridge is detached from the thin filament; this occurs as a molecule of adenosine triphosphate (ATP) binds to the myosin head. The bound ATP molecule is rapidly split, and the bridge resumes its original shape and is thereafter ready to attach again to the actin filament for a new cycle of activity (d). Each working cycle of the cross-bridge thus requires the hydrolysis of one molecule of ATP which, accordingly, serves as the immediate source of energy for the contractile process (see further Woledge et al., 1985). The ATP consumed is continuously replenished. This is partly achieved by reutilizing the breakdown products, adenosine diphosphate (ADP) and inorganic phosphate (P_i), for formation of ATP. However, accumulation of ADP, P_i and H^+ does occur during excessive exercise and this has an unfavourable effect on the performance of the cross-bridges and is a cause of muscle fatigue (see further below).

According to the cross-bridge hypothesis (Huxley, 1957) bridges are thought to act as independent force generators, i.e. the performance of any one bridge is assumed to be uninfluenced by the activity of other bridges. The number of cross-bridges formed is determined by the degree of activation of the contractile system (governed by calcium ions, see above) and by the amount of overlap between the thick and thin filaments. Bridges attach to the thin filament in a position where they are able to produce active force, and if the filaments are restrained from sliding (which can be achieved by holding the sarcomere length constant by feedback control) the bridges will remain in a force-producing position as long as they are attached to the thin filament. However, some turnover of bridges does occur even under isometric (constant length) conditions, i.e. bridges dissociate spontaneously and are replaced by new ones keeping the total number of attached bridges at a given level. This results in there being some energy expenditure even during a purely isometric action when no work is produced by the muscle.

When the ends of the muscle are free to move, the force produced by the cross-bridges make the thin filaments slide towards the centre of the thick filaments. The sliding movement decreases the probability of cross-bridge formation since the myosin bridges will be exposed to a potential binding site for a shorter time as the filaments slide. Thus, as a muscle is allowed to shorten at progressively higher speeds (which is achieved by decreasing the load on the muscle), the number of attached bridges is steadily reduced. By this mechanism the muscle is able to adjust the number of active cross-bridges (and therefore its energy expenditure) to precisely match the load that is lifted during shortening.

Due to the movement of the filaments some of the attached bridges will come into a braking position and counteract the sliding motion. When the load on the muscle is reduced to zero, the number of braking cross-bridges is just equal to the number of bridges that are in a pulling (force producing) position. The distribution between pulling and braking cross-bridges will always be such that no net force

is created for the sliding movement (Huxley, 1957). This ensures that the muscle shortens at a constant velocity. If a net force for the sliding movement were to arise, due to a mismatch between pulling and braking bridges, the muscle would accelerate throughout the shortening phase, a behaviour that would tend to make the body movements jerky and probably less precise.

Contractile performance of striated muscle

The length–tension relation

It has been known for a long time that a muscle's capacity to produce force depends on the length at which the muscle is held, maximum force being delivered near the length that the muscle normally takes up in the body. This length dependence of the contractile performance has attracted much interest in recent years as it has become clear that the relationship between force and sarcomere length provides information of relevance to the elucidation of the sliding-filament mechanism of muscle contraction. A study of the sarcomere length–tension relation, however, is made difficult by the fact that the sarcomere pattern is not uniform within a muscle fibre but varies substantially from one region to another along the fibre. In order to eliminate this problem, techniques have been developed that enable recording of isometric force from merely a part of the intact fibre. Gordon et al. (1966) were first to present such a method. With their 'spot-follower' technique these authors were able to length-clamp a 7–10-mm portion of a muscle fibre during a tetanus, in this way excluding the end regions of the fibre from force recording. Later experiments (Edman & Reggiani, 1984, 1987) have demonstrated, however, that there is a need to length-clamp a considerably smaller fibre segment (c. 0.5 mm in length) to eliminate the error in the length–tension measurement that may arise from non-uniform sarcomere behaviour.

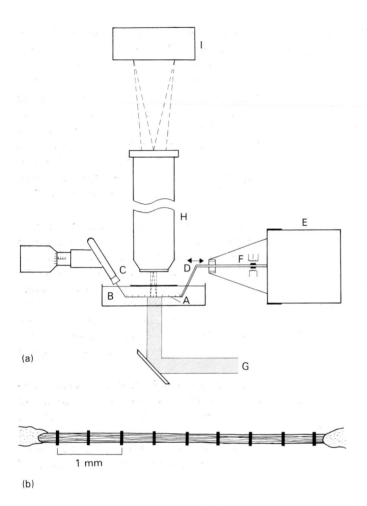

(a)

(b)

Fig. 6.5 (a) Apparatus for recording force and movement in discrete short segments of intact single muscle fibre. A, single muscle fibre; B, muscle chamber filled with saline; C, force transducer; D, shaft movable in the horizontal plane; E, electromagnetic puller; F, transducer for recording movements of shaft D; G, path for laser beam; H, monocular microscope; I, stage above the microscope onto which an image of fibre (and markers) is projected. A photodiode assembly positioned in the plane of the image records the distance between adjacent markers. (b) Drawing of a single muscle fibre with markers attached on the surface.

Figure 6.5 illustrates the approach used for length-clamping a discrete, short segment of an isolated muscle fibre (for further details, see Edman & Höglund, 1981 and Edman & Reggiani, 1984). Illustrated is a single fibre (A) that is mounted horizontally in physiological saline (B) between a force transducer (C) and the shaft (D) of an electromagnetic puller (E). The fibre is stimulated by means of two platinum plate electrodes (not illustrated) that are placed along either side of the fibre in the bath. Discrete segments, approximately 0.5 mm in length, are defined by thin opaque markers that are firmly attached to the upper surface of the fibre. The relative position of any two adjacent markers (outlining one segment) can

be measured with a high degree of accuracy by means of a photoelectric recording device (I). For length-clamping a given segment the puller (E) is commanded to adjust the overall length of the fibre in such a way that the segment's length is maintained constant throughout the contraction. For this manoeuvre the puller is continuously guided by the signal that is provided by the photoelectric device. It is possible in this way to keep the sarcomere length of a small fibre segment very nearly constant (to within 0.1%) during a tetanus. The clamped segment is thus neither shortening nor lengthening during contraction. The tension recorded from the fibre under these conditions is therefore the true isometric force

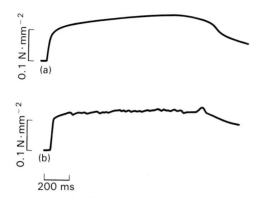

Fig. 6.6 Tetanic force recorded in a single muscle fibre from a frog at 2.95-μm sarcomere length. (a) Conventional recording with the ends of the fibre fixed. Note continuous creep of tension indicating non-uniform behaviour of sarcomeres along the fibre. (b) Recording from a short segment held at constant length during contraction by servo mechanism described in Fig. 6.5. Note constant force production indicating uniform sarcomere behaviour within the short segment.

of the length-clamped segment. Typically, the force so produced remains quite stable during the tetanus period as is illustrated in Fig. 6.6 (record b).

The relationship between maximum tetanic force and sarcomere length is illustrated in Fig. 6.7. The curve is based on measurements from short length-clamped segments, as described above, and can therefore be supposed to reflect the mechanical performance of a uniform sarcomere population of the fibre. It can be seen that maximum force is attained near a sarcomere length of 2.0 μm and that force is progressively reduced above and below this length. The measured force approaches zero when the sarcomeres are extended to 3.6–3.7 μm.

The sarcomere length–tension relation described above differs in some respects from the polygonal length–tension curve that was originally derived by Gordon et al. (1966). The new data show that the length–tension relation has no distinct plateau between 2.0 and 2.2 μm sarcomere length (see comparison of curves in Fig. 6.8). Furthermore, the length–tension relation has a smoother shape than postulated earlier.

Assuming that active force is proportional to the degree of overlap between the thick and thin filaments, the length–tension relation can be used to estimate the average functional length of the A- and I-filaments and the variability of overlap between them. The results of

Fig. 6.7 Variation of maximum tetanic force with sarcomere length. Insets show degree of filament overlap at four different sarcomere lengths. The dashed line shows extrapolation to abscissa of the steep portion of the length–tension relation. The intersection of the dashed line with the abscissa shows the sarcomere length at which the majority of the A- and I-filaments are in end-to-end position. For further information, see text. (From Edman & Reggiani, 1987.)

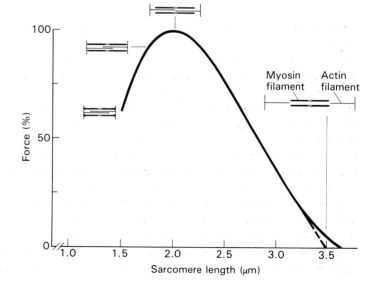

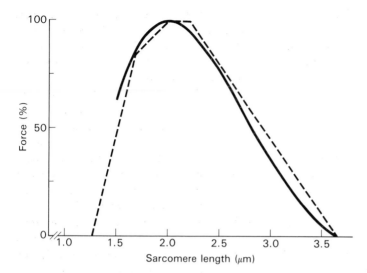

Fig. 6.8 The length–tension relation shown in Fig. 6.7 (——) compared with with the classic polygonal length–tension curve (— — —) described by Gordon *et al.* (1966).

such an analysis (for details, see Edman & Reggiani, 1987) suggests that in frog skeletal muscle the thick and thin filaments have a mean length of 1.55 and 1.94 μm respectively, and that the amount of overlap between the two sets of filaments within a fibre cross-section varies with a standard deviation of 0.21 μm. The filament lengths so derived agree closely with the values of the A- and I-filament lengths (1.55 and 1.92–1.96 μm respectively) that have been presented by Page (1968) and Huxley (1973) on the basis of electron microscopical measurements. The variation in filament overlap is partly due to imperfect alignment of the filaments and accounts for the smooth shape of the length–tension curve.

It is instructive to consider the relative position of the thick and thin filaments at some representative points along the length–tension curve. As is illustrated in Fig. 6.7 (insets), the A- and I-filaments are in end-to-end position at the sarcomere length (approximately 3.5 μm) where active force is close to zero. At 2.0 μm sarcomere length, on the other hand, the ends of the I-filaments are at the centre of the A-filament. This degree of overlap would consequently provide the maximum number of active cross-bridges in line with the finding

The overlap situation becomes more difficult to interpret as the sarcomere length is reduced below 2.0 μm (ascending limb of the length–tension curve). By shortening the sarcomeres below optimum length, for instance to 1.8 μm, the I-filaments will pass into the opposite half of the sarcomere causing double filament overlap, as is shown in Fig. 6.7. The functional significance of the double overlap cannot be assessed at the present time, but it is reasonable to suppose that the phenomenon is causally related to the decline in active force that occurs at these lengths (for further discussion, see Edman & Reggiani, 1987). At sarcomere lengths shorter than 1.7 μm the thick filaments will be compressed when coming up to the Z-discs (Fig. 6.7). This will counteract further sliding and markedly reduce the force produced by the fibre at these lengths.

Incomplete activation of the muscle fibre is yet another possible cause of the decline in tension at very short lengths. As demonstrated by Taylor and Rüdel (1970) the centre of the fibre may not become fully activated at lengths shorter than approximately 1.6 μm due to failure of the inward spread of the action potential under these conditions. However, this complication does not seem to be of any concern within the range of sarcomere lengths considered here. This is indicated by the fact that increasing the release of activator calcium in the fibre (by addition of caffeine) does not affect the length–tension curve depicted in Fig. 6.7 (Edman & Reggiani, 1987).

The force–velocity relation

As already pointed out, muscle has an inherent capacity to adjust its active force to precisely match the load that is experienced during shortening. This remarkable property, which distinguishes muscle from a simple elastic body, is based on the fact that active force continuously adjusts to the speed at which the contractile system moves. Thus, when the load is small, the active force can be made correspondingly small by increasing the speed of shortening appropriately. Conversely, when the load is high, the muscle increases its active force to the same level by reducing the speed of shortening sufficiently. Fenn and Marsh (1935) were first to demonstrate that there exists a given relationship between active force and velocity of shortening. Hill (1938) further characterized the force–velocity relation and he emphasized the importance of this parameter in the study of muscle function. The force–

velocity relation has attracted much new interest in recent years after it had been demonstrated (Huxley, 1957) that this relationship is consistent with the cross-bridge mechanism of muscle contraction.

Figure 6.9 shows the classic load– or force–velocity curve that was published by Hill (1938). It shows the inverse relationship between force and velocity of shortening in an isolated *whole* sartorius muscle of the frog. Hill demonstrated that this relationship had a hyperbolic shape and he provided a general formula for its description that has been widely used in muscle physiology. The maximum speed of shortening (V_{max}) can be seen to occur when the load is zero. Maximum force (P_0), on the other hand, is produced when the muscle is stationary, i.e. neither shortening nor lengthening.

Experiments of single muscle fibres (Edman *et al.*, 1976; Edman, 1988) have demonstrated that the force–velocity relation has a more complex shape than that observed in whole muscle. As illustrated in Fig. 6.10, the force–velocity relation contains *two* distinct curvatures, each one with an upward concavity. The two curvatures are located on either side of a breakpoint near 75% of isometric force, P_0.

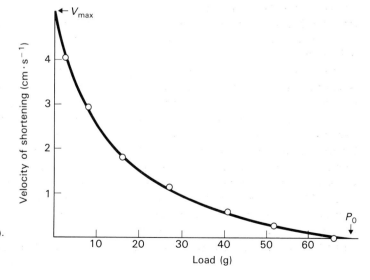

Fig. 6.9 Relation between force and velocity of shortening measured in a whole sartorius muscle of the frog. The equation for the curve, which is a single hyperbola, is given by Hill (1938). For further information, see text. (From Hill, 1938.)

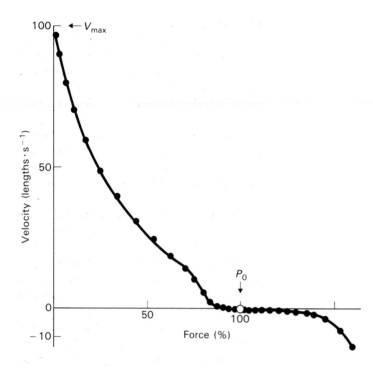

Fig. 6.10 Relation between force and velocity of shortening recorded in a single muscle fibre of the frog. Note that the force–velocity relation has two distinct curvatures on either side of a break point near 75% of P_0. When the load exceeds the isometric force (P_0), the muscle lengthens, i.e. the velocity assumes a negative value. (From Edman, 1988.)

When the load exceeds P_0 the muscle begins to lengthen (eccentric action) as indicated by the negative velocities in Fig. 6.10. However, the force–velocity curve can be seen to be remarkably flat in the force range around P_0. For instance, as the load is increased from 0.9 to 1.2 P_0, a 30% change in load, the velocity of shortening or elongation is altered by less than 2% of V_{max}. The flat region of the force–velocity relation around P_0 is of great significance to muscle function in that it promotes stability within the contractile system. For instance, a muscle that is loaded above its own P_0 value (this may occur during jumping or downstair walking) will nevertheless be able to withstand the load quite well, i.e. the muscle will not yield appreciably. Due to the low speed of lengthening the total length change that the sarcomeres will undergo during the eccentric action will be relatively small. Only when the load is raised by more than 40–50% above P_0 will the muscle elongate at a high speed (see Fig. 6.10).

The force–velocity relation is likely to reflect the kinetic properties of the cross-bridges and attempts have been made to evaluate the various steps in the cross-bridge cycle using the information provided by the force–velocity curve (e.g. Huxley, 1957; Eisenberg & Hill, 1978). There is reason to believe that V_{max} expresses the maximum cycling rate of the cross-bridges. In support of this view, V_{max} has been found to correlate well with the maximum rate of splitting of ATP within the contractile system. This was first demonstrated in studies of whole muscles (Bárány, 1967) and later, in a more quantitative way (Edman et al., 1988), by comparing V_{max} and myofibrillar ATPase activity in isolated single muscle fibres (Fig. 6.11).

If V_{max} represents the maximum speed at which the cross-bridges are able to cycle, V_{max} may be presumed to be independent of the actual number of bridges that interact with the thin filaments. By way of comparison, a light carriage pulled by only one or two horses would reach the same maximum speed as one pulled by many horses. Maximum speed of

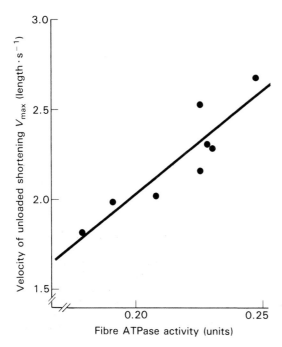

Fig. 6.11 Relation between myofibrillar ATPase activity and maximum speed of shortening, V_{max}, recorded in single muscle fibres. (From Edman *et al.*, 1988.)

shortening would thus be expected to remain constant at different degrees of overlap between the thick and thin filaments and also at different states of activation of the contractile system. These predictions have been verified experimentally as illustrated in Fig. 6.12. Here V_{max} is compared with the tetanic force as the sarcomere length is changed from 1.7 to 2.7 μm. It can be seen that whereas the tetanic force varies considerably, the maximum speed of shortening remains constant over this wide range of sarcomere lengths. Thus, in contrast to the fibre's ability to produce force, the maximum speed of shortening does not depend on the number of myosin bridges that are able to interact with thin filament. Figure 6.13 shows that V_{max} is likewise independent of the degree of activation of the contractile system. These findings thus fully support the sliding-filament model and the theory of independent force generators (Huxley, 1957).

Various muscles in the body differ considerably with respect to their maximum speed of shortening (see for example Buchthal & Schmalbruch, 1980). There is reason to believe

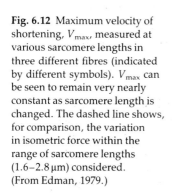

Fig. 6.12 Maximum velocity of shortening, V_{max}, measured at various sarcomere lengths in three different fibres (indicated by different symbols). V_{max} can be seen to remain very nearly constant as sarcomere length is changed. The dashed line shows, for comparison, the variation in isometric force within the range of sarcomere lengths (1.6–2.8 μm) considered. (From Edman, 1979.)

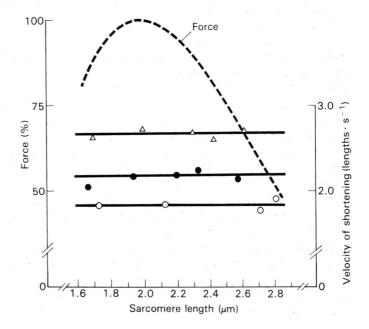

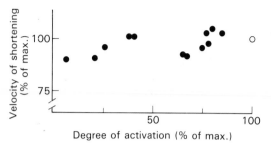

Fig. 6.13 Maximum speed of shortening, V_{max}, recorded at different degrees of activation of single muscle fibres. $\bigcirc$, V_{max} during tetanus, i.e. at full activation. $\bullet$, measurements of V_{max} during twitch contractions representing various degrees of submaximal activation as indicated on abscissa. Note that V_{max} remains virtually constant as activation is changed. (From Edman, 1979 (Table 1).)

that these differences are based on structural heterogeneity of the contractile proteins among the muscles resulting in different kinetic properties of the myofilament system (for references, see Edman *et al.*, 1985). Individual fibres within a muscle generally exhibit marked differences with respect to their shortening characteristics. This is most pronounced in mammalian and avian muscles in which different types of fibres, fast twitch and slow twitch fibres, are regularly found to coexist. Predominance of one particular fibre type determines whether a muscle will acquire fast or slow properties.

Recent studies have demonstrated that the differentiation of the kinetic properties within a muscle extends to *below* fibre level. This is indicated by the finding that both V_{max} and the shape of the force–velocity relation vary substantially from one part to another along the fibre (Edman *et al.*, 1985). Typically, as illustrated in Fig. 6.14, V_{max} varies by 10–45% along the length of a frog muscle fibre. The variation in V_{max} *within* a given fibre may in some cases be as large as that recorded *among* different fibres in a muscle. Each fibre has a unique pattern of V_{max} differences. It is of interest to note, however, that there is a clear trend for V_{max} to decrease towards the distal end of the fibre in the body (see Fig. 6.15).

The experimental evidence suggests that the segmental differences in shortening velocity reflect regional differences in myosin isoform composition along the fibre (Edman *et al.*, 1988). The rationale behind this heterogeneity in function is unclear, but it may be thought to reflect a subcellular adaptation mechanism. A muscle fibre generally spans the entire length of the muscle and the various parts of the fibre may encounter different working conditions when the muscle operates *in situ* in the body. For instance, the passive resistance to shortening may vary along the fibre due to differences in the amount of connective tissue that holds the fibres together. Furthermore, the distal part of a muscle undergoes a larger translation

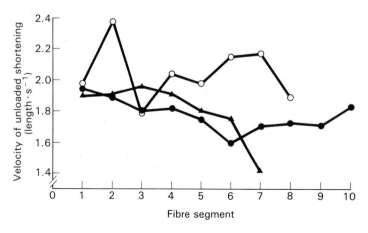

Fig. 6.14 Maximum velocity of shortening, V_{max}, recorded in consecutive segments of three individual muscle fibres (indicated by different symbols). The segments are approximately 0.8 mm in length and are numbered from one tendon insertion to the other in the respective fibre. Note that V_{max} is markedly different along the fibres and that each fibre has a unique velocity pattern. (From Edman *et al.*, 1985.)

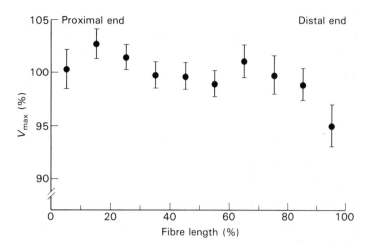

Fig. 6.15 V_{max} of individual fibre segments related to the fibre's orientation in the body. The length of each fibre is normalized to 100%. Data points are mean values (±SE of mean) based on measurements in 14 fibres. Note decline of V_{max} towards the distal fibre end. (From Edman *et al.*, 1985.)

during shortening than does the proximal part. By adjusting the myosin isoform composition in the various regions appropriately the fibre may be able to compensate for any local differences in the passive resistance to shortening that it may experience *in situ* in the body.

Deactivation by shortening

Skeletal muscle that shortens during activity loses temporarily some of its contractile strength. This depressant effect of shortening has been demonstrated both in muscle *in situ* in the body (Joyce *et al.*, 1969) and in isolated whole muscle (Jewell & Wilkie, 1960), and the phenomenon has been explored in considerable detail in isolated single muscle fibres (Edman & Kiessling, 1971; Edman, 1975, 1980).

Figure 6.16 illustrates the depressant effect of active shortening in an isolated muscle fibre of the frog. The two superimposed myograms, A and B, show the development of force during a partially fused tetanus at a sarcomere length of 2.05 μm, i.e. near optimum length. The responses to the respective stimuli are seen as humps in the records and are referred to as twitches. In myogram A the entire contraction is performed at 2.05-μm sarcomere spacing. In myogram B, on the other hand, the contraction is initiated at a longer sarcomere length, 2.55 μm, and the fibre is allowed

to shorten to 2.05 μm during the first twitch period. As can be clearly seen in Fig. 6.16, the active force is greatly depressed after shortening. The peak force of twitch no. 2 in myogram B is thus considerably lower than the force attained in the first twitch of myogram A. This is significant since tension starts from zero level in both cases. The reduced tension in twitch no. 2 of myogram B thus represents a true depression of the fibre's ability to produce force due to preceding shortening. Even twitch no. 3 of myogram B can be seen to be lower than the first twitch in myogram A. It should be noted, however, that the depressant effect of shortening is gradually diminished as contraction goes on; the effect has virtually disappeared by the end of the tetanus period.

The time needed for the movement effect to disappear is remarkably constant from fibre to fibre as is shown in Fig. 6.17. Although the initial force depression varies in different fibres, depending on the amount of shortening used, a time period of almost 1 s is requried for the effect to die away in each case.

The magnitude of force depression depends on the degree of activation of the contractile system when the movement occurs. The movement effect is large during a single twitch or during a *partially* fused tetanus, i.e. under conditions when the contractile system is not fully activated (see Fig. 6.16). On the other

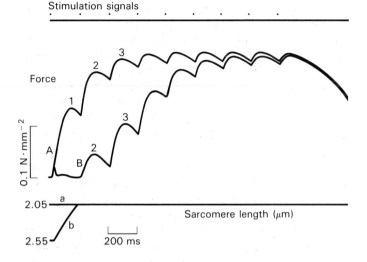

Stimulation signals

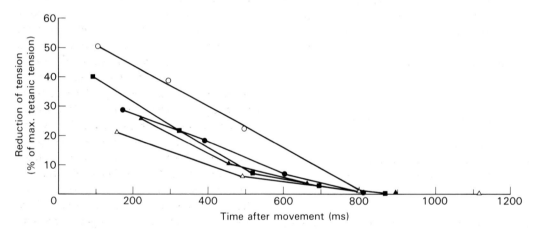

Fig. 6.16 Depressant effect of shortening during partially fused tetanus of a frog muscle fibre. The superimposed myograms A and B show force development at 2.05-μm sarcomere length. In myogram B contraction is initiated at 2.55-μm sarcomere length and the fibre is allowed to shorten to 2.05 μm during the first twitch cycle as indicated by record b underneath. The first few twitch cycles in myograms A and B are numbered for identification in the text, where a full description is given.

Fig. 6.17 Time course of disappearance of the depressant effect of active shortening during incompletely fused tetanus. Results of five experiments (indicated by different symbols) with various degrees of force depression after shortening.

hand, the effect is quite small when the movement occurs during a completely fused tetanus (Edman, 1980). Since muscle activity *in vivo* is based on partially fused tetani, it is reasonable to suppose that force depression by shortening does play a part in daily life. The effect is also likely to influence the results in certain branches of athletics. In weightlifting, for instance, the muscles' capacity to lift the load can be presumed to decline progressively while the lifting occurs. However, after a brief (1–2 s)

pause the muscles will have regained their contractile strength again. The movement effect may serve as a safety mechanism to prevent overuse of the muscles.

It is now possible to conclude that the movement effect is caused by a change within the myofilament system itself. This is indicated by the fact that the depressant effect of shortening also appears in skinned fibres, i.e. preparations in which the contractile machinery can be directly controlled by varying the calcium concentration in the surrounding medium. The results of such studies suggest strongly (Ekelund & Edman, 1982) that active shortening causes a transitory change of the binding site for calcium on the thin filament. This leads to a decrease in the amount of calcium that is bound to the regulatory proteins, and this in turn reduces the degree of activation of the contractile system. In line with this view it is possible to counteract the depressant effect of active shortening in a skinned muscle fibre by increasing the calcium concentration around the myofibrils sufficiently (Ekelund & Edman, 1982). The decrease in calcium affinity of the binding sites is likely to be a direct consequence of the actin–myosin interaction during shortening as discussed in detail elsewhere (Edman, 1975, 1980; Ekelund & Edman, 1982). On this basis then the depressant effect of shortening may be regarded as an integral part of the sliding-filament process.

Cellular mechanisms of muscle fatigue

Muscle fatigue may be defined as a reversible decrease in contractile strength that occurs after long-lasting or repeated muscular activity. There is reason to believe that human fatigue is a complex phenomenon that includes failure at more than one site along the chain of events that leads to stimulation of the muscle fibres (Edwards, 1981). It is thus conceivable that

human fatigue involves a 'central' component that puts an upper limit to the number of command signals that are sent to the muscles. There is little doubt, however, that muscle fatigue also involves a 'peripheral' component. In fact, part of the muscle's failure to produce force is likely to be caused by a change in the myofilament system itself. This is strongly suggested by the fact that the contractile performance of an isolated muscle fibre is greatly dependent on its preceding mechanical activity. The following account will deal with this 'peripheral' effect of muscle fatigue.

Figure 6.18 shows the characteristic changes in active force that occur when a muscle fibre is fatigued by frequent activation. Myogram A illustrates a control tetanus; before this recording the fibre had been stimulated to produce a 1-s isometric tetanus at 15-min intervals until constant responses were obtained. Myogram B shows, for comparison, an isometric tetanus after development of fatigue; in this case the fibre had been stimulated to produce a tetanus once every 15 s over a time period of several minutes. It can be seen that reducing the resting interval between contractions (from 15 min to 15 s) leads to a decrease in the force output during the tetanus. The total amplitude of the tetanus is thus markedly reduced by fatiguing stimulation. Furthermore, force develops less rapidly in the fatigued state, and the fibre requires a longer time to relax. These changes in the contractile performance are fully

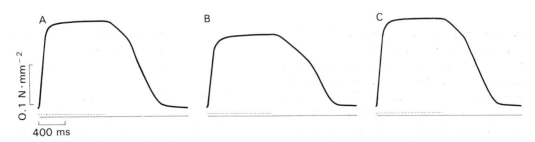

Fig. 6.18 Effects of fatigue on force development during tetanus in a frog muscle fibre. Myogram A shows tetanus during the control period, when intervals between the tetani were 15 min; myogram B shows tetanus after fatiguing stimulation, when intervals between the tetani were 15 s; myogram C shows the return to control stimulation protocol, when intervals between the tetani were 15 min. (From Edman & Mattiazzi, 1981.)

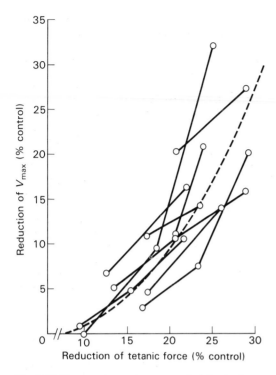

Fig. 6.19 Decrease in maximum speed of shortening (ordinate) in relation to force depression (abscissa) during fatigue of single muscle fibres. Each set of data connected by a solid line is from a single fibre. The dashed line is the calculated mean of all data points. (From Edman & Mattiazzi, 1981.)

reversed after return to the control stimulation protocol (myogram C, Fig. 6.18).

Fatiguing stimulation does not merely affect the muscle's capacity to produce force, it also reduces the speed of shortening of the muscle (Edman & Mattiazzi, 1981). The latter effect is illustrated in Fig. 6.19, which shows the simultaneous changes in tetanic force and maximum speed of shortening, V_{max}, at different degrees of fatigue in single muscle fibres. It can be seen that as fatigue develops (indicated by the decrease of tetanic force, abscissa), the maximum speed of shortening is also steadily reduced (ordinate). This is a relevant finding as it suggests that muscle fatigue involves a change of the kinetic properties of the cross-bridges.

Further information about the molecular mechanism of fatigue has been obtained by studying muscle stiffness. This measurement provides an index of the number of myosin cross-bridges that are attached to the thin filaments (Ford *et al.*, 1977). Muscle stiffness is measured by applying a fast and very small length change to an isolated fibre during activity while recording the corresponding change in force. In principle the approach is the same as that used for testing stiffness of a rubber band: when the stiffness is high there is a large increase in tension as the rubber band is stretched; when the stiffness is small the tension response to the stretch is correspondingly small.

Muscle stiffness is found to be only slightly changed during fatigue. For example, a 25% decrease in the muscle's ability to produce force is associated with merely 9% reduction in muscle fibre stiffness. These findings suggest that the force deficit during fatigue is only partly due to fewer attached cross-bridges. The major portion of the force decline is attributable to *reduced force output of the individual bridge*.

In summary, the following changes in cross-bridge function are likely to occur during muscle fatigue: (i) a slight decrease in the number of interacting cross-bridges; (ii) reduced force output of the individual cross-bridge; and (iii) reduced speed of cycling of the bridges during muscle shortening. There is reason to believe that all three changes are ultimately caused by accumulation of breakdown products of the ATP hydrolysis within the fibre. Sustained muscular activity leads to increased concentrations of ADP, P_i and H^+ (e.g. Edwards *et al.*, 1975; Dawson *et al.*, 1978, 1980), and these products affect force production and speed of shortening in a way that is fully compatible with the changes observed in fatigue (for references and further discussion, see Edman & Lou, 1990). Of the three products, increased H^+ concentration would seem to be of particular importance for the development of muscle fatigue. This is suggested by the finding that the contractile changes observed during fatigue can all be simulated remarkably well by lowering the intracellular pH (Edman & Mattiazzi, 1981; Curtin & Edman, 1989; Edman & Lou, 1990).

It should finally be pointed out that the above changes in mechanical performance refer to experimental conditions where there is no failure of activation of the contractile system (see further Edman & Lou, 1990). Impairment of the excitation–contraction coupling may occur, however, if the muscle is subjected to an extreme fatiguing programme, i.e. with contractions induced at 1–2-s intervals (see, for instance, Eberstein & Sandow, 1963; Lännergren & Westerblad, 1986). Under such conditions there will be a failure of the inward spread of the action potential along the T-tubules, and the interior of the muscle fibre will therefore be inadequately activated (Gonzalez-Serratos et al., 1981; Lou & Edman, 1990). It still remains uncertain, however, whether a stimulation programme intense enough to cause such a failure of activation can ever be achieved under in vivo conditions in the body.

References

Bárány, M. (1967) ATPase activity of myosin correlated with speed of muscle shortening. *Journal of General Physiology*, **50**, 197–218.

Buchthal, F. & Schmalbruch, H. (1980) Motor unit of mammalian muscle. *Physiological Reviews*, **60**, 90–142.

Curtin, N.A. & Edman, K.A.P. (1989) Effects of fatigue and reduced intracellular pH on segment dynamics in 'isometric' relaxation of frog muscle fibres. *Journal of Physiology*, **413**, 159–74.

Dawson, M.J., Gadian, D.G. & Wilkie, D.R. (1978) Muscular fatigue investigated by phosphorus nuclear magnetic resonance. *Nature*, **274**, 861–6.

Dawson, M.J., Gadian, D.G. & Wilkie, D.R. (1980) Mechanical relaxation rate and metabolism studied in fatiguing muscle by phosphorus nuclear magnetic resonance. *Journal of Physiology*, **299**, 465–84.

di Prampero, P.E. (1985) Metabolic and circulatory limitations to VO_{2max} at the whole animal level. *Journal of Experimental Biology*, **115**, 319–32.

Ebashi, S. (1980) Regulation of muscle contraction. *Proceedings of the Royal Society B*, **207**, 259–86.

Ebashi, S. & Endo, M. (1968) Calcium ion and muscle contraction. *Progress in Biophysics and Molecular Biology*, **18**, 125–83.

Eberstein, A. & Sandow, A. (1963) Fatigue mechanisms in muscle fibres. In E. Gutman & P. Hnik (eds) *The Effect of Use and Disuse on Neuromuscular Functions*, pp. 515–26. Nakladatelstvi Ceskoslovenske akademie ved Praha, Prague.

Edman, K.A.P. (1975) Mechanical deactivation induced by active shortening in isolated muscle fibres of the frog. *Journal of Physiology*, **246**, 255–75.

Edman, K.A.P. (1979) The velocity of unloaded shortening and its relation to sarcomere length and isometric force in vertebrate muscle fibres. *Journal of Physiology*, **291**, 143–59.

Edman, K.A.P. (1980) Depression of mechanical performance by active shortening during twitch and tetanus of vertebrate muscle fibres. *Acta Physiologica Scandinavica*, **109**, 15–26.

Edman, K.A.P. (1988) Double-hyperbolic force–velocity relation in frog muscle fibres. *Journal of Physiology*, **404**, 301–21.

Edman, K.A.P. & Höglund, O. (1981) A technique for measuring length changes of individual segments of an isolated muscle fibre. *Journal of Physiology*, **317**, 8–9.

Edman, K.A.P. & Kiessling, A. (1971) The time course of the active state in relation to sarcomere length and movement studied in single skeletal muscle fibres of the frog. *Acta Physiologica Scandinavica*, **81**, 182–96.

Edman, K.A.P. & Lou, F. (1990) Changes in force and stiffness induced by fatigue and intracellular acidification in frog muscle fibres. *Journal of Physiology*, **424**, 133–49.

Edman, K.A.P. & Mattiazzi, A. (1981) Effects of fatigue and altered pH on isometric force and velocity of shortening at zero load in frog muscle fibres. *Journal of Muscle Research and Cell Motility*, **2**, 321–34.

Edman, K.A.P., Mulieri, L.A. & Scubon-Mulieri, B. (1976) Non-hyperbolic force–velocity relationship in single muscle fibres. *Acta Physiologica Scandinavica*, **98**, 143–56.

Edman, K.A.P. & Reggiani, C. (1984) Redistribution of sarcomere length during isometric contraction of frog muscle fibres and its relation to tension creep. *Journal of Physiology*, **351**, 169–98.

Edman, K.A.P. & Reggiani, C. (1987) The sarcomere length–tension relation determined in short segments of intact muscle fibres of the frog. *Journal of Physiology*, **385**, 709–32.

Edman, K.A.P., Reggiani, C. & te Kronnie, G. (1985) Differences in maximum velocity of shortening along single muscle fibres of the frog. *Journal of Physiology*, **365**, 147–63.

Edman, K.A.P., Reggiani, C., Schiaffino, S. & te Kronnie, G. (1988) Maximum velocity of shortening related to myosin isoform composition in frog skeletal muscle fibres. *Journal of Physiology*, **395**, 679–94.

Edwards, R.H.T. (1981) Human muscle and fatigue. In R. Porter & J. Whelan (eds) *Ciba Foundation Symposium 82: Human Muscle Fatigue: Physiological Mechanisms*, pp. 1–18. Pitman Medical, London.

Edwards, R.H.T., Hill, D.K. & Jones, D.A. (1975) Metabolic changes associated with the slowing of relaxation in fatigued mouse muscle. *Journal of Physiology*, **251**, 287–301.

Eisenberg, E. & Hill, T.L. (1978) A cross-bridge model of muscle contraction. *Progress in Biophysics and Molecular Biology*, **33**, 55–82.

Ekelund, M. & Edman, K.A.P. (1982) Shortening induced deactivation of skinned fibres of frog and mouse striated muscle. *Acta Physiologica Scandinavica*, **116**, 189–99.

Fenn, W.O. & Marsh, B.S. (1935) Muscular force at different speed of shortening. *Journal of Physiology*, **85**, 277–97.

Ford, L.E., Huxley, A.F. & Simmons, R.M. (1977) Tension responses to sudden length change in stimulated frog muscle fibres near slack length. *Journal of Physiology*, **269**, 441–515.

Gonzales-Serratos, H., Garcia, M., Somlyo, A., Somlyo, A.P. & McClellan, G. (1981) Differential shortening of myofibrils during development of fatigue. *Biophysical Journal*, **33**, 224a.

Gordon, A.M., Huxley, A.F. & Julian, F.J. (1966) The variation in isometric tension with sarcomere length in vertebrate muscle fibres. *Journal of Physiology*, **184**, 170–92.

Hanson, J. & Huxley, H.E. (1953) The structural basis of the cross-striations in muscle. *Nature*, **172**, 530–2.

Hasselbach, W. (1953) Elektronmikroskopische Untersuchungen an Muskelfibrillen bei totaler und partieller Extraktion des L-Myosins. *Zeitschrift für Naturforschung*, **8b**, 449–54.

Hill, A.V. (1938) The heat of shortening and the dynamic constants of muscle. *Proceedings of the Royal Society B* **126**, 136–95.

Huxley, A.F. (1957) Muscle structure and theories of contraction. *Progress in Biophysics and Biophysical Chemistry*, **7**, 255–318.

Huxley, A.F. & Niedergerke, R. (1954) Structural changes in muscle during contraction: interference microscopy of living muscle fibres. *Nature*, **173**, 971–3.

Huxley, H.E. (1953) Electron-microscope studies of the organization of the filaments in striated muscle. *Biochimica et Biophysica Acta*, **12**, 387.

Huxley, H.E. (1963) Electron microscope studies on the structure of natural and synthetic protein filaments from striated muscle. *Journal of Molecular Biology*, **7**, 281–308.

Huxley, H.E. (1973) Molecular basis of contraction in cross-striated muscle. In G. Bourne (ed.) *The Structure and Function of Muscle, Vol. 1*, 2nd edn, pp. 301–87. Academic Press, New York

Huxley, H.E. & Hanson, J. (1954) Changes in the cross-striations of muscle during contraction and stretch and their structural interpretation. *Nature*, **173**, 973–7.

Jewell, B.R. & Wilkie, D.R. (1960) The mechanical properties of relaxing muscle. *Journal of Physiology*, **152**, 30–47.

Joyce, G.C., Rack, P.M.H. & Westbury, D.R. (1969) The mechanical properties of cat soleus muscle during controlled lengthening and shortening movements. *Journal of Physiology*, **204**, 461–74.

Lännergren, J. & Westerblad, H. (1986) Force and membrane potential during and after fatiguing, continuous high-frequency stimulation of single *Xenopus* muscle fibres. *Acta Physiologica Scandinavica*, **128**, 359–68.

Lou, F. & Edman, K.A.P. (1990) Effects of fatigue on force, stiffness and velocity of shortening in frog muscle fibres. *Acta Physiologica Scandinavica*, **140**, 24A.

Page, S. (1968) Fine structure of tortoise skeletal muscle. *Journal of Physiology*, **197**, 709–15.

Squire, J. (1981) *The Structural Basis of Muscular Contraction*. Plenum Press, New York.

Taylor, S.R. & Rüdel, R. (1970) Striated muscle fibers: inactivation of contraction induced by shortening. *Science*, **167**, 882–4.

Woledge, R.C., Curtin, N.A. & Homsher, E. (1985) *Energetic Aspects of Muscle Contraction*. Academic Press, London.

Chapter 6B

Skeletal Muscle Architecture and Performance

ROLAND R. ROY AND V. REGGIE EDGERTON

Introduction

The two most reliable and reproducible indices of the functional capacities of a skeletal muscle are its maximum force potential and its maximum rate of shortening determined under maximal stimulation conditions. The architectural design of the skeletal muscle has a significant impact on these functional properties. For example, imagine two muscles having similar masses and biochemical profiles. Under maximal stimulation conditions and under identical biomechanical constraints, the relative proportion of half sarcomeres arranged either in series or in parallel will dictate the relative priority of force and displacement in each muscle. In the past decade, the combination of refined morphological techniques and renewed interest in structure–function interrelationships in mammalian skeletal muscle have resulted in dramatic advances in the identification and understanding of the critical motor control issues at the muscle, motor unit and muscle fibre levels (see Stein, 1982; Edgerton, 1983a, b; Windhorst et al., 1989, for a discussion of some of these issues). In the present chapter, some of these issues are addressed. The concepts and data relate principally to studies of the mammalian hindlimb. An excellent review on the theoretical effects of muscle architecture–function interrelationships was published by Gans and Bock in 1965. In the last decade, several reviews in the general area of muscle architecture have been published (Partridge &

Benton, 1981; Gans, 1982; Edgerton et al., 1983a, 1986b; Otten, 1988; Peters, 1989).

Skeletal muscle structure–function relationships

Maximum force production

The maximum force that a muscle can generate is directly related to its physiological cross-sectional area (PCSA) (Close, 1972; Josephson, 1975; Spector et al., 1980; Brand et al., 1981; Edgerton et al., 1986a; Powell et al., 1984). Under in situ conditions where the muscle is tested physiologically and then removed:

$$PCSA = \frac{(muscle\ mass)\ (cosine\ \theta)}{(fibre\ length)\ (muscle\ density)}$$

where: muscle mass is the wet weight of the muscle; θ is the angle of fibre pinnation; fibre length is the mean fibre length within the muscle; and muscle density may be considered to be a constant, i.e. $1.067\ g \cdot cm^{-3}$.

Under in vivo conditions, it appears that the PCSA of an individual muscle or muscle group can be estimated non-invasively with reasonable accuracy from the following formula:

$$PCSA = \frac{muscle\ volume}{fibre\ length}$$

where: muscle volume is determined non-invasively (see below); and fibre length is estimated from the relatively consistent fibre

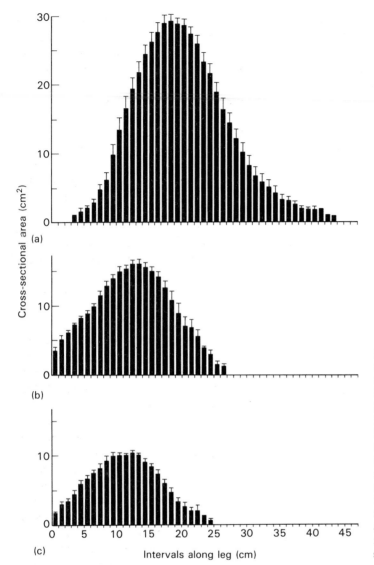

Fig. 6.20 Anatomical cross-sectional areas of the soleus (a), and the medial (b) and lateral (c) heads of the gastrocnemius using MRI techniques determined at 1-cm intervals along the length of the leg. Each bar represents the mean ± standard deviation for 12 subjects. For consistency, slice no. 1 was identified for each subject by the proximal edge of the patella. Note that the maximum cross-sectional area is at a different level for each muscle. (From Fukunaga *et al.*, submitted.)

length to muscle length ratios reported for dissected muscles (see below).

Comparison of physiological and anatomical cross-sectional areas (PCSA and ACSA, respectively)

Theoretically, the ACSA of an individual muscle is determined by the largest cross-sectional area along the length of that muscle. In practice, however, this measure is not as simple to determine as one might expect. In many instances, the ACSA is calculated from the largest girth of a muscle group, with the assumption that this single measure represents the summation of the maximum CSAs for each muscle in the functional group. In reality, the ACSA of individual muscles vary significantly along their proximo-distal axes and, within a functional group of muscles, the maximum ACSAs of individual muscles are often at different levels. For example, the ACSA of the triceps surae in humans corresponds to the maximum ACSA of the soleus, but not of the medial and lateral heads of the gastrocnemius

(Fig. 6.20). A similar relationship is illustrated for the flexor muscles of the arm in Figure 4 of Edgerton *et al.* (1986a). Thus, these arrangements result in significant miscalculations of the maximum CSA of a muscle group when ACSA is used.

Unfortunately, the ACSA is used often to estimate changes in and sometimes even to reflect the absolute maximum force potential of a muscle *in vivo*. There are numerous problems, however, associated with this measurement. For example, even if torque measurements were to take into account moment arms, this method of determining CSA of a muscle precludes any comparisons across muscles because of the variations in fibre lengths as well as muscle shape. Since muscle density is relatively constant as is the muscle fibre to muscle length ratios, a much more reliable and non-invasive technique to estimate CSA is to determine the actual volume of the muscle. Recently, we have used magnetic resonance imaging (MRI) techniques to reconstruct in three-dimensions the individual muscles of the human leg (Fukunaga *et al.*, submitted). Cross-sectional images were taken at 1-cm intervals from just above the knee to the calcaneus. Individual muscles or muscle groups were identified and outlined in serial cross-sections. The sections were then arranged in 3-D and the muscle volumes calculated. These procedures make it feasible to estimate non-invasively changes in muscle mass, e.g. before and after alterations in muscle use such as immobilization and space-flight. In spite of the accuracy in determining muscle volumes, however, fluid distribution changes could have a significant effect on these measures. For example, atrophied muscle particularly seems to accumulate fluid readily (Herbert *et al.*, 1988). The significance of this potential problem is being studied at the moment.

Estimate of fibre lengths

Assuming biochemical consistency across fibres, the length of a muscle fibre, i.e. the number of half sarcomeres in series, deter-

mines the rate of shortening of that fibre. The determination of the length of individual fibres within a muscle is somewhat controversial. One issue appears to be the distinction between a fibre defined as an anatomical vs. a functional entity. For example, based on the inspection of connective tissue interfaces along the length of 'presumed' fibres isolated by conventional maceration techniques, Loeb *et al.* (1987), Richmond and Armstrong (1988), and Gordon *et al.* (1989) have reported that most fibres in a variety of mammalian muscles are ~2cm long. Rarely did they find fibres longer than 3.0cm in cat hindlimb or neck muscles. This finding is in contrast with a multitude of reports that show fibres extending much longer lengths, albeit using techniques that were not as specific for identifying connective tissue intercepts (for example see Table 6.1 and Alexander & Vernon, 1975; Spector *et al.*, 1980; Brand *et al.*, 1981; Sacks & Roy, 1982; Powell *et al.*, 1984; Roy *et al.*, 1984a,b; Huijing, 1985; Lieber & Blevins, 1989; Friederich & Brand, 1990). The controversy appears to be whether these long fibres are actually comprised of a series of shorter fibres that may or may not be innervated by the same motoneurone and, therefore, may or may not be innervated as a functional unit. Implications for such an arrangement are indicated by the longitudinal strips of activation recorded from the cat sartorius during electrical stimulation of intramuscular nerve branches (Loeb, *et al.*, 1987). This conclusion is further supported by the observation that the maximum force potential of a muscle can be predicted quite accurately from the PCSA, even in muscles that have fibres that are much longer than 2cm (Spector *et al.*, 1980; Powell *et al.*, 1984). More direct measurements of functional fibre lengths have been determined via glycogen depletion and subsequent reconstruction of the fibres within a motor unit (see below).

Angle of fibre pinnation considerations

Theoretically, the maximum force and velocity potential of a muscle fibre could be compro-

Table 6.1 Architectural properties of selected human muscles

Muscle	Muscle mass (g)	Muscle length (ML) (mm)	Fibre length (FL) (mm)	FL/ML ratio	PCSA* (cm^2)
Study 1					
FDS IP (6)	6.0 ± 1.1	93 ± 8	32 ± 3	0.34 ± 0.02	1.81 ± 0.83
FDS ID (9)	6.6 ± 0.8	119 ± 6	38 ± 3	0.32 ± 0.01	1.63 ± 0.22
FDS IC (6)	12.4 ± 2.1	207 ± 11	68 ± 3	0.33 ± 0.03	1.71 ± 0.28
FDS L (9)	16.3 ± 2.2	183 ± 12	61 ± 4	0.34 ± 0.01	2.53 ± 0.34
FDS R (9)	10.2 ± 1.1	155 ± 8	60 ± 3	0.39 ± 0.02	1.61 ± 0.18
FDS S (9)	1.8 ± 0.3	103 ± 6	42 ± 2	0.42 ± 0.01	0.40 ± 0.05
FDP I (9)	11.7 ± 1.2	149 ± 4	61 ± 2	0.41 ± 0.02	1.77 ± 0.16
FDP L (9)	16.3 ± 1.7	200 ± 8	68 ± 3	0.34 ± 0.01	2.23 ± 0.22
FDP R (9)	11.9 ± 1.4	194 ± 7	65 ± 3	0.33 ± 0.01	1.72 ± 0.18
FDP S (9)	13.7 ± 1.5	150 ± 5	61 ± 4	0.40 ± 0.02	2.20 ± 0.30
FPL (9)	10.0 ± 1.1	168 ± 10	45 ± 2	0.24 ± 0.01	2.08 ± 0.22
Study 2					
Br (8)	16.6 ± 2.8	175 ± 8	121 ± 8	0.69 ± 0.06	1.33 ± 0.22
PT (8)	15.9 ± 1.7	130 ± 5	36 ± 1	0.28 ± 0.01	4.13 ± 0.52
PQ (8)	5.2 ± 1.0	39 ± 2	23 ± 2	0.58 ± 0.02	2.07 ± 0.33
EDCI (8)	3.1 ± 0.5	114 ± 3	57 ± 4	0.49 ± 0.02	0.52 ± 0.08
EDCL (5)	6.1 ± 1.2	112 ± 5	59 ± 4	0.50 ± 0.01	1.02 ± 0.20
EDCR (7)	4.7 ± 0.8	125 ± 11	51 ± 2	0.42 ± 0.02	0.86 ± 0.13
EDCS (6)	2.2 ± 0.03	121 ± 8	53 ± 5	0.43 ± 0.03	0.40 ± 0.06
EDQ (7)	3.8 ± 0.7	152 ± 9	55 ± 4	0.36 ± 0.01	0.64 ± 0.10
EIP (6)	2.9 ± 0.6	105 ± 7	48 ± 2	0.46 ± 0.02	0.56 ± 0.11
EPL (7)	4.5 ± 0.7	138 ± 7	44 ± 3	0.31 ± 0.02	0.98 ± 0.13
PaL (6)	3.8 ± 0.8	134 ± 12	52 ± 3	0.40 ± 0.03	0.69 ± 0.17
Study 3					
FCR (5)	10.9 ± 1.7	164 ± 4	51 ± 2	0.31 ± 0.01	1.99 ± 0.27
FCU (5)	15.4 ± 1.3	228 ± 16	42 ± 2	0.19 ± 0.01	3.42 ± 0.23
ECRB (5)	13.8 ± 0.9	127 ± 10	48 ± 4	0.38 ± 0.03	2.73 ± 0.18
ECRL (5)	11.8 ± 1.2	94 ± 7	76 ± 6	0.82 ± 0.04	1.46 ± 0.11
ECU (5)	13.6 ± 3.3	182 ± 6	51 ± 3	0.28 ± 0.01	2.60 ± 0.71
Study 4					
BBs (4)	26.5 ± 4.5	213 ± 7	164 ± 12	0.77 ± 0.07	1.62 ± 0.41
BBl (4)	39.8 ± 8.8	245 ± 10	193 ± 17	0.84 ± 0.04	2.18 ± 0.76
B (4)	64.5 ± 19.0	201 ± 5	144 ± 23	0.71 ± 0.09	4.69 ± 1.78
TB (4)	198.0 ± 38.1	237 ± 9	76 ± 6	0.32 ± 0.03	23.85 ± 2.92
Study 5					
RF (3)	84.3 ± 13.8	316 ± 6	66 ± 2	0.21 ± 0	12.73 ± 1.95
VL (3)	219.5 ± 56.1	324 ± 14	66 ± 1	0.20 ± 0.01	35.35 ± 6.17
VM (3)	175.3 ± 41.3	335 ± 14	70 ± 3	0.21 ± 0.01	22.13 ± 4.28
VI (3)	159.6 ± 59.4	329 ± 15	68 ± 5	0.21 ± 0.01	22.30 ± 8.75
Sm (3)	107.5 ± 12.5	262 ± 1	63 ± 5	0.24 ± 0.02	16.87 ± 1.49
BFl (3)	128.3 ± 28.1	342 ± 13	85 ± 5	0.25 ± 0.02	12.83 ± 2.76
BFs (3)	—	271 ± 11	139 ± 3	0.52 ± 0.03	—
St (2)	76.9 ± 7.7	317 ± 4	158 ± 2	0.50 ± 0	5.35 ± 0.95
Sol (1)[†]	215.0	308	20	0.06	58.0
MG (3)[‡]	100.4 ± 9.4	248 ± 10	35 ± 2	0.14 ± 0.01	22.75 ± 2.57
LG (3)[‡]	49.5 ± 4.6	217 ± 11	51 ± 6	0.23 ± 0.01	10.73 ± 1.03

Table 6.1 *Continued*

Muscle	Muscle mass (g)	Muscle length (ML) (mm)	Fibre length (FL) (mm)	FL/ML ratio	PCSA* (cm^2)
Plt (3)	5.3 ± 1.9	85 ± 15	39 ± 7	0.47 ± 0.03	1.20 ± 0.36
FHL (3)	21.5 ± 3.3	222 ± 5	34 ± 2	0.15 ± 0.01	5.27 ± 0.58
FDL (3)	16.3 ± 2.8	260 ± 15	27 ± 1	0.11 ± 0	5.07 ± 0.70
PeL (3)	41.5 ± 8.5	286 ± 17	39 ± 3	0.14 ± 0.01	12.33 ± 2.86
PB (3)	17.3 ± 2.5	230 ± 13	39 ± 4	0.17 ± 0.01	5.70 ± 1.01
TP (3)	53.5 ± 7.3	254 ± 26	24 ± 4	0.09 ± 0.01	20.77 ± 3.02
TA (3)	65.7 ± 10.3	298 ± 12	77 ± 8	0.26 ± 0.02	9.87 ± 1.45
EDL (3)	35.2 ± 3.6	355 ± 13	80 ± 8	0.22 ± 0.02	5.57 ± 0.60
EHL (3)	12.9 ± 1.6	273 ± 2	87 ± 8	0.32 ± 0.03	1.77 ± 0.22
Sar (3)	61.7 ± 14.4	503 ± 27	455 ± 19	0.90 ± 0.02	1.70 ± 0.31
Gr (3)	35.3 ± 7.4	335 ± 20	277 ± 12	0.83 ± 0.02	1.77 ± 0.29
AM (3)	229.3 ± 32.0	305 ± 12	115 ± 8	0.38 ± 0.01	18.17 ± 2.29
AL (3)	63.5 ± 15.7	229 ± 12	108 ± 2	0.48 ± 0.02	6.83 ± 1.92
AB (3)	43.8 ± 8.4	156 ± 12	103 ± 6	0.66 ± 0.04	4.67 ± 0.97
Pec (3)	26.4 ± 6.0	123 ± 4	104 ± 1	0.85 ± 0.04	2.9 ± 0.59
Pop (2)	20.1 ± 2.4	108 ± 7	29 ± 7	0.27 ± 0.04	7.90 ± 1.14

Data were selected from our and Dr R.L. Lieber's laboratories because of the similarity in the determination of the architectural properties of cadaveric muscles (see Alexander & Vernon, 1975; Brand *et al.*, 1981; Huijing *et al.*, 1985; Friederich & Brand, 1990 for comparative data). All values are means ± standard errors of the mean. The number of cadavers used for each muscle is given in parentheses.
* PCSA, physiological cross-sectional area.
† Data based on one cadaver from Wickiewicz *et al.* (1983) but fibre lengths verified in two additional cadavers in our laboratory.
‡ MG and LG relative muscle mass and PCSA values derived from values determined from two additional cadavers.
Muscle abbreviations are: FDS, flexor digitorum superficialis to IP (index, proximal belly), ID (index, distal belly), IC (index, combined bellies), L (long), R (ring) and S (small) fingers; FDP, flexor digitorum profundus to I, L, R and S fingers; FPL, flexor pollicis longus; Br, brachioradialis; PT, pronator teres; PQ, pronator quadratus; EDC, extensor digitorum communis to I, L, R and S fingers; EDQ, extensor digiti quinti; EIP, extensor indicis proprious; EPL, extensor pollicis longus; PaL, palmaris longus; FCR, flexor carpi radialis; FCU, flexor carpi ulnaris; ECRB, extensor carpi radialis brevis; ECRL, extensor carpi radialis longus; ECU, extensor carpi ulnaris; BBs, biceps brachii short head; BBI, biceps brachii long head; B, brachialis; TB, triceps brachii; RF, rectus femoris; VL, vastus lateralis; VM, vastus medialis; VI, vastus intermedius; Sm, semimembranosus; BFI, biceps femoris long head; BFs, biceps femoris short head; St, semitendinosus; Sol, soleus; MG, medial gastrocnemius; LG, lateral gastrocnemius; Plt, plantaris; FHL, flexor hallucis longus; FDL, flexor digitorum longus; PeL, peroneus longus; PB, peroneus brevis; TP, tibialis posterior; TA, tibialis anterior; EDL, extensor digitorum longus; EHL extensor hallucis longus; Sar, sartorius; Gr, gracilis; AM, adductor magnus; AL, adductor longus; AB, adductor brevis; Pec, pectineus; Pop, popliteus.
Study 1: from Jacobson *et al.* (in press); study 2: from Lieber *et al.* (in press); study 3: from Lieber *et al.* (1990); study 4: from Edgerton *et al.* (1986a); study 5: from Wickiewicz *et al.* (1983).

mised as a function of the cosine of the angle of pinnation from the line of pull at the tendon (Alexander & Vernon, 1975; Gans, 1982; Sacks & Roy, 1982; Huijing & Woittiez, 1985). However, in most muscles in the human at a resting length, the angles of pinnation measured in one dimension are relatively small (<10°) and, thus, do not appear to have a significant effect on these functional properties (Wickiewicz *et al.*, 1983, 1984; Edgerton *et al.*, 1986a; Lieber *et al.*, in press; Jacobson *et al.*, in press). It should be emphasized, however, that based on recent data from Otten (1988) and Hoffer *et al.* (1989) that large and variable changes in the angle of pinnation along the length of a contracting muscle can occur during normal movements. These considerations warrant further study.

One consequence of fibre pinnation within a muscle of a given volume is that it allows for more sarcomeres to be arranged in parallel at the expense of sarcomeres arranged in series, and thus enhances the maximum force producing capability of the muscle (Josephson, 1975; Gans, 1982; Sacks & Roy, 1982; Edgerton et al., 1987). A less obvious consequence is that the range of excursion through which a pinnated muscle operates at an efficient sarcomere length is greater than that of a non-pinnated muscle, assuming that the fibre lengths are the same in the two muscles (Gans & Bock, 1965; Muhl, 1982). Thus, a muscle that has pinnated fibres can utilize the length–tension relationship more effectively than if the muscle fibres were arranged in parallel to the line of muscle action.

Compartmentalization

The distinction between a functional and an anatomical muscle also has become complicated as further details of the architecture of muscles and their innervation has become evident. A number of mammalian skeletal muscles have been shown to be compartmentalized, i.e. subdivided into anatomical compartments each having a separate primary nerve branch and showing some sensory (reflex) partitioning (see Windhorst et al., 1989 for a recent review). Individual compartments within a muscle can have very different fibre type distributions and the cross-sectional area of each compartment can vary independently along the proximo-distal axis of the muscle (English & Letbetter, 1982). This arrangement across compartments within a muscle is similar to that described above for muscles within a functional group. The mechanical consequences of this architectural arrangement are unknown at this time. From a motor control aspect, individual compartments can be recruited independently (English, 1984) and thus may function as separate entities.

Motor unit structure–function considerations

The basic unit of motor control is the motor unit, i.e. a motoneurone and all of the fibres that it innervates. Based on isometric twitch contraction time, fatiguability and the presence or absence of 'sag', motor units can be classified into fast fatiguable (FF), fast intermediate (FI), fast fatigue resistant (FR) and slow (S) categories (Burke et al., 1973; Burke, 1981). Further, using a combination of physiological and metabolic properties, muscle fibres can be classified as fast glycolytic (FG), fast oxidative glycolytic (FOG) and slow oxidative (SO) (Peter et al., 1972). Although the fibres within a motor unit are variable in size and metabolic properties, the degree of variability is less than that found in fibres across motor units in the same region of the muscle (Edgerton et al., 1985; Martin et al., 1988).

During a motor task, a pool of motor units will generally be recruited in a stereotypical order, i.e. recruitment of motor units will be ordered relative to some parameter reflecting Henneman's 'size principle' of recruitment (Burke, 1981; Henneman & Mendell, 1981; Edgerton et al., 1983b). Generally, the order of motor unit recruitment will be from 'small' to 'large', even among motor units of the same type within the same muscle. The size of motor units is reflected in several parameters including maximum force and fatiguability of the muscle unit, motoneurone size and axonal conduction velocity (Botterman & Cope, 1988).

Within a muscle, motor units vary widely in their maximum force potential and in their specific tension, i.e. tension per unit cross-sectional area (Burke, 1981; Bodine et al., 1987). Based on a relatively small amount of data, these tension parameters appear to be related, in part, to the unit type. For example, in a muscle that has a mixture of unit types, generally, the slow units are smaller, produce less tension and have a lower specific tension than the fast units (Burke, 1981; Bodine et al., 1987). However, it is becoming apparent that some architectural influences, i.e. how fibres of a unit are spatially organized, may be equally important to consider (Burke & Tsairis, 1973; Bodine et al., 1988; Edgerton et al., 1989; Bodine-Fowler et al., 1990; Ounjian et al., in press).

Motor unit architecture

Localization and spatial distribution of motor unit fibres within the muscle cross-section

The fibres of a motor unit are distributed within a localized region of the muscle cross-section. For example, Bodine et al. (1988) and Bodine-Fowler et al. (1990) have shown that the territory of individual motor units in the tibialis anterior of the cat occupies between 8 and 24% of the total muscle cross-section, with the S units generally having the smallest territory sizes. In similar calculations for the homogeneously slow cat soleus, motor unit territory sizes appear to be somewhat larger, ranging between 41 and 76%. Spatial pattern analyses of the fibres within the territory indicate that the distribution of the fibres is not different from random (based on Monte Carlo distributions), although there are some indications that there are local (short) and long-distance factors operating to keep the fibres in small subclusters that may be related to the branching patterns of the axons during development. The significance of the spatial distribution of the fibres of a motor unit relates to those phenomena that may influence the choice of establishing nerve–muscle interconnections. A second aspect of the location and extent of the territory of individual motor units may be how the forces are transmitted from the contractile elements to the tendons (see below).

Muscle fibre lengths and shape

The anatomical length of individual fibres appears to be highly dependent on the methods of maceration used to isolate the fibres (see discussion above). Consequently, we feel that a more accurate measure is the functional fibre length, i.e. the length of fibres determined from glycogen depleted motor units. Briefly, motor units are isolated using standard ventral root teasing techniques, and the fibres of the unit depleted of their glycogen by repetitive stimulation (methods described in Bodine et al., 1987). The depleted fibres are then identified in serial cross-sections of the muscle and followed throughout their length. Based on our initial results (Ounjian et al., in press), it appears that the fibre lengths within a fascicle of a unit are relatively consistent, whereas the mean fibre lengths across units within a muscle can vary significantly. For example, mean fibre lengths within a fascicle in five cat tibialis anterior fast motor units varied from 8.8 to 48.5 mm. The mean fibre lengths in two slow units were 35.9 and 45.5 mm. Some fibres reached lengths of 58 mm in both the fast and slow units.

The majority of the fibres within a fascicle of the fast units did not extend from one tendinous insertion to another tendinous insertion, i.e. the fibres terminated mid-fascicularly, usually at one end and sometimes at both ends. Further, the ends of the fibres terminating mid-fascicularly invariably tapered, i.e. showed a progressive decrease in cross-sectional area along their length (e.g. see Fig. 6.21). In many cases, the fibres terminated in a fine point with no apparent extension distally into a connective tissue interface. This type of fibre structure has been observed in macerated preparations in a variety of muscles as described and reviewed recently by Loeb et al. (1987). In contrast, the majority of the fibres of the two S units studied spanned the distance between the connective tissue inscriptions demarcating the fascicle and terminated as blunt endings into the connective tissue interface. The differences between fast and slow fibres in their basic architectural design are presumed to have a significant impact on their functional capabilities.

Muscle fibre–connective tissue interfaces

The presence of fibres that do not have a firm anchorage into a connective tissue interface at both ends of a fascicle introduces a newly recognized level of complexity in the transmission of forces from sarcomeres to the tendons of insertion. How the forces generated by the relatively large amount of contractile elements at one end are transmitted along the length of a tapering fibre (i.e. decreasing in the number of contractile elements in parallel) to the tendinous insertion is unknown at the present time. There are indications that forces can be transmitted to adjacent fibres (Street, 1983; Shear & Bloch, 1985). Proteins have been identified that are organized in repeating units that appear to be related to sarcomeric structure. For example, it has been suggested that spectrin links the sarcomeric contractile elements to the sarcolemma (Menold & Repasky, 1984; Terracio *et al.*, 1989). Approximately three times as much spectrin is found in slow than fast muscle and this difference has been interpreted to imply that α-spectrin is responsive to the physiological state of a fibre. Other studies have suggested that the sarcolemma is attached at periodic intervals to the extracellular matrix, thus providing a means of transferring forces from sarcomeres to adjacent fibres (Street, 1983; Shear & Bloch, 1985; Terracio *et al.*, 1989).

Functional significance of motor unit architecture

The newly discovered features of motor unit muscle fibre architecture raises several questions that previously may have been considered of little importance, if considered at all. For example, muscle fibres within the same motor unit can be arranged such that some fibres are arranged in parallel while others seem to be staggered in an in-series arrangement. The overall effect of this longitudinal and cross-sectional area distribution is a gradual tapering of the overall shape of the motor unit territory. Data from the cat tibialis anterior suggest that

although an in-series arrangement of fibres of a motor unit occurs, the territory of a motor unit can extend almost the entire length of the muscle (Fig. 6.21). This extended territory does not appear to be due to end-to-end attachments of fibres within the same motor unit. Rather, it appears that fibres of a motor unit are spatially arranged so that they are not usually in direct anatomical contact (Ounjian *et al.*, in press).

The complex 3-D arrangement of fibres within and across motor units must affect the mechanical output of the whole muscle or, at least, of the net effect of the interaction of subpopulations of motor units (see Demieville & Partridge, 1980; Partridge & Benton, 1981 for discussion). For example, if the fibres of two motor units are arranged in series and the two units are recruited simultaneously, both will contribute to displacement. The force produced by one unit, however, would be as much as if both were activated. In contrast, if the fibres of two units are arranged in parallel, then the force, but not the displacement, of the two units would be additive. The recruitment of one unit could even reduce the force incurred by a previously activated unit if it were anatomically organized so that relatively long fibres in the second unit recruited unloaded shorter parallel fibres in the first unit recruited. Such mechanical interactions could explain, at least in part, the non-linear force addition of recruited units reported by Clamann and Schelhorn (1988).

Based on the limited number of motor units that have been studied architecturally, it appears that many combinations of arrangements of fibres among units could provide an almost infinite number of possible patterns of forces and displacements by a muscle. Thus, it now seems evident that simply knowing the recruitment order of a unit and its maximum force is insufficient to accurately predict the mechanical output of a motor unit *in vivo*. Under *in vivo* conditions one must also know the anatomical arrangement of fibres of units that mechanically interact with the unit in question.

The significance of the effects of motor unit

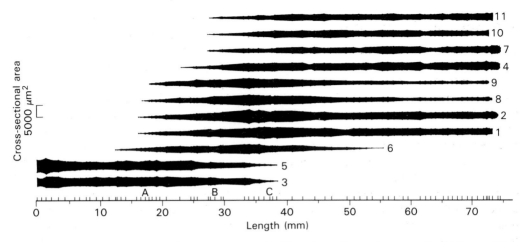

Fig. 6.21 The cross-sectional area and relative position of 11 fibres from a fast motor unit in the tibialis anterior muscle from a cat. The fibres were identified in serial cross-sections stained for glycogen content following glycogen depletion via repetitive stimulation (see Bodine *et al.*, 1987 and Ounjian *et al.*, in press, for methods). All the fibres were located in a single well-defined fascicle of the muscle. Note that the fibres do not necessarily begin and end at the same level along the longitudinal axis of the muscle. Also note the tapering, i.e. the decrease in fibre cross-sectional area, at one or both ends of each fibre. A, B, and C highlight the changes in the number and cross-sectional area of the fibres along the length of the muscle. The hashmarks on the bottom scale indicate the location of each serial section used in the reconstruction of the fibres. On the length scale, zero is the most proximal location of the muscles.

mechanical interactions may be in the stress–strain properties. The higher the forces produced by a fibre or group of fibres, the greater the strain imposed on the tissues arranged in series with the contractile components. The strain that occurs in the serially-arranged tissues will be dependent on the state of activation of the muscles fibres arranged in series, as well as the level of force produced by the motor unit. Varying stress–strain relationships are important to consider for two reasons. First, these relationships can affect the force, velocity and temporal features of activated motor units. Second, the strain imposed on a tissue may be a factor in the occurrence of muscle injury. It is generally believed that strains can occur during muscle actions which will cause damage (rupture) to the connective tissue within muscle, to the muscle fibres and/or to the musculotendinous junctions (Garrett & Tidball, 1987).

An excellent example of the complex stress–strain relationships that might occur in the interactions of motor units in skeletal muscle has been demonstrated in the semitendinosus

muscle of the cat (Bodine *et al.*, 1982; Edgerton *et al.*, 1987; Hutchison *et al.*, 1989). This muscle is somewhat unique in that almost all fibres in this long tubular muscle are limited by a connective tissue inscription located about one-third along its length from the proximal end, thus anatomically dividing the muscle into two compartments arranged in series. Each compartment has a separate nerve trunk and the muscle components of the motor units are clearly located in one or the other end, never in both. However, it seems that this anatomical separation in the muscle has been ignored in the evolution of the nervous system. For example, the motor pools of the two ends of the muscle are anatomically indistinguishable with respect to the projection frequency of the Ia fibres from spindles from both ends of the muscle to the respective motor pools (Botterman *et al.*, 1983). That is, the spindles project to motoneurones that innervate the opposite end (heteronymous) as frequently as they project to their own (homonymous) motoneurones. There must be some functional distinctions in the nervous system, however, since during normal locomotion motor units in both ends seem to be recruited simultaneously. The level of recruitment, however, is not of the same magnitude at both ends (English & Weeks, 1987; Hutchison *et al.*, 1989).

The serially arranged compartments of the semitendinosus are reflected in the contractile properties of the whole muscle (Bodine *et al.*, 1982). For example, the maximum tetanic tension produced when either end is maximally stimulated individually is similar to when both ends are stimulated simultaneously. In contrast, the displacement characteristics, i.e. length changes in both ends, vary markedly depending on whether one or both ends are stimulated (Bodine *et al.*, 1982; Edgerton *et al.*, 1987). These interrelationships are affected by the load on the muscle. For example, with a minimal load, the displacement at the distal tendon when the proximal end is stimulated is about one-third as much as when both ends are activated simultaneously. However, if the proximal end is stimulated while there is a relative high load on the tendon, there will be shortening in the stimulated compartment and lengthening of about the same amount in the distal end with little overall effect on the whole muscle length. The inverse effect occurs when the distal end is stimulated alone, i.e. the passive proximal end lengthens. The importance of these data lie in the fact that the two ends of the semitendinosus may represent the stress–strain events that occur routinely between two fibres attached in series. Therefore, the semitendinosus may serve as a very useful and readily accessible model for the study of fibre-to-fibre mechanical interactions.

A better understanding of the *in vivo* interactive properties of the two compartments of the semitendinosus may also provide some clues as to the role of muscle design patterns on the recruitment and stress–strain relationships of fibres within and among motor units. Is there a high incidence of 'hamstring pulls' or 'strains' because of these complex designs? Are there injuries related to unusual recruitment patterns, e.g. uneven levels of activation of fibres among motor units arranged in series? What are the weak links (tissues that are excessively stretched) in the fibre-to-fibre, fibre-to-fascicle and fibre-to-tendon interfaces?

Muscle design and joint torques

The mass, length, shape, fibre length and the manner in which fibres within a muscle interface differs markedly across muscles. Thus, it is apparent that predictions of joint torques based on simple anatomical CSAs of muscle, even when combined with best estimates of moment arms, are uniformly unsatisfactory. At the very least, a reasonable estimate of the following variables are needed to predict maximal joint torques: muscle mass, muscle length, fibre length, fibre length to muscle length ratio (see Table 6.1) and moment arm. To obtain even these data, assumptions must be made that limit the accuracy of the predictions of muscle forces. For example, fibre lengths cannot be measured *in vivo*. Muscle length, however, can be measured and since the fibre-to-muscle length ratio for an individual muscle seems to be relatively constant across individuals (Table 6.1), fibre length can be estimated using non-invasive imaging techniques, e.g. MRI. Some caution must be used when assuming that the fibre length to muscle length ratio is constant for a given muscle, however, since this assumption is based on data from a limited number of cadavers and may not reflect differences that may be unique to a culture. Using serial scans of MRI images, the volume of a muscle can be measured and the mass estimated based on a muscle density of $1.067\,\mathrm{g}\cdot\mathrm{cm}^{-3}$ (Mendez & Keys, 1960). Although this muscle density value seems to be quite constant across a variety of muscles and species, it may be misleading in circumstances in which a muscle becomes oedematous (Herbert *et al.*, 1988). In effect, muscle volume could be markedly affected by fluid redistribution, while the density of the cytoplasm of the muscle fibres could be normal.

In estimating the force potential of a muscle

group, the mechanical features of the musculo-skeletal system can be a major determinant of the resultant torques (Lieber & Boakes, 1988a,b). The use of MRI in estimating moment arms seems to be feasible (Rugg *et al.*, 1990). More direct estimates made in the frog illustrate the large magnitude of error that can be made in estimating torques with small variations in moment arm lengths (Lieber & Boakes, 1988a,b). Regardless of the preciseness required and the potential error in moment arm measurements or estimates in efforts to identify muscle forces, accurate measures of this parameter also have a significant impact on problems related to surgical manipulations of muscles, tendons and bones, to the design of prostheses and to the evaluation of the relative importance of neural control and muscle performance in a variety of neuromuscular disorders.

Another limiting factor in matching the maximal torque that a subject can produce with the PCSA of the musculature is the uncertainty of the level of activation of a muscle or muscle group relative to its maximum potential. It appears that the level of activation that can be achieved voluntarily in a muscle relative to its maximum varies among subjects and even within the same subject at various test times. There is considerable controversy regarding the issue as to whether large muscle groups can be stimulated so that all muscle fibres contract maximally simultaneously. Theoretically, maximal electrical stimulation could circumvent this key problem, but there are many technical factors that complicate this approach. For example, it must be assumed that the PCSA of a muscle is equivalent to the sum of the CSAs of all of the fibres within the muscle. Consequently, if two or more fibres are functionally arranged in series, but anatomically appear as multiple short fibres, then the PCSA will be overestimated.

In spite of the remaining uncertainties of estimating the mechanical potential of a muscle by using imaging technology, more variables can be obtained non-invasively and probably more accurately now than ever before. Based on a combination of non-invasive imaging,

physiological testing and the integration of anatomical design features of individual muscles, a consensus is evolving that the tension per cross-sectional area of human skeletal muscle is in the range of 23 to $42\,N \cdot cm^{-2}$ (see Edgerton *et al.*, 1986a for a review). Further, this range of specific tension values is similar to that found in other mammalian species (Spector *et al.*, 1980; Powell *et al.*, 1984; Roy *et al.*, 1984c).

Is prevalence of muscle injury related to muscle design?

Muscle injuries occur often even during routine daily activities and are even more likely to occur during strenuous exercise (Garrett, 1990). The nature of these muscle injuries and/or pain responses to exercise differs substantially from injury to injury as do their aetiologies. Although many of these injuries are referred to as 'muscle strains', are they? Assuming that strain contributes to injury and since strain occurs routinely in normal movement, the issue of tissue injury relates more specifically to when the strain of muscle fibres, connective tissue and their interfaces become excessive. The conditions under which excess muscle strain occurs in highly trained athletes provide few clues as to their cause. During movements that have been performed routinely for months, severe muscle pain and injury may occur suddenly. This phenomenon is poorly understood.

If tissue strain indeed is a contributing factor to 'muscle strains', then which tissues are being excessively strained and why did it occur? Obviously an understanding of the stress–strain properties of the musculoskeletal system *in vivo* during normal movements is essential to answer this complex question. Presently, this information is virtually impossible to obtain. Significant progress, however, can and is being made toward understanding the aetiology of at least some types of muscle strains. Forces in individual muscles and movements at single joints can be monitored in normal, routine movements, even in humans (Gregor *et al.*, 1987; Komi *et al.*, 1987). Further, imaging techniques are being developed that can localize damaged muscle tissue (Shellock *et al.*, 1991). Both of these techniques should be helpful, at least in further understanding the more macro levels of strain injuries.

A third approach that seems likely to contribute to a better understanding of muscle injury is the detailed morphological and biochemical characterization of the junctions of muscle fibres and tendons, i.e. the myotendinous junction. This particular approach already has proven to be productive. It is becoming clear that the myotendinous junction is particularly susceptible to strain-induced injury (Garrett & Tidball, 1987). Clear morphological abnormalities are evident at the myotendinous junction after excessive strain (pull to failure) of the rabbit tibialis anterior tendon complex (Garrett & Tidball, 1987). Whether the muscle is active or not does not appear to make a difference as to where tissue failure occurs when the muscle tendon complex is pulled to failure. However, the amount of energy that can be absorbed before failure is greater when the muscle is active compared to inactive (Safran *et al.*, 1988). Further, there is evidence from computed tomography studies that strains tend to occur at myotendinous junctions in human hamstring muscles (Garrett, 1990). The complexity of the architecture of hamstrings, however, precludes any firm conclusion on this issue since it is not clear where the myotendinous junctions are located in these complex muscles. There also is some evidence to suggest that the myotendinous junctions of atrophied muscle fibres are more susceptible to strain injury than those in normal sized fibres in the frog (Tidball, 1984; Tidball & Chan, 1989) and the rabbit (Garrett, 1990). These data are consistent with the long-held view that the 'trained' state of a muscle can affect the incidence of musculo-skeletal injuries.

Other recent studies suggest that strain injuries can occur during normal but fatiguing exercise and can persist for weeks in humans (Garrett, 1990; Shellock *et al.*, 1991). Evidence that tissue strain contributes to muscle injury is the fact that severe pain was developed in muscles when high forces were imposed on the muscle, particularly during loading conditions in which the activated muscles are lengthened rather than shortened. This may be related to the fact that the force that a muscle can produce is significantly higher during maximally active lengthening, or it may be related to the rate at which forces rise when the active muscle is stretched. As noted previously, higher forces will result in a higher strain in the associated tissues. The role of fatigue as a contributing factor to muscle injury is largely unknown.

As can be gathered from the above discussion of muscle injury, the present understanding of the nature and aetiology of muscle pain is superficial at best. Tissue strain is being implicated as a contributing factor to the occurrence of muscle injury, but it remains uncertain as to which events or combination of events result in injury. However, progress is being made toward a better understanding of the stress–strain elements that contribute to the mechanical output of motor units and muscles. These studies have led to the identification of the tissue sites that are susceptible to injury, e.g. the myotendinous junctions, and reasons to implicate tissue strain as a contributing factor to many musculocutaneous injuries.

Acknowledgements

We would like to thank all of our co-workers over the past decade that have contributed significantly to the work presented in this manuscript. We also thank Dr R.L. Lieber and Mr D.J. Pierotti for their critique of the manuscript. Special thanks are given to Dr R.L. Lieber and colleagues for providing us with some of the data presented in Table 6.1. A large portion of this work was supported by NIH Grant NS16333.

References

Alexander, R.M. & Vernon, A. (1975) The dimensions of knee and ankle muscles and the forces they exert. *Journal of Human Movement Studies*, **1**, 115–23.

Bodine, S.C., Garfinkel, A., Roy, R.R. & Edgerton, V.R. (1988) Spatial distribution of motor unit fibers in the cat soleus and tibialis anterior muscles: Local interactions. *Journal of Neuroscience*, **8**, 2142–52.

Bodine, S.C., Roy, R.R., Eldred, E. & Edgerton, V.R. (1987) Maximal force as a function of anatomical features of motor units in the cat tibialis anterior. *Journal of Neurophysiology*, **57**, 1730–45.

Bodine, S.C., Roy, R.R., Meadows, D.A., Zernicke, R.F., Sacks, R.D., Fournier, M. & Edgerton, V.R. (1982) Architectural, histochemical, and contractile characteristics of a unique biarticular muscle: the cat semitendinosus. *Journal of Neurophysiology*, **48**, 192–201.

Bodine-Fowler, S., Garfinkel, A., Roy, R.R. & Edgerton, V.R. (1990) Spatial distribution of muscle fibers within the territory of a motor unit. *Muscle and Nerve*, **13**, 1133–45.

Botterman, B.R. & Cope, T.C. (1988) Maximum tension predicts relative endurance of fast-twitch motor units in the cat. *Journal of Neurophysiology*, **60**, 1215–26.

Botterman, B.R., Hamm, T.M., Reinking, R.M. & Stuart, D.G. (1983) Distribution of monosynaptic Ia excitatory post-synaptic potentials in the motor nucleus of the cat semitendinosus muscle. *Journal of Physiology*, **338**, 379–93.

Brand, P.W., Beach, R.B. & Thompson, D.E. (1981) Relative tension and potential excursion of muscles in the forearm and hand. *Journal of Hand Surgery*, **3**, 209–19.

Burke, R.E. (1981) Motor units: Anatomy, physiology, and functional organization. In J.M. Brookhart & V.B. Mountcastle (eds) *Handbook of Physiology, Section 1. The Nervous System, Vol. 2, Motor Control, Part 2*, pp. 345–422. American Physiological Society, Bethesda.

Burke, R.E., Levine, D.N., Tsairis P. & Zajac, F.E. (1973) Physiological types and histochemical profiles in motor units of the cat gastrocnemius. *Journal of Physiology*, **234**, 723–48.

Burke, R.E. & Tsairis, P. (1973) Anatomy and innervation ratios of motor units of cat gastrocnemius. *Journal of Physiology*, **234**, 749–65.

Clamann, H.P. & Schelhorn, T.B. (1988) Nonlinear force addition of newly recruited motor units in the cat hindlimb. *Muscle and Nerve*, **11**, 1079–89.

Close, R.I. (1972) Dynamic properties of mammalian skeletal muscle. *Physiological Reviews*, **52**, 129–97.

Demieville, H.N. & Partridge, L.D. (1980) Probability of peripheral interaction between motor units and implications for motor control. *American Journal of Physiology*, **238**, R119–R137.

Edgerton, V.R., Bodine, S.C. & Roy, R.R. (1987) Muscle architecture and performance: Stress and strain relationships in a muscle with two compartments arranged in series. In P. Marconnet & P.V. Komi (eds) *Medicine and Sport Sciences: Muscular Function in Exercise and Training, Vol. 26*, pp. 12–23. Karger, Basel.

Edgerton, V.R., Martin, T.P., Bodine, S.C. & Roy, R.R. (1985) How flexible is the neural control of muscle properties? *Journal of Experimental Biology*, **115**, 393–402.

Edgerton, V.R., Roy, R.R. & Apor, P. (1986a) Specific tension of human elbow flexor muscles. In B. Saltin (ed.) *Biochemistry of Exercise*, pp. 487–500. Human Kinetics, Champaign, Illinois.

Edgerton, V.R., Roy, R.R., Bodine, S.C. & Sacks, R.D. (1983a) The matching of neuronal and muscular physiology. In K.T. Borer, D.W. Edington & T.P. White (eds) *Frontiers of Exercise Biology*, pp. 51–70. Human Kinetics, Champaign, Illinois.

Edgerton, V.R., Roy, R.R. & Gregor, R.J. (1989) Motor unit architecture and interfiber matrix in sensorimotor partitioning (peer commentary). *Behavioral Brain Sciences*, **12**, 651–2.

Edgerton, V.R., Roy, R.R., Gregor, R.J., Hager, C.L. & Wickiewicz, T. (1983b) Muscle fibre activation and recruitment. In H. Knuttgen, J. Vogel & J. Poortmans (eds) *Biochemistry of Exercise, International Series of Sport Sciences, Vol. 13*, pp. 31–49. Human Kinetics, Champaign, Illinois.

Edgerton, V.R., Roy, R.R., Gregor, R.J. & Rugg, S. (1986b) Morphological basis of skeletal muscle power output. In N.L. Jones, N. McCartney & A.J. McComas (eds) *Human Muscle Power*, pp. 43–64. Human Kinetics, Champaign, Illinois.

English, A.W. (1984) An electromyographic analysis of compartments in cat lateral gastrocnemius during unrestrained locomotion. *Journal of Neurophysiology*, **52**, 114–25.

English, A.W. & Letbetter, W.D. (1982) Anatomy and innervation patterns of cat lateral gastrocnemius and plantaris muscles. *American Journal of Anatomy*, **164**, 67–77.

English, A.W. & Weeks, O.I. (1987) An anatomical and functional analysis of cat biceps femoris and semitendinosus muscles. *Journal of Morphology*, **191**, 161–75.

Friederich, J.A. & Brand, R.A. (1990) Muscle fiber architecture in the human lower limb. *Journal of Biomechanics*, **23**, 91–5.

Fukunaga, T., Roy, R.R., Shellock, F.G., Hodgson, J.A., Lee, P.L., Kwong-Fu, H. & Edgerton, V.R. Physiological cross-sectional area of human leg muscles based on magnetic resonance imaging. *Journal of Orthopaedic Research* (submitted).

Gans, C. (1982) Fiber architecture and muscle function. *Exercise and Sport Sciences Reviews*, **10**, 160–207.

Gans, C. & Bock, W.J. (1965) The functional significance of muscle architecture—a theoretical analysis. *Ergebnisse der Anatomie und Entwickelungs Geschicte*, **38**, 115–42.

Garrett, W.E., Jr (1990) Muscle strain injuries: clinical and basic aspects. *Medicine and Science in Sports and Exercise*, **22**, 436–43.

Garrett, W.E. Jr & Tidball, J. (1987) Myotendinous junction: Structure, function, and failure. In S.L.Y. Woo & J.A. Buckwalter (eds) *Injury and Repair of Musculoskeletal Soft Tissues*, pp. 171–207. American Academy of Orthopaedic Surgeons and National Institute of Arthritis and Musculoskeletal and Skin Diseases.

Gordon, D.C., Hammond, C.G.M., Fisher J.T. & Richmond, F.J.R. (1989) Muscle-fiber architecture, innervation, and histochemistry in the diaphragm of the cat. *Journal of Morphology*, **201**, 131–43.

Gregor, R.J., Komi, P.V. & Jarvinen, M. (1987) Achilles tendon forces during cycling. *International Journal of Sports Medicine*, **8** (suppl.), 9–14.

Herbert, M.E., Roy, R.R. & Edgerton, V.R. (1988) Influence of one-week hindlimb suspension and intermittent high load exercise on rat muscles. *Experimental Neurology*, **102**, 190–8.

Henneman, E. & Mendell, L.M. (1981) Functional organization of motoneuron pool and its input. In J.M. Brookhart & V.B. Mountcastle (eds) *Handbook of Physiology, Section 1, The Nervous System, Vol. 2, Motor Control, Part 2*, pp. 423–507. American Physiological Society, Bethesda.

Hoffer, J.A., Caputi, A.A., Pose, I.E. & Griffiths, R.I. (1989) Roles of muscle activity and load on the relationship between muscle spindle length and whole muscle length in the freely walking cat. In J.H.J. Allum & M. Hulliger (eds) *Progress in Brain Research, Vol. 80*, pp. 75–85. Elsevier Science Publishers, Amsterdam.

Huijing, P.A. (1985) Architecture of the human gastrocnemius muscle and some functional consequences. *Acta Anatomica*, **123**, 101–7.

Huijing, P.A. & Woittiez, R.D. (1985) Length range, morphology and mechanical behaviour of rat gastrocnemius muscle during isometric contraction at the level of the muscle and muscle tendon complex. *Netherlands Journal of Zoology*, **35**, 505–16.

Hutchison, D.L., Roy, R.R., Bodine-Fowler, S., Hodgson, J.A. & Edgerton, V.R. (1989) EMG amplitude in the proximal and distal compartments of the cat semitendinosus during various motor tasks. *Brain Research*, **479**, 56–64.

Jacobson, M.D., Fazeli, B.M., Botte, M.J. & Lieber, R.L. Architectural evaluation of the flexor digitorum superficialis to profundus transfer. *American Society of Surgery of the Hand* (in press).

Josephson, R.K. (1975) Extensive and intensive factors determining the performance of striated muscle. *Journal of Experimental Zoology*, **194**, 135–54.

Komi, P.V., Salomen, M., Jarvinen, M. & Kokko, O. (1987) *In vivo* registration of Achilles tendon forces in man. I. Methodological development. *International Journal of Sports Medicine*, **8** (suppl.), 3–8.

Lieber, R.L. & Blevins, F.T. (1989) Skeletal muscle architecture of the rabbit hindlimb: Functional implications of muscle design. *Journal of Morphology*, **199**, 93–101.

Lieber, R.L. & Boakes, J.L. (1988a) Sarcomere length and joint kinematics during torque production in frog hindlimb. *American Journal of Physiology*, **254**, C759–C768.

Lieber, R.L. & Boakes, J.L. (1988b) Muscle force and moment arm contributions to torque production in frog hindlimb. *American Journal of Physiology*, **254**, C769–C772.

Lieber, R.L., Fazelli, B.M. & Botte, M.J. (1990) Architecture of selected wrist flexor and extensor muscles. *Journal of Hand Surgery*, **15A**, 244–50.

Lieber, R.L., Fazeli, B.M. & Botte, M.J. Architecture of selected muscles of the arm and forearm. *Journal of Hand Surgery* (in press).

Loeb, G.E., Pratt, C.A., Chanaud, C.M. & Richmond, F.J.R. (1987) Distribution and innervation of short, interdigitated muscle fibers in parallel-fibered muscles of the cat hindlimb. *Journal of Morphology*, **191**, 1–15.

Martin, T.P., Bodine-Fowler, S., Roy, R.R., Eldred, E. & Edgerton, V.R. (1988) Metabolic and fiber size properties of cat tibialis anterior motor units. *American Journal of Physiology*, **255**, C43–C50.

Mendez, J. & Keys, A. (1960) Density and composition of mammalian muscle. *Metabolism*, **9**, 184–8.

Menold, M.M. & Repasky, E.A. (1984) Heterogeneity of spectrin distribution among avian muscle fiber types. *Muscle and Nerve*, **7**, 408–14.

Muhl, Z.F. (1982) Active length–tension relation and the effect of muscle pinnation on fiber lengthening. *Journal of Morphology*, **173**, 285–92.

Otten, E. (1988) Concepts and models of functional architecture in skeletal muscle. *Exercise and Sport Sciences Reviews*, **16**, 89–137.

Ounjian, M., Roy, R.R., Eldred, E., Garfinkel, A., Payne, J., Armstrong, A., Toga, A. & Edgerton, V.R. Physiological and developmental implications of motor unit anatomy. *Journal of Neurobiology* (in press).

Partridge, L.D. & Benton, L.A. (1981) Muscle, the motor. In J.M. Brookhart, V.B. Mountcastle, V.B. Brooks & S.R. Geiger (eds) *Handbook of Physiology, Section 1, The Nervous System*, pp. 43–106. American Physiological Society, Bethesda.

Peter, J.B., Barnard, R.J., Edgerton, V.R., Gillespie, C.A. & Stempel, K.E. (1972) Metabolic profiles of three fiber types of skeletal muscle in guinea pigs and rabbits. *Biochemistry*, **11**, 2627–34.

Peters, S.E. (1989) Structure and function in vertebrate skeletal muscle. *American Zoology*, **29**, 221–34.

Powell, P.L., Roy, R.R., Kanim, P., Bello, M.A. & Edgerton, V.R. (1984) Predictability of skeletal muscle tension from architectural determinations in guinea pig hindlimbs. *Journal of Applied Physiology*, **57**, 1715–21.

Richmond, F.J.R. & Armstrong, J.B. (1988) Fiber architecture and histochemistry in the cat neck muscle, biventer cervicis. *Journal of Neurophysiology*, **60**, 46–59.

Roy, R.R., Bello, M.A., Powell, P.L. & Simpson, D.R. (1984a) Architectural design and fiber-type distribution of the major elbow flexors and extensors of the monkey (*Cynomolgus*). *American Journal of Anatomy*, **171**, 285–93.

Roy, R.R., Powell, P.L., Kanim, P. & Simpson, D.R. (1984b) Architectural and histochemical analysis of the semitendinosus muscle in mice, rats, guinea pigs, and rabbits. *Journal of Morphology*, **181**, 155–60.

Roy, R.R., Sacks, R.D., Baldwin, K.M., Short, M. & Edgerton, V.R. (1984c) Interrelationships of contraction time, V_{max}, and myosin ATPase after spinal transection. *Journal of Applied Physiology*, **56**, 1594–1601.

Rugg, S.G., Gregor, R.J., Mandelbaum, B.R. & Chiu, L. (1990) *In vivo* moment arm calculations at the ankle using magnetic resonance imaging (MRI). *Journal of Biomechanics*, **23**, 495–501.

Sacks, R.D. & Roy, R.R. (1982) Architecture of the hind limb muscles of cats: Functional significance. *Journal of Morphology*, **173**, 185–95.

Safran, M.R., Garrett W.E. Jr, Seaber A.V., Glisson R.R. & Ribbeck, B.M. (1988) The role of warmup in muscular injury prevention. *American Journal of Sports Medicine*, **16**, 123–9.

Shear, C.R. & Bloch, R.J. (1985) Vinculin in subsarcolemmal densities in chicken skeletal muscle: Localization and relationship to intracellular and extracellular structures. *Journal of Cell Biology*, **101**, 240–56.

Shellock, F., Fukunaga, T., Mink, J.H. & Edgerton, V.R. (1991) Acute effects of exercise on MR imaging of skeletal muscle: concentric vs eccentric actions. *American Journal of Roentgenology*, **156**, 765–8.

Spector, S.A., Gardiner, P.F., Zernicke, R.F., Roy, R.R. & Edgerton, V.R. (1980) Muscle architecture and force–velocity characteristics of cat soleus and medial gastrocnemius: Implications for motor control. *Journal of Neurophysiology*, **44**, 951–60.

Stein, R.B. (1982) What muscle variable(s) does the nervous system control in limb movements? *Behavioral and Brain Sciences*, **5**, 535–77.

Street, S.F. (1983) Lateral transmission of tension in frog myofibers: A myofibrillar network and transverse cytoskeletal connections are possible transmitters. *Journal of Cellular Physiology*, **114**, 346–64.

Terracio, L., Gullberg, D., Rubin, K., Craig, S. & Borg, T.K. (1989) Expression of collagen adhesion proteins and their association with the cytoskeleton in cardiac myocytes. *Anatomical Record*, **223**, 62–71.

Tidball, J.G. (1984) Myotendinous junction: Morphological changes and mechanical failure associated with muscle cell atrophy. *Experimental and Molecular Pathology*, **40**, 1–12.

Tidball, J.G. & Chan, M. (1989) Adhesive strength of single muscle cells to basement membrane at myotendinous junctions. *Journal of Applied Physiology*, **67**, 1063–9.

Wickiewicz, T.L., Roy, R.R., Powell, P.L. & Edgerton, V.R. (1983) Muscle architecture of the human lower limb. *Clinical Orthopaedics and Related Research*, **179**, 275–83.

Wickiewicz, T.L., Roy, R.R., Powell, P.L., Perrine, J.J. & Edgerton, V.R. (1984) Muscle architecture and force–velocity relationships in humans. *Journal of Applied Physiology*, **57**, 435–43.

Windhorst, U., Hamm, T.M. & Stuart, D.G. (1989) On the function of muscle and reflex partitioning. *Behavioral and Brain Sciences*, **12**, 629–81.

Chapter 6C

Mechanical Muscle Models

PETER A. HUIJING

Characteristics of muscle to be studied

In considering the properties of muscle that need explanation, there are a number of factors that determine the value of maximal force generated by a given muscle or muscle–tendon complex.

1 Force–length characteristics.
2 Force–velocity characteristics.
3 Excitation characteristics.
4 Characteristics of fatiguability.

In this chapter we will only consider the first two factors and thus assume that the muscles studied are all maximally active and do not fatigue during this activity.

Mechanical muscle models

Scientific muscle models are considered as a quantitative description of (aspects of) muscular performance. Most of the time these models have an heuristic function, i.e. they are used to explain and understand quantitatively effects of certain mechanisms that are operational in muscle. Consequently, muscle models incorporate sometimes extensive simplifications of reality.

In principle, it should be possible to incorporate so many aspects of muscular function in a model as to describe reality almost completely. However, since the actual values of model parameters are very frequently unknown and thus have to be estimated, the value of such very complex models is usually

rather limited. Only in very rare cases are such models usable for actual prediction of muscle performance. In most other cases, the simplifications incorporated may be very extensive and the most simple models are usually the best, considering the heuristic aims. The models to be described and used in this chapter are assigned to the latter category.

Mechanics of muscles and muscle–tendon complexes

All mechanical models of muscle, in some way, relate mechanical performance of whole muscle or muscle–tendon complex to that of the basic entity of contractile function within the system of reference that is applied. Sometimes these basic entities are rather abstract and sometimes they have a readily recognizable morphological identity. The former type of model aims to give a phenomological, but quantitative, description of aspects of muscle performance regardless of its structural units, while the latter tries to identify and describe quantitatively the effects and contributions of such elements of muscle as fibres, aponeuroses and tendons.

Morphologically based models

Sarcomere, myofilaments and cross-bridges

Figure 6.22 shows a schematic representation of a sarcomere, which involves interdigitating thick and thin filaments (e.g. Huxley, 1972). The sliding filament theory of contraction states

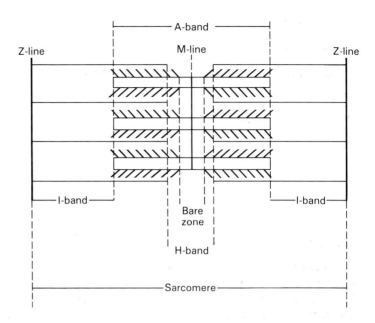

Fig. 6.22 Schematic representation of a sarcomere.

that the length of the myofilaments is constant and does not contribute to shortening of the sarcomere. The only way the sarcomere can change length is by the sliding of filaments relative to each other.

Cross-bridge models of force and motion generation

A complete consideration of cross-bridge models would take us far beyond the scope of this chapter and therefore we will only consider the most simple elements of cross-bridge behaviour. For a critical review of cross-bridge theory the reader is encouraged to study the review by Pollack (1983), who stressed the need to keep approaching the cross-bridge theory critically, with an open eye for inconsistencies. We believe that this approach is a valuable one, but it is good scientific practice that a theory is used until proven inadequate. This has not happened as yet for the cross-bridge theory of contraction (Huxley, 1988).

Cross-bridges are structures that are part of the thick filaments of muscle. They are attached to the backbone of these filaments in such a way as to enable them to attach to sites on the thin filaments that are in their vicinity (Fig.

6.23). At any time during activity of the muscle, some cross-bridges are attached to the thin filaments but others are in a process of detachment or are detached and moving towards new attachment sites. Attached cross-bridges undergo some form of structural deformation that leads to force generation. Shortening is obtained by cyclic repetition of cross-bridge attachment and detachment involving subsequent attachment sites on the thin filament, within reach of a cross-bridge (Fig. 6.23). Shortening occurs by a cyclic occurrence of the following events. Attachment of cross-bridges to the thin filaments is followed by some configurational change of the cross-bridge that causes it to pull the thin filament along the thick filament. Subsequently, the cross-bridge detaches and swings back to its original orientation, from where the next cycle may start. For other details of cross-bridge function, see Chapter 3.

All cross-bridges are functionally identical, act independently and the probability of attachment or detachment is influenced by local environmental conditions only, e.g. calcium ion concentration. It is assumed that active muscle force originates from cross-bridges

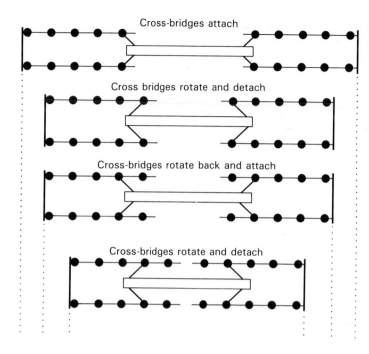

Fig. 6.23 Schematic representation of events occurring in sarcomere shortening. The circles drawn on the thin filaments represent potential locations of cross-bridge attachment.

exclusively. As a consequence of the above, active force generated at any time is dependent on the number of parallel cross-bridges that are attached to the thin filaments. The first quantitative statement to this effect was made by Huxley (1957). For more modern versions of such models the reader is referred to Zahalak (1981, 1986).

Effects of parallel and series arrangement of sources of force and displacement

Figure 6.24a shows a representation of an in-series arrangement of force and displacement generators (cross-bridges). Regarding force, the characteristic of such an arrangement is that the force generated by one unit has to be maintained and transmitted by the next unit so that they can be considered as a pair: the force of the whole structure is equal to the force of one unit. The force exerted by the half sarcomere is equal to the sum of the forces of the attached cross-bridges. If the force exerted by these cross-bridges is to be transmitted to the other Z-disc of the sarcomere, an equal number of cross-

bridges should be attached in the other half of the sarcomere. Each of the cross-bridges within one half of a thick filament are arranged in series with cross-bridges in the complementary half of the sarcomere.

Any displacement caused by the units has to be added in order to obtain the displacement of the whole structure. The shortening of the half sarcomere is equal to the shortening caused by any cross-bridge in one cycle of attachment and detachment multiplied by the number of cycles completed.

If a parallel arrangement of pairs of units is considered (Fig. 6.24b), the forces can be seen to act independently of each other, so that the total force is equal to the sum of the forces of the units. However, the total displacement is equal to that of one unit.

Similar arguments can be made for whole sarcomeres (Fig. 6.25).

Sarcomere length–force characteristics

If a sarcomere is maintained at such lengths that no overlap occurs between its filaments,

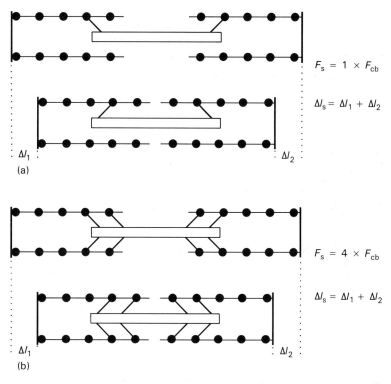

$$F_s = 1 \times F_{cb}$$

$$\Delta l_s = \Delta l_1 + \Delta l_2$$

Δl_1 Δl_2

(a)

$$F_s = 4 \times F_{cb}$$

$$\Delta l_s = \Delta l_1 + \Delta l_2$$

Δl_1 Δl_2

(b)

Fig. 6.24 Schematic representation of effects of in series (a) and parallel (b) arrangement of cross-bridges within a sarcomere. F_s indicates the force exerted by the sarcomere, F_{cb} indicates the force exerted by one cross-bridge and Δl_s is the length change of the sarcomere. (a) Two cross-bridges arranged in series; (b) four parallel pairs of cross-bridges.

activation of the sarcomere will not lead to force production. At the sarcomere length at which some overlap begins, some force can be generated. This length will be referred to as maximal sarcomere length of active force exertion (l_{sam}). If the activation of the sarcomere is performed at shorter sarcomere lengths, the overlap will be increased and thus the number of cross-bridges that can maximally attach. As a consequence, at shorter sarcomere lengths, isometric maximal force will be higher until the overlap is such that all cross-bridges can find an attachment site on the thin filament. A linearly increasing force rising to an optimum value, as predicted by the sliding filament theory, was indeed found (Gordon *et al.*, 1966a,b; Edman & Reggiani, 1987). The sarcomere length at which this active optimal force is encountered

is referred to as sarcomere optimum length (l_{so}).

If the sarcomere is brought to even shorter length, the sliding filament theory predicts that isometric activation of the sarcomere would yield optimal force as well, since the number of potential cross-bridges that can attach to sites on the thin filament remains constant only if geometrical relationships are considered. However, measurements indicate that actual maximal force decreases with shorter sarcomere length. There are two possibilities to explain this phenomenon.

1 Despite the fact that overlap remains optimal, an unknown factor prevents attachment of an increasing number of cross-bridges with decreasing sarcomere length, so that fewer cross-bridges can attach.

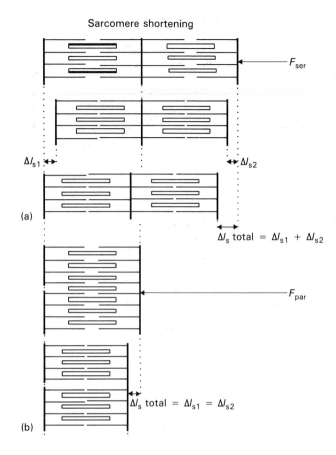

Sarcomere shortening

F_{ser}

Δl_{s1} Δl_{s2}

(a)

Δl_s total $= \Delta l_{s1} + \Delta l_{s2}$

F_{par}

Δl_s total $= \Delta l_{s1} = \Delta l_{s2}$

(b)

Fig. 6.25 Schematic representation of effects of in series and parallel arrangement of sarcomeres. F_{ser} and F_{par} indicate the forces exerted by two sarcomeres arranged in series and parallel, respectively; Δl_s indicates the length changes of the sarcomeres, and Δl_s total, the length change of the arrangement of sarcomeres.

2 All potential cross-bridge attachments are made but some unknown mechanism generates an opposing force, which increases with decreasing sarcomere length. At a particular sarcomere length the net force exerted will be zero. Some suggestions for possible mechanisms have been made (e.g. Gordon *et al.*, 1966a,b; Otten, 1987).

As the exact nature of mechanisms indicated above are unknown, no unequivocal choice can be made between these two hypotheses as yet. The shortest sarcomere length at which active force generation approaches zero is referred to as sarcomere active slack length (l_{sas}).

A very simple model is used here to calculate l_{sam} and l_{so} on the basis of filament length parameters (Fig. 6.26) (Huijing *et al.*, 1989; Heslinga & Huijing, 1990). Considering the lack

of understanding of the mechanism of decreasing force at shorter sarcomere lengths, further assumptions have to be made for prediction of l_{sas} and the pattern of decrease of maximal force with decreasing sarcomere length. For modelling purposes it is assumed that from l_{so} to l_{sas} a parabolic decrease of force was found, and that l_{sas} coincides with a value of 90% of the thick filament length.

Even though myofilament parameters may vary somewhat between species and between different muscles of one species (Granzier *et al.*, 1984), muscles are modelled below that are built of sarcomeres with filament length parameters as shown in Table 6.2 and sarcomere length–force characteristics as shown in Fig. 6.26b.

It should be kept in mind that the length–

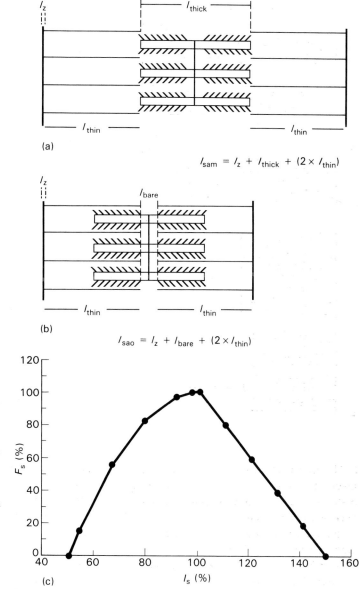

Fig. 6.26 Schematic representation of the model used to estimate (a) sarcomere active maximal length (l_{sam}) and (b) sarcomere active optimum length (l_{sao}) on the basis of filament length parameters. (c) Normalized sarcomere length–force characteristics calculated on the basis of filament length parameters: l_s represents sarcomere length normalized for sarcomere optimum length, and F_s the maximal force exerted by the sarcomere at a given length.

force curve is constructed by connecting points obtained for maximal isometric measurements at different lengths.

Sarcomere force–velocity characteristics

Force–velocity curves are constructed on the basis of measurements in which the effect of velocity on force exerted by the sarcomere is studied. In order to exclude any length effects, contractions are performed at different velocities and as the target length is achieved, the force is measured. Consequently, such force–velocity relations can be made for any length of the sarcomere length range of active force exertion. Figure 6.27 shows an example of the

Table 6.2 Filament length parameters (μm) for sarcomeres of modelled muscles and calculated normalized sarcomere lengths

l_z	l_{thin}	l_{thick}	l_{bare}	l_{sas} (%)	l_{sam} (%)
0.05	1.32	1.60	0.16	50.53	150.53

sarcomere force–velocity curve for optimum length. If the velocity approaches zero, an isometric action yielding optimal force is obtained. The decreased maximal force at higher velocities can be understood intuitively as follows. If the sarcomere is to shorten faster, the cycling rate of cross-bridges will have to be increased. This means that at any moment fewer cross-bridges can be attached and can contribute to force production; thus the sarcomere can exert less force at increasing velocities of shortening. The maximal velocity of contraction is obtained if no force has to be exerted, i.e. almost all cross-bridges are cycling rather than staying attached to exert force.

For purposes of modelling it is assumed that the standard sarcomeres, of which the model muscles are built, have a maximal shortening velocity of $20 \times l_{so} \cdot s^{-1}$ and that their normalized force–velocity characteristics at optimum length appear as shown in Fig. 6.27. At lengths other than l_{sao} (sarcomere active

optimum length), this maximum velocity is constant unless extreme sarcomere lengths are studied (Edman, 1979). For the purposes of simplicity, in our model we will assume a constant maximal velocity at all sarcomere lengths. In addition, it is assumed that the factors determining the shape of the force–velocity relationship are not affected by sarcomere length. This means that the sarcomere force–velocity curve is determined by two factors: isometric force depending on sarcomere length and maximal velocity. The normalized relationship between sarcomere force and velocity is then independent of sarcomere length and Fig. 6.27 can be used as a basis for our model.

Fibre models

A number of sarcomeres arranged in series is called a myofibril. A human myofibril may contain up to many thousands of sarcomeres in series (e.g. Huijing, 1985). According to the rules for series arrangement described above (Fig. 6.25), the force generated by a myofibril is equal to the force generated by one sarcomere of the fibril. Shortening of the fibril is equal to the summed shortening of the sarcomeres. This means that the length range of force exertion is increased but not the force when comparing sarcomere to fibril characteristics.

From a purely biomechanical view, muscle

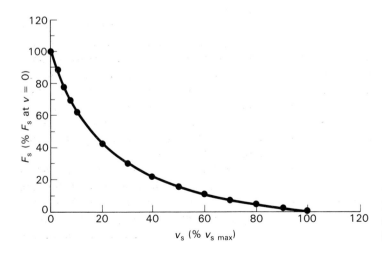

Fig. 6.27 Assumed normalized sarcomere force–velocity characteristics. v_s represents sarcomere shortening velocity normalized for maximal sarcomere shortening velocity; F_s represents maximal force exerted by the sarcomere at a given length and force, normalized for maximal isometric force at the given length.

fibres may be considered as a collection of myofibrils arranged in parallel, and thus as a collection of sarcomeres arranged in parallel as well as in series.

It is clear that on the basis of number of sarcomeres arranged in series and in parallel within a muscle fibre, the force–length and force–velocity curves may be estimated on the basis of sarcomere characteristics. This is true if the sarcomeres in a fibre behave in a uniform fashion. There is some evidence that this is not quite true.

1 Not all sarcomeres of a fibre act at exactly equal lengths, sarcomeres at the ends of fibres being somewhat shorter than those in the middle of the fibre.

2 Not all sarcomeres operate at identical velocities.

However, for our purposes we will neglect these effects. Normalized fibre characteristics should then be equal to normalized sarcomere characteristics (see Figs 6.26 and 6.27). Fibre characteristics obtained this way are often used as input for modelling whole muscle.

Muscle models: muscles of uniform morphology, not incorporating elastic properties

Most muscles may be considered as a collection of fibres arranged in parallel. In some muscle also, series arrangements of muscle fibres exist, but such arrangements will not be considered within the scope of this chapter. Generally, muscle fibres attach to tendon plates or apo-neuroses, which are continuous with the more rounded tendons that run outside of the muscle. The arrangement of fibres within the muscle with respect to each other and with respect to the aponeuroses is generally referred to as muscle architecture. Two types of archi-tecture may be distinguished.

1 Fibres are arranged in such a way that they run parallel, or nearly so, to the line of pull of the muscle. This category is referred to as parallel-fibred muscles.

2 Fibres are arranged at an angle relative to the line of pull of the muscle. In such muscles the fibres are shorter than the muscle. This category is referred to as pennate muscles.

Mechanics of parallel-fibred muscles

In principle, for parallel-fibred muscle, mech-anical features are governed by the same prin-ciples of series and parallel arrangement as was explained for sarcomeres. As muscles are thought of as a collection of fibres arranged in parallel to each other and to the line of pull of the muscle, the length range of force exer-tion of the fibre and the muscle will be equal. Obviously, the magnitude of the force exerted by a fibre and the muscle, at a given length, will differ as the muscle force is equal to the sum of the forces generated by the individual fibres. Therefore, the force–length relationships have similar length ranges, and force–velocity characteristics have similar ranges of velocity for parallel-fibred muscles and their fibres.

Mechanics of pennate muscles

The mechanics of pennate muscle are far more complicated than those of parallel-fibred muscles mainly because of two factors.

1 The geometry of the muscle influences the relationship of fibre and muscle length changes.

2 Fibre force is exerted in a different direction than muscle force.

In order to understand mechanics of pennate muscle, the free body diagram of the apo-neurosis is studied, i.e. all relevant forces acting on the aponeurosis are considered (Fig. 6.28). It is assumed that the force, F_f, which represents the vector sum of all forces gen-erated in individual fibres, is located at the middle of the aponeurosis and points in the direction of the fibres.

F_p indicates the force that is produced as a consequence of pressure created within the muscle as a consequence of activity. This vector is perpendicular to the aponeurosis but its location is unknown. A third force is the muscle

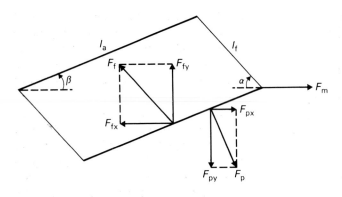

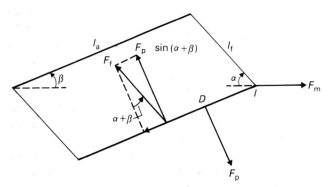

Fig. 6.28 Free body diagram of aponeurosis. l_f and l_a represent the length of the fibre and aponeurosis, respectively; α and β, the angle with the line of pull of the muscle of fibres and aponeuroses, respectively; and F_f, F_p, F_m, the fibre force, pressure-related force and muscle force, respectively. I indicates the point of attachment of the tendon to the muscle, and D the point of application of the pressure-related force.

force, F_m, which points in the longitudinal direction of the muscle from its point of application, I. In a quasistatic approach to the problem the sum of the vectors in the indicated x and y directions should be equal to zero:

$$\Sigma F_x = F_m - F_f \cos \alpha + F_p \cos (90 - \beta) = 0 \quad (1)$$
$$= F_m - F_f \cos \alpha + F_p \sin \beta = 0 \quad (2)$$
$$\Sigma F_y = F_f \sin \alpha - F_p \cos \beta = 0. \quad (3)$$

From equation (3) it follows that:

$$F_p = F_f \sin \alpha / \cos \beta. \quad (4)$$

Combining equations (4) and (1) yields:

$$F_m - F_f \cos \alpha + F_f \sin \alpha \sin \beta / \cos \beta = 0, \quad (5)$$

and thus

$$F_m = F_f (\cos \alpha - \sin \alpha \sin \beta / \cos \beta) \quad (6)$$
$$= F_f (\cos \alpha \cos \beta - \sin \alpha \sin \beta)/(\cos \beta). \quad (7)$$

As

$$\cos \alpha \cos \beta - \sin \alpha \sin \beta = \cos (\alpha + \beta)$$
$$F_m = F_f (\cos (\alpha + \beta)/\cos \beta) \quad (8)$$

or

$$F_f/F_m = (\cos \beta / \cos (\alpha + \beta)). \quad (9)$$

Force exerted on the aponeurosis, F_a, in its longitudinal direction can be calculated as:

$$F_a = F_f \cdot \cos (\alpha + \beta) = F_m \cdot \cos \beta. \quad (10)$$

Further analysis leads to an interesting conclusion regarding intramuscular pressure. Also in the quasistatic analysis the sum of moments with respect to point I should equal zero (Fig. 6.28). Thus

$$(F_f \sin (\alpha + \beta) \cdot \tfrac{1}{2} l_a) - (F_p \cdot l_{ID}) = 0. \quad (11)$$

From equations (4) and (9) it follows that the distance between point I and point D (l_{ID}) equals

$$l_{ID} = \tfrac{1}{2} l_a \sin (\alpha + \beta) \cos \beta / \sin \alpha. \quad (12)$$

From equation (10) it is concluded that l_{ID} cannot be equal to $\tfrac{1}{2} l_a$ (aponeurosis length). This indicates that fibre force and pressure force do not have their point of application at the same

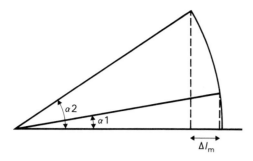

Fig. 6.29 Illustration of the effects of changing fibre angle on muscle length. If fibre angle could be changed without changing fibre length, this would result in a change of muscle length indicated by Δl_m.

location on the aponeurosis. This can only be explained if a gradient is found for intramuscular pressure.

Effects of muscle geometry

If pennate muscles are considered as solid bodies, any length change of the fibres would not be accompanied by an equal length change of the muscle. However, simultaneous with changing of fibre length a change of fibre angle is encountered. If the fibre shortens, the constancy of the muscle volume causes the fibre to rotate at its attachments to the aponeuroses to an increased fibre angle. That such an increase of fibre angle contributes to shortening of the muscle may be illustrated in the following, completely hypothetical, example. Suppose that a fibre could change its angle without any change of fibre length (Fig. 6.29). As a consequence of the angle increase the muscle would be shorter. Note that the magnitude of this effect increases as initial fibre angle is increased. As early as the seventeenth century, some workers in the field of muscle morphology were aware of these phenomena (see Kardel, 1990) but such information was not widespread and disappeared from the current body of knowledge until very recently. As a consequence these insights had to be rebuilt, first with respect to single fibre behaviour in pennate muscle (Benninghoff & Rollhäuser, 1952; Gans & Bock, 1965) and finally incor-

porated in muscle models on the effects of geometry on muscular function of pennate muscles (Huijing & Woittiez, 1984, 1985; Woittiez et al., 1984; Otten, 1988), for which muscle fibres were placed between two aponeuroses.

If a fibre could shorten as well as increase its angle, the effect of these events would be that the length change of the muscle as a function of change of fibre length and fibre angle equals the sum of these effects separately. Considering the angles encountered in pennate muscles the enhancing effects of fibre angle changes on muscle length changes will be greater than the decremental effects of having a fibre angle. We thus encounter evidence that length changes of pennate muscle is increased with respect to length changes of the fibres of that muscle. Quantification of the combined effects of angle effects can be obtained by considering the energetics of the muscle (Otten, 1988). The work performed by fibres as a consequence of very small changes of fibre length can be calculated as follows:

$$W_f = \int F_f dl_f \qquad (13)$$

and similarly that of muscle equals

$$W_m = \int F_m dl_m, \qquad (14)$$

where dl_f and dl_m are length changes chosen to be so small that forces may be considered unchanged. As long as the aponeurosis is not changing its length, work delivered by the fibres and muscle have to be equal. Thus it follows that:

$$dl_f/dl_m = F_m/F_f. \qquad (15)$$

Substituting equation (9) yields:

$$dl_f/dl_m = \cos(\alpha + \beta)/\cos\beta. \qquad (16)$$

Note that this fraction is always smaller than 1 for the range of angles found in muscles (0–50°), but that at small values of angle α the deviation from 1 will be neglible unless the value for β is large. This means that the increased muscle length changes as a consequence of fibre angle, and aponeurosis angle

Table 6.3 Architectural variables of modelled pennate muscles

Muscle	Volume (cm^3)	l_{mo} (cm)	l_{fo} (cm)	l_a (cm)	α (degrees)	β (degrees)
Pen1	1000	24.0	10	14.9	18	12
Pen2	1000	21.1	10	11.6	14	12
Pen3	1000	18.0	10	8.4	10	12

increases are compensated for in the model by changes of muscle force in such a way that total mechanical energy is unchanged by the processes incorporated in the model.

Table 6.3 shows morphological variables of modelled muscles; note that fibre lengths are identical. Figure 6.30 shows a comparison of dynamics of morphology for these muscles and some functional consequences; note that the length range of active force exertion is strongly influenced by muscle architecture. The length range of active force exertion is determined by the following factors: (i) changes of fibre length, which are highly dependent on number of sarcomeres in series; (ii) changes of fibre angle; and (iii) changes of aponeurosis angle.

As the length changes of the fibre occur in a certain time, and the length changes of the muscle in the same time, a similar ratio will be found for velocities of contraction of fibre and muscle:

$$v_f/v_m = \frac{dl_f/dt}{dl_m/dt},\qquad (17)$$

therefore

$$v_f/v_m = \cos(\alpha + \beta)/\cos\beta. \qquad (18)$$

Figure 6.31 shows a comparison of force–velocity characteristics of the modelled muscles; note that at optimum length the functional effects of differences of muscle architecture on force–velocity characteristics are rather limited. However, at short muscle lengths sizeable differences are introduced. For the modelled muscles, Fig. 6.31c shows the magnitude of architectural effects on contraction velocity as a function of muscle length.

Effects of inhomogeneous morphology

In the preceding section muscles were modelled as uniformly built structures. However, it is well known that in real life variation in morphology is encountered when comparing different locations within a muscle. For several human muscles, as well as those of experimental animals, force–length relationships have been found (Huijing *et al.*, 1986, 1987, 1989; Herzog & ter Keurs, 1989; Heslinga & Huijing, 1990) with such length ranges of active force generation that they could not be explained on the basis of number of sarcomeres in series within the fibres, even if effects of muscle architecture were taken into consideration. This initiated a search for other factors influencing muscle force–length characteristics (e.g. Huijing, 1988; Huijing *et al.*, 1989), which is still in its initial phase. Some effects of variation of the morphology of these elements will be considered below.

Variation within sarcomeres

Variations are encountered in filament lengths of different sarcomeres within one muscle, particularly for the thin filaments (Robinson & Winegrad, 1979; Traeger & Goldstein, 1983). Functional effects have not been considered as yet in any detail, but a qualitative analysis shows that particularly the descending part of the sarcomere force–length relationship (i.e. at lengths greater than l_{so}) will be affected by shorter thin filament lengths.

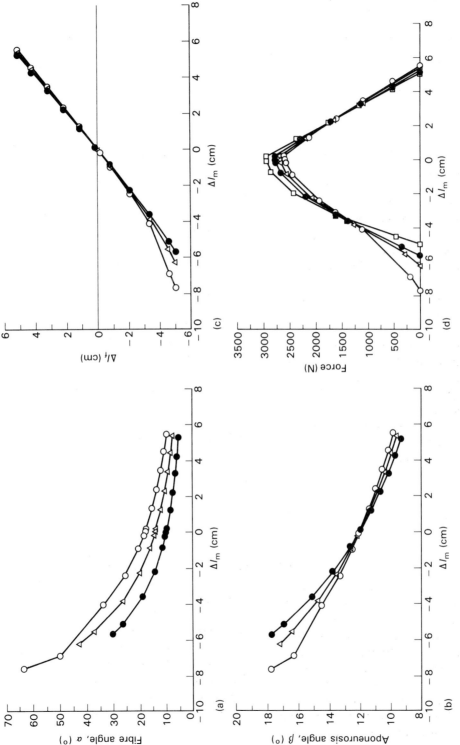

Fig. 6.30 Changes of muscle geometry and muscle length–force characteristics for the modelled muscles. (a) Changes of fibre angle, (b) aponeurosis angle, and (c) fibre length as a function of changes of muscle length. (d) The length–force characteristics are shown for the modelled muscles as well as for the identical fibres of which these muscles are composed. Note that at optimum length, aponeurosis angles and fibre length are identical but fibre angle is varied. Note also for (a) that if fibre angle is increased at the optimum length then the maximal change of fibre angle with muscle shortening is increased as well. For the pennate muscle (Pen1) with the greatest angle changes, the largest length range of active force exertion was encountered (d). ○, Pen1; △, Pen2; ●, Pen3; □, fibres.

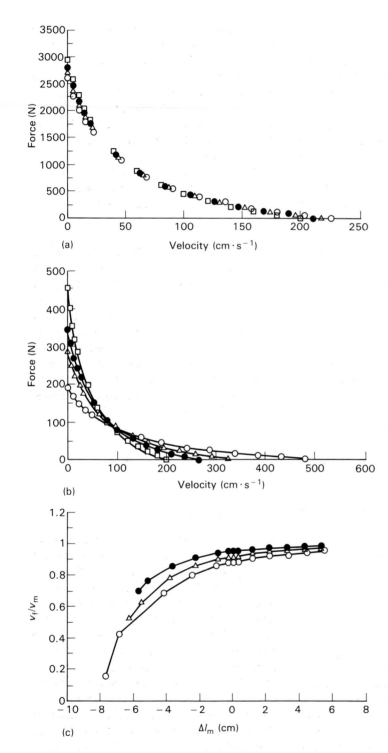

Fig. 6.31 Force–velocity characteristics of modelled muscles and their identical fibres (a) at optimum length and (b) short fibre length (55% of fibre optimum length). Note that at short fibre length considerable differences occur as a consequence of differences of muscle geometry. (c) Effects of muscle geometry, and changes thereof, on shortening velocity in the modelled muscles. The ratio of fibre and muscle shortening velocity calculated according to equation (17) is expressed as a function of changes of muscle length from optimum length.

Variation within fibres

Variations are encountered in the sarcomere lengths along the length of a fibre. This seems to be the case particularly in young animals (Goldspink, 1968), but also in adults a small fraction of the sarcomeres, located at the ends of the fibre, will have shorter sarcomere length than those encountered in the middle parts of the fibre (Huxley & Peachy, 1961; Gordon *et al.*, 1966a,b; Julian & Morgan, 1979). These properties have been the subject of discussion because they could lead to instabilities at the descending part of the force–length curve (see Sugi & Pollack, 1979). The sarcomeres with the shorter length would generate more force and thus stretch the longer sarcomeres, which would cause them to generate even less force, so that the process would rapidly repeat itself and no force could be exerted since the sarcomeres with the longest sarcomere length would be stretched to their maximal length of active force exertion. A collection of sarcomeres in series could then not sustain any force. In reality this does not occur, so obviously this effect must be compensated for by other mechanisms. Morgan (1985) suggested that passive force generated by the sarcomere (a longer sarcomere would mean increased force) and differences between concentric and eccentric force–velocity characteristics could be such mechanisms.

One effect of this distribution of sarcomere lengths within a fibre would be to increase the length range of active force generation of the fibre.

Variation within muscles

Effects of distribution of fibre length and angle. Not all fibres of a muscle contain the same number of sarcomeres (e.g. Huijing, 1985). In parallel-fibred muscles, such a distribution of fibre length would lead to a certain widening and altered shape of the muscle force–length relationship: as the shorter fibres reach their slack lengths the longer fibres can still exert force. At any length the muscle force will be equal to the summed forces of the fibres. In pennate muscle, such a distribution may have a smaller effect since increased fibre length must be compensated by decreased fibre angles if the distance between the tendon plates is to remain constant. This decreased fibre angle will lead to diminished contributions of fibre angle changes to muscle length changes. From this point it is also clear that, given equal fibre lengths, distribution of fibre angles within a muscle will affect the width and shape of the force–length relationship.

Effects of distribution of fibre optimum lengths. Up to this point in our reasoning, it has been implicitly assumed that the optimum length of all fibres coincided at one muscle length as well. However, there are indications that this may not always be true. Experimentally, some evidence has been found by studying force–length characteristics of motor units by selectively stimulating their axons (Stephens *et al.*, 1975). An example of effects of such variation is shown in Fig. 6.42 of Chapter 6D.

Models incorporating elastic properties

Phenomenological models

The impact of this type of muscle modelling can be most clearly described by considering the Nobel prize winning work of A.V. Hill. The so-called Hill model (Hill, 1970) incorporates as a basic element of muscle function the *contractile element* (CE) (Fig. 6.32). This element is the basis of all active behaviour of muscle. In the most simple form of the model it is connected in series with a passive element, which has the characteristics of a spring. Obviously, this does not mean that springs may actually be found within the muscles but that the behaviour of the muscle can be understood if the elastic characteristics of unidentified muscle parts are represented as springs. In the previous

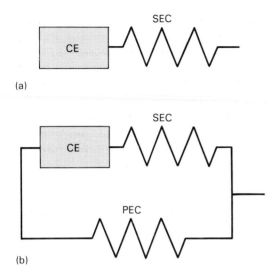

Fig. 6.32 Schematic representation of the Hill model. (a) The most simple form of the model describing active muscle characteristics; (b) model describing active as well as passive muscle characteristics. In these models all contractile activity is concentrated in the contractile element (CE) and all elastic characteristics in the series elastic component (SEC) or parallel elastic component (PEC) depending on their location relative to CE.

paragraphs of this chapter, morphological behaviour of the muscle was studied without considering the effects of elastic tissues within the muscle. Here, the effects of muscle morphology are neglected. This means that particularly aspects of a parallel-fibred muscle–tendon complex can be described accurately with this approach.

The element in series with the contractile element is called the *series elastic component* (SEC) (Fig. 6.32). The most important aspect of the characteristics of the SEC is that it is conservative, i.e. any mechanical energy delivered by the CE will be taken up by the SEC, and returned to the surroundings as the SEC returns to its original condition. In real muscle some of the mechanical energy delivered by the CE may be lost, but in most cases this amount of energy is rather limited so that this simplification does not influence the results to a great extent. This simplification does limit the use of

this model in one way: the history of activity cannot influence performance in the model while in reality this is indeed the case, e.g. eccentric actions.

Mechanics of elements in series indicate two important aspects.

1 Unless inertia has a sizeable effect, the force exerted by the CE should at all times be equal to the force maintained in the SEC.

2 Lengthening or shortening of the CE and of SEC must be added to obtain total lengthening or shortening of the complex. A similar situation exists for velocity of lengthening or shortening of the CE and SEC.

The CE is considered to have force–length as well as force–velocity characteristics that are qualitatively similar to those described for sarcomeres or fibres. This means that at the onset of a contraction, even if the CE could be activated instantly, development of force would follow much more slowly. This can be illustrated for an isometric action of the CE–SEC complex, i.e. total length is kept constant during the contraction. Any force generation by the CE is accompanied by stretching of the SEC, and thus a shortening of the CE. Below CE optimum length this would lead to a decrease of force accompanied by a simultaneous decrease of SEC length. Such sequences will lead to a steady equilibrium at a particular force and CE and SEC length. The attainment of this equilibrium will take some time so that the build-up of muscle force will be slower than that of an isolated CE. A second effect of having elastic elements within the muscle can be illustrated for non-isometric action of the complex. Starting at the final equilibrium of an isometric action at optimum force, if the complex is allowed to shorten force will decrease, because of the force–length and force–velocity characteristics of the CE. As a consequence of the decreasing force SEC length will decrease as well and the total shortening velocity of the complex will be equal to the sum of the shortening velocities of the CE and SEC. If a situation could be created in which the CE force fell very rapidly, e.g. by simultaneously deactivating the CE to a certain extent, the contribution to shortening velocity by the SEC would be much higher than that of the CE. This situation may be compared to that of a sling shot: if the force on the elastic element (the sling) is suddenly decreased by releasing it, all elastic energy stored in it is used to propel the projectile in a certain direction. If at the same time the hand holding the sling shot is moved in the same direction, the projectile will be launched at a velocity that is the sum of the recoil velocity of the sling and the velocity of movement of the hand holding the sling shot.

In order to include explanations of behaviour of passive muscle as well, a third element is often included in the model: *parallel elastic component* (PEC). The PEC is the source of opposing forces encountered when trying to elongate a passive muscle. It is arranged in parallel to the CE and prevents a non-active CE from being torn apart by external forces. If the CE becomes active it will generate so much force compared to that of the PEC that the latter is negligible. The PEC will then be exposed only to small amounts of external force and shorten.

The beauty of a model as described above is that it is very simple and thus can easily illustrate functional behaviour of muscle. A difficulty is that the SEC and CE are only concepts and not physical structures that one can find within the muscle. Cross-bridges are not

equivalent to the CE since they contain elastic characteristics as well as contractile ones. A second contributor to SEC characteristics are the tendinous tissues of a muscle, which cannot be distinguished within the Hill model. By studying isolated fibres (e.g. Blangé *et al.*, 1972) it became clear that a small part of the SEC can be located within the cross-bridges and a major part in the tendinous tissues. Recent estimates made for intact rat muscle (Ettema & Huijing, 1990) indicate that approximately 85% of elastic length changes obtained between zero and optimum force are located in the tendinous tissues and the remaining part is located intracellularly.

Hill-type models incorporating some aspects of muscle morphology

For reasons of simplicity, intracellular (cross-bridges) and intramuscular (aponeurosis) contributions to the SEC are frequently not considered and all compliance of the modelled muscle is assigned to the extramuscular tendon (e.g. Zahalak, 1981; Bobbert *et al.*, 1986a,b). Sometimes the tendon is represented as a morphologically identifiable structure but the muscle to which the tendon is connected is modelled phenomenologically (Zajac *et al.*, 1986a,b,c; Ingen Schenau *et al.*, 1988). Use of these models yields information on the effects of fibres and tendons on the functional

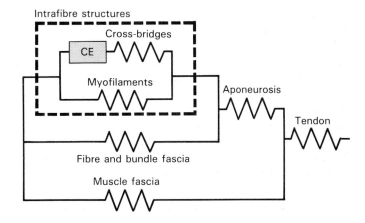

Fig. 6.33 Schematic representation of muscle models incorporating morphologically identifiable entities as fibres, aponeurosis, tendon and several types of fascia. The intrafibre structures are still represented as a phenomenological model despite the fact that some likely morphological units are indicated as intracellular bearers of SEC (cross-bridges) and PEC (myofilaments) characteristics. CE, contractile element.

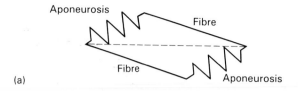

(a)

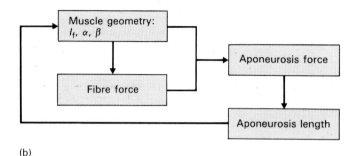

(b)

Fig. 6.34 (a) Schematic representation of a model of pennate muscle incorporating aspects of muscle architecture as well as elastic behaviour of aponeurosis. (b) A flow chart of iterated calculations of muscle geometry and force.

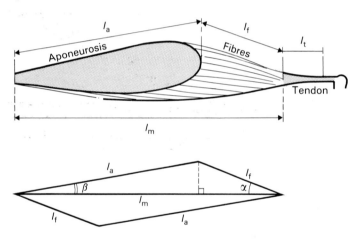

$$l_m = l_a \cos\beta + l_f \cos\alpha$$
$$\Delta l_m = \Delta(l_a \cos\beta) + \Delta(l_f \cos\alpha)$$

Fig. 6.35 Schematic representation of a method describing muscle length changes of a uniformly built muscle as a function of integral contributions of changes of fibre length (l_f) and angle (α) to muscle length (l_m) changes and those of aponeurosis angle (β) and length (l_a) changes. l_t, tendon length.

capabilities of the muscle. Particularly, if these models are run with parameters obtained on the basis of real movement very interesting results can be obtained (Bobbert *et al.*, 1986a,b).

Some of these results will be treated in Chapter 6D.

Figure 6.33 illustrates elements that may be used. It is clear that one of the major advan-

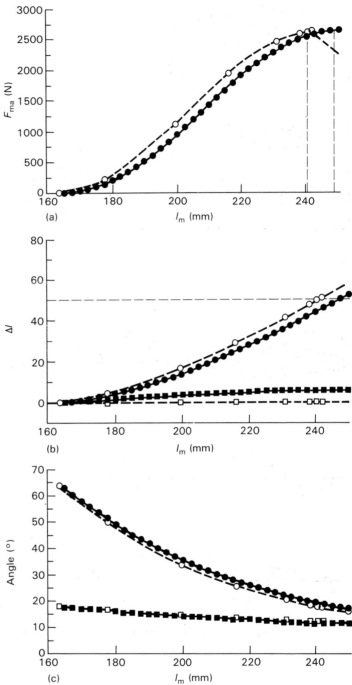

(a)

(b)

(c)

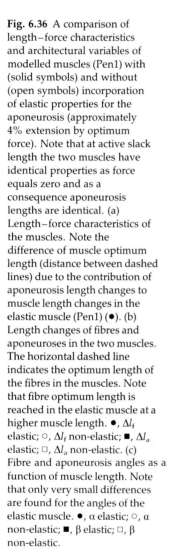

Fig. 6.36 A comparison of length–force characteristics and architectural variables of modelled muscles (Pen1) with (solid symbols) and without (open symbols) incorporation of elastic properties for the aponeurosis (approximately 4% extension by optimum force). Note that at active slack length the two muscles have identical properties as force equals zero and as a consequence aponeurosis lengths are identical. (a) Length–force characteristics of the muscles. Note the difference of muscle optimum length (distance between dashed lines) due to the contribution of aponeurosis length changes to muscle length changes in the elastic muscle (Pen1) (●). (b) Length changes of fibres and aponeuroses in the two muscles. The horizontal dashed line indicates the optimum length of the fibres in the muscles. Note that fibre optimum length is reached in the elastic muscle at a higher muscle length. ●, Δl_f elastic; ○, Δl_f non-elastic; ■, Δl_a elastic; □, Δl_a non-elastic. (c) Fibre and aponeurosis angles as a function of muscle length. Note that only very small differences are found for the angles of the elastic muscle. ●, α elastic; ○, α non-elastic; ■, β elastic; □, β non-elastic.

tages of the Hill-type approach is lost: the model becomes rather complicated. A great deal of work of this type has been performed by Hatze (e.g. 1981). Unfortunately, the effects of this work on people working in movement sciences has been rather limited.

Muscle models incorporating muscle morphology and elastic behaviour

Models of this type are more complex because they involve not only interactions between muscle geometry and fibre length as major determinants of muscle force, but also between exerted force and muscle geometry. Only a few examples of these types of models are known, e.g. Hatze, 1981; Otten, 1988. The model used in this section (Fig. 6.34) was developed by Ettema and Huijing (unpublished observations). In this model, force exerted by the fibres is calculated on the basis of fibre length, assuming fibre length–force characteristics. Calculations of force exerted on the aponeurosis is based on the mechanics shown above. Assuming aponeurosis length-force characteristics, a new aponeurosis length is calculated. Using this length a new muscle geometry is calculated and the whole process iterated until stable results are obtained. Thinking about muscles in this way allows the possibility

of comparing the modelled behaviour of parts of the muscle (e.g. aponeurosis) with its actual behaviour during muscle activity as observed in experiments.

To evaluate experimental results a system is then needed to describe not only length and angle changes of components of muscle but also to quantify their contributions to muscle length changes. The principles of such an approach (Heslinga & Huijing, 1990) are described for modelled muscle, Pen1 (Fig. 6.35). It is clear that muscle length is made up of two components: the length of the fibre and that of the aponeurosis projected onto the line of pull of the muscle:

$$l_m \text{ (fibre)} = l_f \cos \alpha \qquad (19)$$
$$l_m \text{ (apo)} = l_a \cos \beta, \qquad (20)$$

where l_m (fibre) and l_m (apo) indicate those parts of the muscle length as determined by the fibre and aponeurosis respectively.

This means that any change of muscle length can be quantified in terms of changes of these two projected lengths:

$$\Delta l_m = \Delta l_m \text{ (fibre)} + \Delta l_m \text{ (apo)}. \qquad (21)$$

Figure 6.36 shows force–length characteristics for the modelled muscle. It is clear that the length range between muscle active slack length and optimum length is increased because of

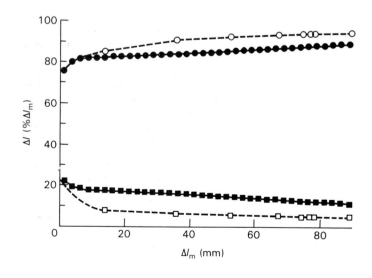

Fig. 6.37 Relative contributions (calculated according to the method shown in Fig. 6.35) of changes of fibre length and angle and of aponeurosis length and angle, to changes of muscle length. A comparison is made for muscles Pen1, modelled with an aponeurosis with and without elastic properties. $l_f \cos (\alpha)$: ●, elastic; ○, non-elastic; $l_a \cos (\beta)$: ■, elastic; □, non-elastic.

the contributions of the elastic aponeurosis to muscle length changes. As a consequence fibre length does not have to change as much to obtain a given muscle length change. Figure 6.36b shows that fibre optimum length is found at a shorter muscle length if a constant (i.e. non-elastic) aponeurosis is modelled. Only minor differences of fibre angle were found between these two muscles (Fig. 6.36c). The integral contributions of fibre length and angle changes to changes of muscle length as well as those of aponeurosis length and angle changes are shown in Fig. 6.37 for muscle Pen1 modelled with and without elastic aponeuroses. Note that as a consequence of elastic properties the contributions of aponeurosis characteristics are somewhat more important and those of fibre characteristics somewhat decreased. Force–velocity characteristics of muscles incorporating elastic aponeuroses are strongly influenced by contributions from these structures. Effects of elastic behaviour will be treated in Chapter 6D.

References

Benninghoff, A. & Rollhäuser, H. (1952) Zur inneren Mechanik des gefiederten Muskels (On the internal mechanism of pennate muscle). *Pflüger's Archiv*, **254**, 527–48.

Blangé, T., Stienen, G.J.M. & Kramer, A.E.J.L. (1972) Elasticity as an expression of cross-bridge activity in rat muscle. *Pflüger's Archiv*, **336**, 277–88.

Bobbert, M.F., Huijing, P.A. & van Ingen Schenau, G.J. (1986a) A model of human triceps surae muscle–tendon complex applied to jumping. *Journal of Biomechanics*, **19**, 887–98.

Bobbert, M.F., Huijing, P.A. & van Ingen Schenau, G.J. (1986b) An estimation of power output and work done by human triceps surae muscle–tendon complex in jumping. *Journal of Biomechanics*, **11**, 899–906.

Edman, K.A.P. (1979) The velocity of unloaded shortening and its relation to sarcomere length and isometric force in vertebrate muscle fibres. *Journal of Physiology*, **291**, 143–59.

Edman, K.A.P. & Reggiani, C. (1987) The sarcomere length tension relation determined in short segments of intact muscle fibres of the frog. *Journal of Physiology*, **385**, 709–32.

Ettema, G.J.C. & Huijing, P.A. (1990) Contribution to compliance of series elastic component by tendinous structures and cross-bridges in rat muscle–tendon complexes. In G.J.C. Ettema (ed.) *Series Elastic Properties and Architecture of Skeletal Muscle in Isometric and Dynamic Constructions*, pp. 33–51. Free University Press, Amsterdam.

Gans, C. & Bock, W.J. (1965) The functional significance of muscle architecture—a theoretical analysis. *Ergebnisse der Anatomie und Entwickelungs Geschichte*, **38**, 115–42.

Goldspink, G. (1968) Sarcomere length during postnatal growth of mammalian muscle fibres. *Journal of Cell Science*, **3**, 539–48.

Gordon, A.M., Huxley, A.F. & Julian, F.J. (1966a) Tension development in highly stretched vertebrate muscle fibres. *Journal of Physiology*, **184**, 143–69.

Gordon, A.M., Huxley, A.F. & Julian, F.J. (1966b) The variation in isometric tension with sarcomere length in vertebrate muscle fibres. *Journal of Physiology*, **184**, 170–92.

Granzier, H.L.M., ter Keurs, H.E.D.J. & Akster, H.A. (1984) The force sarcomere length relations of two perch muscle fiber types that have thin filaments of different length. *Biophysical Journal*, **45**, 155.

Hatze, H. (1981) *Myocybernetic control models of skeletal muscle: Characteristics and applications.* University of South Africa, Muckleneuk, Pretoria.

Herzog, W. & ter Keurs, H.E.D.J. (1989) Force–length relation of *in vivo* human rectus femoris muscles. *Pflüger's Archiv*, **411**, 642–7.

Heslinga, J.W. & Huijing, P.A. (1990) Effects of growth on architecture and functional characteristics of adult rat gastrocnemius muscle. *Journal of Morphology*, **206**, 119–32.

Hill, A.V. (1970) *First and Last Experiments in Muscle Mechanics.* Cambridge University Press, Cambridge.

Huijing, P.A. (1985) The architecture of the human gastrocnemius muscle and some functional consequences. *Acta Anatomica*, **123**, 101–7.

Huijing, P.A. (1988) Determinants of length range of active force exertion. In G. Harris & C. Walker (eds) *Proceedings of the Annual Conference of IEEE Engineering in Medicine and Biology Society*, Vol. 10, Part 4, pp. 1665–6. Publishing Service IEEE, New York.

Huijing, P.A., Greuell, A.E., Wajon, M.H. & Woittiez, R.D. (1987) An analysis of human isometric voluntary plantar flexion as a function of knee and ankle angle. In G. Bergman, R. Kolbel & R.A. Rohlmann (eds) *Biomechanics: Basic and Applied Research*, pp. 662–7. Nijhoff, Dordrecht.

Huijing, P.A., van Lookeren Campagne, A.H.H. & Koper, J.F. (1989) Muscle architecture and fibre characteristics of rat gastrocnemius and semimembranosus muscles during isometric contraction. *Acta Anatomica*, 135, 46–52.

Huijing, P.A., Wajon, M.H., Greuell, A.E. & Woittiez, R.D. (1986) Muscle excitation during voluntary maximal plantar flexion: A mechanical and electromyographic analysis. In G.V. Kondraske & C.J. Robinson (eds) *Proceedings of the VIII Conference of IEEE Engineering in Medicine and Biology Society, Vol. I*, pp. 637–9. Publishing Service IEEE, Piscataway, New Jersey.

Huijing, P.A. & Woittiez, R.D. (1984) The effect of architecture on skeletal muscle performance: a simple planimetric model. *Netherlands Journal of Zoology*, 34, 21–32.

Huijing, P.A. & Woittiez, R.D. (1985) Notes on planimetric and three-dimensional muscle models. *Netherlands Journal of Zoology*, 35, 521–5.

Huxley, A.F. (1957) Muscle structure and theories of contraction. *Progress in Biophysics and Biophysical Chemistry*, 7, 255–318.

Huxley, A.F. (1988) Muscular contraction. *Annual Review of Physiology*, 50, 1–16.

Huxley, A.F. & Peachy, L.D. (1961) The maximal length for contraction in vertebrate striated muscle. *Journal of Physiology*, 156, 150–65.

Huxley, H.E. (1972) Molecular basis of contraction in cross-striated muscles. In G.H. Bourne (ed.) *The Structure and Function of Muscle*, p. 387. Academic Press, New York.

Ingen Schenau, G. J. van, Bobbert, M.F., Ettema, G.J., de Graaf, J.B. & Huijing, P.A. (1988) A simulation of rat EDL force output based on intrinsic muscle properties. *Journal of Biomechanics*, 21, 815–24.

Julian, F.J. & Morgan, D.L. (1979) Intersarcomere dynamics during fixed end tetanic contractions of frog muscle fibres. *Journal of Physiology*, 293, 365–78.

Kardel, T. (1990) Niels Stensen's geometrical theory of muscle contraction (1667): a reappraisal. *Journal of Biomechanics*, 23, 953–65.

Morgan, D.L. (1985) From sarcomeres to whole muscle. *Journal of Experimental Biology*, 115, 69–78.

Otten, E. (1987) Optimal design of vertebrate and insect sarcomeres. *Journal of Morphology*, 191, 49–63.

Otten, E. (1988) Concepts and models of functional architecture in skeletal muscle. *Exercise and Sport Sciences Reviews*, 16, 89–137.

Pollack, G.H. (1983). The cross-bridge theory. *Physiological Reviews*, 63, 1049–113.

Robinson, T.F. & Winegrad, S. (1979) The measurement and dynamic implications of thin filament lengths in heart muscle. *Journal of Physiology*, 286, 607–19.

Stephens, J.A., Reinking, R.M. & Stuart, D.G. (1975) The motor units of cat medial gastrocnemius: Electrical and mechanical properties as a function of muscle length. *Journal of Morphology*, 146, 495–512.

Sugi, H. & Pollack, G.H. (eds) (1979) *Cross-bridge Mechanism in Muscle Contraction*, pp. 292–3. University Park Press, Baltimore.

Traeger, L. & Goldstein, M.A. (1983) Thin filaments are not of uniform length in rat skeletal muscle. *Journal of Cell Biology*, 96, 100–3.

Woittiez, R.D., Huijing, P.A., Boom, H.B.K. & Rozendal, R.H. (1984) A three dimensional muscle model: a quantified relation between form and function of skeletal muscles. *Journal of Morphology*, 182, 95–113.

Zahalak, G.I. (1981) A distribution moment approximation for kinetic theories of muscle contraction. *Mathematical Bioscience*, 55, 89–114.

Zahalak, G.I. (1986) A comparison of the mechanical behavior of the cat soleus muscle with a distribution moment model. *Journal of Biomechanical Engineering*, 108, 131–40.

Zajac, F.E., Stevenson, P.J. & Topp, E.L. (1986a) A dimensionless musculotendon actuator model for use in computer simulations of body coordination: static properties. In P. Allard & M. Gagnon (eds) *Proceedings of the North American Congress on Biomechanics*, pp. 245–6. Montreal.

Zajac, F.E., Topp, E.L. & Stevenson, P.J. (1986b) A dimensionless musculotendon model. In G.V. Kondraske & C.J. Robinson (eds) *Proceedings of the VIII Conference of IEEE Engineering in Medicine and Biology Society, Vol. I*, pp. 601–3. Publishing Service IEEE, Piscataway, New Jersey.

Zajac, F.E., Topp, E.L. & Stevenson, P.J. (1986c) Musculotendon actuator models for use in computer studies and design of neuromuscular stimulation systems. In *Proceedings of the 9th Annual Conference on Rehabilitation Technology (RESNA)*, Minneapolis, 23–26 June, 1986, pp. 442–4.

Chapter 6D

Elastic Potential of Muscle

PETER A. HUIJING

Introduction

The study of functional effects of elastic properties of muscles received its first major stimulus with the work of Hill (for a review of this work see Hill, 1970). Further impetus was generated by Cavagna and co-workers and Alexander and co-workers. For details the reader is referred to a book on this subject (Alexander, 1988b) as well as review articles (Cavagna, 1977; Shorten, 1987; Alexander, 1988a).

In this chapter some of the mechanisms relevant for the determination of the elastic potential of muscle will be considered and distinguished from other effects. In addition, an analysis of human jumping with regard to elastic potential will be made. Information regarding elastic effects in other human movement may be obtained from the literature: for walking and running see the work of Hof (Hof *et al.*, 1983; Hof & van den Berg, 1986; Hof, 1990) and for running that of Alexander (1988a).

Characteristics of the series elastic component

The part of muscular elastic elements that are most important for functioning of active muscle is the series elastic component (SEC). As the major part of this component is located in the tendinous tissues of muscle we will consider some fundamental SEC characteristics on the basis of these tissues. In most muscles these tissues are represented in the form of intramuscular tendon plates and extramuscular tendons (Fig. 6.38). Some concepts will be illustrated on the basis of relevant properties of the tendon, since these properties can be determined in isolated material so that interaction between muscle and tendinous tissues does not influence the results.

Length–force characteristics of isolated tendon

A lot of experimental work has been performed on the characteristics of isolated tendons (for references see Butler *et al.*, 1979). The tendon behaves as a non-linear elastic structure (e.g. Simonsen *et al.*, 1988). Some non-elastic properties, as apparent from small differences of force–length characteristics when force is increased and when force is decreased (e.g. Ker, 1981), are not considered in this chapter. An example of tendon force–length characteristics is shown in Fig. 6.39. In this figure, which is based on data of Woo (1981), length of the tendon is shown up to values of force at which the tendon–bone complex fails and breaks. It is clear that the right-hand part of the curve of Fig. 6.39a does not describe normal function (even though ruptures of tendons under high forces are not unknown in human movement). If the part of the curve well away from tendon failure is considered, it should be noted that at low forces very small changes

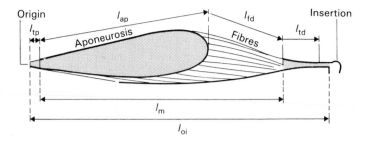

Fig. 6.38 Schematic representation of the muscle–tendon complex and its elements. l_{tp} and l_{td}, length of the proximal and distal tendons respectively; l_{fd}, length of distal muscle fibres; l_{ap}, length of the proximal aponeurosis or tendon plate. Note that the distal tendon plate, which is continuous with the distal tendon cannot be seen in the figure as it is located under the fibres of the muscle. l_m, length of the muscle; l_{oi}, length of muscle–tendon complex.

of force may have relatively large effects on tendon length. At somewhat higher levels of force, the slope of the curve (i.e. dF/dl) is increased, indicating an increased stiffness of the tendon. With still higher forces this increases up to a point after which a constant stiffness is encountered until failure sets in. This constant stiffness is supposed to represent stiffness of the collagen material from which the tendon is constructed. The increasing tendon stiffness found with increasing force at lower force levels is explained by the fact that collagen fibrils are not aligned with the line of pull in the tendon but are arranged in a network at some angle with the line of pull. Higher forces will align the fibrils with the line of pull and collagen material properties will become apparent. Many biological structures show qualitatively similar non-linear force–length characteristics (e.g. Fung, 1981).

Disregarding plastic deformation (i.e. history-dependent behaviour of tendons, e.g. Ker, 1981), tendons may be considered as conservative, i.e. all energy involved in stretching the tendon will be stored as potential energy and released completely as the force exerted on the tendon is allowed to decrease to zero. This is true because viscous properties (i.e. velocity-dependent behaviour) are negligible. As a consequence, force–velocity characteristics of tendons are not very important as velocity of length change is predominantly

determined by the velocity at which changes of force exerted on the tendon are imposed.

The above means that tendons are considered to have unique force–length characteristics and that the energy that can be stored as elastic energy equals:

$$W_t = \int F_t \, dl_t \qquad (1)$$

where W_t indicates the work performed on the tendon by stretching it, F_t is the force by which the tendon is stretched, and dl_t the length change of the tendon. If tendon length or change thereof is plotted versus force exerted, the result of calculations according to equation (1) can be visualized as the area between the force–length curve and the length axis (see also Fig. 6.39a). It should be noted that the value of W is maximized if sizeable length changes of the tendon are caused by large forces. However, for the higher range of forces the tendon is rather stiff. This causes the amount of energy stored to be limited unless the tendon is exposed to very high changes of force. In real life these increased ranges of force can only be obtained in muscles acting eccentrically, i.e. an external force stretches the active muscle–tendon complex to higher lengths, causing active forces higher than isometric optimum force, followed by a concentric action in which the forces drop rapidly. Such sequences of contraction are often referred to as stretch–shortening cycles.

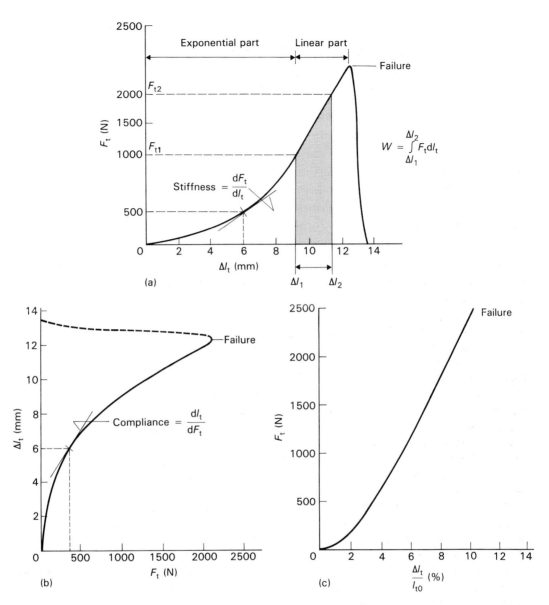

Fig. 6.39 Force–length characteristics of the tendon. (a) Force is plotted as a function of length change from the length the tendon assumes if no force is exerted on it (l_{t0}). (b) The same curve is plotted with length as a function of force. The same data is plotted in two different ways to illustrate the concepts of stiffness and compliance. The curve consists of an exponential part and a linear part, which are indicated in (a). The shaded area in (a) is a measure for energy stored in the tendon if force is increasing from F_{t1} to F_{t2}, which accompanies a length change equal to $\Delta l_1 - \Delta l_2$. (c) Force is represented as a function of tendon length changes normalized for l_{t0}. The figures are based on the data of Woo (1981) obtained for swine digital flexor tendons. The points marked with failure indicate failure of the tendon–bone connection.

The potential energy stored in a tendon or other elastic structure can be released by decreasing force exerted on the structure. If this is done slowly the energy will become available slowly; if this is done at a rapid rate the energy will be released fast. The amount of energy released per unit of time is called power. Power can be calculated as:

$$P_t = dW_t/dt = F_t \cdot v_t \qquad (2)$$

where F_t represents force exerted on the tendon and v_t the velocity of length change of the tendon.

An important functional effect of elastic elements is that muscle fibres can store energy in the tendon at a relatively low rate, allowing the occurrence of high levels of force because of force–velocity characteristics. Subsequently, the tendon acts as an energy pool, which can be applied to obtain high velocities of movement and thus high power output without imposing these high velocities on muscle fibres.

Location of elements of SEC

The SEC is thought to be located in the tendinous structures and the cross-bridges of the muscle fibres (Morgan, 1977; Proske & Morgan, 1984, 1987). As properties of tendinous structures and cross-bridges may be influenced independently it is important to be able to distinguish these two parts of the SEC. Only then is it possible to determine properly the characteristics and role of the SEC under various simple as well as complex loading conditions.

Experiments on the characteristics of isolated extramuscular tendons can only yield limited information regarding this matter, because most muscle–tendon complexes incorporate a sheet-like intramuscular tendon plate (aponeurosis). Jewell and Wilkie (1958) found a significant part of length changes of tendinous structures to occur at the aponeurosis. Rack and Westbury (1984) developed a method, using firing rate of muscle spindles, to examine properties of the entire tendinous structure.

Their results indicated equal normalized values of stiffness for tendon and aponeurosis. On the other hand, Proske and Morgan (1987) emphasized the possibility that aponeurosis properties may be different from those of tendon. Such differences could be possibly related to the complicated junction with the muscle fibres or differences of the form in which the material is arranged (round tendon versus plate-like aponeurosis).

Rather different values for the relative contribution of tendinous structures and cross-bridges to SEC length changes were reported. With respect to this, it should be noted that the amount of tendinous tissues may vary considerably with muscle architecture. Muscles composed of fibres that are almost as long as the muscle (belly) generally will be in series with relatively small amounts of tendinous tissues. Jewell and Wilkie (1958) found that tendinous structures accounted for half of the extension of SEC in frog sartorius muscle. Bressler and Clinch (1974) report that in their preparations of toad sartorius muscle the SEC is mainly located in the cross-bridges. Morgan (1977) found a similar contribution for cat soleus muscle, but a contribution of about 90% was found for the tendinous structures of gastrocnemius medialis of the kangaroo (Morgan et al., 1978). Recent observations (Ettema & Huijing, 1990b) on rat extensor digitorum longus and gastrocnemius medialis muscles showed that approximately 85% of elastic SEC extension by optimum muscle force occurred in tendinous tissues. For muscles having sizeable angles of pennation, the remainder of the extension is obtained from intracellular components as well as relatively small component related to fibre angles, which has been referred to as angular compliance (Ettema & Huijing, 1990a).

Determination of SEC force–length characteristics

It is clear that determination of force–length characteristics of the SEC and its intracellular

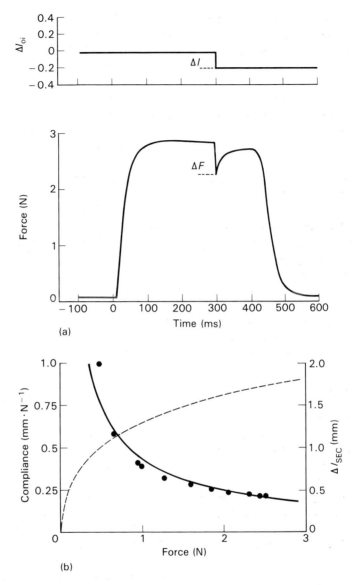

(a)

(b)

Fig. 6.40 Example of a force and length tracing of an experiment on rat EDL (extensor digitorum longus) muscle involving a very small but rapid length step imposed on the active muscle–tendon complex that causes a decrease of force (ΔF). The ratio of Δl_{oi} and ΔF is taken as an estimate for compliance (dl/dF) of the whole series elastic component (SEC), on the assumption that the length change imposed is so rapid that contractile elements of the muscle cannot contribute. (b) Data points for compliance obtained by a series of experiments as shown in (a) at different levels of force exerted by the muscle as a consequence of different levels of excitation. The solid line indicates the curve fitted through these data points and the dashed line the result of integration of the solid curve with respect to force up to the level of optimum force—the extension of the SEC, for which the scale is indicated on the right.

parts as well as of tendon and aponeurosis are of major importance for the estimation of elastic potential of muscle. Direct measurement of SEC force–length characteristics is not possible so that these characteristics have to be estimated from experimental results on whole muscle. For this purpose values for compliance (i.e. dl/dF) of the whole muscle–tendon complex are determined during activity. Note that compliance is the inverse of stiffness (Fig. 6.39b) and that integration with respect to force will yield the total elastic length change (extension) of the object under study. Figure 6.40 shows an example of application of such methods for rat extensor digitorum longus muscle.

Several methods for determining skeletal muscle compliance have been described in the literature. Three of these methods have been reported briefly by Bahler (1967) and Close (1972): (i) the quick release method; (ii) a method using fast constant velocity releases; and (iii) a method calculating compliance from the force–time curve of an isometric tetanic contraction.

Values for extension of the SEC by optimum muscle force generally obtained using these methods are in the order of 2–4% of the length at zero force (e.g. Wilkie, 1956; Bobbert et al., 1986c; Ettema & Huijing, 1989). Only Bahler (1967), using complicated extrapolation methods, reported values up to 10%. Rack and Westbury (1984), using quite different methods, found values of stiffness of the tendinous component compatible with the lower values of stretch on exertion of optimum muscle force.

Tendinous structures in active muscle–tendon complexes

Methods used to determine integral stiffness of all tendinous structures of the muscle–tendon complex (i.e. tendons and aponeuroses) were developed and applied by Morgan (1977) and Rack and Westbury (1984). These experiments provide information about the contribution of the tendon–aponeurosis complex to compli-

ance of the total SEC. Rack and Westbury (1984), who imposed small sinusoidal variations of length of the tendinous component while keeping active muscle fibres at constant length, compared their results with compliance measurements on tendon, and concluded that normalized compliance of the aponeurosis was similar to that of tendon and thus that differences of absolute values of compliance found should be explained by the differences of elastic material arranged in series in these structures. In contrast, Proske and Morgan (1987) concluded that differences of compliance between free tendon and aponeurosis may exist. Morphometric methods involving photography of aponeurosis and tendons of active muscles were applied recently (Huijing & Ettema, 1988/89; Ettema & Huijing, 1989) to study length behaviour of tendon or aponeurosis in active muscle. These studies yielded results for aponeurosis characteristics rather different from those reported for the SEC and for tendon in the literature. For isometric and slow concentric muscle actions, relatively large aponeurosis length changes (of the order of 10%) were found, while decreasing force of maximally active muscle from its optimum value to low values by changing muscle length. Isometric excitation of the muscle at its optimum length, involving similar changes of muscle force but no changes of muscle length, produced aponeurosis length changes in the order of 4%.

To explain these different values of the length changes, Huijing and Ettema (1988/89) concluded that, during actions involving sizeable changes of muscle length, a shift of the aponeurosis force–length curve along its length axis occurred. It was suggested that muscle length itself could be an important factor influencing aponeurosis length, by means of shifting the aponeurosis force–length curve (Ettema & Huijing, 1989) and thus introducing additional, but *non-elastic*, length change (Huijing & Ettema, 1988/89). The concept involves on the one hand a unique curve relating aponeurosis *length change* to exerted force thus describing elastic behaviour of the apo-

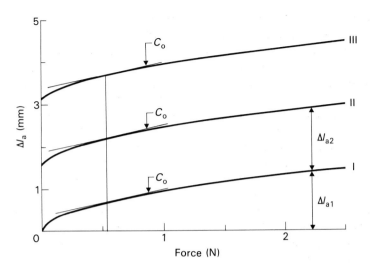

Fig. 6.41 Schematic representation of the hypothesis of shifting aponeurosis force–length characteristics (Ettema & Huijing, 1989). Changes of aponeurosis length are plotted as a function of force exerted on it. Elastic behaviour of the aponeurosis is represented by each force–length curve (I–III). Note that for a given level of force, compliance ($C_o = dl/dF$) of the aponeurosis takes on a given value. Length change Δl_{a1} represents the elastic length change for the indicated increase of force. If this hypothesis is correct, a second (non-elastic) length change of the aponeurosis (Δl_{a2}) is caused by some (as yet unknown) mechanism related to changing muscle length. As a consequence the total length change of the aponeurosis would equal the sum of these two.

Fig. 6.42 Schematic representation of the concept of distribution of fibre optimum lengths with respect to muscle length. Five different groups of fibres (I–V) are assumed, which have an identical number of sarcomeres in series. The physiological cross-sectional area of each group of fibres differs resulting in different levels of force for each group. The sum of these forces for any given muscle length equals muscle force if the modelled muscle is a parallel-fibred one. Note that the width of the muscle force–length relation is wider than that of its fibres.

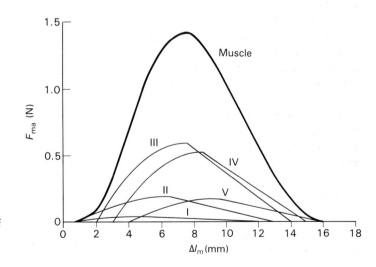

neurosis, and on the other hand the occurrence of muscle length-dependent non-elastic length changes of the aponeurosis (Fig. 6.41). This idea was reinforced by results indicating that for a given level of force, regardless of whether it was obtained by varying muscle length or by using submaximal excitation at muscle optimum length, similar values of total SEC compliance were found while aponeurosis length (determined by using macrophotography) varied considerably with muscle length in these experiments (Ettema & Huijing, 1989). Recent modelling work indicates that an alternative explanation has to be considered as well (Bobbert *et al.*, 1990). Indications can be found that muscle may be built inhomogeneously with respect to aspects of architecture. One of these aspects involves a distribution of fibre optimum lengths with respect to muscle length, i.e. not all fibre optimum length coincide with muscle optimum length (e.g. Fig. 6.42) (Stephens *et al.*, 1975; Huijing, 1988; Huijing *et al.*, 1989). As a consequence, force exerted on the aponeuroses by a particular muscle fibre could be zero even though muscle force is not equal to zero. It is clear that such phenomena would severely complicate the study of aponeurosis force–length relationships. Assuming the first hypothesis to be correct, it is conceivable that this could have consequences for muscular energetics. However, this would not be likely if the second hypothesis has to be adopted. Further experimental and modelling work on these phenomena are clearly needed to be able to draw unequivocal conclusions about functional implications of these effects.

Effects of elastic tendinous structures in stretch–shortening cycles

Stretch–shortening cycles of active muscles are common in daily movement (e.g. Hof *et al.*, 1983; Komi, 1984, 1986; Gregor *et al.*, 1988; see also Chapter 6E).

In order to illustrate most clearly the effects of having elastic tendinous tissues in series with muscle fibres, experiments on rat muscles *in situ* will be considered in which experimental conditions can be controlled in detail. The results of such experiments are compared for two conditions: (i) isometric build-up of force followed by a concentric action; and (ii) pre-stretch conditions in which muscles are excited near the end of a pre-stretch period, which is followed by a concentric phase of similar length range of the muscle–tendon complex. This pre-stretch condition resembles more closely patterns of excitation of natural movement (de Haan *et al.*, 1989; Ettema *et al.*, 1990a) than

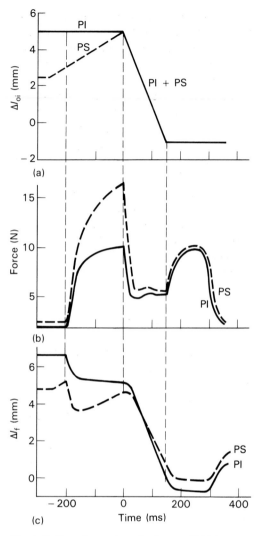

Fig. 6.43 Experimental results for a rat EDL (extensor digitorum longus) muscle undergoing a stretch–shortening cycle (PS) in comparison to an isometric contraction followed by an identical shortening (PI). Variables are shown as a function of time. Shortening was performed at constant speed (isokinetic contraction). (a) shows the history of changes of the muscle–tendon complex length. The first dashed line indicates the onset of excitation of the muscles, the second the onset and the third the end of shortening. Note that force exerted by the PS muscles during shortening (b) is considerably elevated with respect to PI muscles and that the drop of force on shortening is considerably increased as well. Some differences of fibre length are apparent in (c).

the classical experiments in which the muscle was excited first and made to perform an eccentric action before acting concentrically (e.g. Cavagna *et al.*, 1968, 1981, 1985; Cavagna & Citterio, 1974; Edman *et al.*, 1978).

Figure 6.43a shows that muscle–tendon complex length changes in the concentric phase of the action are identical in the pre-isometric and pre-stretch conditions. The force generated in the pre-stretch action is considerably higher during the stretch phase than during the isometric phase, which leads to a higher initial force at the onset of the concentric phase. During all of the concentric phase, force of the pre-stretch action remains higher than during the pre-isometric action. An important aspect within the scope of elastic potential is the fact that the force drop in the first part of the concentric phase is much enhanced for the pre-stretch action as compared to the isometric action. As length change is identical in these two conditions, it is clear that more work (calculated according to equation (1)) is performed in the concentric phase of the pre-stretch action (see also de Haan *et al.*, 1989; Ettema *et al.*, 1990a). The results of a recent study (Ettema *et al.*, 1990b) show that effects of pre-stretch on positive work output of a muscle–tendon complex can be explained on the basis of three mechanisms.

Release of additional elastic energy

Additional elastic energy is released in the enhanced recoil after pre-stretch. The relative contribution to total work of this extra recoil depends strongly on the actual conditions of the contraction performed. In some conditions it explains completely work enhancement of the muscle–tendon complex, while in other conditions a substantial effect of two other mechanisms may be involved.

Interaction effects between lengths of tendinous structures and muscle fibres

The increased intial force in the concentric phase of a pre-stretch contraction will have secondary effects as well, which will be referred to as interaction effects between tendinous structures and muscle fibres.

1 As the length of the tendinous tissues is increased because of the additional force, for a given muscle–tendon complex length fibres will be shorter. The opposite situation applies as well. If force drops, for example as a consequence of a high shortening velocity (muscle force–velocity characteristics), for a given muscle–tendon complex length tendinous tissues will decrease and muscle fibres will increase in length.

2 Due to the increased drop of force the velocity originating from the recoil of tendinous tissues will be increased (due to release of additional elastic energy). Given a certain velocity of shortening of the muscle–tendon complex, the muscle fibres will shorten more slowly.

These differences of fibre length and fibre velocity, which can be seen in Fig. 6.43c, may have either a negative or positive effect on work output, depending on actual conditions. For example, if fibres operate somewhat above their optimum length, this effect will bring them closer to their optimum length allowing a higher level of force (positive effect on work). If this effect brings fibres to lengths smaller than their optimum length, it would decrease force exerted and have a negative effect on work output. Similar arguments can be made for the interaction effects on fibre velocity in relation to their velocity at which optimum power is generated.

Potentiation of contractile material

If the concentric phase of pre-isometric and pre-stretch actions are performed isotonically (i.e. at constant force, after an initial very fast decrease, Fig. 6.44), extra release of elastic energy cannot play a role to explain extra work performed by the muscle–tendon complex. In order to obtain isotonic conditions muscle length is manipulated. As a consequence differences of fibre length are introduced (Fig. 6.44c).

However, enhanced isotonic shortening after

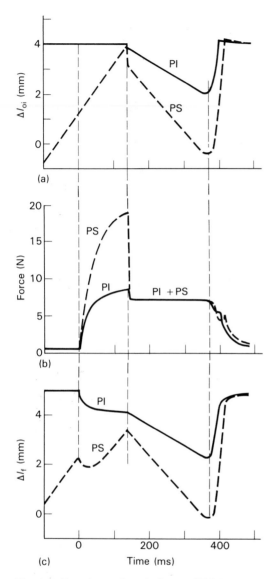

(a)

(b)

(c)

Fig. 6.44 Experimental results for a rat EDL (extensor digitorum longus) muscle undergoing a stretch–shortening cycle (PS, pre-stretch) in comparison to an isometric contraction followed by shortening at identical forces (PI, pre-isometric). Variables are shown as a function of time. Shortening of the muscle was performed at constant force (isotonic contraction) in order to eliminate differences of length of tendinous tissues and thus differences in release of elastic energy. (a) shows the history of changes of muscle–tendon complex length. The first dashed line connecting panels indicates the onset of excitation of the muscles, the second the onset and the third the end of shortening. Note the higher velocity of shortening for PS, indicative of a higher power and work output.

pre-stretch found at lengths above optimum length cannot be explained completely by differences of muscle fibre length between pre-stretch and pre-isometric actions (Ettema *et al.*, 1990b). This means that the CE force–velocity curve must have been shifted towards higher velocities for a given load. This feature is referred to as potentiation. As a detailed description of potentiation is beyond the scope of this chapter, since it does not seem to be related to elastic properties, the reader is referred to literature on this subject (Cavagna *et al.*, 1968, 1985; Cavagna & Citterio, 1974; Edman *et al.*, 1978; Sugi & Tsuchiya, 1981).

It is clear that in the study of elastic potential of muscle, the considerations indicated above should be taken into account. As a consequence, particular attention should be paid to elastic recoil of tendinous tissues as well as interaction effects on fibre length and contraction velocity.

Potential of series elastic behaviour in human movement

In order to illustrate effects of elasticity the role of human m. triceps surae in jumping will be studied in some detail. Figure 6.45 illustrates methods employed and some biomechanical results for one leg in a two-legged countermovement vertical jump. These results are obtained by non-invasive methods. If information is necesary about functioning of individual muscles in the performance of such movements data are also needed about some morphological aspects of these muscles. An important variable is moment arm, i.e. the distance between the axis of rotation and the force vector. If values of moment arm are known, the results of Fig. 6.45 may be expressed in terms of variables pertaining to muscle function (Fig. 6.46): length change of the muscle–tendon complexes and its velocity as well as muscle force.

These values can then be used in modelling simplified representations of the muscles (Fig. 6.47). These time histories of muscle–tendon complex length are imposed on the model,

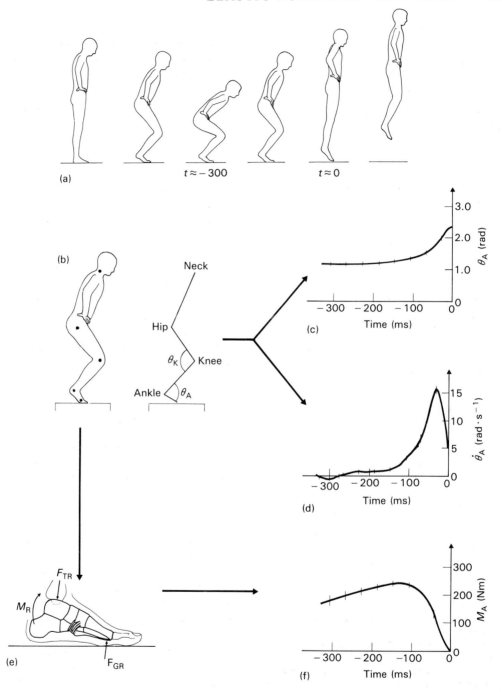

Fig. 6.45 Schematic representation of methods and some results of experiments on human vertical jumps. (a) Representation of images obtained on high speed film (100 frames · s^{-1}) of a subject jumping from a force platform. Results are plotted for the push-off phase of the jump ($t = -300$ to $t = 0$ approximately). (b) Using markers on the body, film data was reduced to stick diagrams for measurement of joint angles and angular velocity. (c, d) These results are shown for the ankle joint. (e) Using data of ground reaction force (F_{GR}) obtained with the force platform, the moment around the ankle was calculated (f). These results are further analysed in Fig. 6.46.

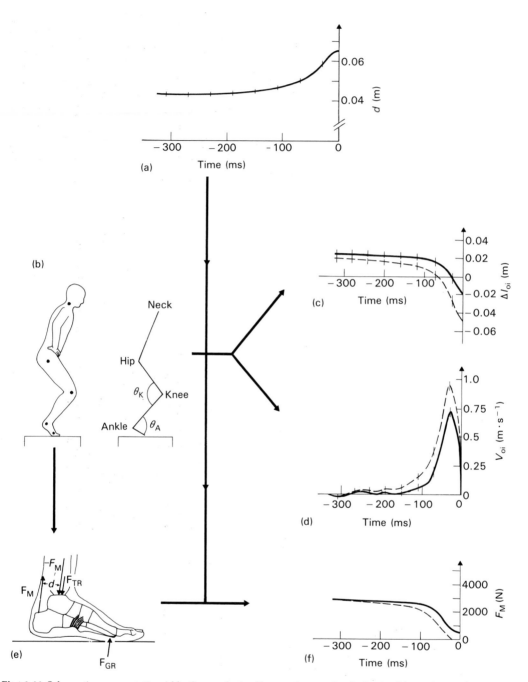

Fig. 6.46 Schematic representation of further analysis of human jumps. On the basis of data relating changes of joint angle to changes of muscle–tendon complex length (Grieve *et al.*, 1978) the moment arm of soleus and gastrocnemius muscles may be estimated (Bobbert *et al.*, 1986a,b) for the ankle joint (a) and knee joint (not shown). Given these relations the analysis can be extended to:
1 Film analysis (b) (results shown for the ankle joint in Fig. 6.45c,d) is converted to results for changes of muscle–tendon complex length (c) and the linear velocity creating these changes (d).
2 Ground reaction force analysis (e) (results shown for the ankle joint in Fig. 6.45f) can be converted to force exerted by the individual muscles (f).
Solid and dashed lines represent results for gastrocnemius and soleus muscles respectively.

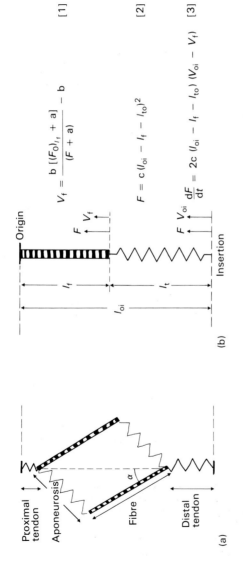

$$V_f = \frac{b\,[(F_0)_{l_f} + a]}{(F + a)} - b \qquad [1]$$

$$F = c(l_{oi} - l_f - l_{to})^2 \qquad [2]$$

$$V_{oi}\frac{dF}{dt} = 2c\,(l_{oi} - l_f - l_{to})\,(V_{oi} - V_f) \qquad [3]$$

where:

l_{oi}	is distance between origin and insertion,
l_f	is length of muscle fibres,
l_t	is length of tendon,
l_{to}	is length of tendon when exerted force is zero,
V_{oi}	is velocity with which origin approaches insertion,
V_f	is shortening velocity of muscle fibres,
F_f	is exerted force,
F_0	is isometric force at fibre optimum length,
$(F_0)_{l_f}$	is isometric force at some fibre length (l_f) different from optimum,
c	is a constant,
a	is the physiological constant in Hill's equation that is proportional to muscle cross-sectional area,
b	is the physiological constant in Hill's equation that is proportional to muscle fibre optimum length.

Fig. 6.47 Schematic representation of the muscle model used. (a) A schematic representation of a pennate muscle (e.g. m. gastrocnemius). (b) The morphological features are reduced in the muscle model. As only fibres and tendinous tissues are present in the model, only fibre force–length and force–velocity characteristics (equation 1) are dealt with in addition to tendon force–length characteristics (equation 2). Equation 3 describes the force of the modelled muscle in time. (c) Two such modelled muscles (m. gastrocnemius and m. soleus) mounted in a model leg and using data shown in Fig. 6.46c,d; the parameters of the model are set so that moment and force exerted at the ankle are in agreement with the results of measurements shown in Fig. 6.46f.

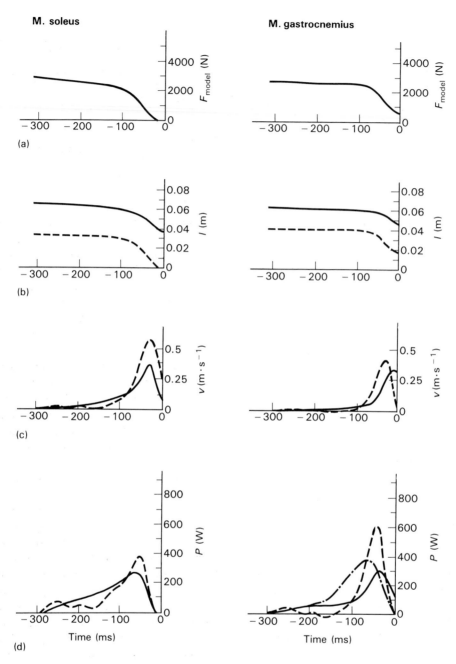

Fig. 6.48 Results of model calculations are shown for the human jump for soleus muscles (left panel) and gastrocnemius muscles (right panel). Using results for the change of length of the muscle–tendon complexes as well as their velocities (shown in Fig. 6.46c,d), changes of fibre length and tendon length (b) as well as their velocities (c) were calculated. The product of instantaneous values of velocity and force (a) equals the power delivered at the ankle by fibres and tendons (d). During push-off the knee is extended as well, which causes the whole gastrocnemius muscle–tendon complex to move upwards at a certain velocity. This movement aids plantar flexion. The product of instantaneous values of this velocity and muscle force equals power transported from knee to ankle joint (—·—). ——, fibre; – –, tendon.

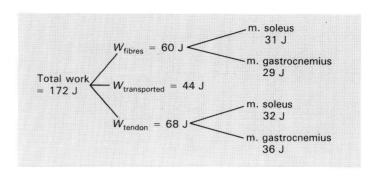

Fig. 6.49 Work performed by one leg during push-off in vertical counter-movement jumping. The sources of the energy are indicated on the basis of model calculations for soleus and gastrocnemius muscles. An elastic stretch by optimum force of 8% was assumed.

in which changes of muscle–tendon complex length and its velocity are assigned to muscle and tendon fibres on the basis of length force and force–velocity characteristics. The triceps surae (i.e. soleus and gastrocnemius) muscle–tendon complex was modelled (Bobbert *et al.*, 1986a,b) by simplifying it to a collection of muscle fibres and tendon fibres, thereby neglecting effects of pennation (Fig. 6.47a,b). In this case we only have to deal with muscle fibre length–force and force–velocity properties as well as tendon force–length characteristics. Figure 6.48 shows results of such model calculations. It is clear that the soleus muscle is exposed to increased length changes and velocities compared to the gastrocnemius muscle. This is caused by the fact that gastro-cnemius length changes accompanying ankle angle changes are counteracted by length changes accompanying knee angle changes. For soleus muscle, being a mono-articular muscle, this is not the case. To consider ener-getics of the muscle–tendon complex, power generation (i.e. energy delivered per unit of time) at the ankle was calculated by multipli-cation of instantaneous values of force and velocity for both muscle fibres and tendon (Fig. 6.48). It is clear that during the end of the push-off phase more power may be delivered by the tendon than by the muscle fibres for both gastrocnemius and soleus muscles. Such a feature is also apparent if the sources of the work delivered in the push-off phase is considered (Fig. 6.49). Most of the mechanical work performed originates from elastic energy

released from the tendon fibres during the push-off as a consequence of decreasing muscle force. It must of course be recognized that at an earlier time most of this energy also originated from a muscular source: during the counter-movement, not shown in the graphs, the tendon fibres are stretched by high forces possible because of eccentrically acting muscle fibres.

During the push-off the muscle fibres also contribute substantial energy to the movement. A third source of energy is indicated as well: transport of energy from the knee to the ankle joint by means of the gastrocnemius muscle. Work delivered by knee extensor muscles is used to create movement (plantar flexion) in the ankle. As this is not related to elastic properties of muscle, this feature will not be considered any further here, despite its import-ance for human movement (Gregoire *et al.*, 1984; Bobbert *et al.*, 1986a,b; Bobbert & van Ingen Schenau, 1988). It should be noted that such modelling as described above requires knowledge of the magnitude of a great number of variables, which are usually not known for human muscles for the obvious reason that human muscles are not usually accessible for controlled experimentation. The values of these variables were estimated. Therefore, the results presented in this paragraph should not be con-sidered as exact values that variables exhibit during human jumping, but as an indication of their order of magnitude and as an illustration of mechanisms that are active. Considering the above it is clear that elastic energy plays a very

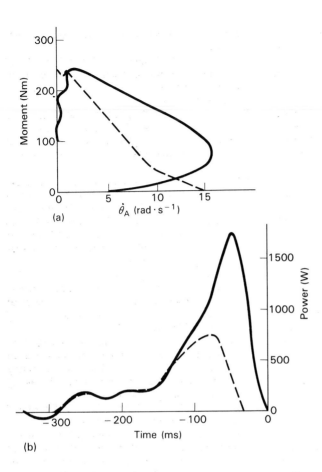

Fig. 6.50 (a) Angular velocity–moment curves for the ankle joint during the push-off phase of jumping. The solid line indicates experimental results and the dashed line results of model calculations in which the calf muscles are modelled without any elastic potential. Note sizeable differences of velocity for a given level of moment exerted. These differences between the curves must be explained on the basis of elastic potential. (b) The solid line shows power production at the ankle calculated for experimental results and the dashed line for modelled muscles without any elastic potential. Power was calculated by multiplying instantaneous values of moment and angular velocity shown in (a).

important role in human movement. This can also be illustrated with the use of Fig. 6.50. It shows a diagram relating angular velocity of the ankle to moment exerted around this joint. It provides experimental results in addition to model results for jumping in which triceps surae muscle was modelled without any elastic properties. Due to the elastic potential of triceps surae, particularly at the higher velocity of movement occurring during push-off, a 100% increase of moment exerted around the ankle is shown. This corresponds to high levels of power actually measured at the ankle. If muscle did not have elastic potential this power would have been much lower (Fig. 6.50b).

This is due to two main reasons also indicated in previous paragraphs.

1 Velocity contributions by the elastic structures allow, for a given level of muscle force, a much higher velocity.

2 Due to length interaction effects of elastic structures and muscle fibres, for a given velocity of movement a higher force may be delivered as the fibres operate at an increased length and lower velocity.

It is likely that explosive movements such as jumping and throwing could not be performed adequately without the elastic potential of muscle–tendon complexes.

It should be noted that some elastic potential for movement may also be found in tissues other than that of muscle (Alexander, 1988a).

References

Alexander, R. McN. (1988a) The spring in your step: the role of elastic mechanisms in human running. In G. de Groot, A.P. Hollander, P.A. Huijing & G.J. van Ingen Schenau (eds) *Biomechanics XI-A*, pp. 17–25. Free University Press, Amsterdam.

Alexander, R. McN. (1988b) *Elastic Mechanisms in Animal Movement*. Cambridge University Press, Cambridge.

Bahler, A.S. (1967) Series elastic component of mammalian skeletal muscle. *American Journal of Physiology*, **213**, 1560–4.

Bobbert, M.F., Brand, C., de Haan, A., Huijing, P.A., Ingen Schenau, G.J. van, Rijnsburger, W.H. & Woittiez, R.D. (1986c). Series-elasticity of tendinous structures of rat EDL. *Journal of Physiology*, **377**, 89P.

Bobbert, M.F., Ettema, G.J.C. & Huijing, P.A. (1990) The force–length relationship of a muscle tendon complex: Experimental results and model calculations. *European Journal of Applied Physiology*, **61**, 323–9.

Bobbert, M.F., Huijing, P.A. & Ingen Schenau, G.J. van (1986a) A model of the human triceps surae muscle–tendon complex applied to jumping. *Journal of Biomechanics*, **19**, 887–98.

Bobbert, M.F., Huijing, P.A. & Ingen Schenau, G.J. van (1986b) An estimation of power output and work done by the human triceps surae muscle–tendon complex in jumping. *Journal of Biomechanics*, **19**, 899–906.

Bobbert, M.F. & Ingen Schenau, G.J. van (1988) Coordination in vertical jumping. *Journal of Biomechanics*, **21**, 249–62.

Bressler, B.H. & Clinch, N.F. (1974) The compliance of contracting skeletal muscle. *Journal of Physiology*, **237**, 477–93.

Butler, D.L., Grood, E.S., Noyes, F.R. & Zernicke, R.F. (1979) Biomechanics of ligaments and tendons. *Exercise and Sport Sciences Reviews*, **6**, 125–81.

Cavagna, G.A. (1977) Storage and utilization of elastic energy in skeletal muscle. *Exercise and Sport Sciences Reviews*, **5**, 89–129.

Cavagna, G.A. & Citterio, G. (1974) Effect of stretching on the elastic characteristics and the contractile component of frog striated muscle. *Journal of Physiology*, **239**, 1–14.

Cavagna, G.A., Citterio, G. & Jacini, P. (1981) Effects of speed and extent of stretching on the elastic properties of active frog muscle. *Journal of Experimental Biology*, **91**, 131–43.

Cavagna, G.A., Dusman, B. & Margaria, R. (1968) Positive work done by a previously stretched muscle. *Journal of Applied Physiology*, **24**, 21–32.

Cavagna, G.A., Mazzanti, M., Heglund, N.C. & Citterio, G. (1985) Storage and release of mechanical energy by active muscle: a non-elastic mechanism? *Journal of Experimental Biology*, **115**, 79–87.

Close, R.I. (1972) Dynamic properties of mammalian skeletal muscles. *Physiological Reviews*, **52**, 129–97.

Edman, K.A.P., Elzinga, G. & Noble, M.I.M. (1978) Enhancement of mechanical performance by stretch during tetanic contractions of vertebrate skeletal muscle fibres. *Journal of Physiology*, **281**, 139–55.

Ettema, G.J.C. & Huijing, P.A. (1989) Properties of tendinous structures and series elastic component of EDL muscle–tendon complex of the rat. *Journal of Biomechanics*, **22**, 1209–15.

Ettema, G.J.C. & Huijing, P.A. (1990a) Architecture and elastic properties of the series elastic element of muscle tendon complex. In J. Winters & S. Woo (eds) *Multiple Muscle Systems*, pp. 57–68. Springer, New York.

Ettema, G.J.C. & Huijing, P.A. (1990b) Contribution to compliance of series elastic component by tendinous structures and cross-bridges in rat muscle–tendon complexes. In G.J.C. Ettema (ed.) *Series Elastic Properties and Architecture of Skeletal Muscle in Isometric and Dynamic Constructions*, pp. 33–51. Free University Press, Amsterdam.

Ettema, G.J.C., Huijing, P.A., Ingen Schenau, G.J. van & Haan, A. de (1990a) Effects of prestretch at the onset of stimulation on mechanical work of rat gastrocnemius muscle–tendon complex. *Journal of Experimental Biology*, **152**, 333–51.

Ettema, G.J.C., van Soest, A.J. & Huijing, P.A. (1990b) The role of series elastic structures in prestretch induced work enhancement during isotonic and isokinetic contractions. *Journal of Experimental Biology*, **154**, 121–36.

Fung, Y.C. (1981) *Biomechanics. Mechanical Properties of Living Tissues*. Springer, New York.

Gregoire, L., Veeger, H.E., Huijing, P.A. & Ingen Schenau, G.J. van (1984) Role of mono- and biarticular muscles in explosive movements. *International Journal of Sports Medicine*, **5**, 301–5.

Gregor, R.J., Roy, R.R., Whiting, W.C., Lovely, R.G., Hodgon, J.A. & Edgerton, V.R. (1988) Mechanical output of the cat soleus during treadmill locomotion: *in vivo* vs *in situ* characteristics. *Journal of Biomechanics*, **21**, 721–32.

Grieve, D.W., Pheasant, S. & Cavanagh, P.R. (1978) Prediction of gastrocnemius length from knee and ankle joint posture. In E. Asmussen & K. Jorgenson (eds) *Biomechanics VIA*, pp. 405–12. University Park Press, Baltimore.

Haan, A. de, Ingen Schenau, G.J. van, Ettema, G.J., Huijing, P.A. & Lodder, M. (1989) Efficiency of rat medial gastrocnemius muscle in contractions with and without an active prestretch. *Journal of Experimental Biology*, **141**, 327–41.

Hill, A.V. (1970) *First and Last Experiments in Muscle Mechanics*. Cambridge University Press, Cambridge.

Hof, A.L. (1990) Effects of muscle elasticity in walking and running. In J. Winters & S. Woo (eds) *Multiple Muscle Systems*, pp. 591–607. Springer, New York.

Hof, A.L. & Berg, J.W. van den (1986) How much

energy can be stored in human muscle elasticity? *Human Movement Science*, **5**, 107–14.

Hof, A.L., Geelen, B.A. & Berg, J.W. van den (1983) Calf muscle moment, work and efficiency in level walking; role of series elasticity. *Journal of Biomechanics*, **16**, 523–37.

Huijing, P.A. (1988) Determinants of length range of active force exertion. In G. Harris & C. Walker (eds) *Proceedings of the Annual Conference of IEEE Engineering in Medicine and Biology Society, Vol. 10, Part 4*, pp. 1665–6. Publishing Service IEEE, Piscataway, New Jersey.

Huijing, P.A. & Ettema, G.J.C. (1988/89) Length characteristics of aponeurosis in passive muscle and during isometric and dynamic contractions of rat gastrocnemius muscle. *Acta Morphologica Neerlando-Scandinavica*, **26**, 51–62.

Huijing, P.A., van Lookeren Campagne, A.H.H. & Koper, J.F. (1989) Muscle architecture and fibre characteristics of rat gastrocnemius and semimembranosus muscles during isometric contraction. *Acta Anatomica*, **135**, 46–52.

Jewell, B.R. & Wilkie, D.R. (1958) An analysis of the mechanical components in frog's striated muscle. *Journal of Physiology*, **143**, 515–40.

Ker, R. (1981) Dynamic tensile properties of the plantaris tendon of sheep (*Ovis aries*). *Journal of Experimental Biology*, **93**, 283–302.

Komi, P.V. (1984) Physiological and biomechanical correlates of muscle function: effects of muscle structure and stretch–shortening cycle on force and speed. *Exercise and Sports Sciences Reviews*, **12**, 81–121.

Komi, P.V. (1986) The stretch–shortening cycle and human power output. In N.L. Jones, N. McCartney & A.J. McComas (eds) *Human Muscle Power*, pp. 27–39. Human Kinetic, Champaign, Illinois.

Morgan, D.L. (1977) Separation of active and passive components of short-range stiffness of muscle.

American Journal of Physiology, **232**, C45–C49.

Morgan, D.L., Proske, U. & Warren D. (1978) Measurement of muscle stiffness and the mechanism of elastic storage of energy in hopping kangaroos. *Journal of Physiology*, **282**, 253–61.

Proske, U. & Morgan, D.L. (1984) Stiffness of cat soleus muscle and tendon during activation of part of the muscle. *Journal of Neurophysiology*, **52**, 459–68.

Proske, U. & Morgan, D.L. (1987) Tendon stiffness: methods of measurement and significance for the control of movement. A review. *Journal of Biomechanics*, **20**, 75–82.

Rack, P.M.H. & Westbury, D.R. (1984) Elastic properties of the cat soleus tendon and their functional importance. *Journal of Physiology*, **347**, 479–95.

Shorten, M.R. (1987) Muscle elasticity and human performance. In B. van Gheluwe & J. Atha (eds) *Current Research in Sport Sciences. Medicine and Sports Science, Vol. 25*, pp. 1–18. Karger, Basel.

Simonson, E.B., Edgerton V.R. & Bojsen-Moller, F. (1988) In G. de Groot, A.P. Hollander, P.A. Huijing & G.J. van Ingen Schenau (eds) *Biomechanics XI-A*, pp. 31–7. Free University Press, Amsterdam.

Stephens, J.A., Reinking, R.M. & Stuart, D.S. (1975) The units of cat medial gastrocnemius: Electrical and mechanical properties of as a function of muscle length. *Journal of Morphology*, **146**, 495–512.

Sugi, H. & Tsuchiya, T. (1981) Enhancement of mechanical performance in frog muscle fibres after quick increases in load. *Journal of Physiology*, **319**, 239–52.

Wilkie, D.R. (1956) Measurement of the series elastic component at various times during a single twitch. *Journal of Physiology*, **134**, 527–30.

Woo, S.L.-Y. (1981) The effects of exercise on the biomechanical and biochemical properties of swine digital flexor tendons. *Journal of Biomechanical Engineering*, **103**, 51–6.

Chapter 6E

Stretch–Shortening Cycle

PAAVO V. KOMI

The nature of the stretch–shortening cycle

In Chapter 1 muscle exercises were classified primarily into static and dynamic types. The classification used in Table 1.1 (p. 4) cannot, however, be used to describe the natural form of muscle function. Muscular exercises seldom involve pure forms of isolated isometric, concentric or eccentric actions. This is because the body segments are periodically subjected to impact forces (Fig. 6.51), as in running or jumping, or because some external force such as gravity lengthens the muscle. In these phases the muscles are acting eccentrically, and concentric action follows. By definition of eccentric action, the muscles must be active during the stretching phase. The combination of eccentric and concentric actions forms a natural type of muscle function called a *stretch–shortening cycle* or SSC (Norman & Komi, 1979; Komi, 1984).

The purpose of SSC is to make the final action (concentric phase) more powerful than that resulting from the concentric action alone. Since Cavagna *et al.* (1965) introduced the basic mechanisms of work enhancement when an isolated muscle was subjected to active stretch (eccentric action) prior to its shortening (concentric action), considerable scientific work has been devoted to explain the detailed mechanisms of force and power potentiation in SSC. Most of the work has come from experiments with isolated muscle preparations or from

mechanical muscle models. These experiments have increased our understanding of this phenomenon, which was simply called elastic potentiation. For details of the current mechanisms of performance potentiation the reader is referred to Chapter 6D.

In vivo demonstration of SSC in natural human locomotion

Whole body exercise involves many joints and groups of muscles. In this complex but well coordinated act each muscle makes its own contribution, usually in the form of SSC action. Identification of SSC for an individual muscle in a particular exercise is often very difficult, and sometimes even impossible. Direct measurements require knowledge of instantaneous forces and changes in muscle–tendon lengths. Methods to calculate length changes separately in muscular and tendon components are not very reliable, and therefore the length is usually expressed for the total segment including both muscular and tendinosus material.

Direct *in vivo* measurement of force requires implantation of a force transducer around the tendon (Fig. 6.52). *In vivo* registration has been applied primarily in animal experiments and has produced considerable information on the mechanical behaviour of the Achilles tendon (AT), e.g. in cat locomotion (Walmsley *et al.*, 1978). A method which directly records forces on human AT using an implanted transducer has been reported recently (Komi *et al.*, 1987b;

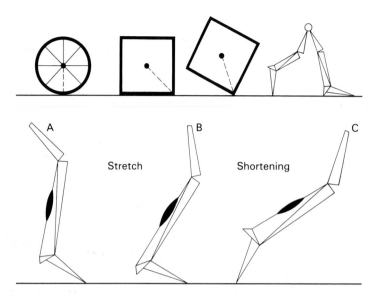

A   Stretch   B   Shortening   C

Fig. 6.51 Human walking and running do not resemble the movement of a rotating wheel, where the centre of gravity is always directly above the point of contact and perpendicular to the line of progression. Instead they resemble the action of a 'rolling' cube and have considerable impact loads when contact takes place with the ground. Before contact the muscles are preactivated (A) and ready to resist the impact, during which they are stretched (B). The stretch phase is followed by a shortening (concentric) action (C). The lower part of the figure demonstrates the SSC, which is the natural form of muscle function. (From Komi, 1984.)

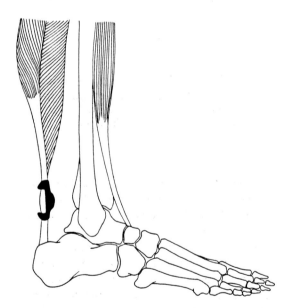

Fig. 6.52 Schematic diagram showing the position of the 'buckle' transducer around the Achilles tendon.

Komi, 1990). This *in vivo* technique utilizes either an E-form or a buckle-type transducer, of which the latter has proven to be more convenient. The transducer is implanted under local anaesthesia around the AT of adult

volunteers. After appropriate calibration procedures the subjects can perform normal unrestricted locomotion including walking, running at different speeds, hopping, jumping and bicycling. In some cases even maximal efforts were performed without any discomfort. All movements were performed either on a long force platform or on a bicycle which had special force transducers on the pedals. Electromyograph (EMG) activities were registered from the major leg muscles. AT force (ATF) and EMGs were telemetred, and all the signals were stored on magnetic tape. The entire measurement lasted 2–3 hours, after which the transducer was removed. Each performance was also filmed at 100 frames $\cdot$ s^{-1} so that the percent changes of the lengths of the gastrocnemius and soleus muscles could be estimated (Grieve *et al.*, 1978). This estimation was then used to calculate the force–length and force–velocity curves for the two muscles. It must be emphasized that in this analysis the force values represent the two muscles simultaneously because AT is a common tendon for both of them.

Figure 6.53 presents typical results (Komi *et al.*, unpublished observations) of the occur-

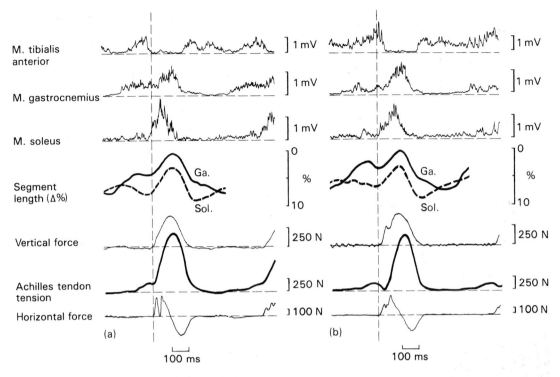

Fig. 6.53 A representative record of the Achilles tendon force and segmental length changes of the gastrocnemius (Ga.) and soleus (Sol.) muscles together with Fz and Fy ground reaction forces and selected EMG activities when the subject was running along a long force platform. The vertical line indicates the beginning of the ground contact as well as of the stretch–shortening cycle (SSC) of the muscles. The upward and downward deflections of the segmental length changes signify, respectively, stretching (eccentric) and shortening (concentric) phases of the cycle. (a) Ball running; (b) heel running.

rence of SSC in gastrocnemius and soleus muscles separately during running. There are several important features to be noted. First, the changes in muscle–tendon length are very small during the stretching phase. This suggests that the conditions favour the potential utilization of short-range stiffness in the muscle (Rack & Westbury, 1974). Second, the segmental length changes in these two muscles take place in phase in both the lengthening and shortening parts of the SSC. This is typical for running and jumping; it has considerable importance because the transducer measures forces of the common tendon for the two muscles. The situation is not so simple in other activities, such as bicycling (Gregor *et al.*, 1991), where the length changes are more out of

phase in these two muscles. The third important feature of the example in Fig. 6.53 is that the form of the AT force curve, resembles that of a bouncing ball.

The force–length and force–velocity curves can then be computed on the basis of the curves, as presented in Fig. 6.53. It must be emphasized that in this analysis the force values represent the two muscles simultaneously, because AT is a common tendon for both of them.

Figure 6.54 presents an analysis for the force–length and force–velocity curves during the contact phase in running. The force–length curve demonstrates a very sharp increase in force during the stretching phase, which is characterized by a small change in length. The

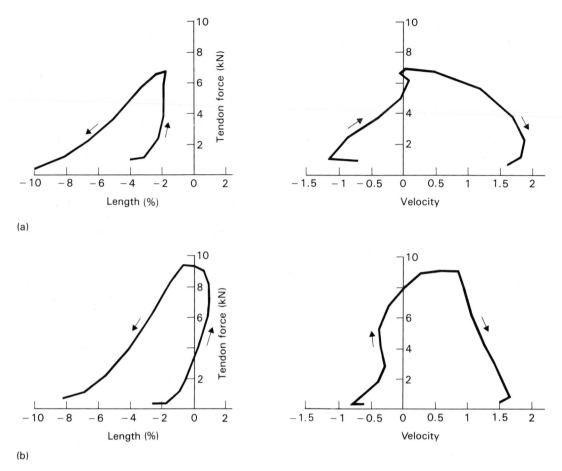

Fig. 6.54 Instantaneous force–length and force–velocity curves of the gastrocnemius muscle for SSC when the subject ran at two different velocities: (a) 9.02 m · s^{-1}; (b) 5.78 m · s^{-1}. The upward deflection signifies stretching (eccentric action) and the downward deflection shortening (concentric action) of the muscle.

right-hand side of the figure shows the force–velocity comparison demonstrating high potentiation during the stretching phase (concentric action). If these curves are compared with the force–velocity curves obtained with isolated muscle preparations (e.g. Hill, 1938) or with human forearm flexors (e.g. Komi, 1973) the dissimilarities are evident. It must be noted that these force–length and force–velocity curves are instantaneous plots during the SSC and may therefore represent more truly the behaviour of the muscles during natural movements. If the subject is running on two occasions at similar speeds, the analysis gives

remarkably similar results. Running at near maximum speed (9.02 m · s^{-1}) seemed to result in a lower peak ATF, but the length change in the eccentric phase was much smaller (Fig. 6.54a). The utilized muscle length estimates have shown that running and jumping are not the only activities where SSC can be identified. Recent evidence (Gregor et al., 1987, 1991) has demonstrated that the gastrocnemius and soleus muscles also function in bicycling in SSC, although the stretching phases are not as apparent as in running or jumping.

The in vivo measurement technique for humans has been developed following reports on animal experiments (e.g. Sherif *et al.*, 1983). Many of these animal studies have included similar parameters to those used in our human studies, such as muscle length, force and EMG. The most relevant report for comparison with present human experiments is that by Gregor *et al.* (1988); they measured mechanical outputs of the cat soleus muscle during treadmill locomotion. In this study the results indicated that the force generated at a given shortening velocity during late stance phase was greater, especially at higher speeds of locomotion, than the output generated at the same shortening velocity *in situ*. Thus both animal and human *in vivo* force experiments seem to give similar results with regard to the force–velocity relationships during SSC. Although the present human experiments cannot include some of the *in situ* measurements of Gregor *et al.* (1988), the form of the curves in Fig. 6.54 clearly indicate performance potentiation in the concentric phase of SSC.

The difference between the force–velocity curve and the classical curve in isolated muscle preparations (e.g. Hill, 1938) or in human experiments (e.g. Wilkie, 1950; Komi, 1973) may be due to natural differences in muscle activation levels between the two types of activities; this, however, can only partly explain the deviations. While the *in situ* preparations may primarily measure the shortening properties of the contractile elements in the muscle, natural locomotion, primarily utilizing SSC action, involves controlled release of high forces, caused primarily by the eccentric action. This high force favours storage of elastic strain energy in the muscle–tendon complex. A portion of this stored energy can be recovered during the subsequent shortening phase and used for performance potentiation. Both animal and human experiments seem therefore to agree that natural locomotion with primarily SSC muscle action may produce muscle outputs which can be very different to the conditions of isolated preparations, where activation levels are held constant and storage of strain energy is limited.

Mechanical efficiency of SSC exercise

If mechanical outputs of the muscle are enhanced in SSC action the logical consequence should be that the work efficiency is enhanced as well. Mechanical efficiency (ME) has been studied for almost a century and the textbooks of physiology have until recently referred to ME as varying between 20 and 25%. Experiments conducted primarily during the last two decades have shed some doubts on such a relatively low level of ME which varies only slightly. It is now known that the different forms of muscle action have different ME, and that the velocity of shortening or stretching influences its value (e.g. Margaria, 1968; Kaneko *et al.*, 1984; Aura & Komi, 1986a). In addition the SSC alone may introduce very different loading conditions and subsequently different ME.

Conventionally, mechanical efficiency of work (ME) is the ratio of external work performed to the extra energy production:

$$\text{ME} = \frac{W \times 100}{E - e}$$

where E is the gross energy output, e is the resting metabolic rate and W is the external work performed.

To examine the ME values of either isolated eccentric or concentric exercises, or their combination, the sledge apparatus (Fig. 6.55) was constructed. The apparatus consists of: (i) a sledge ($m = 33$ kg) to which the subject is fixed in a sitting position; (ii) a 'slide' on which the sledge runs along the slow-friction aluminium track; and (iii) the force-plate placed perpendicular to the sliding surface (for details see Kaneko *et al.*, 1984; Aura & Komi, 1986a,b; Komi *et al.*, 1987a). The relationship between enengy expenditure and mechanical work was shown to be linear in a small range of shortening velocities of the concentric exercise (Kaneko *et al.*, 1984), but when the movement velocity was increased (Aura & Komi, 1986b) this linearity was no longer true. For this reason ME of concentric exercise was not constant, but

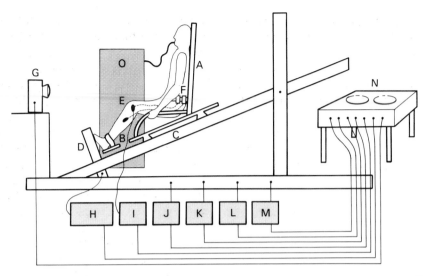

Fig. 6.55 The sledge apparatus and other necessary equipment used to investigate the mechanical efficiency of isolated concentric and eccentric exercises and SSC exercise. A, sledge; B, ankle support; C, aluminium slide bars; D, force plate; E, electric goniometer; F, EMG–telemetry transmitters; G, audio signal; H, amplifier, force; I, amplifier, 'Elgon'; J–M, EMG–telemetry receiving units; N, FM recorder Racal 7 DS; O, oxygen-4-analyser. For details see Aura and Komi (1986b).

decreased with increasing shortening velocities. In eccentric exercise, ME increased in all subjects when mechanical work was increased, and in some individuals it reached values over 60% (Aura & Komi, 1986a, Kyröläinen *et al.*, 1990). The evidence suggests that the ME of eccentric exercise is very high but not constant and that great variation between individuals is characteristic. The high efficiency can be improved by increasing stretch velocity, and it can be obtained with low motor unit activation. However, in concentric exercise EMG, energy expenditure and mechanical work change in parallel in slow muscle actions, but increasing shortening velocities will modify these relationships.

Pre-stretching of an active muscle during SSC exercise probably also influences the ME of the positive work phase (concentric action) of the cycle. Accepting that negative work does not have a constant efficiency value, then investigation of the ME of SSC exercise must be preceded by first defining that the ME of pure eccentric exercise is exactly the same in stretch-ing velocity and amplitude as the one to be used in SSC exercise. This method was applied in the sledge apparatus described above by Aura and Komi (1986a). Maximum concentric exercise (W_{max}) was defined as the energy level which the subject is able to exert in one pure concentric action. For each subject the positive work intensity was always kept at 60% of W_{max}, and the preceding eccentric action was varied from day to day. SSC actions were repeated 80 times on each situation at a rate of one every 3 s.

At the beginning of each exercise cycle the sledge was released from a certain distance corresponding to the specific energy level. The height of dropping varied the potential energy of the sledge–subject system and subsequently varied the negative (kinetic) work done during the breakdown. Within each exercise the dropping height was constant, but was varied between exercises, being 20–120% of W_{max}. During contact with the force-plate the subject resisted the downward movement (negative work), and immediately after stopping the sledge (knee angle 90%) the legs were extended to perform positive work. The effort in positive work was controlled so that the change in the potential energy of the sledge–subject system corresponded to 60% of W_{max}. When the sledge had reached its highest position, two assistants checked that the starting position corresponded to the specific energy level of the negative work. The mechanical efficiencies of the pure negative and pure positive work were measured individually for all of the subjects 1 or 2 days prior to the actual SSC exercises. The formulae for calculating ME during SSC exercises are given elsewhere (Aura & Komi, 1986a).

Figure 6.56 shows how the efficiency of positive work increases in SSC exercise when the pre-stretch load (negative work) is increased. The results therefore suggest that the efficiency of the constant concentric action can be changed considerably by modifying the preceding eccentric stretch load.

The most recent experiments (Oksanen *et al.*, 1990) have questioned the accuracy of estimating the ME of the positive work (W_{pos}) phase in the SSC. In our earlier studies (Aura & Komi, 1986a; Kyröläinen *et al.*, 1990), the calculation of W_{pos} of ME in the SSC was based on the assumption that the eccentric phase of SSC exercise was the same as in the respective pure

eccentric condition. However, EMG activity levels demonstrated that in isolated forms of eccentric action, the EMGs were much lower than in the comparable eccentric phase in the SSC exercise. Thus despite the apparently same mechanical work, the energy expenditure must have been different. This will naturally have introduced errors in the calculation of ME of W_{pos} in the SSC and the final result will probably be an overestimation. Higher EMG values would imply higher energy expenditure when the two types of eccentric phases, which have the same mechanical work, are compared with each other. However, the use of the sledge apparatus in studying ME of the entire SSC as well as of its two phases is certainly an improvement over the other attempts, which have used a constant value of −1.2 (or 120%) (Margaria, 1968) for the eccentric phase ME and then applied it to the calculation of ME in more practical type exercises (e.g. Bosco *et al.*, 1982; Ito *et al.*, 1983).

Fatigue and training adaptation of SSC exercises

Fatigue has been examined quite extensively in isolated forms of isometric, concentric or

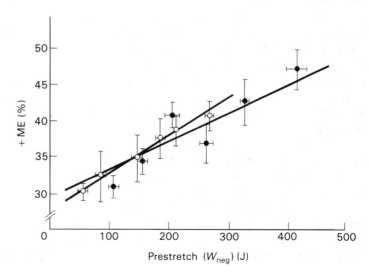

Fig. 6.56 The mechanical efficiency of positive work (+ME) in SSC exercise, related to the pre-stretch intensity (W_{neg}). The subjects performed SSC exercises on a sledge apparatus (Fig. 6.55), in which the take-off (positive work) was always at the same point on the slide bars, but the dropping distance (pre-stretch intensity) was varied on different test days. For details see Aura and Komi (1986b). ●, Male; ○, female.

eccentric actions. Because SSC is probably the only natural form of muscle function, it could be of interest to know how repeated SSCs are receptive to fatigue and how the fatigue phenomenon can be characterized in different parts of the cycle. Unfortunately, however, the literature lacks comprehensive efforts in this regard. The stretch reflex components are expected to play an important role in situations where stretching loads are high or efficient stretch–shortening behaviour is necessary. Under these conditions muscle stiffness must be well coordinated to meet external loading conditions. The sledge apparatus shown in Fig. 6.55 can be used for fatigue experiments using SSCs. In the study by Gollhofer *et al.* (1987a,b), normal healthy men performed 100 sub-maximal SSCs so that they were lying on the sledge with their heads toward the force-plate. The exercise was then performed with their arms. The results showed that during 100 SSCs fatigue was characterized by increases in the contact times for both the eccentric and concentric phases of the SSC (Fig. 6.57).

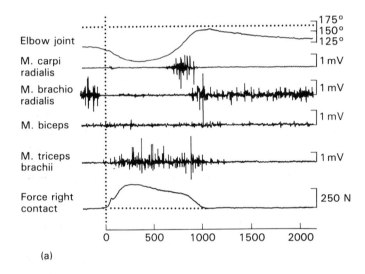

(a)

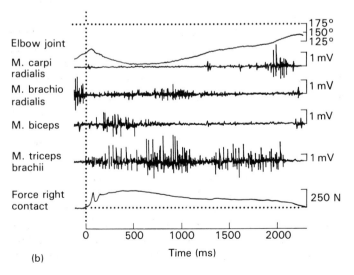

(b)

Fig. 6.57 Influence of exhaustive stretch–shortening cycle (SSC) exercises using the arms on EMG records and force–time curves. The subject performed 100 repeated SSCs on a special sledge apparatus (Fig. 6.55), and was lying with the head towards the force plate. Note the increased period of hand contact on the force plate between the first (a) and last (b) of the SSCs. Similarly, the initial force peak during contact increased with increasing fatigue. (From Gollhofer *et al.*, 1987b.)

Fig. 6.58 The subject in Fig. 6.57 also performed maximal SSC (high drops against the force plate) before (a) and immediately after (b) 100 exhaustive SSCs. The initial force peaks and subsequent drops increased dramatically due to fatigue. Rectified EMG records suggest augmentation of the short and medium latency reflex components (the first two shaded areas in the EMG records) during the test immediately following the fatiguing SSC exercise. (From Gollhofer *et al.*, 1987b.)

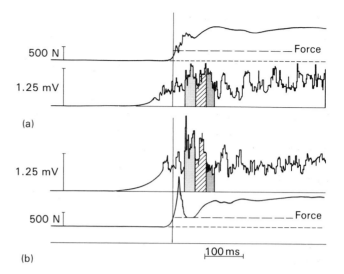

The force–time curves during contact on the platform were influenced by fatigue so that the initial force peak became higher and the subsequent initial drop of force more pronounced. More interestingly, however, the reflex contribution to sustain the repeated stretch loads became enhanced, especially when measured during the maximal drop-test condition before, and immediately after, the fatigue loading (Fig. 6.58). Thus in a non-fatigue state, the muscles are able to damp the impact in the SSC by a smooth force increase and by a smooth joint motion. However, repeated damping movements followed by the concentric action may eventually become so fatiguing that the neuromuscular system changes its 'stiffness' regulation. This change is characterized especially by a high impact force peak followed by a rapid temporary force decline. The enhanced stretch reflex contribution during fatigue could be interpreted to imply attempts of the nervous system to compensate by increasing activation of the loss of the muscles' contractile force to resist repeated impact loads. Recent studies on marathon running (Komi *et al.*, 1986; Nicol *et al.*, 1991a,b) have confirmed observations of laboratory tests which show that the ground reaction force curves, both during running and in special drop jump tests, imply reduced tolerance to stretch loads as well as loss in the recoil characteristics of the muscles.

It is, however, not known what could trigger the enhanced reflex contribution. One possible candidate could be accumulation of the metabolic products which induce acidosis in the milieu surrounding Ia-afferent nerve terminals. This hypothesis follows the observation of Fujitsuka (1979) that modulated Ia-afferent discharges in stretched muscle spindles of isolated frog muscle increased up to twice the value for normal pH conditions when the pH value in the extracellular medium was lowered by 0.1–0.2.

It may not be surprising that the mechanism of SSC fatigue is not well understood. What is astonishing, however, is the fact that the literature lacks comprehensive coverage of the mechanistic events which occur when the muscles are trained for several weeks or months using controlled SSC exercises. There is no doubt that special jumping exercises which utilize the SSC have beneficial effects on strength and power (e.g. Komi *et al.*, 1982). Chapters 9A, 9B and 18 deal partially with the problems of utilizing jumping exercises in power training. In addition to metabolic stimuli in the muscular tissue, training with SSC exercise specifically loads the components related to stiffness regulation. One of the main purposes of strength and power training is to improve muscle stiffness, especially in the explosive type of force production. It has been proposed (Komi, 1986) that the influence of the length-feedback component (facilitatory reflex), which originates from the muscle spindles, can be enhanced through training. This would improve muscle stiffness during the important stretching phase of the SSC. When the role of the inhibitory force-feedback component (from the Golgi tendon organs) can be simultaneously decreased, the final result is a further increase in muscle stiffness. This would allow the muscle to tolerate greater stretch loads, possibly store more elastic energy, and improve power as well as ME. In this regard Kyröläinen *et al.* (1991) have demonstrated that a 16-week SSC training improved ME. The greatest changes in ME occurred during higher pre-stretch intensities. The ME values changed from $49.3 \pm 12.9\%$ to $55.4 \pm 12.1\%$ ($P < 0.5$) in pure eccentric exercise with the legs as measured on the sledge apparatus. In SSC the corresponding overall ME, including the concentric phase, changed from $39.5 \pm 4.6\%$ to $46.1 \pm 5.0\%$ ($P < 0.1$). After training the subjects preactivated their leg extensor muscles earlier, before the impact, thus adding to the possibility of increased power during the braking (eccentric) phase. These observations look promising in explaining the possible potential of training with SSC exercises. Further research projects are, however, needed before conclusive evidence for comprehensive understanding of SSC training is available.

References

Aura, O. & Komi, P.V. (1986a) Mechanical efficiency of pure positive and pure negative work with special reference to the work intensity. *International Journal of Sports Medicine*, **7**, 44.

Aura, O. & Komi, P.V. (1986b) Effects of prestretch intensity on mechanical efficiency of positive work and on elastic behavior of skeletal muscle in stretch–shortening cycle exercise. *International Journal of Sports Medicine*, **7**, 137.

Bosco, C., Ito, A., Komi, P.V., Luhtanen, P., Rahkila, P., Rusko, H. & Viitasalo, J.T. (1982) Neuro-muscular function and mechanical efficiency of human leg extensor muscles during jumping exercise. *Acta Physiologica Scandinavica*, **114**, 543–50.

Cavagna, G.A., Saibene, F.P. & Margaria, R. (1965) Effect of negative work on the amount of positive work performed by an isolated muscle. *Journal of Applied Physiology*, **20**, 157.

Fujitsuka, N. (1979) The effects of extracellular pH changes on sensory nerve terminals in isolated frog muscle spindle (In Japanese). *Journal of the Physiological Society of Japan*, **4**, 21.

Gollhofer, A., Komi, P.V., Fujitsuka, N. & Miyashita, M. (1987a) Fatigue during stretch–shortening cycle exercises. II. Changes in neuromuscular activation patterns of human skeletal muscle. *International Journal of Sports Medicine*, **8** (suppl.), 38–47.

Gollhofer, A., Komi, P.V., Miyashita, M. & Aura, O. (1987b) Fatigue during stretch–shortening cycle exercise. I. Changes in mechanical performance of human skeletal muscle. *International Journal of Sports Medicine*, **8**, 71–8.

Gregor, R.J., Komi, P.V., Browing, R.C. & Järvinen, M (1991) A comparison of the triceps surae and residual muscle moments at the ankle during cycling. *Journal of Biomechanics*, **24**, 287–97.

Gregor, R.J., Komi, P.V. & Järvinen, M. (1987) Achilles tendon forces during cycling. *International Journal of Sports Medicine*, **8** (suppl.), 9–14.

Gregor, R.J., Roy, R.R., Whiting, W.C., Hodgson, J.A. & Edgerton, V.R. (1988) Force–velocity potentiation in cat soleus muscle during treadmil locomotion. *Journal of Biomechanics*, **21**, 721–32.

Grieve, D.W., Pheasant, S. & Cavanagh, P.R. (1978) Prediction of gastrocnemius length from knee and ankle joint posture. In E. Asmussen & K. Jorgensen (eds) *Biomechanics VI-A*, pp. 405–12. University Park Press, Baltimore.

Hill, A.V. (1938) The heat and shortening of the dynamic constant of muscle. *Proceedings of the Royal Society London B*, **126**, 136–95.

Ito, A., Komi, P.V., Sjödin, B., Bosco, C. & Karlsson J. (1983) Mechanical efficiency of positive work in running at different speeds. *Medicine and Science in Sports and Exercise*, **4**, 299–308.

Kaneko, M., Komi, P.V. & Aura, O. (1984) Mechanical efficiency of concentric and eccentric exercises performed with medium to fast contraction rates. *Scandinavian Journal of Sports Sciences*, **6**(1), 15.

Komi, P.V. (1973) Measurement of the force–velocity relationship in human muscle under concentric and eccentric contractions. In *Medicine and Sport, Vol. 8, Biomechanics III*, pp. 224–9. Karger, Basel.

Komi, P.V. (1984) Physiological and biomechanical correlates of muscle function: effects of muscle structure and stretch–shortening cycle on force and speed. In R.L. Terjung (ed.) *Exercise and Sport Sciences Reviews, Vol. 12*, pp. 81–121. Collamore Press, Lexington, Mass.

Komi, P.V. (1986) Training of muscle strength and power: interaction of neuromotoric, hypertrophic, and mechanical factors. *International Journal of Sports Medicine*, **7** (suppl.), 10.

Komi, P.V. (1990) Relevance of *in vivo* force measurements to human biomechanics. *Journal of Biomechanics*, **23** (suppl. 1), 23–34.

Komi, P.V., Hyvärinen, T., Gollhofer, A. & Mero, A. (1986) Man–shoe surface interaction: special problems during marathon running. *Acta Univ. Oulu [A]*, **179**, 69–72.

Komi, P.V., Kaneko, M. & Aura, O. (1987a) EMG activity of the leg extensor muscles with special reference to mechanical efficiency in consentric and eccentric exercises. *International Journal of Sports Medicine*, **8** (suppl.), 22.

Komi, P.V., Karlsson, J., Tesch, P., Suominen, H. & Heikkinen, E. (1982) Effects of heavy resistance and explosive type strength training methods on mechanical, functional and metabolic aspects of performance. In P.V. Komi (ed.) *Exercise and Sport Biology*, pp. 90–102. Human Kinetics, Champaign, Illinois.

Komi, P.V., Salonen, M., Järvinen, M. & Kokko, O. (1987b) *In vivo* registration of Achilles tendon forces in man. I. Methodological development. *International Journal of Sports Medicine*, **8** (suppl.), 3–8.

Kyröläinen, H., Komi, P.V. & Kim, D.H. (1991) Effects of power training on neuromuscular performance and mechanical efficiency. *Scandinavian Journal of Medicine and Science in Sports* (in press).

Kyröläinen, H., Komi, P.V., Oksanen, P., Häkkinen, K., Cheng, S. & Kim, D.H. (1990) Mechanical efficiency of locomotion in females during different kinds of muscle action. *European Journal of Applied Physiology*, **61**, 446–52.

Margaria, R. (1968) Positive and negative work performance and their efficiencies in human locomotion. *Internationale Zeitschrift fuer Angewande Physiologie*, **25**, 339–51.

Nicol, C., Komi, P.V. & Marconnet, P. (1991a) Fatigue effects of marathon running on neuromuscular performance. I. Changes in muscle force and stiffness characteristics. *Scandinavian Journal of Medicine and Science in Sports*, **1**, 10–17.

Nicol, C., Komi, P.V. & Marconnet, P. (1991b) Fatigue effects of marathon running on neuromuscular performance. II. Changes in force, integrated electromyographic activity and endurance capacity. *Scandinavian Journal of Medicine and Science in Sports*, **1**, 18–24.

Norman, R.W. & Komi, P.V. (1979) Electromyographic delay in skeletal muscle under normal movement conditions. *Acta Physiologica Scandinavica*, **106**, 241.

Oksanen, P., Kyröläinen, H., Komi, P.V. & Aura, O. (1990) Estimation of errors in mechanical efficiency. *European Journal of Applied Physiology*, **61**, 473–8.

Rack, P.M. & Westbury, D.R. (1974) The short range stiffness of active mammalian muscle and its effect on mechanical properties. *Journal of Physiology*, **240**, 331.

Sherif, M.H., Gregor, R.J., Liu, M., Roy, R.R. & Hager, C.L. (1983) Correlation of myoelectric activity and muscle force during selected cat treadmill locomotion. *Journal of Biomechanics*, **16**, 691–701.

Walmsley, B., Hodgson, J.A. & Burke, R.-E. (1978) Forces produced by medial gastrocnemius and soleus muscles during locomotion in freely moving cats. *Journal of Neurophysiology*, **41**, 1203.

Wilkie, D.R. (1950) The relation between force and velocity in human muscle. *Journal of Physiology*, **110**, 249.

Chapter 7A

Anthropometric Factors

KURT TITTEL AND HEINZ WUTSCHERK

Introduction

Strength is the physical basis for movement or acceleration of freely moving bodies (dynamic effect) or for deformation of immobile ones (static effect). Because of the hierarchical structure related to biotic systems an athlete's muscular strength depends upon somatic and morphological structures (Malina, 1975), which as well as being strength developing are strength transmitting and controlling (regulating) systems. There are, however, methodological limitations that result from specifics of the somatic and morphological procedures that are used when quantitative aspects of strength are investigated.

Muscular strength is causally defined by the contractility of the muscle fibres, varying in their morphological, physiological and biochemical (energetic) capacities. Contractile effects are transmitted to the skeletal system by the tight, collagenous components of connective tissues (tendons, ligaments); the spring-angle of the muscular fibres and the tendinous origin or point of attachment modify the level and amount of strength since they determine the lengths of the power or load levers. In any motor action, however simple, different morphological structures are always cooperating, so that athletic performance, where submovements are combined in a complicated manner, are based upon an interaction of agonistic and antagonistic muscle groups forming 'muscle slings' (Tittel, 1988, 1990). The complexity of all motor activities explains why athletic movements have been described rather simply so far. The structural exploration of strength capacity requires, therefore, further use of probability statistics, permitting the simplification (feature reductions, intercorrelations) and the investigation of subaspects (structural levels, subsystems). Substantial sport–anthropometric questions are, therefore, related to the effects of somatic variabilities upon the variance of athletic results.

Terminology

In sports, maximal muscular strength and power capacities represent essential elements of physical performance. Their characteristics consist in the athlete's ability to overcome resistances or external forces (friction forces, momentum at sport apparatus, gravity) by extremely high muscular tensions (Schnabel & Thiess, 1986; Neumann & Schüler, 1989). Strength itself is determined by the level of neural activation, which provides a better synchronization of the motor units, particularly during the early stages of adaptation. Its value is temporally relevant (Fukunaga, 1976; Komi, 1986; Komi & Häkkinen, 1988). 'Maximal strength' represents the skeletal musculature's capacity to voluntarily develop very great forces. However, they are necessary in their extreme form only in weightlifting sports where they approach the measurable athletic result. This maximal expression of strength is clearly reflected in a weightlifter's somatotypical features (see below) and becomes particularly visible by the extraordinarily high body-mass/body-height indices. For weightlifting it is important that the strength applied by the athlete is focused upon overcoming the very high external resistance (weight of the barbell). The 'load range' varies between 80 and 100% of the maximal strength. In other events, also termed 'maximal strength sports' (throwing or shot-putting in athletics, wrestling, rowing, etc.), there are not only additional performance factors (force–lever relations, coordinative abilities) that come into play, but also specific competitive conditions. These athletes' somatotypical shapes are particularly determined by the type and amount of external resistance to be overcome because of the varying strength requirements. This should be taken into account when strength training programmes are to be established.

External resistances can be constant or variable in their masses; they might be inanimate objects (sport apparatus) or an athletic opponent. These are the reasons why the mass characteristics of throwers or shot-putters differ from those of weightlifters, and both of these differ from combat sports (athletic opponent). In weightlifting, the amount of external resistance equals the value that can just be overcome physically by maximal muscular tension. These resistances are much less, however, in the throwing or shot-putting events, so that the somatotypical features of these athletes vary according to the mass of the apparatus (7.25 kg in shot-putting, 0.8 kg in javelin throwing).

Maximal strength sports are not, therefore, a homogeneous group. Terms like 'power events' or 'strength endurance' reflect this fact. Indeed, it could not be otherwise, since an athlete's muscular strength is the only active structural element, and the irrefutable basis for any motor activity. Required strength is determined to an overwhelming extent by the force–time or force–velocity principles. Seen this way, maximal strength in sports is a rela-

tive strength. This term includes various definitions, for example: (i) the relation between the muscle strength to be produced and the athlete's body mass; (ii) the relation between the maximally achievable strength an the level necessary for the specific event; and (iii) the relation between the strength reached by the athlete and his/her genetically–typologically possible level.

Maximal strength sports are generally acyclic. In some of the cyclic events that also demand high levels of strength capacity, e.g. rowing, the time factor must be added, causing the strength effort per motor cycle to decline clearly below the maximal strength value resulting from Hill's equation. Sport methodology allows for this situation by combining two diverging abilities: strength and endurance. In an anthropometric system of categories where the strength direction represents a first structural principle (centripetal, centrifugal), and the resistance characteristics (constant, variable, opponent) a second structural principle, the corresponding categories will come into existence by the strength characteristics. This makes it obvious that no formal limitations exist (Fig. 7.1).

Methodology

There are uncertainties in the quantitative registration of somatic or morphological equivalents (structures) of muscular strength. Functional–morphological test procedures (to assess the muscle fibre's spectrum, cross-section or surfaces as the size and frequency of cell nuclei) and neurophysiological analyses (to record integrated electromyographic activities) have been primarily laboratory methods. In contrast, anthropometry and somatometry, which the following concentrates upon, offer advantages for field and large-scale studies because of their simplicity, although the range of methods shows limitations in validity, making the original strength-determining structures only indirectly accessible. This is also true with the somatotypical measures,

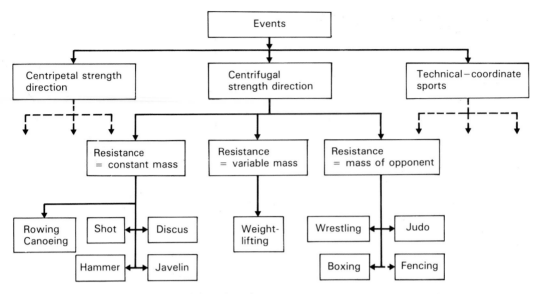

Fig. 7.1 Categories of sports from an anthropological view.

the variability of which causes the maximal strength capacity of an athlete to vary. The following somatotype measures should be regarded as features that are correlatively connected with maximal strength.

1 The circumferences of limbs. We should, however, take into consideration that agonistically and antagonistically acting muscular groups are also included in the measured values as are osseous or subcutaneous fat tissues. It seems important to relate circumferential measurements to those strength values that are most closely connected with these structures (e.g. hand strength: lower arm, hand, and finger musculature).

2 The total body mass as that of individual tissues (body composition) or body segments. Conclusions regarding the total strength of the body ('absolute strength') measurable by specific tests or by summing-up substrengths are admissible.

3 The muscle mass, the proper structural element of muscular strength, can be estimated anthropometrically (Matiegka, 1921). Using the body's total mass instead of its muscle mass, it is postulated that the first will change at the

same direction and amount as does the muscle mass. However, this is only true when the mass of the other tissues stays constant (body composition).

4 Surfaces and diameters as variations of muscular origins and attachments; meaning that power and load levers vary. However, none of the procedures applied so far, e.g. xero-radiography, computer tomography, can be counted as routine.

Relations between somatotypical features and maximal strength

Although only the somatotypical feature 'muscle mass' causally determines the maximal muscular strength, the 'total body mass' is the somatic equivalent to strength. It shapes the phenotype and can easily be determined. However, we may suppose from the high correlation coefficients between body and muscular masses that the variations of body mass tend to correspond to those of the muscle mass, so that conclusions may be drawn from the body mass for variations in maximal strength.

The vast majority of findings presented so far have confirmed this.

Mathematical relation between body mass and maximal strength

A large number of results are related to the issue termed by Lietzke (1956) as the hypothesis of the 'two-third strength', which assumes that changes of muscular strength are proportional to the muscle's diameter and thus to body height $(BH)^2$, those of the body mass (BM) to BH^3, and thus to the muscular strength of $BM^{2/3}$ ($BM^{0.667}$). This function has been included in many publications (Abramovskij, 1968; Tumanjan & Martirosov, 1976; Michailov *et al.*, 1981). Croucher *et al.* (1984) calculated lower exponents from data with weightlifters: 16.21 $BM^{0.557}$ in the clean-and-jerk, and 12.57 $BM^{0.581}$ in the snatch.

From two-event performances and the body mass of weightlifters participating in the 1986 European Championships, a polynomial equation resulted as the best approximation:

$$\text{two-event performance} = 89.19 + 8.974\,\text{BM} - 0.036\,\text{BM}^2, \quad (1)$$

which corresponds to the function of Croucher *et al.* mentioned already (30 $BM^{0.58}$). Even when a higher exponent is assumed (26.5 $BM^{0.61}$) a comparable approximation will result with variations of −20 or −18, +18 or +15, −12 or −22 kg in both functions at two-event performances. The function as calculated by Wutscherk (1990) is more exact: $[168 \times (\text{BM} - 43)^{0.24}]$.

A linear relation between strength and body mass as assumed by Vorobjev (1981) seems, therefore, unlikely. It might exist in restricted ranges of values as clarified in a graphic representation (Fig. 7.2) comparing measured data with lines calculated by Sabo *et al.* (1979). Performance data and body mass values of the six best weightlifters of every weight category participating in the 1980 Olympic Games (Fig. 7.3) illustrate the non-linearity of relations between two-event results (muscular strength)

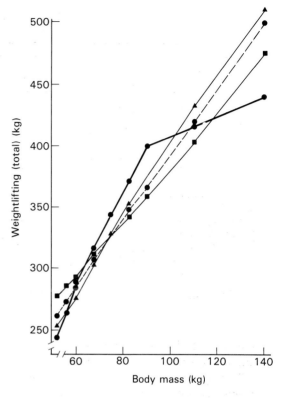

Fig. 7.2 Approximation of equations to real performances in two events (weightlifting). ●———●, real performance curve; ▲———▲, $y = k \cdot d^2$; ■———■, $y = a + bx$; ●-----●, $y = (c_1 \mathrm{e}^{-\frac{cx}{2}} + c_3)\,x$, where c_1, c_2, c_3 are constants and x is body mass.

and body mass in a convincing manner (Lathan, 1987).

The influence of body height upon muscular strength

Two-event performances in weightlifting certainly represent the maximum of achievable physical strength, so that it seems justified to call this performance 'maximal strength'. The subdivision of these athletes into weight categories also displays variations in BH since, so far, variations of BM have been assumed as being proportional to BH^3. High correlation coefficients ($r = 0.955$: Tittel & Wutscherk, 1972;

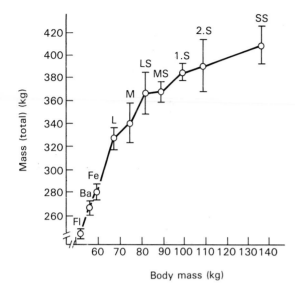

Fig. 7.3 Relationship between the total mass lifted and the body mass in two events of the six best weightlifters of each category in the 1980 Olympic Games. Fl, fly-weight; Ba, bantam-weight; Fe, feather-weight; L, light-weight; M, middle-weight; LS,light-heavy-weight; MS, middle-heavy-weight; 1.S, 1st heavy-weight; 2.S, 2nd heavy-weight; SS, super-heavy-weight. (From Lathan, 1987.)

Lathan, 1987) exist between the two somato-type features, BH and BM. Thus, maximal strength does not only require the adaptation-ally conditioned maximal muscle hypertrophy but is also genetically–typologically condi-tioned, as BM is enlarged with increasing BH. Muscle mass increases with enlarging BM, and so the 'absolute' body strength is increasing, too. These are the reasons why such non-linear relations are found as between BH and BM (equation 2) and two-event performance and BH (equation 3), as between BM and two-event result (equation 1). The following polynomial equations adapting optimally to the measured values have been calculated from the data of the best (European) weightlifters:

$$y_{BM} = 1708.34 - 21.67 \, BH + 0.071 \, BH^2 \quad (2)$$

$$y_{\text{2-event performance}} = -3512.88 + 38.670 \, BH$$
$$- 0.098 \, BH^2. \quad (3)$$

Representation of the maximal strength capacity in the coordinate system of body height and body mass

Maximal strength capacity is expressed in the coordinate system of body mass (y) and height (x) by the location of the point of intersection of both the somatotype features (Fig. 7.4). The relation between the three features (two-event performance, BH and BM) becomes obvious when it can be shown, by applying two ab-scissa (BH and two-event performance), that the two coordinates resulting do not cor-respond with each other in their non-linear progressions. It should, therefore, be assumed that the function for the relation BM/BH (equation 2) can reflect maximal strength capacities when no strength values are avail-able.

It is clear from those values of throwers and shot-putters included from athletics as well as from those of judokas, that other functions for the relation BH/BM must be valid in other maximal strength sports. Related sport-specific equations are, however, missing as are the cor-responding generally comparable values of strength capacity. The assumption that the progression of sport-specific maximal strength values approaches that of the relation BH/BM offers, therefore, another opportunity to assess an athlete's preconditions for his (or her) maximal strength capacities. However, this re-quires the non-distorted evaluation of indi-vidual deviations from their average functions. This has not been possible with indices that have been applied so far, e.g. BM/BH, BM/BH², BM/BH³, $\sqrt[3]{BM/BH}$, BH/$\sqrt[3]{BM}$ (Kopf, 1962).

All the quotients requiring linearity change dramatically in relation to the differing BH between the weightlifters' categories (Table 7.1) since the function applied does not correspond to the real progression of the value-couple. Using real progressions, however (equations 2, 3), calculating the mean values of BM and two-event performance and relating the per-centage values of the measured data to them, the quotients registered in all the weight cat-

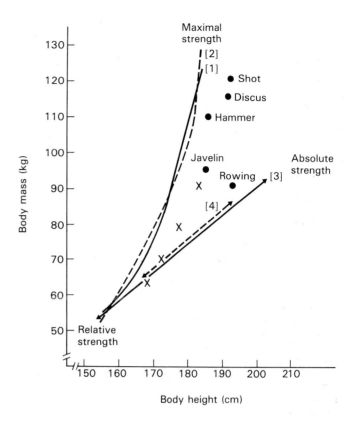

Fig. 7.4 Location of maximal strength sports in the coordinates of body height and body mass. [1], [2], [3], [4] refer to equations in the text; x, judoka.

egories reach about 100% (Table 7.1). Such a procedure is confirmed by the fact that the relative values of BM and two-event performance stay roughly equal and do not increase from one category to another. Some variability is maintained; this can be blamed partly on the inaccuracy of the equations, but mainly upon the varying constitutional adaptations of the athlete. 'Performance reserves' become immediately visible when the latter fact is stressed. Submasses of the body ('compartments' of body mass, i.e. depot fat, lean body mass, muscle mass, osseous mass and, perhaps, 'rest masses') must be assessed to include them in an improvable athletic shape. There are only a few available procedures but these are simple and very practical; however, they necessitate permanent calibration. Submasses of the body can be determined as follows:

1 Depot fat components should be calculated by applying tabloid equations (Parízková, 1962).

2 Muscle mass (kg) results (according to Matiegka, 1921) from:

$$L \times r^2 \times k,$$

where L = body height, and r = mean value of the radii from four diameters of limbs

$$= \frac{\bar{x} \text{ diameters}}{2\pi},$$

$$\bar{x} \text{ diameters} = \sum_{1-4}\text{diameters} - \sum_{1-4}\frac{\text{skin folds}}{2},$$

and $k = 6.5$.

3 The osseous mass (kg) results (according to Matiegka, 1921) from:

$$L \times o^2 \times k,$$

where L = body height, o = mean value from four limb diameters, and $k = 1.2$.

Table 7.1 Body height (BH), body mass (BM) and performance in weightlifting (1986 European Championships)

Category	Body height (cm)	Body mass (kg)	Body mass[1] (kg)	Relative body mass BM/BH (g/cm)	%[2]	%[3]	Performance total kg	%[4]	Total/BM (kg/kg)
<52	156.3	54.5	56.4	331	93	97	292	94	5.18
56	158.0	59.2	57.5	353	98	103	300	100	5.22
60	157.0	61.8	56.8	379	107	109	335	106	5.90
67.5	163.1	68.5	63.3	410	110	108	356	101	5.62
75	167.5	76.3	71.3	444	115	107	378	100	5.30
82.5	170.1	82.3	77.3	475	122	107	405	101	5.24
90	176.4	89.7	95.8	504	124	94	423	100	4.42
100	177.7	98.6	100.3	550	135	98	440	99	4.39
110	180.0	105.4	108.9	585	142	97	448	98	4.11
>110	183.5	123.2	123.4	706	160	100	472	101	3.82

1, BM calculated from equation (2); 2, BM% of a 'normal' population, from equation (4a); 3, real BM/calculated BM (from equation 2); 4, real performance/calculated performance (from equation 1).

For a 'normal' population other relations are valid for the interrelations between somatotype features and maximal strength. This seems to be reasonable since non-athletes do not possess the hypertrophy of skeletal muscles aimed at by imposing high loads. The term 'maximal' is related to the 'possible' level of a non-trained subject but not to the strength capacity he/she could reach by adaptation. The terms 'absolute strength' or 'total physical strength' correspond better to this situation than maximal strength does. There are many reasons why convincing findings are not available; among others the expected age-differentiated versatility, so that data from students' groups are used rather frequently. It seems, at first sight, astonishing that only low correlation coefficients have been found between absolute strength and body mass (e.g. also from Bale *et al.*, 1984, 1985). Their findings are congruent, however, and therefore gain some interpretation. Unexpected findings (Press & Komarova, 1974) stated that athletic performance in discus throwing with top-class athletes is much more dependent on BM than in younger athletes, who are somato-typically closer to the non-athlete (because of their incomplete training condition) than to

the top-class thrower. With non-athletes, the progression of BH and BM can, therefore, also be accepted as an indicator for absolute strength. It has, obviously, a linear character (Fig. 7.4), as demonstrated, for example, by the body-height differentiated tables of Möhr (1981). These values correspond to the 'optimal weight' for the medium type (Ott, 1963), as expressed in a regression equation:

Men: $y_{BM} = -69.6 + 0.8x$; e.g.

$$BH_{175} = 70.4 \, BM \quad (4a)$$

Women: $y_{BM} = -39.2 + 0.6x$; e.g.

$$BH_{165} = 59.8 \, BM \quad (4b)$$

where x = body height.

Optimal ranges for slim or strong types are different from each other but not for age groups. It might not, therefore, be surprising to see varying empirical data, e.g. for 18 to 25-year-old male and female subjects as registered by Greil (personal communication, 1983):

Men: $y_{BM} = -72.5 + 0.826x$; e.g.

$$BH_{175} = 72.0 \, BM \quad (5a)$$

Women: $y_{BM} = -58.0 + 0.709x$; e.g.

$$BH_{165} = 56.0 \, BM \quad (5b)$$

where x = body height.

We could summarize that the relations between the linear and the mass criteria and strength show a non-linear character in the maximal strength events. A linear progression may, however, be assumed for a normal population. Correspondingly, all those values relative to a normal population are inaccurate in maximal strength sports. They are expressed in the relative values of weightlifting, increasing from one category to another. It seems to be recommendable to utilize sport-specific curves, whereas weightlifters' strength dynamics or the calculated relations between BH and BM may be assumed when such data are not available.

Strength capacity and somatotype

According to the various growth tendencies of human beings, which are also expressed in strength-determining individual criteria, e.g. in body mass, different somatotypes have been defined. There are two procedures of assessment favoured in sports: that of Heath and Carter (1967) based upon that of Sheldon *et al.* (1940) and Parnell (1954), and that of Conrad (1963) where the so-called scheme of coordinates is applied with the metric and plastic indices used as ranking values. The advantage of both procedures lies in their metric basis, their disadvantage (like other schemes, too) in formalistic approaches concerning the type-determining criteria (Grimm, 1966), and the global causality claim (Seršantov, 1978). What findings can be reached, for example, by transforming the sum of three skinfolds into a scale of endomorph components or the quotient, $BH/\sqrt[3]{BM}$, in a scale of ectomorph components as compared with the analysis of the criteria within their real spectrum of distribution? This shows equally that differences exist between groups of various somatotypes regarding their individual criteria. These differences cause, as far as can be correlated with the corresponding ability, the relationship between the somatotype and its strength capacity. This opinion is also held, if not explicitly, by Bale *et al.* (1984, 1985) resulting from their presentations of strength capacities and somatotypes. They have concluded from the individual criteria characterizing the single types that 'the body mass represents an important factor of strength'.

Essential aspects of the correlative connection between somatotype and strength capacity have been demonstrated in the individual findings of Bale *et al.*, the data for which they collected from male or female students from so-called fitness groups. The mesomorph component showed the strongest effects in both the sexes when their fat component (!) and their lean body masses were higher than average. The endo-mesomorph group, termed according to rather formal aspects, showed the highest strength values, but also greatest body mass data. Indeed, the ranking order of body mass proceeds synchronously with the ranking order of 'total strength' in the groups (Table 7.2). This work resulted in the authors' conclusions mentioned earlier. A high level of muscle mass and fat mass above average must be the characteristics of an endo-mesomorph grouping when the mesomorph component (Heath & Carter, 1967) has been assessed according to the 'muscularity-scale', and that of the endomorph to the 'fat-scale'. As will be confirmed later, there are (according to Conrad, 1963) pyknomorph (~endomorph) somatotypes possessing muscular and fat masses far above average even during childhood and adolescence. However, contrasting tendencies can also be registered, i.e. fat components above average at low muscular portions. It is, therefore, not surprising that the mean strength values plainly differentiate between the somatotypes on the one hand (Table 7.2), while on the other hand the correlation coefficients based upon individual values are very low, e.g. $r_{BM\,mesomorph} = 0.18$, $r_{BM\,endomorph} = 0.10$, $r_{BM\,ectomorph} = 0.15$. Other published findings show higher coefficients (0.32–0.44) (Thorsen, 1964; Laubach & Conville, 1966).

This situation is also valid for the range in top-class athletes. On the one hand, relatively constant mean positions of the somatotype can

Table 7.2 Somatotypical differences in strength of female students (after Bale *et al.*, 1985)

| Somatotype | Body height (cm) | Body mass (kg) | Rank | Strength (N) | | | | | Rank |
				Grip right	Grip left	Back	Leg	Total	
1 Central—balanced	164.3	55.2	3	324	291	753	2311	3680	3
2 Endo-mesomorph	162.3	67.8	1	361	324	818	2430	3930	1
3 Endo-ectomorph	168.9	54.3	4/5*	313	282	726	2272	3594	4
4 Endomorph	166.8	64.6	2	335	306	802	2273	3715	2
5 Ectomorph	170.7	54.3	4/5	322	293	693	1435	2743	5

*4/5 = joint rank of 4 and 5.

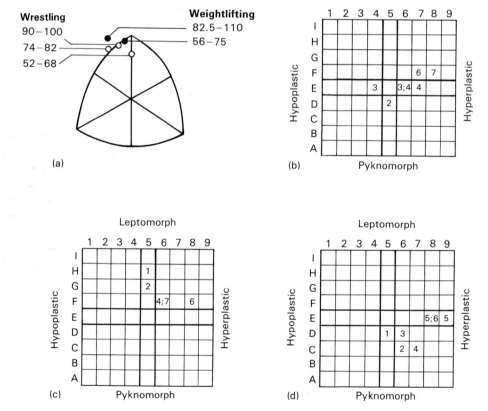

Fig. 7.5 Somatotypes of sportsmen in maximal strength sports. (a) Mean values of body weight of wrestlers and weightlifters (from de Garay *et al.*, 1974; method from Heath & Carter, 1967). (b–d) Individual values of participants in the 1986 European Championships: (b) GDR team; (c) French team; (d) Bulgarian team. (Data for (b)–(d) from Herm & Schulze, 1987.)

be seen. On the other, correlation coefficients gained in judo for example are not sufficient to explain the variance of athletic results by somatotype features (Wutscherk, 1981). Coefficients for body mass and result show variations in the individual weight categories from $r = 0.12$ to 0.45. Nevertheless, the somatotype of the athlete in the maximal strength sports stays relatively unchanged (Fig. 7.5). Viewing Heath and Carter's or Conrad's presentations on somatotypes it is obvious that the mesomorph component of the procedure utilized by the first authors parallels only partly the hyperplastic shaping stated by the latter author (Tittel & Wutscherk, 1978).

Somatotypically conditioned differences of strength capacities in children and adolescents

Muscle mass is thus the essential structural element of strength capacity. It can be determined quantitatively by anthropometric measurements. A question can be raised as to how far the somatotype differentiates strength capacities during childhood and adolescence. This question can be answered with the results of comprehensive anthropometric studies made with school pupils in the township of Leipzig.

Somatotypical differences in absolute body mass

Somatotypes have been established for children and adolescents according to Conrad's procedure (1963) and adjusted to the childrens' and adolescents' age groups (Wutscherk, 1983). Instead of the nine categories originally used five newly created categories seemed to be sufficient for differentiation: category 1, leptomorph; category 2, lepto-metromorph; category 3, metromorph; category 4, metropyknomorph; and category 5, pyknomorph.

Results

Leptomorph children and adolescents have lower body masses from 7 to 18 years of age than pyknomorphs (Fig. 7.6). Group differences found in the 7-year-olds were maintained even in the oldest groups (18 years old). Synchronously with the differences of body mass all the other submasses of the body (body mass compartments) were differentiated. The average amount of body depot fat, but also the mean values of muscle and osseous masses, were increased remarkably at greater body mass, i.e. with the tendency to pyknomorphy. In agreement with the findings of Bale *et al.* (1984, 1985) strength capacities above average levels should, therefore, be expected with pyknomorph children and adolescents.

Somatotypical differences in relative body mass

During growth, body masses cannot be directly compared because of body height differences. Body height/body mass indices having been applied so far for compensation are mathematically inaccurate, as mentioned above. Therefore, the functions between BM and BH have been newly calculated and utilized as the mathematical basis for further assessments. Non-linear connections have been found (Fig. 7.7) for the total body mass as well as for the submasses (compartments) of the body, as follows:

1 Body mass (y):

Boys: $y = 107.68 - 1.6622x + 0.008x^2$
Girls: $y = 124.84 - 1.938x + 0.0091x^2$.

2 Lean body mass (y):

Boys: $y = 79.65 - 1.26x + 0.006x^2$
Girls: $y = 28.13 - 0.55x + 0.004x^2$.

3 Muscle mass (y):

Boys: $y = 54.16 - 0.87x + 0.004x^2$
Girls: $y = 4.72 - 0.15x + 0.0014x^2$.

4 Osseous mass (y):

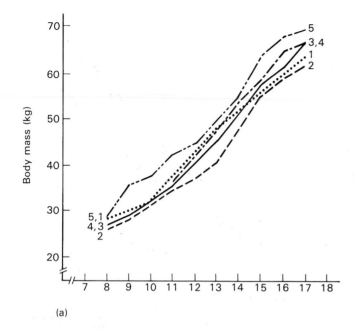

(a)

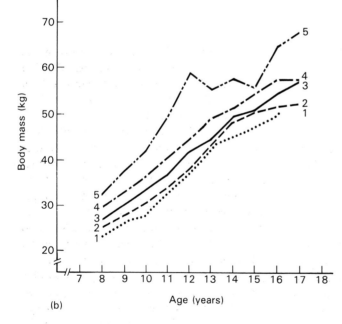

(b)

Age (years)

Fig. 7.6 Mean values of body mass for boys (a) and girls (b) aged 7 to 18 years, divided into somatotypes.
⋯⋯⋯, category 1 (leptomorph);
— — —, category 2 (leptomesomorph);
——, category 3 (metromorph);
— ▬ —, category 4 (metropyknomorph);
—·—·—, category 5 (pyknomorph) (cf. Fig. 7.5b–d: I, H, category 1; G,F, category 2; E, category 3; D,C, category 4; B,A, category 5).

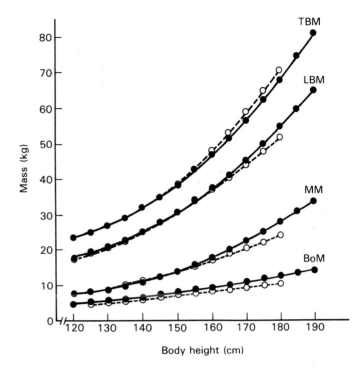

Fig. 7.7 Relationships of body height, total body mass (TBM), lean body mass (LBM), muscle mass (MM) and bone mass (BoM) (according to Wutscherk *et al.* 1988; Wutscherk & Schulze, 1988). ●——●, boys 7–18 years of age (●); ○——○, girls 7–18 years of age (○).

Boys: $y = -1.18 - 0.11x + 0.00048x^2$
Girls: $y = -9.12 + 0.12x - 0.00007x^2$.

Where x = body height.

The values resulting from these equations are mean values for a given body height and termed normal body, normal muscle, or normal osseous mass (= 100%) (Wutscherk *et al.*, 1988; Wutscherk & Schulze, 1988). The relative masses (%) are defined by:

$$\frac{\text{Individual value (kg)}}{\text{Normal mass (kg)}} \times 100.$$

This procedure has several advantages: it does not distort in lower or higher ranges of BH, and the relative masses concerned are universally comparable, e.g. between BH ranges, age groups as well as between the relative masses of individual compartments.

Results

From leptomorph to pyknomorph somatotypes the relative masses become larger. All relative masses (total body mass, lean body mass, muscle mass) differentiate between the five categories of the metric index at a level of about 5% (Table 7.3), except the osseous mass (where differences are about 2.5%).

Clarke's (1971) longitudinal investigations demonstrated the strength-promoting effects of mesomorph shapes with children and adolescents and the strength-reducing effects by ectomorph components of the somatotype. These results are verified by our own findings by relating the influence of the somatotype to the differences of the relative muscle mass, which is much higher with pyknomorph subjects than with leptomorphs. The partly positive effects of endomorphy upon strength can also be explained by the fact that pyknomorph children not only possess more depot fat (degree of the endomorph component) but, what is more important, also show a high relative muscle mass. The pyknomorph somatotype should therefore be suited for strength capacity as body mass (in sports with weight

Table 7.3 Mean values of relative body masses of boys and girls aged 7–16 years (categories 1 to 5, see text)

	Boys					Girls				
	1	2	3	4	5	1	2	3	4	5
1 Body mass	90.5	94.5	99.5	106.0	112.0	88.5	94.5	99.5	108.0	118.0
2 Lean body mass	91.2	96.6	99.3	105.0	106.9	90.3	95.2	99.9	105.9	112.7
3 Muscle mass	88.7	95.0	100.2	105.4	110.1	88.7	94.2	101.1	106.7	112.5
4 Bone mass	95.4	98.0	100.3	103.2	105.2	96.6	97.7	100.6	103.4	105.2
5 Fat*	19.0	18.4	19.8	20.9	24.5	20.1	22.1	22.7	24.4	26.9
Totals: 1–3	90	95	100	105	110	90	95	100	105	>112
4	95	97.5	100	102.5	105	95	97.5	100	102.5	105

*Per cent of body mass (kg).

Table 7.4 Body height and relative body mass of the finalists at the 1988 Seoul Olympic Summer Games

Event	Body height (cm)			Relative body mass (%)			
	Mean	Variation	Winner	Mean	Variation	Winner	Difference*
Athletics (men)							
Shot	194.0	186–200	194	145.3	136.0–162.0	140.2	−5.1
Discus	195.3	190–202	194	134.3	126.2–140.8	126.2	−8.1
Hammer	188.7	180–193	180	135.5	130.0–134.4	134.4	−1.1
Javelin	188.9	184–196	196	117.7	103.0–130.0	120.4	2.7
Athletics (women)							
Shot	180.8	174–188	188	134.5	121.0–153.4	134.5	0
Discus	180.4	175–188	178	129.1	119.8–146.3	119.8	−9.3
Javelin	172.8	168–180	172	109.6	91.6–132.0	98.4	−11.2
Rowing (men)	193.3	182–205	—	107.6	95.9–121.3	—	—
Rowing (women)	176.6	168–188	—	111.4	98.9–119.8	—	—
Weightlifting (kg)							
<52.0	153.4	148–162	152	102.8	90.0–113.5	113.5	10.7
56.0	160.6	152–168	155	101.1	90.9–111.5	102.9	1.8
60.0	162.0	158–167	160	105.6	93.7–116.2	106.2	0.6
67.5	165.3	160–170	166	110.4	100.9–113.9	109.2	−1.2
75.0	168.6	164–170	170	117.6	115.6–121.8	120.5	2.9
82.5	171.4	168–175	169	122.9	116.4–129.6	129.6	6.7
90.0	172.6	168–180	168	131.4	127.8–138.9	138.9	7.5
100.0	179.1	176–184	178	135.5	127.7–140.4	137.4	1.9
110.0	183.8	173–194	180	142.2	133.5–149.5	147.8	5.6
>110.0	184.1	178–190	185	168.0	144.7–194.7	159.4	−8.8
Judo (kg)							
<60.0	165.4	157–172	172	97.9	88.2–107.1	88.2	−9.7
65.0	168.8	164–178	168	104.5	97.8–110.6	100.3	−4.2
71.0	179.0	168–182	170	101.6	93.4–109.9	109.9	8.3
78.0	179.5	175–188	180	108.5	104.0–115.4	110.2	1.7
86.0	178.3	166–186	186	117.9	108.6–136.0	108.6	−9.3
95.0	183.6	178–194	182	122.4	111.0–133.2	125.0	2.6
>95.0	187.6	180–198	180	153.3	118.8–192.2	192.2	38.9

*Difference between winner and mean value.

Table 7.5 Variations in measurements of body height and body mass of 14 weightlifters (personal communications, 1986 and 1988).

Number	Country	Body height*	Body mass
1	GDR	+	−
1	Austria	−	0
1	Romania	+	−
2	Bulgaria	0, +	+ +
2	Italy	0	+
3	Hungary	+ +	− −, 0, +
1	France	+	+ +
3	FRG	− −	+ + +
SD		3.6 cm[†]	6.5 kg[‡]

*0, no difference; +, + +, + + +, increasing differences; −, − −, − − −, decreasing differences.
[†] Partly aimed weight reductions visible.
[‡] In general the differences in body height were too large.

categories) and body height (in throwing or shot-putting events) can cause other disadvantages. The varying concepts, as used by several countries, for the selection of talented children (e.g. for weightlifting) can be seen from Fig. 7.5b–d. It is especially impressive that the rather successful Bulgarian lifters are clearly pyknomorph shaped, even in the lighter weight categories. Theoretically, all those children and adolescents who show values of relative muscle mass beyond 100% during these phases of life should be suited for strength sports.

The phenotype of athletes in maximal strength sports

The athlete's phenotype is still the most frequent, though not sufficient, form of explanation for athletic performance variations. Here the demonstration of differences in BH and BM are dominant, partly because of methodical practicability and partly because of the intercorrelation between these two criteria and the remaining body dimensions. Maximal strength requires maximally developed musculature, the quantity of which can be assessed by various somatic features. Therefore, athletes from maximal strength sports have basically above

average body masses, which can be characterized by a considerable BH, as required by the sport concerned (Tittel & Wutscherk, 1972). They range, therefore, consistently above the regression line in the coordinate system of BH and BM, where the line represents the mean progression of BH and BM within a normal population (Fig. 7.4). This spectrum is limited by a line resulting from the relations between BH, BM and performance in the two weightlifter's events. Data collected from the most successful athletes (participants of the Seoul Olympic Games 1988) confirm this (Table 7.4). Body mass has been entered in this table in the same way as the procedure applied with the children and adolescents, i.e. in per cent of normal BM (100%), as the relative BM. It is, however, well known that the values of BH and BM of Olympic participants are personal descriptions given by these athletes. To check their accuracy, data from 14 weightlifters have been compared with those measured by Herm and Schulze (1987) during the 1986 European Championships. There are some differences that can be traced, to some extent, to subjective inaccuracies (e.g. with BH), but also partly to changes in measurements (changes of weight categories); nevertheless, differences are astonishingly high (Table 7.5).

A more comprehensive description of an athlete's features is not very instructive because very often they are based upon varying methods of measurement. It is frequently also not clear how the deviations from the mean values should be interpreted. This also restricts the statements of the otherwise impressive presentations of findings gained from Olympic participants (Correnti & Zauli, 1964; Tanner, 1964; de Garay et al., 1974). It is necessary that individual values are evaluated when these data are used. Mean values are impressive, but a positive trend of performance is not always expressed by them. For example, the individual values of the best weightlifters from three countries (Table 7.6) point to areas where possible reserves might be found for progress (e.g. body masses), although they do not provide an explanation for the variety of dif-

Table 7.6 Size of weightlifters in the 1986 European Championships

Category no. (kg)	Body mass (kg)	Body height (cm)	Lengths Arm (cm)	Leg (cm)	Diameters Shoulder (cm)	Chest (transv.) (cm)	Chest (sag.) (cm)	Circumferences Chest (cm)	Epicond. (cm)	BM/BH (g/cm)	Relative BM (%)	ST	Muscle mass (%)	Fat (%)	Bone mass (%)
GDR															
2 (56.0)	59.0	156.0	66.9	81.8	37.5	29.0	19.7	88.5	28.2	378	107.3	D5	55.1	8.5	15.8
3 (60.0)	61.0	157.0	67.4	82.8	37.8	29.3	17.8	92.5	28.3	389	109.3	E4	54.6	6.9	15.4
3 (60.0)	63.5	157.5	66.0	82.3	38.8	29.9	17.7	94.0	29.1	403	113.0	E6	54.3	7.7	15.7
4 (67.5)	67.3	164.4	73.3	88.0	37.6	29.1	19.0	100.5	29.3	409	108.7	E6	53.7	8.4	15.8
4 (67.5)	70.0	163.1	69.8	87.8	40.8	31.5	18.0	102.0	30.3	429	115.3	E7	53.2	9.6	16.0
6 (82.5)	81.6	176.2	77.4	95.9	40.3	30.9	18.6	104.0	30.1	463	114.7	F7	54.5	11.0	14.7
7 (90.0)	90.8	178.6	76.3	91.3	40.0	29.4	20.3	103.5	32.0	508	124.2	F8	53.7	11.0	15.1
8 (100.0)	100.8	178.7	78.5	96.1	43.6	32.1	22.5	113.0	32.5	564	137.8	D9ᵤ	53.2	15.2	14.1
10 (>110.0)	128.3	179.8	84.2	96.8	46.0	35.7	26.2	131.0	34.7	714	173.4	ᵤA9	47.4	17.0	12.6
France															
1 (<52.0)	53.0	161.5	69.0	81.7	38.3	25.7	15.7	83.0	27.2	309	89.2	H5	53.0	8.9	17.2
2 (56.0)	59.2	161.2	70.5	85.0	36.9	26.5	17.1	94.0	29.5	365	100.0	G5	51.8	9.7	16.6
4 (67.5)	66.7	172.6	74.9	91.4	38.5	29.2	19.5	96.0	28.4	386	97.7	F6	53.1	8.6	15.6
6 (82.5)	83.9	176.3	76.3	92.3	41.9	30.9	19.8	101.0	30.0	476	117.8	F8	48.7	11.1	14.2
7 (90.0)	87.8	168.9	73.6	88.5	41.9	27.3	20.9	103.0	32.6	520	134.4	F6	55.2	11.4	15.4
7 (90.0)	90.5	182.0	79.2	96.5	43.5	31.0	19.1	100.5	30.9	497	119.1	G9ᵤ	54.9	9.5	14.4
8 (100.0)	96.0	178.6	82.3	94.5	44.1	31.1	22.3	111.0	33.4	538	131.3	E9ᵤ	54.2	12.2	15.5
9 (110.0)	102.2	174.6	76.7	92.0	43.0	33.1	21.5	117.5	33.1	585	146.2	D9ᵤ	50.3	18.5	14.0
Bulgaria															
1 (52.0)	56.0	150.0	57.1	75.8	38.3	28.2	18.3	93.0	27.7	373	111.6	D5	46.8	11.6	15.4
2 (56.0)	60.0	155.5	69.2	83.1	37.8	29.1	19.7	97.0	28.5	386	109.9	C6	49.8	10.6	15.8
3 (60.0)	59.6	150.0	62.5	75.1	38.3	30.5	16.3	93.0	29.6	397	118.7	D6	51.9	10.4	16.6
4 (67.5)	70.0	161.2	70.8	87.4	38.8	29.5	20.5	98.0	28.9	434	118.2	C7	51.3	9.8	14.4
5 (75.0)	74.5	159.6	72.4	84.4	42.1	29.4	18.4	97.0	30.4	467	128.7	E9	55.7	10.2	14.9
5 (75.0)	74.5	169.5	73.9	88.0	39.5	28.7	18.2	101.0	30.9	439	113.2	E8	54.4	12.0	16.2
6 (82.5)	82.0	171.2	77.9	93.0	40.6	31.0	19.2	101.0	31.4	479	122.0	E8	51.1	11.1	15.5

BH, body height; BM, body mass; sag., sagittal; ST, somatotype; transv., transverse; ᵤ outside the coordinate system.

ferences in criteria. In category 4 (up to 67.5 kg), those athletes belonging to the European top-ranking group, have striking differences in their total leg lengths (82.3, 91.4 and 87.4 cm, respectively). Such variability points vigorously to the fact that athletic capacity, which is co-determined by maximal strength, is multi-variately conditioned so that the relationships of the determining features become more important and an optimal athletic technique provides for a finite number of effective possibilities because of the multiplicity of features (Wutscherk & Tittel, 1981).

Summary

Applying anthropometric and morphological procedures it is possible to assess essential elements of an athlete's strength capacities. The maximal strength of an athlete is sport-specific from a quantitative aspect, whereas the values and features of weightlifters define the upper limitations. In this sport the relations between strength and somatotype features are non-linear and can be mathematically described. Comparable strength values for other maximal strength sports are lacking, as well as for the total population. From the far-reaching coincidence of relationships between BH, BM and performance in two-event weightlifting it is recommended that muscular development, the precondition for strength performances, is assessed from the relationship between BH and BM. It should be regarded that, in a proper sense, tendency and level of muscle mass should be expressed by BM. It is possible, and recommended, to determine the latter by means of anthropometric methods.

The somatotype has an influence upon the level of maximal strength that can be reached; whereas the mesomorph component is the strength-enhancing factor in Heath and Carter's system, as compared to the hyperplastic shape and tendency to pyknomorphy in Conrad's. Somatotypes also vary, however, in strength-determining criteria so that the type's effects finally result from the intercorrelation between the individual features.

The developmental progress of body masses (total BM, lean BM, muscle mass, osseous mass, depot fat), being determinants of strength development, have been presented for age periods from 7 to 18 years of age. Evidence could be found that these body masses are somatotypically developed, allowing for conclusions on further levels of strength capacities as early as childhood or adolescence. New, mathematically more precise methods have been introduced (normal BM, relative BM) to evaluate BM independently of height.

The data presented at the end regarding BH and BM relationships of world-best athletes, as well as the individual criteria of the best European weightlifters, demonstrate, among other things, the adaptational effects achieved by athletic training in the maximal strength sports. It is, thus, not only possible to recognize certain aspects of aptitude for maximal strength sports rather early when anthropometric and morphological procedures are applied, but also to follow up and to influence the development of strength-determining criteria during the progress of training activities.

References

Abramovskij, I.N. (1968) Zavisimost mezdu siloj, vesom i rostom sports-mena. *Teorija i praktika fizičeskoj kul'tury*, **31**, 17–19.

Bale, P., Colley, E. & Mayhew, J.L. (1984) Size and somatotype correlates of strength and physiological performance in adult male students. *Australian Journal of Science and Medicine in Sport*, **16**, 2–6.

Bale, P., Colley, E. & Mayhew, J.L. (1985) Relationship among physique, strength and performance in women students. *Journal of Sports Medicine and Physical Fitness*, **25**, 98–103.

Clarke, H.H. (1957) Relationship of strength and anthropometric measures to physical performances involving the trunk and legs. *Research Quarterly for Exercise and Sport*, **28**, 223–39.

Conrad, K. (1963) *Der Konstitutionstypus*. Springer, Berlin.

Correnti, V. & Zauli, B. (1964) *Olimpionici 1960*. Tipolitografie Marves, Rome.

Croucher, J.S. (1984) An analysis of world weight-lifting records. *Research Quarterly for Exercise and Sport*, **55**, 285–8.

de Garay, L., Levine, J. & Carter, J.E.L. (1974) *Genetic*

and *Anthropological Studies of Olympic Athletes.* Academic Press, New York.

Fukunaga, T. (1976) Die absolute Muskelkraft und das Muskelkrafttraining. *Sportarzt-Sportmedizin,* **27,** 255–8.

Grimm, H.H. (1966) *Grundriß der Konstitutionsbiologie und Anthropometrie.* Volk & Gesundheit, Berlin.

Heath, B.H. & Carter, J.E.L. (1967) A modified somatotypological method. *American Journal of Physical Anthropology,* **27,** 57–74.

Herm, K.P. & Schulze, S. (1987) Results of anthropometrical examinations during the 1986 European Weightlifting Championships. *World Lifting,* **1,** 46–8.

Komi, P.V. (1986) Training of muscle strength and power: Interaction of neuromotoric, hypertrophic, and mechanical factors. *International Journal of Sports Medicine,* **7**(suppl.), 10–15.

Komi, P.V. & Häkkinen, K. (1988) Strength and power training. In A. Dirix, H. Knuttgen & K. Tittel (eds) *The Olympic Book of Sports Medicine,* pp. 181–93. Blackwell Scientific Publications, Oxford.

Kopf, H. (1962) Über die Fehlerhaftigkeit und Korrekturmöglichkeit bestehender Quotientendefinitionen in der Medizin und Biologie unter besonderer Berücksichtigung des respiratorischen Quotienten. *Zeitschrift für Biologie,* **113,** 161–72.

Lathan, H. (1987) *Die Bedeutung ausgewählter organismischer Leistungsvoraussetzungen bei der Entwicklung sportlicher Höchstleistungen in der Sportart Gewichtheben.* Medical Dissertation B, Academy for Medical Professional Training, Berlin.

Laubach, L.L. & McConville, J.T. (1966) Muscle strength, flexibility, and body size of adult males. *Research Quarterly for Exercise and Sport,* **37,** 384–92.

Lietzke, M.H. (1956) Relation between weightlifting totals and body weight. *Scientific American,* **124,** 486–7.

Malina, R.M. (1975) Anthropometric correlates of strength and motor performance. *Exercise and Sport Sciences Reviews,* **3,** 249–72.

Matiegka, J. (1921) The testing of physical efficiency. *American Journal of Physical Anthropology,* **4,** 223–30.

Michailov, V.V., Zatsiorskij, V.M. & Geselevic, V.A. (1981) Untersuchungen über die Abhängigkeit der funktionellen Möglichkeiten der Sportler von ihrem Körpergewicht. *Medizin und Sport,* **21,** 169–73.

Möhr, M. (1981) Die Beurteilung der Körpermasse. *Medizin und Sport,* **21,** 85–9.

Neumann, G. & Schüler, K.P. (1989) *Sportmedizinische Funktionsdiagnostik.* Sportmedizinische Schriftenreihe, Vol. 25. Barth, Leipzig.

Ott, H. (1963) Normalgewicht und Optimalgewicht. *Ernährungsumschau,* **10,** 49–52.

Parízková, J. (1962) *Rozvoj aktivni hmoty a tuku u deti a mladeje.* Státni zdravotnické nahladatelství, Praha.

Parnell, R.W. (1954) Somatotyping by physical anthropometry. *American Journal of Physical Anthropology,* **12,** 209–39.

Press, T.N. & Komarova, A.D. (1974) Vzaimosvjaz' sportivnogo resul'tata i urovna razvitija fiziceskich kacestv u junich sportsmenok-meta-tel'nic. *Teorija i praktika fizičeskoj kul'tury,* **37,** 36–8.

Sabo, H., Maslobojev, J.V. & Mezei, I. (1979) Issledovanie zavisimosti moscnosti ot vesa stangistov. *Teorija i praktika fizičeskoj kul'tury,* **42,** 9–12.

Schnabel, G. & Theiss, G. (1986) *Grundbegriffe des Trainings.* Sportverlag, Berlin.

Seršantov, W.F. (1978) *Einführung in die Methodologie der modernen Biologie.* Fischer, Jena.

Sheldon, W.H., Stevens, S.S. & Tucker, W.B. (1940) *The Varieties of Human Physique.* Harper & Brothers, New York.

Tanner, J.M. (1964) *The Physique of Olympic Athletes.* Allen & Unwin, London.

Thorsen, M.A. (1964) Body structure and design. Factors in the motor performance of college women. *Research Quarterly for Exercise and Sport,* **35,** 418–32.

Tittel, K. (1988) Coordination and balance. In A. Dirix, H. Knuttgen & K. Tittel (eds) *The Olympic Book of Sports Medicine,* pp. 194–211. Blackwell Scientific Publications, Oxford.

Tittel, K. (1990) *Beschreibende und funktionelle Anatomie des Menschen.* ll. Aufl. Fischer, Jena-Stuttgart.

Tittel, K. & Wutscherk, H. (1972) *Sportanthropometrie.* Sportmedizinische Schriftenreihe, Vol. 6. Barth, Leipzig.

Tittel, K. & Wutscherk, H. (1978) Vorzüge und Grenzen der Conradschen Methode in der Sportanthropometrie. *Medizin und Sport,* **18,** 11–18.

Tumanjan, G.S. & Martirosov, E.G. (1981) *Telosl_oženie i sport.* Fizkul'tura i Sport, Moscow.

Vorobjev, A.W. (1981) *Tjaželaja atletika.* Fizkul'tura i Sport, Moscow.

Wutscherk, H. (1981) *Grundlagen der Sportanthropometrie.* Deutsche Hochschule für Körperkultur, Leipzig.

Wutscherk, H. (1983) Aussagen und Möglichkeiten körperbautypologischer Bestimmungen bei jugendlichen Sportlern. *Ärztliche Jugendkunde,* **74,** 330–4.

Wutscherk, H., Schmidt, H. & Schulze, S. (1988) Vorschlag zur Bewertung der Körpermasse bei Kindern und Jugendlichen. *Medizin und Sport,* **28,** 177–82.

Wutscherk, H. & Schulze, S. (1988) Vorschläge zur Erhöhung der Körpermassen-Beurteilung. *Medizin und Sport,* **28,** 209–15.

Wutscherk, H. & Tittel, K. (1981) Zum Problem des Sporttyps. *Medizin und Sport,* **21,** 40–3.

Wutscherk, Th. (1990) *Programm zur Berechnung kurvenlinearer Funktionen.* Unpublished manuscript.

Chapter 7B

Mechanical Basis of Strength Expression

JAMES G. HAY

Joint mechanics

When a muscle is activated, it exerts force on each of its points of attachment. Thus, for example, when the biceps brachii is activated, it exerts forces at its attachments to the coracoid process and supraglenoid tuberosity of the scapula, to the bicipital tuberosity of the radius and, via the bicipital aponeurosis, to the ulna (Fig. 7.8a).

These forces tend to translate the points of attachment in the direction in which the forces act, and to rotate them about the intervening joint or joints (Newton's second law). Thus the force exerted on the bicipital tuberosity in Fig. 7.8a tends to translate that bony prominence and to rotate it about a transverse axis through the elbow joint.

In general, the location of the axis about which the bones forming a joint rotate shifts as the motion progresses. The location of the axis at any instant during the course of the motion is called the *instantaneous axis of rotation*.

The magnitude (or amount) of the rotational tendency is known as the *moment* of the force and is equal to the product of the force and the distance between its line of action and the instantaneous axis, a distance known as the *moment arm* (Fig. 7.8b).

Because the maximum force that a muscle can exert is a function of its length (force–length relationship), and because the length of the moment arm of the muscle changes during the course of a joint motion, the maximum

moment the muscle can exert also changes during the motion. In short, the maximum moment that a muscle can exert is a function of the joint configuration.

Joint motions are rarely produced by the action of a single muscle. Instead, a group of muscles, e.g. the elbow flexor muscles, act together to produce the motion. However, because the moment exerted by each of the muscles of such a group varies with the angle of the joint, the sum (or *resultant*) of all these moments also varies with the angle of the joint.

If the end of a segment involved in a joint motion is fixed in position, and the muscles responsible for that motion are activated maximally, a force is exerted by the segment against the fixture. In reaction, the fixture exerts an equal and opposite reaction against the end of the segment (Newton's third law). Because the segment concerned is in equilibrium, i.e. it is not linearly or angularly accelerated, the sum of all the forces acting on it, and the sum of all the moments acting on it, are both equal to zero. Taking elbow flexion as an example once again (Fig. 7.9), this means that the sum of the moments about the instantaneous axis of the elbow due to the actions of the biceps, brachialis and brachio-radialis muscles, and the moments due to the other forces acting at or across the elbow joint (moments exerted by other muscles, by ligaments, by the contact between the humerus and ulna bones, and by the weight of the forearm-and-hand segment, for instance) are exactly matched by the con-

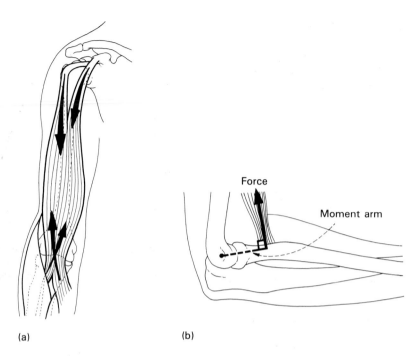

Force

Moment arm

(a)   (b)

Fig. 7.8 (a) An active biceps brachii muscle exerts forces on the structures to which it is attached. (b) The moment of the force exerted via the biceps brachii tendon about the instantaneous centre of rotation of the elbow is equal to the product of that force and the moment arm.

trary moment due to the force exerted by the fixture on the forearm segment.

Finally, if this latter moment is measured, or if the force and moment arm are measured, the resultant elbow moment can readily be determined. It is equal, and opposite in direction, to (i) the measured moment, or (ii) the product of the force and the moment arm.

Strength curves

Definition

The term *strength curve* is used to refer to a plot of the resultant moment exerted about an axis through a joint (or the external force exerted) vs. an appropriate measure of the joint configuration (Fig. 7.10).

The choice of dependent variable (moment or force) is most frequently dictated by the avail-

able, or preferred, measurement device; and the choice of independent variable (joint configuration) by the investigator's personal convictions concerning the most appropriate or convenient convention for defining joint angles. In this latter respect, there are two conventions in common use: the *included joint angle*, i.e. the smaller of the two relevant angles between the two segments defining a joint; and the *anatomical joint angle*, i.e. the angle through which the joint would have to be moved to take it from the anatomical position to the position of interest. Thus, for elbow flexion, the two angles are as shown in Fig. 7.11.

The resultant moment at the joint is often referred to as the resultant muscle moment or, even more simply, as the muscle moment. Such usage assumes that all the other, non-muscular (or passive) contributions to the resultant moment at the joint—the moments of bone-on-

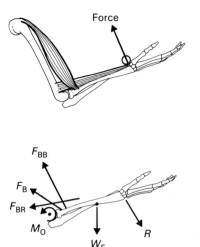

Force

F_{BB}

F_B

F_{BR}

M_o

W_F

R

Fig. 7.9 With the forearm and hand in equilibrium, the sum of the moments about the instantaneous centre due to the forces exerted by the biceps brachii (F_{BB}), the brachio-radialis (F_{BR}), and the brachialis (F_B) muscles, and the moments due to the forces exerted by other structures (M_o), is equal to the sum of the moments due to the weight of the forearm-and-hand segment (W_F) and the reaction force (R).

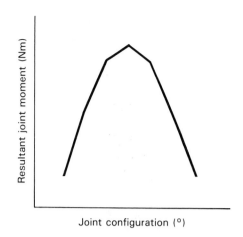

Resultant joint moment (Nm)

Joint configuration (°)

Fig. 7.10 A strength curve is a plot of the resultant moment about an axis through a joint vs. an appropriate measure of joint configuration.

bone, ligament, cartilage and joint capsule forces—sum to zero, or that their sum is so small that it can be ignored without a significant loss in accuracy. The validity of this assumption is rarely tested in the context of studies involving strength curves.

In some instances, the resultant joint moment is referred to as the moment due to the action of a specific group of muscles, e.g. the elbow flexor moment. This usage involves another poorly substantiated assumption, i.e. that there is no antagonistic muscle activity involved and thus no antagonistic muscle contribution to the resultant moment at the joint. Electromyographic data that would support or reject this assumption are rarely gathered in studies involving the determination of strength curves.

One can only conclude that, unless the passive contribution to a resultant joint moment is found to be negligible throughout the range of the joint motion involved, the expression 'resultant muscle moment', or 'muscle moment',

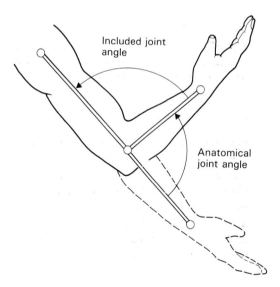

Included joint angle

Anatomical joint angle

Fig. 7.11 Anatomical and included joint angles used to designate joint configuration.

should not be used. And, unless it is also established that there is no antagonistic muscle activity, the expression '(agonistic muscle group) moment' should not be used. Indeed, given the complexities involved, a strong case can be made for using the term 'resultant joint moment' exclusively.

Forms

Strength curves have three basic forms: *ascending*, in which the force or moment increases as the joint angle increases; *descending*, in which the force or moment decreases as the joint angle increases; and *ascending–descending*, in which the force or moment first increases and then decreases as the joint angle increases (Fig. 7.12). Although one might also imagine a descending–ascending curve, there have been no reports to date of the existence of such a curve.

There are several factors that determine the form of the strength curve for a given joint motion. These include (i) the convention used in describing the joint angle, (ii) the relationship between the length of a muscle and the maximum force that it is capable of exerting, (iii) the relationship between the joint angle and the moment arm of the muscle, and (iv) the contributions that moments due to passive structures, and to the activity of antagonistic muscles, make to the resultant joint moment.

The distinction between ascending and descending strength curves rests on the convention used in describing the joint angle. Thus, for example, the ascending strength curve reported for knee flexion when the force or moment is plotted against the included joint angle (Kulig *et al.*, 1984) becomes a descending strength curve when the force or moment is plotted against the anatomical joint angle (Fig. 7.13).

In all those cases in which an ascending or descending strength curve has been reported, the force or moment increased as the length of the agonistic muscles increased. Because this is exactly what might be expected from a consideration of the force–length relationship in muscles, it is tempting to explain such findings solely in terms of this relationship. Such an explanation should be avoided because it takes no heed of the the contributions that changes in the moment arm, the moments due to passive forces and the moments due to antagonistic muscle activity made to the resultant joint

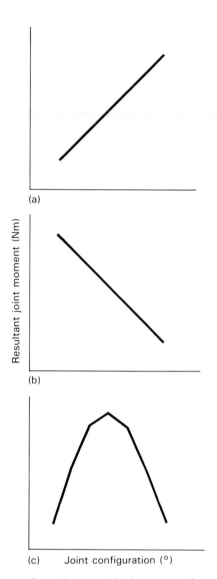

Fig. 7.12 Strength curves take three general forms: (a) ascending; (b) descending; and (c) ascending–descending.

moment. While some of these contributions might well have been trivial, the contributions of others might equally well have been significant, at least at some points within the range of joint motion tested.

In those cases in which an ascending–descending curve has been reported, the

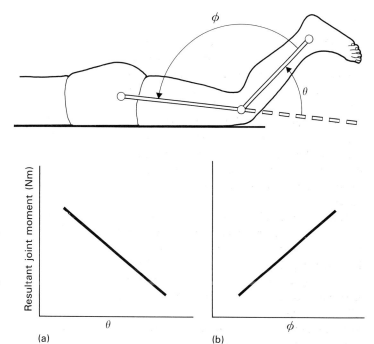

Fig. 7.13 A knee flexion strength curve is either ascending (a) or descending (b), depending on how the joint configuration is defined.

ascending part of the curve indicated that the force or moment increased as the length of the muscle increased. The comments made in the preceding paragraph thus apply equally well to this ascending part of the ascending–descending curve.

The descending part of reported ascending–descending strength curves has indicated that the force or moment decreased as the length of the involved muscles increased. This is exactly the opposite of what would be expected from a consideration of the force–length relationship alone. It must therefore be concluded that changes in (i) the moment arms of the involved agonist muscles, (ii) the moments due to passive structures, or (iii) the moments due to antagonistic muscle activity, are more influential in determining the form of the strength curve for that part of the joint motion, than are changes in the lengths of the agonist muscles. And of these alternatives, it is a decrease in the moment arm as the joint angle increases that appeals as the dominant influence in deter-

mining the form of this part of the strength curve.

The forms of the strength curves for selected joint motions are summarized in Table 7.7.

Measurement

Exercise condition

Strength curves are most commonly based upon data gathered under isometric conditions. The term strength curve is also used with reference to data gathered under so-called isokinetic conditions, i.e. under conditions in which the joint angle is assumed to change at some preselected constant rate. Numerous studies have shown, however, that isokinetic dynamometers do not provide a constant rate of change of the joint angle, i.e. a constant angular velocity, throughout their range of motion. Instead, they exhibit one or more of the following deviations from this desired constant rate: an initial period of acceleration up to the preselected rate, a period whose duration

Table 7.7 Forms (ascending, descending or ascending–descending) for selected joint motions. For flexion-extension, the included joint angle was used. For abduction-adduction, the angle between the line of the segment and the line of the torso increased from 0°, when the two lines were parallel, to c. 180°, when the segment was maximally adducted

Joint	Motion	Form of representative curve
Shoulder	Flexion	Descending
	Extension	Ascending–descending
	Abduction	Descending
	Adduction	Ascending–descending
Elbow	Flexion	Ascending–descending
	Extension	Descending; ascending–descending*
Hip	Flexion	Ascending; ascending–descending*
	Extension	Descending; ascending–descending*
	Abduction	*Descending*; ascending–descending*
	Adduction	Ascending
	Internal rotation	Ascending
	External rotation	Descending
Knee	Flexion	*Ascending*; ascending–descending*
	Extension	Descending; *ascending–descending*

*Results of different authors conflict. Where the results of a clear majority of the authors are in agreement, that form is italicized.

increases with the preselected rate; an 'overshoot' that exceeds the preselected rate by 11–500%; and oscillations following the initial overshoot (Osternig, 1986).

In accord with the force–velocity relationship, the absolute values of the moments recorded under isometric conditions are generally greater than those recorded under concentric isokinetic conditions. And, while strength curves obtained for the same joint motion under isometric and isokinetic conditions are generally of the same form, i.e. ascending, descending or ascending–descending, the accelerative effects just described result in the joint angle at which the peak moment is recorded varying with the preselected angular velocity of joint motion. For example, Thorstensson *et al.* (1976) have reported results for the mean anatomical knee angles at which the peak torque was recorded for a knee extension exercise performed at five different preselected rates (Table 7.8).

Dependent variable

Early investigators made use of cable tensiometers, load cells, and custom-built force-measurement systems. These investigators almost invariably used the force exerted at the distal end of the segment of interest as the dependent variable. Later investigators have relied almost exclusively on commercially available strength-testing and training machines such as the Biodex, Cybex, Kin-Com, Lido and Merac. These machines are typically designed for the measurement of single-joint exercises and call for the alignment of the joint axis—an approximation of the average location of the joint axis for the exercise concerned—with the axis of the rotating arm of the machine against which forces are exerted by the subject. The dependent variable used in these cases is almost invariably the resultant joint moment or torque, the latter of which terms appears to be preferred by equipment manufacturers.

Table 7.8 Mean anatomical knee angles at which peak torque was recorded

Angular velocity ($° \cdot s^{-1}$)	Angle at which peak torque recorded (°)*
15	66.2
30	63.4
60	61.0
90	58.3
180	54.7

*From Thorstensson *et al.* (1976).

Validity

If the data gathered are to have any value at all, it is imperative that the device used measures what it purports to measure. For example, the torque recorded by the device must be equal to the resultant joint moment sought. The validity of the device can easily be established in the isometric case by suspending a known weight at a known distance from the axis of the rotating arm and comparing the recorded torque with the product of the weight and the distance (or moment arm). A similar comparison can be made in the isokinetic case. In the latter instance, however, it is necessary to obtain some record of the angular position vs. time history of the rotating arm of the device so that the computed moment–time curve can be correctly synchronized with the recorded torque–time curve.

Position and alignment

Because the human body contains many muscles that cross two or more joints, the positions of the joints adjacent to the one under consideration can be expected to have an influence on the strength curve being measured. For example, the knee extension strength curve obtained when the subject is in a back-lying position differs from that obtained when the subject is in an upright seated position (Fig. 7.14).

The extent to which the location of the joint axis coincides with the axis of the rotating arm of the measurement device influences the validity of the results obtained. In those cases where the instantaneous axis of the joint moves only a little during the joint motion, the error due to misalignment of the axes may be quite small. Conversely, in those cases where it moves a great deal, e.g. in some motions of the shoulder and ankle (Rothstein *et al.*, 1987), the error due to misalignment may be substantial. In either case, care should be exercised in aligning the axes in such a way as to minimize the error.

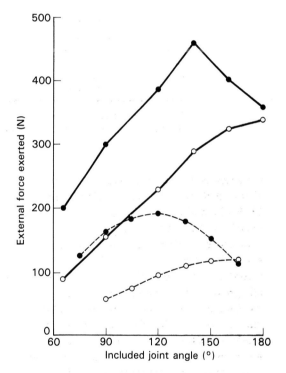

Fig. 7.14 The position of adjacent joints influence both the magnitude of the external forces recorded and the form of the strength curve. Mean knee extension curves are shown for 10 men, 10 women and 20 children (solid lines) by Williams and Stutzmann (1959) and for eight women (broken lines) by Houtz *et al.* (1957). In a seated position (●) the included hip joint angle was *c.* 90–100°; in a supine position (○), *c.* 180°. Thigh, shank and foot orientations were the same in both seated and supine positions.

Stabilization

Humans required to exert the maximum force of which they are capable during the performance of a given exercise are remarkably resourceful in locating muscle groups, in addition to those that are primarily responsible for the motion involved, to contribute to the effort. If useful strength measurements are to be obtained, the contributions from these extraneous sources must be eliminated. To this end, the muscles that might contribute in this way must be rendered ineffective by strapping down (or otherwise fixing the positions of) the relevant segments on which they act. This process, known as stabilizing the subject, requires careful pilot work in which the possibilities are explored and effective stabilizing solutions found. It is only rarely that the operation manuals supplied by the manufacturers of strength-measuring equipment contain adequate solutions to this fundamental problem.

Protocol

An examination of published studies in which strength curves have been reported reveals a marked lack of consistency in the protocols used to obtain the data defining the strength curve. Thus, for example, the number of joint angles tested ranges from as few as three (Singh & Karpovich, 1968) to as many as 13 (Wehr, 1964); and the time between consecutive trials from 10 s (Graves *et al.*, 1989) to 2 min (Johnson *et al.*, 1990).

Furthermore, the impact that each variation in protocol has on the strength curves ultimately obtained is largely unknown. However, what is known suggests that the protocol should allow the subject to become familiar with the testing device, and to warm up adequately before being tested. The protocol should also include testing of a large enough number of joint angles to permit the form of the strength curve to be clearly defined, and a small enough number to minimize the adverse effects of fatigue. The protocol used by Graves *et al.*

(1989) and Manning *et al.* (1990) appears to meet these latter requirements well. In these studies, the subjects were tested at eight different joint angles through the range of motion in two sessions at least 48 hours apart. In one of these sessions, the subject was tested at anatomical knee angles starting at 9° and ending at 110°; and in the other, starting at 110° and ending at 9°. The mean values for all subjects, for each of these orders of testing (Fig. 7.15), showed clearly the influence that fatigue exerts on the strength curve obtained. The mean values recorded towards the end of the order were below the corresponding mean values recorded near the beginning of the order.

Reliability

The reliability of the torque measures taken for the purpose of establishing a strength curve are a function of the reliability of the measurement device, something that is easy to establish using a known weight and measures of the moment arm; the reliability of the operator, which depends on experience and skill with respect to such matters as alignment and stabilization; and the reliability of the subject, which appears to depend on such things as the subject's health status, sex, and motivation. The reliability of the measurements taken is not addressed as frequently (and, in many instances, not as rigorously) as it deserves. It is clear, nonetheless, that it is the reliability of the operator and, even more so, the reliability of the subject that are the main sources of variation in the measurements obtained. (Note: for a thorough discussion of the reliability of isometric and isokinetic torque measures, the reader is referred to Mayhew & Rothstein, 1985.)

Uses

Clinical

Strength curves are used routinely in clinical settings to characterize the present status of

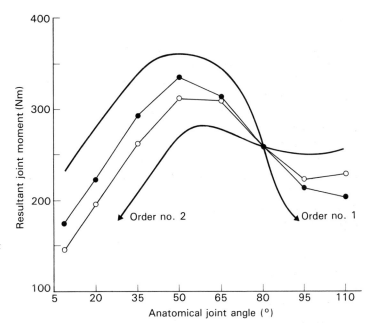

Fig. 7.15 Fatigue influences the magnitudes of the resultant joint moment. For each order of testing, the mean knee extension values recorded for the final joint angles were significantly less than for the reverse order. (From Graves *et al.*, 1989.) ●, Mean values for order no. 1; ○, mean values for order no. 2.

patients for purposes of exercise prescription and for subsequent monitoring of the rehabilitation process (Garrett & Duncan, 1988). Their possible use as an aid in diagnosis has also been discussed (Davies, 1987). Serious concern has been expressed, however, that their use in these instances has not been supported by strong, scientific evidence. Rothstein *et al.* (1987) have stated, for example, that '... some clinicians are using torque curves to plan treatments and to determine their patient's pathological condition. In the absence of data, such conclusions may be irresponsible'.

At the heart of the problem identified here is the reliability of the measurements upon which strength curves are based. If variation in measurements of the joint torque from trial to trial or day to day exceeds the changes due to rehabilitation (or the differences due to injury or disease), the use of strength curves as a means of monitoring a patient's progress (or as a means of diagnosing the cause or causes of a patient's condition) cannot be supported. On the other hand, if the reliability of measurement is high, both of these uses of strength curves might well be highly beneficial in a clinical setting.

Equipment design

Strength curves have also been used in the design of strength-training equipment. The development of strength-training machines in the 1960s was accompanied, it was claimed, by the development of mechanisms that provided resistance according to the capacity of the involved muscles to exert force (Garhammer, 1989). This meant that, for single-joint exercises, the resistance was said to vary in accord with the strength curve for the exercise concerned. A knowledge of the form of the strength curve for a given exercise was thus a prerequisite to the design of such a mechanism. (One commonly used mechanism, a variable radius cam, is shown in Fig. 7.16.)

The basis for the design of mechanisms for multiple-joint exercises, for which similar claims have been made, is less obvious because strength curves for multiple-joint exercises have yet to be reported.

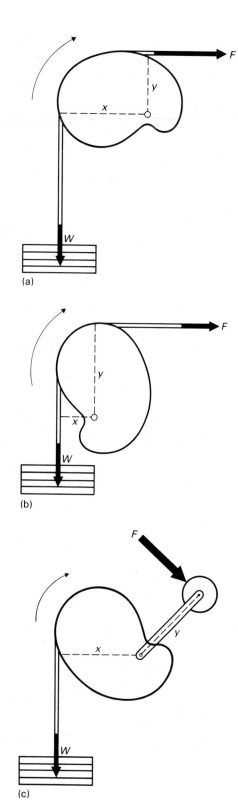

The validity of the claims for a matching of the resistance to the capacity of the involved muscles has frequently been called into question. First, because it was apparently not feasible to design a variable resistance mechanism that could be adapted to match well the capacities of subjects of different sexes and anthropometric dimensions, the variable resistance offered by these machines was based on average values (Garhammer, 1989). Second, the results of several studies have indicated that the resistance offered via the cams used in some machines do not match average strength curves (Harman, 1983; Fleming, 1984; Hughes, 1986).

Incidentally, it should perhaps be noted here that variable resistance machines were developed on the assumption that existing strength-training procedures demanded a maximum effort from the muscles only at that point in the range of motion where they were weakest, the so-called 'sticking point', and that improved strength development would result from taxing the muscles to capacity throughout the range. Training studies designed to test the validity of this notion have repeatedly failed to demonstrate that variable resistance exercise holds an advantage over traditional methods (Atha, 1981; Silvester et al., 1981/1982; Manning et al., 1990).

Research

Strength curves have been used in research projects designed to provide normative data for clinical purposes (Schlinkman, 1984; Ivey et al., 1985); and to determine the effects of different training regimes (Graves et al., 1989). They have also been used as input data to math-

Fig. 7.16 Applied force (*F*) and weight force (*W*) have changing moment arms (*x* and *y*, respectively): (a) at points in the range where a large *F* can be generated, $y < x$; (b) at points in the range when only small forces can be exerted $y > x$ (from Stone & O'Bryant, 1987). In some designs (c) the moment arm of the applied force is constant; and the moment of the weight changes.

ematical models of musculoskeletal function and as a means to validate a mathematical model. In this regard, Delp *et al.* (1990a) used published data on strength curves for the hip, knee, ankle and subtalar joints to validate a mathematical model of the lower extremity used to study the consequences of tendon transfer surgeries. Delp *et al.* (1990b) also used a published strength curve for hip abduction to validate a similar model to evaluate the efficacy of differing pelvic osteotomies.

References

Atha, J. (1981) Strengthening muscle. *Exercise and Sport Sciences Reviews*, **9**, 1–73.

Clark, H.H. (1966) *Muscular Strength and Endurance in Man*, pp. 37–51. Prentice-Hall, Inc., Englewood Cliffs, NJ.

Davies, G.J. (1987) *A Compendium of Isokinetics in Clinical Usage and Rehabilitation Techniques*. S & S Publishers, Onalaska, WI.

Delp, S.L., Bleck, E.E., Zajac, F.E. & Bollini, G. (1990b) Biomechanical analysis of the Chiari Pelvic Osteotomy. *Clinical Orthopaedics*, **254**, 189–98.

Delp, S.L., Loan, J.P., Hoy, M.G., Zajac, F.E., Topp, E.L. & Rosen, J.M. (1990a) An interactive graphics-based model of the lower extremity to study orthopaedic surgical procedures. *IEEE Transactions on Biomedical Engineering*, **37**, 757–67.

Fleming, L.K. (1984) *Accommodation capabilities of Nautilus machines to human strength curves*. Masters thesis, University of Alabama, Birmingham.

Garhammer, J. (1989) Weight lifting and training. In C.L. Vaughan (ed.) *Biomechanics of Sport*, pp. 169–211. CRC Press, Boca Raton, FL.

Garrett, W.E. & Duncan, P.W. (1988) Muscle rehabilitation. In T.R. Malone (ed.) *Muscle Injury and Rehabilitation*, p. 49. Williams & Wilkins, Baltimore.

Graves, J.E., Pollock, M.L., Jones, A.E., Colvin, A.B. & Leggett, S.H. (1989) Specificity of limited range of motion variable resistance training. *Medicine and Science in Sports and Exercise*, **21**, 84–9.

Harman, E. (1983) Resistive torque analysis of five Nautilus exercise machines. *Medicine and Science in Sports and Exercise*, **15**, 113.

Houtz, S., Lebow, M. & Beyer, F. (1957) Effect of posture on strength of the knee flexor and extensor muscles. *Journal of Applied Physiology*, **11**, 475–80.

Hughes, C.J. (1986) *Resistive torque capabilities of the Nautilus cam under static and dynamic conditions*. Masters thesis, Springfield College, Massachusetts.

Ivey, F.M., Calhoun, J.H., Rusche, K. & Bierschenk, J. (1985) Isokinetic testing of shoulder strength: Normal values. *Archives of Physical Medicine and Rehabilitation*, **66**, 384–6.

Johnson, J.H., Colodyny S. & Jackson, D. (1990) Human torque capability versus machine resistive torque for four Eagle resistance machines. *Journal of Applied Sport Science Research*, **4**, 83–7.

Kulig, K., Andrews, J.G. & Hay, J.G. (1984) Human strength curves. *Exercise and Sport Sciences Reviews*, **12**, 417–66.

Manning, R.J., Graves, J.E., Carpenter, D.M., Leggett, S.H. & Pollock, M.L. (1990) Constant vs. variable resistance knee extension training. *Medicine and Science in Sports and Exercise*, **22**, 397–401.

Mayhew, T.P. & Rothstein, J.M. (1985) Measurement of muscle performance with instruments. In J.M. Rothstein (ed.) *Measurement in Physical Therapy*, pp. 57–102. Churchill Livingstone, New York.

Osternig, L.R. (1986) Isokinetic dynamometry: Implications for muscle testing and rehabilitation. *Exercise and Sport Sciences Reviews*, **14**, 45–80.

Rothstein, J.M., Lamb, R.L. & Mayhew, T.P. (1987) Clinical uses of isokinetic measurements. *Physical Therapy*, **67**, 1840–4.

Schlinkman, B. (1984) Norms for high school football players derived from Cybex data reduction computer. *Journal of Orthopaedic and Sports Physical Therapy*, **5**, 243–5.

Silvester, L.J., Stiggins, C., McGown, C. & Bryce, G.R. (1981/1982) The effect of variable resistance and free-weight training programs on strength and vertical jump. *National Strength and Conditioning Assocation Journal*, **3**, 30–3.

Singh, M. & Karpovich, P.V. (1968) Strength of forearm flexors and extensors. *Journal of Applied Physiology*, **25**, 177–80.

Stone, M.H. & O'Bryant, H.S. (1987) The biomechanics of lifting. In *Weight Training: A Scientific Approach*, p. 84. Bellwether Press, Minneapolis.

Thorstensson, A., Grimby, G. & Karlsson, J. (1976) Force–velocity relations and fiber composition in human knee extensor muscles. *Journal of Applied Physiology*, **40**, 12–16.

Wehr, R.W. (1964) *The relationship between selected joint angles of selected movements and human strength values*. Doctoral dissertation, Florida State University, Tallahassee.

Williams, M. & Stutzmann, L. (1959) Strength variation through the range of joint motion. *Physical Therapy*, **39**, 145–52.

PART 3

MECHANISMS OF ADAPTATION IN STRENGTH AND POWER TRAINING

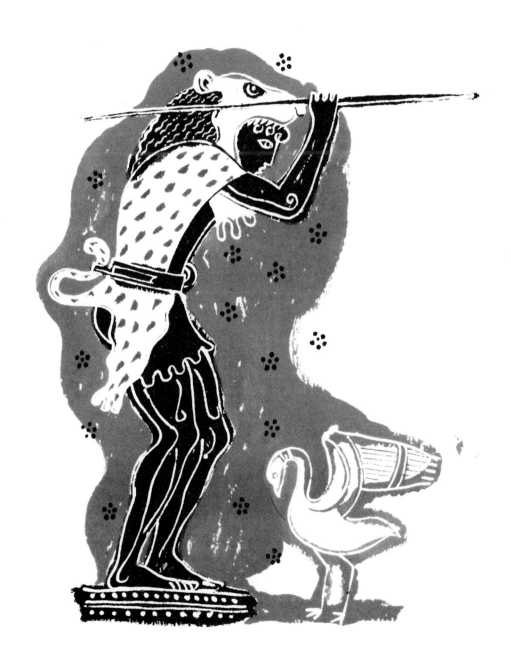

Chapter 8A

Cellular and Molecular Aspects of Adaptation in Skeletal Muscle

GEOFFREY GOLDSPINK

Skeletal muscle is a tissue that possesses an intrinsic ability to adapt to the type of physical activity it is required to perform. Adaptation takes place during normal growth and as a response to exercise training. This chapter is concerned with the cellular and molecular mechanism involved in adaptation for increased power output. With the emergence of methods that enable us to study changes in gene expression, we can now begin to understand adaptation in terms of levels of transcription and translation of individual genes and subsets of genes. This will enable us to obtain an understanding that will range from the whole tissue to the gene level and to design athletic training and/or rehabilitation exercise regimes accordingly. With the effort that is now being expended in the sequencing of the entire human genome it may be possible, sometime in the future, to predict which people have the genetic potential to become world-class athletes. This would inevitably involve formulating a new code of ethics.

Cellular and molecular basis of muscle power

Means by which muscle shortens and produces force

The process by which muscle converts chemical energy into mechanical work has attracted the attention of many physicists, biochemists and physiologists. This is a brief overview as more detailed accounts can be found in cell biology and physiology textbooks.

Muscle is made up of cellular units called muscle fibres, which are 20–100 μm in diameter. The muscle fibres contain rod-like contractile structures, myofibrils, which are about 1 μm in diameter. These are made up of protein filaments arranged in units called sarcomeres (Fig. 8.1). Each sarcomere consists of one set of thick (myosin) filaments and two sets of thin (actin) filaments, and during the contraction of muscle the thin filaments are pulled in over the thick filaments so that each sarcomere shortens. The means by which the filaments slide over each other has not been completely elucidated. However, it is known that there are projections from the thick (myosin) filaments called myosin cross-bridges. Each cross-bridge is an independent force generator, which interacts with a thin filament and pulls it towards the centre of the sarcomere. The cross-bridge then detaches from the thin filament and has to be reprimed by adenosine triphosphate (ATP) before it can go through another cycle of force generation. Some of our work has shown that the rate at which cross-bridge work in different muscles varies considerably depending on the kind of muscle and the kind of activity it is adapted for (Goldspink, 1977b, 1981, 1984).

As mentioned, during contraction the thin filaments slide over the thick filaments, which results in the shortening of each sarcomere and this happens all along the length of the

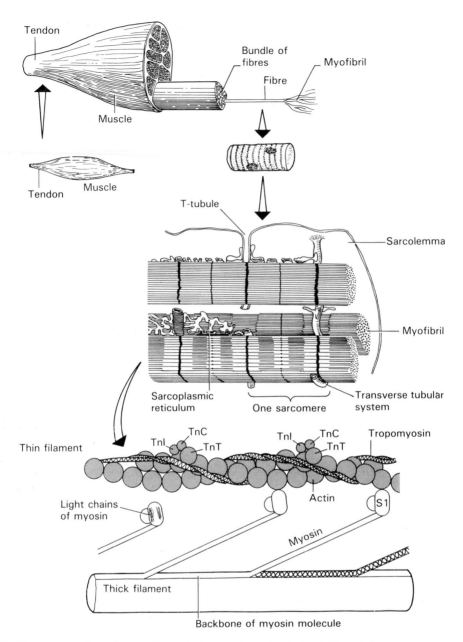

Fig. 8.1 The structure of muscle from the whole tissue to the molecular level. The cellular units or muscle fibres contain contractile elements called myofibrils, which in skeletal and cardiac muscle are striated. The striations are due to the presence of thick (myosin) and thin (actin) filaments. These protein filaments are arranged in units called sarcomeres, which shorten during contraction by the sliding of the thin filaments over the thick filaments. This sliding movement is brought about by the myosin cross-bridges, which act as independent force generators. Movement of the thin filaments commences when calcium binds to the troponin complex (TnI, TnT, TnC), which is believed to pull the tropomyosin to one side to reveal active sites on the actin filament. The other requirement is that the myosin cross-bridges are charged with ATP. The cross-bridge is the part of the myosin heavy chain molecule that projects from the thick filament. The end of the cross-bridge terminates in two globular heads (S1 fragment) that contain the ATPase and the actin binding sites. The rate at which the cross-bridge works is mainly determined by the ATPase activity of the type of myosin heavy chain that constitutes the cross-bridge. Also associated with the S1 are two myosin light chains that are believed to modify the cross-bridge cycle time to some extent.

myofibrils, hence the muscle as a whole shortens. The biochemistry of muscular contraction is very interesting, and if we look at the proteins that make up the thick and thin filaments (Fig. 8.1) we find that not only does the system possess a means of generating force but also a mechanism for 'switching on' and 'switching off' the contractile apparatus. The thin actin filaments of the sarcomere are rather like a double pearl necklace that is twisted into a spiral or helix. Decorating these thin filaments are regulatory complexes made up of proteins, tropomyosin and troponins I, T and C. When calcium ions bind with the troponin complex this causes a conformational change in the complex, which results in the tropomyosin being pulled to one side. When the tropomyosin position is changed, active sites are exposed that allow the myosin cross-bridges to interact with thin filaments. The cross-bridges go through repeated cycles of activity until calcium is withdrawn and sequestered by the sarcoplasmic reticulum or until ATP levels are depleted.

Ultrastructural and molecular determinants of muscle strength

Strength can be defined as the maximum force that a muscle can develop during a single contraction. At the ultrastructural level this is related to the number of myosin cross-bridges in parallel that can interact with the actin filaments and generate force. As mentioned, each myosin cross-bridge is an independent force generator. When primed with ATP and activated by calcium ions it will go through a cycle of attachment to the actin, force generation and then a detachment phase. The force generation cycle differs for different types of muscle depending on what kind of heavy chain protein constitutes the myosin cross-bridge, and there is some evidence that not all types of cross-bridges generate the same amount of force. Also, only a percentage of cross-bridges may be activated even during a maximum contraction, hence these are two

other factors that must be borne in mind when trying to explain maximum force at the fundamental level.

For most practical purposes it is convenient to relate the maximum force developed to the muscle fibre cross-sectional area. Providing the myofibrillar content of the fibres does not differ markedly, this is a reasonably accurate way of predicting the force that a muscle can develop. It is often more convenient to relate strength to muscle cross-sectional area. However, it must be realized that this is more imprecise because the percentage of extracellular space and the arrangement of muscle fibres varies from muscle to muscle. With regard to the former, it seems that one of the earliest responses to strength training is for a consolidation of the tissue as the muscle fibres increase in girth at the expense of extracellular spaces. That is to say, the initial response is for the muscle fibre cross-sectional area to increase without a commensurate increase in muscle cross-sectional area taking place. With regard to the latter point, the fibre arrangements in different muscles differ according to whether the muscle is designed for high force generation or for high rate shortening (Fig. 8.2). In order to increase the effective cross-sectional area of muscles such as those in the lower leg, the muscle fibres are arranged in a chevron fashion. These are referred to as pennate or multipennate muscles. A necessary consequence of this type of arrangement is that the muscle fibres will be relatively shorter and this means that the muscle will have a lower *overall* slow rate of shortening.

Ultrastructural and molecular determinants of velocity of shortening

As mentioned above, the overall rate of shortening of the muscle is, in part, determined by the number of sarcomeres in series. It is also determined by the intrinsic velocity (v_{max}) of shortening of the sarcomeres. When activated the sarcomeres contract and have an additive effect, so that the more of them that there are in

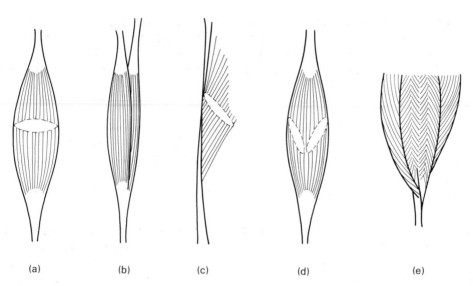

(a)   (b)   (c)   (d)   (e)

Fig. 8.2 The different arrangements of fibres within muscles of the body: muscles adapted for high overall rate of shortening have parallel fibres and are arranged in a fusiform manner (a, b). The fibres in muscles adapted for high force generation are arranged in a chevron-like fashion, which provides a larger effective fibre cross-sectional area, shown by the area encircled by the dotted lines. These are referred to as pennate (c), bipennate (d) or multipennate (e) muscles.

series and the higher their v_{max}, the more rapid the overall rate of shortening of the fibre. Because the overall rate of shortening is partly determined by length, it is necessary to express the v_{max} as the rate of shortening per sarcomeres or per muscle length. As mentioned the v_{max} also depends on the velocity of shortening of each sarcomere, which in turn is dependent on the predominant type of myosin that the cross-bridges are made of.

The individual myosin molecule consists of two heavy chains, which are wound around each other except for their globular heads or S1 regions. Part of the double-stranded region forms the backbone (LMM) that is embedded in the myosin filament. The heavy meromyosin (HMM) forms the cross-bridge and terminates in the S1 head region. The S1 part of the myosin heavy chain contains the actin attachment site and the ATPase site, which are believed to be important elements of the contractile mechanism that determine the cross-bridge cycle and hence the maximum velocity of shortening (v_{max}). The HMM part of the myosin heavy chain that projects from the filament is hinged so it can swing out and allow the S1 head to attach to the active site on the thin filament. The S1 heads apparently walk or flick the thin filament along, resulting in sarcomere shortening. The rate of shortening of each sarcomere depends on the number of cross-bridges that can reach the actin filaments; therefore the initial overlap of the filaments (sarcomere length) is important. There are two myosin light chains associated with the S1 head and these apparently modify the rate of shortening to some extent. Single fibre contraction studies, in which the myosin light chains have been switched, indicate that they can modify the rate of shortening by up to 20% but this is to be regarded as fine tuning compared with the several hundred percent that exist between the v_{max} of different types of fast and slow muscle fibres. Other proteins, such as the regulatory proteins troponins and tropomyosin, exist as different fast and slow isoforms and are involved in the fine tuning of the contractile system. The question arises as to what determines the kind of myosin and hence what kind of sarcomeres a muscle fibre should produce. This will be dealt with later under gene regulation of contractile proteins during muscle fibre differentiation and development.

Muscle power and different muscle fibre-phenotype

A common misuse of the term power is to use it when one really means force: power = work done (force × distance) per unit time. As mentioned above, muscle strength can be defined as the maximum force produced in a single tetanic contraction. Muscles are often used to produce repeated contraction, e.g. running. In this case we need to think in terms of power output. Power combines the two parameters mentioned above, i.e. force and velocity; the higher and more rapid the force generation, the greater the power output. As we shall see there are different types of muscle fibres, some of which are adapted for a high power output over a short period (fast glycolytic type IIb), while others are adapted for a high power output over a longer period of time (fast, oxidative, glycolytic type IIa). Both of these fibre types possess a type of myosin and other contractile proteins that produce a short cross-bridge cycle time and develop force very rapidly. However, the latter type (IIa) have more mitochondria and a more oxidative metabolism so they are capable of sustaining the high power output over a longer period. The other major type of fibre found in mammalian muscles is the slow oxidative, type I fibre that has a type of myosin and other contractile proteins which result in a slow cross-bridge cycle. This makes these fibres more efficient and more economical for producing slow repetitive movements and sustaining isometric force but not for generating power (Goldspink, 1977b). The type I fibre is particularly numerous in postural muscle such as the soleus, which is a muscle that is activated virtually all the time during standing, walking

and running. During any activity, except perhaps ballistic movements, the slow fibres are recruited first. When the power or force requirements increase, the fast type II fibres have to be recruited to provide the necessary power output.

Adaptation for increased force generation

Muscle fibre hypertrophy and myofibrillar proliferation

The number of muscle fibres apparently does not increase during postnatal growth or as a result of exercise training at reasonable intensity levels. However, the mean cross-sectional area of the existing fibres does increase considerably. Studies on laboratory animals indicate that the total number of fibres is indirectly, genetically determined. It is about the same in males and females but the ultimate muscle fibre size attained in the male is greater than in the female. This is, no doubt, due to the influence of testosterone and other hormones.

The increase in fibre cross-sectional area is associated with a large increase in the myofibrillar content of the fibres. This involves a process by which a myofibril undergoes longitudinal splitting into two or more daughter myofibrils. In this way the myofibrillar mass becomes subdivided as it increases in volume and this allows the sarcoplasmic reticulum and transverse tubular systems to invade the mass and to come into close juxtaposition with the actin and myosin filaments. The longitudinal splitting of existing myofibrils apparently occurs because there is a built-in mismatch between the actin and myosin lattice so that the actin filaments are slightly displaced as they run from the Z-disc (square lattice) to the A-band (hexagonal lattice). This displacement or oblique pull of the actin filaments causes a mechanical stress to occur in the centre of each Z-disc that results in splitting of the myofibril (Goldspink, 1971) (Fig. 8.3). Splitting tends to be more complete in fast contracting fibres and

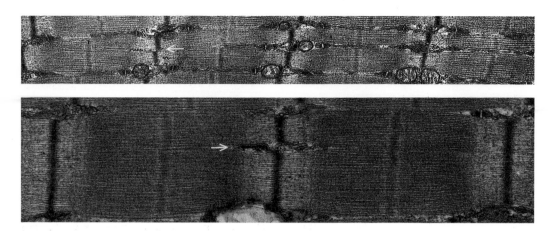

(a)

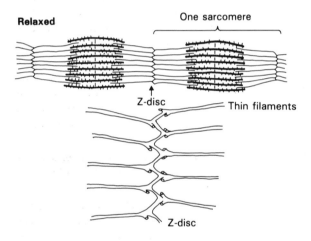

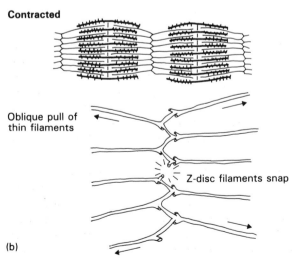

(b)

Fig. 8.3 (a) Longitudinal sections showing myofibrils in the process of splitting as seen under the electron microscope. The top section shows a myofibril that has divided on the left hand side. The lower section is a myofibril that has just commenced to split with intact Z-discs on each side of the ripped disc. Already elements of the SR and T systems can be seen in the fork of the split. (b) The mechanism of longitudinal splitting appears to depend on the oblique pull of peripheral actin filaments. This arises because of a mismatch in the actin and myosin filament lattices. The obliqueness increases as the myofibrils grow and increase in girth. When force is developed, this oblique pull of the actin filaments results in a mechanical stress being set up in the centre of the Z-disc, which causes it to rip. This is repeated all along the myofibril resulting in two daughter myofibrils.

therefore the myofibrils in these fibres are small and punctate. In slow-contracting fibres splitting is often incomplete and therefore the myofibrils appear branched in longitudinal section. An increase in the total number of myofibrils within existing fibres occurs during growth and during hypertrophy in response to overload. The maximum force production of a muscle is related to the myofibril cross-sectional area so that the physiological significance of this type of adaptation is apparent. However, we still need to ask what biochemical changes are occurring in an overloaded muscle that causes it to respond by producing more myofibrillar proteins.

Optimization of sarcomere length for force development

During postnatal development there is a considerable increase in the length of muscles and this results from the constituent fibres adding on sarcomeres serially. Studies with radioactive precursors have shown that the new sarcomeres are added on at the ends of the existing myofibrils (Williams & Goldspink, 1971). The functional significance of the sarcomere addition is apparent since the velocity of contraction and the force developed by a muscle are dependent on the number of cross-bridges that can be engaged between actin and myosin filaments. As stated above, this depends on the overlap of these filaments within the sarcomere and the only way initial sarcomere length can be adjusted is by changing the sarcomere number in series (Fig. 8.4). As the limb bones grow, the fibres are apparently stretched out to a point where there would be no overlap of the thick and thin filaments, were it not for the addition of new sarcomeres.

The number of sarcomeres in series is important in determining not only the distance through which the muscle can shorten but also the sarcomere length at which it can produce maximum power. Sarcomere number is not fixed, even in adult muscle, being capable of either increasing or decreasing (Tabary *et al.*,

1972: Williams & Goldspink, 1973) (Fig. 8.4). Regulation of sarcomere number is considered to be an adaptation to changes in the functional length of the muscle. These length-associated changes can be induced when the working length of the muscle is experimentally altered (Oudet & Petrovic, 1981) or where there is postural misalignment (Kendall *et al.*, 1952). Similar effects are observed during immobilization. In muscle immobilized in the shortened position, sarcomeres are lost and the remaining sarcomeres are altered to a length that enables the muscle to develop its maximum tension at the length which corresponds to the immobilized position (Williams & Goldspink, 1978). In muscles immobilized in the lengthened position, sarcomeres are added on and this results in sarcomere length being reduced as compared with non-adapted muscle fixed in a similar position. Maximum tension again is found to be developed at an increased functional length, which corresponds to the immobilized position. When the cast is removed sarcomere number returns to normal within a few days.

The regulation of sarcomere number to allow adjustment of sarcomere length would imply that the muscle fibre monitors sarcomere length in some way, either at a particular joint angle or over a range of angles. The sarcomere length would then be adjusted by adding or subtracting sarcomeres resulting in a decrease or increase in sarcomere length, respectively. The significant factor for the monitoring of sarcomere length may be the amount of tension along the myofibril and/or the myotendon junction, with high tension leading to an addition of sarcomeres and low tension to a substraction of sarcomeres (Herring *et al.*, 1984). The internal tension sensing may involve the cytoskeletal elements that form the scaffold on which the thick and thin filaments are assembled and in particular the protein titin, which is believed to transmit force through the sarcomere. Normal muscle functions at many lengths and obviously sarcomere length can be optimum for force production at only one joint

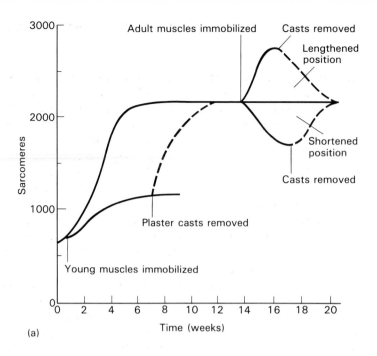

(a)

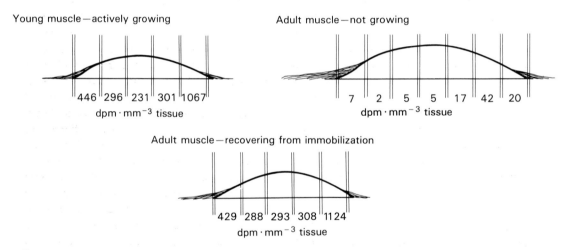

Fig. 8.4 (a) Summarizes data for the addition of sarcomeres along existing myofibrils during the normal growth of a muscle (mouse soleus). Also given are data for immobilization of a muscle in a young animal where the production of sarcomeres is suppressed. However, when the plaster cast is removed sarcomeres are produced at a very rapid rate until the normal number is attained within a week or so. In the adult animal, immobilization of the muscle in its lengthened position results in the addition of 20 or 30% more sarcomeres, whilst holding the muscle in a shortened position results in 20% loss of sarcomeres in series. This adaptation to a new functional length is reversible and when the plaster cast is removed the sarcomere number in series soon returns to normal. (b) The incorporation of radioactively labelled adenosine into the newly formed actin filaments in a young actively growing muscle, in an adult muscle that is not growing in length or in girth, and in an adult muscle that is recovering from a period of immobilization in the shortened position. The data were obtained by sectioning the muscle from end to end and placing batches of sections in a scintillation counter. Some sections were mounted on microscope slides and used to estimate the volume of tissue in each batch so that the radioactivity could be expressed as disintegrations per minute (dpm) per mm^3 of tissue. Note that the end regions of the fibres are the most heavily labelled in young and adult muscle recovering from the shortened position. This and other evidence indicates that the new sarcomeres are added onto the ends of the existing myofibrils.

angle. It seems likely that sarcomere number is regulated so as to achieve optimum sarcomere length at the muscle length at which most force (active and passive) is normally exerted.

Hypertrophy, protein synthesis and the importance of stretch

There are two main ways in which proteins are accumulated during growth or exercise training. One way is to increase the rate at which proteins are synthesized. The other is to decrease the rate at which they are broken down. Even in adult muscle, proteins are constantly being synthesized and broken down and the turnover, or half-life, of the contractile proteins is probably of the order of 7–15 days. The soluble sarcoplasmic proteins have an even shorter half-life. A process in which more than half of the contractile proteins are broken down and replaced every 7 days or so would seem to be rather wasteful. However, the process enables the muscle to replace damaged proteins and confers a certain adaptability for changing the type of protein at certain stages of development and under certain physiological conditions. Also, reutilization of amino acids takes place so the process is expensive in terms of energy but not in supply of amino acids.

All types of muscle fibres are capable of undergoing hypertrophy but they do not usually undergo hypertrophy to the same extent. Also, it appears that they use different strategies for the secretion of protein. With fast fibres the synthesis rate is increased, and with slow fibres the degradation rate is decreased. The fast contracting fibres are recruited only infrequently (for rapid power movements or high intensity isometric contractions) but when they are recruited and 'overloaded' they tend to undergo hypertrophy very readily. Selective hypertrophy of the fast fibres can be regarded as an adaptation for increased power production under situations when all or most of the fibres are being recruited. Slow fibres may also increase in size as a response to frequent recruitment, but to a lesser extent than the fast

fibres. In repetitive low-intensity exercise and postural activity, the fast fibres may hardly ever be recruited. Under these conditions they may atrophy at the same time as the slow fibres are undergoing some hypertrophy, for example during long distance running or cycling (Fig. 8.5). Thus, there is a selective response depending on the type of training. The other way muscle fibres respond to repetitive type training is to produce more mitochondria and oxidative enzymes. Accompanying this there is also an increase in the number of capillaries per fibre (Hoppler & Lindstedt, 1985). Both the slow-contracting and the fast-contracting fibres may respond by increasing their oxidative enzyme levels (Goldspink & Waterson, 1971). This type of adaptation therefore confers increased fatigue resistance on the muscle and hence an increased aerobic power output.

The question is often asked as to whether hyperplasia (increase in cell numbers) occurs as well as hypertrophy (increase in cell size) in response to strenuous exercise training. In general, experiments using normal types of exercise have not shown any change in the total number of fibres (Goldspink & Ward, 1979). However, partially splitting muscle fibres, not to be confused with splitting myofibrils, can be observed in surgically overloaded muscle (Vaughan & Goldspink, 1979). It is therefore possible that muscle fibre splitting may lead to hyperplasia, e.g. under conditions of repeated, incremental exercise. For this to be regarded as an adaptive phenomenon rather than a pathological change, the splitting would have to be complete and resulting fibres innervated. The question of muscle fibre hyperplasia and hypertrophy is discussed in Chapter 8B.

The degree of atrophy in disused muscle is affected by the amount of stretch placed on the muscle. Stretching the soleus muscle for 3 or 5 days produced marked changes in protein turnover. Increases in protein synthesis have been found in stretched muscle when measured *in vivo* (Booth & Seider, 1979; Goldspink *et al.*, 1983; Goldspink & Goldspink, 1986) or *in vitro* (Goldspink, 1977a). Such changes have

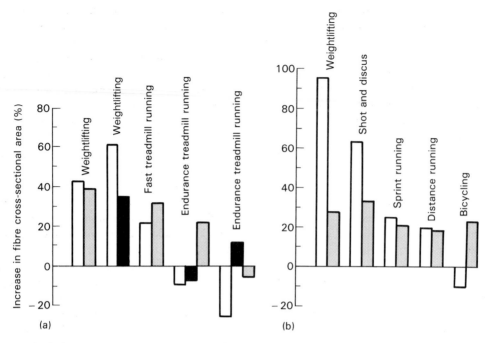

Fig. 8.5 The data presented here shows the ability of different muscle fibre types to undergo hypertrophy in response to different types of exercise. (a) Data from experiments on laboratory rodents with the change in fibre size being expressed as percentage increase over the control values. (b) Data for human subjects using quadriceps biopsy tissue by Professor Bengt Saltin's group. The fibre size is expressed as a percentage difference to a sedentary person. In both the animal and the human situations weightlifting induced the greatest hypertrophy in all fibre types with the greatest increase occurring in the fast glycolytic fibres. Interestingly, slow repetitive exercise resulted in atrophy of the fast glycolytic and a modest hypertrophy of the more fatigue resistant fibres (slow and the fast oxidative fibres). This illustrates that one way the properties of a muscle adapt during exercise training is to change the cross-sectional area of a muscle fibre types by selective hypertrophy or atrophy □, fast glycolytic fibres; ■, fast oxidative fibres; ▨, slow oxidative fibres.

been detected as early as 6 hours after the imposition of stretch in both normally innervated and denervated muscles; the latter pointing to a passive myogenic response rather than any active component triggered by sensory receptors within the stretched muscle. Thus the effect of stretch is to significantly increase the rate of muscle protein synthesis as well as to increase the number of sarcomeres in series.

The therapeutic applications of stretch therefore should be borne in mind when designing regimes for rehabilitation or improved athletic performance.

Connective tissue and changes in muscle stiffness

Other types of cells in addition to muscle cells respond to mechanical stress including bone cells, skin cells and fibroblasts. These, and also perhaps muscle cells, are induced to secrete extra collagen when subjected to an overload situation (Williams & Goldspink, 1984). Certainly the collagen framework of muscle can be rapidly remodelled in response to changed functional length as well as overload. As discussed, the loss of sarcomeres and reduction in muscle fibre length that occurs when muscles are working at a shortened length is accompanied by an increase in muscle stiffness (Tabary et al., 1972). Length/passive tension curves for muscles immobilized in a shortened position are steeper than those for control muscle and this is the case even when allowances are made for the shorter lengths of the immobilized muscles (Goldspink & Williams, 1979). Biochemical analysis of hydroxyproline (which can be considered to occur exclusively in collagen and which can therefore be used to calculate collagen content) demonstrates that during immobilization in the shortened position there is an increase in the proportion of collagen to muscle fibre tissue (Williams & Goldspink, 1984). It should be noted that this is only a proportional increase; indeed there is a total loss of collagen but an even greater loss of muscle fibre tissue. The connective tissue component can also be investigated in detail using sections stained selectively for collagen, and computerized image analysis can be used to convert the optical image into a digitized signal (Fig. 8.6). Following immobilization of a muscle in its shortened position, the proportion of both endomysium and perimysium is increased (Williams & Goldspink, 1984). This presumably explains why the muscle is stiffer. The events that occur during the first few days of immobilization are particularly interesting. An increase in the relative amount of perimysium occurs after only 2 days of immobilization in the shortened position; indeed before there is evidence of loss of sarcomeres. Interestingly, stretch causes the muscle fibres to become longer by addition of sarcomeres but thickening of the connective tissue does not occur although there must be an increase in total amount of collagen in the longer muscles.

When muscle is immobilized in the shortened position it is subjected not only to lack of stretch but also to lack of activity and either or both could result in connective tissue remodelling. Experiments on rabbit muscle using immobilization combined with electrical stimulation have gone some way towards determining the relative importance of these two parameters (Fig. 8.7). Immobilization in the shortened position combined with electrical stimulation subjects the muscle to contractile activity whilst eliminating passive stretch. Such muscles show a loss of serial sarcomeres but no connective tissue changes, implying that lack of activity is an important factor in connective tissue remodelling.

It is interesting to note that stimulation alone causes a reduction in serial sarcomere number. This is probably due to the fact that stimulation causes the muscle to be held in a more shortened position than normal, i.e. the muscle is working at and adapting to a reduced length. Therefore, sarcomere loss is apparently associated with reduced functional length rather than reduced contractile activity. The changes that occur in immobilized muscles have important implications for the treatment and rehabilitation of people whose limbs are subjected to a period of disuse following injury. This is because the range of joint movement is reduced both by the shortening of the muscle fibres and by loss of muscle. Experiments have therefore been carried out to determine whether short periods of stretch are effective in preventing the changes in muscle connective tissue and sarcomere number. Very short periods of stretch (15 min every second day) are found to be sufficient to maintain normal muscle connective tissue (Williams, 1988).

Molecular regulation of muscle fibre type, growth, hypertrophy and atrophy

Muscle is a tissue in which gene expression is regulated to a large extent by mechanical signals. Mammalian muscles consist of populations of slow contracting, oxidative, fibres that are adapted for slow repetitive movements and semi-isometric postural activity. They also possess populations of fast contracting fibres that are required for rapid powerful movements. As well as having a higher mitochondrial content than the fast fibres, the slow fibres have different contractile protein isoforms. Using

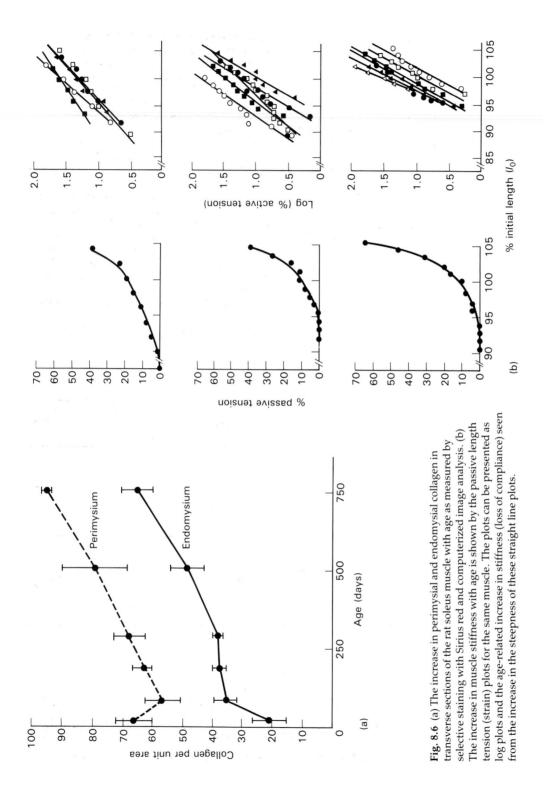

Fig. 8.6 (a) The increase in perimysial and endomysial collagen in transverse sections of the rat soleus muscle with age as measured by selective staining with Sirius red and computerized image analysis. (b) The increase in muscle stiffness with age is shown by the passive length tension (strain) plots for the same muscle. The plots can be presented as log plots and the age-related increase in stiffness (loss of compliance) seen from the increase in the steepness of these straight line plots.

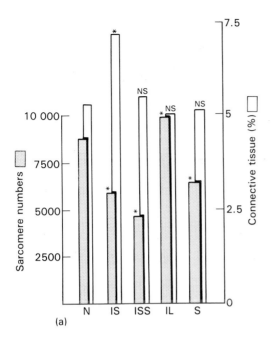

(a)

Fig. 8.7 (a) Summarized data for the change in sarcomere number and connective collagen concentration in different conditions of stretch and stimulation. Sarcomere number changes are induced by the functional length changes (length at which the muscle is habitually held) whilst collagen changes seem to be a response to lack of stimulation (movement). N, normal; IS, immobilized and shortened; ISS, immobilized, shortened and stimulated; IL, immobilized and lengthened; S, stimulated only. Using the paired t test, the change in sarcomere number and the change in connective tissue concentration compared to normal are shown by *, $P < 0.01$; NS, not significant. (b) Physiological plots of active and passive tension for muscles that have been immobilized in the shortened position for 3 weeks (○) and for normal muscles (●). The active tension data show that the initial length at which the muscle develops maximum force is shifted by the change in the serial sarcomere number. The passive tension plots in the immobilized shortened muscles are stiffer and develop tension at a much shorter length, which reflects the restructuring of the connective tissue in these muscles.

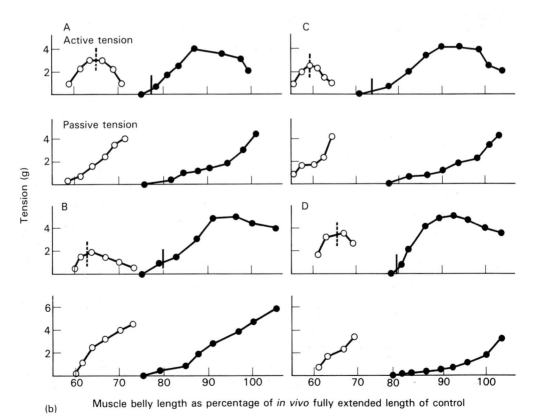

(b) Muscle belly length as percentage of *in vivo* fully extended length of control

electrical stimulation to control force generation and limb immobilization to alter the degree of stretch, the author's laboratory has studied the role of physical activity in determining fast and slow muscle fibre phenotype (Williams *et al.*, 1986). Changes in gene expression were detected by analysing RNA in hybridization studies employing cDNA probes specific for fast and slow myosin heavy chain genes (Goldspink & Scutt, 1989; Goldspink *et al.*, 1991). The skeletal myosin heavy chain genes belong to a family of genes that are arranged in tandem on chromosome 17 in man (chromosome 11 in the rat). The cardiac muscle myosin genes, for which there are two isoforms α and β, are on chromosome 14 in man. There are at least five isoform genes for the skeletal myosin heavy chains and these are expressed in the sequence: embryonic, neonatal, adult fast, adult fast oxidative, and adult slow.

As a result of overload in the stretched position, the fast contracting tibialis anterior muscle in an adult rabbit is induced to synthesize a lot of protein and to grow by as much as 30% within a period as short as 4 days. This very rapid hypertrophy was found to be associated with a 250% increase in the RNA content of the muscle and a change in the species of mRNA produced. Both stretch alone and electrical stimulation alone caused some activation of the slow type and repression of the fast-type genes. However, a more complete switch in myosin heavy chain gene expression was achieved when these mechanical stimuli were combined and when higher frequencies of stimulations were used. This leads to the conclusion that muscle fibre adult phenotype is determined by stretch and force generation (passive plus active tension) and that this is controlled at the level of gene transcription. The regulation of growth, however, is probably limited by the rate of translation of the message into protein. In this context it is interesting to note that the ribosomal density is increased very significantly during hypertrophy. It also decreases significantly during postnatal growth in line with the slowing of muscle develop-

ment. It therefore appears that the translational process, which is known to be much slower than the transcriptional process, is the rate-determining step in hypertrophy. Certainly, the 250% increase in ribosomal RNA during the rapid hypertrophy of an adult muscle means that extra ribosomes are available to translate the message, whatever it may be. Therefore, the rapid synthesis of more ribosomes seems to be the first step in producing muscle fibre hypertrophy.

Adaptation for increased velocity or economy

Adjustment to optimum sarcomere length

It follows that the velocity of contraction of a muscle is dependent or the initial sarcomere length and hence the number of myosin cross-bridges that can engage as well as the predominant type of cross-bridge. The way sarcomere length and sarcomere number are adjusted during growth has been described above. These adjustments are all in scale with the changes in skeleton dimensions. In the adult there seems to be little scope for adjustment during normal athletic training. However, if the muscle is not habitually put through its normal range of excursion then problems may arise. For instance, the wearing of high-heeled shoes can cause the gastrocnemius and soleus muscles to shorten by losing sarcomeres and remodelling their connective tissue. This results in the Achilles tendon being pulled off the bone when the adapted shortened muscle is then required to go through the normal range of lengthening (eccentric) actions.

Determination of muscle fibre phenotype cross-sectional area

As mentioned above there are fast contracting fibres that are adapted for high power output and slow contracting fibres that are adapted for performing slow movements efficiently and developing isometric force economically. The slow fibres apparently have a higher maximum efficiency of converting ATP into work than the fast fibres. In order for the slow fibres or the fast fibres to achieve their maximum efficiency, their intrinsic rate of shortening has to be matched to the rate to which they are required to shorten (Fig. 8.8). Therefore, the slow fibres with the slow myosin cross-bridges are much more efficient for producing the slow repetitive contractions required for, say, long distance running. They are also more economical for developing and maintaining isometric force or semi-isometric force as their slow cross-bridge cycle time means that attachment phase (when no ATP is being used) is much longer than it is for fast muscle. In endurance events, when it is important to maintain power output, the training has to be directed towards increasing the percentage of slow type contractile proteins and more mitochondria. In explosive power events it is important to increase the total amount of fast type myosin. There are two ways in which the contractile properties and hence the energy efficiency of a muscle can be altered during training. These include the interconversion of fibres, for example fast into slow, and the selective hypertrophy of a given fibre type. Basically, these may represent the same mechanism, as fibres do not exist as discrete types but as a continuum. Indeed, all fibres have a mixture of the different contractile protein isoforms, but in fast fibres there is a predominance of the fast myosin heavy chain and other fast contractile protein isoforms. This resolves down to which isoform genes are induced and which are repressed. So far our studies have indicated that the fast adult genes are the default genes. However, when the muscle is subjected to stretch or to repeated stimulation it will express the slow adult genes. There may be a window of a certain time period needed for switching on the slow genes so that they are only switched on by long bursts of activity. The cellular signals for the muscle gene switching are not understood, but these may include changed metabolite or calcium levels.

Age-related changes at the cellular and molecular levels

Decline in muscle function with age

During this century the age structure of society has changed, so that the percentage of old people alive today is much higher than ever before. As life expectancy increases, so will the number of persons with locomotory handicaps, unless of course, commensurate strides are made in medical research and health care. For this reason, it is important to understand ageing in skeletal muscle and the locomotor system. The decrease in muscle mass and muscular performance with advancing age has been documented by a number of workers (e.g. Grimby & Saltin, 1983). To what extent this decline in performance is a consequence of the change in activity of people with age and vice versa is difficult to quantify. At the turn of the century most of the population in the developed countries made their living by carrying out manual tasks. Now only a small percentage do so, and with the advance of the 'hi tech' revolution this percentage will drop even further. The relationship between physical exercise and the ageing process is therefore an important area that needs further study. The increasing cost of health care emphasizes the need for a preventative approach to medicine; otherwise a disproportionate amount of the wealth of a country will be used in caring for its increasing proportion of infirm, elderly citizens. Hence, it can be argued that the prime goal of ageing research should be to prolong the active period of life rather than life expectancy *per se*. The loss of mobility and the ability to perform basic physical tasks coupled with the increased reliance on other people have profound psychological implications for some ageing individuals. In this context, a study of the functional changes in the locomotor system with age is of prime importance.

Increased usage of skeletal muscle as a result of endurance training is known to bring about morphological (Green *et al.*, 1984),

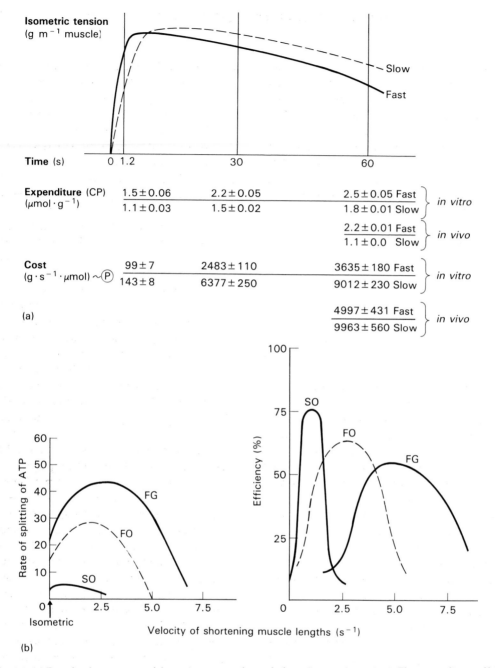

Fig. 8.8 (a) Data for the ecomony of the maintenance of muscle force (isometric tension). The expenditure of high energy phosphate (CP) and the cost of producing and maintaining isometric force are given for fast and slow type muscles. Values are given for muscles treated with iodoacetate and nitrogen. Also given are values for muscles in which replenishment of ATP and CP can proceed. Note that the slow muscle uses considerably less energy for developing and particularly for maintaining isometric force. (b) Summarizes data for the expenditure of fast glycolytic (FG) fast oxidative (FO) and slow oxidative (SO) muscle during isotonic contractions at different shortening velocities. Also shown on the right is the efficiency of doing work for these three types of muscle. The slow fibres are seen to have a higher maximum efficiency providing they are shortening at about one muscle length per second. At velocities above this they become very inefficient and contribute very little to the work produced by the muscle. The fast contracting fibres are responsible for the power output at the higher rates of shortening and they also have optimum velocities with regard to efficiency of converting high energy phosphate into work.

physiological (Salmons & Vrbova, 1969) and biochemical (Vihko *et al.*, 1978) changes depending upon the duration and intensity of the exercise stimulus. However, these effects have been found to be less pronounced in ageing muscle in laboratory animals (Silberman *et al.*, 1983) and humans (Larsson, 1982). Ageing rats exercise less in voluntary exercise programmes and models have been proposed that indicate a 'threshold age' beyond which exercise training following a sedentary life may even be deleterious rather than beneficial (Pollock *et al.*, 1974).

Muscle stiffness

Ageing changes are known to occur in connective tissue and a considerable amount of research has been directed towards characterizing the changes that occur in skin and those associated with joints. It is surprising that so little attention has been paid to the possibility of age-related muscle fibrosis and in particular age–exercise interactions. Collagen is known to decrease in solubility and to become more crosslinked with age, and evidence is available of molecular differences between collagen synthesized in young and old animals. Immobilization is known to increase collagen turnover and deposition in ligaments and thus increase the stiffness of joints.

It has been shown that there is an appreciable increase in collagen content of muscle with age and this is associated with thickening of the endomysium and perimysin (see Fig. 8.6). Experiments involving the exercising of old animals suggests that the age-related fibrosis is reduced by regular exercise. This provides a basis for understanding how moderate exercise helps to maintain muscle suppleness with age.

The future

As mentioned in the introduction, a great deal of scientific effort is now being directed towards sequencing the human genome. Once all the genes have been catalogued, this will inevitably lead to study of the differences

between individuals. As performance of any athletic event involves many different parameters involving several body systems, e.g. central nervous system, cardiovascular, muscle, etc., it is unlikely that predictions of performance will be made on this basis, at least for many years to come. However, emerging methods in molecular biology do offer the prospect of optimizing training regimes by assessing alterations in gene expression. By attaching synthetic DNA (oligonucleotides) probes to each end of a specific gene sequence, it is possible to amplify that particular DNA sequence by a million times within a couple of hours using the polymerase chain reaction (PCR). The specific probes act as primers for the DNA polymerase enzyme that replicates the gene, inserting labelled nucleotide bases, which are also in the reaction mixture. The procedure requires that the tissue sample or extract be heated first to 90 °C to separate the two strands of DNA. It is then cooled to 40 °C to allow the probes (primers) to anneal and then warmed to 70 °C for replication. This is achieved by a programmed water bath and by the use of a special TAQ DNA polymerase, which is thermostable so it does not have to be replenished for each temperature cycle. A million labelled copies of the gene can then result from 20 cycles of strand separation, probe hybridization and replication. Not only can this method be used to detect the presence of a given gene but it can be used to measure the expression of that gene in a given tissue by detecting the mRNA (gene transcript). For this purpose the RNA is first converted by reverse transcriptase and this is then amplified in the usual way. The PCR needs very little tissue and is therefore suitable for detecting the presence of a particular gene using a blood cell smear or for assessing gene expression in, say, muscle biopsy samples.

In situ hybridization is another method that is sensitive and which has the advantage that the expression of a specific gene can be detected in a given muscle fibre type. In our laboratory (Fig. 8.9) we use specific cRNA rather than cDNA probes as these can be generated with

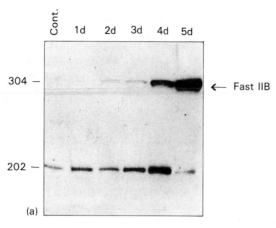

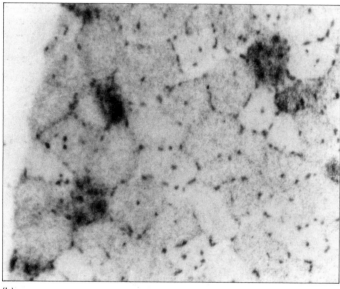

(a)

(b)

Fig. 8.9 Two molecular biology methods that can be used to detect changes in gene expression during training and in damaged muscle. (a) Hybridization procedure involving S1 nuclease blotting using a cDNA probe for fast type IIB myosin heavy chain. In this experiment the soleus muscle was immobilized in the shortened position and this slow muscle, which does not normally synthesize fast IIB myosin, commenced to transcribe the fast gene after only 2 days. (From Loughna *et al.*, 1990.) (b) *In situ* hybridization using a probe to the collagen III gene on dystrophic muscle. The advantage of this approach is that cell-specific gene expression can be detected with great sensitivity so that it can be used on biopsy sections.

high specific levels of labelling (radioactive or biotin label). Also, the sensitivity of cRNA to mRNA is 10 times greater than cDNA to mRNA. This procedure we believe is very suitable for use on muscle biopsy sections, which can also be stained using monoclonal antibodies, etc. In this way athletic and re-habilitation training regimes can be optimized for power production or for endurance.

Acknowledgements

Whilst this chapter was being written the author's salary was paid by the Wellcome Trust, London.

References

Booth, F.W. & Seider, M.J. (1979) Early changes in skeletal muscle protein synthesis after im-mobilization of rats. *Journal of Applied Physiology*, **49**, 974–7.

Goldspink, D.F. (1977a) The influence of immobiliza-tion and stretch on protein turnover of rat skeletal muscle. *Journal of Physiology*, **264**, 267–82.

Goldspink, D.F., Garlick, P.J. & McNurlan, M.A. (1983) Protein turnover measured *in vivo* and *in vitro* in muscles undergoing compensatory growth and subsequent denervation atrophy. *Biochemical Journal*, **210**, 89–98.

Goldspink, D.F. & Goldspink, G. (1986) The role of passive stretch in retarding muscle atrophy. In W.A. Nix & G. Vrbova (eds) *Electrical Stimulation and Neuromuscular Disorders*, pp. 91–100. Springer Verlag, Berlin.

Goldspink, G. (1971) Ultrastructural changes in striated muscle fibres during contraction and growth with particular reference to the mechanism of myofibril splitting. *Journal of Cell Science*, **9**, 123–38.

Goldspink, G. (1977b) Muscle energetics. In R. McN. Alexander & G. Goldspink (eds) *Mechanics and Energetics of Animal Locomotion*, Chapter 3. Chapman & Hall, London.

Goldspink, G. (1981) Design of muscle for locomotion and maintenance of posture. *Trends in Neurosciences*, **39**, 218–21.

Goldspink, G. (1984) Alterations in myofibril size and structure during growth. In L. Peachy, R. Adrian & S.R. Gerzer (eds) *Handbook of Physiology. Skeletal Muscle*, pp. 539–54. American Physiological Society, Bethesda.

Goldspink, G. & Scutt, A. (1989) Stretch and isometric tension induce rapid changes in gene expression in adult skeletal muscle. *Journal of Physiology*, **415**, 129p.

Goldspink, G., Scutt, A., Martindale, J., Jaenicke, T., Turay, L. & Gerlach, G.-F. (1991). Stretch and force generation induce rapid hypertrophy and isoform gene switching in adult skeletal muscle. *Biochemical Society Transactions*, **19**, 368–73.

Goldspink, G. & Ward, P.S. (1979) Changes in rodent muscle fibre types during post-natal growth, undernutrition and exercise. *Journal of Physiology*, **296**, 453–69.

Goldspink, G. & Waterson, S.E. (1971) The effect of growth and inanition on the total amount of Nitro-blue tetrazolium deposited in individual muscle fibres of fast and slow skeletal muscle. *Acta Histochemica*, **40**, 16–22.

Goldspink, G. & Williams, P.E. (1979) The nature of the increased passive resistance in muscle following immobilization of the mouse soleus muscle. *Journal of Physiology*, **289**, 55p.

Green, H.J., Klug, G.A. & Reichmann, H. (1984) Exercise-induced fibre type transitions with regard to myosin parvalbumin and sarcoplasmic reticulum in muscles of the rat. *Pflügers Archiv*, **400**, 432–8.

Grimby, G. & Saltin, B. (1983) The ageing muscle. *Clinical Physiology*, **3**, 209–18.

Herring, S.W., Grimm, A.F. & Grimm, B.R. (1984) Regulation of sarcomere number in skeletal muscle: a comparison of hypotheses. *Muscle and Nerve*, **7**, 161–73.

Hoppeler, H. & Lindstedt, S.L. (1985) Malleability of skeletal muscle in overcoming limitations: structural elements. *Journal of Experimental Biology*, **115**, 355–64.

Kendall, H.O., Kendall, F.P. & Boynton, D.A. (1952) In M.D. Baltimore (ed.) *Posture and Pain*, pp. 103–24. Williams & Wilkins, Baltimore.

Larsson, L. (1982) Physical training effects on muscle morphology in sedentary males at different ages. *Medicine and Science in Sports and Exercise*, **14**, 203–6.

Loughna, P.T., Izumo, S., Goldspink, G. & Nadal-Ginard, B. (1990) Rapid changes in sarcomeric myosin heavy chain gene and alpha-actin expression in response to disuse and stretch. *Development*, **109**, 217–23.

Oudet, C.L. & Petrovic, A.G. (1981) Regulation of the anatomical length of the lateral pterygoid muscle in the growing rat. *Advances in Physiological Sciences*, **24**, 115–21.

Pollock, M.L., Miller, H.S. & Wilmore, J. (1974) Physiological characteristics of champion American track athletes 40–75 years of age. *Journal of Gerontology*, **29**, 649.

Salmons, S. & Vrbova, G. (1969) The influence of activity on some contractile characteristics of mammalian fast and slow muscles. *Journal of Physiology*, **201**, 535–49.

Silberman, M., Finkelbrand, S. & Weiss, A. (1983) Morphometric analysis of aging skeletal muscle following endurance training. *Muscle and Nerve*, **6**, 136–42.

Tabary, J.C., Tabary, C., Tardieu, C., Tardieu, G. & Goldspink, G. (1972) Physiological and structural changes in the cat's soleus muscle due to immobilization at different lengths by plaster cast. *Journal of Physiology*, **224**, 231–44.

Vaughan, H.S. & Goldspink, G. (1979) Fibre number and fibre size in a surgically overloaded muscle. *Journal of Anatomy*, **129**, 293–303.

Vihko, V., Salminen, A. & Rantamaki, J. (1978) Oxidative and lysosomal capacity of mice after endurance training of different intensities. *Acta Physiologica Scandinavica*, **104**, 74–81.

Williams, P.E. (1988) Effect of intermittent stretch on immobilized muscle. *Annals of the Rheumatic Diseases*, **47**, 1014–16.

Williams, P.E. & Goldspink, G. (1971) Longitudinal growth of striated muscle fibres. *Journal of Cell Science*, **9**, 751–67.

Williams, P.E. & Goldspink, G. (1973) The effect of immobilization on the longitudinal growth of striated muscle fibres. *Journal of Anatomy*, **116**, 45–55.

Williams, P.E. & Goldspink, G. (1978) Changes in sarcomere length and physiological properties in immobilized muscle. *Journal of Anatomy*, **127**, 459–68.

Williams, P.E. & Goldspink, G. (1984) Connective tissue changes in immobilized muscle. *Journal of Anatomy*, **138**, 343–50.

Williams, P., Watt, P., Bicik, V. & Goldspink, G. (1986) Effect of stretch combined with electrical stimulation on the type of sarcomeres produced at the ends of muscle fibres. *Experimental Neurology*, **93**, 500–9.

Chapter 8B

Hypertrophy or Hyperplasia

J. DUNCAN MacDOUGALL

Introduction

Skeletal muscle is an extremely dynamic tissue with an impressive capacity to adapt both anatomically and physiologically to a wide range in functional demands. It is well known that when adult muscles are caused to act at intensities that exceed 60–70% of their maximum force generating capacity, adaptations occur that result in an increase in total muscle size (cross-sectional area) and strength. Theoretically, an increase in muscle size could occur as a result of an increase in fibre size, an increase in fibre numbers, and/or an increase in interstitial connective tissue.

The fact that increases in muscle fibre size occur in response to a functional overload such as resistance training has been well established in humans (MacDougall et al., 1979, 1980; McDonagh & Davies, 1984; Tesch, 1987) and other mammals (Gonyea & Ericson, 1976; Timson et al., 1985). While it is known that the major contributor to muscle growth up until early infancy is an increase in fibre numbers (Goldspink, 1974; Mastaglia, 1981; Malina, 1986), the possibility that this process might contribute to training-induced hypertrophy in adulthood is considerably more controversial. There have been very few investigations of the effects of resistance training on interstitial connective tissue but since it occupies a relatively small proportion of the total muscle volume its potential for making a major contribution to changes in muscle size is limited.

A number of experimental models have been used in order to stimulate muscle hypertrophy. These include animal models involving ablation, tenotomy or denervation of synergists (Goldberg, 1967; Gollnick et al., 1981; Timson et al., 1985), chronic passive stretch of a muscle or muscle group (Sola et al., 1973; Holly et al., 1980; Alway et al., 1989b) and heavy resistance training or weightlifting. Discussion in this chapter will, for the most part, be confined to the hypertrophy response to resistance training as would be performed by the strength and power athlete or bodybuilder.

Hypertrophy of muscle fibres in response to strength training

Fibre area

In adult subjects heavy resistance training results in an increase in cross-sectional area of both type I and type II fibres. The magnitude of this increase varies considerably and is dependent upon a number of factors including the individual's responsiveness to training (MacDougall, 1986a), the intensity and duration of the training programme and the training status of the subject prior to commencement of the programme. Over a number of longitudinal resistance training studies, where we have obtained needle biopsies from young adults before and after a training programme, we have observed wide variations in changes in fibre area. These have ranged from no significant

230

change in area of either fibre type in vastus lateralis of young men and women following 6 months of training (Sale *et al.*, 1990) to an increase of 33% in type II and 27% in type I fibre areas in a group of previously untrained young men who trained their triceps brachii for 6 months (MacDougall *et al.*, 1979). In a study where 14 older men (60–70 years) performed resistance training for 3 months, type II fibre area in biceps brachii was found to increase by 30% and type I by 14% (Brown *et al.*, 1988). In a cross-comparison study, fibre areas for biceps brachii in a group of elite bodybuilders were found to be approximately 58% (type II) and 39% (type I) larger than those of untrained age-matched controls (MacDougall *et al.*, 1984).

In a recent study where 15 postmenopausal women (52–68 years) trained for 11 months, total muscle cross-sectional area of the elbow flexors (as determined by CT scan) increased by approximately 20% (Moroz *et al.*, 1990) but, using the same technique, we were unable to detect any increase in muscle size in a group of prepubescent boys (9–11 years) who underwent similar training for 5 months (Ramsay *et al.*, 1990).

Changes in fibre area according to fibre type

Although strength training results in an increase in cross-sectional area of all fibre types, most studies indicate that a greater relative hypertrophy occurs in the type II units (Thorstensson, 1976; MacDougall *et al.*, 1979; Tesch *et al.*, 1985; Staron *et al.*, 1989). Since both fibre types are probably equally recruited in the performance of a maximal or near-maximal contraction, the greater hypertrophy of the type II fibres may reflect a greater *relative* involvement of these high threshold units than would normally occur during daily activity.

Conversion of fibre types with training

Although a recent study has reported conversion of type II subunits in human skeletal muscle following heavy resistance training

(Staron *et al.*, 1989), it is unlikely that such training alters the proportions of type I and type II fibres. This conclusion is based on our finding of no change in the percentage of these fibre types following 6 months of intensive training (MacDougall *et al.*, 1980) as well as our finding of the same percentage fibre type in triceps and biceps of elite bodybuilders as that of untrained subjects, despite 6–8 years of training by the bodybuilders (MacDougall *et al.*, 1982, 1984) (see Fig. 8.10).

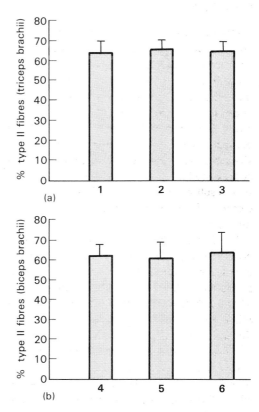

Fig. 8.10 (a) Percent type II fibres in triceps brachii of male subjects before (1: *n* = 9) and after (2: *n* = 9) 6 months of heavy-resistance training and after 6 weeks of immobilization of the elbow joint (3:*n* = 8). (b) Percent type II fibres in biceps brachii in a group of untrained controls (4:*n* = 13), a group of intermediate bodybuilders (5: *n* = 7) and a group of elite bodybuilders (6: *n* = 5). Values are means ± 1 SD. (From MacDougall, 1986a.)

Other changes

The proportion of interstitial connective tissue remains quite constant over a wide range of muscle sizes, as indicated by biopsies from biceps of elite and novice bodybuilders and untrained controls. We have estimated the volume density of non-contractile tissue to be approximately 13% of the total muscle volume, of which approximately 6% is collagen (as indicated by Gomori trichrome staining) and 7% other tissue (MacDougall *et al.*, 1984). These data indicate that increases in fibre size due to resistance training are accompanied by a proportional increase in interstitial connective tissue. Thus, while the absolute amount of connective tissue increases with strength training, this can only be considered as having a minor effect on changes in total muscle size.

Unlike endurance training, resistance training has little or no effect on the capillary-to-fibre ratio. When expressed as capillary density (capillaries $\cdot$ mm^{-2}), in studies where training has resulted in a significant increase in fibre area, this value decreases, presumably due to the dilution effect of increased contractile protein (MacDougall, 1986b). Similar findings have been noted in cross-sectional studies that have compared weight- and power-lifters with untrained subjects (Tesch *et al.*, 1984). A possible exception may occur in muscles of bodybuilders who perform lower intensity and higher volume training than other strength athletes. In such subjects, Tesch and co-workers (1986) have noticed capillary densities similar to that of untrained individuals.

Changes in muscle ultrastructure

Electron microscopic investigations of the training-induced hypertrophy process in human muscle reveal that the increase that occurs in fibre area is directly related to an increase in both the myofibril area and the myofibril number, with no change in myofibril packing density (MacDougall, 1986b). With training, actin and myosin filaments are added to the periphery of the myofibrils, thus creating larger myofibrils without altering filament packing density or cross-bridge spacing. Since total fibre area increases to a greater extent than does average myofibril area, it is apparent that myofibril numbers also increase (MacDougall, 1986b). This increase in myofibril number is thought to be the result of longitudinal 'splitting', as has been shown to occur with normal postnatal growth in young animals (Goldspink, 1970, 1974). This splitting may be a mechanical process, which results from discrepancies between the A- and I-band lattice spacing. When the myofibril achieves a critical size and strength, forceful contractions are thought to cause tearing or rupturing of the connective tissue in the Z-discs, which are transmitted along the myofibril to result in two or more 'daughter myofibrils' of the same length (Goldspink, 1970) (Fig. 8.11).

The increase in contractile protein dilutes the mitochondrial proportion of the fibre resulting in a significant decrease in mitochondrial volume density (MacDougall *et al.*, 1979; Lüthi *et al.*, 1986). Sarcoplasmic reticulum and T-tubule volume density, on the other hand, increase in proportion to the change in myofibrillar volume so that its relative volume density remains constant for both fibre types and the time-related contractile properties are unaltered (Alway *et al.*, 1989a).

Hyperplasia of skeletal muscle fibres

Fibre proliferation during development

Mammalian skeletal muscle develops embryonically from the mesoderm. Repeated mitotic division gives rise to millions of mononucleated cells known as myoblasts. By approximately the fourth week of gestation, groups of myoblasts align and begin to fuse together to form the multinucleated myotubes that will eventually become mature muscle fibres. The process continues until birth and perhaps a few months after birth. Since the peripherally located nuclei of the myotubes are incapable

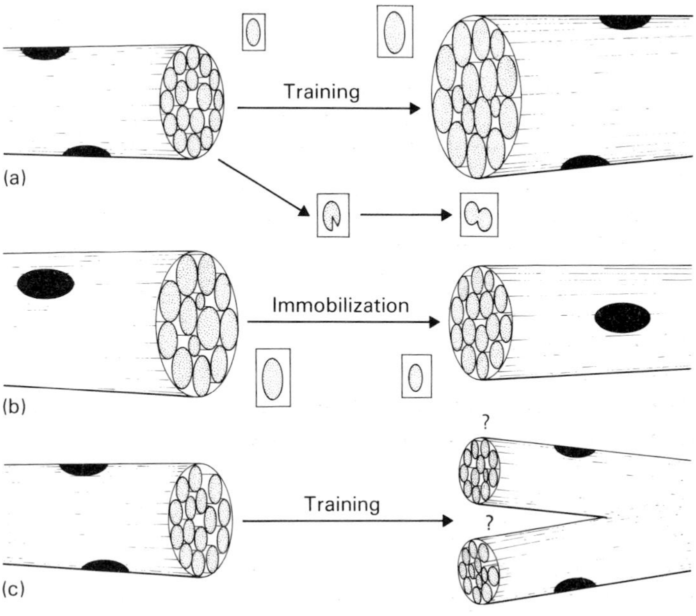

Fig. 8.11 A model for changes in muscle size that occur in response to strength training and immobilization. (a) With training, cross-sectional fibre area increases in direct proportion to the increases in myofibril size and number. (b) With immobilization, fibre area decreases in proportion to the decrease in myofibril size. (c) Training-induced fibre splitting has been postulated to occur in certain species but it is unlikely that it occurs in adult humans. (From MacDougall, 1986b.)

of further mitotic division at this stage, it is generally thought that, by birth (or shortly thereafter), total muscle fibre number is fully established (Fischman, 1972; Mastaglia, 1981; Malina, 1986).

Postnatal muscle growth is the result of an increase in fibre area and length. The increase in muscle length is the result of the addition of sarcomeres to the ends of the fibre and continues until bone growth is complete. The increase in fibre area and length is accompanied by a proportional increase in the number of myonuclei. These nuclei are thought to be derived from satellite cells (Moss & LeBlond, 1971; Goldspink, 1974; Malina, 1986), which in turn are considered to be derived from populations of myoblasts that did not fuse to form myotubes during prenatal development (White & Esser, 1989).

Hyperplasia of fibres in neonatal muscle

Several investigators have reported numerical increases in muscle fibres during early neonatal growth in certain species such as the rat (Chiakulus & Pauly, 1965; Rayne & Crawford,

1975). Various mechanisms have been proposed to account for such hyperplasia.

1 *De novo* formation of fibres from residual myoblasts.

2 Longitudinal splitting of or budding from existing fibres.

3 Lengthening of short fibres that did not previously traverse the full length of the muscle.

4 Separation and further growth of immature fibres previously enclosed within the basement membrane of fibres at a more advanced stage of development (Mastaglia 1981).

Electron microscopic investigations of developing neonatal muscle in rats indicate that the first two mechanisms do not occur and that what appears to be an addition of fibre numbers can be accounted for by the latter two processes (Ontell & Dunn, 1978; Mastaglia, 1981).

Hyperplasia of fibres in adult muscle?

Since the work by Morpurgo in 1897, who trained dogs on a running wheel, it has generally been accepted that the fibre content of adult mammalian skeletal muscle remains constant and that muscle growth occurs exclusively through enlargement of the existing fibres. In the 1970s, however, a series of studies appeared which suggested that compensatory and training-induced growth in chicken, cat and rat muscle may be the result of both hypertrophy of existing fibres and the addition of new fibres (Reitsma, 1969; Hall-Craggs, 1970; Sola *et al.*, 1973; Gonyea *et al.*, 1977; Gonyea, 1980).

In 1981, Gollnick and colleagues challenged these latter studies and suggested that methodological errors associated with the method of estimation of fibre numbers from histological sections may have biased their interpretation. Utilizing a technique by which all of the fibres in a muscle were isolated and counted, these authors (Gollnick *et al.*, 1981) concluded that, in rats, muscle enlargement caused by ablation of a synergist and treadmill running could be completely accounted for by hypertrophy of the existing fibres without the addition of more fibres. This was corroborated by a subsequent study using mice (Timson *et al.*, 1985). Use of running as a training mode differs considerably, however, from the heavy resistance training that was used in many of the studies that have reported hyperplasia and indeed, using the same fibre counting technique as Gollnick and co-workers, a significant 9% increase in fibre numbers has been found in cats, following heavy weightlifting (Gonyea *et al.*, 1986). A 52% increase in fibre numbers of latissimus dorsi has also recently been demonstrated in adult quail where a heavy weight was suspended from one wing for a period of 30 days (Alway *et al.*, 1989b).

Fibre hyperplasia in humans

The extent to which hyperplasia might occur in muscles of humans who participate in heavy resistance training is equally controversial. Indirect evidence based on measurement of fibre size (MacDougall *et al.*, 1982; Tesch & Larsson, 1982) and estimations of fibre num-

bers per motor unit (Larsson & Tesch, 1986) suggest that some bodybuilders possess more muscle fibres than untrained subjects. In such instances, however, it must be recognized that the greater fibre numbers may have been inherited and may not be the result of training-induced hyperplasia. Because of the methodological difficulties in determining muscle fibre numbers in humans it is difficult to resolve this issue.

Using an *in vivo* method for estimating fibre numbers we examined biceps brachii in 25 young males, of whom five were elite bodybuilders, seven were intermediate calibre bodybuilders and 13 were age-matched untrained controls (MacDougall *et al.*, 1984). Muscle fibre numbers were determined from measurements of total muscle area (CT scanning) and fibre area (from needle biopsies) with the assumption that since most fibres of biceps extend from origin to insertion, measurement of cross-sectional area at the belly of the muscle includes all fibres. Since biceps is a muscle that is trained by bodybuilders to achieve maximum hypertrophy, it is particularly suited for investigation of possible hyperplasia. It was our hypothesis that, if heavy resistance training induces an increase in fibre number, the biceps of such individuals should show evidence of hyperplasia in comparison to control subjects.

The data indicated that while total fibre numbers in biceps brachii ranged from approximately 172 000 to 419 000 fibres, the average number of fibres was the same for each group (Fig. 8.12). Since both groups of bodybuilders had trained their biceps to achieve maximum hypertrophy for a minimum of 6 years and yet had the same number of fibres as the untrained control subjects, we concluded that such training does not result in a significant net increase in fibre numbers. We also found that, within each group, there was a tendency for the subjects with the largest muscles to also have a higher than average number of fibres. Thus, although muscle size is primarily determined by the size of the individual fibres, it is also

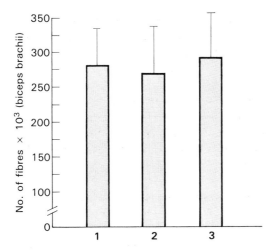

Fig. 8.12 Estimated fibre number in biceps brachii for a group of untrained controls (1: $n = 13$), a group of intermediate bodybuilders (2: $n = 7$) and a group of elite bodybuilders (3: $n = 5$). Values are means ± 1 SD. (From MacDougall, 1986a.)

affected by the genetically determined number of fibres.

Muscle satellite cells and the hypertrophy process

The term 'satellite cell' was first used by Mauro (1961) to describe a type of non-functioning, reserve cell that occurs outside the muscle fibre plasma membrane but within the basal lamina. At the light microscope level such cells appear as normal myonuclei but are visible at the electron microscope level since myonuclei occur within the plasma membrane. It is thought that these satellite cells are derived from a population of myoblasts that do not fuse to form myotubes and functional fibres during embryonic development (White & Esser, 1989).

Satellite cells occur most frequently in the muscles of younger animals and decrease in frequency with ageing (Schultz, 1989; White & Esser, 1989). In healthy adult humans, satellite cell nuclei constitute approximately 4 ($\pm$2)% of all myonuclei detected in cross-sectional electron micrographs (Schmalbruch & Hellhammer,

1976). The cells remain quiescent until muscle homeostasis is altered to the point where they become stimulated to undergo rapid proliferation through mitotic division.

In addition to being the source for adding myonuclei to muscle fibres as they increase in area and length with maturity, they are known to play an important role in the regeneration of injured fibres (Bischof, 1989; Schultz, 1989). When a traumatic injury such as a crush lesion occurs to a muscle fibre, satellite cells on the injured fibre are activated to undergo mitotic proliferation and to migrate along the length of the fibre to the site of the injury. They then fuse to form a multinucleated myotube, which matures into a new muscle fibre through a process similar to that which occurs during fetal development. In such a manner, a new muscle fibre is formed to replace the necrotic fibre (Schultz, 1989). It should also be noted that Schultz and colleagues have determined that, with injury, activation of satellite cells is confined to those on the damaged fibre, with little or no recruitment of satellite cells occurring from non-damaged fibres (Schultz et al., 1986). Thus it appears that the regeneration process is simply one of replacement, with no net addition of fibre number.

Satellite cell activation with exercise and training

Satellite cell proliferation has been shown to occur as a result of eccentric treadmill running in rats (Darr & Schultz, 1987), concentric resistance training in cats (Giddings et al., 1985), compensatory muscle hypertrophy in mice (James, 1973) and cycling training in humans (Appell et al., 1988). Appell and colleagues (1988) have also noted the presence of developing myotubes in trained muscles (monopedal cycling) compared to untrained muscles in humans. They interpret their data as evidence for new fibre formation and fibre hyperplasia through training-induced activation of satellite cells.

An alternative interpretation could be that

satellite cells are activated by exercise-induced damage to certain fibres, as has been shown to occur with forceful muscular contractions (Giddings *et al.*, 1985), especially if there is an eccentric component to the exercise (Fridén *et al.*, 1983). Possible support for this interpretation is furnished by the relatively high incidence of abnormal fibres, as evidenced by the presence of central nuclei, angulated shape and very small area, which are found in elite bodybuilders who are undergoing intensive training (MacDougall *et al.*, 1982). Thus, the extent to which the 'new' fibres reported by Appell and colleagues (1988) represent replacement of damaged fibres, as opposed to a net increase in fibre numbers, is not known. If the degree of damage must be sufficient to cause fibre necrosis before satellite cell proliferation can occur, then it would appear that the process is a 'one-for-one' replacement that does not result in an increase in total fibre numbers.

On the other hand, if satellite cells can be activated to proliferate and to fuse to form new myotubes as the result of 'mild damage', which does not result in fibre death (Bischof, 1989), then one must accept that a mechanism for the formation of additional numbers of fibres does exist in adult skeletal muscle. In support of this, it should be noted that satellite cell proliferation, in the absence of apparent fibre necrosis, has been observed with compensatory hypertrophy in overloaded chicken muscle (Kennedy *et al.*, 1988) and muscle that has been subjected to only slight mechanical compression (Teräväinen, 1970).

Summary

Heavy resistance training results in an increase in cross-sectional area of skeletal muscle fibres. This increase is a direct result of increased contractile protein, as evidenced by an increase in both myofibril area and numbers. Interstitial connective tissue also increases in proportion to the increase in fibre area.

While some investigators have suggested that strength training may also result in an increase in fibre numbers in adult muscle, the general belief is that fibre number is established at birth (or shortly thereafter) and that no net increase occurs as a result of training. Mammalian skeletal muscle possesses a population of reserve or satellite cells, which, when activated, can trigger a sequence of events that result in the replacement of damaged fibres with new fibres. Thus a mechanism clearly exists for the generation of new fibres in the adult animal. In some species and with certain perturbations, such as chronic passive stretch of wing muscles of the quail, this process results in an increased number of fibres as well as an increased fibre size. In humans who perform traditional heavy resistance training, however, the process appears to be only one of replacement of necrotic fibres, so that there is no significant increase in the net number of muscle fibres. It thus appears that, until further evidence, one must accept that the increase in muscle size that occurs in humans in response to heavy resistance training is caused exclusively by the increase in fibre and connective tissue area, with no addition in fibre numbers.

References

Alway, S.E., MacDougall, J.D. & Sale, D.G. (1989a) Contractile adaptations in the human triceps surae after isometric exercise. *Journal of Applied Physiology*, **66**, 2725–32.

Alway, S.E., Winchester, P.K., Davis, M.E. & Gonyea, W.J. (1989b) Regionalized adaptations and muscle fiber proliferation in stretch-induced enlargement. *Journal of Applied Physiology*, **66**, 771–81.

Appell, H.J., Forsberg, S. & Hollmann, W. (1988) Satellite cell activation in human skeletal muscle after training: evidence for muscle fiber neoformation. *International Journal of Sports Medicine*, **9**, 297–9.

Bischoff, R. (1989) Analysis of muscle regeneration using single myofibers in culture. *Medicine and Science in Sports and Exercise*, **21** (suppl.), S164–S172.

Brown, A.B., McCartney, N., Moroz, D., Sale, D. & MacDougall, J.D. (1988) Strength training effects in aging. *Medicine and Science in Sports and Exercise*, **20**, S80.

Chiakulus, J.J. & Pauly, J.E. (1965) A study of post

natal growth of skeletal muscle in the rat. *Anatomical Record*, **152**, 55–62.

Darr, K.C. & Schultz, E. (1987) Exercise-induced satellite cell activation in growing and mature skeletal muscle. *Journal of Applied Physiology*, **63**, 1816–21.

Fischman, D.A. (1972) Development of striated muscle. In G.H. Bourne (ed.) *The Structure and Function of Muscle: Structure Part 1, Vol. 1*, pp. 75–148. Academic Press, New York.

Fridén, J., Sjöstrom, M. & Ekblom, B. (1983) Myofibrillar damage following intense eccentric exercise in man. *International Journal of Sports Medicine*, **3**, 170–6.

Giddings, C.J., Neaves, W.B. & Gonyea, W.J. (1985) Muscle fiber necrosis and regeneration induced by prolonged weight-lifting exercise in the cat. *Anatomical Record*, **211**, 133–41.

Goldberg, A.L. (1967) Work-induced growth of skeletal muscle in normal and hypophysectomized rats. *American Journal of Physiology*, **213**, 1193–8.

Goldspink, G. (1970) The proliferation of myofibrils during muscle fiber growth. *Journal of Cell Science*, **6**, 593–603.

Goldspink, G. (1974) Development of muscle. In G. Goldspink (ed.) *Growth of Cells in Vertebrate Tissues*, pp. 69–99. Chapman & Hall, London.

Gollnick, P.D., Timson, B.F., Moore, R.L. & Reidy, M. (1981) Muscle enlargement and number of fibers in skeletal muscle of rats. *Journal of Applied Physiology*, **50**, 939–43.

Gonyea, W., Erickson, G.C. & Bonde-Peterson, F. (1977) Skeletal muscle fiber splitting induced by weight lifting exercise in cats. *Acta Physiologica Scandinavica*, **99**, 105–9.

Gonyea, W.J. (1980) Role of exercise in inducing increases in skeletal muscle fiber number. *Journal of Applied Physiology*, **48**, 421–6.

Gonyea, W.J. & Ericson, G.C. (1976) An experimental model for the study of exercise-induced skeletal muscle hypertrophy. *Journal of Applied Physiology*, **40**, 630–3.

Gonyea, W.J., Sale, D., Gonyea, F. & Mikesky, A. (1986) Exercise induced increases in muscle fiber number. *European Journal of Applied Physiology*, **55**, 137–141.

Hall-Craggs, E.C.B. (1970) The longitudinal division of overloaded skeletal muscle fibers. *Journal of Anatomy*, **107**, 459–70.

Holly, R.G., Barnett, J.G., Ashmore, C.R., Taylor, R.G. & Molé, P.A. (1980) Stretch-induced growth in chicken wing muscles: A new model of stretch hypertrophy. *American Journal of Physiology*, **7**, C62–C71.

James, N.T. (1973) Compensatory muscular hypertrophy in the extensor digitorum longus of the

mouse. *Journal of Anatomy*, **116**, 57–65.

Kennedy, J.M., Eisenberg, B.R., Reid, S.K., Sweeney, L.J. & Zak, R. (1988) Nascent muscle fiber appearance in overloaded chicken slow-tonic muscle. *American Journal of Anatomy*, **181**, 203–15.

Larsson, L. & Tesch, P.A. (1986) Motor unit fiber density in extremely hypertrophied skeletal muscles in man. *European Journal of Applied Physiology*, **55**, 130–6.

Lüthi, J.M., Howald, H., Classen, H., Rösler, K., Vock, P. & Hoppeler, H. (1986) Structural changes in skeletal muscle tissue with heavy-resistance exercise. *International Journal of Sports Medicine*, **7**, 123–7.

McDonagh, M.J.N. & Davies, C.T.M. (1984) Adaptive response of mammalian muscle to exercise with high loads. *European Journal of Applied Physiology*, **52**, 139–55.

MacDougall, J.D. (1986a) Adaptability of muscle to strength training—a cellular approach. In B. Saltin (ed.) *Biochemistry of Exercise VI, Vol. 16*, pp. 501–13. Human Kinetics, Champaign, Illinois.

MacDougall, J.D. (1986b) Morphological changes in human skeletal muscle following strength training and immobilization. In N.L. Jones, N. McCartney & A.J. McComas (eds) *Human Muscle Power*, pp. 269–88. Human Kinetics, Champaign, Illinois.

MacDougall, J.D., Elder, G.C.B., Sale, D.G., Moroz, J.R. & Sutton, J.R. (1980) Effects of strength training and immobilization on human muscle fibers. *European Journal of Applied Physiology*, **43**, 25–34.

MacDougall, J.D., Sale, D.G., Alway, S.E. & Sutton, J.R. (1984) Muscle fiber number in biceps brachii in bodybuilders and control subjects. *Journal of Applied Physiology*, **57**, 1399–1403.

MacDougall, J.D., Sale, E.G., Elder, G.C.B. & Sutton, J.R. (1982) Muscle ultrastructural characteristics of elite powerlifters and bodybuilders. *European Journal of Applied Physiology*, **48**, 117–26.

MacDougall, J.D., Sale, D.G., Moroz, J.R., Elder, G.C.B., Sutton, J.R. & Howald, H. (1979) Mitochondrial volume density in human skeletal muscle following heavy resistance training. *Medicine and Science in Sports*, **11**, 164–6.

Malina, R.M. (1986) Growth of muscle tissue and muscle mass. In F. Falkner & J.M. Tanner (eds) *Human Growth. A Comprehensive Treatise, Vol. 2*, pp. 77–99. Plenum Press, New York.

Mastaglia, F.L. (1981) Growth and development of the skeletal muscles. In J.A. Davis & J. Dobbing (eds) *Scientific Foundations of Paediatrics*, pp. 590–620. Heinemann, London.

Mauro, A. (1961) Satellite cell of skeletal muscle fibers. *Journal of Biophysical and Biochemical Cytology*, **9**, 493–5.

Moroz, D.E., Sale, D.G., Webber, C.E. & MacDougall,

J.D. (1990) The effect of strength and endurance training on bone in post menopausal women. *Medicine and Science in Sports and Exercise*, **22**, S64.

Morpurgo, B. (1897) Überaktivitäts-Hypertrophie der willkürlichen Muskeln. *Virchows Archiv für Pathologische Anatomie und Physiologie*, **15**, 522–54.

Moss, F.P. & LeBlond, C.P. (1971) Satellite cells as the source of nuclei in muscles of growing rats. *Anatomical Record*, **170**, 421–36.

Ontell, J. & Dunn, R.F. (1978) Neonatal muscle growth: A quantitative study. *American Journal of Anatomy*, **152**, 539–56.

Ramsay, J., Blimkie, C.J.R., Sale, D., MacDougall, D., Smith, K. & Garner, S. (1990) Effects of 20 weeks of resistance training on muscle morphology, voluntary strength and evoked contractile properties in prepubertal boys. *Medicine and Science in Sports and Exercise*, **22**, 605–14.

Rayne, J. & Crawford, G.N.C. (1975) Increase in fiber numbers of the rat pterygoid muscles during postnatal growth. *Journal of Anatomy*, **119**, 347–57.

Reitsma, W. (1969) Skeletal muscle hypertrophy after heavy exercise in rats with surgically reduced muscle function. *American Journal of Physical Medicine*, **48**, 237–59.

Sale, D.G., MacDougall, J.D., Jacobs, I. & Garner, S. (1990) Interaction between concurrent strength and endurance training. *Journal of Applied Physiology*, **68**, 260–70.

Schmalbruch, H. & Hellhammer, U. (1976) The number of satellite cells in normal human tissue. *Anatomical Record*, **185**, 279–88.

Schultz, E. (1989) Satellite cell behavior during skeletal muscle growth and regeneration. *Medicine and Science in Sports and Exercise*, **21** (suppl.), S181–S186.

Schultz, E., Jaryszak, D.L., Gibson, M.C. & Albright, D.J. (1986) Absence of exogenous satellite cell contribution to regeneration of frozen skeletal muscle. *Journal of Muscle Research and Cell Motility*, **7**, 361–7.

Sola, O.M., Christensen, D.L. & Martin, A.W. (1973) Hypertrophy and hyperplasia of adult chicken anterior latissimus dorsi muscles following stretch with and without denervation. *Experimental Neurology*, **41**, 76–100.

Staron, R.S., Malicky, E.S., Leonardi, M.J., Falkel, J.E., Hagerman, F.C. & Dudley, G.A. (1989) Muscle hypertrophy and fast fiber type conversions in heavy resistance trained women. *European Journal of Applied Physiology*, **60**, 71–9.

Teräväinen, H. (1970) Satellite cells of striated muscle after compression injury so slight as not to cause degeneration of the muscle fibers. *Zeitschrift fur Zellforsch*, **103**, 320–7.

Tesch, P.A. (1987) Acute and long-term metabolic changes consequent to heavy-resistance exercise. *Medicine and Science in Sports and Exercise*, **26**, 67–87.

Tesch, P.A. & Larsson, L. (1982) Muscle hypertrophy in bodybuilders (1982) *European Journal of Applied Physiology*, **49**, 301–6.

Tesch, P.A., Thorrson, A. & Kaiser, P. (1984) Muscle capillary supply and fiber type characteristics in weight and power lifters. *Journal of Applied Physiology*, **56**, 35–8.

Tesch, P.A., Häkinen, K. & Komi, P.V. (1985) The effect of strength training and detraining on various enzyme activities. *Medicine and Science in Sports and Exercise*, **17**, 245.

Thorstensson, A. (1976) Muscle strength, fiber types and enzyme activities in man. *Acta Physiologica Scandinavica*, **433** (suppl.), 1–44.

Timson, B.F., Bowlin, B.K., Dudenhoeffer, G.A. & George, J.B. (1985) Fiber number, area and composition of mouse soleus muscle following enlargement, *Journal of Applied Physiology*, **58**, 619–24.

White, T.P. & Esser, K.A. (1989) Satellite cell and growth factor involvement in skeletal muscle growth. *Medicine and Science in Sports and Exercise*, **21** (suppl.), S158–S163.

Chapter 8C

Short- and Long-Term Histochemical and Biochemical Adaptations in Muscle

PER A. TESCH

Acute adaptations to strength exercise

Strength exercise is always performed intermittently (see Chapter 17). Thus a sequence or a set of coupled concentric and eccentric muscle actions is typically followed by a short rest period and then repeated two to four times. Training with very heavy loads that are performed with a few number of repetitions only is usually followed by relatively long rest periods. For exercise sessions utilizing less heavier loads and where sets comprise approximately 12–15 repetitions carried out until muscular failure, the period of rest between sets is typically shorter or less than 2 min. A complete exercise session may comprise up to 10–12 different exercises.

Oxygen uptake during a session involving the large muscle groups of the lower limbs while performing the leg press or the squat exercises average 50–60% of maximal aerobic power in strength trained (Fig. 8.13; Tesch, 1987) or untrained (Fig. 8.14; Tesch et al., 1990a) men. The energy turnover for exercises activating smaller muscle mass, such as when performing upper-body exercises, therefore must be lower.

Despite the apparently low oxygen uptake all available major energy sources are mobilized during a strength exercise session that is aimed at increasing muscle mass. Adenosine triphosphate (ATP) and creatine phosphate and glycogen contents decreased in response to 30 min of exercise performed at a calculated power output of approximately 200 W. There were also marked increases in blood lactate concentration and in the intramuscular lactate, glucose, glucose-6-phosphate and glycerol 3-phosphate contents, indicating a high rate of anaerobic glycolysis (Table 8.1; Tesch et al., 1986). Although anaerobic–non-glycolytic and glycolytic energy sources were utilized there was evidence of lipids being mobilized as substrate as well. Thus, plasma concentration of glycerol increased and most individuals showed decreased muscle triglyceride content after exercise (Table 8.1; Essén-Gustavsson & Tesch, 1990).

It seems plausible though that strength exercise can be executed solely at the expense of the available ATP and creatine phosphate stores (Keul et al., 1978) providing very few muscle actions are performed in a sequence and that there is ample time allowed for during the recovery that follows. A regimen relying on lower resistance, higher number of repetitions, and short recovery periods during exercise sessions would call for greater reliance upon anaerobic–glycolytic and oxidative metabolism (Fig. 8.15; Tesch et al., 1986). Hence, the plasma lactate levels are higher during such an exercise regimen compared to that carried out with higher load and lower number of repetitions (Kraemer et al., 1987). It is not known to what extent the metabolic stress *per se* influences the desired adaptations such as increases in muscle mass or strength.

239

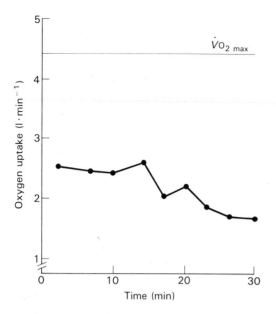

Fig. 8.13 Oxygen uptake during a 30-min heavy-resistance training session in strength-trained men (*n* = 8). They performed four sets (6–12 repetitions per set) each of front and back squat, leg press and leg extension. Each set lasted approximately 30 s and was followed by a 60-s rest period. Expired gas was collected repeatedly using the Douglas bag technique. Each data point represents measurements performed during exercise and the subsequent rest period. (From Tesch, 1987; for details see also Tesch *et al.*, 1986.)

From studies of the selective glycogen depletion pattern using standard histochemical staining procedures it appears that forces below 20% of maximum voluntary isometric force can be sustained by the recruitment of slow twitch muscle fibres only (Gollnick *et al.*, 1974). To produce higher forces fast twitch muscle fibres are brought into play as evidenced by a progressively greater rate of glycogen loss when the level of sustained tension is increased. Accordingly, one would expect a more marked decrease in glycogen content of both fibre types in response to a session of strength exercise typical for weight trainees carried out with loads equal to 70–90% of the maximum load lifted. After performing 20 sets of 6–12 repetitions each of four different quadriceps exercises (see Tesch *et al.*, 1986), there was a greater decrease in glycogen content of fast than slow twitch muscle fibres. At cessation of exercise, no slow twitch fibres, but 15% of the fast twitch fibres examined were glycogen voided (Fig. 8.16; Tesch, unpublished results). Although strenous strength training, appears not to exhaust the glycogen stores the high rate of glycogen utilization may be sufficient to deplete certain muscle fibres. This in turn may limit the ability to perform multiple daily exercise sessions.

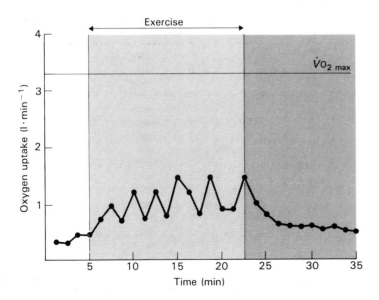

Fig. 8.14 Oxygen uptake before, during and after supine leg press exercise in untrained men (*n* = 8). They performed five sets of (6–12 repetitions per set). Each set was followed by 3 min of rest. Expired gas was collected continuously and oxygen uptake analysed using an on-line system. Each data point represents the mean value for every 2.5-min period. (From Tesch *et al.*, 1990a.)

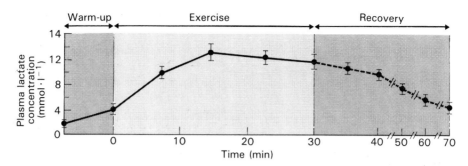

Fig. 8.15 Plasma lactate concentration before and during strength exercise and during recovery. For details see Fig. 8.14. (From Tesch *et al.*, 1986.)

Long-term adaptations to strength exercise

Most effective strength training programmes produce increased muscle cross-sectional area mainly due to an increase in myofibrillar protein content (see Chapter 8B). In response to short-term training programmes, however, appreciable increases in muscular strength and strength-related performances are possible with no or minute concomitant muscle hyper-

trophy. This is important to keep in mind when discussing the specific metabolic adaptations that occur in response to strength training because some of the changes described below occur secondary to the training-induced muscle hypertrophy.

Fibre type composition

There is substantial evidence at hand to suggest that endurance training may induce a shift in

Table 8.1 Muscle metabolite contents (mmol·kg^{-1} d.w.) and plasma metabolite concentrations (mmol·l^{-1}) before (after warm-up) and at cessation of 30 min of strength exercise comprising four sets (6–12 repetitions per set) each of front and back squat, leg press and leg extension. Subjects were bodybuilders ($n = 9$). Differences ($P < 0.05$) between mean values are denoted by *. (From Tesch *et al.*, 1986 and Essén-Gustavsson & Tesch, 1990.)

	Pre-exercise	Post-exercise	Difference
Muscle			
ATP	24.8	19.7	*
Creatine phosphate	89.5	45.8	*
Creatine	50.8	100.0	*
Glucose	1.5	8.2	*
Glucose-6-phosphate	1.8	16.7	*
Glycerol-3-phosphate	5.7	14.1	*
Lactate	22.7	79.5	*
Glycogen	690	495	*
Triglyceride	23.9	16.7	$P > 0.05$
Plasma			
Free fatty acids	0.22	0.22	$P > 0.05$
Glycerol	0.02	0.1	*
Glucose	4.2	5.5	*
Lactate	3.8	11.7	*

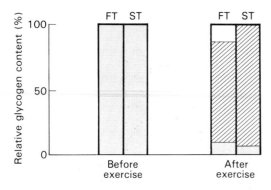

Fig. 8.16 Relative glycogen content of fast twitch (FT) and slow twitch (ST) fibres before and after heavy-resistance exercise. Both fibre types showed no glycogen depletion before exercise. After exercise 15% of the FT fibres were glycogen depleted (□), 77% were moderately filled (▨) and only 8% completely filled (□). Among ST fibres 95% were moderately filled and 5% filled. For details see Fig. 8.14. (From Tesch, unpublished results.)

fibre type composition promoting transformation of fast to slow twitch fibres (cf. Saltin & Gollnick, 1983). Although trained muscles of successful Olympic weightlifters and power-lifters and other power athletes typically possess a predominance of fast twitch fibres (Gollnick *et al.*, 1972; Prince *et al.*, 1976; Staron *et al.*, 1984; Tesch *et al.*, 1984; Tesch & Karlsson, 1985), it is unlikely that this is the result of the specific training carried out by these athletes. In bodybuilders, a wide range in fibre type composition of vastus lateralis, deltoideus, biceps brachii and triceps brachii muscles have been reported (MacDougall *et al.*, 1982; Schantz, 1982, 1983; Tesch & Larsson, 1982; Dudley *et al.*, 1986; Larsson & Tesch, 1986; Essén-Gustavsson & Tesch, 1990).

There are no studies providing results suggesting that strength training will increase the fast twitch fibre percentage. Studies are available, however, that evidently show a marked shift of fast twitch b (type IIb) to fast twitch a (type IIa) fibres with weight training similar to the response shown after endurance training. In bodybuilders the lateral vastii muscle (Essén-Gustavsson & Tesch, 1990) and the deltoid

muscle (Schantz & Källman, 1989) show very few fast twitch b fibres. Also, in response to strength programmes emphasizing supine leg press exercise and resulting in marked muscle hypertrophy, fast twitch a percentage increased at the expense of decreased fast twitch b percentage in females (Staron *et al.*, 1989) and males (Fig. 8.17; Dudley & Tesch, unpublished results). These results, based on conventional histochemical staining procedures, have to be confirmed by studies using more recently applied techniques to assess the myosin heavy chain isoform pattern (Klitgaard *et al.*, 1990).

Capillary supply

Numerous studies have demonstrated that the capillary supply, either expressed as capillaries per fibre or as capillaries per mm^2, increases in response to endurance training. Likewise, endurance-trained athletes show greater capillary density than sedentaries (cf. Saltin & Gollnick, 1983). In contrast to strength training, endurance training does not produce muscle hypertrophy. An increase in muscle fibre size *per se* therefore will decrease capillary density. Most effective strength training regimens are associated with increases in muscle cross-sectional area as a result of increases in individual muscle fibre size. Assuming no capillary neoformation one would expect capillary density to decrease in proportion to the increase in muscle fibre size in response to strength training. In concordance, successful Olympic weightlifters and power-lifters show lower capillary density than non-trained subjects (Tesch *et al.*, 1984). Thus, whereas the number of capillaries per fibre of m. vastus lateralis is equal in lifters and non-athletes, capillaries per unit muscle area is markedly lower in lifters. Bodybuilders relying on a different training regimen, however, show somewhat greater capillaries per fibre and similar capillaries per unit area as non-athletes (Schantz, 1982; Tesch *et al.*, 1984; Schantz & Källman, 1989; Essén-Gustavsson & Tesch, 1990). Thus, in the light of the greater

Fig. 8.17 The percentage of slow twitch (ST) and fast twitch a (FTa) and fast twitch b (FTb) fibres of m. vastus lateralis before (□) and after (□) 19 weeks of heavy resistance and after 8 weeks of detraining (▨). Subjects trained 2 days each week and performed 4–5 sets of the supine leg press and knee extension exercises to failure with 6–12 repetitions per set; 3 min of rest occurred between sets. Mean values different from pretraining values are denoted by * ($P < 0.05$). (From Dudley & Tesch, unpublished results.)

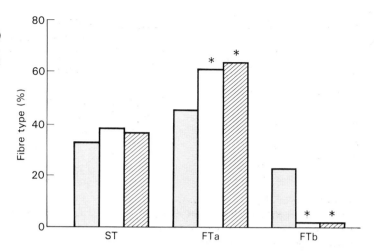

capillaries per fibre, a certain capillary proliferation of m. quadriceps femoris may occur in these athletes. In the non-postural m. triceps brachii of bodybuilders, however, a pattern similar to that observed in the vastus lateralis of lifters (Tesch *et al.*, 1984) has been demonstrated. Lifters and bodybuilders have been compared with regard to capillary supply of m. vastus lateralis and m. triceps brachii (Dudley *et al.*, 1986). In both muscles bodybuilders showed greater capillaries per fibre than lifters indicating that capillary proliferation may occur in both postural and non-postural muscles in response to strength training emphasizing high repetition training systems. No changes in capillary density were observed following short-term strength-training programmes of 6–12 weeks duration (Tesch *et al.*, 1983; Lüthi *et al.*, 1986; Tesch *et al.*, 1990b).

Interestingly, and in part contradictory to the hypothesis outlined above, two studies of longer duration showing impressive increases in muscle mass produced mainly by supine leg press exercise, both men and women showed increases in capillaries per fibre but in capillary per unit area as well (Fig. 8.18; Staron *et al.*, 1989; Dudley & Tesch, unpublished results). This may suggest that adaptive responses are possible that are of similar nature to those attained by endurance training. The discrep-

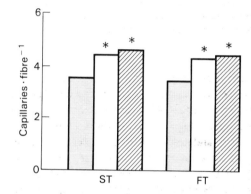

Fig. 8.18 Capillaries per fibre of ST and FT fibres of m. vastus lateralis before (□) and after (□) 19 weeks of strength training and after 8 weeks of detraining (▨). For details see Fig 8.17. Mean values different from pretraining values are denoted by * ($P < 0.05$). (From Dudley & Tesch, unpublished results.)

ancy from the results obtained in earlier studies is however difficult to explain.

From the data available it therefore appears that strength training emphasizing high-load, low-repetition exercises, will not necessarily result in capillary neoformation. When pronounced hypertrophy of individual muscle fibres occurs, the capillary density rather decreases. More intense training regimens, emphasizing moderately high load and larger number of repetitions per set, may induce capillary proliferation. Nevertheless, the hypertrophic effect may counteract, or more likely, be greater with the net result being maintained or decreased capillary density.

Mitochondrial density

Observations on lower mammals have suggested exercise-induced muscle hypertrophy to be associated with a proportional increase in mitochondrial volume (Seiden, 1976). Studies of strength-trained athletes have, however, demonstrated reduced mitochondrial density of the trained muscles (MacDougall et al., 1982; Alway et al., 1988). This finding, albeit not being a consistent observation (Staron et al., 1984), have found support in that mitochondrial volume density decreased in parallel with increases in muscle mass in subjects conducting a strength training regimen over 6–8 weeks (Fig. 8.19; MacDougall et al., 1979; Lüthi et al., 1986). A decrease in mitochondrial density

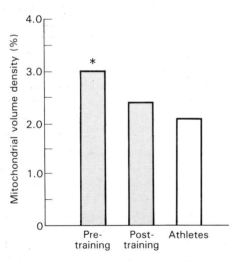

Fig. 8.19 Mitochondrial volume density of m. triceps brachii before and after 6 months of strength training; muscle fibre size increased by 30%. Values for athletes (bodybuilders and power-lifters) are shown for comparison. * denotes a difference from values obtained after short-term (post-training) or long-term (athletes) heavy-resistance training. (From MacDougall et al., 1979.)

secondary to exercise-induced muscle hypertrophy is commensurate with the observations (see below) of attenuated oxidative enzyme content in muscles of athletes training for strength or power.

Enzyme content

Aerobic–oxidative enzymes

Heavy-load strength training does not enhance the activity of enzymes involved in aerobic–oxidative metabolism (Komi et al., 1982; Houston et al., 1983; Tesch et al., 1987, 1990b). Thus the contents of succinate dehydrogenase, malate dehydrogenase or citrate synthase or 3-hydroxyacyl-CoA dehydrogenase (HAD), favouring lipid oxidation, remained unchanged or even decreased somewhat in response to programmes that induced substantial increases in muscular strength. These results are supported by the demonstration of normal or 'subnormal' oxidative enzyme activities in strength- or power-trained athletes (Gollnick et al., 1972; Apple & Tesch, 1989; Schantz & Källman, 1989; Tesch et al., 1989a; Essén-Gustavsson & Tesch, 1990). The difference in enzyme activity between fast and slow twitch fibres that is typically observed in untrained or endurance-trained populations was also present in strength-trained athletes. In these athletes, however, the citrate synthase and HAD activity of slow twitch fibres was lower than in sedentaries. Interestingly, bodybuilders demonstrated higher citrate synthase activity of fast twitch fibres than Olympic weightlifters or power-lifters. Hence, the high repetition strategy practised by bodybuilders obviously produces more favourable adaptations with regard to aerobic metabolism than the heavy-resistance low-repetition regimens often practised by lifters.

Anaerobic–non-glycolytic enzymes

Enzymes favouring contractility or fast ATP replenishment, for example ATPase, creatine kinase or myokinase, have been suggested to have physiological implications in athletic events requiring speed, strength or power. It is unlikely, however, that strength training provokes meaningful increases in 'contractile' enzyme content although myokinase have been shown to increase somewhat in response to explosive or strength training (Thorstensson *et al.*, 1976a; Komi *et al.*, 1982). However, these are not consistent findings. These studies, for example, did not report an increase in ATPase or creatine kinase contents and there are several studies that do not show evidence of enhanced content of anaerobic–non-glycolytic enzymes in response to strength training (Thorstensson *et al.*, 1976b; Häkkinen *et al.*, 1981; Houston *et al.*, 1983; Tesch *et al.*, 1987, 1990b).

Anaerobic–glycolytic enzymes

Endurance training programmes typically do not enhance anaerobic–glycolytic enzyme activity and to produce such changes exercise has to be carried out at work loads exceeding maximal aerobic power (cf. Saltin & Gollnick, 1983). The activities of phosphofructokinase or lactate dehydrogenase are unaffected by heavy-resistance training (Thorstensson *et al.*, 1976a; Komi *et al.*, 1982; Houston *et al.*, 1983; Tesch *et al.*, 1987, 1990b). Strength-trained athletes, however, show slightly higher glycolytic activity, e.g. lactate dehydrogenase, of fast twitch fibres than sedentaries (Tesch *et al.*, 1989a). This difference may simply reflect the limited use of fast twitch fibres in sedentaries, not a specific training response, because strength- or endurance-trained athletes and moderately active 'non-athletes' (Apple & Tesch, 1989) demonstrated similar lactate dehydrogenase activity of fast and slow twitch fibres. Similar results were reported in mixed tissue samples from a non-postural muscle, e.g. m. deltoideus. Thus, bodybuilders, swimmers and physically active students showed similar levels of phosphofructokinase (Schantz & Källman, 1989).

Muscle substrate levels

Glycogen content

Resting glycogen content of skeletal muscle increases in response to endurance training and this adaptation appears to occur following strength training as well. Thus, in the triceps brachii muscle of individuals who had trained for 5 months using variable resistance the glycogen content increased by 35% (MacDougall *et al.*, 1977). Also, the vastus lateralis muscle of bodybuilders showed more than 50% higher glycogen content than typically noticed in non-athletes (Tesch *et al.*, 1986). Glycogen content was, however, not enhanced in response to 3 months of quadriceps training (Tesch *et al.*, 1990b).

ATP and creatine phosphate content

Bouts of strength exercise lower ATP and creatine phosphate stores (see above) with partial or complete resynthesis between bouts (Tesch *et al.*, 1989b). This acute metabolic response may then provide the adaptive stimuli for increased storage capacity of high energy phosphate compounds. Substantial increases in the resting phosphagen levels of the triceps brachii muscle have been shown after 5 months of strength training that produced marked increases in elbow extensor strength and fibre size (MacDougall *et al.*, 1977, 1979). In contrast, 3 months of quadriceps training three times a week comprising 48–60 maximal voluntary muscle actions per session did not alter resting ATP and creatine phosphate stores (Tesch *et al.*, 1990b). Since this latter study produced only a small insignificant increase in muscle fibre size, it could be argued that increases in ATP and creatine phosphate contents only occur providing there is a concomitant increase in myofibrillar protein content. This hypothesis could, however, be disputed by the finding of normal ATP and creatine phosphate levels in athletes possessing marked muscle hypertrophy of m. vastus lateralis (Tesch *et al.*, 1986). It could only be speculated whether these conflicting findings reflect different responses between postural and non-postural muscles.

Lipid content

There is uncertainty whether endurance training promotes increased content of lipids stored in the muscle (cf. Saltin & Gollnick, 1983). Likewise, it is not clear whether or not strength training stimulates an increase in lipid content. The triglyceride content of the quadriceps muscle of bodybuilders is not different compared to that of untrained populations (Essén-Gustavsson & Tesch, 1990) and bodybuilders showed similar lipid volume fraction as sedentary or active controls (Alway et al., 1988). The findings of lower lipid content in the quadriceps of lifters (Staron et al., 1984) and the observation of an increase in the lipid volume density of the triceps muscle (McDougall et al., 1979) but not of the quadriceps muscle (Lüthi et al., 1986) in response to heavy-resistance training may imply different responses between muscles or the influence of type of training.

Myoglobin content

Myoglobin has an important role for oxygen transport within skeletal muscle. Thus myoglobin facilitates oxygen extraction. Although slow twitch muscle fibres typically contain more myoglobin than fast twitch fibres endurance training does not promote an increase in myoglobin content of human skeletal muscle (cf. Saltin & Gollnick, 1983). Because myoglobin content increased in parallel with a decrease in oxidative enzyme content secondary to muscle atrophy induced by immobilization (Jansson et al., 1988), there are reasons to believe that myoglobin content would decrease following a strength training regimen. Myoglobin content has been measured in the vastus lateralis muscle before and after a 16-week strength training programme that induced a 20% increase in muscle fibre size. The data suggested that muscle hypertrophy was paral-

leled by a corresponding decrease in myoglobin content (Fig. 8.20; Sylvén et al., unpublished results). During detraining, muscle fibre size decreased and this effect was accompanied by an increase in myoglobin content. Provided there is an increase in muscle fibre size these results suggest that long-term strength exercise may reduce the potential for skeletal muscle to extract oxygen. Such an effect would probably decrease aerobic work capacity.

Conclusions

Strength training promotes few favourable and some unfavourable metabolic adaptations. The occurrence and the magnitude of these effects are influenced by the type, intensity and dur-

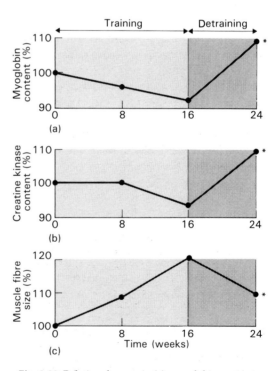

Fig. 8.20 Relative changes in (a) myoglobin content, (b) creatine kinase content, and (c) muscle fibre size in m. vastus lateralis in response to 16 weeks of heavy-resistance training followed by 8 weeks of detraining. Changes ($P < 0.05$) from week 16 to 24 are denoted *. (For details see Häkkinen et al., 1981; from Sylvén et al., unpublished results.)

ation of training. It is clear, for example, that the metabolic adaptations are different when comparing programmes comprising high load–low repetitions or light load–high repetitions or if the programme is of such a duration and intensity that it will induce muscle hypertrophy or not.

Likewise, the initial state of training will influence the metabolic response. Results obtained in studies examining prepubertal children, untrained women or aged populations for example, therefore should be interpreted with caution and should not be regarded as reflecting 'classical' responses to heavy-resistance training. Similarly, the adaptations shown in weight-trained athletes may not apply to strength training programmes.

Some of the confusion concerning the metabolic adaptations taking place in response to strength training stems from the fact that results have been reported from studies where the training performed had been termed 'strength', 'weight' or 'heavy-resistance' training although they have not induced meaningful increases in strength or muscle mass. When prescribing exercises for athletes, physically active or inactive or aged populations or those undergoing rehabilitation, this is a serious consideration.

References

Alway, S.E., MacDougall, J.D., Sale, D.G., Sutton, J.R. & McComas, A.J. (1988) Functional and structural adaptations in skeletal muscle of trained athletes. *Journal of Applied Physiology*, **64**, 1114–20.

Apple, F.S. & Tesch, P.A. (1989) CK and LD isozymes in human single muscle fibers in trained athletes. *Journal of Applied Physiology*, **66**, 2717–20.

Dudley, G.A., Tesch, P.A., Fleck, S.J., Kraemer, W.J. & Baechle, T.R. (1986) Plasticity of human muscle with resistance training. *Anatomical Record*, **214**, 4.

Essén-Gustavsson, B., & Tesch, P.A. (1990) Glycogen and triglyceride utilization in relation to muscle metabolic characteristics in men performing heavy-resistance 3 exercise. *European Journal of Applied Physiology*, **61**, 5–10.

Gollnick, P.D., Armstrong, R.B., Saubert IV, C.W., Piehl, K. & Saltin, B. (1972) Enzyme activity and fiber composition in skeletal muscle of untrained and trained men. *Journal of Applied Physiology*, **33**, 312–19.

Gollnick, P.D., Karlsson, J., Piehl, K. & Saltin, B. (1974) Selective glycogen depletion in skeletal muscle fibres of man following sustained contractions. *Journal of Physiology*, **241**, 59–67.

Häkkinen, K., Komi, P.V. & Tesch, P.A. (1981) Effect of combined concentric and eccentric strength training and detraining on force–time, muscle fiber and metabolic characteristics of leg extensor muscles. *Scandinavian Journal of Sports Science*, **3**, 50–8.

Houston, M.E., Froese, E.A., Valeriote, St P., Green, H.J. & Ranney, D.A. (1983) Muscle performance, morphology and metabolic capacity during strength training and detraining. A one leg model. *European Journal of Applied Physiology*, **51**, 25–35.

Jansson, E., Sylvén, C., Arvidsson, I. & Eriksson, E. (1988) Increase in myoglobin content and decrease in oxidative enzyme activities by leg muscle immobilization in man. *Acta Physiologica Scandinavica*, **132**, 515–17.

Keul, J., Haralambie, G., Bruder, M. & Gottstein, H.J. (1978) The effect of weight lifting exercise on heart rate and metabolism in experienced weight lifters. *Medicine and Science in Sports and Exercise*, **10**, 13–15.

Klitgaard, H., Zhou, H. & Richter, E. (1990) Myosin heavy chain comparison of single fibres from m. biceps brachii of male bodybuilders. *Acta Physiologica Scandinavica*, **140**, 175–80.

Komi, P.V., Karlsson, J., Tesch, P.A., Suominen, H. & Heikkinen, E. (1982) Effects of heavy resistance and explosive-type strength training methods on mechanical functional and metabolic aspects of performance. In P.V. Komi (ed.) *Exercise and Sport Biology*, International Series on Sports Sciences, Vol. 12, pp. 90–102. Human Kinetics, Champaign, Illinois.

Kraemer, W.J., Noble, B.J., Clark, M.J. & Culver, B.W. (1987) Physiologic responses to heavy-resistance exercise with very short rest periods. *International Journal of Sports Medicine*, **8**, 247–52.

Larsson, L. & Tesch, P.A. (1986) Motor unit fibre density in extremely hypertrophied skeletal muscles in man. *European Journal of Applied Physiology*, **55**, 130–6.

Lüthi, J.M., Howald, H., Claassen, H., Rösler, K., Vock, P. & Hoppeler, H. (1986) Structural changes in skeletal muscle tissue with heavy-resistance exercise. *International Journal of Sports Medicine*, **7**, 123–7.

MacDougall, J.D., Sale, D.G., Elder, G.C.B. & Sutton, J.R. (1982) Muscle ultrastrucutral characteristics of elite powerlifters and bodybuilders.

European Journal of Applied Physiology, **48**, 117–26.

MacDougall, J.D., Sale, D.G., Moroz, J.R., Elder, G.C.B., Sutton, J.R. & Howald, H. (1979) Mitochondrial volume density in human skeletal muscle following heavy resistance training. *Medicine and Science in Sports*, **11**, 164–6.

MacDougall, J.D., Ward, G.R., Sale, D.G. & Sutton, J.R. (1977) Biochemical adaptation of human skeletal muscle to heavy resistance training and immobilization. *Journal of Applied Physiology*, **43**, 700–3.

Prince, F.P., Hikida, R.S. & Hagerman, F.C. (1976) Human muscle fiber types in power lifters, distance runners and untrained subjects. *Pflügers Archiv*, **363**, 19–26.

Saltin, B. & Gollnick, P.D. (1983) Skeletal muscle adaptability: significance for metabolism and performance. In L. Peachy, R. Adrian & S.R. Gerzer (eds) *Handbook of Physiology. Skeletal Muscle*, pp. 555–631. American Physiological Society, Bethesda.

Schantz, P. (1982) Capillary supply in hypertrophied human skeletal muscle. *Acta Physiologica Scandinavica*, **114**, 635–7.

Schantz, P. (1983) Capillary supply in heavy-resistance trained non-postural human skeletal muscle. *Acta Physiologica Scandinavica*, **117**, 153–5.

Schantz, P.G. & Källman, M. (1989) NADH shuttle enzymes and cytochrome b5 reductase in human skeletal muscle: effect of strength training. *Journal of Applied Physiology*, **67**, 123–7.

Seiden, D. (1976) A quantitative analysis of muscle cell changes in compensatory hypertrophy and work-induced hypertrophy. *American Journal of Anatomy*, **145**, 459–68.

Staron, R.S., Hikida, R.S., Hagerman, F.C., Dudley, G.A. & Murray, T.F. (1984) Human skeletal muscle fiber type adaptability to various workloads. *Journal of Histochemistry and Cytochemistry*, **32**, 146–52.

Staron, R.S., Malicky, E.S., Leonardi, M.J., Falkel, J.E., Hagerman, F.C. & Dudley, G.A. (1989) Muscle hypertrophy and fast fiber type conversions in heavy resistance-trained women. *European Journal of Applied Physiology*, **60**, 71–9.

Tesch, P.A. (1987) Acute and long-term metabolic changes consequent to heavy-resistance exercise. *Medicine and Sport Science*, **26**, 67–89.

Tesch, P.A., Buchanan, P. & Dudley, G.A. (1990a) An approach to counteracting long-term microgravity-induced muscle atrophy. *The Physiologist*, **33** (1) (suppl.), 77–9.

Tesch, P.A., Colliander, E.B. & Kaiser, P. (1986) Muscle metabolism during intense, heavy-resistance exercise. *European Journal of Applied Physiology*, **55**, 362–6.

Tesch, P.A., Hjort, H. & Balldin, U.I. (1983) Effects of strength training on G tolerance. *Aviation Space and Environmental Medicine*, **54**, 691–5.

Tesch, P.A. & Karlsson, J. (1985) Muscle fiber types and size in trained and untrained muscles of elite athletes. *Journal of Applied Physiology*, **59**, 1716–20.

Tesch, P.A., Komi, P.V. & Häkkinen, K. (1987) Enzymatic adaptations consequent to long-term strength training. *International Journal of Sports Medicine*, **8** (suppl.), 66–9.

Tesch, P.A. & Larsson, L. (1982) Muscle hypertrophy in bodybuilders. *European Journal of Applied Physiology*, **49**, 301–6.

Tesch, P.A., Thorsson, A. & Colliander E.B. (1990b) Effects of eccentric and concentric resistance training on skeletal muscle substrates, enzyme activities and capillary supply. *Acta Physiologica Scandinavica*, **140**, 575–80.

Tesch, P.A., Thorsson, A. & Essén-Gustavsson, B. (1989a) Enzyme activities of FT and ST muscle fibers in heavy-resistance trained athletes. *Journal of Applied Physiology*, **67**, 83–7.

Tesch, P.A., Thorsson, A. & Fujitsuka, N. (1989b) Creatine phosphate in fiber types before and after exhaustive exercise. *Journal of Applied Physiology*, **66**, 1756–9.

Tesch, P.A., Thorsson, A. & Kaiser, P. (1984) Muscle capillary supply and fiber type characteristics in weight and power lifters. *Journal of Applied Physiology*, **56**, 35–8.

Thorstensson, A., Hultén, B., Döbeln, W. von & Karlsson, J. (1976a) Effect of strength training on enzyme activities and fibre characteristics in human skeletal muscle. *Acta Physiologica Scandinavica*, **96**, 392–8.

Thorstensson, A., Karlsson, J., Viitasalo, J.H.T., Luthanen, P. & Komi, P.V. (1976b) Effect of strength training on EMG of human skeletal muscle. *Acta Physiologica Scandinavica*, **98**, 232–6.

Chapter 9A

Neural Adaptation to Strength Training

DIGBY G. SALE

Introduction

The most noticeable effect of strength training in athletes, apart from the increase in strength itself, is an increase in muscle size. Since a larger muscle can generate greater force, muscle enlargement is an adaptation to strength training which makes an important contribution to the increase in strength that occurs. In training programmes that continue over several months or years the upper limit of strength increases is determined by the ability of the athlete to continue to respond to training by increasing muscle size. As the upper limit of strength increase is approached increases in muscle size and consequently strength are very difficult to achieve (Hakkinen, 1985). This difficulty and the associated lack of progress and frustration may explain the strong temptation to use anabolic steroids to stimulate further increases in muscle size and strength (Sale, 1988).

However, strength performance is determined not only by the size of the involved muscles, but also by the ability of the nervous system to appropriately activate the muscles (Fig. 9.1). A sport or athletic movement considered to require a high level of strength can be likened to a skilled act. The muscles mainly responsible for producing the large force in the intended direction of movement, called the agonists, must be fully activated. Muscles that assist in coordinating the movement, called synergists, must be appropriately activated.

Finally, muscles that produce force in the opposite direction to that of the agonists, called antagonists, must be appropriately activated. Thus the control by the nervous system of the muscles involved in common strength-training exercises such as the squat and the bench press is very complex. It is therefore not unreasonable to expect that when an unfamiliar exercise is introduced into the strength-training programme of an athlete, the early increase in strength, assessed as increased performance in the training exercise, is due in part to adaptive changes in the nervous system that optimize control of the muscles involved in the exercise. Adaptive changes in the nervous system in response to training are referred to as neural adaptation.

Possible mechanisms of neural adaptation

Increased activation of agonists

The basic functional unit of a muscle is called a *motor unit*. A motor unit consists of a motor nerve cell (commonly called a motoneurone) and the muscle fibres it innervates. Each motor unit contains a few to several hundred muscle fibres. Muscles contain a few hundred thousand muscle fibres; thus, each muscle is comprised of a few to several hundred motor units. For an agonist muscle to produce its greatest possible force, all of the motor units in the muscle must be activated (recruited).

249

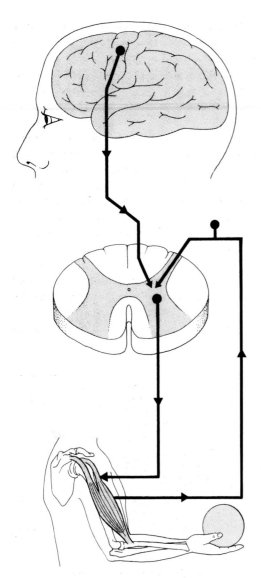

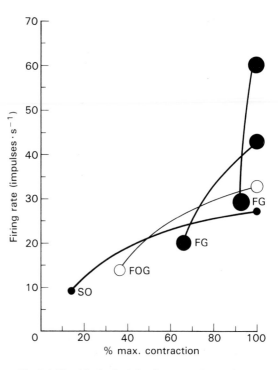

Fig. 9.1 Control of muscle by the nervous system. Voluntary strength performance is determined not only by the quantity and quality of the involved muscle mass, but also by the ability of the nervous system to effectively activate the muscles. Nervous system adaptations to strength training may improve the central command of the muscles (brain control) and enhance certain reflex responses (schematic segment of spinal cord is shown).

Fig. 9.2 The 'size' principle of motor unit recruitment is illustrated. Motor units are recruited in order according to size as a voluntary contraction increases from zero force to a maximal voluntary force level (100% maximum contraction). The recruitment threshold and range of firing rates for four representative motor units are shown. Bear in mind that this is a sample of four motor units from a muscle that contains a total of at least a few hundred units. The relatively small slow twitch oxidative (SO) motor unit is recruited at a low force level, i.e. it has a low threshold force for being recruited. At the other extreme the largest high threshold fast twitch glycolytic (FG) motor unit is not recruited until the exerted force exceeds 90% of maximum. In between are another lower threshold FG unit and a fast twitch oxidative glycolytic (FOG) motor unit. Note that as the force of contraction exceeds the recruitment threshold of a motor unit, its firing rate increases. In a true maximal voluntary contraction, all motor units are recruited and all units are firing at a rate high enough to produce the maximum possible force from their muscle fibres. Fast twitch units require higher firing rates to attain maximum force because of their faster contractile response. (From Hannerz, 1974.)

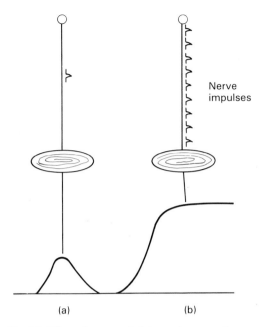

Nerve impulses

(a)   (b)

Fig. 9.3 Effect of motor unit firing rate on muscle force. If a motoneurone were to discharge a single nerve impulse down its axon to its constituent muscle fibres, the response would be a brief, low force twitch contraction (a). In contrast, if the motoneurone sent a high frequency 'train' of impulses down to the muscle fibres, i.e. a high firing rate, the response would be a much stronger and longer tetanic action (b). In human muscles the force of a high frequency tetanic action is about 10 times greater than that of a twitch contraction. In voluntary contractions motoneurones rarely if ever fire a single impulse; nevertheless, by varying its firing rate a motor unit can vary its force output over about a 10-fold range (see also Fig. 9.4).

Some so-called 'high threshold' motor units are recruited only when a person makes a maximal voluntary effort in performing the contraction (Fig. 9.2). Indeed, many untrained athletes (i.e. unfamiliar with a strength-training exercise) may not be able to recruit the highest threshold motor units; in other words, they are not able to fully activate the agonist muscles. In the early phase of training with the new exercise the athlete may acquire the ability to recruit the high threshold motor units, thus achieving increased activation of agonists and increased muscle force.

Maximal force output from a muscle requires more than recruitment of all motor units. When the central nervous system recruits a motor unit, it can make the motor unit 'fire' at different frequencies (Fig. 9.3). Firing frequency or rate refers to the number of nerve impulses (excitations) per second that the muscle fibres of a motor unit receive from their motoneurone. Motor units fire at rates ranging from about 10 to 60 impulses $\cdot$ s^{-1}. The greater the level of excitation of the motoneurones by the central nervous system, the greater the firing rates of the motor units. As illustrated in Fig. 9.4 a change in the firing rate causes a marked change in a motor unit's force output; an increase in frequency causes an increase in force. Figure 9.2 shows that higher threshold motor units have higher firing rates. Thus the maximum force output from an agonist muscle requires not only that all motor units be

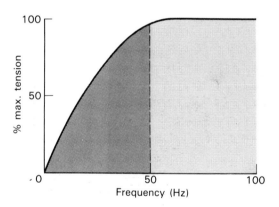

Fig. 9.4 Force–frequency curve. When the force produced by stimulating a muscle at different frequencies (simulating different motor unit firing rates) is plotted, a force–frequency curve is produced. Note that there is a range of frequencies over which relatively small changes in frequency cause large changes in force (per cent maximum tension). At the higher frequencies the opposite applies: only small increases in force are obtained despite large increases in frequency. Thus, doubling the frequency from 50 to 100 impulses $\cdot$ s^{-1} (frequency expressed in hertz in figure) brings almost no increase in force. The normal 'working' range of firing for motor units is about 10–60 Hz, a range over which there is a large variation in force output.

recruited but also that all units are firing at a sufficiently high rate to produce maximum force. Therefore, increased activation of agonists as a neural adaptation to strength training could take the form of recruitment of high threshold units not previously recruitable, or increased firing rates of units.

Electromyographic studies

Electromyography is a method of recording and quantifying the electrical activity produced by the muscle fibres of activated motor units. If electromyographic (EMG) recordings are made from an agonist muscle during maximal voluntary contractions, before and after a training programme, an increase in the quantity of recorded EMG (called integrated EMG or IEMG) would generally indicate that more motor units have been recruited, that motor units are firing at higher rates, or that some combination, of the two adaptations has occurred. An increased IEMG has been recorded after strength training involving weightlifting (Moritani & deDvries, 1979; Häkkinen & Komi, 1983, 1986; Häkkinen *et al.*, 1985a), isometric actions (Komi *et al.*, 1978), 'isokinetic' concentric actions (Narici, *et al.*,

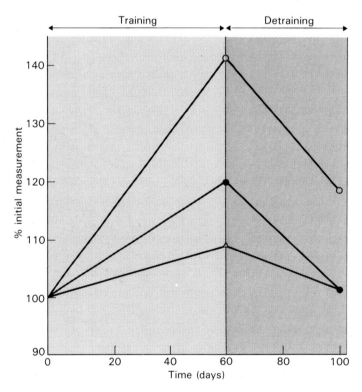

Fig. 9.5 Effects of 60 days of strength training and 40 days of detraining on knee extension isometric strength (MVC) (●), quadriceps integrated EMG (IEMG) (○), and quadriceps muscle cross-sectional area (CSA) (△). Training was 10 isokinetic knee extensions at 2.09 rad · s^{-1}, done 4 days per week. Note that strength increased more than muscle size after training, suggesting that part of the increase in strength was caused by neural adaptations, as evidenced by the increase in IEMG. Not so easy to explain is why strength did not increase at least as much as IEMG, because one might expect the increase in strength to equal the sum of the neural (IEMG) and muscle (CSA) adaptations. Part of the increase in IEMG may have been due to muscle hypertrophy, because larger muscle fibres would tend to produce larger action potentials. (From Narici *et al.*, 1990.)

1990), and 'explosive' jumping (Häkkinen *et al.*, 1985b). The results of the most recent of these studies are shown in Fig. 9.5. Analysis of IEMG has also revealed a possible neural adaptation to high stretch loads, as encountered by athletes doing 'plyometric' exercise. In jumping down to the floor from a height of 110 cm (drop jumps) an untrained person responds with a period of inhibition (reduced agonist activation) during the eccentric action phase after landing (stretch load). In contrast, a trained jumper

responds with a period of facilitation (increased agonist activation) (Fig. 9.6). The facilitation in the jumper may be an adaptation of certain reflex responses. This adaptation may be specific to certain stretch loads (Fig. 9.7).

Another EMG method that has been applied to strength-training studies is called reflex potentiation. In this method reflex EMG responses are elicited during maximal voluntary contractions. The greater the voluntary effort and hence the motor unit activation, the greater the potentiation of the reflex response. Strength-training studies have demonstrated an increase in reflex potentiation after training

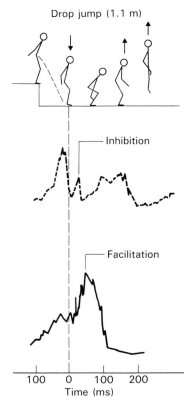

Fig. 9.6 EMG recordings from the gastrocnemius muscle during drop jumps in an untrained subject (----) and in a trained jumper (——). During the eccentric phase of high stretch load (to immediate right of vertical dashed line at time 0), the untrained subject responded with a period of inhibition. In contrast, the trained jumper responded with a period of facilitation. The facilitation in the jumper may reflect a neural adaptation to training that is related to reflex responses. (From Schmidtbleicher & Gollhofer, 1982.)

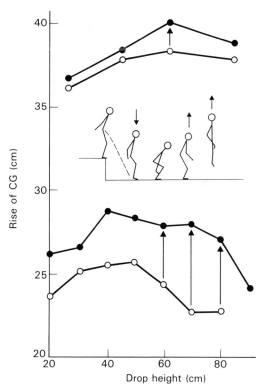

Fig. 9.7 Comparison of drop jump performance in athletes (●) and control subjects (○). At the top, male volleyball players excelled over control subjects only at one particular drop jump height, perhaps reflecting a neural adaptation to a specific stretch load. At the bottom, the female gymnasts outperformed the control subjects at all drop heights but most particularly at the highest stretch loads. (From Komi, 1984.)

(Milner-Brown *et al.*, 1975; Sale *et al.*, 1983a). Cross-sectional studies have shown reflex potentiation to be enhanced in weightlifters (Milner-Brown *et al.*, 1975; Sale *et al.*, 1983b) and sprinters (Upton & Radford, 1975). Like the IEMG method, the reflex potentiation method cannot distinguish the relative contributions of increased recruitment and increased firing rates to the increase in motor unit activation.

The EMG methods discussed so far usually employ surface recording electrodes (electrodes taped to the skin overlying the muscle). These electrodes cannot directly record the firing rates of individual motor units. A more demanding and invasive technique is to insert needle or fine wire electrodes into the muscle. This technique does allow single motor unit recordings to be made. By analogy, a surface electrode could be likened to a microphone placed over the centre of a soccer field. It can record the roar of the crowd but cannot register what individual crowd members are saying. The intramuscular electrode can be likened to a microphone placed close to the mouth of a single crowd member. Although the background roar can still be heard, it is possible to hear what the single crowd member is saying, i.e. record the firing rate of individual motor units. Unfortunately, single motor unit recordings have never been undertaken in a strength-training study. However, two relevant observations have been made. In a fatigue study, some subjects were unable to fire high threshold units at rates necessary for maximum force output. After repeated experiments these subjects were then able to achieve higher firing rates; at this point their voluntary force matched the force evoked by tetanic (high frequency) stimulation. The repeated experiments, which consisted of sustaining maximal contractions, could be considered a form of strength training. This training also increased the time (from a few seconds to about 20 s) that the highest threshold motor units could be kept active (recruited) in sustained maximal contractions (Grimby *et al.*, 1981). A second recent observation has been a decrease in maximum firing rates of motor units following a period of limb immobilization in a cast (Duchateau & Hainaut, 1990). Thus it seems that maximum firing rates can be increased by training but decreased by periods of disuse.

Bilateral deficit

Many common strength-training exercises require simultaneous activation of both limbs. Examples are squat, leg press, bench press, and

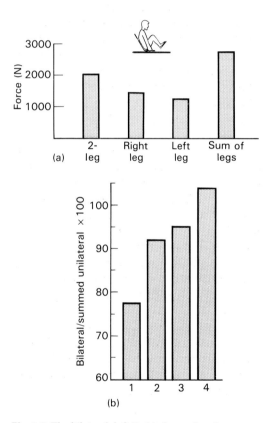

Fig. 9.8 The bilateral deficit. (a) shows that the bilateral (2-leg) force is less than the sum of the left and right legs acting alone (summed unilateral). (b) shows that training with bilateral contractions, as done for example by rowers, may reduce or eliminate the bilateral deficit. The vertical scale expresses bilateral force as a percentage of summed unilateral force. (From Secher, 1975.) 1, controls ($n = 6$); 2, club oarsmen ($n = 11$); 3, national oarsmen ($n = 22$); 4, international oarsmen ($n = 7$).

overhead press. It has been found that when untrained subjects attempt such bilateral movements, the total force produced is less than the sum of the forces produced by the left and right limbs acting alone (Henry & Smith, 1961; Coyle *et al.*, 1981; Ohtsuki, 1981, 1983; Vandervoort *et al.*, 1984, 1987; Van Soest *et al.*, 1985; Howard & Enoka, 1987). This bilateral deficit (Fig. 9.8) is associated with a reduction in IEMG (in comparison to the same muscles active in the unilateral condition) in agonists (Ohtsuki, 1983; Vandervoort *et al.*, 1984; Howard & Enoka, 1987). The bilateral deficit is greater in some movements than others (Vandervoort *et al.*, 1987) and may be absent (Kroll, 1965) in others.

If the bilateral deficit involves depressed activation of the involved agonists, the possibility is raised that strength training with bilateral movements may overcome the bilateral deficit by increasing the activation of agonists in the bilateral condition. The bilateral deficit may be absent in athletes who train with bilateral movements. For example, rowers have little or no bilateral deficit, and the most elite rowers actually perform better in the bilateral than unilateral condition (Fig. 9.8). The same is true for weightlifters, whereas cyclists, who train with alternating or reciprocal movements, display the bilateral deficit (Howard & Enoka, 1987). Short-term training studies have also demonstrated a reduction of the bilateral deficit (Enoka, 1988).

The reduction or elimination of the bilateral deficit could thus be considered a neural adaptation to strength training, that takes the form of an increased ability to activate agonists in bilateral movements.

Rate of force development

The discussion so far has focused on how increased activation of agonist muscles could increase strength, i.e. the peak force of a maximal voluntary contraction. Equally important to athletic performance is the ability to develop force rapidly. In many athletic movements only a fraction of a second is available to develop the greatest possible force. In these movements a high rate of force development is a limiting factor to success. For example, ski jumpers were found not to have greater leg extension peak force than untrained men, but the jumpers were able to achieve their peak force more rapidly (Komi, 1984). A related phenomenon is the so-called velocity specificity in strength training. Training with high velocity movements increases high velocity strength relatively more than low velocity strength, and vice versa (Caiozzo *et al.*, 1981; Coyle *et al.*, 1981; Kanehisa & Miyashita, 1983; Duchateau & Hainaut, 1984; Rosler *et al.*, 1986; Narici *et al.*, 1990). Part of the velocity specific training effect could be related to adaptive changes in the muscle, such as an increase in maximal muscle shortening velocity after high velocity training (Duchateau & Hainaut, 1984). There is also evidence that neural adaptations may be involved. For example, 'explosive' jump training caused a specific increase in the rate of onset of motor unit activation, as revealed by surface electromyography (Häkkinen *et al.*, 1985b).

Various possible neural mechanisms can be identified that might contribute to the velocity specific training effect. The organization and central command for the most rapid ballistic muscle actions differ from that of slow actions (Desmedt & Godaux, 1979), and these differences could be accentuated by specific low or high velocity training. Agonist muscles exhibit a premovement silence (PMS), i.e. little or no motor unit activity is present, just prior to ballistic (brief, high velocity) actions. The PMS occurs most often in maximal ballistic efforts but is not always present. The PMS may be a learned rather than an automatic response to ballistic tasks (Mortimer *et al.*, 1987), leaving open the possibility that increased frequency of occurrence of PMS may be a neural adaptation to high velocity training. The PMS may increase the rate of force development and peak force of ballistic actions in two ways. The brief silent period may bring all motoneurones into a non-refractory state, allowing them all to be more readily recruited and brought to the maximum possible firing rates. The PMS may also, by inducing a brief stretch–shortening cycle, increase the rate of force development and peak force of the ensuing ballistic action (Walter, 1988).

The importance of motoneurone firing rate to the force output of a motor unit has already been pointed out; up to a certain frequency an increase in firing rate increases the force of contraction. But EMG recordings from single motor units have shown that in maximal voluntary contractions motor units may begin to fire at rates well in excess of those needed to achieve maximum isometric force. For example, motor units may fire at 100 impulses · s^{-1} (i.e. 100 Hz) for about 100 ms at the onset of a maximal contraction, even though maximum isometric force can be attained at a rate of 50 Hz (Grimby et al., 1981). The high rate of 100 Hz will, however, increase rate of force development (Fig. 9.9). The highest motor unit firing rates have been recorded in maximal ballistic actions, where rates as high as 120 Hz have been observed (Desmedt & Godaux, 1977). A neural adaptation to high velocity training may consist of an acquired ability to increase the maximum motor unit firing rates in ballistic actions. An increase in maximum motor unit firing rates may have been responsible for the more rapid onset of EMG observed after explosive jump training (Fig. 9.10).

Selective recruitment of motor units within agonists

In general, the recruitment of motor units within a muscle is governed by the 'size' principle, i.e. motor units are recruited in order according to their size (Fig. 9.2). This pattern is most readily seen when the force of a muscle contraction is gradually increased from zero force to the maximum value. The smaller slow twitch motor units are recruited first, followed by the larger fast twitch units. There is some evidence, however, that apparent violations of the size principle may sometimes occur. For

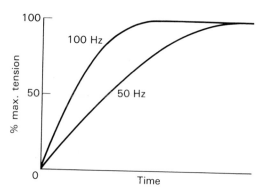

Fig. 9.9 Effect of high frequency stimulation on rate of force development. Stimulation at 100 Hz produced a greater rate of force development but no greater peak *isometric* force than at 50 Hz (see also Fig. 9.4). Thus the very high motor unit firing rates observed at the onset of ballistic contractions (100–120 Hz) serve to increase the rate of force development of ballistic contractions. Such high rates would also increase the peak force of *dynamic* actions done at high velocity.

example, the larger fast twitch motor units may be preferentially recruited over the smaller slow twitch units when rapid ballistic muscle actions are performed. It is also possible that in muscles that can contribute to more than one joint movement (e.g. biceps brachii contributes to elbow flexion and forearm supination), certain subpopulations of motor units may be selectively activated to carry out specific movements. These two departures from the size principle could be related, respectively, to neural adaptations related to specificity of velocity and movement pattern in strength training.

Velocity and action type specificity

Although there is also evidence to the contrary (Desmedt & Godaux, 1977), high threshold fast twitch motor units have been shown to be preferentially activated in brief, rapid concentric (muscle shortening) actions in which the intent is to relax quickly (Grimby & Hannerz, 1977). It has also been demonstrated that fast twitch motor units are preferentially recruited

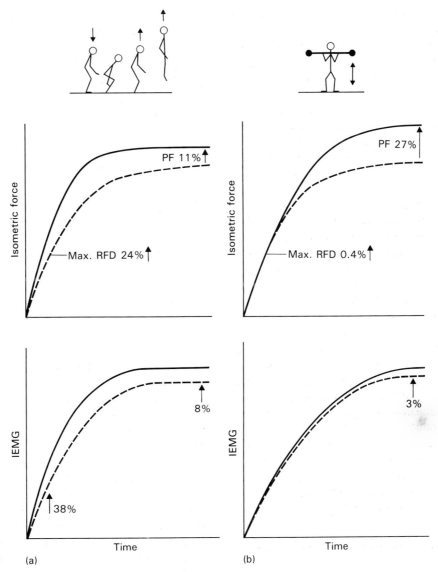

Fig. 9.10 (a) Effect of explosive jump training on isometric strength and motor unit activation (IEMG). The top panel shows that rate of force development (max. RFD) increased more (24%) than peak force (PF, 11%). Similarly, the bottom panel shows that the maximum rate of onset of EMG increased more (38%) than the peak EMG (8%). The greater increases related to rate of force development may reflect specific neural adaptations to explosive training. (b) By comparison heavy-resistance weight training produced the opposite pattern of results. (From Häkkinen *et al.*, 1985a,b, and redrawn with permission from Sale, 1988.) ----, pre-training; ——, post-training.

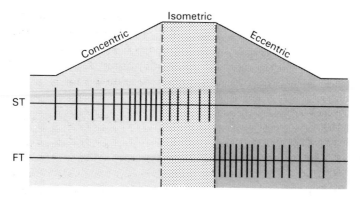

Fig. 9.11 Effect of action type on motor unit recruitment pattern. Recordings were made from a low threshold slow twitch (ST) and a high threshold fast twitch (FT) motor unit in the gastrocnemius muscle when the muscle was acting as an agonist in a shortening (concentric) action to raise a weight, an isometric action to hold the weight still briefly, and in a lengthening (eccentric) action to lower the weight back down again. This movement pattern is typical of weight training exercises. Note that the ST unit was preferentially activated during the concentric and isometric phases, whereas the FT unit was preferentially activated during the eccentric phase. The selective activation of the FT unit was most pronounced when the eccentric action was done relatively quickly. (From Nardone *et al.*, 1989.)

in eccentric (muscle lengthening) actions performed at moderate to high velocities (Fig. 9.11). It is possible that a neural adaptation to high velocity training consists of an accentuation of the preferential activation of fast twitch motor units.

Movement pattern specificity

It has often been observed in strength-training studies that the magnitude of measured increases in strength depends on how similar the strength test is to the actual training exercise (Sale & MacDougall, 1981). For example, if athletes were to train their legs by doing the squat exercise, the increase in strength measured as maximal squatting strength would be much greater than strength increases measured in isometric leg press or knee extension tests (Fig. 9.12). This specificity of movement pattern in strength training probably reflects the role of learning and coordination (Rutherford & Jones, 1986). Improved coordination would take the form of the most efficient activation of all of the involved muscles, and the most efficient activation of

motor units within each muscle. In regard to the latter, there is evidence that certain motor units in a muscle may be preferentially recruited when a muscle is engaged in a particular task (Desmedt & Godaux, 1981; Ter Harr Romeny *et al.*, 1982, 1984). For example, motor units in the lateral portion of the long head of the biceps are preferentially activated when this muscle is engaged in elbow flexion, whereas motor units in the medial portion are preferentially activated in forearm supination (Fig. 9.13). The recruitment thresholds of motor units in a muscle are also influenced by the type of muscle action associated with a movement. In elbow flexion, biceps motor units have a lower threshold in slow concentric and eccentric actions than isometric actions; in contrast, the reverse is true for brachialis (Tax *et al.*, 1989). These different recruitment patterns are related more to central command than sensory feedback (Tax *et al.*, 1990). The recruitment thresholds of motor units of a muscle active in a movement may also be affected by changes in joint angle (van Zuylen *et al.*, 1988). Herein may be the basis of part of the neural adaptations related to specificity of joint angle

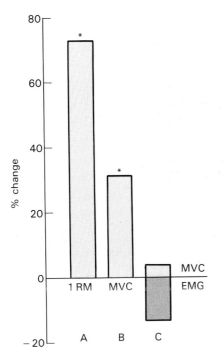

Fig. 9.12 Specificity of movement pattern in strength training. Subjects trained their legs with the barbell squat exercise for 8 weeks. There was a large increase (*, significant change) in specific weightlifting strength (A) (1 RM = one repetition maximum) but much smaller increases in non-specific isometric leg press (B) and knee extension strength (C). EMG was measured only in the knee extension test (C) and did not change with training. Perhaps increases would have been observed had measurements been made during the squat and leg press movements. (Based on Thorstensson et al., 1976a,b, and redrawn with permission from Sale, 1988.) MVC, maximal voluntary contraction.

observed in strength training (Thépaut-Mathieu et al., 1988; Kitai & Sale, 1989).

Selective activation of agonists within a muscle group

In the previous section it was shown that action velocity, action type, and movement pattern could affect motor unit recruitment within a muscle. The same is true for muscles within a group. Some muscles in a functional group may be preferentially activated over others

depending on velocity and type of action, and on movement pattern. Some neural adaptations to strength training may consist of alterations in the nature of the preferential activation of muscles within a group.

Velocity and action type specificity

Fast muscles, i.e. those with a relatively high proportion of fast twitch motor units, may be preferentially activated over slow muscles in the execution of high velocity movements. The evidence (in humans) on this point to date is confined to the soleus and gastrocnemius muscles of the calf. In stationary cycling, gastrocnemius is preferentially activated over soleus at the higher pedalling speeds (Duchateau et al., 1986). The gastrocnemius is also preferentially activated in hopping (Moritani et al., 1990). In moderate force concentric and eccentric actions, soleus is preferentially activated in the concentric phase, while gastrocnemius is preferentially activated in the eccentric phase (Fig. 9.14). The latter pattern is accentuated at higher lengthening velocities (Nardone & Schiepatti, 1988).

Movement pattern specificity

There are many complex interactions among muscles that act at a joint (Buchanan et al., 1989). The coordination and relative activation of muscles is task specific (Tax et al., 1990), and the central nervous system may activate 'task groups' that consist of parts of different muscles (Loeb, 1985). At the elbow joint, for example, biceps is more readily activated than brachialis in dynamic actions, whereas the reverse is true for isometric actions (Tax et al., 1989). The activity of muscles acting at the hip and knee joints is altered depending on whether they are involved in single or multijoint movements (Yamashita, 1988). The relative contributions of muscles through a range of movement depends on the joint angle. At a particular angle, muscles with a greater mechanical advantage may be preferentially

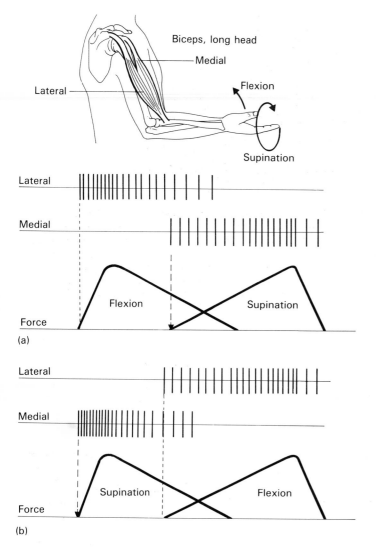

Fig. 9.13 Effect of movement
pattern on motor unit
recruitment. The biceps can act
as an agonist in elbow flexion
and forearm supination. (a)
shows that when a flexion force
is first developed the motor unit
in the lateral portion of the long
head of the biceps is
preferentially recruited over the
unit in the medial portion. As the
subject reduces the flexion force
and begins to develop a
supination force, the medial unit
is preferentially activated. (b)
shows that when the order of
producing flexion and supination
forces is reversed, so is the order
of preferential activation.
Selective activation of motor
units within a muscle depending
on the task, may be related to the
specificity of movement pattern
that has been observed in
strength training. (From Ter Harr
Romeny *et al.*, 1984.)

activated (van Zuylen *et al.*, 1988). It is quite possible that when a particular movement is repeated many times over a period of weeks or months, as happens is strength-training programmes, alterations occur in the complex interactions among muscles, with the result that performance is enhanced.

Co-contraction of antagonists

Contraction of agonists (prime movers in a task) may be associated with simultaneous contraction of their antagonists (muscles that produce force and movement in the opposite direction). This co-contraction of antagonists is quite common, particularly when the agonist contraction is strong and/or rapid (Freund & Budingen, 1978; Smith, 1981; Baratta *et al.*, 1988; Corcos *et al.*, 1989), and when the task requires precision or when subjects are untrained in the task (Person, 1958). Co-contraction of antagonists would seem to be counterproductive, particularly in a strength task, because the opposing torque developed

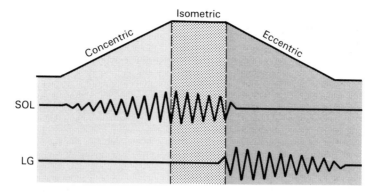

Fig. 9.14 Effect of action type on muscle activation. Recordings are made from soleus (SOL) and lateral gastrocnemius (LG) muscles of the calf when the muscles are acting as agonists in a shortening (concentric) action to raise a weight, an isometric action to hold the weight still briefly, and in a lengthening (eccentric) action to lower the weight back down again. This movement pattern is typical of weight training exercises. Note that the soleus was preferentially activated during the concentric and isometric phases, whereas the lateral gastrocnemius was preferentially activated during the eccentric phase. The selective activation of the LG was most pronounced when the eccentric action was done relatively quickly. (From Nardone & Schieppati, 1988.)

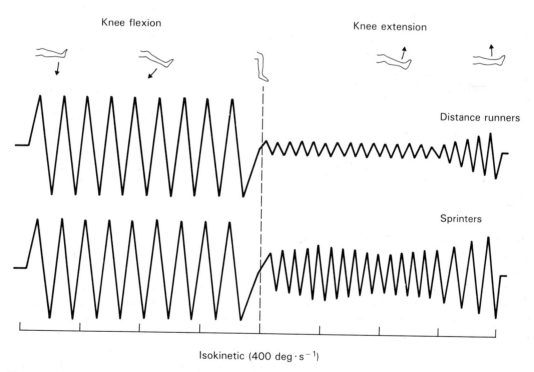

Fig. 9.15 Schematic representation of knee flexor EMG during alternate rapid knee extension and flexion on an isokinetic dynamometer. In the extension phase when the flexors were acting as antagonists, flexor activity was greater in sprinters than distance runners. The difference in flexor activity may reflect specific neural adaptation to training. (From Sale, 1988, based on data of Osternig *et al.*, 1986.)

by the antagonists would decrease the net torque in the intended direction of movement. For example, in maximal knee extensions the antagonist knee flexors will generate torque equal to about 10% of total extensor torque (Baratta *et al.*, 1988). There is even evidence that antagonist co-contraction may impair, by reciprocal inhibition, the ability to fully activate agonists (Tyler & Hutton, 1986).

What then are the functions of the co-contraction of antagonists? In strong contractions, antagonist contraction may assist ligaments in maintaining joint stability (Baratta *et al.*, 1988). Antagonist co-contraction may be part of the coordination of a movement. For example, biceps is an agonist for supination of the forearm. However, biceps also acts to

flex the elbow. To prevent unwanted elbow flexion, triceps (antagonist) must be activated to neutralize the flexor torque (van Zuylen *et al.*, 1988; Jongen *et al.*, 1989). Antagonist co-contraction is prominent in high velocity (ballistic) actions (Corcos *et al.*, 1989), where it may provide stabilization, precision, and a braking mechanism (Lestienne, 1979; Marsden *et al.*, 1983; Wierzbicka *et al.*, 1986). Finally, the apparently detrimental inhibition of agonists caused by antagonist co-contraction may be a protective mechanism in activities involving strong or rapid contractions (Tyler & Hutton, 1986).

There have been few studies that have examined the effect of training on patterns of antagonist co-contraction. In a cross-sectional

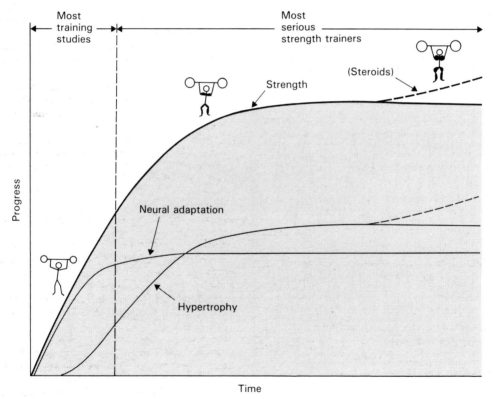

Fig. 9.16 The relative roles of neural and muscular adaptation to strength training. In the early phase of training neural adaptation predominates. This phase also encompasses most training studies. In intermediate and advanced training, progress is limited to the extent of muscular adaptation that can be achieved, notably hypertrophy; hence the temptation to use anabolic steroids when it becomes difficult to induce hypertrophy by training alone. (Redrawn with permission from Sale, 1988.)

study sprinters showed a greater degree of antagonist co-contraction than distance runners when performing high velocity knee extensions (Fig. 9.15). In contrast, strength and power athletes vs. endurance athletes had less knee flexor co-contraction during slow knee extensions designed to stretch the knee flexors (Osternig et al., 1990). Athletes with hypertrophied quadriceps show less co-contraction of knee flexors during low velocity isokinetic knee extensions than control subjects, but if athletes are given specific knee flexion training exercises, flexor co-contraction increases to control levels within a few weeks (Baratta et al., 1988). Further research is needed to clarify the roles of altered co-contractions of antagonists as neural adaptations to strength training.

Conclusion

There is no doubt that neural adaptation plays an important role in the overall adaptation to strength training. When a new training exercise is introduced into the programme, neural adaptation will predominate in the first several weeks of training as the athlete masters the coordination necessary to perform the exercise efficiently. Other adaptations, such as the ability to fire motor units at very high rates to achieve maximal rate of force development, may require a longer period of training to attain and be lost more rapidly during detraining. In the long term over months and years the ability to elicit adaptations in muscle may be the limiting factor to further improvement in performance (Fig. 9.16). Even at this stage, however, the role of the nervous system should not be ignored. The desired muscle adaptations, whether increased strength or rate of force development, will critically depend on the way the muscles are activated by the nervous system during training.

References

Baratta, R., Solomonow, M., Zhou, B.H., Letson, D., Chuinard, R. & D'Ambrosia, R. (1988) Muscular

coactivation. The role of the antagonist musculature in maintaining knee stability. *American Journal of Sports Medicine*, **16**, 113–22.

Buchanan, T.S., Roval, G.P. & Rymer, W.Z. (1989) Strategies for muscle activation during isometric torque generation at the human elbow. *Journal of Neurophysiology*, **62**, 1201–12.

Caiozzo, V.J., Perrine, J.J. & Edgerton, V.R. (1981) Training-induced alterations of the *in-vivo* force–velocity relationship of human muscle. *Journal of Applied Physiology: Respiratory, Environmental, and Exercise Physiology*, **51**, 750–4.

Corcos, D.M., Gottlieb, G.L. & Agarwal, G.C. (1989) Organizing principles for single-joint movements. II. A speed sensitive strategy. *Journal of Neurophysiology*, **62**, 358–68.

Coyle, E.F., Feiring, D.C., Rotkis, T.C., Cote, R.W., Lee, W. & Wilmore, J.H. (1981) Specificity of power improvements through slow and fast isokinetic training. *Journal of Applied Physiology: Respiratory, Environmental, and Exercise Physiology*, **51**, 1437–42.

Desmedt, J.E. & Godaux, E. (1977) Ballistic contractions in man: characteristic recruitment patterns of single motor units of the tibialis anterior muscle. *Journal of Physiology*, **264**, 673–93.

Desmedt, J.E. & Godaux, E. (1979) Voluntary motor commands in human ballistic contractions. *Annals of Neurology*, **5**, 415–21.

Desmedt, J.E. & Godaux, E. (1981) Spinal motoneuron recruitment in man: rank deordering with direction but not with speed of voluntary movement. *Science*, **214**, 933–6.

Duchateau, J. & Hainaut, K. (1984) Isometric or dynamic training: differential effects on mechanical properties of a human muscle. *Journal of Applied Physiology*, **56**, 296–301.

Duchateau, J. & Hainaut, K. (1990) Effects of immobilization on contractile properties, recruitment and firing rates of human motor units. *Journal of Physiology*, **422**, 55–65.

Duchateau, J., Le Bozec, S. & Hainaut, K. (1986) Contributions of slow and fast muscles of triceps surae to a cyclic movement. *European Journal of Applied Physiology*, **55**, 476–81.

Enoka, R.M. (1988) Muscle strength and its development. New perspectives. *Sports Medicine*, **6**, 146–68.

Freund, H.J. & Budingen, H.J. (1978) The relationship between speed and amplitude of the fastest voluntary contractions of human arm muscles. *Experimental Brain Research*, **31**, 1–12.

Grimby, L. & Hannerz, J. (1977) Firing rate and recruitment order of toe extensor motor units in different modes of voluntary contraction. *Journal of Physiology*, **264**, 865–79.

Grimby, L., Hannerz, J. & Hedman, B. (1981) The fatigue and voluntary discharge properties of single motor units in man. *Journal of Physiology*, **316**, 545–54.

Häkkinen, K. (1985) Factors influencing trainability of muscular strength during short term and prolonged training. *National Strength and Conditioning Association Journal*, **7**, 32–7.

Häkkinen, K., Alen, M. & Komi, P.V. (1985a) Changes in isometric force- and relaxation-time, electromyographic and muscle fibre characteristics of human skeletal muscle during strength training and detraining. *Acta Physiologica Scandinavica*, **125**, 573–85.

Häkkinen, K. & Komi, P.V. (1983) Electromyographic changes during strength training and detraining. *Medicine and Science in Sports and Exercise*, **15**, 455–60.

Häkkinen, K. & Komi, P.V. (1986) Training-induced changes in neuromuscular performance under voluntary and reflex conditions. *European Journal of Applied Physiology*, **55**, 147–55.

Häkkinen, K., Komi, P.V. & Alen, M. (1985b) Effect of explosive type strength training on isometric force- and relaxation-time, electromyographic and muscle fibre characteristics of leg extensor muscles. *Acta Physiologica Scandinavica*, **125**, 587–600.

Hannerz, J. (1974) Discharge properties of motor units in relation to recruitment order in voluntary contraction. *Acta Physiologica Scandinavica*, **91**, 374–84.

Henry, F.M. & Smith, L.E. (1961) Simultaneous vs. separate bilateral muscular contractions in relation to neural overflow theory and neuromuscular specificity. *Research Quarterly*, **32**, 42–6.

Howard, J.D. & Enoka, R.M. (1987) Interlimb interactions during maximal efforts. *Medicine and Science in Sports and Exercise*, **19**, 53.

Jongen, H.A.H., Denier van der Gon, J.J. & Gielen, C.C.A.M. (1989) Inhomogeneous activation of motoneurone pools as revealed by co-contraction of antagonistic human arm muscles. *Experimental Brain Research*, **75**, 555–62.

Kanehisa, H. & Miyashita, M. (1983) Specificity of velocity in strength training. *European Journal of Applied Physiology*, **52**, 104–6.

Kitai, T.A. & Sale, D.G. (1989) Specificity of joint angle in isometric training. *European Journal of Applied Physiology*, **58**, 744–8.

Komi, P.V. (1984) Physiological and biomechanical correlates of muscle function: effects of muscle structure and stretch–shortening cycle on force and speed. *Exercise and Sport Sciences Reviews*, **12**, 81–121.

Komi, P.V. (1986) Training of muscle strength and power: interaction of neuromotoric, hypertrophic and mechanical factors. *International Journal of Sports Medicine*, **7** (suppl.), 10–16.

Komi, P.V., Viitasalo, J., Rauramaa, R. & Vihko, V. (1978) Effect of isometric strength training on mechanical, electrical and metabolic aspects of muscle function. *European Journal of Applied Physiology*, **40**, 45–55.

Kroll, W. (1965) Central facilitation in bilateral versus unilateral isometric contractions. *American Journal of Physical Medicine*, **44**, 218–23.

Lestienne, F. (1979) Effects of inertial load and velocity on the braking process of voluntary limb movements. *Experimental Brain Research*, **35**, 407–18.

Loeb, G. (1985) Motoneurone task groups: coping with kinematic heterogeneity. *Journal of Experimental Biology*, **115**, 137–46.

Marsden, C.D., Obeso, J.A. & Rothwell, J.C. (1983) The function of antagonist muscle during fast limb movement in man. *Journal of Physiology*, **335**, 1–13.

Milner-Brown, H.S., Stein, R.B. & Lee, R.G. (1975) Synchronization of human motor units: possible roles of exercise and supraspinal reflexes. *Electroencephalography and Clinical Neurophysiology*, **38**, 245–54.

Moritani, T. & deVries, H.A. (1979) Neural factors vs. hypertrophy in time course of muscle strength gain. *American Journal of Physical Medicine and Rehabilitation*, **58**, 115–30.

Moritani, T., Oddsson, L. & Thorstensson, A. (1990) Differences in modulation of the gastrocnemius and soleus H-reflexes during hopping in man. *Acta Physiologica Scandinavica*, **138**, 575–6.

Mortimer, J.A., Eisenberg, P. & Palmer, S.S. (1987) Premovement silence in agonist muscles preceding maximum efforts. *Experimental Neurology*, **98**, 542–54.

Nardone, A., Romano, C. & Schieppati, M. (1989) Selective recruitment of high-threshold human motor units during voluntary isotonic lengthening of active muscles. *Journal of Physiology*, **409**, 451–71.

Nardone, A. & Schieppati, M. (1988) Shift of activity from slow to fast muscle during voluntary lengthening contractions of the triceps surae muscles in humans. *Journal of Physiology*, **395**, 363–81.

Narici, M.V., Roi, G.S., Landoni, L., Minetti, A.E. & Cerretelli, P. (1990) Changes in force, cross-sectional area and neural activation during strength training and detraining of the human quadriceps. *European Journal of Applied Physiology*, **59**, 310–19.

Ohtsuki, T. (1981) Decrease in grip strength induced by simultaneous bilateral exertion with reference to finger strength. *Ergonomics*, **24**, 37–48.

Ohtsuki, T. (1983) Decrease in human voluntary isometric arm strength induced by simultaneous bilateral exertion. *Behavioral Brain Research*, **7**, 165–78.

Osternig, L.R., Hamill, J., Lander, J.E. & Robertson,

R. (1986) Co-activation of sprinter and distance runner muscles in isokinetic exercise. *Medicine and Science in Sports and Exercise*, **18**, 431–5.

Osternig, L.R., Robertson, R.N., Troxel, R.K. & Hansen, P. (1990) Differential responses to proprioceptive neuromuscular facilitation (PNF) stretch techniques. *Medicine and Science in Sports and Exercise*, **22**, 106–11.

Person, R.S. (1958) An electromyographic investigation of coordination of the activity of antagonist muscles in man during the development of a motor habit. *Pavlov Journal of Higher Nervous Activity*, **8**, 13–23.

Rosler, K., Conley, K.E., Howald, H., Gerber, C. & Hoppeler, H. (1986) Specificity of leg power changes to velocities used in bicycle endurance training. *Journal of Applied Physiology*, **61**, 30–6.

Rutherford, O.M. & Jones, D.A. (1986) The role of learning and coordination in strength training. *European Journal of Applied Physiology*, **55**, 100–5.

Sale, D.G. (1988) Neural adaptation to resistance training. *Medicine and Science in Sports and Exercise*, **20**, (suppl.), S135–S145.

Sale, D.G. & MacDougall, D. (1981) Specificity in strength training: a review for the coach and athlete. *Canadian Journal of Applied Sports Science*, **6**, 87–92.

Sale, D.G., MacDougall, J.D., Upton, A.R.M. & McComas, A.J. (1983a) Effect of strength training on motoneuron excitability in man. *Medicine and Science in Sports and Exercise*, **15**, 57–62.

Sale, D.G., Upton, A.R.M., McComas, A.J. & MacDougall, J.D. (1983b) Neuromuscular function in weight-trainers. *Experimental Neurology*, **82**, 521–31.

Schmidtbleicher, D. & Gollhofer, A. (1982) Neuromuskuläre Untersuchungen zur Bestimmung individueller Belastungsgrössen für ein Teifsprungtraining. *Leistungssport*, **12**, 298–307.

Secher, N.H. (1975) Isometric rowing strength of experienced and inexperienced oarsmen. *Medicine and Science in Sports*, **7**, 280–3.

Smith, A.M. (1981) The coactivation of antagonist muscles. *Canadian Journal of Physiology and Pharmacology*, **59**, 733–47.

Tax, A.A.M., Denier van der Gon, J.J., Gielen, C.C.A.M. & Kleyne, M. (1990) Differences in central control of m. biceps brachii in movement tasks and force tasks. *Experimental Brain Research*, **79**, 138–42.

Tax, A.A.M., Denier van der Gon, J.J., Gielen, C.C.A.M. & Tempel, C.M.M. van den (1989) Differences in the activation of m. biceps brachii in the control of slow isotonic movements and isometric contractions. *Experimental Brain Research*, **76**, 55–63.

Ter Harr Romeny, B.M., Denier van der Gon, J.J. & Gielen, C.A.M. (1982) Changes in recruitment order of motor units in the human biceps muscle. *Experimental Neurology*, **78**, 360–8.

Ter Harr Romeny, B.M., Denier van der Gon, J.J. & Gielen, C.A.M. (1984) Relation between location of a motor unit in the human biceps brachii and its critical firing levels for different tasks. *Experimental Neurology*, **85**, 631–50.

Thépaut-Mathieu, C., Van Hoecke, J. & Maton, B. (1988) Myoelectrical and mechanical changes linked to length specificity during isometric training. *Journal of Applied Physiology*, **64**, 1500–5.

Thorstensson, A., Hulten, B., Von Doblen, W. & Karlsson, J. (1976a) Effect of strength training on enzyme activities and fibre characteristics in human skeletal muscle. *Acta Physiologica Scandinavica*, **96**, 392–8.

Thorstensson, A., Karlsson, J., Viitasalo, J.H.T., Luhtanen, P. & Komi, P.V. (1976b) Effect of strength training on EMG of human skeletal muscle. *Acta Physiologica Scandinavica*, **98**, 232–6.

Tyler, A.E. & Hutton, R.S. (1986) Was Sherrington right about co-contractions? *Brain Research*, **370**, 171–5.

Upton, A.R.M. & Radford, P.F. (1975) Motoneuron excitability in elite sprinters. In P.V. Komi (ed.) *Biomechanics V-A*, pp. 82–7. University Park Press, Baltimore.

Van Soest, A.J., Roebroeck, M.E., Bobbert, M.F., Huijing, D.A. & Ingen Schenau, G.J. van (1985) A comparison of one-legged and two-legged countermovement jumps. *Medicine and Science in Sports and Exercise*, **17**, 635–9.

van Zuylen, E.J., Gielen, C.C.A.M. & Denier van der Gon, J.J. (1988) Coordination and inhomogeneous activation of human arm muscles during isometric torques. *Journal of Neurophysiology*, **60**, 1523–48.

Vandervoort, A.A., Sale, D.G. & Moroz, J. (1984) Comparison of motor unit activation during unilateral and bilateral leg extension. *Journal of Applied Physiology: Respiratory, Environmental and Exercise Physiology*, **56**, 46–51.

Vandervoort, A.A., Sale, D.G. & Moroz, J.R. (1987) Strength–velocity relation and fatiguability of unilateral versus bilateral arm extension. *European Journal of Applied Physiology*, **56**, 201–5.

Walter, C.B. (1988) The influence of agonist premotor silence and the stretch–shortening cycle on contractile rate in active skeletal muscle. *European Journal of Applied Physiology*, **57**, 557–82.

Wierzbicka, M.M., Wiegner, A.W. & Shahani B.T. (1986) Role of agonist and antagonist muscles in fast arm movements in man. *Experimental Brain Research*, **63**, 331–40.

Yamashita, N. (1988) EMG activities in mono- and bi-articular thigh muscles in combined hip and knee extension. *European Journal of Applied Physiology*, **58**, 274–7.

Chapter 9B

Time Course of Adaptations during Strength and Power Training

TOSHIO MORITANI

Introduction

Before describing the time course of adaptations in neural activation and morphological changes during strength training, a brief review of neuromuscular physiology will be provided. A motor unit (MU) consists of a motoneurone in the spinal cord and the muscle fibres it innervates (Burke, 1981). The number of MUs per muscle in humans may range from about 100 for a small hand muscle to 1000 or more for large limb muscles (Henneman & Mendell, 1981). It has also been shown that different MUs vary greatly in force-generating capacity, i.e. a 100-fold or more difference in twitch force (Stephens & Usherwood, 1977; Garnett et al., 1979). In voluntary contractions, force is modulated by a combination of MU recruitment and changes in MU activation frequency (rate coding) (Milner-Brown et al., 1973; Tanji & Kato, 1973; Kukulka & Clamann, 1981; Moritani & Muro, 1987). The greater the number of MUs recruited and their discharge frequency, the greater the force will be. During MU recruitment the muscle force, when activated at any constant discharge frequency, is approximately $2-5\,kg \cdot cm^{-2}$, and in general is relatively independent of species, gender, age and training status (Ikai & Fukunaga, 1970; Close, 1972; Alway et al., 1990).

The electrical activity in a muscle is determined by the number of MU recruited and their mean discharge frequency of excitation, i.e. the same factors that determine muscle force (Woods et al., 1978; Bigland-Ritchie, 1981; Moritani et al., 1986a; Moritani & Muro, 1987). Thus, direct proportionality between electromyogram (EMG) and force might be expected. Under certain experimental conditions, these proportionalities can be well demonstrated by recording the smoothed rectified or integrated EMG (IEMG) (Lippold, 1952; deVries, 1968; Seyfert & Kunkel, 1974; Milner-Brown & Stein, 1975; Moritani & deVries, 1978, 1979; Woods et al., 1978) and reproducibility of EMG recordings are remarkably high, e.g. the test–retest correlation ranging from 0.97 to 0.99 (Komi & Buskirk, 1970, 1972; Moritani & deVries, 1978, 1979). However, the change in the surface EMG should not automatically be attributed to changes in either MU recruitment or excitation frequencies as the EMG signal amplitude is further influenced by the individual muscle fibre potential, degree of MU discharge synchronization, and fatigue (Milner-Brown, et al., 1975; Jessop & Lippold, 1977; Bigland-Ritchie et al., 1979; Bigland-Ritchie, 1981; Moritani et al., 1985, 1986b). None the less, carefully controlled studies have successfully employed surface EMG recording techniques and demonstrated the usefulness of IEMG as a measure of muscle activation level under a variety of experimental conditions (Komi & Buskirk, 1972; Komi et al., 1978; Moritani & deVries, 1979, 1980; Häkkinen & Komi, 1983, 1985; Häkkinen et al., 1985, 1987; Moritani et al., 1987; Sale, 1988).

Time course of muscle strength gain: neural factors vs. hypertrophy

It is a common observation that repeated testing of the strength of skeletal muscles results in increasing test scores in the absence of measurable muscle hypertrophy (Bowers, 1966; deVries, 1968; Coleman, 1969). Such increasing test scores are typically seen in daily or even weekly retesting at the inception of a muscle strength training regimen. In some cases, several weeks of intensive weight training resulted in significant improvement in strength without a measurable change in girth (deVries, 1968; Komi et al., 1978). It has also been shown that when only one limb is trained, the paired untrained limb improves significantly in subsequent retests of strength but without evidence of hypertrophy (Coleman, 1969; Ikai & Fukunaga, 1970; Moritani & deVries, 1979, 1980; Houston et al., 1983). Rasch and Morehouse (1957) demonstrated strength gains from a 6-week training in tests when muscles were employed in a familiar way, but little or no gain in strength was observed when unfamiliar test procedures were employed. These data suggest that the higher scores

in strength tests resulting from the training programmes reflected largely the acquisition of skill (Rutherford & Jones, 1986).

All of the above findings support the importance of 'neural factors', which although not yet well defined, certainly contribute to the display of maximal muscle force that we call strength. On the other hand, a strong relationship has been demonstrated both between absolute strength and the cross-sectional area of the muscle (Rodahl & Horvath, 1962; Close, 1972) and between strength gain and increase in muscle girth or cross-sectional area (Ikai & Fukunaga, 1970). It is quite clear, therefore, that human voluntary strength is determined not only by the quantity (muscle cross-sectional area) and quality (muscle fibre types) of the involved muscle mass, but also by the extent to which the muscle mass has been activated (neural factors) (see Fig. 9.17).

A reasonable hypothesis for describing the time course of strength gain with respect to its two major determinants is that suggested by De Lorme and Watkins (1951) who postulated that: 'The initial increase in strength on progressive resistance exercise occurs at a rate far greater than can be accounted for by morphological

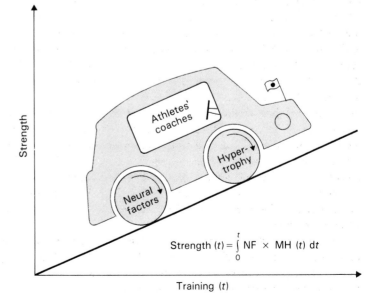

Fig. 9.17 A schematic representation showing the basic mechanisms for muscle strength gain during training. Muscle strength can be increased by neural adaptations (NF) and muscle hypertrophy (MH) during training with variable contributions at any given point in time (t).

$$\text{Strength } (t) = \int_0^t \text{NF} \times \text{MH} (t) \, dt$$

changes within the muscle. These initial rapid increments in strength noted in normal and disuse-atrophied muscles are, no doubt, due to motor learning... It is impossible to say how much of the strength increase is due to morphological changes within the muscle or to motor learning'.

We now have available EMG instrumentation and methodology that make it possible to separate muscle activation level (motor learning) from hypertrophic effects (morphological changes) as described by deVries (1968) and Moritani and deVries (1979, 1980). Our experimental results that showed an increase in IEMG after weight training is illustrated in Fig. 9.18. In the trained arm, the increase in strength was associated with both an increase in IEMG and an increase in muscle size. The contralateral untrained arm also showed an increase in strength but this was associated only with an increase in IEMG, indicating that the so-called 'cross education or cross-training' effect was the result of neural adaptation. In this case, there was no change in force per given muscle

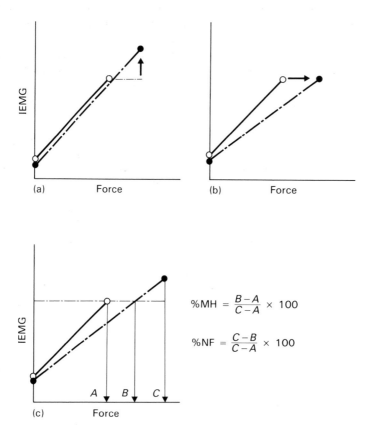

$$\%MH = \frac{B-A}{C-A} \times 100$$

$$\%NF = \frac{C-B}{C-A} \times 100$$

Fig. 9.18 Schema for evaluation of percent contributions of neural factors (NF) and muscle hypertrophy (MH) to the gain of strength. If strength gain is brought about by 'neural factors' such as learning to disinhibit, then we would expect to see increases in maximal activation without any change in force per fibre or motor units innervated as shown in (a). On the other hand, if strength gain were entirely attributable to muscle hypertrophy, then we would expect the results shown in (b). Here the force per fibre (or per unit activation) is increased by virtue of the hypertrophy but there is no change in maximal IEMG. (c) shows our method for evaluation of the percent contributions of the two components when both factors may be operative in the course of strength training. (From Moritani & deVries, 1979.) ○—○, before training; ●---●, after training.

activation level (E/F ratio). When hypertrophy of muscle fibres took place with training, the motor unit activation required to produce a given force decreased.

Figure 9.19 illustrates the time course of strength gain with respect to the calculated percent contributions of neural factors and hypertrophy. The results clearly demonstrate that the neural factors played a major role in strength development at early stages of strength gain and then hypertrophic factors gradually dominated over the neural factors in the contribution to the strength gain. The strength gain seen for the untrained contralateral arm flexors provide further support for the concept of cross-education. It is reasonable to assume that the nature of this cross-education effect may entirely rest on the neural factors presumably acting at various levels of the nervous system, which could result

in increasing the maximal level of muscle activation. Our subsequent study (Moritani & deVries, 1980) with older men (mean age of 70 years) demonstrated that the old subjects achieved the strength gain by virtue of neural factors, as indicated by the increases in the maximal IEMG in the absence of hypertrophy. It is suggested that the training-induced increase in the maximal level of muscle activation (neural factors) through greater MU discharge frequency and/or MU recruitment may be the only mechanism by which the aged subjects increase their strength in the absence of any significant evidence of hypertrophy. Data illustrated in Fig. 9.20 further support this assumption on the basis that there seems to be a very close association between the rate of increase in the maximal IEMG and the subsequent increase in the maximal strength in the aged subjects (Moritani, 1981). These results

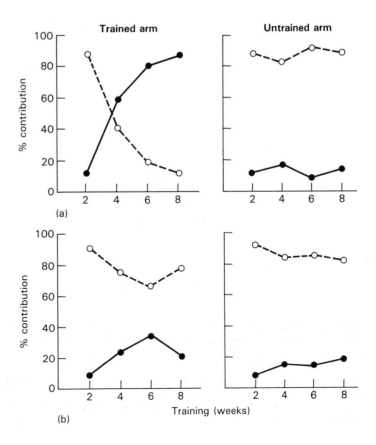

Fig. 9.19 The time course of strength gain showing the percent contributions of neural factors (○–––○) and hypertrophy (●—●) in the trained and contralateral untrained arms of (a) young and (b) old subjects. (From Moritani & deVries, 1980.)

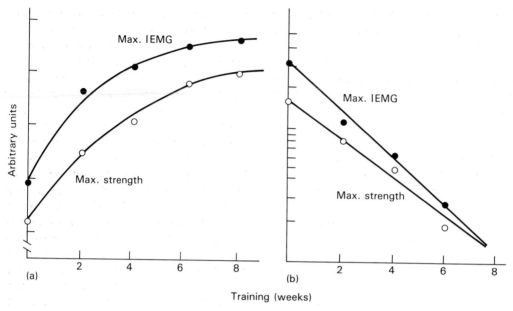

Fig. 9.20 Training curves (time course of changes) of the maximal strength (○) and maximal IEMG (●) of the old subjects' trained arm (a) and their plots on semi-logarithmic coordinates (b). Note the close association between changes in max. IEMG and maximal strength. (From Moritani, 1981.)

are entirely consistent with those reported by Komi *et al.*, (1978) who have demonstrated that changes in IEMG and force takes place almost in parallel during the course of 12 weeks of training. Häkkinen *et al.* (1981) demonstrated that the subject trained with high-intensity loads of combined concentric and eccentric actions showed an accelerated increase in force together with the parallel increase in IEMG during the first 8 weeks of training while showing minor muscle fibre hypertrophy. Greater muscle hypertrophy of both slow and fast twitch fibres was observed during the last 8 weeks of training that resulted in further strength gain with no significant change in the IEMG. Subsequent studies (Häkkinen *et al.*, 1981, 1985, 1987; Häkkinen & Komi, 1983, 1985; Houston *et al.*, 1983; Davies *et al.*, 1985; Komi, 1986; Jones & Rutherford, 1987; Davies *et al.*, 1988; Narici *et al.*, 1989; Ishida *et al.*, 1990) have confirmed these observations and provided evidence for the concept that in strength training the increase in voluntary neural drive accounts for the larger proportion of the initial

strength increment and thereafter both neural adaptation and hypertrophy takes place for further increase in strength, with hypertrophy becoming the dominant factor (Moritani & deVries, 1979; Häkkinen *et al.*, 1981).

Interestingly, there has been some evidence suggesting that strength development can be achieved by involuntary contractions initiated by electrical stimulation (Nowakowska, 1962; Eriksson *et al.*, 1981; Romero *et al.*, 1982). However, these experiments resulted in considerably smaller strength gains than the values found in normal voluntary training. Since the motor pathways are probably minimally involved in electrical training, it seems likely that a training stimulus resided in the muscle tissue itself and hence the hypertrophic factor was the principal constituent for strength development. More recent studies (McDonagh & Davies, 1984; Davies *et al.*, 1985) have indicated that the muscle training using electrically evoked actions (80 maximal isometric tetani for 10 s) produced no increase in maximal voluntary strength, suggesting that neural drive has to be present in the training in order to produce large increases in maximal voluntary strength.

A new approach to the study of training is to obtain the changes in electrically evoked muscular forces. These forces are obviously independent of volition and should represent the force generating capacity of the muscle fibres themselves, not the level of neural drive (McDonagh & Davies, 1984; Davies et al., 1985; Ishida et al., 1990). Davies et al. (1985) have shown that isometric strength training for 8 weeks resulted in a 33% increase in maximal strength, but electrically evoked tetanic tension increased only 11%. Recent work from our laboratory (Ishida et al., 1990) has also demonstrated a similar discrepancy between increases in maximal strength and electrically evoked twitch parameters. These data fit well with other data that indicate a discrepancy between increases in the cross-sectional area of muscle tissue and the increases in maximal strength following high force training (Ikai & Fukunaga, 1970; Komi et al., 1978; Moritani & deVries, 1979; Häkkinen et al., 1981, 1985; Jones & Rutherford, 1987; Davies et al., 1988; Narici et al., 1989). These findings again strongly support the hypothesis that the increase in maximal voluntary strength in the early stages of training is due to a change in voluntary neural drive to the muscle tissue.

There are two studies (Thorstensson et al., 1976b; Cannon & Cafarelli, 1987), which failed to show an increase in IEMG after high force training. Thorstensson et al. (1976) employed the barbell squat exercise and showed a large increase in weightlifting strength while observing no increase in isometric knee extension strength. It was this last movement that IEMG recorded and showed no change. Cannon and Cafarelli (1987) have shown an approximately 15% increase in maximal voluntary strength of adductor pollicis muscle after 5 weeks of training and have observed no change in neural drive (EMG). They also observed a significant increase in maximal voluntary strength of the untrained contralateral muscles with no change

in EMG amplitude. They sugested that their data did not reveal some unspecified increase in neural drive but rather a more responsive group of hypertrophied muscles. However, their argument seems to fail to explain the significant strength gain observed in the untrained contralateral muscles, as these muscles are unlikely to possess responsive groups of 'hypertrophied' muscles. It has also been shown that the adductor pollicis muscle is largely composed of type I fibres (Johnson et al., 1973) and the rate coding (MU firing frequency modulation) might be the only mechanism for increasing force above 50% maximal voluntary strength, as no MUs are recruited above this level of force (Kukulka & Clamann, 1981; Moritani et al., 1986a). One would, therefore, expect a greater degree of synchronization of MU activity for this small hand muscle, which in turn should result in increasingly large oscillations in the surface EMG. On this basis and a considerable amount of evidence for neural adaptations presented in this section, it is very difficult to explain the dissociation between the increase in maximal strength and the surface EMG amplitude. Further studies with intramuscular MU spike recordings are definitely needed for elucidating the nature of strength gain without accompanying increased neural drive.

Strength-training studies are typically carried out for a period of 5–20 weeks and have shown that the early increases in voluntary strength are associated mainly with neural adaptation, with hypertrophy beginning to occur at the latter stage of training as described (see Fig. 9.16, Chapter 9A). Serious athletes, however, train over a period of many months or years. Häkkinen et al. (1985) have studied the effects of strength training for 24 weeks with intensities ranging between 70 and 120% of maximal voluntary force. The increase in strength correlated with significant increase in the neural activation (IEMG) of the leg extensor muscles during the most intensive training months along with significant enlargement of fast twitch fibre area. During subsequent detraining a great decrease in the maximal strength was correlated with the decrease in maximal IEMG of the leg extensors. It was suggested that selective training-induced hypertrophy could contribute to strength development but muscle hypertrophy may have some limitations during long-term strength training, especially in highly trained subjects. This suggestion has recently been confirmed by a 1-year training study indicating the limited potential for strength development in elite strength athletes (Häkkinen *et al.*, 1987).

Time course of muscle power development

The development of muscular power is of great importance in sports events requiring a high level of force and speed. Significant correlations have been demonstrated among the force–velocity characteristics, muscle mechanical power and muscle fibre composition in human knee extensor muscles (Thorstensson *et al.*, 1976a; Tihanyi *et al.*, 1982). Faulkner *et al.* (1986) have recently studied the contractile properties of bundles of muscle fibres from human skeletal muscles. It was found that the peak power output of fast twitch fibres was fourfold greater than that of slow twitch fibres due to a greater

shortening velocity for a given afterload. When the composite power curve for the mixed muscle was studied, the fast twitch fibres contributed 2.5 times more than the slow twitch fibres to the total power.

Training effect of different loads on the force–velocity relationship and mechanical power output in human muscles has been extensively studied by Kaneko and his colleagues (Kaneko, 1970, 1974; Kaneko *et al.*, 1983). For example, Kaneko (1974) studied the time course of changes in the force–velocity and mechanical power output with respect to different training intensities [e.g. 0, 30, 60, 100% F_o (maximal strength)] for a period of 20 weeks. This study showed significantly large initial improvements in the force–velocity curve and corresponding mechanical power outputs as a result of muscle power training (see Fig. 9.21). Kaneko *et al.* (1983) also demonstrated the 'specificity' of muscle power training effect; i.e. the training by maximal contractions with 0% F_o was found to be most effective for improving the maximal velocity tested with no external load, while 100% F_o training improved maximal strength most. It was concluded that different training loads could bring about specific modifications of the force–velocity relationship, and that the load

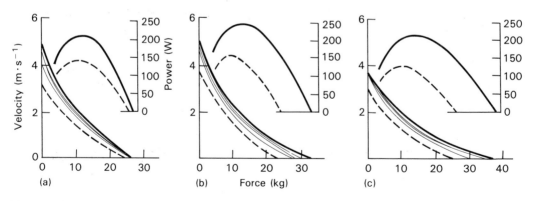

Fig. 9.21 The time course of changes in the force–velocity (concave) and force–power (convex) relationships during muscle power training with different loads. (a) 0% F_o; (b) 30% F_o; (c) 100% F_o. (From Kaneko, 1974.) ---, before training; — after 20 weeks of training.

30% F_o was most effective in improving maximal mechanical power output. In these and other studies (Moffroid & Whipple, 1970; Caiozzo et al., 1981; Coyle et al., 1981), no EMG recording was made so that it was not possible to determine the effects of muscle power training on maximal muscle activation level and other possible neural adaptations.

We have recently investigated the effects of short-term 30% F_o muscle power training upon the force–velocity, power and electrophysiological parameters (Moritani et al., 1987). The right biceps brachii muscle was trained by pulling a load equivalent to 30% F_o with maximal effort, 30 times per day, three times per week for a period of 2 weeks. The surface and intramuscular EMGs from the long and short heads were recorded simultaneously and analysed by means of frequency power spectrum and MU amplitude–frequency histogram techniques, respectively (Moritani et al., 1985, 1986b). Figure 9.22 represents a typical set of computer outputs showing the raw EMG signals recorded from the biceps brachii long and short head muscles and the corresponding power spectral parameters. It was found that the level of muscle activation as determined by RMS (root mean square EMG amplitude) values increased dramatically at any given load after training. On the other hand,

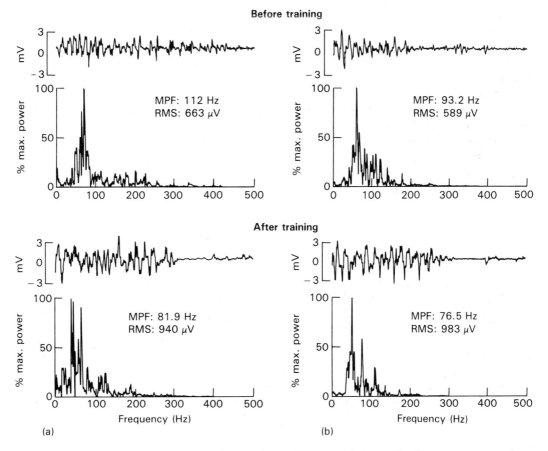

Fig. 9.22 A typical set of computer outputs showing the raw EMGs and corresponding frequency power spectra observed for the biceps brachii short (a) and long head (b) muscles before (above) and after (below) training. (From Moritani et al., 1987.)

MPF (mean power frequency), which reflects the frequency component of the recorded action potentials, markedly shifted toward lower frequency bands as a result of large, low-frequency EMG oscillations due possibly to better summation (synchronization) of the underlying action potentials.

To further elucidate the possibility of synchronous muscle activation patterns or association in the time and frequency domains, cross power spectra and cross-correlation coefficients were obtained between the action potentials recorded from the short and long head muscles at the pre- and post-training periods. Figures 9.23 and 9.24 represent the typical changes observed. It seems apparent that two action potential waveforms have little association in the amplitude and waveform patterns at the pretraining stage, revealing a maximal cross-correlation coefficient (R_{xy} of 0.40 (see Fig. 9.23). However, very similar action potential waveforms with much higher amplitude were obtained after the training, which increased R_{xy} to 0.91 (Fig. 9.24). This suggests a greater muscle activation and more synchronous MU activities after training (Milner-Brown et al., 1975). This may lead to an increased oscillation in the surface EMG, which may even approach the area of the maximal evoked M waves (mass action potential), indicating that all MUs are now fully synchronized (Bigland-Ritchie, 1981). Group data

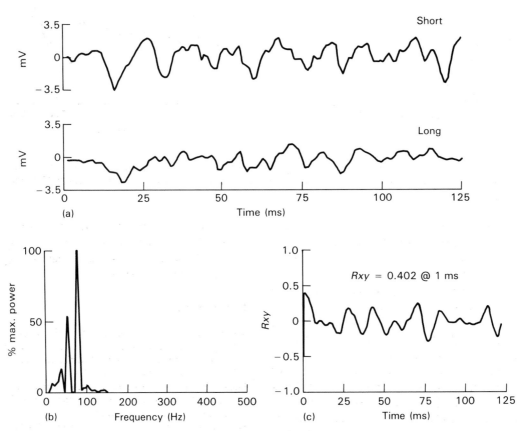

(a)

(b)   Frequency (Hz)

$Rxy = 0.402$ @ 1 ms

(c)   Time (ms)

Fig. 9.23 A typical set of action potential recordings from the biceps brachii short and long head muscles (a) and the corresponding cross-spectra (b) and cross-correlation (c) coefficients obtained before training. (From Moritani et al., 1987.)

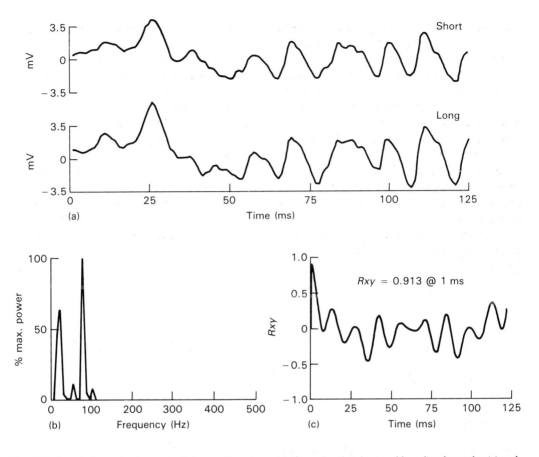

Fig. 9.24 A typical set of action potential recordings from the biceps brachii short and long head muscles (a) and the corresponding cross-spectra (b) and cross-correlation (c) coefficients obtained after training. (From Moritani *et al.*, 1987.)

indicated that there were highly significant increases in the maximal power output, RMS and R_{xy} together with the significant decrease in MPF after the training in all load conditions. These data strongly suggest that the short-term training-induced shifts in force–velocity relationship and the resultant mechanical power output might have been brought about by the neural adaptations in terms of greater muscle activation levels and more synchronous activation patterns. It should be of particular interest for athletic coaches if real-time analyses of surface EMG spectral parameters together with cross-correlation coefficients become available, as then muscle activation level and synchronization patterns can be available to

the trainees for immediate feedback. Whether or not this new approach for training may prove to be superior to the traditional training methods needs to be investigated.

References

Alway, S.E., Stray-Gundersen, J., Grumbt, W.H. & Gonyea, W.J. (1990) Muscle cross sectional area and torque in resistance-trained subjects. *European Journal of Applied Physiology*, **60**, 86–90.

Bigland-Ritchie, B. (1981) EMG/force relations and fatigue of human voluntary contractions. *Exercise and Sport Sciences Reviews*, **9**, 75–117.

Bigland-Ritchie, B., Jones, D.A. & Woods, J.J. (1979) Excitation frequency and muscle fatigue: Electrical responses during human voluntary and stimulated contractions. *Experimental Neurology*, **64**, 414–27.

Bowers, L. (1966) Effects of autosuggested muscle contraction on muscle strength and size. *Research Quarterly*, **37**, 302–12.

Burke, R.E. (1981) Motor units: anatomy, physiology and functional organization. In V. B. Brooks (ed.) *Handbook of Physiology. Section 1, Vol. II*, pp. 345–422. American Physiological Society, Bethesda.

Caiozzo, V.J., Perrine, J.J. & Edgerton, V.R. (1981) Training-induced alterations of the *in vivo* force–velocity relationship of human muscle. *Journal of Applied Physiology*, **51**, 750–4.

Cannon, R.J. & Cafarelli, E. (1987) Neuromuscular adaptations to training. *Journal of Applied Physiology*, **63**, 2396–402.

Close, R.I. (1972) Dynamic properties of mammalian skeletal muscles. *Physiological Reviews*, **52**, 129–97.

Coleman, E.A. (1969) Effect of unilateral isometric and isotonic contractions on the strength of the contralateral limb. *Research Quarterly*, **40**, 490–5.

Coyle, E.F., Feiring, D.C., Rotkis, T.C., Cote III, R.W. & Wilmore, J.H. (1981) Specificity of power improvements through slow and fast isokinetic training. *Journal of Applied Physiology*, **51**, 1437–42.

Davies, C.T., Dooley, P., McDonagh, M.J.N. & White, M. (1985) Adaptation of mechanical properties of muscle to high force training in man. *Journal of Physiology*, **365**, 277–84.

Davies, J., Parker, D.F., Rutherford, O.M. & Jones, D.A. (1988) Changes in strength and cross sectional area of the elbow flexors as a result of isometric strength training. *European Journal of Applied Physiology*, **57**, 667–70.

De Lorme, T.L. & Watkins, A.L. (1951) *Progressive Resistance Exercise*. Appleton Century Inc., New York.

deVries, H.A. (1968) Efficiency of electrical activity as a measure of the functional state of muscle tissue. *American Journal of Physical Medicine*, **47**, 10–22.

Eriksson, E., Häggmark, T., Kiessling, K.H. & Karlsson, J. (1981) Effect of electrical stimulation on human skeletal muscle. *Journal of Sports Medicine*, **2**, 18–22.

Faulkner, J.A., Claflin, D.R. & McCully, K.K. (1986) Power output of fast and slow fibers from human skeletal muscles. In N.L. Jones, N. McCartney & A.J. McComas (eds) *Human Muscle Power*, pp. 81–94. Human Kinetics, Champaign, Illinois.

Garnett, R.A.F., O'Donovan, M.J., Stephens, J.A. & Taylar, A. (1979) Motor unit organization of human medial gastrocnemius. *Journal of Physiology*, **287**, 33–43.

Häkkinen, K., Alen, M. & Komi, P.V. (1985) Changes in isometric force- and relaxation-time, electromyographic and muscle fiber characteristics of human muscle during strength training and detraining. *Acta Physiologica Scandinavica*, **125**, 573–85.

Häkkinen, K. & Komi, P.V. (1983) Electromyographic changes during strength training and detraining. *Medicine and Science in Sports and Exercise*, **15**, 455–60.

Häkkinen, K. & Komi, P.V. (1985) Effect of explosive type strength training on electromyographic and force production characteristics of leg extensor muscles during concentric and various stretch shortening cycle exercises. *Scandinavian Journal of Sports Science*, **7**, 65–76.

Häkkinen, K., Komi, P.V., Alen, M. & Kauhanen, H. (1987) EMG, muscle fiber and force production characteristics during 1 year training period in elite weight-lifters. *European Journal of Applied Physiology*, **56**, 419–27.

Häkkinen, K., Komi, P.V. & Tesch, P. (1981) Effect of combined concentric and eccentric strength training and detraining on force-time, muscle fiber and metabolic characteristics of leg extensor muscles. *Scandinavian Journal of Sports Science*, **3**, 50–8.

Henneman, E. & Mendell, L.M. (1981) Functional organization of motoneurone pool and its inputs. In V.B. Brooks (ed.) *Handbook of Physiology, Section 1, Vol. II*, pp. 423–507. American Physiological Society, Bethesda.

Houston, M.E., Froese, E.A., Valeriote, St. P. & Green, H.J. (1983) Muscle performance, morphology and metabolic capacity during strength training and detraining: A one leg model. *European Journal of Applied Physiology*, **51**, 25–35.

Ikai, M. & Fukunaga, T. (1970) A study on training effect on strength per unit cross-sectional area of muscle by means of ultrasonic measurements. *Internationale Zeitschrift fur Angewandte Physiologie*, **28**, 173–80.

Ishida, K., Moritani, T. & Itoh, K. (1990) Changes in voluntary and electrically induced contractions during strength training and detraining. *European Journal of Applied Physiology*, **60**, 244–8.

Jessop, J. & Lippold, O.C.J. (1977) Altered synchronization of motor unit firing as a mechanism for long-lasting increases in the tremor of human hand muscles following brief, strong effort. *Journal of Physiology*, **269**, 29P–30P.

Johnson, M.A., Polgar, J., Weightman, D. & Appleton, D. (1973) Data on the distribution of fiber types in thirty-six human muscles. An autopsy study. *Journal of Neurological Sciences*, **18**, 111–29.

Jones, D.A. & Rutherford, O.M. (1987) Human muscle strength training: The effects of three different regimes and the nature of the resultant changes. *Journal of Physiology*, **391**, 1–11.

Kaneko, M. (1970) The relationship between force, velocity and mechanical power in human muscle. *Research Journal of Physical Education* (Japan), **14**, 141–5.

Kaneko, M. (1974) *The Dynamics of Human Muscle* (In Japanese). Kyorinshoin, Book Company, Tokyo.

Kaneko, M., Fuchimoto, T., Toji, H. & Suei, K. (1983) Training effect of different loads on the force–velocity relationship and mechanical power output in human muscle. *Scandinavian Journal of Sports Sciences*, **5**, 50–5.

Komi, P.V. (1986) Training of muscle strength and power: Interaction of neuromotoric, hypertrophic and mechanical factors. *International Journal of Sports Medicine*, **7**, 10–15.

Komi, P.V. & Buskirk, E.R. (1970) Reproducibility of electromyographic measurements with inserted wire electrodes and surface electrodes. *Electromyography*, **4**, 357–67.

Komi, P.V. & Buskirk, E.R. (1972) Effect of eccentric and concentric muscle conditioning on tension and electrical activity of human muscle. *Ergonomics*, **15**, 417–34.

Komi, P.V., Viitasalo, J.T., Rauramaa, R. & Vihko, V. (1978) Effect of isometric strength training on mechanical, electrical and metabolic aspects of muscle function. *European Journal of Applied Physiology*, **40**, 45–55.

Kukulka, C.G. & Clamann, H.P. (1981) Comparison of the recruitment and discharge properties of motor units in human brachial biceps and adductor pollicis during isometric contractions. *Brain Research*, **219**, 45–55.

Lippold, O.C.J. (1952) The relation between integrated action potentials in a human muscle and its isometric tension. *Journal of Physiology*, **117**, 492–9.

McDonagh, M.J.N. & Davies, C.T.M. (1984) Adaptive response of mammalian skeletal muscle to exercise with high loads. *European Journal of Applied Physiology*, **52**, 139–55.

Milner-Brown, H.S. & Stein, R.B. (1975) The relation between the surface electromyogram and muscular force. *Journal of Physiology*, **246**, 549–69.

Milner-Brown, H.S., Stein, R.B. & Lee, R.G. (1975) Synchronization of human motor units: possible roles of exercise and supraspinal reflexes. *Electroencephalography and Clinical Neurophysiology*, **38**, 245–54.

Milner-Brown, H.S., Stein R.B. & Yemm, R. (1973) The orderly recruitment of human motor units during voluntary isometric contractions. *Journal of Physiology*, **230**, 359–70.

Moffroid, M.T. & Whipple, R.H. (1970) Specificity of speed of exercise. *Physical Therapy*, **50**, 1692–9.

Moritani, T. (1981) Training adaptations in the muscles of older men. In E.L. Smith & R.C. Serfass (eds) *Exercise and Aging: The Scientific Basis*, pp. 149–66. Enslow Publishers, New Jersey.

Moritani, T. & deVries, H.A. (1978) Reexamination of the relationship between the surface integrated electromyogram (IEMG) and force of isometric contraction. *American Journal of Physical Medicine*, **57**, 263–77.

Moritani, T. & deVries, H.A. (1979) Neural factors versus hypertrophy in the time course of muscle strength gain. *American Journal of Physical Medicine*, **58**, 115–30.

Moritani, T. & deVries H.A. (1980) Potential for gross muscle hypertrophy in older men. *Journal of Gerontology*, **35**, 672–82.

Moritani, T. & Muro (1987) Motor unit activity and surface electromyogram power spectrum during increasing force of contraction. *European Journal of Applied Physiology*, **56**, 260–5.

Moritani, T., Muro, M., Ishida, K. & Taguchi, S. (1987) Electromyographic analyses of the effects of muscle power training. *Journal of Medicine and Sports Sciences* (Japan), **1**, 23–32.

Moritani, T., Muro, M., Kijima, A. & Berry, M.J. (1986a) Intramuscular spike analysis during ramp force output and muscle fatigue. *Electromyography and Clinical Neurophysiology*, **26**, 147–60.

Moritani, T., Muro, M., Kijima, A., Gaffney, F.A. & Persons, D. (1985) Electromechanical changes during electrically induced and maximal voluntary contractions: Surface and intramuscular EMG responses during sustained maximal voluntary contraction. *Experimental Neurology*, **88**, 484–99.

Moritani, T., Muro, M. & Nagata, A. (1986b) Intramuscular and surface electromyogram changes during muscle fatigue. *Journal of Applied Physiology*, **60**, 1179–85.

Narici, M.V., Roi, G.S., Landoni, L., Minetti, A.E. & Cerretelli, P. (1989) Changes in force, cross-sectional area and neural activation during strength training and detraining of the human quadriceps. *European Journal of Applied Physiology*, **59**, 310–19.

Nowakowska, A. (1962) Influence of experimental training by electrical stimulation of skeletal muscle. *Acta Physiologica Polonica*, **12**, 32–8.

Rasch, P.J. & Morehouse, L.E. (1957) Effect of static and dynamic exercise on muscular strength and hypertrophy. *Journal of Applied Physiology*, **11**, 29–34.

Rodahl, K. & Horvath, S.M. (1962) *Muscle as a Tissue*. McGraw-Hill Book Company Inc., New York.

Romero, J.A., Sanford, T.L., Schroeder, R.V. & Fahey, T.D. (1982) The effects of electrical stimulation of normal quadriceps on strength and girth. *Medicine and Science in Sports and Exercise*, **14**, 194–7.

Rutherford, O.M. & Jones, D.A. (1986) The role of learning and coordination in strength training. *European Journal of Applied Physiology*, **55**, 100–5.

Sale, D.G. (1988) Neural adaptation to resistance training. *Medicine and Science in Sports and Exercise*, **20**, S135–S145.

Seyfert, S. & Kunkel, H. (1974) Analysis of muscular activity during voluntary contraction of different strengths. *Electromyography and Clinical Neurophysiology*, **14**, 323–30.

Stephens, J.A. & Usherwood, T.P. (1977) The mechanical properties of human motor units with special reference to their fatiguability and recruitment threshold. *Brain Research*, **125**, 91–7.

Tanji, J. & Kato, M. (1973) Firing rate of individual motor units in voluntary contraction of abductor digiti minimi in man. *Experimental Neurology*, **40**, 771–83.

Thorstensson, A., Grimby, G. & Karlsson, J. (1976a) Force–velocity relations and fiber composition in human knee extensor muscles. *Journal of Applied Physiology*, **40**, 12–16.

Thorstensson, A., Karlsson, J., Viitasalo, J.H.T., Luhtanen, P. & Komi, P.V. (1976b) Effect of strength training on EMG of human skeletal muscle. *Acta Physiologica Scandinavica*, **98**, 232–6.

Tihanyi, J., Apor, P. & Fekete, G.Y. (1982) Force–velocity–power characteristics and fiber composition in human knee extensor muscles. *European Journal of Applied Physiology*, **48**, 331–43.

Woods, J.J., Jones, D.A. & Bigland-Ritchie, B. (1978) Components of the surface EMG during stimulated and voluntary contractions. *Medicine and Science in Sports and Exercise*, **10**, 67.

Chapter 10

Connective Tissue and Bone Response to Strength Training

MICHAEL H. STONE

Introduction

Strength training is used extensively to enhance performance, prevent injuries, improve general fitness, increase muscle size, and in rehabilitation programmes (Stone & Wilson, 1985; Stone, 1990). Considering the uses of strength training and its effects on muscle it is reasonable to believe that strength training may have marked effects on connective tissue. However, objective data concerning the effects of strength training on connective tissue is scarce. Some information is available on the effects of endurance training or weighted exercise training on connective tissue and bone mineral incorporation. The potential effects of strength training on connective tissue can be inferred from these studies. Because connective tissue provides a basic framework and supportive structure, and force conveying network, an understanding of how exercise and training affects connective tissue is of major importance.

Anatomical and biochemical characteristics

Connective tissue is made up of collagen, elastin or reticular cells, and fibres. These cells and fibres are embedded in a ground substance containing tissue fluid and various metabolites. The ground substance contains relatively large amounts of aminopolysaccharides or glycoproteins giving it a gelatinous characteristic. Collagen is the major fibre in all types of con-

nective tissue comprising about 30% of total body protein (Van Pilsum, 1982; Viiduk, 1986).

Collagen molecules consist of three chains each in a left-handed helix of approximately 100 residues. These three chains are wound around each other in a right-handed helix with glycine residues at crossing points occurring at every third residue. The approximate formula is X-Y-Gly. Most of the amino acid residues are glycine (33%); hydroxyproline makes up about 15% and proline 12%. Collagen molecules form fibrils that are staggered in a parallel manner and range from 10–200 nm depending upon the type of collagen. Each molecule is displaced from adjacent molecules by 0, 1, 2, 3 or 4 axial stagger lengths of 234 ± 1 residues (Schultz, 1982). The staggered nature of collagen molecules results in banding with electron microscopy (Fig. 10.1).

The cyclic nature of the amino acid residues (X-Y-Gly) results in increased stability by limiting rotation. Additional amino acids may act as hydrophobically charged clusters and occupy the X or Y positions. Specific genes code for the basic structure of collagen chains (Shultz, 1982). At least five different types of collagen exist with different organ distribution (Table 10.1).

Additional stabilization can be achieved by post-translational crosslinking. Crosslinks are formed by the oxidation of lysyl side chains to aldehydes and eventual formation of aldol bridges between collagen fibrils (Viiduk, 1986). Crosslinking increases with age.

279

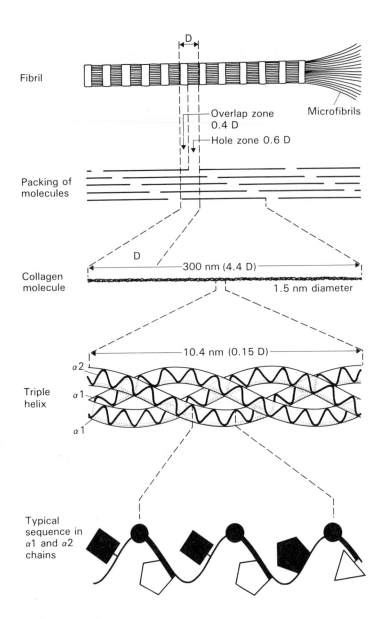

Fibril

Overlap zone
0.4 D

Hole zone 0.6 D

Microfibrils

Packing of
molecules

Collagen
molecule

D

300 nm (4.4 D)

1.5 nm diameter

Triple
helix

10.4 nm (0.15 D)

$\alpha 2$

$\alpha 1$

$\alpha 1$

Typical
sequence in
$\alpha 1$ and $\alpha 2$
chains

Fig. 10.1 Structure of collagen.

Mechanical properties of connective tissue

The development of stress–strain curves has been a valuable tool in studying the mechanical properties of connective tissue. The stress–strain curve can be developed from a load–deformation curve where load is expressed as units of cross-sectional area and deformation is expressed as units of original length (Viiduk, 1986). Typically, the point of failure (σ max) or the energy absorbed to the point of failure have been important variables in comparing tissue strength (Fig. 10.2).

Stress–strain curves can be either passive or active. For example, ligament or tendon strength can be examined passively by simple stretching to failure. Active stress–strain curves

Table 10.1 Collagen species

Type	Distribution	Form	Characteristics
1	Bone, tendon, skin, dentin, ligament, fascia, arteries, uterus	$[a1(I)]_2a2$	Hybrid composed of two chains low in hydroxylysine and glycosylated hydroxylysine
2	Cartilage	$[a1(II)]_3$	High in hydroxylysine, glycosylated hydroxylysine
3	Skin, arteries, uterus	$[a1(III)]_3$	High in hydroxylysine, low in hydroxylysine disulphide bonds
4	Basement membrane	$[a1(IV)]_3$	Large globular regions, high in hydroxylysine, glycosylated hydroxylysine
5	Basement membrane, lens capsule	aA and aB	Similar to IV

can be accomplished using muscle–tendon preparations where the muscle is electrically stimulated at the appropriate time (Garret *et al.*, 1987).

Effects of physical training on connective tissue

Large amounts of connective tissue exist around and within muscle including the epimysium, perimysium, and endomysium. Connective tissue also makes up tendons and ligaments. This connective tissue is responsible for either conveying force from the muscle to the bone-lever system or providing additional supportive strength, as occurs with ligaments.

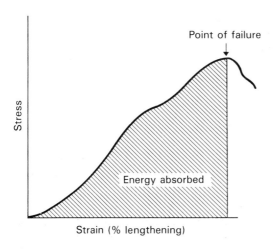

Fig. 10.2 Stress–strain curve for connective tissue.

Adaptations of connective tissue to exercise and training include a variety of morphological and biochemical changes.

Biochemical alterations

Exercise, particularly high force eccentric exercise, places considerable stress on muscle and on connective tissue. Prolonged endurance training (24-hour run) resulted in increased serum concentrations of enzymes associated with synthesis of type III collagen (Takala *et al.*, 1976). Eccentric exercise, which produces delayed muscle soreness, has been associated with increased serum concentrations of hydroxyproline (Abraham, 1977). Forced elongation of rat muscle caused considerable structural damage as well as an infiltration of lymphoid cells. Within 5 days proteoglycan localization was apparent suggesting regeneration of damaged connective tissue (Fritz & Stauber, 1988; Stauber *et al.*, 1988). These data suggest that exercise, especially strength training, may damage connective tissue as well as muscle and that tissue damage may be important in regeneration (see tissue injury below).

Training can also produce marked effects on connective tissue. Most of the training studies have been short-term endurance exercise protocols and have examined the effects of training on tendons and ligaments. Endurance training produced increased nuclei number and tendon weights in young mice but no change in tendon weight of adult mice (Ingelmark, 1948). Ligament weights have shown increases in male but not in female adult rats (Tipton *et al.*, 1975b). Endurance training can also increase the aerobic enzyme activity and rate of collagen synthesis in animal tendons (Tipton *et al.*, 1974). Eight weeks of endurance training increased the collagen content (46%) of immature rooster Achilles tendons, but did not affect DNA, dry tendon weight, or proteoglycan concentration (Curwin *et al.*, 1988). Additionally, fewer (50%) pyridinoline crosslinks were present in the trained tendons compared to controls. These results suggest that the training caused a greater matrix–collagen turnover in growing roosters resulting in reduced maturation of tendon collagen (Curwin *et al.*, 1988). Hydroxyproline is found as a constant fraction of collagen (Van Pilsum, 1982). Because hydroxyproline is found in few other tissues (elastin and complement), which are not associated with tendons or ligaments, its measurement may reflect changes in the collagen content of connective tissue (Viiduk, 1986). Hydroxyproline concentration was unchanged in the tendons of young mice (Kiiskinen & Heikkinen, 1976) or the ligaments of adult rats (Tipton *et al.*, 1970) but was increased in adult dogs (Tipton *et al.*, 1975a). Training-induced changes in hydroxyproline concentration should be viewed with caution. Apparent changes in hydroxyproline may be a result of actual hydroxyproline loss or gain within the connective tissue, or it could represent changes (loss or gain) in other tissue components. Therefore, changes in hydroxyproline concentration would represent changes in tissue state but not necessarily the nature of the change (Viiduk, 1986).

Compensatory hypertrophy models or chronic stretch do not reflect the same chronic adaptations as resistive training. Differential effects on connective tissue are possible because of differences in the exercise intensity between endurance training and compensatory hypertrophy models of training or chronic stretch. Muscle connective tissue sheaths (epimysium, perimysium, endomysium) are a primary component accounting for muscle tensile strength, the viscoelastic properties of muscle, and the framework for conveying muscle force to the tendons and bone (Fleck & Falkel, 1986). Endurance training did not increase total collagen content in these sheaths in adult rats (Kovanen, *et al.*, 1980, 1984). However, compensatory rat plantaris hypertrophy (Turto *et al.*, 1974) did show increased collagen content as did loading the intact chicken wing (Laurent *et al.*, 1978).

MacDougall *et al.* (1984) estimated the total collagen and other non-contractile protein content of biceps among untrained subjects and two groups of bodybuilders. The proportion of collagen was similar in untrained, novice and elite groups, with collagen representing 69% and 7% being identified as other tissue. This suggests a stable relative collagen content but an increased total collagen content as a result of bodybuilding. The increased total collagen content likely represents an increase in muscle sheath strength.

The possibility of a general systemic response of connective tissue is supported by several observations in both animals and humans. Hydroxyproline concentration increased in the skin of immature and adult mice as a result of endurance training (Kiiskinen & Heikkinen, 1976; Suominen *et al.*, 1978). Skin elasticity was observed to be enhanced following 8 weeks of physical training in 69-year-old men and women (Suominen *et al.*, 1977, 1978). Strength training has been shown to stimulate endomysial connective tissue in young men (Brzank & Peiper, 1986).

Mechanical alterations

While disuse and inactivity cause atrophy and weakening of connective tissue, physical training can increase maximum tensile strength and the amount of energy absorbed before failure (Stone, 1988). Physical activity returns damaged tendons and ligaments to normal tensile strength values faster than complete rest (Tipton *et al.* 1975b). Endurance training causes increased maximum tensile strength in isolated tendons, and in bone–tendon and bone–ligament preparations (Elliot & Crawford, 1965; Viiduk, 1968; Tipton *et al.*, 1974).

Care must be taken in interpreting much of the animal data on connective tissue strength. Trained animals are typically compared to untrained caged animals. Confinement may reduce connective tissue size and maximum tensile strength; therefore, training may simply return tissue properties to unconfined values (Butler *et al.*, 1978; Stone, 1988). Additionally, the strain rates used in these studies were below normal physiological rates, making generalizations back to intact unconfined animals difficult (Butler *et al.*, 1978).

The flexor muscles of most adult animals produce higher maximum force outputs than the extensor muscles (Elliot & Crawford, 1965). Flexor tendons of adult pigs have a greater maximum tensile strength and contain more collagen than tendons from extensor muscles, and can store more elastic energy (Woo *et al.*, 1982; Shadwick, 1990). Developmentally, this suggests that the forces encountered by these tendons at least partially influence the collagen content and maximum tensile strength at maturation. After physical training, extensor muscle tendons increased collagen content and stiffness, reaching values similar to the flexor tendons (Woo *et al.*, 1982). This suggests that strengthening of muscle may affect gains in connective tissue maximum tensile strength and elastic energy storage capabilities.

The stress placed on tendons as a result of voluntary muscle contraction has been estimated to be 30% of the maximum tensile strength (Hirsch, 1974). This leaves a 200% safety margin. During normal intact functioning in which both concentric and eccentric actions occur, about 50% of the safety margin is used (Alexander, 1981). The safety margin may be increased during fast rates of loading as a result of locking the viscous components of tissue (Noyes, 1977). The nature of tissue failure is also a function of strain rate (Noyes, 1977). At very slow strain rates, failure occurs at the junction of bone–tendon or bone–ligament. At faster strain rates,

failure occurs at the tendon or ligament. If the junction fails, the tendon or ligament is not being tested. When muscle–tendon preparations are being tested, failure occurs at the belly of the muscle or most often at the muscle–tendon junction, regardless of strain rates (Garret *et al.*, 1987; Safran *et al.*, 1988).

Connective tissue subjected to a constant stress elongates with time (stress-relaxation), resulting in a fall in tension below initial values (Laban, 1962). Similar phenomena occur in muscle–tendon preparations (Safran *et al.*, 1988). Warm-up afforded by isometric action prior to stretching (at physiological strain rates) elongated the muscle–tendon unit to a greater length and required more force at failure than muscles not warmed up (Safran *et al.*, 1988). The warm-up stretches the muscle–tendon unit resulting in an increased length at a given load; this places less tension on the muscle–tendon junction and reduces injury potential. Similar increases in stress relaxation have been shown to occur in rabbit tendons as a result of exercise (Viiduk, 1968). Essentially, the safety margin is increased by warm-up.

Muscle force may also be important in extending the safety margin before failure of the muscle–tendon junction. A greater force at failure and a greater absorbance of energy before failure of the muscle–tendon junction results from both tetanic and wave-summated muscle action in various rabbit muscle tendon preparations (Garret *et al.*, 1987). The authors suggest that stored elastic energy and the force of eccentric action were important factors in increasing the amount of energy absorbed prior to failure. It is possible that increased eccentric muscle action force resulting from strength training may further improve energy absorbance and reduce injury potential.

These data suggest that physical training, particularly strength training, may alter the properties of tendons and ligaments such that they are larger, stronger, and more resistant to injury. It should be noted that certain drugs commonly used in medicine or athletics may have profound effects on tendon and ligament strength. Corticosteroids are used to treat a variety of inflammatory problems such as tendinitis and bursitis. Corticosteroids are catabolic in nature and may cause atrophy, wasting, and weakening of connective tissue, especially if injected directly into a tendon or ligament. Tendon rupture may have occurred as a result of the use of these drugs (Chechick *et al.*, 1982). Anabolic steroids are used by strength/power athletes to enhance performance. Some evidence suggests that anabolic steroids change the biomechanics of connective tissue such that a tendon or ligament may have a decreased tensile strength, regardless of training (Wood *et al.*, 1988), thus increasing the injury potential.

Bone mineral density and bone mass

Bone acts as structural support and as a lever system in transferring muscle force into loco-motion and other physical activities. It is a storage depot for phosphorus and calcium. Bone is a plastic material, changing density, mass, and form according to stresses en-countered in development (Falch, 1982). Bone density and bone mass are related to the strength of the tissue.

Weightlessness and immobilization

Weightlessness (Vogel & Whittle, 1976) and immobilization (Hanson *et al.*, 1975) can cause profound loss of bone density and mass. Immobilization causes a marked increase in urinary calcium excretion, which reflects the loss of bone material (Falch, 1982). Low in-tensity exercise does not reduce the amount of urinary calcium lost in otherwise immobilized subjects. Standing at attention for 3 hours decreased urinary calcium loss but physical activity performed lying down or in a wheel-chair did not (Falch, 1982). These data suggest that the antigravity muscles must be activated to maintain or enhance bone density and mass. Fleck and Falkel (1986) suggest that resistive training may activate the antigravity muscles.

Significance of increased bone mass

An important consideration is whether or not physical training can enhance bone mineral density and strengthen bone tissue to greater levels than development alone. Stronger bones may be of benefit for several reasons. Stronger bones may protect against injury as a result of daily work tasks or athletic competition. The loss of bone tissue (osteoporosis) occurs with the ageing process; if bone density and maximum tensile strength can be enhanced before the osteoporotic process begins then complications can be minimized.

Fitness level

The level of athlete and type of physical activity may also influence bone density. Cross-sectional comparisons of physically active men and women generally suggest that a positive relationship exists between physical activity level and bone density and mass. Chow *et al.* (1986) and Pocock *et al.* (1986) have shown that bone density of the lumbar vertebra and femur are related to measures of fitness including maximum muscular strength and aerobic power ($\dot{V}O_{2max}$). Additionally, some evidence suggests that childhood physical activity may have a marked subsequent influence on adult bone density (McCulloch *et al.*, 1990). How-ever, not all training programmes necessarily produce the same result (Stone, 1988).

Several cross-sectional studies suggest that physical activity can affect increased bone mineral density (Helela, 1969; Dalen & Olsen, 1974; Chow *et al.*, 1986; Stillman *et al.*, 1986). It may be expected that the dominant limbs of athletes are subjected to higher stress and more total work than non-dominant limbs, and this may be reflected in differences in bone mineral incorporation and bone densities and mass. The humerus of the dominant arm in tennis players has been shown to have a greater mass (Jones *et al.*, 1977) and bone width and mineral content (Montoye *et al.*, 1980). Similar results have been reported for baseball players (Watson, 1974). Among various athletes the femur of the dominant leg also shows higher bone density than the non-dominant leg (Nilsson & Westlin, 1971).

Aerobic training

Cross-sectional studies of highly trained aerobic athletes have produced mixed results as to the effects of aerobic activities, particularly jogging, on bone density. Male long distance runners (>64 km per week) had similar tibial and radial bone densities, but significantly lower vertebral bone densities compared to sedentary or moderately (<64 km per week) trained runners (Bilanin et al., 1989). Young (13.1 years) male and female distance runners compared to untrained age-, height- and weight-matched controls (Rodgers et al., 1990), were shown to have significantly lower mid-ulnar length (15.9 vs. 17.0 cm), bone mineral density (0.67 vs. 0.76 g·cm^{-1}) and mineral/width (0.57 vs. 0.62 g · cm^{-2}). Bone mineral density was more affected in males than in females. Buchanan et al. (1988) studied 30 women aged 18 to 22 years. The groups examined were sedentary ($n = 11$), eumenorrhoeic athletes ($n = 10$), and amenorrhoeic/oligomenorrhoeic athletes ($n = 9$). None of the women trained with resistance training. No significant differences in lumbar spine densities were found between groups. However, the amenorrhoeic/oligomenorrhoeic group did have the lowest bone density. The authors concluded that hormone profile was an important factor in bone density status. Similar findings have been reported by Moen et al. (1990) for lumbar spine bone density among female distance runners (15–18 years). Bone density and bone mass may be adversely affected by amenorrhoea regardless of the volume, intensity or type of exercise (Olsen, 1989).

Longitudinal studies generally reflect the results of the cross-sectional studies. Non-resistive training programmes have shown increases toward normal bone density in degenerated bone (Goodship et al., 1979). Dalen and Olsen (1974) did not find that aerobic training affected bone mineral content in office workers over 3 months. Marguiles et al. (1986) examined the effects of military training on tibial bone density in 259 infantry recruits over 14 weeks. The average increase in bone density was 5.2% for the right leg and 11.1% for the left leg. However, 41% of the original 268 recruits did not complete the training course and the increase in bone density was related to the training time completed. Many of those not finishing dropped out because of stress fractures. Williams et al. (1984) found that male runners averaging 141 km per week had a greater bone density of the calcaneus compared to runners averaging 65 km or less per week.

Among postmenopausal women, aerobic dance was more effective in reducing bone loss over a 6-month period than was walking (White et al., 1984). Chow et al. (1987) divided 58 women into three groups: control ($n = 19$), aerobic dance ($n = 19$), and aerobic dance plus very low intensity strength training with hand-held weights ($n = 20$). After 1 year results suggest that bone density had increased in the combined exercise group, showed little change in the aerobic dance group, and showed a small reduction in the controls. This suggests that combined aerobic and strength exercise is more effective in remodelling bone. Differences in the effect of aerobic training on bone mineral density may be influenced by the degree of weight-bearing and the volume and intensity of training.

Strength training

Nilsson and Westlin (1971) examined the bone density of the lower limb in different athletic groups including nine international level athletes. Bone densities were greater in international athletes compared to lower level athletes who possessed greater bone densities than untrained controls. Additionally, it was shown that sports requiring repeated high force movements, such as weightlifting and throwing events, had higher bone densities than distance runners and soccer players. Swimmers (non-weight-bearing exercise) had the lowest bone densities (Nilsson & Westlin, 1971). Twelve males regularly engaged in resistance training for at least 1 year were compared to 50 age-matched controls (19–50 years). Resistance training was associated with increased bone mineral density (g · cm^{-2}) at the lumbar spine (1.35 vs. 1.22), trochanter (0.99 vs. 0.96) and femoral neck (1.18 vs. 1.02), but not at mid radius (0.77 vs. 0.77), suggesting that resistance training is associated with increased bone density at weight-bearing but not non-weight-bearing sites (Colletti *et al.*, 1989). Granhed *et al.* (1987) demonstrated that among eight power-lifters the calculated force applied at L3 (3rd lumbar) and the total load lifted during training over the previous year were related to the bone mineral content of the spine. Compressive forces on L3 ranged from 18 to 36.4 kN. The bone mineral content was highly correlated to training load ($r = 0.82$). Among junior (17.4 years) elite weightlifters, Conroy *et al.* (1990) demonstrated bone mineral density, compared to reference data (20–39 years), to be 113% (spine L2–4) and 134% (proximal femur neck) greater. Additionally, significant relationships were found between bone mineral density at the spine, femur neck, trochanter, and Ward's triangle and maximum lifting ability in the snatch, clean and jerk, and total (snatch plus clean and jerk).

Over a 5-month period, partner-assisted and body weight-resistive training in postmenopausal women caused a 3.8% increase in the distal radius, with the control group decreasing 1.9% (Simkin *et al.*, 1987). Twelve months of weight training produced a significant increase in lumbar bone density compared to controls in premenopausal women (Gleeson *et al.*, 1990). Although this weight training programme did not directly load the spine, exercises were performed that caused contraction in the muscles with direct attachments to the spine. Lane *et al.* (1988) compared aerobic training (jogging) with weight training over a 5-month period. When considering programme adherence, the weight training produced significantly better increases in lumbar bone density than the aerobic group. The importance of intensity of exercise and

weight-bearing was pointed out by Martin *et al.* (1981). Beagles were exercised on a treadmill at 3.3 k.p.h. for 75 min, 5 days per week for 71 weeks. The dogs wore weighted jackets, the weight of which was increased up to approximately 130% of the dogs body mass by week 23 and was held constant for the remaining 48 weeks. The rate of bone mineral incorporation in the tibia was enhanced compared to sedentary controls. Previous research with no weighted jackets showed no effect on bone density or rate of mineral incorporation (Martin *et al.*, 1981). Weight training, particularly with a weight-bearing component, can substantially alter bone mineral density.

Potential connective tissue enhancement mechanisms

Tissue injury

Exercise, especially exercise with a large eccentric action component, causes muscle damage (Ebbling & Clarkson, 1989). Very long-term running (24 hours) effected changes, likely to be injury to collagen synthesizing cells, resulting in elevated serum concentrations of galactosylhydroxylysyl glucosyltransferase (S-GGT) and serum type III procollagen amino-terminal propeptide (S-PRO(III)-N-P) (Takala *et al.*, 1976). Neither the change in concentration in S-GGT or S-PRO-(III)-N-P corresponded with changes in serum CPK (creatine phosphokinase) or LDH (lactate dehydrogenase). The S-GGT returned to normal after exercise but the S-PRO-(III)-N-P continued to increase (40%) after exercise. This would likely stimulate type III collagen synthesis.

High forces associated with eccentric actions cause considerable stress to the muscle and connective tissue. Products of collagen injury and damage as a result of exercise may act as chemotactic agents for monocytes to transfer from blood to muscle (Armstrong *et al.*, 1983). Upon entering an injured area monocytes transform into macrophages, which have a phagocytic function. The invading cells may be a consequence rather than a cause of damage and are acting to remove damaged cellular components (Jones *et al.*, 1986). The invading cells may have myogenic activity (Stauber *et al.*, 1988). Proteoglycans, components of connective tissue that are influenced by the muscle damage process, are important in regulating the myogenic process (Fritz & Stauber, 1988). Thus, connective tissue may have a regulatory as well as a structural role in the damage and repair process (Ebbling & Clarkson, 1989).

Growth promoting peptides may also play a role in connective tissue regeneration and growth. Mitogens that promote muscle regeneration after damage have been indentified (Bishoff, 1986). Other growth promoting molecules may exist that affect growth of connective tissue. Resistance training, having a high eccentric component and causing muscle damage, could promote the production of such mitogens.

Bone mineral incorporation stimulus

Remodelling is a function of stress and strain encountered by bone. The adaptation of bone is modified by various factors including nutritional, hormonal, and functional strain. It has been suggested that a 'minimum effective strain' exists, which is the lowest strain necessary to maintain balanced remodelling and to preserve bone at relatively constant values (Frost, 1986). However, magnitude is only one factor contributing to the functional strain that is a stimulus for bone remodelling. Three factors that modify bone are the magnitude of strain, the strain rate, and the distribution of the strain (Lanyon, 1987).

Small strains will not contribute to effective bone remodelling regardless of distribution (Lanyon, 1987). These factors may explain the relatively small changes in bone associated with aerobic training (low intensity of exercise). Additionally, amenorrhoeic women, with low oestrogen concentrations, performing aerobic training may experience two problems. First, the aerobic training may not be of sufficient intensity to adequately effect bone remodelling, and the low oestrogen concentrations may reduce calcium reabsorption.

Strength training may more adequately satisfy the criteria for bone remodelling. Furthermore, the strain rate may be particularly important in bone remodelling. Exercise designed to increase peak bone mass and density or prevent decreases, such as those occurring with age, should involve high strain rates, but need be of relatively short duration. Certain types of strength/power training such as Olympic style weightlifting training, which includes various fast movements as well as whole body exercises, may provide a high magnitude of strain, and varied strain distribution and high strain rates.

Hormonal influences

Exercise and training can cause marked changes in blood hormones (Terjung, 1980; Stone, 1990). Anabolic hormones including testosterone and growth hormone can increase as a result of exercise (including strength exercises) of appropriate intensity (Terjung, 1980; Stone, 1991). The testosterone/cortisol ratio may reflect the relative anabolic state (Häkkinen *et al.*, 1985). Appropriate resistance training may increase this ratio, which may induce increases in lean body mass, including connective tissue (Häkkinen *et al.*, 1985). Over-training may reduce this ratio as well as affect other hormones, e.g. oestrogen, which could adversely effect connective tissue growth and maintenance (Stone, 1990; Stone *et al.*, 1991). It is of interest that high volumes of endurance training have been associated with decreased bone density in men and women (Bilanin *et al.*, 1989; Michel *et al.*, 1989).

Testosterone, insulin, other hormones, minerals and vitamins directly related to bone mineral deposition may also be stimulated by resistance training. Males weight training for 1 year were found to have increased serum Gla protein and serum vitamin D concentrations, both markers of bone formation, compared to controls (Bell *et al.*, 1988). Hormone number and sensitivity may also affect connective tissue. Endocrine as well as autocrine and paracrine mechanisms may also be active in connective tissue metabolism.

Summary

Evidence suggests that physical activity can modify connective tissue. It appears that to most effectively stimulate connective tissue growth: (i) the intensity of the exercises used must be high; (ii) antigravity muscles should be active, especially for axial bone remodelling; and (iii) load-bearing activities may be most effective in stimulating bone formation. Furthermore, overtraining may adversely affect connective tissue growth.

Acknowledgement

The author is indebted and grateful to Travis Triplett and Brian Conroy for their assistance in preparing this manuscript.

References

Abraham, W.M. (1977) Factors in delayed muscle soreness. *Medicine and Science in Sports*, **9**, 11–20.

Alexander, R.Mc. (1981) Factors of safety in the structure of animals. *Scientific Progress*, **67**, 109–30.

Armstrong, R.B., Ogilvie, R.W. & Schwane, J.A. (1983) Eccentric exercise-induced injury to rat skeletal muscle. *Journal of Applied Physiology*, **54**, 80–93.

Bell, N.H., Godsen, R.N., Henry, D.P., Shary, J. & Epstein, S. (1988) The effects of muscle-building exercise on vitamin D and mineral metabolism. *Medicine and Science in Sports and Exercise*, **20**, S215.

Bilanin, J.O., Blanchard, M.S. & Russek-Cohen, E. (1989) Lower vertebral bone density in male long distance runners. *Medicine and Science in Sports and Exercise*, **21**, 66–70.

Bishoff, R. (1986) A satellite cell mitogen from crushed adult muscle. *Developmental Biology*, **15**, 140–7.

Brzank, K.D. & Peiper, K.S. (1986) Effect of intensive strength building exercise training on the fine structure of human skeletal muscle capillaries. *Anatomischer Anzeiger*, **161**, 243–8.

Buchanan, J.R., Myers, C., Lloyd, T., Leuenberger, P. & Demers, L.M. (1988) Determinants of trabecular bone density in women: The role of androgens, estrogens and exercise. *Journal of Bone and Mineral Research*, **3**, 673–80.

Butler, D.L., Grood, E.S., Noyes, F.R. & Zernicke, R.F. (1978) Biomechanics of ligaments and tendons. *Exercise and Sports Sciences Reviews*, **6**, 125–81.

Chechick, A., Amit, Y., Israeli, A. & Horozowski, H. (1982) Recurrent rupture of the achilles tendon induced by corticosteroid injection. *British Journal of Sports Medicine*, **16**, 89–90.

Chow, R.K., Harrison, J.E., Brown, C.F. & Hajek, V. (1986) Physical fitness effect on bone mass in postmenopausal women. *Archives of Physical Medicine and Rehabilitation*, **67**, 231–4.

Colletti, L.A., Edwards, J., Gordon, L., Shary, J. & Bell, N.H. (1989) The effects of muscle building exercise on bone mineral density of the radius, spine, and hip in young men. *Calcified Tissue International*, **45**, 12–14.

Conroy, B.P., Kraemer, W.J., Dalsky, G.P., Miller, P.D., Fleck, S.J., Kearney, J.T., Stone, M.H., Warren, B. & Maresh, C.M. (1990) Bone mineral density in elite junior weightlifters. *Medicine and Science in Sports and Exercise*, **22**, S77.

Curwin, S.L., Vailas, A.C. & Wood, J. (1988) Immature tendon adaptation to strenuous exercise. *Journal of Applied Physiology*, **65**, 2297–301.

Dalen, N. & Olsen, K.E. (1974) Bone mineral content and physical activity. *Acta Orthopaedica Scandinavica*, **45**, 170–4.

Ebbling, C.B. & Clarkson, P.M. (1989) Exercise-induced muscle damage and adaptation. *Sports Science*, **7**, 207–34.

Elliot, D.H. & Crawford, G.N.C. (1965) The thickness and collagen content of tendon relative to strength and cross-sectional area of muscle. *Proceedings of the Royal Society of London B*, **162**, 137–46.

Falch, J.A. (1982) The effects of physical activity on the skeleton. *Scandinavian Journal of Social Medicine*, (suppl. 29), 55–8.

Fleck, S.J. & Falkel, J.E. (1986) Value of resistance training for the reduction of sports injuries. *Sports Medicine*, **3**, 61–8.

Fritz, V.K. & Stauber, W.T. (1988) Characterization of muscles injured by forced lengthening. II. Proteoglycans. *Medicine and Science in Sports and Exercise*, **20**, 354–61.

Frost, H.M. (1986) *The Intermediate Organization of the Skeleton*. CRC Press, Boca Raton.

Garret, W.E., Safran, M.R., Seaber, A.V., Glisson, R.R. & Ribbeck, B.M. (1987) Biomechanical comparison of stimulated and nonstimulated skeletal muscle pulled to failure. *American Journal of Sports Medicine*, **15**, 448–54.

Gleeson, P.G., Protas, E.J., Leblanc, A.D., Schneider, V.S. & Eveans, H.J. (1990) Effects of weight lifting on bone mineral density in premenopausal women. *Journal of Bone and Mineral Research*, **5**, 153–8.

Goodship, A.E., Lanyon, L.E. & McFie, H. (1979) Functional adaptations of bone to increased stress. *Journal of Bone and Joint Surgery*, **61A**, 539–46.

Granhed, H., Jonson, R. & Hansson, T. (1987) The

loads on the spine during extreme weightlifting. *Spine*, **12**, 146–9.

Häkkinen, K., Pakarinen, A., Markku, A. & Komi, P.V. (1985) Serum hormones during prolonged training of neuromuscular performance. *European Journal of Applied Physiology*, **53**, 287–93.

Hanson, T.H., Roos, B.O. & Nachemson, A. (1975) Development of osteopenia in the fourth lumbar vertebrae during prolonged bedrest after operation for scoliosis. *Acta Orthopaedica Scandinavica*, **46**, 621–30.

Helela, T. (1969) Variations of thickness of cortical bone in two populations. *Annals of Clinical Research*, **1**, 227–31.

Hirsch, G. (1974) Tensile properties during tendon healing. *Acta Orthopaedica Scandinavica* (suppl. 153).

Ingelmark, B.E. (1948) Der Bau der sehnen wahrend verschiederaltersperioden und unter wechselendes funktionellen bedigngungen. I. *Acta Anatomica*, **6**, 113–40.

Jones, D.A., Newham, D.J., Round, J.M. & Tolfree, S.E.J. (1986) Experimental human muscle damage: Morphological changes in relation to other indices of damage. *Journal of Physiology*, **375**, 435–48.

Jones, H.H., Priest, J.D., Hayes, W.C., Tichnor, C.C. & Nagel D.A. (1977) Humeral hypertrophy in response to exercise. *Journal of Bone and Joint Surgery*, **59**A, 204–8.

Kiiskinen, A. & Heikkinen, H. (1976) Physical training and connective tissue in young mice. *British Journal of Dermatology*, **95**, 525–9.

Kovanen, V., Suominen, H. & Heikkenen, E. (1980) Connective tissue of fast and slow skeletal muscle in rats—effects of endurance training. *Acta Physiologica Scandinavica*, **108**, 173–80.

Kovanen, V., Suominen, H. & Heikkenen, E. (1984) Collagen of fast twitch and slow twitch muscle fibers in different types of rat skeletal muscle. *European Journal of Applied Physiology*, **52**, 235–42.

Laban, M.M. (1962) Collagen tissue: Implications of its response to stress *in vitro*. *Archives of Physical Medicine and Rehabilitation*, **43**, 461–6.

Lane, N., Bevier, W., Bouxsein, M., Wiswell, R., Careter, D. & Marcus, R. (1988) Effect of exercise intensity on bone mineral. *Medicine and Science in Sports and Exercise*, **20**, S51.

Lanyon, L.E. (1987) Functional strain in bone tissue as an objective and contolling stimulus for adaptive bone remodeling. *Journal of Biomechanics*, **2**, 1083–93.

Laurent, G.J., Sparrow, M.P., Bates, P.C. & Millward, D.J. (1978) Collagen content and turnover in cardiac and skeletal muscles of the adult fowl and the changes during stretch induced growth. *Biochemistry Journal*, **176**, 419–27.

McCulloch, R.G., Baily, D.A., Houston, C.S. & Dodd, B.L. (1990) Effects of physical activity, dietary calcium intake, and selected lifestyle factors on bone density in young women. *Canadian Medical Association Journal*, **142**, 221–32.

MacDougall, J.D., Sale, D.G., Alway, S.E. & Sutton, J.R. (1984) Muscle fibre number in biceps brachii in body builders and control subjects. *Journal of Applied Physiology*, **57**, 1399–403.

Margulies, J.K., Simkin, A., Leichtor, I., Bivas, A., Steinberg, R., Stein, M., Kashtan, H. & Milgrom, C. (1986) Effects of intense physical activity on the bone mineral content in the lower limbs of young adults. *Journal of Bone and Joint Surgery*, **68A**, 1090–3.

Martin, R.K., Albright, J.P., Clark, W.R. & Niffnegger, J.A. (1981) Load-carrying effects on the adult beagle tibia. *Medicine and Science in Sports and Exercise*, **13**, 343–9.

Michel, B.A., Bloch, D.A. & Fries, J.F. (1989) Weight-bearing exercise, overexercise, and lumbar bone density over age 50 years. *Archives of Internal Medicine*, **149**, 2325–9.

Moen, S., Sanborn, C., Bonnick, S., Keizer, H., Dimarco, N., Ben-Ezra, V. & Gench, B. (1990) Lumbar bone density in female distance runners. *Medicine and Science in Sports and Exercise*, **22**, S77.

Montoye, H.J., Smith, E.L., Fardon, D.F. & Howley, E.T. (1980) Bone mineral in senior tennis players. *Scandinavian Journal of Sports Science*, **2**, 26–32.

Nilsson, B.E. & Westlin, N.E. (1971) Bone density in athletes. *Clinical Orthopaedics*, **77**, 179–82.

Noyes, F.R. (1977) Functional properties of knee ligaments and alterations induced by immobilization: A correlative biomechanical and histological study in primates. *Clinical Orthopaedics*, **123**, 210–42.

Olsen, B.R. (1989) Exercise induced amenorrhea. *American Family Physician*, **39**, 213–21.

Pocock, N.A., Eisman, J.A., Yeates, M.G., Sambrook, F.N. & Eberl, S. (1986) Physical fitness is a major determinant of femoral neck and lumber spine bone mineral density. *Journal of Clinical Investigation*, **78**, 618–21.

Rodgers, C.D., Vanheest, J.L., Nowak, J.L., Van Huss, W.D., Heusner, W.W. & Seefeldt, V.D. (1990) Bone mineral content in young endurance-trained male and female runners. *Medicine and Science in Sports and Exercise*, **22**, 576.

Safran, M.R., Garret, W.E., Seaber, A.V., Glisson, R.R. & Ribbeck, B.M. (1988) The role of warmup in muscular injury prevention. *American Journal of Sports Medicine*, **16**, 123–9.

Shadwick, R.E. (1990) Elastic energy storage in tendons: Mechanical differences related to function and age. *Journal of Applied Physiology*, **68**, 1033–40.

Shultz, R.M. (1982) Proteins II. In T.M. Devlin (ed.)

Biochemistry with Clinical Correlations, pp. 124–32. John Wiley & Sons, New York.

Simkin, A., Ayalon, J. & Leichter, I. (1987) Increased trabecular bone density due to bone loading exercises in postmenopausal women. *Calcified Tissue International*, **40**, 59–63.

Stauber, W.T., Fritz, B.K., Vogelbach, D.W. & Dahlmann, B. (1988) Characterization of muscles injured by forced lengthening. I. Cellular infiltrates. *Medicine and Science in Sports and Exercise*, **20**, 345–53.

Stillman, R.J., Lohman, T.G., Slaughter, M.H. & Massey, B.H. (1986) Physical activity and bone mineral incorporation content in women aged 30 to 85 years. *Medicine and Science in Sports and Exercise*, **18**, 576–80.

Stone M.H. (1988) Implications for connective tissue and bone alterations resulting from resistance exercise training. *Medicine and Science in Sports and Exercise*, **20**, S162–S168.

Stone, M.H. (1990) Muscle conditioning and muscle injuries. *Medicine and Science in Sports and Exercise*, **22**, 457–62.

Stone M.H., Keith, R.E., Kearney, J.T., Fleck, S.J., Wilson, G.D. & Triplett, N.T. (1991) Overtraining: a review of the signs, symptoms and possible causes. *Journal of Applied Sports Science Research*, **5** (1), 35–50.

Stone, M.H. & Wilson, G.D. (1985) Selected physiological effects of weight-training. *Medical Clinics of North America*, **69** (1), 109–22.

Suominen, H., Heikkinen, E., Moiso, H. & Viljama, K. (1978) Physical and chemical properties of skin in habitual trained and sedentary 31 to 70 year old men. *British Journal of Dermatology*, **99**, 147–54.

Suominen, W.T., Heikkinen, E. & Parkatti, T. (1977) Effect of eight weeks physical training on muscle and connective tissue of the m. vastus lateralis in 69-year old men and women. *Journal of Gerontology*, **32**, 33–7.

Takala, T.E., Vuori, J., Antinen, H., Vaanen, K. & Myllyla, R. (1976) Prolonged exercise causes an increase in the activity of galactosyl hydroxylysyl glucosyltransferase and in the concentration of type III procollagen amino propeptide in human serum. *Pflügers Archiv*, **407**, 500–3.

Terjung, R. (1980) Endocrine response to exercise. *Exercise and Sport Science Reviews*, **7**, 153–80.

Tipton, C.M., James, S.L., Merger, J.W. & Tcheng, T.K. (1970) Influence of exercise on strength of medial collateral knee ligaments of dogs. *American Journal of Physiology*, **218**, 894–902.

Tipton, C.M., Martin, R.K., Matthes, R.D. & Carey, R.A. (1975a) Hydroxyproline concentrations in ligaments from trained and non-trained dogs. In H. Howald & J.R. Purtmans (eds) *Metabolic Adaptations to Prolonged Physical Training*, pp. 262–7. Birkhauser Verlag, Basel.

Tipton, C.M., Matthes, R.D., Maynard, J.A. & Carey, R.A. (1975b) The influence of physical activity on ligaments and tendons. *Medicine and Science in Sports*, **7**, 165–75.

Tipton, C.M., Matthes, R.D. & Sandage, D.S. (1974) *In situ* measurements of junction strength and ligament elongation in rats. *Journal of Applied Physiology*, **37**, 758–62.

Turto, H., Lindy, S. & Holme, J. (1974) Protocollagen proline hydroxylase activity in work-induced hypertrophy of rat muscle. *American Journal of Physiology*, **226**, 63–5.

Van Pilsum, J.F. (1982) Metabolism of individual tissues. In T.M. Devlin (ed.) *Biochemistry with Clinical Correlations*, pp. 1050–2. John Wiley & Sons, New York.

Viiduk, A. (1968) Elasticity and tensile strength of the anterior cruciate ligament in rabbits as influenced by training. *Acta Physiologica Scandinavica*, **74**, 372–80.

Viiduk, A. (1986) Adaptability of connective tissue. In B. Saltin (ed.) *Biochemistry of Exercise VI*, pp. 545–62. Academic Press, London.

Vogel, J.M. & Whittle, M.W. (1976) Bone mineral content changes in the skylab astronauts. *American Journal of Roentgenology*, **126**, 1296.

Watson, R.C. (1974) Bone growth and physical activity in young males. International Conference on Bone Mineral Measurements, US Department of Health, Education, and Welfare, Publication NIH 75-683, pp. 380–5.

White, M.K., Martin, R.B., Yeater, R.A., Butcher, R.L. & Radin, E.L. (1984) The effects of exercise on postmenopausal women. *International Orthopedics*, **7**, 209–14.

Williams, J.A., Wagner, J., Wasnich, R. & Heilburn, L. (1984) The effects of long distance running upon appendicular bone mineral content. *Medicine and Science in Sports and Exercise*, **16**, 223–7.

Woo, S.L.Y., Gomex, M.A., Woo, Y.K. & Akeson, W.H. (1982) Mechanical properties of tendons and ligaments. II. The relationship between immobilization and exercise on tissue remodeling. *Biorheology*, **19**, 397–408.

Wood, T.O., Cooke, P.H. & Goodship, A.E. (1988) The effect of exercise and anabolic steroids on the mechanical properties and crimp morphology of the rat tendon. *American Journal of Sports Medicine*, **16**, 153–8.

Chapter 11

Endocrine Responses and Adaptations to Strength Training

WILLIAM J. KRAEMER

Strength and power training presents a potent exercise stimulus to the musculoskeletal system. This type of exercise stress activates a wide variety of physiological mechanisms involved with the activation of muscle and chronic adaptations to training. One of the physiological systems that has been shown to be responsive to acute heavy resistance exercise is the neuroendocrine system (Kraemer, 1988). Furthermore, chronic training adaptations in the endocrine system have been related to improved force production (Häkkinen, 1989).

Hormonal increases in response to resistance exercise take place in a physiological environment that is quite unique to this type of exercise stress. Significant amounts of force are produced by the muscle cell membrane due to the heavy external loads being lifted. Additionally, tissue repair mechanisms are activated as a part of the recovery and remodelling process after each exercise session. This appears to be especially true when eccentric actions are utilized in the exercise session (Clarkson & Tremblay, 1988). Thus, such tissue conditions consequent to strength exercise may provide suitable sites of interaction for various hormonal increases that are observed during and following resistance exercise. A variety of hormonal mechanisms (see Chapter 4) could theoretically influence the growth and remodelling process of various body tissues (e.g. muscle, bone and other connective tissue) over the course of a strength training programme.

The exercise stimulus in resistance exercise is made up of a combination of variables that have been previously described in detail (Fleck & Kraemer, 1987; Kraemer et al., 1988; Kraemer & Fleck, 1988; Kraemer & Baechle, 1989). In general, the exercise choice dictates the mode of muscle action, the musculature used, and other biomechanical aspects of each exercise. The order of exercise influences the metabolic demands and the fatigue state of the muscle prior to the start of an exercise. The load utilized for the exercise defines the motor unit recruitment patterns, the metabolic demands, and the velocity of movement. The number of sets helps to determine the volume (sets × repetitions × load) of strength exercise. And finally, the length of the rest periods between sets and exercises affects the metabolic demands, load utilized, and recovery status of the muscle.

Each of these five programme variables interact to define an acute exercise stimulus for a strength exercise protocol. Therefore, the neuroendocrine responses and adaptations would be linked to the configuration of the specific resistance exercise stimulus, e.g. choice of exercise, order of exercise, load, etc. Many different protocols are possible when dealing with the various combination of acute programme variables. The magnitude of the hormonal response will be related to the specific configuration of the chosen exercise protocol, e.g. short rest.

It is interesting to note that programme variation (e.g. periodization methods that change the exercise stimulus configuration over time) has been shown to be very effective in eliciting superior strength/power performance gains (Stowers *et al.*, 1983; Stone & O'Bryant, 1987; O'Bryant *et al.*, 1988). Using different exercise protocols results in different hormonal responses and such differences probably influences the adaptational mechanisms during a strength training programme (Kraemer, 1988). Figure 11.1 is a schematic sequence of events that would involve neuroendocrine mechanisms in resistance training.

The mechanisms of hormonal interaction with muscle tissue (Chapter 4) are based on several factors. First, when exercise acutely increases the blood concentrations of hormones, regardless of mechanism, a greater probability of interaction with receptors is possible. Second, since adaptations to heavy resistance exercise are 'anabolic' in nature, the recovery mechanisms involved are related to tissue remodelling and repair. Third, mistakes in exercise prescriptions can result in a greater catabolic effect (e.g. overtraining) or an exercise programme that is ineffective. Accordingly, hormonal mechanisms will either adversely affect tissue development or minimally activate

mechanisms that augment the adaptational changes initiated by the neural recruitment and the force production demands of high intensity strength exercise. The gestalt of such mechanisms is what is thought to stimulate the phenomenon of exercise-induced hypertrophy and subsequent increases in muscular strength and power. The various hormonal mechanisms probably respond differentially in trained and untrained individuals (Häkkinen, 1989). In addition, certain hormonal mechanisms may not be fully operational (e.g. testosterone) in both males and females. It now appears that a wide array of hormonal mechanisms with differential effects based on programme design, strength/power fitness level, gender, genetic predisposition, and adaptational potential appear to provide a myriad of possible adaptation strategies needed for the maintenance or improvement of muscle size, strength, and power (Kraemer, 1988; Häkkinen, 1989).

A number of physiological mechanisms may contribute in varying degrees to the increases in peripheral blood concentrations of hormones. These include shifts in fluid volumes, changes in extrahepatic clearance rates, changes in

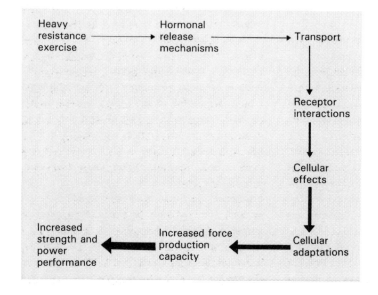

Fig. 11.1 Schematic flow chart of events involving the neuroendocrine system from the heavy resistance exercise stimulus to increased strength performance.

hepatic clearance rates secondary to hepatic blood flow, hormonal degradation, venous pooling of blood, and receptor interactions. All of these mechanisms interact with secretion rates and receptor-binding turnover. Thus, gradient changes in concentration in the various localized biocompartments appear a plausible way in which receptor interactions can be enhanced in response to strength exercise without dramatic changes in hormonal secretory rates.

It should be remembered that hormonal secretions respond to homeostatic alterations to bring a physiological function back into 'normal' or functional ranges (Galbo, 1983). Thus, changes in hormonal release can reflect the state of adaptational response. These homeostatic mechanisms of the neuro-endocrine system can be activated in response to an acute resistance exercise stress or be altered after a chronic period of resistance training (Kraemer, 1988). The mechanisms that mediate such acute homeostatic changes typically respond with a sharp increase or decrease in hormonal concentrations in response to acute strength exercise stress in order to regulate a physiological variable. Conversely, a more subtle increase or decrease usually occurs in the chronic resting hormonal concentrations in response to resistance training and helps to mediate the homeostatic regulation of various physiological adaptations. The neuroendocrine adaptations can be expressed at a number of levels within the various biocompartments and these are shown Fig. 11.2. This could include adaptations in synthesis and storage, transport mechanisms, hepatic and extrahepatic clearance rates, degradation, fluid shifts, receptor affinity and maximal binding, cellular effector changes (e.g. activation of tyrosine kinases) and in nuclear binding sites.

Testosterone

Increases in peripheral blood concentrations of total testosterone have been observed during and following many types of high intensity exercise (Galbo, 1983; Stone et al., 1984). The possible actions of testosterone in anabolic actions have been previously reviewed (Chapter 4). It appears that its role in augmentation of other hormonal mechanisms in growth promoting actions may be of primary interest. Since testosterone increases have been observed after even endurance exercise, variations in its action may be due to differences in the cellular environment consequent to strength exercise.

In males, several factors appear to influence the acute serum concentrations of total testosterone and may play a role in determining if significant serum increases are observed during or following exercise. Several basic exercise and experimental factors can influence the responses of serum testosterone concentrations.
1 The use of large muscle group exercises (e.g. deadlift, leg press) with heavy resistance (85–95% 1 RM), and a moderate to high volume of exercise achieved with multiple sets or multiple exercises.
2 The time course of blood sampling around an exercise protocol is also very important as it provides a physiological window to view the effects of strength exercise stress. Due to the intermittent nature of resistance exercise, samples are typically obtained immediately following the exercise stress. In the case of evaluating longer recovery periods, e.g. hours, care has to be observed so diurnal variations are controlled, e.g. windowed into time of day.
3 The pre-exercise concentrations will ultimately affect the acute exercise responsivity of a hormone to strength exercise stress and determine the magnitude of change. It is important that specific windows are utilized with the day, training phase and/or during the menstrual cycle.

Increases in serum total testosterone appear to occur when blood is sampled before and immediately after exercise protocols that utilize large muscle group exercise, e.g. deadlift vs. bench press (Fahey et al., 1976; Guezennec et al., 1986). When blood is sampled over a longer

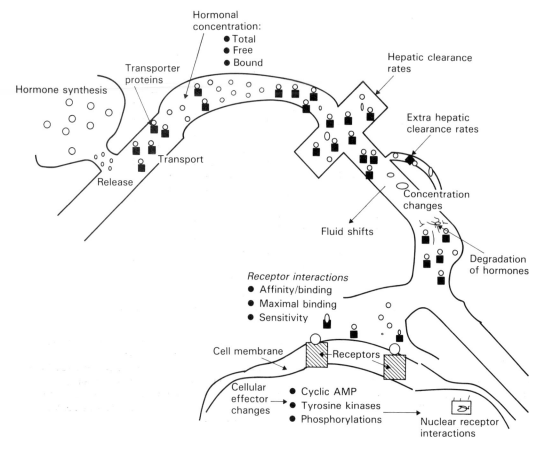

Fig. 11.2 Factors that can theoretically reflect training-related adaptations in the neuroendocrine system.

duration (e.g. >4 hours) and not immediately surrounding the exercise stress, other factors, e.g. diurnal variations or recovery phenomena, can affect the magnitude or direction of the acute stress response. This can make interpretations difficult when trying to evaluate the acute exercise changes. Possible rebounds or decreases in testosterone blood values over time may reflect augmentation or depression of diurnal variations (Kraemer *et al.*, 1990).

Various acute postexercise responses of serum total testosterone concentrations to various resistance exercise protocols are presented in Fig. 11.3. A wide variety of exercise protocols has been shown to elicit changes in response to acute exercise stress. The lack of

changes can typically be attributed to one of the previously discussed factors.

Fahey *et al.* (1976) were unable to demonstrate significant increases in high-school-aged males in serum concentrations of total testosterone. A recent report by Fry *et al.* (1990) suggests that increases may occur if the strength training experience of the high-school-aged males, i.e. 14–18 years, is 2 years or more. This initial report supports the possibility that resistance exercise training may alter physiological release and/or concentrating mechanisms of the hypothalamic–pituitary–testicular axis in younger males. Only recently have more advanced resistance exercise training programmes in younger children become acceptable in

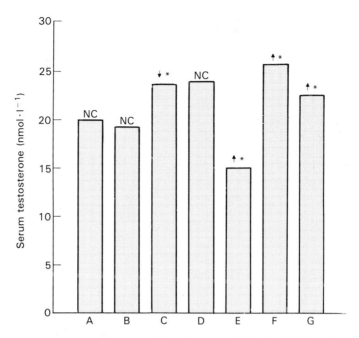

Fig. 11.3 Testosterone responses to various strength exercise protocols. *, $P < 0.05$ from the corresponding resting or pre-exercise value; ↑ or ↓ signify direction of change; NC, no change from rest. A, 1 set of bench presses, maximal number at 70% 1 RM (1 repetition maximum) (Guezennec *et al.*, 1986); B, 6 sets of 8 repetitions of bench press-ups at 70% 1 RM (Guezennec *et al.*, 1986; C, full Olympic exercise workout (second day) (Häkkinen *et al.*, 1988a); D, full Olympic exercise workout (first day) (Häkkinen *et al.*, 1988a); E, 3 sets of four exercises at 80% 1 RM (Weiss *et al.*, 1983); F, 5 sets of deadlifts at 5 RM—unskilled participants (Fahey *et al.*, 1976); G, 5 sets of deadlifts at 5 RM—skilled participants (Fahey *et al.*, 1976).

both the scientific and medical communities (Kraemer *et al.*, 1989). The consistent use of a wide range of advanced protocols may influence the responses of testosterone in younger males. Exactly how this is related to pubertal growth and development remains to be studied.

Scant data are available concerning the acute exercise responses of free testosterone. Primarily from the work of Häkkinen and co-workers (1987a,b, 1988a,b), they have observed that free testosterone remains unaltered or decreases after resistance exercise training sessions. The 'free hormone hypothesis' supports the idea that only the free hormone is transported into the target tissues. Still, the validity of such a hypothesis has not been established and it appears that the 'bound' hormone could sig-

nificantly influence the rate of hormone delivery and thus have a great deal of physiological significance (Ekins, 1990). The role, regulation, and interaction of binding proteins with the ligand and binding protein–ligand complex with the receptor presents even more intriguing complex possibilities. In fact, the binding protein may act as hormone itself and have a biological activity (Rosner, 1990). The biological role of various binding proteins appears to be an important factor with tissue interactions (Hammond, 1990; Rosner 1990). This importance has again been reflected in studies by Häkkinen and co-workers (1987a,b, 1988a,b). Their observations have demonstrated that changes in sex hormone-binding globulin (SHBG) and SHBG/testosterone ratios are correlated to isometric leg strength and have reflected the patterns of force production improvements in leg musculature.

Training adaptations

Comparing subjects with little strength exercise training experience and subjects who had at least 2 years experience, Fahey *et al.* (1976) were unable to demonstrate any significant differences in serum testosterone concentrations before or after an exercise protocol consisting of 5 sets of 5 repetition maximum (RM) deadlifts. This suggested that the hypothalamic–pituitary–testicular axis appears similarly responsive after maturation in adult males. Conversely, Häkkinen *et al.* (1988b) have demonstrated that over the course of 2 years of training in elite weightlifters, increases in resting serum testosterone concentrations do occur. This was concomitant to increases in follicle stimulating hormone (FSH) and luteinizing hormone (LH). While the testosterone changes showed remarkable similarities to the patterns of strength changes, the SHBG/testosterone ratio mirrored strength changes even more closely. It is interesting to hypothesize that in athletes where little adaptive potential exists for changes in muscle hypertrophy, i.e. highly trained strength athletes, changes in testosterone cybernetics may be a part of a more advanced adaptive strategy to increase force production capabilities of muscle. This may occur via potentiation of other hormonal mechanisms in tissue development or by the enhancement of neural factors (Florini, 1985, 1987). Such differences in adaptational strategies appear essential to provide for further gains in performance over the course of a long-term training programme. This may reflect the interplay of different neural and hypertrophic factors involved in mediating strength and power changes as training time is extended into years (Sale, 1988).

Growth hormone

Growth hormone (GH) has been found to be

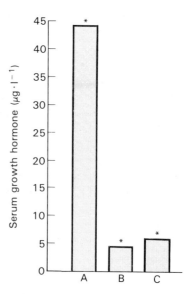

Fig. 11.4 Post exercise serum growth hormone responses following various exercise protocols. *, $P <$ 0.05 from the corresponding pre-exercise values. A, Olympic lifting workout at 70–85% 1 RM (Lukaszewska *et al.*, 1976); B, 7 sets of 7 at 85% 7 RM (Van Helder *et al.*, 1984); C, Olympic lifting training session (first day) at 70–100% 1 RM (Häkkinen *et al.*, 1988c).

responsive to a variety of exercise stressors including resistance exercise (Galbo, 1983; Kraemer, 1988). It has been shown that GH increases in response to breath holding and hyperventilation alone (Djarouva *et al.*, 1986) in addition to hypoxia (Sutton, 1977). Similar stimulatory mechanisms may be operational to varying extents during resistance exercise. Increases in GH in response to resistance exercise are shown in Fig. 11.4. It is important to note that not all strength exercise protocols demonstrate increases in serum GH concentrations. In an investigation by Van Helder *et al.* (1984) they observed that when a light load (28% of 7 RM) was utilized with a high number of repetitions in each set, no changes were observed in the serum concentrations of GH. This suggests that in resistance exercise a threshold exists for intensity (i.e. load) to elicit a significant stimulatory response of the hypothalamic–pituitary axis in response to resistance exercise. It further underscores the concept that there are various types of resistance exercise protocols that do not alter the peripheral concentrations of GH. Resistance loads utilized can span a wide continuum and operationally define the resistance exercise protocols. Thus, it may be characterized as a very light, e.g. 15 RM, to a very heavy, e.g. >10 RM, resistance exercise protocol. Typically, heavy resistance exercise protocols utilize loads ranging from 1 to 10 RM (Fleck & Kraemer, 1987). Loads that are lighter while increases in strength are observed, are typically directed toward improving local muscular endurance

rather than maximal strength and power (Atha, 1981; Fleck & Kraemer, 1987). In more advanced strength training programmes periodization techniques are used that vary the loads and the volume (sets × repetitions × loads) of exercise over the course of training (Fleck & Kraemer, 1987; Stone & O'Bryant, 1987). Therefore, it appears that depending upon load and volume of exercise differential GH responses occur.

In a study by Kraemer et al. (1990) it was demonstrated that GH increases are differentially sensitive to various strength exercise protocols (see Fig. 11.5). When the intensity utilized was 10 RM, high total work (approx.

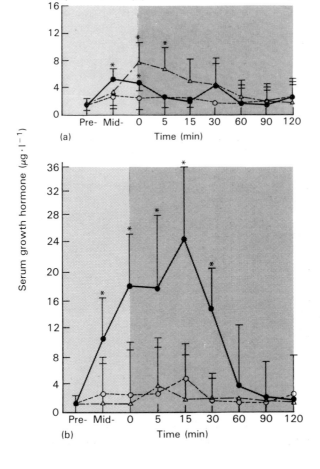

Fig. 11.5 Serum growth hormone responses to various strength exercise protocols. All exercise sessions consisted of eight identically ordered resistance exercises, which exercised each of the main muscle groups of the body. (a) Series 1 (lower total work) was a 5-repetition maximum (RM) based workout of 3–5 sets per exercise; this made up the primary workout (●). Total work for the load control (5–10 RM) (○) and the rest control (3 min reduced to 1 min) (△) was identical to the primary workout. (b) Series 2 (higher total work, same exercises and order): the primary workout was 3 sets of 10 RM for the eight identical exercises (●). Again, total work for the load control (10–5 RM) (○) and the rest control (1 min increased to 3 min) (△) were identical. *, $P < 0.05$ from corresponding resting value. (Adapted from Kraemer et al., 1990.)

60 000 J), and when the length of the rest periods used were short (1 min), significant increases were observed in serum concentrations of GH. The most dramatic increases were demonstrated in response to a decrease in rest period length (1 min) when the duration of exercise was longer (10 RM vs. 5 RM). With such differences being related to the exercise configuration (e.g. rest period length) of the exercise session, it appears greater attention needs to be given to programme design variables when evaluating physiological adaptations to strength training. Future studies will need to explore the use of various exercise protocols and various combinations to determine where muscle tissue hypertrophy and strength/power adaptations are optimized for individuals of different training levels.

Training adaptations

The changes in GH with training have not been extensively studied but observations of normal resting levels of GH in elite lifters suggests that alterations in resting levels are not a plausible mechanism of chronic adaptation (Häkkinen et al., 1988a,b). This is consistent with the dynamic feedback mechanisms GH is involved with and its roles in the homeostatic control of various dynamic variables, e.g. glucose. It is more likely that differences in feedback mechanisms, changes in receptor sensitivities, insulin-like growth factor potentiation, diurnal variations, and/or maximal exercise concentrations may mediate and be representative of GH alterations with resistance training.

Insulin-like growth factors (somatomedins)

Scant data are available concerning the acute responses of insulin-like growth factors (IGF) to exercise. Variable responses in serum concentrations of IGF-I have been observed consequent to endurance exercise (Jahreis et al., 1989; Suikkari et al., 1989). Again, Kraemer et al. (1990) have shown that almost all resistance

exercise protocols show temporal increases in IGF-I, i.e. somatomedin C, at some point during or following strength exercise protocols (see Fig. 11.6). Systematic alterations in circulatory responses of IGF to various types of exercise protocols appear to be closely related to regulatory factors of IGF release and transport (Blum et al., 1989). As discussed in Chapter 4, transport protein binding of IGF, with release when receptors become available, probably contributes to a more complex regulation of serum IGF concentrations. Evaluation of serum changes over longer periods may be necessary to evaluate specific effects and relationships to GH in the serum (Florini et al., 1985).

Training adaptations

Responses of IGF-I to strength training remain unknown. Similar to GH, training-induced adaptations in IGF will probably be reflected in a variety of release, transport, and receptor interaction changes. Such adaptations remain to be examined in response to exercise training and more specifically strength exercise.

Adrenal hormones

Because of the catabolic role attributed to cortisol, a significant interest in its potential as a whole body marker of tissue breakdown or catabolism has been observed. Furthermore, the testosterone/cortisol ratio (T/C) has been used in the attempt to mark anabolic/catabolic status of the body (Häkkinen et al., 1985). While such markers are attractive conceptually, the use of serum cortisol and the T/C ratio has only met with limited success in predicting or monitoring changes in strength/power capabilities. Still, the important role of cortisol in catabolic actions in muscle tissue in vivo and its subsequent effects on muscle force production cannot be ignored. The use of cortisol as an overt marker of such catabolic actions in healthy individuals remains somewhat elusive and requires further study in its application.

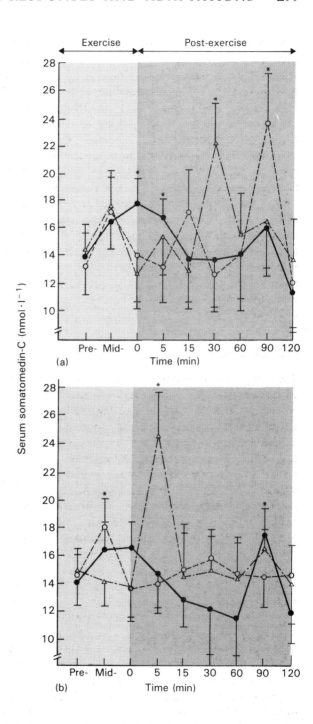

Fig. 11.6 Serum somatomedin-C (IGF-I) responses to various strength exercise protocols. Exercise parameters are described in Fig. 11.5. *, $P < 0.05$ from corresponding resting value. (From Kraemer *et al.*, 1990.)

Application problems are probably associated with a multiplicity of roles for cortisol and other hormones. It is interesting to note that acute resistance exercise stress that produces in-creases in anabolic hormones concomitantly stimulates increase in cortisol too (Skierska *et al.*, 1976; Kraemer *et al.*, 1987, 1990, 1991). This acute cortisol response may reflect a combination of factors including the metabolic intensity of the exercise stress and the need to maintain glucose availability (Galbo, 1983). In addition, the changes in glucocorticoid binding in tissue that is structurally disrupted in response to heavy resistance exercise may result. It is very probable that vast differences are observed in the physiological role of cortisol in acute versus chronic exercise responses to resistance exercise. Acutely, cortisol may reflect the metabolic stress of the exercise and in chronic aspects be primarily involved with tissue homeostasis involving protein metabolism (Florini, 1987). Thus, its role in overtraining, detraining or injury may be critical, as muscle tissue atrophy as well as decreases in force production capabilities are observed (MacDougall, 1986).

Catecholamines appear to reflect the acute demands and physical stress of the strength exercise protocol (Kraemer et al., 1987; Maresh et al., 1989). A high intensity, short rest (i.e. 10 s to 60 s between sets and exercises) heavy resistance exercise routine (10 exercises, 3 sets, 10 RM) typically utilized by bodybuilders for development of strength and hypertrophy maintained plasma noradrenaline, adrenaline, and dopamine increases for 5 min into recovery (Kraemer et al., 1987). Such data demonstrates how different configurations of an exercise stimulus can produce dramatic physiological stress of which only highly trained individuals can perform or tolerate.

Training adaptations

High-intensity endurance training has been shown to increase the ability of an individual to secrete greater amounts of adrenaline during maximal exercise (Kjaer & Galbo, 1988). How strength training affects catecholamine responses to exercise remains unclear. Investigations have shown acute increases in catecholamines and it has been suggested that training reduces adrenaline responses to a single bench press exercise protocol (Guezennec et al., 1986). Since the role of catecholamines,

more specifically adrenaline, is involved with metabolic control and force production, in addition to helping to potentiate other hormonal response mechanisms (e.g. testosterone, IGF), stimulation of the sympatho-adrenal secretion is probably one of the first neuro-endocrine mechanisms to become operational in response to resistance exercise. These roles reflect the classic stress response of the adrenal medulla and provide important signal cues to a myriad of endocrine feedback loops (Carmichael, 1986).

Other hormones

While insulin, thyroid hormones, and other hypopituitary hormones (e.g. β-endorphin) have all been implicated in growth, repair, and exercise stress mechanisms, few data are available concerning their responses and adaptations to resistance exercise or training. Due to the relatively tight homeostatic control surrounding both insulin and thyroid hormone secretion, alterations in circulating resting concentrations of these hormones due to chronic training adaptations would not be expected. It is more likely that changes in sensitivity of the receptors and binding interactions would be affected. As demonstrated by Pakarinen et al. (1988), only slight non-significant decreases were observed in serum concentrations of total and free T_4 after 20 weeks of strength training. The permissive effects of such hormones in metabolic control, amino acid synthesis, and augmentation of other hormonal release mechanisms are the essence of such interactions with strength training.

Additionally, few data are available concerning the responses of β-endorphin or other endogenous opioid peptides to resistance exercise. One study has demonstrated that increases in peripheral plasma concentrations of β-endorphin are possible (Elliot et al., 1984). In a study by Borer et al. (1986), using a golden hamster animal model, their data also suggest that endogenous opioid peptides may be in some way involved with exercise-induced increases in muscle cell hypertrophy. Still, a direct mechanism has not been elucidated. Several possibilities exist involving interactions and potentiation of other hormones in the hypothalamic–pituitary axis. Influences at receptor sites of GH and IGF are also attractive hypotheses for mechanisms of action but such roles have not yet been demonstrated. Still, it is interesting to speculate that endogenous opioid peptides may be involved with mechanisms that allow the performance of strenuous training sessions as well as with the adaptations and recovery process from heavy resistance exercise.

Hormonal responses of females to strength exercise

For the most part, the majority of data examining hormonal responses to resistance exercise and training have utilized male subjects. The testosterone hormonal response patterns during growth and development, i.e. maturation, have been classically credited as being responsible for differences in muscular development and strength in males and females. The higher secretion of adrenal androgens in some females has possibly accounted for the individual variations observed when examining resting concentrations, acute exercise, and chronic exercise responses. To date, the majority of studies have shown that females typically do not demonstrate an exercise-induced increase in testosterone consequent to various forms of strength exercise (Fahey et al., 1976; Hetrick & Wilmore, 1979; Weiss et al., 1983; Kraemer et al., 1991). This may vary with individual females when high adrenal androgen release is possible. In one report, changes have been seen in baseline levels of testosterone compared to inactive controls (Cumming et al., 1987). Still, other studies have been unable to demonstrate changes in serum concentrations of testosterone with training (Westerlind et al., 1987). Recently, Häkkinen et al. (1990) have shown that total and free testosterone changes during strength training were correlated with

muscle force production characteristics but no significant increases were observed.

How menstrual phases affect hormonal responses to resistance exercise and training remain unclear. It has been shown that menstrual phase does alter certain hormone concentrations and exercise responses (DeSouza et al., 1989). Kraemer et al. (1991) found that females during the early follicular phase of the menstrual cycle had significantly higher GH concentrations at rest compared to males. Furthermore, when using a heavy resistance exercise protocol that was characterized by longer rest (3 min) and heavy loads (5 RM), GH levels were not increased above the resting concentrations. Conversely, when a short rest (1 min) and moderate resistance (10 RM) exercise protocol was used significant increases in serum GH levels were observed. This suggests that hormonal response patterns to different resistance exercise routines may not be similar over the course of the menstrual cycle due to possible alterations in resting levels (Kraemer et al., 1991). The possibility of periodizing strength training over the course of the menstrual cycle remains to be examined. More research is needed to elucidate any gender-related neuroendocrine adaptational mechanisms. At present, the reduced levels of testosterone and differential resting hormonal levels over the course of the menstrual cycle appear to be the most striking neuroendocrine differences between males and females. How such differences are related to the training adaptations and to the development of muscle tissue and expression of strength and power remains to be demonstrated.

Summary

It is quite evident that hormonal mechanisms are responsive to strength exercise and training (Kraemer, 1988). The specific neuroendocrine mechanisms that mediate physiological adaptations in the development of muscle tissue and subsequent improvement in force production characteristics, i.e. strength and power, remain unclear. It is evident that the intact animal's muscle fibre benefits from the homeostatic and regulatory mechanisms of the neuroendocrine system. Neuroendocrine mechanisms appear to be intimately involved with both the acute exercise response and chronic training adaptations. A greater physiological understanding of muscle hypertrophy and subsequent strength and power performances may well be elucidated by studies that examine the molecular biology of various neuroendocrine mechanisms.

References

Atha, J., (1981) Strengthening muscle. *Exercise and Sport Sciences Reviews*, **17**, 1–73.

Blum, W.F., Jenne, E.W., Reppin, F., Kietzmann, K., Ranke, M.B. & Bierich, J.R. (1989) Insulin-like growth factor I (IGF-I)-binding protein complex is a better mitogen than free IGF-I. *Endocrinology*, **125**, 766–72.

Borer, K.T., Nicoski, D.R. & Owens, V. (1986) Alteration of pulsatile growth hormone secretion by growth-inducing exercise: Involvement of endogenous opiates and somatostatin. *Endocrinology*, **118**, 844–50.

Carmichael, S.W. (1986) *The Adrenal Medulla, Vol. 4.* Cambridge University Press, Cambridge.

Clarkson, P. & Tremblay, I. (1988) Exercise-induced muscle damage, repair, and adaptation in humans. *Journal of Applied Physiology*, **65**, 1–6.

Cumming, D.C., Wall, S.R., Galbraith, M.A. & Belcastro, A.N. (1987) Reproductive hormone responses to resistance exercise. *Medicine and Science in Sports and Exercise*, **19**, 234–8.

DeSouza, M.J., Maresh, C.M., MaGuire, M.S., Kraemer, W.J., Flora-Ginter, G. & Goetz, K.L. (1989) Menstrual status and plasma vasopressin, renin activity, and aldosterone exercise responses. *Journal of Applied Physiology*, **67**, 736–43.

Djarova, T., Ilkov, A., Varbanova, A., Nikiforova, A. & Mateev, G. (1986) Human growth hormone, cortisol, and acid–base balance changes after hyperventilation and breath-holding. *International Journal of Sports Medicine*, **7**, 311–15.

Ekins, R. (1990) Measurement of free hormones in blood. *Endocrine Reviews*, **11**, 5–45.

Elliot, D., Goldberg, L., & Watts W. (1984) Resistance exercise and plasma beta-endorphin/beta-lipotrophin immunoreactivity. *Life Sciences*, **35**, 515–18.

Fahey, T.D., Rolph, R., Moungmee, P., Nagel, J. & Mortar, S. (1976) Serum testosterone, body composition, and strength of young adults. *Medicine and Science in Sports*, **8**, 31–4.

Fleck, S.J. & Kraemer, W.J. (1987) *Designing Resistance Training Programs*. Human Kinetics, Champaign, Illinois.

Florini, J.R. (1985) Hormonal control of muscle cell growth. *Journal of Animal Science*, **61**, 21–37.

Florini, J.R. (1987) Hormonal control of muscle growth. *Muscle and Nerve*, **10**, 577–98.

Florini, J.R., Prinz, P.N., Vitiello, M.V. & Hintz, R.L. (1985) Somatomedin-C levels in health young and old men: relationship of peak and 24 hour integrated levels of growth hormone. *Journal of Gerontology*, **40**, 2–7.

Fry, A.C., Kraemer, W.J., Stone, M.H., Fleck, S.J., Warren, B., Conroy, B.P., Weseman, C.A. & Gordon, S.E. (1990) Acute endocrine responses in elite junior weightlifters (Abstract). *Medicine and Science in Sports and Exercise*, **22** (suppl.), 54.

Galbo, H. (1983) *Hormonal and Metabolic Adaptation to Exercise*. Georg Thieme Verlag, Stuttgart.

Guezennec, Y., Leger, L., Lhoste, F., Aymonod, M. & Pesquies, P.C. (1986) Hormone and metabolite response to weight-lifting training sessions. *International Journal of Sports Medicine*, **7**, 100–5.

Häkkinen, K. (1989) Neuromuscular and hormonal adaptations during strength and power training. *Journal of Sports Medicine and Physical Fitness*, **29**, 9–24.

Häkkinen, K., Komi, P.V., Alén, M. & Kauhanen, H. (1987a) EMG, muscle fibre and force production characteristics during a one year training period in elite weightlifters. *European Journal of Applied Physiology*, **56**, 419–27.

Häkkinen, K., Pakarinen, A., Alén, M., Kauhanen, H. & Komi, P.V. (1987b) Relationships between training volume, physical performance capacity, and serum hormone concentrations during prolonged training in elite weight lifters. *International Journal of Sports Medicine*, **8**, 61–5.

Häkkinen, K., Pakarinen A., Alén, M., Kauhanen, H. & Komi, P.V. (1988a) Daily hormonal and neuromuscular responses to intense strength training in one week. *International Journal of Sports Medicine*, **9**, 422–8.

Häkkinen, K., Pakarinen, A., Alén, M., Kauhanen, H. & Komi, P.V. (1988b) Neuromuscular and hormonal adaptations in athletes to strength training in two years. *Journal of Applied Physiology*, **65**, 2406–12.

Häkkinen, K., Pakarinen, A., Alén, M., Kauhanen, H. & Komi, P.V. (1988c) Neuromuscular and hormonal responses in elite athletes to two successive strength training sessions. *European Journal of Applied Physiology*, **57**, 133–9.

Häkkinen, K., Pakarinen, A., Alén, M. & Komi, P.V.

(1985) Serum hormones during prolonged training of neuromuscular performance. *European Journal of Applied Physiology*, **53**, 287–93.

Häkkinen, K., Pakarinen, A., Kyrolainen, H., Cheng, S., Kim, D.H. & Komi, P.V. (1990) Neuromuscular adaptations and serum hormones in females during prolonged power training. *International Journal of Sports Medicine*, **11**, 91–8.

Hammond, G.L. (1990) Molecular properties of corticosteroid binding globulin and the sex-steroid binding proteins. *Endocrine Reviews*, **11**, 65–79.

Hetrick, G.A. & Wilmore, J.H. (1979) Androgen levels and muscle hypertrophy during an eight-week training program for men/women (Abstract). *Medicine and Science in Sports*, **11**, 102.

Jahreis, G., Hesse, V., Schmidt, H.E. & Scheibe, J. (1989) Effect of endurance exercise on somatomedin-C/insulin-like growth factor I concentration in male and female runners. *Experimental and Clinical Endocrinology*, **94**, 89–96.

Kjaer, M. & Galbo, H. (1988) Effect of physical training on the capacity to secrete epinephrine. *Journal of Applied Physiology*, **64**, 11–16.

Kraemer, W.J. (1988) Endocrine responses to resistance exercise. *Medicine and Science in Sports and Exercise*, **20** (suppl.), S152–S157.

Kraemer, W.J. & Baechle, T.R. (1989) Development of a strength training program. In A.J. Ryan & F.L. Allman (eds) *Sports Medicine*, 2nd edn, pp. 113–27. Academic Press, San Diego.

Kraemer, W.J., Deschenes, M.R. & Fleck, S.J. (1988) Physiological adaptations to resistance exercise implications for athletic conditioning. *Sports Medicine*, **6**, 246–56.

Kraemer, W.J. & Fleck, S.J. (1988) Resistance training: exercise prescription. *Physician in Sportsmedicine*, **16**, 69–81.

Kraemer, W.J., Fry, A.C., Frykman, P.N., Conroy, B. & Hoffman, J. (1989) Resistance training and youth. *Pediatric Exercise Science*, **1**, 336–50.

Kraemer, W.J., Gordon, S.E., Fleck, S.J., Marchitelli, L.J., Mello, R., Dziados, J.E., Friedl, K. & Harman, E. (1991) Endogenous anabolic hormonal and growth factor responses to heavy resistance exercise in males and females. *International Journal of Sports Medicine*, **12**, 228–35.

Kraemer, W.J., Marchitelli, L., McCurry, D., Mello, R., Dziados, J.E., Harman, E., Frykman, P., Gordon, S.E. & Fleck, S.J. (1990) Hormonal and growth factor responses to heavy resistance exercise. *Journal of Applied Physiology*, **69**, 1442–50.

Kraemer, W.J., Noble, B.J., Clark, M.J. & Culver, B.W. (1987) Physiologic responses to heavy-resistance exercise with very short rest periods. *International Journal of Sports Medicine*, **8**, 247–52.

Lukaszewska, J., Biczowa, B., Bobilewixz, D., Wilk, M. & Bouchowixz-Fidelus, B. (1976) Effect of physical exercise on plasma cortisol and growth hormone levels in young weight lifters. *Endokrynologia Polska*, **2**, 149–58.

MacDougall, J. (1986) Morphological changes in human skeletal muscle following strength training and immobilization. In N.L. Jones, N. McCartney & A.J. McComas (eds) *Human Muscle Power*, pp. 269–84. Human Kinetics, Champaign, Illinois.

Maresh, C.M., Kraemer, W.J., Fleck, S.J., Goetz, K.L., Harman, E., Frykman, P.N. & Falkel, J. (1989) Effects of heavy resistance exercise on hemodynamic, stress hormone and fluid regulatory factors. *Medicine and Science in Sports and Exercise*, **21** (suppl.), 37.

O'Bryant, H.S., Byrd, R. & Stone, M.H. (1988) Cycle ergometer performance and maximum leg and hip strength adaptations to two different methods of weight training. *Journal of Applied Sport Science Research*, **2**, 27–30.

Pakarinen, A., Alén, M., Häkkinen, K. & Komi, P. (1988) Serum thyroid hormones, thyrotropin and thyroxine binding globulin during prolonged strength training. *European Journal of Applied Physiology*, **57**, 394–8.

Rosener, W. (1990) The functions of corticosteroid-binding globulin and sex hormone-binding globulin: recent advances. *Endocrine Reviews*, **11**, 81–91.

Sale, D.G. (1988) Neural adaptation to resistance training. *Medicine and Science in Sports and Exercise*, **20**, 135–45.

Skierska, E., Ustupska, J., Biczowa, B. & Lukaszewska, J. (1976) Effect of physical exercise on plasma cortisol, testosterone and growth hormone levels in weight lifters. *Endokrynologia Polska*, **2**, 159–65.

Stone, M.H., Byrd, R. & Johnson, C. (1984) Observations on serum androgen response to short term resistive training in middle age sedentary males. *National Strength and Conditioning Association Journal*, **5**, 40–65.

Stone, M. & O'Bryant, H. (1987) *Weight Training*. Bellwater Press, Minneapolis.

Stowers, T., McMillian, J., Scala, D., Davis, V., Wilson, D. & Stone, M. (1983) The short-term effects of three different strength-power training methods. *National Strength and Conditioning Association Journal*, **5**, 24–7.

Suikkari, A.-M., Koivisto, V.A., Koistinen, R., Seppala, M. & Yki-Jarvinen, H. (1989) Prolonged exercise increases serum insulin-like growth factor-binding protein concentrations. *Journal of Clinical Endocrinology and Metabolism*, **68**, 141–4.

Sutton, J.R. (1977) Effect of acute hypoxia on the hormonal response to exercise. *Journal of Applied Physiology: Respiratory, Environmental and Exercise Physiology*, **39**, 587–92.

Van Helder, W.P., Radomski, M.W. & Goode, R.C. (1984) Growth hormone responses during intermittent weight lifting exercise in men. *European Journal of Applied Physiology*, **53**, 31–4.

Weiss, L.W., Cureton, K.J. & Thompson, F.N. (1983) Comparison of serum testosterone and androsterenione responses to weight lifting in men and women. *European Journal of Applied Physiology*, **50**, 413–19.

Westerlind, K.C., Byrnes, W.C., Freedson, P.S. & Katch, F.I. (1987) Exercise and serum androgens in women. *Physician and Sportsmedicine*, **15**, 87–94.

Chapter 12

Cardiovascular Response to Strength Training

STEVEN J. FLECK

There is a paucity of information concerning the cardiovascular responses and adaptations to strength training. Conclusions concerning these cardiovascular responses are further complicated by several factors, paramount of which is the effect the volume and intensity of training has upon the physiological response and long-term adaptations to strength training. This chapter focuses upon the cardiovascular adaptations at rest and during exercise due to chronic long-term resistance training and the acute response to strength training exercise.

Chronic adaptations at rest (Table 12.1)

Decreased resting heart rate and blood pressure and changes in the blood lipid profile are positive adaptations to training. Changes in cardiac morphology, stroke volume and cardiac output at rest are of interest because they may indicate normal or abnormal cardiac function. In addition, some of these variables are indicators of cardiovascular risk. The effect strength training has upon all of these variables has been investigated to varying degrees using cross-sectional and longitudinal study designs.

Heart rate

Highly strength-trained athletes have average (Fleck, 1988) or lower than average resting heart rates (Stone *et al.*, 1991). Short-term longi-

tudinal studies report significant decreases of from 5 to 12% (Fleck, 1988; Haennel *et al.*, 1989; Stone *et al.*, 1991) and non-significant decreases in resting heart rate (Fleck, 1988; Haennel *et al.*, 1989; Blumenthal *et al.*, 1990; Stone *et al.*, 1991). Although in some studies resting heart rate decreased non-significantly, it is important to note it did decrease. Decreased resting heart rate is normally attributed to a combination of increased parasympathetic and diminished sympathetic tone (Frick *et al.*, 1967; Blomqvist & Saltin, 1983).

Blood pressure

The majority of reports show highly strength-trained athletes to have average or lower than average systolic and diastolic blood pressures (Fleck, 1988; Fleck *et al.*, 1989b; Goldberg, 1989; Stone *et al.*, 1990). In addition, short-term (6–20 weeks) longitudinal studies on males show no change or decreases in systolic and diastolic resting blood pressures (Fleck, 1988; Goldberg, 1989; Stone *et al.*, 1991). Despite this evidence it is a common misconception that strength training causes hypertension. The most likely explanations of hypertension when observed in highly strength-trained athletes are essential hypertension, chronic overtraining, use of androgens or large gains of muscle mass (Stone *et al.*, 1991). Possible explanations for decreased resting blood pressure, when it does occur due to strength training, include decreased body fat, decreased body salt and alterations of the

305

Table 12.1 Adaptations at rest

Heart rate	↓ or no change
Blood pressure	
Systolic	↓ or no change
Diastolic	↓ or no change
Double product	↓ or no change
Stroke volume (absolute)	↑ or no change
Relative to BSA	No change
Relative to LBM	No change
Cardiac systolic function	↑ or no change
Cardiac diastolic function	No change (↑ ?)
Lipid profile	
Total cholesterol	↓ or no change
HDL-C	↑ or no change
LDL-C	↓ or no change

BSA, body surface area; HDL-C, high-density lipoprotein cholesterol; LBM, lean body mass; LDL-C, low-density lipoprotein cholesterol.

sympathoadrenal drive (Fleck, 1988; Goldberg, 1989; Stone et al., 1991).

Double product

The double product (heart rate × systolic blood pressure) is an estimate of myocardial work and is proportional to myocardial oxygen consumption. The resting double product of college-aged males has been shown to decrease in several longitudinal strength training studies (Stone et al., 1991). This indicates a decrease in myocardial oxygen consumption at rest as an adaptation to strength training.

Stroke volume

Changes in absolute resting stroke volume (echocardiographic techniques) of highly strength-trained males are equivocal, with normal and greater than normal values being reported (Fleck, 1988; Effron, 1989). Relative to body surface area or lean body mass differences between athletes and controls are non-existent (Fleck, 1988; Effron, 1989). Increased absolute stroke volume when present is due to a significantly greater diastolic left ventricular diameter and a normal ejection fraction (Fleck, 1988). A short-term longitudinal study also shows absolute stroke volume to be unchanged in a group of weight trainers (Lusiani et al., 1986).

Lipid profile

The effect of strength training on the blood lipid profile is controversial. Male strength-trained athletes have been reported to have normal, higher and lower than normal HDL-C (high-density lipoprotein cholesterol) levels, LDL-C (low-density lipoprotein cholesterol) levels, total cholesterol levels and total cholesterol to HDL-C ratios (Kraemer et al., 1988; Hurley, 1989; Stone et al., 1991). Two reports of the lipid profile of female strength-trained athletes also yield controversial results (Elliot et al., 1987; Morgan et al., 1986). Body-builders do appear to have lipid profiles similar to runners and power-lifters have lower HDL-C and higher LDL-C values than runners when body fat, age and androgen use (which depresses HDL-C levels) are controlled for (Hurley et al., 1984, 1987).

Results of longitudinal training studies are also inconclusive, with reductions in LDL-C levels, reductions in total cholesterol, increases in HDL-C and no significant changes in these measures being reported (Kraemer et al., 1988; Hurley, 1989; Stone et al., 1991). All of the cross-sectional and longitudinal studies can be criticized for one or more of the following reasons: inadequate control of age, diet, training regimes and androgen use of the subjects, use of only one blood sample in determining the lipid profile, no control group, did not account for changes in body composition and did not rule out the possible acute effect of the last training session (Hurley, 1989).

Due to limitations in study design and methodology, conclusions from studies examining the effect of strength training on the lipid profile must be viewed with caution. However, it does appear that strength training can affect the lipid profile in a positive manner. In addition, programmes using predominantly 8–12 repetitions per set of an

Table 12.2 Cardiac morphology adaptations at rest

| | Absolute | Relative to: | |
		BSA	LBM
Wall thickness			
Left ventricle	↑ ↑ ↑*	↑ ↑ or no change	↑ ↑ or no change
Septal	↑ ↑ ↑	↑ ↑ or no change	↑ ↑ or no change
Right ventricle	No change	No change	No change
Chamber volume			
Left ventricle	↑ ↑ or no change	No change	No change
Right ventricle	No change	No change	No change
Left ventricular mass	↑ ↑ ↑ or no change	↑ ↑ or no change	↑ or no change

BSA, body surface area; LBM, lean body mass.
*The number of arrows indicates in an arbitrary fashion the size of the change.

exercise and short rest periods (bodybuilding-type programme) may more positively affect the lipid profile than programmes using predominantly heavy resistances for 1–6 repetitions per set of an exercise and long rest periods between sets and exercises (power-lifting-type programme).

Cardiac wall thickness

Diastolic posterior left ventricular (PWTd) and intraventricular septum (IVSd) are the most commonly determined wall thicknesses using echocardiographic techniques. Measurement of these variables in highly weight-trained males indicate that absolute PWTd and IVSd is increased due to strength training but that the increase is greatly reduced or non-existent if examined relative to body surface area or lean body mass (Table 12.2) (Fleck, 1988). The increased wall thicknesses are due to a training adaptation to the intermittent elevated blood pressures encountered during strength training exercise (Effron, 1989).

It is interesting to note that increased PWTd occurs more frequently than increased IVSd in strength-trained athletes and that the majority of studies reporting greater PWTd in strength-trained athletes than controls involve national/international calibre athletes (Fleck, 1988).

This might indicate that PWTd is affected by calibre of athlete. However, a meta-analysis (a statistical procedure by which data from independent studies can be collectively analysed) indicates absolute IVSd and not PWTd is significantly greater in national/international and regional calibre athletes than in recreational strength trainers (Fleck, 1988).

Short-term (10–20 weeks) longitudinal training studies, using young adult males as subjects, support the concept that strength training can increase left ventricular wall thickness, but that it is not a necessary outcome of training. Longitudinal studies report both increased and no change in PWTd and IVSd (Fleck, 1988; Effron, 1989). This discrepancy is probably due to differences in exercises performed (large vs. small muscle mass), training intensity and training volume.

The amount of left ventricular wall thickening appears to be related to training intensity (Effron, 1989). Therefore, it might be hypothesized that left ventricular wall thickening would be different between bodybuilders, who train predominantly with 6–12 repetition maximum resistances, and weightlifters, who spend a great deal of training time using one to three repetition maximum resistances. One study comparing bodybuilders and weightlifters found that both groups had significantly greater absolute and relative to body surface area and lean body mass PWTD and IVSd than a control group. However, no significant differences between these types of athletes in PWTD and IVSd were found (Deligiannis *et al.*, 1988).

Right ventricular wall thickness has received considerably less attention than left ventricular wall thickness. A recent study using magnetic resonance imaging found no difference in systolic and diastolic right ventricular wall thickness between male junior elite Olympic weightlifters and an age- and weight-matched control group (Fleck *et al.*, 1989b). This suggests that the right ventricle is not exposed to elevated pressures, sufficient to cause hypertrophy of ventricular walls, during strength training exercise.

Conclusions warranted from the present data are that strength training can cause increased left ventricular wall thicknesses, but that it is not a necessary consequence of all strength-training programmes. Increased right ventricular wall thickness does not occur. Increased wall thickness is caused by the intermittent elevated blood pressures encountered during training and is related to the calibre of athlete and to the strength training intensity and volume.

Chamber dimensions

Increased left ventricular systolic and diastolic internal dimensions or volumes is considered to be an indication of a volume overload on the heart as found in endurance athletes. The majority of studies show highly strength-trained males do not have greater left ventricular internal dimensions, in absolute or relative to body surface or lean body mass terms, than control groups (Table 12.2) (Fleck, 1988; Effron, 1989; Stone *et al.*, 1991). The conclusion that left ventricular volumes are not increased due to strength training is supported by results of short-term longitudinal studies that report no change in systolic or diastolic left ventricular volumes (Fleck, 1988; Effron, 1989; Stone *et al.*, 1991).

Increased left ventricular chamber size is due to a volume overload on the heart. Therefore, it might be hypothesized that bodybuilding-type training would have a greater potential to increase chamber size than Olympic or power-lifting type training. This contention is supported by a study reporting bodybuilders, but not weightlifters, to have a greater absolute end-diastolic and systolic volume than a control group (Deligiannis *et al.*, 1988). The differences between the bodybuilders and control group, however, were not present if evaluated relative to body surface area or lean body mass. The bodybuilders, but not the weightlifters, also had a greater right ventricular internal dimension in absolute, relative to body surface area and lean body mass terms than control subjects. This finding is corroborated by a report of no change in right ventricular dimensions in a group of junior elite Olympic weightlifters (Fleck *et al.*, 1989b). Both bodybuilders and weight-lifters have a greater end-systolic left atrium internal dimension in absolute, relative to body surface area and lean body mass terms than control subjects (Deligiannis *et al.*, 1988). Bodybuilders also have significantly greater left atrium internal dimension than weightlifters.

It appears that the majority of strength-training programmes do not cause an increase in cardiac chamber sizes. However, high volume bodybuilding-type programmes may cause increased cardiac chamber sizes.

Left ventricular mass

Either an increase in wall thickness or ventricular size or both can result in increased left ventricular mass (Table 12.2). In a manner similar to wall thickness, absolute left ventricular mass of highly strength-trained athletes is greater than controls in the majority of studies, but the difference is greatly reduced or non-existent when examined relative to body surface area or lean body mass (Fleck, 1988; Stone *et al.*, 1991). Short-term longitudinal training studies support this concept (Fleck, 1988). There is also some data to suggest that national/international calibre athletes have a greater left ventricular mass than athletes of a lesser calibre (Fleck, 1988; Effron, 1989).

Left ventricular mass of bodybuilders and weightlifters is not significantly different (Deligiannis et al., 1988). Both bodybuilder's and weightlifter's PWTd and IVSd are significantly greater than controls, but only bodybuilders have a greater left ventricular end-diastolic volume than controls (Deligiannis et al., 1988). Therefore, it appears that both of these types of training can cause increased left ventricular mass. However, the increased mass due to bodybuilding is a result of both increased chamber size and wall thickness, whereas in weightlifters it is due solely to increased wall thickness.

As with wall thickness, increased left ventricular mass can occur due to strength training. The increased left ventricular mass is related to the intensity of training and perhaps to the calibre of athlete (Fleck, 1988; Effron, 1989; Stone et al., 1991).

Systolic function

Per cent fractional shortening, ejection fraction and velocity of circumferential shortening are commonly determined measures of systolic function using echocardiographic techniques. Per cent fractional shortening has been reported to be significantly greater (32 vs. 37%) in strength-trained athletes than a control group (Colan et al., 1985) and significantly increased (32 to 36%) due to a short-term training period (Kanakis & Hickson, 1980). However, the vast majority of data show strength training to have no effect upon systolic function (Fleck, 1988; Effron, 1989).

Diastolic function

Abnormalities in diastolic function are associated with cardiac hypertrophy due to hypertension and valvular heart disease. Power-lifters, with significantly greater absolute and relative to body surface area left ventricular mass, appear to have normal left ventricular function (Colan et al., 1985; Pearson et al., 1986). In fact

left ventricular peak rate of chamber enlargement (13.6 vs. 16.5 cm · s^{-1}) and peak rate of wall thinning (8.4 vs. 10.6 cm · s^{-1}) and atrial peak filling rate (225 vs. 296 ml · s^{-1}) have been reported to be greater in power-lifters than normal individuals (Colan et al., 1985; Pearson et al., 1986). This indicates an enhancement of left ventricular diastolic function. Power-lifters with a history of long-term androgen use do, however, have decreased left ventricular mean peak filling index (1.88 vs. 2.24) and ratio of peak early to peak atrial velocities (1.76 vs. 2.62) compared to normal values (Pearson et al., 1986). Due to the few studies examining diastolic function in strength-trained athletes, the results must be viewed with caution. However, it does appear that strength training does not affect diastolic function despite an increase in left ventricular mass unless accompanied by long-term androgen use (Fleck, 1988; Effron, 1989).

Acute response

Acute response refers to the cardiovascular response during one strength-training exercise. The acute cardiovascular response to dynamic strength training (Table 12.3) has received little study from the sports science community. This makes drawing conclusions concerning the acute cardiovascular

Table 12.3 Acute response of strength exercise relative to rest

| | Portion of repetition | |
	Concentric	Eccentric
Heart rate	↑	↑
Blood pressure		
Systolic	↑	↑
Diastolic	↑	↑
Intrathoracic pressure	↑	↑
Cardiac output	No change*	↑ *
Stroke volume	No change*	↑ *

* Due to the few studies examining this variable, the conclusion must be viewed with caution.

response to dynamic strength training difficult. However, the following conclusions seem warranted.

Heart rate and systolic and diastolic blood pressures increase substantially during the performance of dynamic heavy strength exercise (Fleck, 1988; Stone *et al.*, 1991). During performance of a two-legged leg press to failure at 95% of one repetition maximum, in which a Valsalva manoeuvre was allowed, pressures of 320/250 mmHg and a heart rate of 170 beats per minute have been reported (MacDougall *et al.*, 1985). The highest heart rate and blood pressures normally occur during the last repetitions of a set to volitional fatigue (Fleck, 1988; Stone *et al.*, 1991). Higher blood pressures occur during the eccentric as opposed to the concentric portion of the repetition (Fig. 12.1) (MacDougall *et al.*, 1985). The heart rate, blood pressure and cardiac output response increase with in-

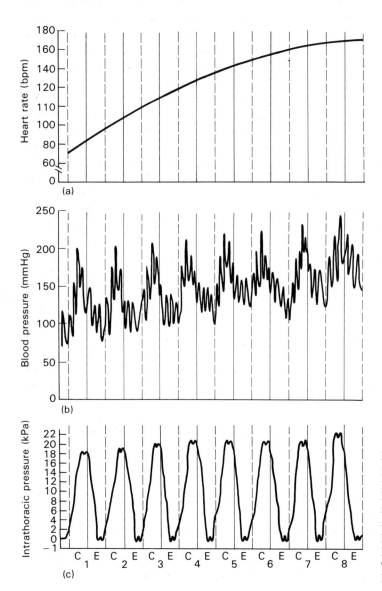

Fig. 12.1 (a) Heart rate, (b) blood pressure, and (c) intrathoracic pressure response to a hypothetical set at 8 repetition maximum of a strength exercise. A Valsalva manoeuvre was performed during the concentric portion of each repetition. C, concentric portion, E, eccentric portion of each repetition.

creased active muscle mass; however, the response is not linear (Fleck, 1988; Fleck *et al.*, 1989a; Stone *et al.*, 1991).

Without performance of a Valsalva manoeuvre mean cardiac output (determined via electrical impedance techniques) is not significantly altered from rest during performance of knee extensions at a 12 repetition maximum resistance (Miles *et al.*, 1987). No change in mean cardiac output is seen due to an increased heart rate coupled with a decreased stroke volume (Miles *et al.*, 1987). This is true even though electrical impedance contractility indices (R–Z interval, Heather index) indicate contractility increased (Miles *et al.*, 1987). However, the cardiac output response during the eccentric and concentric portion of the repetitions is different. Cardiac output is significantly lower during the concentric as compared to the eccentric portion of the exercise (Miles *et al.*, 1987). Heart rate is the same during the eccentric and concentric portions and the difference in cardiac output is due to a smaller stroke volume during the concentric phase (Miles *et al.*, 1987). The cardiac output and stroke volume portion of this study must, however, be viewed with caution due to possible limitations of impedance cardiography during activity (Miles & Gotshall, 1989).

The exact mechanisms resulting in the acute cardiovascular response to dynamic strength-training exercise are not completely elucidated. However, several hypotheses that may affect the pressor response can be advanced. High cardiac outputs can contribute to increased blood pressures. However, as stated above, mean cardiac output is not elevated significantly above rest during knee extension exercise in novice strength-trained subjects (Miles *et al.*, 1987). This is corroborated by a report that cardiac output during strength-training exercises (leg press and knee extension) has an inverse significant relationship to systolic and diastolic blood pressures (Fleck *et al.*, 1989a). Thus it appears that increased cardiac output does not contribute to the increased blood pressures during strength training. In fact the increased blood pressures may limit cardiac output during this type of exercise.

Increased intrathoracic or intra-abdominal pressures may have an impact upon cardiac output and so blood pressure during strength-training exercise (Fleck, 1988). Classically, increased intrathoracic pressures are thought to decrease venous return to the heart and so decrease cardiac output. Intrathoracic pressure has a significant inverse relationship to cardiac output and stroke volume (determined via impedance cardiography) and a significant positive relationship to systolic and diastolic blood pressure during strength-training exercise (Fleck *et al.*, 1989a). Thus it appears that increased intrathoracic pressures may indeed limit venous return and so decrease cardiac output, but at the same time this may cause a build-up of blood in the systemic circulation that may contribute to increased blood pressures. The above line of reasoning indicates that performance of strength-training exercises with a Valsalva manoeuvre, which elevates intrathoracic pressure, would lead to a greater blood pressure response than performance of the exercise without a Valsalva manoeuvre.

Increased intramuscular pressure during strength exercise could result in increased total peripheral resistance and so increased blood pressure. Intramuscular pressures have been measured during static muscular actions and are quite high (quadriceps 92 kPa; Edwards *et al.*, 1972). For blood to flow through a vessel intraluminal pressure must exceed extravascular pressure. Although there is considerable intermuscular variability, even static actions of a moderate nature (40–60% of maximum) can occlude blood flow (Fleck, 1988). Mechanically-induced increases in peripheral resistance are the most probable reason for blood pressures to be higher during the concentric versus the eccentric portion of an exercise (Miles *et al.*, 1987).

The blood pressure response is higher during sets performed to volitional fatigue at 70, 80 and 95% of 100% of one repetition maximum than at 100% or lower percentages of 100% of one repetition maximum (MacDougall *et al.*, 1985; Fleck & Dean, 1987; Fleck *et al.*, 1989a). Sets carried to fatigue at 70–95% of 1 repetition maximum are probably of sufficient duration and intensity to allow both of these factors to influence blood pressure. However, sets above or below this region do not allow both factors to substantially affect the pressor response (Fleck, 1988).

The increased intrathoracic pressure may have a protective function for the cerebral blood vessels (MacDougall *et al.*, 1985). Increased intrathoracic pressure is directly transmitted to the cerebrospinal fluid, and thus the cerebrospinal fluid pressure matches the intrathoracic pressure. The increased intrathoracic pressure during strength training and performance of a Valsalva manoeuvre reduces the transmural pressure across the cerebral vessels and may reduce the risk of damage to these vessels due to the increased blood pressures found during strength-training exercise.

Chronic adaptations during strength exercise

Classical cardiovascular training adaptations are reductions in heart rate and blood pressure at a specified submaximal workload. Few studies have attempted to examine cardiovascular adaptations during work due to strength training.

Maximal systolic and diastolic intra-arterial blood pressures and maximal heart rate during one-armed dumb-bell overhead presses and one-legged knee extensions are lower in male bodybuilders than in sedentary subjects and novice (6–9 months training experience) strength-trained subjects (Fleck & Dean, 1987). Sets of each exercise were performed to volitional fatigue at 100, 90, 80, 70 and 50% of one repetition maximum in this study. Thus the bodybuilders had a lower pressor response at the same relative workload. In addition, because the bodybuilders were stronger than the other two groups they had a lower pressor response at a greater absolute workload.

During arm ergometry at the same absolute workloads bodybuilders have a lower heart rate and lower double product but not systolic or diastolic blood pressures than a group of medical students (Colliander & Tesch, 1988).

Short-term training studies also report positive adaptations in the blood pressure and heart rate response to work. After 12 weeks of strength training time to reach 85% of predicted, maximal heart rate during an incremental load bicycle ergometry test is significantly increased (Blessing *et al.*, 1987). After 16 weeks of strength training, systolic and diastolic blood pressure and the double product but not the heart rate response of adult males and females were significantly lowered during treadmill walking holding hand weights (Goldberg *et al.*, 1988). Cross-sectional and longitudinal data both support the concept that strength training can result in a lower pressor response and lower myocardial oxygen consumption as indicated by a lower double product during work.

Soviet research indicate that weightlifters' cardiac outputs increase 1.5–2 times above resting values during strength exercise activity (Stone *et al.*, 1991). Cardiac output of weightlifters also increases up to $30 l \cdot min^{-1}$ after exercise with stroke volume increasing up to 150–200 ml, while untrained subjects show no significant change in cardiac output during strength training activity (Stone *et al.*, 1991). Cardiac output and stroke volume, but not heart rate, of bodybuilders is significantly greater than that of power-lifters during sets of the back squat at various percentages of 1 repetition maximum to volitional fatigue (Murray *et al.*, 1989). These authors determined stroke volume using impedance cardiography, which has been criticized as a method to determine stoke volume during activity (Miles & Gothshall, 1989). Therefore, the results of this study must be viewed with caution. The above studies do, however, suggest strength training may lead to an adaptation that allows cardiac output to be elevated during strength-training activity. One such adaptation, already discussed, may be decreased blood pressure during activity resulting in a decreased after-load on the left ventricle. The difference between the bodybuilders and the power-lifters may be related to performance of a more forceful Valsalva manoeuvre by the power-lifters, resulting in greater intrathoracic and intra-abdominal pressures. Stroke volume and cardiac output have been shown to be negatively related to intrathoracic pressure during strength training (Fleck et al., 1989a); this could in part explain the lower cardiac output in the power-lifters.

Peak oxygen consumption ($\dot{V}O_{2max}$) on a treadmill or bicycle ergometer is normally considered an indicator of cardiovascular fitness. Heavy strength training is normally not considered to have an impact upon $\dot{V}O_{2max}$. However, $\dot{V}O_{2max}$ of competitive bodybuilders, Olympic weightlifters and power-lifters range from 41 to 55 ml $\cdot$ kg^{-1} $\cdot$ min^{-1} (Fleck & Kraemer, 1987; Kraemer et al., 1988; Stone et al., 1991), which are average to moderately above average values for $\dot{V}O_{2max}$. This could be interpreted to mean that strength training may cause increased $\dot{V}O_{2max}$ in some but not all individuals or that not all strength programmes cause a change in $\dot{V}O_{2max}$. The latter is a more plausible explanation. Such factors as the total training volume, the rest periods between sets and large vs. small muscle mass exercises could account for the differences in $\dot{V}O_{2max}$ among elite strength-trained athletes.

Insight into the effect the type of resistance programme performed can have upon $\dot{V}O_{2max}$ can be gained by examining results from short-term longitudinal studies. Circuit weight training consists of performing sets of exercises of 12–15 repetitions at 40–60% of 1 repetition maximum with 15–30 s rest between sets and exercises (Gettman & Pollock, 1981). This type of training causes a moderate increase in $\dot{V}O_{2max}$ of 4% in men and 8% in women in 8–20 weeks of training (Gettman & Pollock, 1981). More traditional heavy strength training programmes using 3–5 sets of each exercise and 5 repetitions per set result in no change in

$\dot{V}O_{2max}$ (Fahey & Brown, 1973; Hickson et al., 1980). An Olympic style weightlifting training programme does result in moderate gains in absolute (9%) and relative (8%) $\dot{V}O_{2max}$ in an 8-week period (Stone et al., 1983). In this study, during the first 5 weeks of training 3–5 sets of an exercise of 10 repetitions per set and rest periods of 3.5–4 min between sets and exercises, were performed for two training sessions per day on 3 alternate days per week. On 2 days of the week 5 sets of 10 vertical jumps were performed, making a total of 5 training days per week. This period of training resulted in the majority of gain in $\dot{V}O_{2max}$ (39.5–42.4 ml $\cdot$ kg^{-1} $\cdot$ min^{-1}). The next 2 weeks of training were essentially identical to the first 5 weeks except 3 sets of five repetitions per sets of an exercise were performed. This period of training resulted in no further increase in $\dot{V}O_{2max}$. The results of these studies indicate that a large volume of strength-type training can result in moderate gains in $\dot{V}O_{2max}$. However, the increase in $\dot{V}O_{2max}$ brought about by strength training is of a smaller magnitude than the 15–20% gains normally associated with a traditional training programme of running, cycling or swimming.

In conclusion, performance of a strength-training activity does result in a pressor response that has an impact upon the cardiovascular system. In addition, information to date indicates that long-term performance of strength training can result in positive adaptations of the cardiovascular system at rest and

Table 12.4 Adaptations during exercise due to strength training relative to normals

Heart rate	↓
Blood pressure	
Systolic	↓ or no change
Diastolic	↓ or no change
Double product	↓
Cardiac output	↑ or no change*
Stroke volume	↑ or no change*
$\dot{V}O_{2max}$	↑ or no change

*Due to the few studies examining this variable, the conclusion must be viewed with caution.

during work (Table 12.4). The extent of these adaptations may in large part be dependent upon the volume and intensity of strength training performed and this is the area where future research efforts need to focus.

References

Blessing, D., Stone, M., Byrd, R., Wilson, D., Rozenek, R., Pushparani, D. & Lipner, H. (1987) Blood lipid and hormonal changes from jogging and weight training of middle-aged men. *Journal of Applied Sport Science Research*, **1**, 25–9.

Blomqvist, C.G. & Saltin, B. (1983) Cardiovascular adaptations to physical training. *Annual Review of Physiology*, **45**, 169–89.

Blumenthal, J.A., Fredrikson, M., Khun, C.M., Ulmer, R.L., Walsh-Riddle, M. & Appelbaum, M. (1990) Aerobic exercise reduces levels of cardiovascular and sympathoadrenal responses to mental stress in subjects without prior evidence of myocardial ischemia. *American Journal of Cardiology*, **65**, 93–8.

Colan, S., Sanders, S.P., McPherson, D. & Borrow, K.M. (1985). Left ventricular diastolic function in elite athletes with physiologic cardiac hypertrophy. *Journal of the American College of Cardiology*, **6**, 545–9.

Colliander, E.B. & Tesch, P. (1988) Blood pressure in resistance-trained athletes. *Canadian Journal of Sports Science*, **13**, 31–4.

Deligiannis, A., Zahopoulou, E. & Mandroukas, K. (1988) Echocardiographic study of cardiac dimensions and function in weight lifters and body builders. *International Journal of Sports Cardiology*, **5**, 24–32.

Edwards, R.H.T., Hill, D.K. & McDonnell, M.N. (1972) Monothermal and intramuscular pressure measurements during isometric contractions of the human quadriceps muscle. *Journal of Physiology*, **224**, 58–9.

Effron, M.B. (1989) Effects of resistance training on left ventricular function. *Medicine and Science in Sports and Exercise*, **21**, 694–7.

Elliot, D.L., Goldberg, L., Kuehl, K.S. & Katlin, D.H. (1987) Characteristics of anabolic-androgenic steroid-free, competitive male and female bodybuilders. *Physician in Sportsmedicine*, **15**, 169–79.

Fahey, T.D. & Brown, H. (1973) The effects of an anabolic steroid on the strength, body composition, and endurance of college males when accompanied by a weight training program. *Medicine and Science in Sports*, **5**, 272–6.

Fleck, S.J. (1988) Cardiovascular adaptations to resistance training. *Medicine and Science in Sports and Exercise*, **20**, S146–S151.

Fleck, S.J. & Dean, L.S. (1987) Resistance-training experience and the pressor response during resistance exercise. *Journal of Applied Physiology*, **63**, 116–20.

Fleck, S.J., Falkel, J., Harman, E., Kraemer, W.J., Frykman, P., Maresh, C.M., Goetz, K.L., Campbell, D., Roesenstein, M. & Roesenstein, R. (1989a) Cardiovascular responses during resistance training (Abstract). *Medicine and Science in Sports and Exercise*, **21**, S114.

Fleck, S.J., Henke, C. & Wilson, W. (1989b) Cardiac MRI of elite junior Olympic weight lifters. *International Journal of Sports Medicine*, **10**, 329–33.

Fleck, S.J. & Kraemer, W.J. (1987) *Designing Resistance Training Programs*. Human Kinetics, Champaign, Illinois.

Frick, M.H., Elovainio, R.O & Somer, T. (1967) The mechanism of bradycardia evoked by physical training. *Cardiology*, **51**, 46–54.

Gettman, L.R. & Pollock, M.L. (1981) Circuit weight training: a critical review of its physiological benefits. *Physician in Sportsmedicine*, **9**, 44–60.

Goldberg, A.P. (1989) Aerobic and resistive exercise modify risk factors for coronary heart disease. *Medicine and Science in Sports and Exercise*, **21**, 669–74.

Goldberg, L., Elliot, D.L. & Kuehl, K.S. (1988) Cardiovascular changes at rest and during mixed static and dynamic exercise after weight training. *Journal of Applied Sport Science Research*, **2**, 42–5.

Haennel, R., Teo, K-K., Quinney, A. & Kappagoda, T. (1989) Effects of hydraulic circuit training on cardiovascular function. *Medicine and Science in Sports and Exercise*, **21**, 605–12.

Hickson, R.C., Rosenkoetter, M.A. & Brown, M.M. (1980) Strength training effects on aerobic power and short-term endurance. *Medicine and Science in Sports and Exercise*, **12**, 336–9.

Hurley, B.F. (1989) Effects of resistance training on lipoprotein-lipid profiles: a comparison to aerobic exercise training. *Medicine and Science in Sports and Exercise*, **21**, 689–93.

Hurley, B.F., Hagberg, J.M., Seals, D.R., Ehsani, A.A., Goldberg, A.P. & Holloszy, J.O. (1987) Glucose tolerance and lipid-lipoprotein levels in middle-aged powerlifters. *Clinical Physiology*, **7**, 11–19.

Hurley, B.F., Seals, D.R., Hagberg, J.M., Goldberg, A.C., Ostrove, S.M., Holloszy, J.O., Wiest, W.G. & Goldberg, A.P. (1984) High-density-lipoprotein cholesterol in bodybuilders v powerlifters. *Journal of the American Medical Association*, **252**, 507–13.

Kanakis, C. & Hickson, C. (1980). Left ventricular responses to a program of lower-limb strength training. *Chest*, **78**, 618–21.

Kraemer, W.J., Deschenes, M.R. & Fleck, S.J. (1988) Physiological adaptatations to resistance exercise implications for athletic conditioning. *Sports Medicine*, **6**, 246–56.

Lusiani, L., Ronsisvalle, G., Bonanome, A., Castellani, V., Macchia, C. & Pagnan, A. (1986). Echocardiographic evaluation of the dimensions and systolic properties of the left ventricle in freshman athletes during physical training. *European Heart Journal*, **7**, 196–203.

MacDougall, J.D., Tuxen, D., Sale, D.G., Moroz, J.R. & Sutton, J.R. (1985) Arterial blood pressure response to heavy resistance exercise. *Journal of Applied Physiology*, **58**, 785–90.

Miles, D.S. & Gotshall, R.W. (1989) Impedance cardiography: noninvasive assessment of human central hemodynamics at rest and during exercise. *Exercise and Sports Sciences Reviews*, **17**, 231–64.

Miles, D.S., Owens, J.J., Golden, J.C. & Gothsall, R.W. (1987) Central and peripheral hemodynamics during maximal leg extension exercise. *European Journal of Applied Physiology*, **56**, 12–17.

Morgan, D.W., Cruise, R.J., Girardin, B.W., Lutz-Schneider, V., Morgan, D.H. & Qi, W.M. (1986) Hdl-c concentrations in weight-trained, endurance-trained, and sedentary females. *Physician in Sportsmedicine*, **14**, 166–81.

Murray, T.F., Falkel, J.E. & Fleck, S.J. (1989) Differences in cardiac output responses between elite power lifters and body builders during resistance exercise (Abstract). *Medicine and Science in Sports and Exercise*, **21**, S114.

Pearson, A.C., Schiff, M., Mrosek, D., Labovitz, A.J. & Williams, G.A. (1986) Left ventricular diastolic function in weight lifters. *American Journal of Cardiology*, **58**, 1254–9.

Stone, M.H., Fleck, S.J., Triplett, N.R. & Kraemer, W.J. (1991) Physiological adaptations to resistance training exercise. *Sports Medicine*, **11**, 210–31.

Stone, M.H., Wilson, G.D., Blessing, D. & Rozenek, R. (1983) Cardiovascular responses to short-term Olympic style weight-training in young men. *Canadian Journal of Applied Sport Sciences*, **8**, 134–9.

PART 4

SPECIAL PROBLEMS IN STRENGTH AND POWER TRAINING

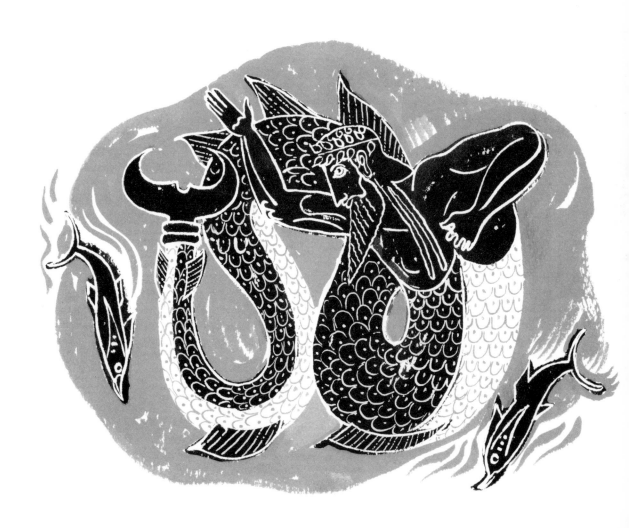

Chapter 13

Age-Related Changes in Strength and Special Groups

SIEGFRIED ISRAEL

Introduction

Strength is an indispensible precondition for any movement. The coordinated control of the body mass against the force of gravity permanently requires an adequate amount of strength. In addition, lifting, holding and carrying loads need strength. These conditions apply to all age groups.

The generation of strength is bound to the action of muscles. The musculature, the biological basis of strength development, is the largest system of the body. In early adulthood about 35% (women) to 40% (men) of the body mass of normal weight persons consists of muscle tissue. Therefore, because of its quantity, the muscle system must have a notable influence on a multitude of physiological (and also pathological) events, on the general state of the body, and also on ageing processes.

A muscle can grow or atrophy depending on its use. Muscle tissue responds to adaptive stimuli; the quantity and quality of a muscle change according to the imposed demands. It is an everyday observation and experience that high demands for strength cause hypertrophy and that low demands are followed by atrophy, with a subsequent weakness of the affected muscles.

The adaptability (trainability) of the muscles changes during the course of life. The existing strength potential has to be evaluated with respect to use und disuse of the musculature. Further, constitutional factors, e.g. fibre composition and hormonal factors, have to be taken into account.

Prepubertal age

Experiments have shown that some endurance-induced adaptations can be transferred from pregnant animals to the embryo, e.g. relative bradycardia, heart enlargement, smaller fat cells; these adaptations are obviously caused by blood-borne signals. Comparable experiments with strength training have not yet been carried out, but beneficial adaptational influences on the offspring is probable.

Only about 20% of the body mass of a newborn child is muscle tissue. The infant is weak, and the strengthening of the muscles in the first months takes place by spontaneous movements particularly of the limbs; these movements should not be limited by tight clothes.

The motor development of the infant proceeds on the basis of an inborn programme that guarantees an optimal outcome of muscular strength. With progressing age the movements become more complex and the trainability of strength becomes evident, e.g. myotonia congenita, a rare congenital disease, is characterized by a considerable strain on all movements resulting in a visibly pronounced muscle hypertrophy at a very young age. Also, children born with handicaps of the limbs demonstrate early hypertrophy to compensate for their deformities. These paradigms prove that the

319

muscle is adaptable (trainable) to strength stimuli in the very early periods of life. It has to be emphasized that the infant and the little child should not be burdened with systematic strength training; quick movements (without additional loading) provide an appropriate stimulus for the development of an optimal amount of muscular strength.

In general, during prepubertal development increase of physical strength takes place as demonstrated in Figs 13.1 and 13.2. There is a continuous increment until fundamental hormonal changes occur in puberty. In the prepubertal phase muscle mass increases parallel to body mass. Moderate strength train-

ing is recommended but higher burdens should be avoided because of the sensitivity of the joint structures, especially of the growth zones (epiphysis) of the bones.

During prepuberty there are no differences between girls and boys with respect to the trainability for strength. Boys have a small genetic advantage, which is completely compensated by the developmental advance of girls. There is no biological basis for a sex-dependent evaluation of strength performances, e.g. in physical education at school. A still existing difference in strength between girls and boys, particularly in the area of shoulders and arms, emerges predominantly

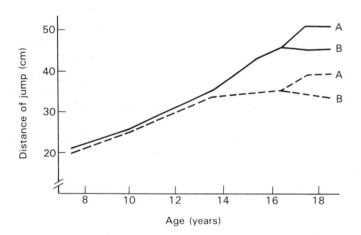

Fig. 13.1 Longitudinal analysis of performance in a jump and reach test. (From Crasselt, 1990.) ——, male; ----, female. A, secondary schoolchildren; B, children in occupational training.

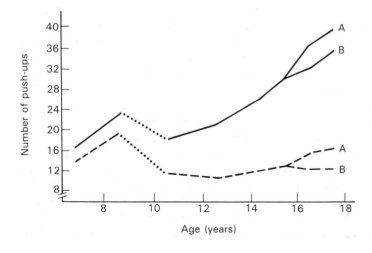

Fig. 13.2 Longitudinal analysis of performance in push-ups (from a kneeling position before, and from a stretched position after, the dotted lines). (From Crasselt, 1990.) ——, male; ---, female. A, secondary schoolchildren; B, children in occupational training.

Table 13.1 Plasma concentration (ng · 100 ml^{-1}) of some sexual hormones during puberty (From Reiter & Root, 1975.)

Age (years)	Oestrone		Oestradiol		Testosterone	
	Female	Male	Female	Male	Female	Male
8–9	20	—	10	—	20	24–30
10–11	20–67	—	10–200	10	10–65	41–60
12–13	20–117	—	20–270	2–30	20–80	131–249
14–15	20–100	—	15–400	5–40	20–85	328–643

for social reasons; it is due to the identification with typical gender roles in education. Girls encounter gravity in the same manner as boys (Fig. 13.1); therefore, no difference in the strength of the legs is evident. But girls use their arms less powerfully than boys; this behaviour causes a relative weakness of the upper extremities (Fig. 13.2). Young female top-class gymnasts are able to perform 40 pull-ups! This example demonstrates what is really possible.

Puberty

All motor properties (strength, endurance, motor skill, etc.) are adaptable throughout life, i.e. these abilities can be improved by training. However, during ontogenesis periods of high trainability ('sensitive phases') can be identified. For males, puberty is a very effective period for the development of strength.

The kinetics of the sexual hormones during puberty are documented in Table 13.1. In the development of strength the male sexual hormones are of outstanding significance because of their anabolic (protein incorporating) component. This effect facilitates the synthesis of muscle protein. During maturation the proportion of muscles increases in boys from 27 to 40% of the body mass. Figures 13.1 and 13.2 demonstrate that with the onset of puberty the strength characteristics of girls and boys diverge markedly. This finding has its basis primarily in a changed hormonal adjustment. In addition, the figures show that the

development of strength potential has a social component at this age, as it depends on the educational level.

Puberty is an important stage for the development of strength; the phase is not a crisis as believed in the past. All-round training should take place (strength from head to toe). Adequate strength training is essential, as rapid growth takes place; the gain in body height may be 10 cm for girls and 12 cm for boys within 1 year. An optimal musculature stabilizes the quickly growing skeleton.

On average girls attain the following proportions of the strength capacity of boys:

11–12 years: 90%
13–14 years: 85%
15–16 years: 75%.

This gender difference has a biological basis, but girls exhibit a socially induced deficit too. Pubertal girls tend to avoid actions that require strength for psychological reasons.

The undisturbed rapid growth during puberty does not call for physical restrictions, but certain precautions in carrying out strength exercises are warranted. The zones of ossification are sensitive and liable to injury and damage. Heavy loads, unilateral burdens or faulty techniques should be avoided in order to take care of the cartilage of the epiphysis. Attention has to be paid to arthromuscular dysbalances and to a possible onset of osteochondrosis. Experience in top performance sport revealed that very hard training in the prepubertal and pubertal period may hamper

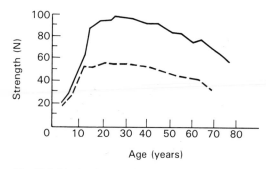

Fig. 13.3 Maximal strength in hand grip. (From Hettinger, 1968.) ——, male; ---, female.

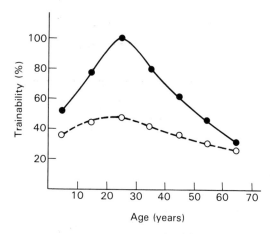

Fig. 13.4 Trainability of strength given as a per cent of the maximum trainability of men. (From Hettinger, 1968.) ——, male; ---, female.

the growth in height. In general, after a reduction of the loading the deficit in height is gradually compensated.

Early adulthood

Figures 13.3 and 13.4 show that strength potential reaches the highest level during this age period. The competent biological structures show a state of good adaptability (trainability), the joints tolerate high loads, and the social situation makes a certain use of strength necessary. At this age period top performances are possible in those kinds of sport that require a maximum of strength and power. Most chapters of this book refer to this age group.

Middle-aged persons (30–60 years)

Again, Figs 13.3 and 13.4 show in general the typical time course of strength abilities after the physical high-performance age. Figures 13.5 and 13.6 complete and deepen the insight in this situation. A continuous decline of the curves is obvious.

The decrement of strength during the course of ageing has to be differentiated according to training activities, gender and body area. Training affects the magnitude of strength significantly. Trained persons (activities in general sport for 2 hours per week) demonstrate that a relatively small amount of exercise is sufficient to exert a beneficial influence on strength quality; the curves of active and inactive persons exhibit a significantly different level (Figs 13.5 and 13.6). A certain divergence of the characteristics can be noted with advancing age. This finding is due to the fact that a small amount of training expands the difference between active and inactive persons with increasing age. The steepness of the curve of the inactive individuals is due to diminishing social need for strength performances. In this connection it is of interest that persons from white-collar professions have the same or even more strength than persons from blue-collar professions (Yokomizo 1985; Nygard *et al.*, 1987); thus, leisure time activities account more for existing strength than professional demands. The level of strength decreases with advancing age because the social need for hard work becomes progressively less.

The decrease of strength with advancing age affects women and men in a different way. In general, the baseline level at an age of 30 years is lower in women than in men. For this reason, the decline of the curve, if expressed in absolute terms, is less steep in women than in men. Nevertheless, in all age periods women and men require more strength for health and well-being.

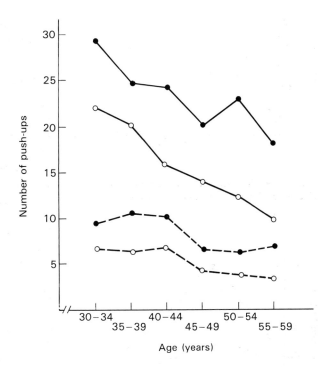

Fig. 13.5 Number of push ups done by people both active (●) and inactive (○) in sport (*n* = 864). ——, male; ----, female.

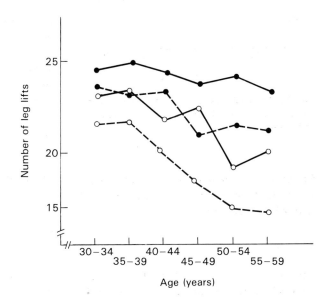

Fig. 13.6 Number of leg-lifts done in 30 s by people both active (●) and inactive (○) in sport (*n* = 864). ——, male; ---, female.

The decline of strength with increasing age differs in dependency of the body region. As Figs 13.5 and 13.6 exhibit, the arms are more affected than the trunk (the legs occupy a medium position). This typical development again has a biological and a social basis; the muscles of the trunk are somewhat more burdened in everyday living than the muscles

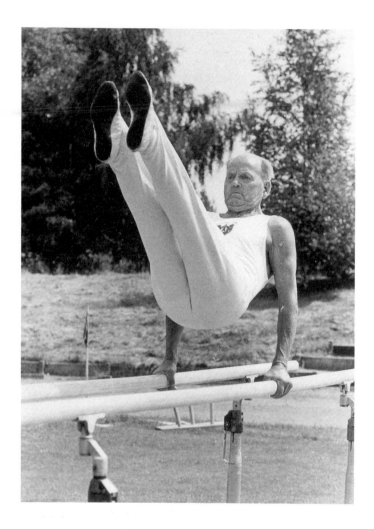

Fig. 13.7 Old gymnast (84 years) still active on the parallel bars.

of arms and shoulders. With respect to the muscles of the trunk, active elderly women even surpass inactive men; this may be an outcome of gymnastics and free exercises, which are preferred by women active in sport.

Advanced age

The knowledge of muscular strength in old age is still limited. However, it is well documented that an adaptability for strength stimuli persists; of course, the trainability decreases gradually.

Muscle biopsy studies by Grimby *et al.* (1982), Larsson (1982) and Aniansson *et al.* (1984) revealed that in old age exercise-induced reversibility of an existing muscular atrophy is possible. Aniansson and Gustafson (1981) found with 69–74-year-old men, after defined strength training, showed a gain in strength that almost equalled the values of young men. All investigators have confirmed that predominantly fast twitch fibres were affected by the hypertrophic increase in cross-sectional area. Commonly, at the onset of regular training in old age, marked atrophy is present so that even low stimuli induce an increase in strength. Sidney and Shephard (1980) found among 60–83-year-old women, after a period of regular hiking, a significant increase in the strength of the knee extensors. Klitgaard *et al.*

(1989) demonstrated that age-related changes in sarcoplasmic reticulum proteins did not occur in strength-trained old subjects. Dobrev (1978) reported that strength training with men beyond 70 years of age yielded a considerable gain of strength; this favourable development was associated with an increase in health (particularly of musculoskeletal status) and in emotional stability (Fig. 13.7).

Older muscles require a relatively long time interval for recovery after a strenuous exertion. The optimal relationship between strength training in particular muscles and general recreation changes in the course of life. In general, fatiguability increases with advancing age. With elderly persons the rest periods during a training session should be extended, and there should be an adequate interval between the sessions.

A growing number of investigations have revealed that with advancing age an irreversible loss of myocytes takes place. This adverse development concerns predominantly the fast twitch fibres. This type of muscle fibre prevails in the generation of strength. The question has to be raised whether this deficit is caused by the natural processes of ageing or whether it is the very last stage of permanent disuse, with the consequence of deconditioning and deterioration. Probably both events are responsible. The conclusion is that old people require appropriate strength stimuli.

Medical implications

Strength training has an essential impact on the quality of the bone tissue; it counteracts atrophy. Carter *et al.* (1987) have proposed a bone maintenance theory. Bone mass and density is regulated by loading; loading conditions induce a hypertrophic response and immobilization causes bone resorption. Atrophy of the bones is associated with increased fragility. Further, the functional integrity of a joint depends markedly on the quality of the competent muscles. Strong muscles are associated with tight ligaments and stable cartilage. In view of the high prevalence of disorders of the joints lifelong exercise-induced strengthening of all constituents of a joint is a major means of stabilizing health in this region. This is important for all age groups and for all joints; the spine and feet deserve special attention.

Well-developed strength helps prevent or moderates the symptoms that originate from degenerative alterations of the joints. Attention has to be directed to those muscles susceptible to atrophic weakening (Janda, 1986; Fig. 13.8). Priority should be given to the deep flexors of the neck, muscles that fix the scapula, abdominal muscles, gluteus muscles, and extensors of the knee. The preferential strengthening of these muscles eliminates disproportions, reduces joint disorders and assures arthromuscular integrity. A long-lasting abnormal strength ratio of agonists and antagonists may be harmful for the joints. Against this background, therefore, a deliberate strengthening programme should be practised already during the early periods of life.

Unjustifiably little attention is paid to the strength of the ventilatory muscles (diaphragm, intercostal muscles). Emphysema and chronic bronchitis are common in old people, and the deliberate strengthening of the ventilatory muscles in all age groups may prevent, moderate or retard this adverse development.

Strength training has selective effects on health-related physical mechanisms. Viitasalo *et al.* (1979) and Juhlin-Dannfelt *et al.* (1979) found a direct correlation between strength and systolic blood pressure. This finding becomes more important with increasing age. The prevalence of intermittent claudication is correlated with the rate of fast twitch fibres (Sjöström *et al.*, 1980). There is initial evidence that strength training does not prevent diabetes mellitus. Therefore, all strength training should be combined with components of endurance. Besides, strength training as practised by bodybuilders is more health-oriented than training in the manner of weightlifters (Tesch, 1988).

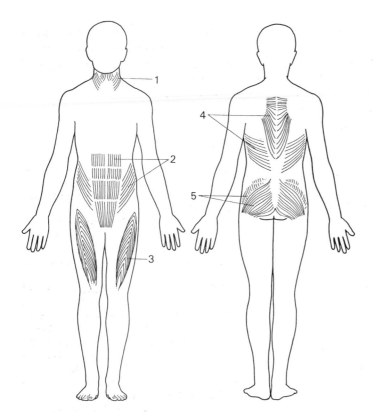

Fig. 13.8 Muscles that tend to atrophic weakening: 1, m. scalenus, m. longus colli, m. rectus capitis ant.; 2, m. obliquus abdominis, m. rectus abdominis; 3, m. vastus medialis, lateralis, intermedius; 4, m. trapezius (pars transversa et ascendus); 5, m. gluteus maximus et medius.

Concluding remarks

Some issues of strength training are of particular significance for children and for elderly and old persons. The upright posture of the human being requires that the postural muscles of the trunk and also of the legs are in a good state. During growth and ageing this musculature is frequently insufficient. The consequences are a hunched posture and premature wear and tear. Goal-oriented strength training is necessary.

Strength training causes well-known adaptations of muscle cells, but it also induces neural adaptations, which play a role in the threshold of response, in the recruitment patterns of the muscle fibres, in the type of excitation in the central nervous system, etc. It is important to aquire these abilities at an early age and to maintain them throughout life. Further, it has been proved that ageing processes of the spinal cord and peripheral nerves proceed relatively slowly in athletic old persons.

Strength training has a marked influence on the phenotype (the bodily shape) of a person; this phenomenon is of importance from puberty to old age. Nowadays, it is of concern for both sexes. The psychological implications are notable; without doubt, self-image and self-confidence are boosted by well-developed strength abilities with their impact on outward appearence.

Between the age of 30 to 70 years muscle mass decreases on average about 30%; the loss of strength is approximately the same. There is no convincing physiological argument for this steep decline. Normal ageing processes account only for a portion of this loss of musculature and strength; atrophy due to inactivity accounts for the greatest amount of muscle loss with age. This negative development for muscles, bones and joints may be avoided to a large extent by adequate and age-related strength training. With advancing age the social needs and individual motivation for the use of strength become less; consequently, there will be an atrophy that is not based on ageing events as they obey the laws of nature, but which reflects the effects of disuse. The weakness and infirmity of elderly and old people, as well as a multitude of problems that originate from the joints, respond in a desirable manner to appropriate strength training. The voluntary and deliberate use of the motor system in daily-life activities and in intentional strength training is able to counteract the loss of muscle mass as observed with increasing age. The vigorous use of muscles, particularly among old people, has a beneficial impact on the essential parameters of health and well-being.

Consideration has to be given to the health-related interplay of strength and flexibility, which have their working point at the joints. This is the reason why these physical properties enter into several interrelationships and why they have to be viewed under common aspects that gain importance with advancing age. Further, stretching of a muscle increases its strength (Vandenburgh, 1987).

Life expectancy is growing. As a consequence, there is much time for the development of deformations, chronic diseases, degeneration and wear and tear. In particular, the joints (their constituents) are affected by these alterations. Strength training, correctly employed exercises and dosage, is in this connection a tool of primary health care. It enhances or preserves the durability, solidity and wear resistance of the tissues forming the joints; further, strength training may reduce the symptoms originating from the above-mentioned pathological deteriorations, and it may even correct some alterations. By this, disturbances, discomfort and pain may be avoided or attenuated.

The weakness and infirmity of old age cannot be explained by ageing processes alone; these features of old age are, to a considerable degree, an expression of insufficient physical activity and the subsequent atrophy. Proper development of strength is, therefore, a means for optimal development in the early periods of life, is a chance to avoid premature ageing, and in elderly people may be regarded as a factor of a low biological age.

References

Aniansson, A. & Gustafsson, E. (1981) Physical training in old men with special reference to quadriceps muscle strength and morphology. *Clinical Physiology*, **1**, 87–98.

Aniansson, A., Ljundberg, P., Rundgren, A. & Wetterquist, H. (1984) Effect of a training programme for pensioners on condition and muscular strength. *Archives of Gerontology and Geriatry*, **3**, 229–41.

Carter, D.R., Fyhrie, D.P. & Whalen, R.T. (1987) Trabecular bone density and loading history: regulation of connective tissue biology by mechanical energy. *Journal of Biomechanics*, **20**, 785–94.

Crasselt, W., Forchel, I., Kroll, M. & Schulz, A. (1990) *Zum Kinder- und Jugendsport—Realitäten, Wünsche und Tendenzen. (Sport of Children and Adolescents—Reality, Expectations, and Tendencies.)* Deutsche Hochschule für Körperkultur, Leipzig.

Dobrev, P. (1978) Znacenieto na silovite upraznenija s tezesti za merfofuncionalnoto razvitie i usu vursenstruvane na organizma na lica v sredna naprednala i starceska vizrast. (The significance of strength training with weights for the morphological and functional development of the body of persons in middle, advanced and old age.) *Vuprosi na fiziceskata kultura*, **23**, 599–603.

Grimby, G., Danneskiold-Samse, W., Hvid, K. & Saltin, B. (1982) Morphology and enzymatic capacity in arm and leg muscles in 78–81-year-old men and women. *Acta Physiologica Scandinavica*, **115**, 125–34.

Hettinger, Th. (1968) *Isometrisches Muskeltraining. (Isometric Muscle Training.)* Georg Thieme Verlag, Stuttgart.

Janda, V. (1986) *Muskelfunktionsdiagnostik. (Functional Diagnostic Tests for Muscles.)* Verlag Volk und Gesundheit, Berlin.

Juhlin-Dannfelt, A., Frisk-Holmberg, M., Karlson, J. & Tesch, P. (1979) Central and peripheral circulation in relation to muscle-fibre composition in normo- and hypertensive men. *Clinical Science*, **56**, 335–40.

Klitgaard, H., Ausoni, S. & Damiani, E. (1989) Sarcoplasmatic reticulum of human skeletal muscle: age-related changes and effect of training. *Acta Physiologica Scandinavica*, **137**, 23–31.

Larsson, L. (1982) Physical training effects on muscle morphology in sedentary males at different ages. *Medicine and Science in Sports and Exercise*, **14**, 203–6.

Nygard, C.-H., Luopajärvi, T., Cedercreutz, G. & Ilmarinen, J. (1987) Musculoskeletal capacity of employees aged 44 to 58 years in physical, mental and mixed types of work. *European Journal of Applied Physiology*, **56**, 555–61.

Reiter, E.O. & Root, A. (1975) Hormonal changes of adolescence. *Medical Clinics of North America*, **59**, 1289.

Sidney, K.H. & Shephard, R.J. (1980) Wahrnehmung von Anstrengungen bei Älteren. (Perception of loads by old people.) *Sportpraxis*, **21**, 125–31.

Sjöström, M., Ängquist, K.A. & Rais, O. (1980) Intermittent claudication and muscle fibre fine structure. Correlation between clinical and morphological data. *Ultrastructure and Pathology*, **1**, 309–26.

Tesch, P.A. (1988) Skeletal muscle adaptations consequent to long-term heavy resistance exercise. *Medicine and Science in Sports and Exercise*, **20**, 132–4.

Vandenburgh, H.H. (1987) Motion into mass: how does tension stimulate muscle growth. *Medicine and Science in Sports and Exercise*, **19**, 142–9.

Viitasalo, J.T., Komi, P.V. & Karvonen, M.J. (1979) Muscle strength and body composition as determinants of blood pressure in young men. *European Journal of Applied Physiology*, **42**, 165–73.

Yokomizo, Y.I. (1985) Measurement of ability of older workers. *Ergonomics*, **28**, 843–54.

Chapter 14

Use of Electrical Stimulation in Strength and Power Training

GARY A. DUDLEY AND ROBERT T. HARRIS

Introduction

Transcutaneous electromyostimulation (EMS) has long been used by clinicians to aid in rehabilitation of patients with limited motor function (Delitto & Robinson, 1989). For example, it has been used in treatment of knee joint injuries such as chondromalacia patellae (Johnson *et al.*, 1977) because reflex inhibition and pain decrease voluntary control. In postoperative patients with immobilized joints or a limited ability to generate force due to pain or neural inhibition, EMS has been shown to retard atrophy and dysfunction (Eriksson & Häggmark, 1979; Gould *et al.*, 1983; Wigerstad-Lossing *et al.*, 1988).

There has been a proliferation of EMS studies involving healthy subjects during the last two decades (for review see Kramer & Mendryk, 1982). Likewise, EMS is beginning to receive attention as a training method for athletes (Delitto *et al.*, 1989). Much of this interest has arisen in response to reports of Jakov Kots' work in the Soviet Union (Kots & Chwilon, 1971). Kots has claimed that a brief programme of high-frequency EMS can produce marked strength gains in highly-trained athletes. Several studies have since been conducted in an apparent effort to duplicate these results (e.g. Currier & Mann, 1983; St Pierre *et al.*, 1986).

In this chapter we will limit the presentation to the use of EMS in the conditioning of elite athletes. For the sake of simplicity, we will discuss the potential use of EMS by endurance and strength/power athletes such as marathon runners and Olympic weightlifters, respectively. These athletes represent the extremes of the spectrum of humans to develop muscular power. The marathon runner maintains an impressive 'steady-state' power output for over 2 hours, which is supported by aerobic metabolism. The Olympic weightlifter, in contrast, uses great muscular strength to develop as much as 15 times more power, but it is only sustained for milliseconds.

This chapter will be presented in four parts: methods of application of EMS, rationale for the use of EMS in conditioning athletes, data supporting the efficacy of EMS in conditioning athletes, and directions for future research. It is hoped that this approach will give some clarity to the 'smorgasbord' of concepts and ideas that presently exist concerning the use of EMS.

Methods of application of EMS

A variety of different stimulation protocols have been used to artificially activate skeletal muscle using EMS. The simplest approach has been to control the pulse duration and frequency and the duration and amplitude of activation. For example, 500-μs rectangular pulses at 20 Hz have been applied via a surface bipolar electrode configuration for 1 s (Hultman *et al.*, 1983). The amplitude of stimulation can be set to induce a force equal to a given percentage of maximal voluntary isometric

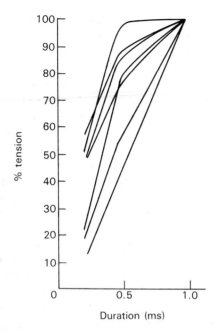

Fig. 14.1 The relationship between pulse duration and relative force during trancutaneous EMS of the knee extensor muscle group. Pulse duration was increased from 200 μs to 1 ms. Square pulses were delivered at 20 Hz and amplitude was held constant at a value that would elicit a force up to 70% of maximal voluntary isometric under optimal conditions. (From Hultman *et al.*, 1983.)

force (Currier & Mann, 1983) or, as is generally done, to subject tolerance (e.g. Laughman *et al.*, 1983).

The influence of altering one of these factors on isometric force development while the others are held at a given value has received some attention. Increasing pulse duration from 200 to 500 μs during 20 Hz stimulation results in markedly increased force (Hultman *et al.*, 1983) (Fig. 14.1). Further increases in pulse duration to 1000 μs have a modest effect. The authors recommended that pulse durations between 500 and 1000 μs be used during EMS for optimal force development, although this has not always been appreciated (Enoka, 1988). The relation between pulse frequency and isometric force is sigmoidal in nature, with tetanic force occurring at about 50 Hz (Davies *et al.*, 1985) (Fig. 14.2b). Likewise, the relation between isometric force and stimulation amplitude is sigmoidal (Davies *et al.*, 1985) (Fig. 14.2a). When amplitude is increased from the threshold of isometric force, rather large increases are required to induce modest increases in force. Thereafter, force increases abruptly with increases in amplitude until a plateau is realized (Fig. 14.2a). The plateau

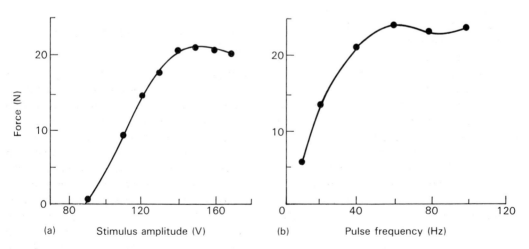

Fig. 14.2 The relationship between the amplitude of stimulation and tetanic force (a) and between pulse frequency and force (b) during transcutaneous EMS of the first dorsal interosseus muscle. Square pulses of 100 μs were used for a duration of 500 ms. The frequency of pulses was 40 Hz in (a). The amplitude of stimulation was supramaximal in (b). (From Davies *et al.*, 1985.)

is not always attained at forces greater than maximal voluntary isometric force (MVIF). In fact, few studies report forces during stimulation that are greater than MVIF.

A major hindrance to force development during EMS appears to be subject intolerance to pain. Along these lines, high-frequency stimulation has been suggested to be more tolerable (Moreno-Aranda & Seireg, 1981a,b). A carrier frequency of 10 000 Hz of a sinusoidal signal is used and modulated at 100 Hz. Moreover, the stimulation is applied with a duty cycle of 20%. The 10 000 Hz indicates that the pulse duration is 100 μs. The 100-Hz modulation indicates that the signal is given in 10-ms blocks. Finally, the duty cycle of 20% indicates that the stimulation is on for the first 2 ms of the 10-ms block. Thus, 20 sinusoidal 100-μs pulses are delivered continuously for the first 2 ms of each 10-ms block. The duration of the tetanic stimulation is around 1–2 s with 4–5 s rest. While this type of stimulation appears to be most tolerant, force development is not optimal, probably because of the short pulse duration.

In an effort to refute or substantiate the work of Kots and Chwilon (1971), several investigators have used medium frequency stimulation. The sinusoidal signal at 2500 Hz is modulated at 50 Hz. What is not obvious is that the signals are given with a 50% duty cycle. Thus, 400-μs pulses are delivered continuously for the first 10 ms of each 20-ms time period. The duration of the stimulation is usually a few seconds. Because the refractory period of motoneurones is around 3 ms (Miller et al., 1981), they are activated at most three times during each 10-ms period or 150 times per second for the fifty 10-ms blocks. In essence, 400-μs signals excite the motoneurones 150 times per second. Likewise, during high-frequency stimulation, the motoneurones are essentially activated by 100-μs duration pulses 100 times per second.

In the few studies where the interest has been to increase the endurance capacity of skeletal muscle, a markedly different stimulation protocol has been used (Scott et al., 1985).

Square wave 50-μs pulses were delivered at 5–10 Hz for 1 hour, three times daily.

Electrodes of a variety of different materials, such as aluminium foil or carbon–conditioned, have been used, generally in the bipolar configuration, for the application of EMS. The negative electrode is generally placed over the motor point of a given muscle or muscle group of interest, while the positive one is placed distally. In the case of the knee extensors, it has been shown that greater force is developed as electrode size increases (Alon, 1985) and that both electrodes need to be placed on this muscle group (Ferguson et al., 1989).

The pain sensations associated with EMS arise due to the non-homogeneity of the electrode–skin interface (Mason & Mackay, 1976). This results in localized areas of low resistance where current densities become large enough to exceed the threshold for damage. Wetting the electrodes prior to application provides a more uniform resistance and reduces occurrence of these 'hot-spots' (Mason & Mackay, 1976). Alternatively leaving the electrodes in place for 30 min prior to stimulation allows accumulation of insensible perspiration, which creates a more homogeneous electrode–skin interface.

Rationale for the use of EMS in conditioning athletes

The practical use of EMS obviously requires that it provide some advantage over voluntary muscle activation. In this regard two lines of reasoning have been proposed. First, it is suggested that neural factors limit force during maximal voluntary efforts. Thus, EMS can provide a more intense contraction to the muscle that is stimulated, and thereby induce greater adaptive responses (Delitto & Snyder-Mackler, 1990). How the EMS-trained muscle that could not be voluntarily activated before EMS is to be voluntarily activated after EMS is not clear (McDonagh & Davies, 1984).

It is generally accepted that the intensity of training, judged by the magnitude of the train-

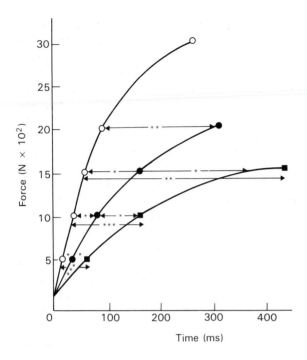

Fig. 14.3 Force plotted as a function of time during the bilateral isometric extension exercise that is similar to a leg press. Force is developed as rapidly as possible on auditory command. The male strength athletes were seven elite bodybuilders and power-lifters (○). The physically active males (●) ($n = 9$) and females (■) ($n = 10$) were not trained but engaged in different types of physical activities (e.g. jogging or weightlifting) one to three times per week. The symbols indicate a significant difference among groups in the time required to develop a given force. *, $P < 0.05$; **, $P < 0.01$; ***, $P < 0.001$. (From Ryushi et al., 1988.)

ing load, is the most important factor for inducing adaptive responses in strength/power athletes (Häkkinen & Keskinen, 1989). It is not so obvious how EMS could provide a greater training stimulus for these individuals. An increased ability to maximally activate skeletal muscle is a fundamental adaptive response to strength training (Komi, 1986). Moreover, strength training increases the rate of activation, and thereby the speed at which a given force can be developed (Fig. 14.3) (Ryushi et al., 1988). Finally, MVIF per unit cross-sectional area of skeletal muscle is markedly greater in strength/power trained athletes than active individuals (Ryushi et al., 1988; Häkkinen & Keskinen, 1989). This has been attributed in part to greater activation in the trained athletes. If strength/power athletes have developed such an impressive ability to activate their trained skeletal muscle, it is not clear how EMS could augment this adaptive response. Thus, it is not obvious how EMS could increase their intensity of training and thereby induce greater strength.

Secondly, the efficacy of EMS for strength training is based on the concept that fast twitch fibres, which are difficult to activate during maximal voluntary isometric efforts, are preferentially stimulated (Delitto & Snyder-Mackler, 1990). It is well known that as the force of voluntary isometric effort is progressively increased, motor units are recruited in a precise orderly manner (Henneman et al., 1965). There is considerable evidence suggesting that the difference in motoneurone size is the physiological basis for this orderly recruitment (for review see Burke, 1981). According to Henneman's 'size principle' the input resistance and thus susceptibility to discharge is inversely related to motoneurone size. Motor units innervated by the smallest alpha-motoneurones are comprised of slow twitch muscle fibres, which are few in number and small in diameter. Conversely, larger motoneurones innervate larger motor units containing fast muscle fibres. This arrangement ensures that for sustained low intensity exercise, small fatigue-resistant motor units are preferentially recruited.

Hultman *et al.* (1983) demonstrated that EMS of the thigh muscles of curarized patients fails to elicit a contraction even when voltage is far in excess of that needed to evoke force before curarization. It is therefore apparent that EMS does not directly activate the muscle. Instead, the stimulation current is propagated along the more excitable terminal nerve branches within the muscle.

Since muscle activation via EMS involves excitation of peripheral nerves and not direct stimulation of the muscle, the question arises as to whether motor units are activated in a specific order. It has been demonstrated that larger motoneurones have a lower threshold of electrical excitability (e.g. Solomonow *et al.*, 1986). This apparently occurs as a result of lower resistance offered by larger motoneurones. The use of EMS via surface electrodes may thus be expected to activate the largest units at the lowest stimulation level. Indeed, two recent reviews have concluded that EMS preferentially activates the large fast twitch motor units and thus occurs in reverse of the normal recruitment order (Enoka, 1988; Delitto & Snyder-Mackler, 1990). This preferential activation of fast motor units is thought (Enoka, 1988; Delitto & Snyder-Mackler, 1990) to be facilitated by afferent input from stimulation of cutaneous afferents, which inhibit motoneurones of slow motor units and excite motoneurones of fast motor units (Garnett & Stephens, 1981). EMS activates the distal motoneurone branches (Hultman *et al.*, 1983). It is, therefore, not clear how reflex inhibition of slow motoneurones via cutaneous afferent stimulation could override this distal motoneurone activation.

Indirect evidence to support this idea is provided by Cabric *et al.* (1988) who demonstrated that 19 days of EMS to the triceps surae for 10 min each day resulted in increases in myonuclei size and mitochondrial fraction. The greatest responses were suggested to occur in fast fibres. Unfortunately, inference that a fibre was a given type was made by indirect morphometric measures. It has recently been suggested, in a case study, that EMS causes preferential glycogen depletion in fast twitch type IIA fibres (Sinacore *et al.*, 1990). Thus, it was suggested that mainly this fibre type was stimulated. This was based on the observation that type IIA fibres showed qualitatively less glycogen staining intensity after than before a single bout of EMS. This observation is difficult to reconcile with the fact that the glycogen content of the mixed fibre biopsy samples was the same before and after stimulation.

Evidence that EMS does not preferentially activate fast twitch fibres has recently been presented by Knaflitz *et al.* (1990). Motor unit recruitment order was assessed by measuring conduction velocity and mean and median power frequency at different relative levels of voluntary or EMS force. Conduction velocity and mean and medium power frequency increase with increasing force during voluntary efforts, indicating the recruitment of progressively larger fibres with higher conduction velocities. It was demonstrated that for both voluntary and EMS-evoked muscle actions conduction velocity and mean and medium power frequency were less at lower force levels, suggesting activation of slower motor units. It was concluded that motor unit activation via EMS does not occur in reverse of the normal recruitment order. This may have occurred because large motor axons do not necessarily have large branches and/or because their motor branches may not have been oriented in the current field to favour activation.

The evidence is not clear, therefore, that EMS preferentially activates fast twitch fibres. If this were the case, it would appear to be advantageous as it has been suggested that the fast twitch fibre composition of a given muscle may ultimately determine the magnitude of the adaptive response to strength training (Häkkinen *et al.*, 1985). It is also obvious, however, that strength/power trained athletes have 'large' fast twitch fibres (Tesch, 1987). In fact, preferential fast twitch fibre hypertrophy is a common adaptive response to strength training (Tesch, 1987). This would suggest that these fibres are recruited during training, and that they respond accordingly. While the large fast twitch motor units may be difficult to activate during isometric efforts, they appear to be preferentially recruited during voluntary eccentric actions (Romanò & Schieppati 1987; Nardone & Schieppati, 1988; Nardone et al., 1989). Thus, it is not difficult to envision their repeated use during the high force repetitions of a weight-training exercise where both eccentric and concentric muscle actions are performed.

It seems that low-frequency long-term EMS might be used to increase the resistance to fatigue in endurance-trained athletes. This type of stimulation in lower mammals has been shown to induce several well-documented changes including an almost complete fast to slow twitch muscle conversion, and a marked increase and decrease in oxidative and glycolytic enzymes, respectively (Pette & Vrbovà, 1985). Moreover, fast twitch fibre degeneration and fibre atrophy occur (Maier et al., 1986). While the latter two responses are not especially attractive, skeletal muscle composed mainly of slow twitch fibres with a high aerobic capacity is characteristic of muscle tissue in endurance-trained athletes. The use of EMS to this end has received little attention. Three hours per day of 5–10-Hz EMS has been shown to increase the resistance to fatigue in tibialis anterior muscle of untrained females (Scott et al., 1985). It should be noted that the well-documented effects of low-frequency long-term stimulation of skeletal muscle of lower mammals has often been erroneously cited to support the use of artificial stimulation in EMS studies designed to increase muscle strength and size (e.g. see Delitto et al., 1989).

Data to support the efficacy of EMS in conditioning athletes

There are few reports of the effects of EMS on strength and muscle size in athletes. To the authors' knowledge, only three such papers exist. The work of Kots and Chwilon (1971) appears to have generated a substantial amount of interest in this ares. Kots suggests that athletes can enjoy strength improvements of 30–40% after only 4–5 weeks of EMS. The stimulation protocol uses medium-frequency EMS like that described above. A sinusoidal 2500-Hz signal modulated at 50 Hz is applied for 10 ms with a 10-ms interval between trains. Ten 10-s contractions are performed per day, 5 days each week for 4–5 weeks. There was a 50-s rest interval between contractions. It is argued that frequencies at this level minimize the sensation of pain, while maximizing force development during the isometric actions (Kots & Chwilon, 1971). It has been suggested elsewhere, however, that EMS at this frequency is in fact quite painful (Moreno-Aranda & Seireg, 1981a,b). It was indicated, but the actual data were not reported, that such EMS allows force development that is 10–30% greater than MVIF.

Unfortunately, Kots and colleagues have not been able to duplicate these results. Strength and muscle size were unchanged or reduced in 10 athletes after seven sessions of EMS (St Pierre et al., 1986). The EMS protocol described above was applied to the knee extensor muscle group during 7 days of the 8-day experiment. The authors indicated that EMS induced an isometric force that was 80–100% of MVIF, but again the actual data for either variable were not reported. Peak torque during isokinetic concentric muscle actions decreased on average by 10%. Interestingly, fast twitch fibre size decreased significantly in the males and did not change in the females. Slow twitch fibre size did not change for either group. These data do not seem to support the use of EMS in the conditioning of athletes.

The most convincing data to date to support the use of EMS in the conditioning of athletes were recently reported in a case study (Delitto et al., 1989). A weightlifter who competed in the 1984 Olympic Games was studied over the course of 3.5 months. Electromyostimulation of the knee extensors during isometric actions was done 3 days per week in conjunction with his normal training during weeks 5 through 8 and weeks 13 and 14. A 2500-Hz triangular wave interrupted at 75 pulses $\cdot$ s^{-1} was used to induce ten 11-s muscle actions per day. Three minutes of rest separated the isometric actions. In essence, 400-μs signals were delivered continuously for about the first 7 ms of each 14-ms time period. Because the refractory period of motoneurones is about 3 ms (Miller *et al.*, 1981), each 11-s isometric muscle action was induced using 400-μs signals delivered at 150 Hz. The amplitude of EMS was set to induce an isometric force equal to on average 112% of MVIF. As is usually the case, neither the stimulated nor voluntary isometric values were reported.

Most notable was that the one repetition maximum for the squat exercise increased about 20 kg during the periods of EMS. The one repetition maximum for the clean and jerk, and snatch also increased with EMS. The magnitude of these responses is impressive, especially in the squat, considering the level of the athlete. Elite weight trainees do not show such increases in strength over 2 years of training (Häkkinen *et al.*, 1988). Moreover, this study of Delitto and colleagues is one of the few studies that has examined and shown increased performance ability as a result of EMS. From the athletes perspective, this is obviously the most important concern.

It is difficult to ascertain the mechanism(s) responsible for the increased weightlifting ability. Both fast and slow twitch fibre size decreased significantly, such that relative fibre area actually decreased about 16%. The authors suggested that hyperplasia may have occurred and actually increased muscle mass. Hyperplasia of such an extent has not been reported for other models of muscle hypertrophy (Gollnick *et al.*, 1981; see also Chapter 8B). Electromyography was not conducted; thus it is not known whether increased neural activation occurred.

Directions for future research

The data to date are not convincing that EMS should be used by strength/power or endurance athletes to enhance their performance. The data in the case study of an elite Olympic weightlifter by Delitto *et al.* (1989) are exciting enough, however, to warrant further research. A well-controlled study to determine if EMS can enhance performance in strength/power athletes is needed. A sufficient number of subjects needs to be used to ensure scientific validity of the data. Control subjects must be used and an effort should be made to delineate the potential placebo effect of EMS *per se*. Moreover, measures of muscular performance during EMS and the competitive sport must be made. Finally, measures of muscle size, muscle performance and neural activation should be made to establish the mechanisms responsible for the adaptive responses, if any, induced by EMS.

Studies also need to be conducted to examine the effect of EMS that is applied during dynamic muscle actions. It has long been known that skeletal muscle of lower mammals activated artificially *in situ* develops force that is markedly greater during eccentric than isometric actions (Katz, 1939). Likewise, we have recently found that with EMS, force of the knee extensor muscle group is about 40% greater during eccentric than isometric muscle actions (Dudley *et al.*, 1990). Eccentric torque developed by the knee extensors during maximal voluntary efforts, in contrast, is not appreciably greater than isometric, at least for untrained individuals (Westing *et al.*, 1988). It should be possible, therefore, to elicit forces with EMS that are markedly greater than maximal voluntary force. Westing *et al.* (1989) have recently shown this to be the case. Electromyostimulation of the knee extensors was applied at an amplitude that resulted in an isometric torque (262 N $\cdot$ m) equal to about 85% of maximal voluntary isometric (306 N $\cdot$ m). The EMS torque (345 N $\cdot$ m) during eccentric actions was greater than maximal voluntary isometric (306 N $\cdot$ m) or eccentric (316 N $\cdot$ m) torque. Because the intensity of training, as judged by the magnitude of load acted against or the force developed during a given muscle action, is an important factor in inducing adaptive responses to strength/power training, EMS during eccentric actions warrants consideration as a training method.

It is well documented that long-term low-frequency stimulation of skeletal muscle in lower mammals results in mainly slow twitch fibres with a high mitochondrial content (Pette & Vrbová, 1985). These characteristics of skeletal muscle appear to be important attributes for successful competition in endurance-type sports. It seems reasonable, therefore, that low-frequency, long-term EMS should be investigated as a conditioning method to enhance the performance ability of these athletes.

Acknowledgements

The graphical assistance of Ms Susan Loffek is gratefully acknowledged. The research reported by the authors and the writing of this paper were supported under NASA contracts NAS10 10285 and NAS10 11624, respectively.

References

Alon, G. (1985) High voltage stimulation: Effects of electrode size on basic excitatory responses. *Physical Therapy*, **65**, 890–5.

Burke, R.E. (1981) Motor units: anatomy, physiology and functional organization. In V.B. Brooks (ed.) *Handbook of Physiology. The Nervous System, Section 1, Vol. II*, pp. 345–422. American Physiological Society, Bethesda.

Cabric, M., Appell, H.J. & Resic, A. (1988) Fine structural changes in electrostimulated human skeletal muscle. *European Journal of Applied Physiology*, **57**, 1–5.

Currier, D.P. & Mann, R. (1983) Muscular strength development by electrical stimulation in healthy individuals. *Physical Therapy*, **63**, 915–21.

Davies, C.T.M., Dooley, P., McDonagh, M.J.N. & White M.J. (1985) Adaptation of mechanical properties of muscle to high force training in man. *Journal of Physiology*, **365**, 277–84.

Delitto, A., Brown, M., Strube, M.J., Rose, S.J. & Lehman, R.C. (1989) Electrical stimulation of quadriceps femoris in an elite weight lifter: A single subject experiment. *International Journal of Sports Medicine*, **10**, 187–91.

Delitto, A. & Robinson, A.J. (1989) Electrical stimulation of muscle: techniques and applications. In L. Snyder-Mackler & A.J. Robinson (eds) *Clinical Electrophysiology: Electrotherapy and Electrophysiologic Testing*, pp. 95–138. Williams & Wilkins, Baltimore.

Delitto, A. & Snyder-Mackler, L. (1990) Two theories of muscle strength augmentation using percutaneous electrical stimulation. *Physical Therapy*, **70**, 158–64.

Dudley, G.A., Harris, R.T., Duvoisin, M.R., Hather, B.M. & Buchanan, P. (1990) Effect of voluntary vs. artificial activation on the relationship of muscle torque to speed. *Journal of Applied Physiology*, **69**, 2215–21.

Enoka, R.M. (1988) Muscle strength and its development, new perspectives. *Sports Medicine*, **6**, 146–68.

Eriksson, E. & Häggmark, T. (1979) Comparison of isometric muscle training and electrical stimulation supplementing isometric muscle training in the recovery after major knee ligament surgery. *American Journal of Sports Medicine*, **7**, 169–71.

Ferguson, J.P., Blackley, M.W., Knight, R.D., Sutlive, T.G., Underwood, F.B. & Greathouse, D.G. (1989) Effects of varying electrode site placements on the torque output of an electrically stimulated involuntary quadriceps femoris muscle contraction. *Journal of Orthopaedic and Sports Physical Therapy*, **11**, 24–9.

Garnett, R. & Stephens, J.A. (1981) Changes in the recruitment threshold of motor units produced by cutaneous stimulation in man. *Journal of Physiology*, **311**, 463–73.

Gollnick, P.D., Timson, B.F., Moore, R.L. & Riedy, M. (1981) Muscular enlargement and number of muscle fibers in skeletal muscles of rats. *Journal of Applied Physiology*, **50**, 936–43.

Gould, N., Donnermeyer, D., Gammon, G., Pope, M. & Ashikaga, T. (1983) Transcutaneous muscle stimulation to retard disuse atrophy after open meniscectomy. *Clinical Orthopaedics and Related Research*, **178**, 190–7.

Häkkinen, K. & Keskinen, K.L. (1989) Muscle cross-sectional area and voluntary force production characteristics in elite strength- and endurance-trained athletes and sprinters. *European Journal of Applied Physiology and Occupational Physiology*, **59**, 215–20.

Häkkinen, K., Komi, P.V. & Alén, M. (1985) Effect of explosive type strength training on isometric force- and relaxation-time, electromyographic and muscle fibre characteristics of leg extensor muscles. *Acta Physiologica Scandinavica*, **125**, 587–600.

Häkkinen, K., Pakarinen, A., Alén, M., Kauhanen, H. & Komi, P.V. (1988) Neuromuscular and hormonal adaptations in athletes to strength training in two years. *Journal of Applied Physiology*, **65**, 2406–12.

Henneman, E., Somjen, G. & Carpenter, D.O. (1965) Functional significance of cell size in spinal motor neurones. *Journal of Neurophysiology*, **28**, 560–80.

Hultman, E., Sjoholm, H., Jaderholm-Ek, I. & Krynicki, J. (1983) Evaluation of methods for electrical stimulation of human skeletal muscle *in situ*. *Pflügers Archiv*, **398**, 139–41.

Johnson, D.H., Thurston, P. & Ashcroft, P.J. (1977) The Russian technique of faradism in the treatment of chondromalacia patellae. *Physiotherapy Canada*, **29**, 266–8.

Katz, B. (1939) The relation between force and speed in muscular contraction. *Journal of Physiology*, **96**, 45–64.

Knaflitz, M., Merletti, R. & DeLuca, C.J. (1990) Inference of motor unit recruitment order in voluntary and electrically elicited contractions. *Journal of Applied Physiology*, **68**, 1657–67.

Komi, P.V. (1986) Training of muscle strength and power: Interaction of neuromotoric, hypertrophic, and mechanical factors. *International Journal of Sports Medicine*, **7**, 10–15.

Kots, Y. & Chwilon, W. (1971) Muscle training with the electrical stimulation method. *Teoriya i Prakitka Fizicheskoi Kultury USSR*, **3/4**.

Kramer, J.F. & Mendryk, S.W. (1982) Electrical stimulation as a strength improvement technique: a review. *Journal of Orthopaedic and Sports Physical Therapy*, **4**, 91–8.

Laughman, R.K., Youdas, J.W., Garrett, T.R. & Chao, E.Y.S. (1983) Strength changes in the normal quadriceps femoris muscle as a result of electrical stimulation. *Physical Therapy*, **63**, 494–9.

McDonagh, M.J.N. & Davies, C.T.M. (1984) Adaptive response of mammalian skeletal muscle to exercise with high loads. *European Journal of Applied Physiology*, **52**, 139–55.

Maier, A., Gambke, B. & Pette, D. (1986) Degeneration–regeneration as a mechanism contributing to the fast to slow conversion of chronically stimulated fast-twitch rabbit muscle. *Cell and Tissue Research*, **244**, 635–43.

Mason, J.L. & Mackay, N.A.M. (1976) Pain sensations associated with electrocutaneous stimulation. *IEEE Transactions on Biomedical Engineering*, **23**, 405–9.

Miller, R.G., Mirka, A. & Maxfield, M. (1981) Rate of tension development in isometric contractions of a human hand muscle. *Experimental Neurology*, **73**, 267–85.

Moreno-Aranda, J. & Seireg, A. (1981a) Electrical parameters for over-the-skin muscle stimulation. *Journal of Biomechanics*, **14**, 579–85.

Moreno-Aranda, J. & Seireg, A. (1981b) Investigation of over-the-skin electrical stimulation parameters for different normal muscles and subjects. *Journal of Biomechanics*, **14**, 587–93.

Nardone, A., Romanò, C. & Schieppati, M. (1989) Selective recruitment of high-threshold human motor units during voluntary isotonic lengthening of active muscles. *Journal of Physiology*, **409**, 451–71.

Nardone, A. & Schieppati, M. (1988) Shift of activity from slow to fast muscle during voluntary lengthening contractions of the triceps surae muscles in humans. *Journal of Physiology*, **395**, 363–81.

Pette, D. & Vrbová, G. (1985) Invited review: Neural control of phenotypic expression in mammalian muscle fibers. *Muscle and Nerve*, **8**, 676–89.

Romanò, C. & Schieppati, M. (1987) Reflex excitability of human soleus motoneurones during voluntary shortening or lengthening contractions. *Journal of Physiology*, **390**, 271–84.

Ryushi, T., Häkkinen, K., Kauhanen, H. & Komi, P.V. (1988) Muscle fiber characteristics, muscle cross-sectional area and force production in strength athletes, physically active males and females. *Scandinavian Journal of Sports Science*, **10**, 7–15.

Scott, O.M., Vrbova, G., Hyde, S.A. & Dubowitz, V. (1985) Effects of chronic low frequency electrical stimulation on normal human tibialis anterior muscle. *Journal of Neurology, Neurosurgery, and Psychiatry*, **48**, 774–81.

Sinacore, D.R., Delitto, A., King, D.S. & Rose, S.J. (1990) Type II fiber activation with electrical stimulation: a preliminary report. *Physical Therapy*, **70**, 416–22.

Solomonow, M., Baratta, R., Shoji, H. & D'Ambrosia, R. (1986) The myoelectric signal of electrically stimulated muscle during recruitment: an inherent feedback parameter for a closed loop control scheme. *IEEE Transactions on Biomedical Engineering*, **33**, 735–45.

St Pierre, D., Taylor, A.W., Lavoie, M., Sellers, W. & Kots, Y.M. (1986) Effects of 2500 Hz sinusoidal current on fibre area and strength of the quadriceps femoris. *Journal of Sports Medicine*, **26**, 60–6.

Tesch, P.A. (1987) Acute and long-term metabolic changes consequent to heavy-resistance exercise. *Medicine and Sport Science*, **26**, 67–89.

Westing, S.H., Seger, J.Y., Karlson, E. & Ekblom, B. (1988) Eccentric and concentric torque–velocity characteristics of the quadriceps femoris in man. *European Journal of Applied Physiology*, **58**, 100–4.

Westing, S.H., Seger, J. & Thorstensson, A. (1989) Does neural inhibition suppress eccentric knee extension torque in man? *Medicine and Science in Sports and Exercise*, **21**, S67.

Wigerstad-Lossing, I., Grimby, G., Jonsson, T., Morelli, B., Peterson, L. & Renstrom, P. (1988) Effects of electrical muscle stimulation combined with voluntary contractions after knee ligament surgery. *Medicine and Science in Sports and Exercise*, **20**, 93–8.

Chapter 15

Clinical Aspects of Strength and Power Training

GUNNAR GRIMBY

General effects of immobilization and reduced muscle activation

Immobilization and reduced muscle activation will result in muscle wasting. Hypotrophy of a specific fibre type may dominate such as hypotrophy of type I (slow twitch) fibres at immobilization with short muscle length, e.g. soleus at a plantar flexed foot after Achilles tendon injury, quadriceps at immobilization with straight knee (Häggmark et al., 1981) or of type II (fast twitch) fibres at a lack of activation of the higher threshold motor units (disuse atrophy).

Muscle strength is in principle proportionate to the cross-sectional area of the musculature, providing a complete activation at maximal effort. In the immobilized or injured state, however, full maximal voluntary activation may not be the case, either as an unspecific effect of disuse (lack of optimal neural drive) or due to reflex inhibition (Stokes & Young, 1984). The condition will be still more complex if there also are soft tissue lesions, which may involve muscle tissue as well as nerves. It is of special importance to identify any inhibitory influence in order to eliminate or reduce such factors.

It is noteworthy that inhibition may be present without any sensation of pain or discomfort. Even mild joint effusion may result in significant reduction in muscle activation (Stokes & Young, 1984). Still more obvious is a painful state, as in the immediate postoperative phase after knee surgery (Arvidsson et al.,

1986b). Monitoring electromyography (EMG) is the direct approach to follow the degree of voluntary muscle activation and its variation with the degree of inhibition. In a clinical situation and for repeated assessments, EMG recordings may, however, not be feasible. Indirect evidence of lack of full muscle activation at strength measurement can be achieved from comparison of the recorded force and the cross-sectional muscle area. If the area cannot be measured by computerized tomography or ultrasound, the clinician should be aware of the limitations of circumference measurements. Up to 25% side difference in thigh muscle cross-sectional area may be masked by increase in other tissue structures (subcutaneous fat) in the injured or immobilized side with muscle atrophy.

A theoretical well-based approach to analyse the degree of maximal voluntary muscle activation is the technique of electrial stimulation with superimposed single twitches. The stimulatory intensity to achieve a maximal single twitch is identified. At submaximal voluntary muscle activation an increase in the recorded force is seen at the twitch stimulation, whereas this is not the case at full voluntary activation of the muscle. The technique has also been demonstrated reliably in transcutaneous stimulation of, for example, the quadriceps muscle (Rutherford et al., 1986b). This approach is rather simple to handle and may therefore be more used in a clinical situation in the future, providing a dynamometer and an electrical stimulator that can deliver single twitches are available. As another alternative stimulation with superimposed short tetanic trains may also be used.

Risks and injury prevention

Overload on muscle, connective tissue and joint structures

MUSCLE SORENESS

During physical training, specifically in an untrained state, minor lesion of the muscle structure and inflammation resulting in muscle soreness is a common problem (for review see, e.g. Ebbeling & Clarkson, 1989). The background of soreness may be several and includes myofibrillar damage localized to the Z-band, membrane damage, oedema, swelling and inflammatory processes. The serum or plasma level of creatine kinase (CK) is elevated, and is considered as an indicator of muscle damage as CK is found almost exclusively in muscle tissue. The muscle function deteriorates and there may even be a reduced muscle strength for a week or more after intensive eccentric exercise. It is possible to distinguish between immediate soreness and delayed soreness. The delayed soreness usually has its maximum about 2 days after the exertion. It is clearly demonstrated that eccentric activities play a dominant role for the delayed soreness. In the untrained individual even a moderate amount of eccentric exercise may result in delayed but also immediate soreness. There is, however, clear evidence that there is an adaptive process so that at repeated training sessions the soreness and concomitant reduction in muscle function will be less (Fridén et al., 1983). Even during the soreness period, moderate activity is advised, as the adaptation response is prior to full recovery and restoration of muscle function. Several hypotheses have been presented to explain the adaptation. Stress-susceptible fibres or susceptible areas within a fibre may be eliminated and then regenerated, muscle fibres

and/or connective tissue may be strengthened by the initial bout of exercise or there may be a more homogeneous recruitment of adjacent muscle fibres belonging to different motor units.

A somewhat different type of soreness and reduced muscle function may occur during very long and intense exercise bouts, probably not related to the muscle tension development but to the total metabolic load. Such exercise-induced symptoms may have several components, one being connected to the production of free radicals resulting in membrane damage. Free radicals are produced in metabolic processes involving oxygen and metabolism of purine nucleotides by the enzyme xanthine oxidase. The production of free radicals may be a factor causing muscle damage also during intermittent resistive type of exercise over a longer period. Research has to be pursued to further understand these processes and the possibility of using free radical scavengers to reduce such effects. Another component may be a direct catabolic effect on the muscle cells, as in extreme conditions of high intensity exercise for a prolonged period.

OVERWORK

Besides the extreme conditions mentioned above with overwork it can be questioned whether overwork phenomena exists even at more moderate training regimes over an extended period. It is well known that intense training, or overtraining, may lead to mood disturbances and reduce the effect of training with decrease in performance. Whether this is actually related to 'pure' structural and functional changes of the musculature is more of an open question.

In the strength-training situation using high resistive exercises, muscle fibre hypertrophy will result, with the size of individual muscle fibres doubling or more. In this process fibre hyperplasia may also occur, even if that is not a main factor of the training-induced increase in muscle volume. Whether muscle fibres during extreme training may proportionately increase their contractile properties is not very well studied. An extreme adaptive situation occurs when a large reduction in the number of motor units is seen, e.g. the post-polio condition, and has demonstrated the marked adaptive potential of the muscle fibre, with hypertrophy up to two to three times normal fibre size (Grimby *et al.*, 1989) without any obvious negative effects at continuous levels of physical activity.

One negative side of extreme muscle fibre hypertrophy is, however, the relatively low mitochondrial activity and capillary density, with increased diffusion distances resulting in reduced endurance capacity for that musculature. Such a negative effect of an extreme strengthening programme may be reduced by adding endurance training to the regime.

CONNECTIVE TISSUE

Overload on connective tissue is associated with the effect of tension development of ligaments healing after injury or surgery. Caution in this respect has mainly been raised for the cruciate ligaments of the knee. Active leg extension exercises create deforming forces on the anterior cruciate ligament from 60 to 0° knee ankle, with the majority of anterior cruciate ligament stress occurring between 30 to 0° (Renström *et al.*, 1986; Silfverskiöld *et al.*, 1988). Few *in vivo* studies have, however, been performed including assessment of cocontraction of the hamstrings and quadriceps muscles. By such a coactivation there is a protective effect on the anterior cruciate ligament graft, as the hamstrings function is synergistic with the anterior cruciate ligament, preventing the anterior tibial displacement produced by the quadriceps activation in the terminal degree of extension of the knee. One of the problems at injury or graft replacement of the ligament may be loss of signals from the mechanoreceptors, which are important for the hamstrings activation. The half-squat exercise could be a 'safe'

way to achieve a combined quadriceps and hamstrings activation. The weight-bearing bend includes concentric as well as eccentric exercises.

JOINT STRUCTURES

Muscle activation will lead to compressive forces of variable degree on joint structures. One way to achieve a high degree of neural activation, and at the same time a rather moderate degree of torque development and, thus, relatively low compressive force of joint structures, is the high velocity isokinetic training principle. Such a training regime has therefore been advocated for neural activation but may have less marked effect on the muscle volume where the produced tension in the muscle is supposed to be the stimulus for protein synthesis. Another way to reduce load on joint structures is to perform exercises without weight-bearing such as on the various dynamometers and by using bicycle or swimming exercises.

Reduction of forces on joint surfaces may, however, sometimes be in conflict to the reduction of load on the ligaments. One such example, which has been discussed, is the increase in patello–femoral joint reaction force at knee angles between 25 and 60°, when on the other hand the strain is less on the anterior cruciate ligaments than at a more extended position.

Injury prevention

The effects of strength training in injury prevention is an important area but with many unanswered questions. It is related to muscle as well as to tendons, ligaments and bone tissue and includes also aspects on proprioceptive function and motor control.

MUSCLE STRENGTH

A number of studies have examined the ratio of muscle strength between agonists and antagonists, especially of the knee joint. The hamstrings quadriceps (H/Q) ratio has been used as indication of the appropriate strength relationship. However, there are several limitations in the use of this ratio. The peak torque does not appear at the same knee angle for knee extension as for knee flexion; thus, comparison of quadriceps and hamstrings torque values should be made at the same knee angle and not with peak torque values. In many reports the type of measurements are not clearly stated. Furthermore, the importance of the ratio may be different in different parts of the range of motion, due to the functional coactivation of quadriceps and hamstrings, as in the terminal phase of extension (Draganich et al., 1989). One main objection is also that when the quadriceps activity is concentric, the hamstrings activity is eccentric. Dvir et al. (1989) have also demonstrated that the ratio between hamstrings eccentric peak torque and quadriceps concentric peak torque could discriminate between an anterior cruciate ligament (ACL)-insufficient knee and the uninjured knee but not the concentric H/Q ratio.

One of the main implications of the coactivation of hamstrings is to prevent anterior tibial displacement. This may amount for up to 20% of maximal activation in the sitting knee extension. Comparable observations during weight-bearing knee extension is not available. The amount of force development speaks, however, in favour of the importance of appropriate motor control, including reflex activation from mechanoreceptors as well as central nervous activation.

Another aspect on the limitation of the H/Q ratio is the large individual differences as reported by Kannus (1988). In ACL-knees as well as in healthy knees a high intersubject variability can be seen in the H/Q ratio. However, the injured knee had higher H/Q ratio than the healthy knee in all subjects. When comparing with standardized knee-scoring scales, the outcome was significantly better in the subject whose H/Q ratio of the injured knee was similar to that of their uninjured knee, but

the absolute H/Q ratio was of no significant importance. Thus, the H/Q ratio comparison should be made with the uninjured side and of concentric quadriceps with eccentric hamstrings torque values. Further consideration should be given to the importance of different knee angles.

Several authors have suggested that screening of H/Q ratios would be of value in predicting athletes at risk for injury, e.g. Parker et al., 1983. However, as emphasized also by Fleck and Falkel (1986) in their review, future studies are needed to understand the relationship between muscular imbalance and injury risks as well as identifying normative values and appropriate measurement procedures.

Studies on upper extremity muscle function have demonstrated that progressive exercise training of wrist extensors and flexors will prevent tennis elbow pain (Kulund et al., 1979). Also, in swimmers the ratio of external rotation muscular endurance/internal rotation muscular endurance was lower in those with shoulder pain than in those without (Fleck & Falkel, 1986) and indicates that strength training of the external rotators may prevent impingement shoulder problems. Several examples of similar benefit of specific strength training programmes to prevent pain and injury may be found.

TENDONS AND LIGAMENTS

As with other structures, tendon and ligaments adapt to physical activity by increased thickness, weight and strength (for review see, e.g. Tipton et al., 1986). When stress is applied to bone–ligament–bone preparations separation will occur at the attachment site of the ligament. Junction strength is not the same in all ligaments and is low in, for example, the medial collateral ligament. Studies on different animals have clearly demonstrated that immobilization will decrease and physical activity increase the strength of connective tissue.

The same effect of activity holds true also for the connective tissue within and around the muscle itself. This represents a major part of the viscoelastic properties of the muscle itself and also acts to protect against overload of the muscle. Strength training can increase the collagen content of the muscle, indicating an increase in strength of the epimysium (the connective tissue around the entire muscle), perimysium (around groups of muscle fibres) and endomysium (surrounding individual muscle fibres).

BONE DENSITY

Much has been discussed on the decline in bone density during inactivity and in ageing. The prevention of the reduction in bone density would be of great importance in reducing the risk of fractures. Not least in connection with space research, the importance of the activation of antigravity muscles to prevent bone mineral loss has been demonstrated. The longitudinal forces on bones are necessary as a stimulus for maintaining bone mineral content, and muscle activity itself is not sufficient to prevent the negative effects of loss of antigravity forces.

There are a number of studies where bone mineral content has been compared in trained and untrained individuals, and it has been demonstrated that athletes who had the greatest strain on the lower limbs had the highest bone mineral content. Even moderate activity is sufficient to produce an increase in bone mineral content compared to sedentary individuals. Specific studies on strength training and bone mineral content are not available, but it must be assumed that resistance training sufficient to activate antigravity muscles will prevent bone mineral loss during immobilization and contribute to the regain in bone mineral content at the subsequent activation.

In women bone mineral density has aroused special interest with its connection to oestrogen levels. The bone density falls at menopause. The importance of maintaining bone mineral density by sports activity in middle-aged women should therefore be stressed, as should the risk for fractures from falls if activities are undertaken without due preparation. High intensity endurance training in young women may cause amenorrhoea and changes in hormone balance leading to reduced bone mineral density. The question may arise whether large amounts of very intense strength training will have similar negative effects or if these effects will be counteracted by sufficient activity of the antigravity muscles, which is likely to be the case in the relatively few number of women engaged in such hard training.

SKELETAL STRESS OF STRENGTH TRAINING

There are some observations that certain sport activities may be harmful to the skeletal system causing injury particularly of the spine. In exercises with heavy lifts it is important that the training is performed with proper technique, so that the compressive stress will not be excessive. However, in follow-up studies on various athletes, spinal abnormalities were overrepresented in those engaged in the more vigorous sports, especially male gymnasts and wrestlers (Swärd et al., 1989).

Muscle strength in follow-up studies after injury

In a number of follow-up studies in athletes at various intervals after their injury, persistent reduction in muscle strength has been demonstrated. There may be several reasons, such as reduced activity due to the injury, remaining inhibition, insufficient training or lack of awareness of a moderate strength reduction. Thus, there are differences whether there still is an insufficient joint function or if there is near or complete recovery after the injury. The possibility of remaining inhibition has already been discussed. The lack of awareness of a remaining strength reduction is connected to the inability to detect moderate (10–20%) side difference in strength, and is found also in athletes who have resumed full athletic training (Grimby et al., 1980). It can be explained by the fact that bilateral maximal force development is not required in many sports, but presumably side differences would be subjectively easier to detect in sports such as rowing or weightlifting, where there is bilateral maximal muscle activation. Athletes, as well as the physician, physiotherapist and trainer, should be aware of non-perceived muscle weakness. The use of objective tests, both functional tests related closely to the specific demands of the sport activity, and dynamometer tests, should be encouraged to demonstrate full recovery before finishing the rehabilitation regime.

Some studies with reports on muscle strength after knee injury will be summarized below to exemplify the documented experience.

With ACL insufficiency due to incomplete tear of the ACL there was a significant reduction in quadriceps but not in hamstrings strength compared to the uninjured side in patients studied on average 11 months after onset of symptoms (Dvir et al., 1989). Hamstrings function can, however, also be dependent on time, as hamstrings endurance measures (total work for 30 consecutive isokinetic maximal actions at π rad $\cdot$ s^{-1}) were reduced in subjects less than 40 months after ACL reconstruction but not later (Harter et al., 1990). The need for long-term rehabilitative programmes is advocated.

In a long-term follow up, 8 years after ACL injury, (Kannus et al., 1987) remaining strength deficit was noted in the quadriceps but also, though less marked, in the hamstrings muscles. Knee strength correlated well with estimates of thigh atrophy and was especially noted at high velocities of muscle action.

Arvidsson et al. (1981) also pointed out that patients operated for knee ligament injuries may not improve muscle function in the operated leg over the years. Thus, the major part of the patients in a follow-up study 5–10 years after surgery had reduced quadriceps torque values. The importance of objectively recording muscle strength was stressed by these authors and many others, as was the need for continuous strength and endurance training as well as avoidance of inhibitory factors. The functional consequences of the maintained reduction in muscle strength can be illustrated by the correlation between the increase in quadriceps and hamstrings strength after ACL reconstruction and the return to functional activities as demonstrated (Arvidsson et al., 1981; Seto et al., 1988).

In follow-up studies interest has also been given to the selective hypotrophy of a specific fibre type in the quadriceps muscle. In an early report (Edström, 1970) hypotrophy of the slow twitch type I fibres was demonstrated in persons with unstable knees especially with remaining pain. Later studies have, however, demonstrated a reduction in type II fibres in relation to type I fibre size (Grimby et al., 1980; Baughner et al., 1984). This could be explained by the activity pattern of the unstable ACL-insufficient knees, which function in stance, walking and other activities of daily living, recruiting mainly type I fibres, but less recruiting of type II fibres which occurs in activities requiring rapid acceleration or deceleration (Baughner et al., 1984). If so, more emphasis should be put on exercise programmes directed at the fast twitch type II fibres.

Treatment aspects

Prevention of reflex inhibition

Of fundamental importance to avoid muscle weakness and subsequently muscle wasting is to prevent reflex inhibition. A typical situation is the knee after injury or in the postoperative phase, but the principal aspects are true for other joints. Two principles for prevention of reflex inhibition are specially emphasized in this review: pain relief and joint position.

PAIN

Reflex inhibition is associated with but not bound to the occurrence of pain. Treatment is at first directed towards the reduction of pain, using analgesics; peroral, local or epidural anaesthesia. The effectiveness of epidural anaesthesia in the immediate postoperative phase in increasing neural activation, as seen from EMG recordings, has been demonstrated by Arvidsson, *et al.* (1986b), but naturally its clinical value for maintaining muscle force has only a limited period of action. Later, non-invasive techniques are needed, with the best documentation concerning the use of transcutaneous electrical nerve stimulation (TENS). Thus, TENS has been shown to be significantly more effective than placebo (Jensen *et al.*, 1985; Arvidson & Eriksson, 1986), but more detailed studies have to be performed to identify the best procedures and modalities to avoid reflex inhibition associated with postinjured/postoperative pain.

JOINT EFFUSION AND JOINT POSITION

It has been clearly demonstrated that even a moderate degree of joint swelling without noticeable pain can create reflex inhibition (Stokes & Young, 1984). The amount of quadriceps inhibition after knee injury is partly dependent on the knee angle, with less inhibition in a flexed than in a full extension position (Shakespeare *et al.*, 1985). A possible reason for the increased inhibition in the extended position may be increased intra-articular pressure. To avoid knee effusion the choice of knee joint position during quadriceps muscle training is important; a knee joint range having the least intra-articular pressure (15–60° of flexion) should be used in resting and training. Different modalities and choice of position have been suggested (see for example Antich & Brewster, 1986) but few have been scientifically tested.

Neural activation

A major problem after immobilization and/or injury is the lack of optimal neural activation, which has already been discussed. Besides prevention of reflex inhibition, the principal treatment modalities are the use of functional oriented training, including those based on neurophysiological principles, dynamometer training, biofeedback and voluntary training

supported with electrical muscle stimulation. The specific effects of various training programmes, such as the limited effects of training to specific joint angles or angular velocities of the exercises used, has to be considered.

FUNCTIONAL TRAINING PRINCIPLES

In so-called functional training programmes, the patient mainly has to activate his/her musculature in normally occurring activities. This means for the knee joint that it aims to enhance dynamic stability including use of proprioceptive information, motor control and appropriate muscle force development. It may start with walking and jumping on two legs, then incorporating different types of balancing and jumping, jogging, running and later sprinting. Strength may improve, as also performance in performance tests, as well as with a strict dynamometer (isokinetic) programme (Tegner, 1990). Such an experience demonstrates the importance of functional training for improving neural activation and motor control. As will be pointed out in connection with training for muscle hypertrophy, combined training programmes may be of optimal benefit. The use of different neurophysiological principles for facilitating the neural activation of the musculature, such as proprioceptive neuromuscular facilitation (PNF), has its original place in the treatment of patients with muscle weakness due to neural lesions or neuromuscular diseases. It has not been used or documented to any great extent in the treatment of sports injuries. Among the general principles, however, that are common is the use of verbal, in certain situations also tactile, stimuli, rhythmic stabilization and the use of coactivation of muscles in naturally occurring synergism, e.g. diagonal movements (Engle & Canner, 1989).

Weakness, even if present (e.g. Lentell *et al.*, 1990), may not be the major functional deficit in chronic ankle instability, where proprioceptive deficits have a greater functional import as shown by several studies. As a consequence when muscle weakness is present proprioceptive activities should be the primary consideration combined with strengthening exercises in the training programme.

DYNAMOMETER TRAINING

With the introduction of new dynamometers, either with the isokinetic principle or with variable resistance, there has been an increased use and knowledge of dynamometer training in different clinical conditions. In addition, dynamometers also including eccentric loading have recently become available. For discriminating the effect on neural activation from that on muscle hypertrophy, reliable measurements of EMG are necessary in addition to strength measurements. For the increase in neural activation, the specificity of joint angle and speed of motion has to be considered, as also the use of the open (as in dynamometers) vs. the closed kinematic chain exercise.

Studies in uninjured as well as injured subjects have demonstrated the dominant role of increased neural activation in the early phase of dynamometer training (e.g. Komi & Buskirk, 1972; Moritani & deVries 1979; Komi, 1984; Sale, 1986; Enoka, 1988). The neural mechanisms in uninjured and in injured subjects include reflex potentiation, motor unit synchronization, improved coordination and learning. Experience from healthy subjects are dealt with in other chapters of this book. Unfortunately, examples in injured subjects that discriminate between increase in muscle strength through neural activation from that due to muscular factors are lacking.

One indirect approach to obtain evidence of the importance of neural factors at dynamometer training is through the specificity of the exercise programme. The speed and angular specific effects have mainly been reported in healthy subjects. Thomeé et al. (1987) could demonstrate in ACL patients 3–12 months after surgery that fast speed isokinetic training gave a larger strength increase at the higher speed than at slower speeds. Also, the

cross-sectional area of the fast twitch type II muscle fibres tended to increase more with a fast training regime than with slow training. The cross-over effects are other examples of neural factors as demonstrated in the study by Grimby et al. (1980) in isokinetic as well as in weight training, with a training effect in both uninjured and injured leg by 6 weeks training about 18 months after surgery.

There are, however, in the literature contradictory observations concerning the specificity of training programmes in postinjured patients, which may be due to different training periods duration and intensity. Ingemann-Hansen and Halkjaer-Kristensen (1985), thus, found no significant difference in training effects when comparing 4 weeks of progressive resistance exercise, maximum isometric action, isokinetic low and high speed actions after 4–6 weeks of immobilization in cast due to knee ligament injuries. However, their subjects started their training as early as 7 days after cast removal and therefore pain and inflammatory reactions might have been limiting factors.

In dynamometer training sufficient muscle activity has to be developed also to recruit the high threshold motor units. Information from healthy subjects (e.g. Gollnick et al., 1974) cannot be transformed directly to patients subject to reflex inhibition as well as to muscle wasting. Relative, and not absolute, activity seems to determine the motor unit recruitment. In a study of patients after leg injury, with about 60% of normal muscle strength and using 30% of actual muscle strength of a muscle, type II fibres were found to be activated at around 20% of normal muscle strength (Hultén et al., 1981) (Fig. 15.1). This is comparable to the relative force (torque) for recruitment of type II fibres in normals (Gollnick et al., 1974).

The importance of voluntary effort to overcome a resistance has recently been especially emphasized when comparing the neural activation with variable resistance dynamometer with that using the isokinetic principle, where the load is directly determined by the effort of the subject. Thus, higher EMG recordings could be

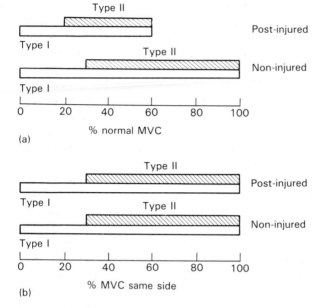

Fig. 15.1 Schematic pattern for recruitment of slow twitch motor units (type I muscle fibres) (□) and fast twitch motor units (type II muscle fibres) (▨) in relation to normal (a) and actual (b) percentage of maximal voluntary contraction (MVC) in postinjured and non-injured sides. For further explanation see text.

noted with a variable resistance dynamometer than with the isokinetic dynamometer, both using maximal effort. This further illustrates the importance of considering different facilitatory techniques to achieve a maximal voluntary muscle activation at the point of training, where the aim is to recruit all types of motor units.

BIOFEEDBACK

Biofeedback can be used in different ways in connection to strength training. A common approach, although not scientifically tested, is to let the subject get visual feedback from the torque recordings on a screen or indicator. The use of EMG biofeedback has been evaluated in a number of studies (Wise *et al.*, 1984; Morrisey, 1989). It has been reported to be more effective than electrical muscle strength stimulation to increase the EMG activity in the vastus lateralis, though more research is needed in this area (Morrisey, 1989).

ELECTRICAL MUSCLE STIMULATION

Electrical muscle stimulation (EMS) in the early phase of strength training or to prevent reduc-

tion in strength by immobilization may have an effect on neural activation—by preventing (TENS effect) or overriding reflex inhibition and by supporting a simultaneous voluntary activation, but is naturally also directed at muscle factors. It must be pointed out that in order to enhance the neural drive to the muscle, EMS has to be combined with voluntary muscle contractions. It has been discussed whether the nerve activation pattern is different in EMS compared with voluntary muscle activation. In the latter, low-threshold slow twitch motor units innervating type I muscle fibres will be activated first, followed by motor units with higher threshold (fast twitch, type II fibres). It has also been clearly demonstrated that with direct nerve stimulation, as applied by implanted electrodes, larger axons belonging to the fast twitch type II muscle fibres will be activated first as they have the lowest threshold of electrical excitability. However, with surface stimulation as used with EMS, there is no convincing evidence that this holds true. In fact, Knaflitz *et al.* (1990) recently showed that with electrical surface stimulation of a muscle, motor unit recruitment order similar to voluntary contraction was most common. This could be explained by changes in the diameter of axonal branches and by geometric factors.

In summary, the order of motor unit activation with EMS depends on three factors at least (Enoka, 1988): (i) the diameter of the motor axon, (ii) the distance between the axon and the active electrode, and (iii) the effect of input to motoneurones from cutaneous afferents activated by EMS.

When used clinically with the highest tolerable stimulating intensity all terminal nerve twigs within a territory will probably be depolarized and this, combined with voluntary muscle activation, leads to contraction of all muscle fibres in the muscle providing the EMS has a sufficient depolarization current amplitude. One clinical use of EMS is to direct muscle activity specifically to a single component or head of a large muscle group, such as training of the vastus medialis (Bohannon, 1983), where selective inhibition has been noted (Wise et al., 1984).

In normal individuals, EMS with or without voluntary contraction has been demonstrated to give equivalent effects with a voluntary muscle training programme only. Some studies in the early phase of postoperative rehabilitation after ACL surgery indicate a more pronounced effect of EMS combined with simultaneous voluntary contractions. Wigerstad-Lossing et al. (1988) could, thus, report that EMS treatment (frequency 30 Hz, on–off time 6/10 s) in patients while immobilized in a cast for 6 weeks could limit strength reduction to about half of that in patients performing voluntary exercises only. Also, the cross-sectional area of the quadriceps muscle was less reduced after EMS plus voluntary contraction than after voluntary contractions only. Daily stimulation of periods at least 4 × 10 min is recommended. Eriksson and Häggmark (1979) and Arvidsson et al. (1986a) could also demonstrate the limitation of muscle wasting by EMS during immobilization, as also did DeLitto et al. (1988) concerning muscle strength. Even EMS without voluntary contraction but with a very long stimulating period (8 hours a day, frequency 50 Hz, on–off time 10/50 s) may limit the reduc-

tion in strength and muscle volume (Morrisey et al., 1985), but the beneficial effect of the simultaneous voluntary activation is lost.

In contrast, some authors report no significant protection in quadriceps strength loss by EMS alone (5 days per week, 1 hour daily at 10 or 50 Hz) (Halkjaer-Kristenson & Ingemann-Hansen, 1985) or by a combination of EMS (8 hours daily, frequency 40 Hz, on–off time 10/36 s) and isometric action for 6 weeks following ACL reconstruction (Sisk et al., 1987).

Most experiences of EMS in postinjured patients are with relatively low frequency (30–50 Hz) rectangular, asymmetric-balanced, biphasic pulses. The highest tolerable stimulating intensity using a constant current apparatus is most commonly used. In healthy subjects a number of reports have appeared in recent years using high-frequency sine-wave stimulators, which are constant-voltage monitored. It has been advocated that this apparatus can give higher tolerable contraction forces, maybe due to less discomfort from skin receptors. Whether this is the case in postoperative subjects remains to be documented. Only a few reports in patients (e.g. DeLitto et al., 1988) are available. However, in healthy well-motivated subjects Grimby and Wigerstad-Lossing (1989) could not document less discomfort or higher contraction forces with high-frequency (2500 Hz in trains of 50 Hz) stimulation than with rectangular low-frequency (30 Hz) stimulation. As nerve depolarization is determined by the strength of the current field, constant-current stimulators may give a more constant stimulus effect than constant-voltage stimulators due to variations in skin resistance. Both type of stimulators may, however, be clinically useful.

Muscle structure

When reflex inhibition is avoided and neural activation is optimal or near optimal, a major effect on muscle structure can be expected. The main emphasis has been placed on muscle hypertrophy, demonstrated by an increased cross-sectional area of the muscle as measured by computerized tomography. Other structural effects with an impact on strength development should also be considered, such as increase in the volume density of contractile proteins or increase in intracellular connective tissue matrix among muscle fibres enhancing the proportion of sarcomere force that can be transmitted to the skeletal system (Enoka, 1988). There is evidence suggesting that changes in quality and quantity of connective tissue through training—and, in an opposite direction, by immobilization—may influence muscle force development. Increased strength of connective tissue may improve the transmission of force from individual sarcomeres with less force dissipating to surrounding tissue. Furthermore, changes in the length of muscle fibres will affect force development. Strength training may, thus, result in an increase in force but not in peak power production, which is the product of force and velocity (Rutherford *et al.*, 1986a).

Little is known about these muscular factors and their importance for strength training in connection with immobilization and injuries. It is, however, clear that simple separation of neural and muscular factors is not possible based only on the relationship between strength values and cross-sectional area measurements. There may be variations in specific tension values (force/muscle cross-sectional area) at various contraction velocities during immobilization and training that are related to several factors, besides variation in neural activation, also to the length of the sarcomere and to the variation in transmission of forces from myofibrils to the selected system (Enoka, 1988). Further attention should be given to collagenous tissue factors, which may have a great impact on eccentric force production or concentric force production after eccentric activity (stretch–shortening cycle; Komi, 1984), where the elastic forces in the muscle tension system play an important role for force development.

The time for tension development after activation (electromechanical delay, EMD) is another aspect of muscle force development, which may also alter with immobilization and training in relation to injuries. It has been demonstrated to increase after injury or surgery (Komi, 1984).

There are principally two ways for increase in the cross-sectional area of the muscle to occur—hyperplasia (increase in number of muscle fibres) and hypertrophy of individual muscle fibres. In normal muscles, there are clear indications that the main factor in muscle mass increase at strength training is hypertrophy of individual muscle fibres, based partly on animal experiments, even if contradictory information on the relatively large importance of muscle fibre hyperplasia has also been reported. In patients with muscle wasting no direct information is available, so it can only be assumed that muscle fibre hypertrophy is dominant here also (provided that there is no direct muscle injury) since evidence of fibre hyperplasia with fibre splitting is rarely reported in histopathological studies.

DIFFERENT TRAINING METHODS

The stimulus for increased protein synthesis is documented to be the tension developed in the myofilaments, which give signals for increased uptake of amino acids (Goldberg *et al.*, 1975). If this is true, then strength training should be carried out with the greatest muscular tension possible.

In the use of dynamometers, biomechanial principles have to be analysed and practically considered by clinicians. In weight training, comparison should be made between the torque produced by the weight and the maximal torque profile of the muscle. Using weight at the ankle or foot in quadriceps training the weight gives its largest torque with a straight knee, whereas the produced maximal load is relatively low and therefore this is not the optimal arrangement for pure muscle mass training. By adapting the arrangements for weight training, as in the quadriceps table training device, the weight torque can be given a maximum at a 60° knee angle, as is the case with the

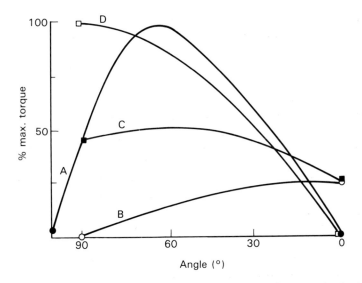

Fig. 15.2 Torque–angle curves with torque given as per cents of the maximal torque value for A, slow maximal isokinetic concentric knee extension; B, maximal tolerated weight placed at the foot at one repeated contraction; C, maximal tolerated weight using 60° angle between the weight-bearing arm and the resistance arm at one repeated contraction; D, maximal tolerated weight using 90° angle between the weight-bearing arm and the resistance arm at one repeated contraction. The placement of the maximum and its relation to the maximal isokinetic contraction with low speed are based on experimental observations by Grimby *et al.* (1980) and Ekholm *et al.* (pers. comm.).

maximal muscle torque curve (using a 60° angle between the weight-bearing arm and resistance arm) (Fig. 15.2) or better still with a 90° angle between the weight-bearing arm and resistance arm. The torque–angle curve produced by the weight will then approximate that produced by maximal knee extension for most of the joint motion.

One of the advantages of isokinetic dynamometers is that, by definition, they give a resistance corresponding to the maximal torque of the muscle at maximal effort. Only at the end of movement will no resistance be given. It is, therefore, to be expected that the training effect in patients with muscle weakness and wasting will be larger with an isokinetic device than with training using a constant weight (Grimby *et al.*, 1980). On the other hand, in newly immobilized patients (Ingemann-Hansen & Halkjaer-Kristensen, 1985) where neural factors may have a larger influence than the developed muscle tension, such a difference could not be noted.

Another approach than the isokinetic principle to achieve a resistance torque–angle curve corresponding to the musculature is to use the variable resistance dynamometer. These machines attempt to accomodate the muscle's changing level of force output through the range of motion by varying the resistance produced by the machine using a specially formed cam. However, in healthy subjects Manning *et al.* (1990) could not report any difference in strength increase over a 10-week training period comparing variable resistance with constant resistance training over the full range of motion. It is noteworthy that the training was slow and also included an eccentric component. Comparable studies in patients with muscle wasting are not available. It could tentatively be assumed that subjects with muscle hypotrophy are more sensitive to optimal torque–angle curve development during training, as increased protein synthesis proportionally has great importance for their regain in strength.

Table 15.1 Summary of aspects on various treatment modalities for muscle weakness

Treatment	Main indications	Advantages	Disadvantages/limitations
Isometric exercise	Limited joint mobility or pain-free range of motion	Easy to implement; choice of specific angles	No training of full range of motion; non-functional except at certain position
Dynamic exercises			
Constant resistance	'Basic' or home training programmes	Concentric and eccentric training exercise; simple equipment	Inefficient matching of muscle and load torque; does not accommodate to pain
Variable resistance	Neurogen and muscle volume training	Exercise through full range of motion; concentric and eccentric exercise	Eccentric exercise cannot be avoided; does not accommodate to pain
Isokinetic concentric	Specific effects at high and low speed; muscle volume training	Voluntary maximum load through range of motion; accommodates to pain; reduced joint compression force at high speed with maintained motor unit recruitment	No load at the end of movement
Isokinetic eccentric	Muscle volume training at relatively good muscle strength	High force development	Muscle soreness when unaccustomed; difficult to accommodate to pain
Transcutaneous electrical nerve stimulation (TENS)	Reduction of pain and reflex inhibition	Easy to apply; repeatable	Practically none
Electrical muscle stimulation (EMS)	Includes TENS effects; support to voluntary training especially during immobilization	Muscle actions also at low degree of voluntary activation	More or less discomfort; no central nervous training effect; relatively expensive apparatus for self-use

Eccentric action will give larger torque values than concentric action (Westing *et al.*, 1988). Neural activation, however, is not larger, as indicated by maximal EMG activity which may be lower at eccentric actions (Komi, 1984). Even if part of this tension is produced by non-contractile elements, the largest stimulus for protein synthesis may be given then by eccentric activity. The strength gain by eccentric training has been studied in healthy individuals with different results. In comparison with other training methods, most studies have not showed much of a difference. Komi and Buskirk (1972) were, however, able to demonstrate the superiority of eccentric training vs. isokinetic concentric training, but with muscle soreness in the eccentric training group. Fortunately, the soreness lessened over the first week of continuous training. In patients with muscle wasting, the specific benefit of eccentric training has still to be established. It would, based on present knowledge and basic principles, be challenged to a greater extent in a phase with optimal neural activation of the muscle, where it could be carefully monitored to avoid muscle soreness. The use of the stretch–shortening cycle to achieve benefits of strength training in other than contractile structures has already been mentioned.

Electrical muscle stimulation would be another tool to enhance muscle tension and, thus, protein synthesis. Evidence has been given that brief periods of transcutaneous electrical stimulation can prevent the fall in protein synthesis at immobilization (Gibson et al., 1989). Presumably also, an increase in protein synthesis would occur by EMS giving high muscle tension. Electrical stimulation superimposed on voluntary contraction demonstrated, on the other hand, that subjects 1–5 years after immobilization for leg injuries were able to maximally activate their quadriceps of both legs (Rutherford et al., 1990). When this is the case EMS can only be looked upon as a support for the already available maximal voluntary muscle activation.

Summary

In clinical situations, it is often not possible to analyse in detail the structural and functional deficits in muscular weakness as reviewed in this chapter. The clinician needs good theoretical knowledge of such factors and should be able to identify the main aims for the strength and power training in a specific situation. The principal aims to consider in the choice of treatment programmes are:
1 To prevent reflex inhibition.
2 To increase the neural activation.
3 To achieve structural changes in the muscle and related tissues.
These aspects are often mixed, but at a specific time one factor may be dominant. In all circumstances it is necessary to abolish and prevent reflex inhibition before effective muscle strength training can be achieved.

Knowledge on the proper use and advantages and disadvantages of various treatment modalities is also necessary. In Table 15.1 common methods are summarized; comments

have been presented earlier in the text. Only one technique should seldom be used and a combination of two or several treatment techniques may be necessary, such as the combination of TENS (EMS) and isometric training in the immobilized phase or the combination of functional and dynamic training in later phases where neural as well as muscular factors will contribute to an increase in muscle strength.

In the postinjury/postsurgical period three phases can often be identified (Grimby & Thomeé, 1988).

A *first phase* with *immobilization*, where to abolish or prevent reflex inhibition and maintain muscle structure and strength dominate.

A *second phase* with *activation*, where neural factors first will dominate giving increase in muscle strength and power without marked concomitant structural changes. The training effects may then be rather specific and limited to the type of exercise in the training programme. The need for several simultaneous training principles is therefore obvious, and training limited to, for example, only isometric exercise in a specific joint angle could only give limited effects. There is also a cross-over effect indicating the use of bilateral training.

In later stages of this phase, where optimal or near-optimal neural activation has been achieved, the main factor in building up strength will be through an increase in muscle volume. Training effects will therefore be less specific for the type of training exercise. This period may often cover a long period after more marked muscle wasting and weakness at postinjury/postsurgery. It may further be complicated by remaining factors giving reflex inhibition, which sometimes may be difficult to avoid. Dynamometer training allowing the possibility for training with maximal effort and stabilizing joint motion is an important part of the training programme, although never excluding more functionally oriented training. Dynamometer training gives easy repeatable resistance without much supervision, but this is also true for the carefully monitored functional training programme.

In the *third phase* with adaptation of *function*, specific functional needs of the patient have to be considered. The training regime should successively include activities similar or identical to the sport activities of the person. In this phase neural factors, which include training of proprioception, precision and flexibility as well as strength and power, will again play a special role. The need for not only muscle strength but also endurance should always be kept in mind, although endurance training is not specially covered in the present review.

There are naturally different training needs for a person active only in recreational sports and for top athletes in strength and power-demanding sports. For certain postinjured persons it is necessary to advise a change in the sports or activity pattern, so that they can be tolerated with the remaining deficiencies in joint stability and muscle strength. Even here the clinician has an important function in analysing the person's capacity and preference, and giving recommendations on suitable physical activities and direct the training in accordance.

References

Antich, T.J. & Brewster, C.E. (1986) Modification of quadriceps femoris muscle exercises during knee rehabilitation. *Physical Therapy*, **66**, 1246–51.

Arvidsson, I., Arvidsson, H., Eriksson, E. & Jansson, E. (1986a) Prevention of quadriceps wasting after immobilization—an evaluation of the effect of electrical stimulation. *Orthopaedics*, **9**, 1519–28.

Arvidsson, I. & Eriksson, E. (1986) Postoperative TENS pain relief after knee surgery: objective evaluation. *Orthopaedics*, **9**, 1346–51.

Arvidsson, I., Eriksson, E., Häggmark, T. & Johnson, R.J. (1981) Isokinetic thigh muscle strength after ligament reconstruction in the knee joint: Result from a 5–10 year follow-up after reconstruction of the anterior cruciate ligament in the knee joint. *International Journal of Sports Medicine*, **2**, 7–11.

Arvidsson, I., Eriksson, E., Knutsson, E. & Arner, S. (1986b) Reduction of pain inhibition on voluntary muscle activation by epidural analgesia. *Orthopaedics*, **9**, 1415–19.

Baughner, W.M., Warren, R.F., Marshall, J.L. & Joseph, A. (1984) Quadriceps atrophy in the anterior cruciate insufficient knee. *American Journal of Sports Medicine*, **12**, 192–5.

Bohannon, R.W. (1983) Effect of electrical stimulation to the vastus medialis muscle in a patient with chronically dislocating patellae. *Physical Therapy*, **63**, 1445–7.

DeLitto, A., Rose, S., McKoven, J.M., Lehman, R.C., Thomas, J.A. & Shively, R.A. (1988) Electrical stimulation versus voluntary exercise in strengthening thigh musculature after anterior cruciate ligament surgery. *Physical Therapy*, **68**, 660–3.

Draganich, L.F., Jaeger, R.J. & Kralj, A.R. (1989) Coactivation of hamstrings and quadriceps during extension of the knee. *Journal of Bone and Joint Surgery*, **71A**, 1075–81.

Dvir, Z., Eger, G., Halperin, N. & Shklar, A. (1989) Thigh muscle activity and anterior cruciate ligament insufficiency. *Clinical Biomechanics*, **4**, 87–91.

Ebbeling, C.B. & Clarkson, P.M. (1989) Exercise-induced muscle damage and adaptation. *Sports Medicine*, **7**, 207–34.

Edström, L. (1970) Selective atrophy of red muscle fibres in the quadriceps in long-standing knee-joint dysfunction. *Journal of Neurological Sciences*, **11**, 551–9.

Engle, R.P. & Canner G.C. (1989) Proprioceptive neuromuscular facilitation (PNF) and modified procedures for anterior cruciate ligament (ACL) instability. *Journal of Orthopaedic and Sports Physical Therapy*, **11**, 230–6.

Enoka, R.M. (1988) Muscle strength and its development. New perspectives. *Sports Medicine*, **6**, 146–68.

Eriksson, E. & Häggmark, T. (1979) Comparison of isometric muscle training and electrical stimulation supplementing isometric muscle training in the recovery after major knee ligament surgery. *American Journal of Sports Medicine*, **7**, 169–71.

Fleck, S.J. & Falkel, J.E. (1986) Value of resistance training for the reduction of sports injuries. *Sports Medicine*, **3**, 61–8.

Fridén, J., Seger, J., Sjöström, M. & Ekblom, B. (1983) Adaptive response in human skeletal muscle subjected to prolonged eccentric training. *International Journal of Sports Medicine*, **4**, 177–83.

Gibson, J.N., Morrison, W.L., Scrimgenour, C.M., Smith, K., Stoward, P.J. & Rennie, M.J. (1989) Effects of therapeutic percutaneous electrical stimulation of atrophic human quadriceps muscle on muscle composition, protein synthesis and contractile properties. *European Journal of Clinical Investigation*, **19**, 206–12.

Goldberg, A.L., Etlinger, J.D., Goldspink, D.F. & Jablecki, C. (1975) Mechanisms of work-induced hypertrophy of skeletal muscle. *Medicine and Science in Sports*, **7**, 248–61.

Gollnick, P.D., Karlsson, J., Piehl, K. & Saltin, B.

(1974) Selective glycogen depletion in skeletal muscle fibres of man following sustained contraction. *Journal of Physiology*, **241**, 59–67.

Grimby, G., Einarsson, G., Hedberg, M. & Aniansson, A. (1989) Muscle adaptive changes in post-polio subjects. *Scandinavian Journal of Rehabilitation Medicine*, **21**, 19–26.

Grimby, G., Gustafson, E., Peterson, L. & Renström, P. (1980) Quadriceps function and training after knee ligament injury. *Medicine and Science in Sports and Exercise*, **12**, 70–5.

Grimby, G. & Thomeé, R. (1988) Principles of rehabilitation after injuries. In H.G. Knuttgen & K. Tittel (eds) *Olympic Book of Sports Medicine, Vol. 1*, pp. 489–508. Blackwell Scientific Publications, Oxford.

Grimby, G. & Wigerstad-Lossing, I. (1988) Comparison of high- and low-frequency muscle stimulators. *Archives of Physical Medicine and Rehabilitation*, **70**, 835–8.

Häggmark, T., Jansson, E. & Eriksson, E. (1981) Fiber type area and metabolic potential of the thigh muscle in man after knee injury and immobilization. *International Journal of Sports Medicine*, **2**, 12–17.

Halkjaer-Kristensen, J. & Ingemann-Hansen, T. (1985) Wasting of the human quadriceps muscle after knee ligament injuries. IV. Dynamic and static muscle function. *Scandinavian Journal of Rehabilitation Medicine* (suppl. **13**), 29–37.

Harter, R.A., Osternig, L.R. & Standifer, L.W. (1990) Isokinetic evaluation of quadriceps and hamstrings symmetry following anterior cruciate ligament reconstruction. *Archives of Physical Medicine and Rehabilitation*, **71**, 465–8.

Hultén, B., Renström, P. & Grimby, G. (1981) Glycogen-depletion patterns with isometric and isokinetic exercise in patients after leg injury. *Clinical Science*, **61**, 35–42.

Ingemann-Hansen, T. & Halkjaer-Kristensen, J. (1985) Physical training of the hypotrophic quadriceps muscle in man. I. The effects of different training programmes on muscular performance. *Scandinavian Journal of Rehabilitation Medicine* (suppl. **13**), 38–44.

Jensen, J.E., Conn, R.C., Hazelrigg, G. & Hewett, J.E. (1985) The use of transcutaneous neural stimulation and isokinetic testing in arthroscopic knee surgery. *American Journal of Sports Medicine*, **13**, 27–33.

Kannus, P. (1988) Knee flexor and extensor strength ratios with deficiency of the lateral collateral ligament. *Archives of Physical Medicine and Rehabilitation*, **69**, 928–31.

Kannus, P., Latvala, K. & Järvinen, M. (1987) Thigh muscle strengths in the anterior cruciate ligament

deficient knee: isokinetic and isometric long-term results. *Journal of Orthopaedic and Sports Physical Therapy*, **9**, 223–7.

Knaflitz, M., Merlitto, R. & DeLuca, C.J. (1990) Inference of motor unit recruitment order in voluntary and electrically elicited contractions. *Journal of Applied Physiology*, **68**, 1657–67.

Komi, P.V. (1984) Physiological and biomechanical correlates of muscle function: Effects of muscle structure and stretch–shortening cycle on force and speed. *Exercise and Sport Sciences Reviews*, **12**, 81–121.

Komi, P.V. & Buskirk, E.R. (1972) Effect of eccentric and concentric muscle conditioning on tension and electrical activity of human muscle. *Ergonomics*, **15**, 417–34.

Kulund, D.N., McCue, F.G., Rockwell, D.A. & Gieck, J.A. (1979) Tennis injuries: prevention and treatment. *American Journal of Sports Medicine*, **3**, 249–53.

Lentell, G.L., Katzman, L.L. & Walteri, M.R. (1990) The relationship between muscle function and ankle stability. *Journal of Orthopaedic and Sports Physical Therapy*, **11**, 605–11.

Manning, R.J., Graves, J.E., Carpenter, D.M., Leggett, S.H. & Pollock, M.L. (1990) Constant vs variable resistance training. *Medicine and Science in Sports and Exercise*, **22**, 397–401.

Moritani, I. & deVries, H.A. (1979) Neural factors versus hypertrophy in the time course of muscle strength gain. *American Journal of Physical Medicine*, **58**, 115–30.

Morrisey, M.C. (1989) Reflex inhibition of thigh muscles in knee injury. Causes and treatment. *Sports Medicine*, **7**, 263–76.

Morrisey, M.C., Brewster, C.E., Shields, C.L. & Brown, M. (1985) The effects of electrical stimulation on the quadriceps during postoperative immobilization. *American Journal of Sports Medicine*, **13**, 40–5.

Parker, M.G., Ruhling, R.O., Holt, D., Barrman, E. & Prayna, M. (1983) Descriptive analysis of quadriceps and hamstrings muscle torque in high-school football players. *Journal of Orthopaedic and Sports Physical Therapy*, **5**, 2–6.

Renström, P., Arms, F.W., Stanwyck, T.F., Johnson, R.J. & Pope, M.H. (1986) Strain within the anterior cruciate ligament during hamstrings and quadriceps activity. *American Journal of Sports Medicine*, **14**, 83–6.

Rutherford, O.M., Craig, C.A., Sargeant, A.J. & Jones, D.A. (1986a) Strength training and power output: transference effects in the human quadriceps muscle. *Journal of Sports Sciences*, **4**, 101–7.

Rutherford, O.M., Jones, D.A. & Newham, D.J. (1986b) Clinical and experimental application of the percutaneous twitch superimposition technique for the study of human muscle activation. *Journal of Neurology, Neurosurgery and Psychiatry*, **49**, 1288–91.

Rutherford, O.M., Jones, D.A. & Round, J.M. (1990) Long-lasting unilateral muscle wasting and weakness following injury and immobilization. *Scandinavian Journal of Rehabilitation Medicine*, **22**, 33–7.

Sale, O.G. (1986) Neural adaptation in strength and power training. In N.L. Jones, N. McCartney & A.J. McComas (eds) *Human Muscle Power*, pp. 289–307. Human Kinetics, Champaign, Illinois.

Seto, J.L., Orofino, A.S., Morrisey, M.C., Medeiros, J.M. & Mason, W.J. (1988) Assessment of quadriceps/hamstring strength, knee ligament stability, functional and sports activity levels five years after anterior cruciate ligament reconstruction. *American Journal of Sports Medicine*, **16**, 170–80.

Shakespeare, D.T., Stokes, M., Sherman, K.P. & Young, A. (1985) Reflex inhibition of the quadriceps after meniscetomy: Lack of association with pain. *Clinical Physiology*, **5**, 137–44.

Silfverskiöld, J.P., Steadman, J.R., Higgins, R.W., Hagerman, T. & Atkins, J.A. (1988) Rehabilitation of the anterior cruciate ligament in the athlete. *Sports Medicine*, **6**, 308–19.

Sisk, T.D., Stralka, S.W., Deering, M.B. & Griffin, J.W. (1987) Effect of electrical stimulation on quadriceps strength after reconstructive surgery of the anterior cruciate ligament. *American Journal of Sports Medicine*, **15**, 215–20.

Stokes, M. & Young, A. (1984) The contribution of reflex inhibition to arthrogenous muscle weakness. *Clinical Science*, **67**, 7–14.

Swärd, L., Hellström, M., Jacobsson, B. & Peterson, L. (1989) Back pain and radiological changes in the thoraco-lumbar spine of athletes. *Spine*, **15**, 124–9.

Tegner, Y. (1990) Strength training in the rehabilitation of cruciate ligament tears. *Sports Medicine*, **9**, 129–36.

Thomeé, R, Renström, P., Grimby, G. & Peterson, L. (1987) Slow or fast isokinetic training after knee ligament surgery. *Journal of Orthopaedic and Sports Physical Therapy*, **8**, 475–9.

Tipton, C.M., Vailas, A.C. & Matthes, R.D. (1986) Experimental studies on the influences of physical activity on ligaments, tendons and joints: A brief review. *Acta Medica Scandinavia*, (suppl. 711), 157–68.

Westing, S.H., Seger, J.Y., Karlsson, E. & Ekblom, B. (1988) Eccentric and concentric torque–velocity characteristics of the quadriceps femoris in man. *European Journal of Applied Physiology*, **58**, 100–4.

Wigerstad-Lossing, I., Grimby, G., Jonsson, T., Morelli, B., Peterson, L. & Renström, P. (1988) Effects of electrical muscle stimulation combined with voluntary contractions after knee ligament surgery. *Medicine and Science in Sports and Exercise*, **20**, 93–8.

Wise, H.H., Fiebert, I.M. & Kater, J.L. (1984) EMG biofeedback as treatment for patellofemoral pain syndrome. *Journal of Orthopaedic and Sports Physical Therapy*, **6**, 95–103.

PART 5

STRENGTH AND POWER TRAINING FOR SPORTS

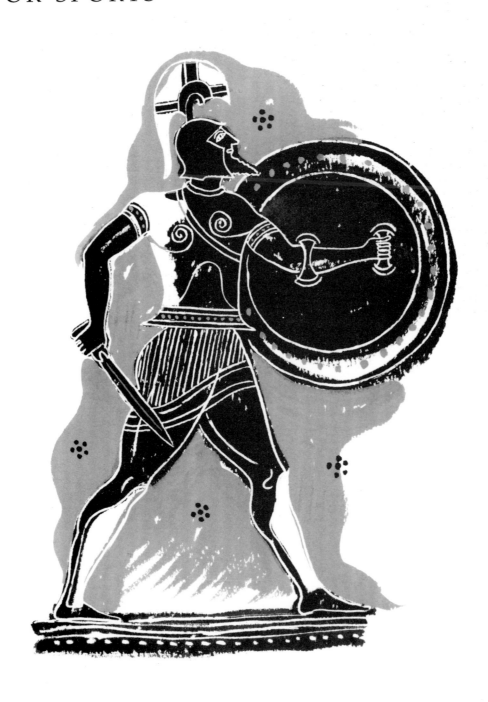

Chapter 16

Training for Weightlifting

JOHN GARHAMMER AND BOB TAKANO

Introduction

Since 1972, two overhead lifts have been contested in the sport of weightlifting, the snatch, and the clean and jerk. The sport is often referred to as Olympic (style) weightlifting since it is contested in the Olympic Games. In the snatch lift, the barbell is lifted in one continuous motion from the competition platform to arms length overhead. The athlete catches the barbell overhead in a deep squat position, and then stands with the barbell in control until a 'down' signal is received from the officials (Fig. 16.1).

The 'clean' phase of the clean and jerk lift is similar to the snatch except that the barbell is lifted to the shoulders rather than overhead and a narrower hand spacing is used on the bar. When the athlete stands from the squat position to finish the clean lift he/she must then 'jerk' the barbell overhead to complete the two-part lift. The jerk is performed starting with the barbell held firmly on the shoulders. The knee and hip joints are slightly flexed and then rapidly extended in a jumping action (rising onto the balls of the feet) to thrust the barbell upward. The lifter then either splits the feet forward and backward, or again quickly flexes the knee and hip joints, to lower the body and catch the barbell at arms length overhead. The feet are then brought together and the legs straightened to hold the barbell under control overhead until the 'down' signal is given by the officials (Fig. 16.2). The above three lifting

movements are performed very rapidly, with the major lifting forces applied to the bar for about 0.8 s in the snatch and clean, and about 0.2 s in the jerk.

The training programmes followed by athletes who compete in weightlifting are based primarily on three principles: specificity of exercise, overload, and variability. Specificity implies the use of training lifts similar to the competitive lifts, performed for low repetitions with near maximal loads, since in competition the goal is to lift the heaviest weight possible in the snatch, and clean and jerk for one repetition. Overload relates to lifting heavier and/or more total weight in workouts than a given athlete is accustomed to. Variability relates to changes and variety in the composition of the training programme in order to avoid physiological and psychological maladaptation problems, commonly referred to as 'overtraining' (Stone *et al.*, 1991). As the following discussion emphasizes, the variability principle leads to some training programme designs that seem to violate the principles of specificity and overload.

Before proceeding with a more detailed presentation of training methods for weightlifting, it must be stated that details of training programme design and content may vary considerably based on the ability level and years of training and competition experience of a given athlete. Thus, most of the remaining content of this article will relate primarily to elite level weightlifters who have trained for the sport

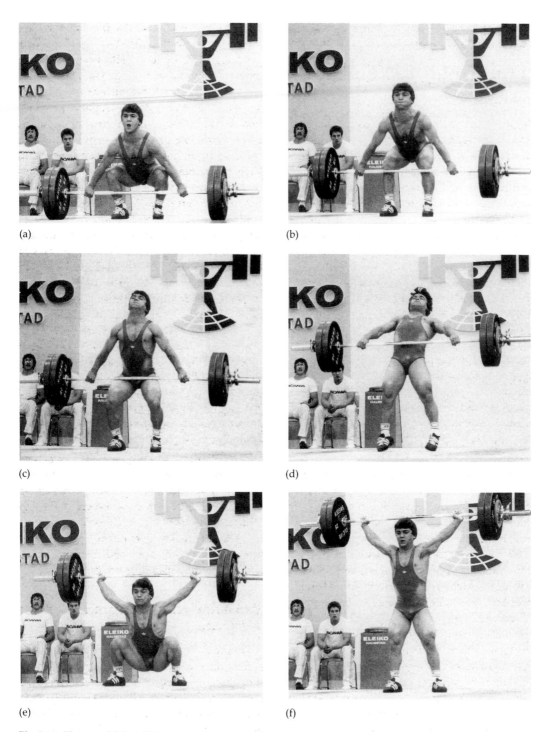

Fig. 16.1 The snatch lift. (a) Start position; (b) end of first pull; (c) start of second pull (power position) after transition from the first pull (note rebending of knees); (d) end of second pull (jump phase); (e) catch position; (f) finish of the lift. (Courtesy of B. Klemens Photos.)

for 3 or more years and who compete at national and international level.

Variability as the key training principle

If specificity and overload were dominant and/or exclusive principles of training, the design of a weightlifter's exercise programme would be rather simple: (i) perform the competitive lifts in low repetitions with maximal weights; and (ii) add a few 'assistance' exercises to emphasize and improve physical qualities associated with proper execution of the competitive lifts, such as speed, strength, and flexibility. Practical experience, however, shows that such a plan fails if followed for any prolonged period of time (several days to several weeks). The reason for failure of such an approach to training is summarized by the term 'overtraining'. Overtraining can involve psychological factors, such as loss of motivation, and/or physiological factors related to muscle fatigue or injury, as well as neural and hormonal changes (Nilsson, 1986; Kuipers & Keizer, 1988; Stone et al., 1991).

Sale (1988) and Enoka (1988) have discussed the importance of neural adaptations for increases in strength, particularly in the early stages of a resistance training programme. Kraemer (1988) has reviewed the responses of the endocrine system to resistive exercise and has pointed out the conflicting research results, likely due to variables such as exercise volume (total number of lifts performed) and intensity (average weight lifted relative to maximum possible), rest intervals, and training status of subjects. As discussed below, Häkkinen and colleagues have performed considerable research on the neural and hormonal responses that occur in elite weightlifters during typical training programmes.

In studies of 1 to 2 years duration Häkkinen et al. (1987, 1988a) found that increases in performance correlated to increases in leg extensor isometric force and integrated electro-myographic (IEMG) activity (neural activation levels), serum testosterone levels and anabolic/catabolic (A/C) hormone ratios (endocrine responses). Short duration studies (Häkkinen et al., 1988b,c) showed that such responses were sensitive to acute intense workout sessions, with IEMG activity and leg extensor isometric force decreasing. Testosterone was found to increase during the second workout session in 1 day but decreased gradually after several days of intense workouts. A single rest day was sufficient to reverse this trend. Results of such research indicates the importance of neural adaptations, even in experienced strength and power athletes, and that neural fatigue (decreased IEMG levels) does occur with intense exercise. Also, endocrine responses could be monitored in elite strength and power athletes during important training periods in order to adjust training intensity to optimal levels, i.e. without causing decreases in serum testosterone levels and A/C ratios, which likely relate to reduced adaptability levels and the possibility of overtraining. A recent article (Häkkinen et al., 1990) suggests that these conclusions are applicable for both male and female athletes.

Thus, variability in quality training programmes for weightlifters can reduce the possibility of overtraining while maintaining reasonable, if not optimal, progress for the athlete. This is possible via periodic oscillations in overload, meaning planned underload or 'unload' training sessions and training weeks, and strategically placed rest days.

Variability vs. biomechanical specificity

A variety of lifting exercises, beyond the competition lifts, are regularly used in the training programme of weightlifters (for an extensive discussion of them see Vorobyev, 1978). This not only permits one to emphasize the development of various physical qualities needed to execute the competition lifts optimally, such as

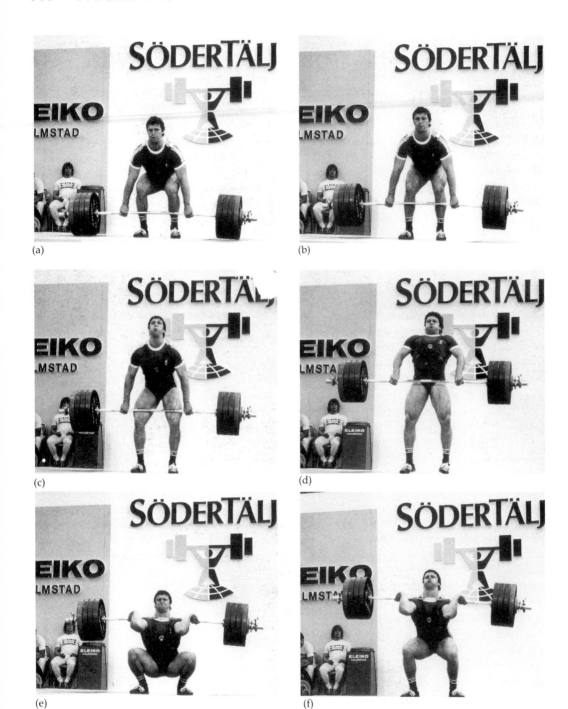

Fig. 16.2 The clean and jerk lift. (a) Start ('lift-off'); (b) middle of first pull; (c) near the start of the second pull; (d) end of the second pull (jump phase); (e) catch position; (f) standing from the catch position (front squat movement); (g) start position for the jerk; (h) bottom of the 'dip' prior to the upward thrust; (i) end of the thrust phase (jump) of the jerk; (j) 'split' catch position; (k) finish of the lift. (Courtesy of B. Klemens Photos.)

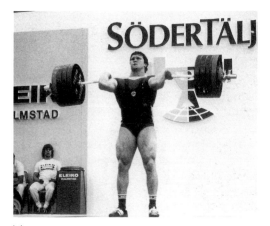

(g)

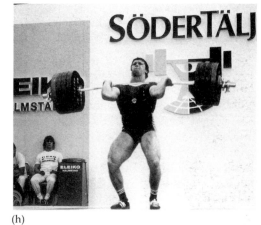

(h)

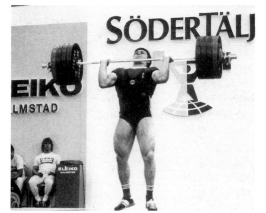

(i)

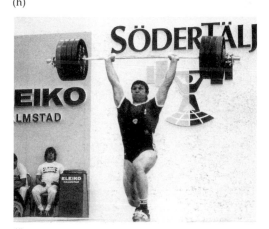

(j)

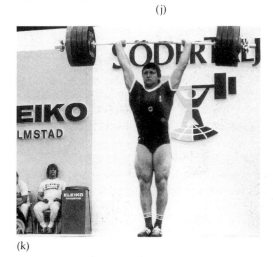

(k)

strength, speed, and flexibility, but permits a biomechanical variation that may help avoid overtraining symptoms caused by movement pattern monotony. The weightlifting coach, however, needs to be aware of how the movement properties of a given 'assistance' exercise differ from that of the actual competition lifts. That is, how does the applied force pattern, bar movement velocity and trajectory profile, range of motion of involved body joints, and mechanical power output of the exercise relate to the physical qualities that are to be developed by the exercise. Also, how do these factors change as the weight of the barbell changes?

A recent review article (Garhammer, 1989) points out that several sport scientists have published data indicating that as barbell weight increases the height to which it is lifted, maximal vertical bar velocity, peak applied vertical force, and/or power output decrease (e.g. Garhammer & Gregor, 1979, 1991; Häkkinen et al., 1984; Garhammer, 1985). Thus, for example, an athlete who needs to be faster should emphasize lower intensity lifts (70–85%) while one who needs to improve strength should emphasize higher intensity lifts (85+%). For a given weight, the same trends in the above parameters have been noted for later repetitions in a multiple repetition sequence (set) (Häkkinen, 1988).

Numerous reports have been published comparing the biomechanical properties of various assistance exercises with the competition lifts. For example, for snatch-related exercises see Frolov et al. (1977), Häkkinen and Kauhanen (1986) and Häkkinen (1988); for clean-related exercises, Medvedjev et al. (1981) and Häkkinen and Kauhanen (1986); for jerk-related exercises, Medvedjev et al. (1982).

The most common snatch-related assistance exercises are the following.
1 Power snatch: very similar to the competition snatch lift but caught overhead with only slight knee and hip flexion rather than in a deep squat position.
2 Snatch pull: similar to the competition snatch lift but the barbell is only pulled to the height of

3 Snatch or snatch pull from the hang: initial barbell position is not on the floor but rather held just above the floor to just above the knees.
4 Snatch or snatch pull from blocks: initial barbell position is above the floor resting on blocks, usually positioning the bar at about knee height.

It is difficult to make general statements about the results of biomechanical comparisons between these assistance exercises and the competition lifts due to the dependence of measured parameters on the weight of the barbell used in any given exercise. However, some specific cases can be discussed.

The maximal weight that can be used in the power snatch by a given athlete is about 80% of the weight of that athlete's maximal competition snatch lift. With this load the barbell will be pulled higher, reach a greater maximum vertical velocity, result in a greater peak applied vertical propulsion force, elicit slightly different IEMG activity from leg extensor muscles, include a higher peak knee angular velocity and greater range of motion at the knee, and result in greater mechanical power output when compared to the competition snatch lift. Power snatches are, therefore, a useful assistance exercise for an athlete who needs to improve speed of movement and speed-strength (power).

Conversely, a snatch pull from the floor may be performed with 10% or more above an athlete's maximum competition snatch weight. With a load on the barbell equal to the maximum competition snatch, it will be pulled to a lower height, reach a lesser maximum vertical velocity, result in a smaller peak applied vertical propulsion force, elicit slightly different IEMG activity from leg extensor muscles, and result in lower mechanical power output when compared to the competition snatch lift. Snatch pulls are, therefore, useful for an athlete who needs to improve strength in the snatch movement pattern.

Biomechanical characteristics of snatch assistance exercises from the hang or from blocks depend on the exact starting position of the bar (e.g. above or below knee level), as well as on load. In general, if the starting position is above knee level the exercise will emphasize the development of speed-strength in the final phase of the snatch pull (upper or top pull). If the starting position is closer to the floor the biomechanical characteristics will be more similar to the snatch pull from the floor.

Essentially identical statements to those for the snatch assistance exercises can be made regarding the clean assistance exercises; namely, the power clean, clean pull, and clean or clean pulls from the hang or from boxes.

The primary assistance exercises for improving the jerk are the following.

1 Jerk: weight taken from supports rather than cleaned from the floor.
2 Jerk from behind the neck (taken from supports).
3 Push or power jerk: barbell thrust upward as in the competition jerk but caught overhead with only slight flexion at the knees and hips.
4 Half-jerk: barbell is thrust upward as in the competition jerk but only to approximately head height; it then falls back to the athlete's shoulders.

Work by Medvedjev *et al.* (1982) indicates that the most important variables related to success in the jerk are the maximum force generated against the ground, time interval to reach maximum force, and the time interval for 'breaking' or stopping the initial descent phase of the movement. The jerk and jerk from behind the neck were determined to be most effective in perfecting jerk technique, while the half-jerk and depth (drop) jumps were best to develop speed-strength. It was also recommended that no more than five to seven jerks be performed per workout with 90% or more of the maximum jerk (the higher the lifter's classification the lower the number of heavy jerks).

General concepts in the training plan for weightlifters

The above discussion presented information that can be helpful to a weightlifting coach when making specific decisions about the content of a training plan. Before detailed examples of actual training programmes used by weightlifters can be presented, a few general concepts in training theory need to be explained.

Matveyev (1972) presented the basic ideas of periodized training programmes. A programme is periodized when it is divided into phases, each of which has primary and secondary goals. In his original model Matveyev suggested the initial phase of a strength–power programme (preparation phase) contain a high volume (many repetitions) with lower intensity (low average weight lifted relative to maximum possible in each movement). As weeks pass the volume decreases and intensity increases. The resulting higher intensity and lower volume represent the characteristics of a competitive phase of training that leads up to an actual competition. Typical high volume (preparatory) phases for weightlifters contain more training sessions per week (6–15), more exercises per workout session (3–6), more sets per exercise (4–8), and more repetitions per set (4–6). Typical high intensity (competition) phases for weightlifters contain fewer training sessions per week (5–12), fewer exercises per workout session (1–4), fewer sets per exercise (3–5), and fewer repetitions per set (1–3). The duration of each phase may be several weeks to several months in length. Two or more complete cycles (preparatory plus competition) may fit into a training year.

Stone *et al.* (1981) have proposed and successfully tested a periodized model of strength–power training with sequential phases that change rather drastically. For example, a phase to increase muscle size (5 sets of 10 repetitions in core exercises), a phase to improve basic strength (3–5 sets of 5 repetitions), a phase to improve speed-strength (3–5 sets of 3 repetitions), and a phase to 'peak' for competition (1–3 sets of 1–3 repetitions). The use of 10 repetitions per set is higher than typically recommended in the early preparation phase but has proved to be successful in a number of studies (e.g. Stone *et al.*, 1982).

The training programme for a weightlifter is

generally planned in terms of a training year. Modifications are made as the actual training year progresses based on specific observed needs of an athlete. The plan begins with a judgement as to how many total lifts (counting all major exercises) should be performed during the year. As an example, 20 000 is a reasonable number for an elite athlete. This total yearly 'volume' is then divided unequally into 12 4-week training months, some of which will be more than double the volume of other months. Each training month then has its volume divided unequally into four weekly volumes. The highest volume week in a given month may have more than twice the lifts of the lowest volume week. Each week then has its volume divided amongst an appropriate number of training sessions, i.e. such that no session has an unreasonably large or small number of lifts. Multiple workout sessions per day are now common among elite weightlifters. A lifter may workout 5 or 6 days per week with 1–3 sessions per day being common. Each session must then be assigned specific lifting exercises based on the particular athlete's strengths and weaknesses. This approach to training programme development provides for extensive variation, which can stimulate progress while minimizing the chances of overtraining. Details related to the above overview of training plan development are discussed by Vorobyev (1978).

The following sections describe examples of training weeks during preparatory and competition months that are representative of two different national programme philosophies.

Training methods

Most of the world's weightlifting training programmes are variations of the models established by Bulgaria and the Soviet Union, the two top programmes in the sport. In recent years both nations have allowed foreign coaches and athletes to participate in their training programmes, thus making this information available to students of the sport. These two programmes and their philosophies are strongly affected by geopolitical factors.

The Soviet Union benefits from the diversity of human types that inhabit this vast geopolitical complex. The geographic distances between training centres create problems that inhibit strict monitoring of training, and allow for a greater degree of variation from the established national philosophies. It also inhibits the frequency of collective training by national team members. There has been some discontinuity within the Soviet Weightlifting Federation in the past decade relative to the development of a standardized training methodology. For example, the position of national coach, largely administrative, has been filled by four men. The financial incentives available for top athletes, however, have allowed the Soviet Union's national team to overcome the inconsistencies of the development structure.

The Bulgarian programme involves a smaller number of carefully selected athletes occupying a much smaller geographic area than the Soviet Union. The 20-year term of service of national coach Ivan Abadjiev provided great continuity with little opportunity for variation. The relatively small size of the country allows the national junior and senior teams to train collectively for a majority of the time.

The two programmes differ philosophically in the longevity expected of their top performers. The Bulgarians expect an athlete to mature quickly, produce high results at a single Olympics, and then, in all probability, to be replaced before the next renewal of the Games. Hence, double Olympic gold medallists are rare. The Soviets expect a lengthier career from their top performers.

Both programmes are designed to train talented athletes with no serious limitations in joint mobility. The technique learned by the athlete during the first year of training is not altered significantly except to account for increases in body weight. The larger battery of exercises employed during the earlier developmental years of training should minimize any imbalances in the development of muscular anatomy.

Those athletes involved in these training programmes must be in sufficiently fit condition to endure the stresses generated. An individual returning from injury rehabilitation, or any other layoff should employ a more diversified programme before undertaking elite level training.

The *K*-value is a derived figure that is used to monitor the intensity of training programmes. The *K*-value can be defined as the average weight lifted per repetition divided by the two-lift total performed at the end of the training cycle. Empirical results indicate that the optimal range of average weight lifted lies between 38 and 42% of the total (Takano, 1990).

Restoration is a necessity for an athlete to train in these types of regimes. Jacuzzi, steam baths, sauna or massage must be employed several times weekly. Nutritional supplementation is also required.

Bulgarian training

The Bulgarian training approach is unique in that it does not deal with percentages of maximum or expected maximum, a procedure common to weightlifting training for at least the last three decades. The battery of primary exercises is limited to only six (snatch, clean and jerk, power snatch, power clean and jerk, front squat and back squat). Training sessions are limited to 45-min periods. This time limit is to ensure that athletes are training only during the period in which the body can maintain elevated blood testosterone levels (Abadjiev, 1989). Two 45-min sessions are combined into a complex around a 30-min rest period during which testosterone levels can be restored.

To begin a complex, the athlete warms up with snatch singles toward a weight near the maximum expected for the date. If the first lift is successful, more weight is added. This procedure is continued through the six attempts. As an alternative, the athlete may take singles at 15, 10, or 5 kg below maximum between the six maximum attempts. Lifting is terminated at the 45-min limitation. The athletes then may recline while listening to music for 30 min. The second session of the complex involves the clean and jerk performed in the same progression pattern. Less time is required since less warm-up is necessary. Front squats with several maximum singles follow the clean and jerks. Lifting is terminated at 45 min.

The same progression pattern is employed for the power snatch, power clean and jerk, and back squat during the Wednesday and Saturday training complexes (Table 16.1).

Table 16.1 Bulgarian preparation week

Monday
Morning
    Session 1: Snatch—singles to 6 maximum efforts
           Rest 30 min
    Session 2: Clean and jerk—singles to 6 maximum efforts
           Front squat—singles to 1–6 maximum efforts
Afternoon
    Repeat morning complex
Evening
    Repeat morning complex

Tuesday
    Repeat Monday's training schedule

Wednesday
Morning
    Session 1: Power snatch—singles to 6 maximum efforts
           Rest 30 min
    Session 2: Power clean and jerk—singles to 6 maximum efforts

Thursday
    Repeat Monday's training schedule

Friday
    Repeat Monday's training schedule

Saturday
    Repeat Wednesday's training schedule

Sunday
Morning
    Session 1: Less formally structured training

Table 16.2 Maxima to determine weights for each exercise

Exercises	Maximum (100%)
Snatch, snatch pull, power snatch, snatch deadlift	Snatch
Clean and jerk, clean pull, power clean, clean deadlift, front squat	Clean and jerk
Press	Press
Good morning	*
Back squat	At least 125% of clean and jerk

*The style of performance will dictate the maximum weight.

Variation seems limited on first inspection, but the following variants are available for the discretion of the supervising coach.

1 Number of maximum lifts per session, day, week.

2 Number of complexes per day.

In addition, the maximum weights for each day will vary with the condition of the athlete. These weights are utilized as indicators for the planning of future training by the supervising coach.

This system requires close supervision. Consequently, the ratio of athletes to coaches must be small. Three coaches are assigned to the 20-man senior team, with the periodic assistance of personal coaches. These coaches must be able to identify characteristics of each phase and make appropriate adjustments in the training.

In the competitive phase the same exercises are used on the same day as in the preparatory weeks. The number of times that the complexes may be performed is reduced to one or two times per day on Monday, Tuesday, Thursday and Friday. The number of times that the weights are reduced and then reloaded to maximum may also be varied during a workout in this phase.

Soviet training

The Soviet system may be even more diversified than it may appear to be on the surface due to the aforementioned geopolitical factors.

The widely dispersed elite level coaches tend to develop and emphasize the successes of their own training methods. This situation may lead to more variation in training programme design, especially when considering the lack of prolonged strong leadership that Bulgaria has enjoyed under national coach Ivan Abadjiev.

The Soviets utilize a greater variety of exercises, more variation of these exercises, and fewer training sessions per day and week. All movements designated as 'hang' are performed from above the knee. Percentages of expected competition maxima are used to designate the intensities of the exercises.

Table 16.2 indicates which maxima are used to determine the weights for each exercise.

The Soviet system also utilizes diversified non-weightlifting activities in what is collectively termed active rest. Active rest normally involves calisthenics, running and jumping drills, swimming, competitive games and similar activities that encourage the development of competitiveness, anaerobic endurance, motive qualities and increased local circulation.

The notation of the accompanying training programmes (Tables 16.3 and 16.4) is:

$$(70\%/3)3$$

where the numerator is the percentage of maximum, the denominator is the number of repetitions per set, the number following the parentheses is the number of sets, and the lack of parentheses indicates a single set.

Table 16.3 Soviet preparation week

Day 1
Morning
1 Press: (60%/3)2, (70%/3)2
2 Snatch: (60%/3)2, (70%/3)3, (80%/2)2
3 Front squat: (60%/4)2, (70%/4)2, (80%/4)2
Afternoon
4 Hang clean and jerk: (60%/3 + 1)3, (70%/3 + 1)2, (80%/3 + 1)3
5 Clean pull: 70%/4, (80%/4)2, (85%/4)2
6 Good morning: (X/8)4

Day 2
Morning
1 Power snatch: (65%/3)3, (75%/3)2, (80%/2)2
2 Power clean and jerk: (60%/3 + 1)2, (70%/3 + 1)2, (80%/2 + 1)3
3 Jerk: (70%/3)2, (80%/2)2
4 Eccentric snatch deadlift: (80%/3)6–20 s
5 Eccentric clean deadlift: (90%/3)6–20 s

Day 3
Active rest

Day 4
Morning
1 Press: 60%/4, 70%/4, (80%/3)2
2 Clean and jerk: (60%/3 + 1)2, (70%/3 + 1)2, (80%/3 + 1)2
3 Back squat: (0%/5)2, (70%/5)2, (80%/5)2
Afternoon
4 Hang snatch: (60%/3)2, (70%/3)2, (75%/2)3
5 Snatch pull: (70%/4)2, 80%/4, (90%/4)2
6 Good morning: (X/8)4

Day 5
Morning
1 Snatch: (60%/3)3, (70%/3)2, (80%/2)2
2 Hang clean and jerk:
3 Snatch pull: (70%/4)2, (80%/4)2, (90%/3)2
4 Front squat: (70%/5)2, (80%/4)2, (905/3)2

Day 6
Morning
1 Power clean and jerk: (60%/3 + 1)2, (70%/3 + 1)2, (80%/2 + 1)2
2 Jerk: 70%/3, (80%/3)2, (90%/2)2
3 Back squat: (70%/5)2, (80%/5)2, (90%/3)2
Afternoon
4 Hang snatch: (60%/3)3, (70%/3)2, (80%/2)2
5 Snatch pull: (60%/4)2, (70%/4)2, 80%/3
6 Slow snatch deadlift: (80%/3)6–10 s up

Day 7
Complete rest

Total repetitions: 582

X, an extremely variable weight from one individual to another, with a varied relationship to either of the two competitive lifts (see also Table 16.2).

Table 16.4 Soviet competitive week

Day 1
Morning
1 Snatch: (70%/3)3, (80%/2)2, (90%/1)2
2 Clean and jerk: (70%/2 + 1)3, (80%/2 + 1)2, (90%/1 + 1)2, (100%/1 + 1)2
3 Jerk: 70%/2, 80%/2, 90%/2, 100%/2
Afternoon
4 Front squat: (70%/3)3, (80%/3)2, (90%/3)2
5 Snatch pull: 60%/3, 70%/3, 80%/3, 90%/2
6 Good morning: (X/8)4

Day 2
1 Power snatch: (60%/3)2, (70%/3)2, (80%/2)2
2 Power clean: (60%/3)2, (70%/3)2, (80%/2)2
3 Clean pull: (80%/3)3, 90%/3, (100%/2)2
4 Back squat: 70%/3, (80%/3)2, 90%/3
5 Press: 60%/3, (70%/3)2

Day 3
Active rest

Day 4
Morning
1 Snatch: (70%/2)2, (80%/2)2, 90%/1
2 Clean and jerk: (70%/2 + 1)3, (80%/2 + 1)3, (90%/1 + 1)2
3 Jerk: 70%/3, 80%/2, (90%/1)2
Afternoon
4 Back squat: 70%/3, (80%/2)2, (90%/2)3
5 Snatch pull: 60%/4, (70%/3)2, (80%/3)2
6 Good morning: (X/8)4

Day 5
1 Hang snatch: 60%/3, (70%/2)2, (80%/2)2, (90%/1)2
2 Clean and jerk: 60%/3 + 1, (70%/2 + 1)2, (80%/2 + 1)2
3 Clean pull: 70%/3, (80%/3)2, (90%/3)2
4 Back squat: (70%/3)2, (80%/3)2, (90%/3)2
5 Press: (70%/3)2

Total repetitions: 324

X, see note to Table 16.3.

The training of women

Women's weightlifting, officially inaugurated in 1987 by the first World's Championships, is rapidly passing through developmental stages. Apparently, there is little or no variation in the training programmes for women from those designed for men, since all training is based on the individual's personal maxima. Blood testosterone levels and societal perceptions of female participation in strength activities appear to be the major factors in considering alterations in training based on gender. The former may have the more significant effect, while the latter should warrant less consideration as greater enlightenment on the subject is realized.

References

Abadjiev, I. (1989) *The Bulgarian Training System* (lecture). National Strength and Conditioning Association study tour, Sofia, Bulgaria.

Enoka, R.M. (1988) Muscle strength and its development. *Sports Medicine*, **6**, 146–68.

Frolov, V., Efimov, N. & Vanagas, M. (1977) Training weights for snatch pulls. *Tyazhelaya Atletika*, pp. 65–7. *Soviet Sports Review*, 1983, **18**, 58–61.

Garhammer, J. (1985) Biomechanical analysis of weightlifting at the 1984 Olympic Games. *International Journal of Sport Biomechanics*, **1**, 122–30.

Garhammer, J. (1989) Weight lifting and training. In C.L. Vaughan (ed.) *Biomechanics of Sport*, pp. 169–211. CRC Publishers, Boca Raton.

Garhammer, J. & Gregor, R. (1979) Force plate evaluations of weightlifting and vertical jumping (Abstract). *Medicine and Science in Sports and Exercise*, **11**, 106.

Garhammer, J. & Gregor, R. (1991) A comparison of propulsive forces for weightlifting and vertical jumping. *Journal of Applied Sports Science Research* (in press).

Häkkinen, K. (1988) A biomechanical analysis of various combinations of the snatch pull exercises. *Journal of Human Movement Studies*, **15**, 229–43.

Häkkinen, K. & Kauhanen, H. (1986) A biomechanical analysis of selected assistance exercises of weightlifting. *Journal of Human Movement Studies*, **12**, 271–88.

Häkkinen, K., Kauhanen, H. & Komi, P.V. (1984) Biomechanical changes in the Olympic weightlifting technique of the snatch and clean and jerk from submaximal to maximal loads. *Scandinavian Journal of Sports Sciences*, **6**, 57–66.

Häkkinen, K., Pakarinen, A., Alen, M., Kauhanen, H. & Komi, P.V. (1987) Relationships between training volume, physical performance capacity, and serum hormone concentrations during prolonged training in elite weight lifters. *International Journal of Sports Medicine*, **8** (suppl.), 61–5.

Häkkinen, K., Pakarinen, A., Alen, M., Kauhanen, H. & Komi, P.V. (1988a) Neuromuscular and hormonal adaptations in athletes to strength training in two years. *Journal of Applied Physiology*, **65**, 2406–12.

Häkkinen, K., Pakarinen, A., Alen, M., Kauhanen, H. & Komi, P.V. (1988b) Daily hormonal and neuromuscular responses to intensive strength training in 1 week. *International Journal of Sports Medicine*, **9**, 422–8.

Häkkinen, K., Pakarinen, A., Alen, M., Kauhanen H. & Komi, P.V. (1988c) Neuromuscular and hormonal responses in elite athletes to two successive strength training sessions in one day. *European Journal of Applied Physiology*, 57, 133–9.

Häkkinen, K., Pakarinen, A., Kyröläinen, H., Cheng, S., Kim, D.H. & Komi, P.V. (1990) Neuromuscular adaptations and serum hormones in females during prolonged power training. *International Journal of Sports Medicine*, **11**, 91–8.

Kraemer, W.J. (1988) Endocrine responses to resistance exercise. *Medicine and Science in Sports and Exercise*, **20** (suppl.), S152–S157.

Kuipers, H. & Keizer, H.A. (1988) Overtraining in elite athletes. *Sports Medicine*, **6**, 79–92.

Matveyev, L.P. (1972) *Periodisienang das Sportlichen Training* (translated into German by P. Tschiene with a chapter by A. Kruger). Beles and Wernitz, Berlin.

Medvedjev, A., Frolov, V., Lukashev, A. & Krasov, E. (1981). A comparative analysis of the clean and clean pull technique with various weights. *Tyazhelaya Atletika*, **10**, 33–5. *Soviet Sports Review*, 1983, **18**, 17–19.

Medvedjev, A.S., Masalgin, N.A., Herrera, A.G. & Frolov, V.I. (1982) Classification of jerk exercises and methods of their use depending upon weightlifters qualification. In *1982 Weightlifting Yearbook*. Fizkultura i Sport, Moscow (translated by Andrew Charniga). Sportivny Press, Livonia, Michigan, pp. 4–9.

Nilsson, S. (1986) Overtraining. In S. Maehium, S. Nilsson & P. Renstrom (eds) *An Update on Sports Medicine*, pp. 97–104. Proceedings of the Second Scandinavian Conference on Sports Medicine, Soria Moria, Oslo, Norway, March 1986.

Sale, D.G. (1988) Neural adapation to resistance training. *Medicine and Science in Sports and Exercise*, **20** (suppl.), S135–S145.

Stone, M.H., Keith, R.E., Kearney, J.T., Fleck, S.J., Wilson, G.D. & Triplett, N.T. (1991) Overtraining: A review of the signs, symptoms and possible causes. *Journal of Applied Sports Science Research*, **5**, 35–50.

Stone, M., O'Bryant, H. & Garhammer, J. (1981) A hypothetical model for strength training. *Journal of Sports Medicine and Physical Fitness*, **21**, 342–51.

Stone, M., O'Bryant, H, Garhammer, J., McMillan, J. & Rozenek, R. (1982) A theoretical model of strength training. *National Strength and Conditioning Association Journal*, **4**, 36–9.

Takano, B. (1990) *K*-value: a tool for determining training intensity. *National Strength and Conditioning Association Journal*, **12**, 60–1.

Vorobyev, A.N. (1978) *A Textbook on Weightlifting* (translated by J. Brice). International Weightlifting Federation, Budapest.

Chapter 17

Training for Bodybuilding

PER A. TESCH

Introduction

During the last decade strength training for non-athletic purposes or general conditioning have become increasingly popular. In parallel the appreciation for bodybuilding as a sport seems to have evolved. Most of the strategies employed in non-competitive strength training have been adopted from those invented and used by bodybuilders. Today both men and women enjoy the benefits of strength training programmes as an aid to increase or maintain muscle mass and strength, reduce body fat and improve physical appearance. It is also becoming more frequently used as an effective therapy in the treatment of various diseases. Similarly, the potential value of strength training in geriatrics to combat muscle atrophy and loss of bone mass has recently been brought to our attention. Training programmes employed to serve any of these purposes should be specifically designed. There is, however, limited scientific data available to indicate how a conditioning programme should be structured or organized to produce optimal gains in muscle mass or strength. It seems reasonable, however, that many of the principles used by bodybuilders in the design of their programmes could be applied for categories of trainees who are not aiming at achieving that level. The purposes of this chapter are firstly to provide some insight with regard to the approaches taken by athletes training for bodybuilding, and secondly to describe some physical and physiological

characteristics of competitive bodybuilders. Although the maintenance of a perfected diet is fundamental to success in competitive bodybuilding, both in the long and the short-term perspective, this issue will not be addressed in this chapter.

Characteristics of bodybuilders

The bodybuilder's ultimate goal is to develop superior muscularity and mass, symmetry and harmony between different body parts, and to enhance muscle density and visual separation of muscles. To do this subcutaneous fat has to be reduced to a minimum. In a contest these qualities are judged during the posing acts. There is, however, no objective way of measuring the athletic ability of a bodybuilder. Both men and women compete in bodybuilding but it is still a controversial issue what criteria should be used to judge female bodybuilders (Fig. 17.1).

Anthropometry

Successful bodybuilders display extraordinary muscularity and mass. Thus, bodybuilders show much greater body weight or lean body mass relative to stature than non-athletes and most other athletic groups (Katch *et al.*, 1980). Enhanced muscle mass has also been documented in that muscle cross-sectional area and individual muscle fibre size is much greater than in other individuals (see Chapter 8B). The

370

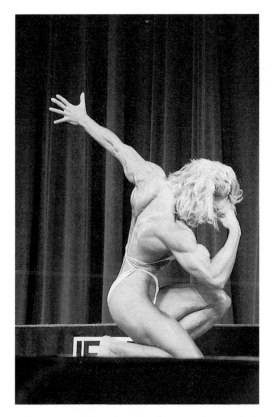

Fig. 17.1 Female bodybuilder performing the pose act. (Courtesy of B & K Sports Magazine.)

girth of arm, chest or lower limbs, for example, is larger (Fig. 17.2) and subcutaneous fat is much lower than in non-athletes. When in peak condition and especially in conjunction with a contest, body fat percentage of national or regional calibre male and female bodybuilders may average less than 6 and 10% respectively (Heyward *et al.*, 1989).

Strength

Due to the increased muscle mass of bodybuilders they also possess enhanced muscular strength and power (Häkkinen *et al.*, 1984). It is, however, not clear whether bodybuilders show greater muscle strength relative to body weight or muscle cross-sectional area than non-trained individuals (Pipes, 1979; Spitler *et al.*, 1980; Tesch & Larsson, 1982; Sale & MacDougall, 1984). Compared to other populations the upper body appears to be more developed than muscle groups of the lower limb (Fig. 17.3). Thus, relative to non-athletes or other strength-trained athletes bodybuilders possess greater arm than leg strength (Sale & MacDougall, 1984). Similarly, the difference in muscle strength between male and female bodybuilders is greater for upper than lower body.

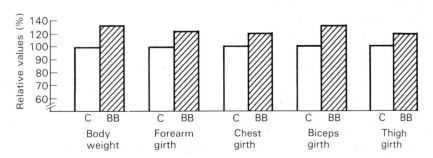

Fig. 17.2 Body weight and forearm, chest, biceps and thigh girths in healthy age- and height-matched non-athletic controls (C) and bodybuilders (BB). The values of BB (▨) are set relative to the values obtained in C (▢). (From Tesch & Lindeberg, 1984, and Colliander & Tesch, 1988.)

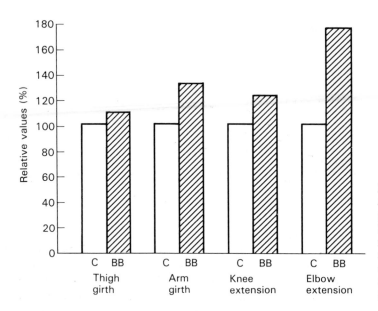

Fig. 17.3 Thigh and arm girths and knee and elbow extension peak torque (0.52 rad · s⁻¹) in healthy, age- and height-matched non-athletic controls (C) and bodybuilders (BB). The values of BB (▨) are set relative to the values obtained C (▢). (From Sale & MacDougall, 1984.)

Aerobic work capacity

Analagous with the concept of specificity of training, bodybuilders do not possess markedly enhanced aerobic power or capacity. Maximal oxygen uptake, expressed in absolute terms, however seems to be greater in bodybuilders than in height-matched physically active, non-athletic men (Häkkinen *et al.*, 1984; Colliander & Tesch, 1988). They do show somewhat increased maximal oxygen uptake relative to body weight or lean body mass (Häkkinen *et al.*, 1984; Colliander & Tesch, 1988) or, owing to the increased body mass, low maximal aerobic power relative to body weight (Spitler *et al.*, 1980; Urhausen *et al.*, 1989). This is not surprising because oxygen uptake during heavy resistance exercise using large muscle groups seldom exceeds 60% of maximal aerobic power (Tesch, 1987; Dudley *et al.*, 1991b; Chapter 8C). Despite possessing excessive muscle mass, these athletes also display limited capacity to sustain standardized submaximal cycle ergometer exercise and low plasma lactate tolerance to such exercise. Thus bodybuilders do not show higher anaerobic threshold or aerobic capacity when performing two-legged

cycle ergometry (Fig. 17.4; Tesch, 1987) or arm-cranking (Tesch & Lindeberg, 1984) exercise than non-athletes. This may simply be explained by the lack of increase in skeletal muscle oxidative capacity in these athletes (see Chapter 8C). The demonstration of lower mitochondrial and oxidative enzyme content and capillary supply shown in power- or strength-trained athletes would suggest a reduction in aerobic work capacity with more intense heavy resistance training that is not seen in bodybuilders. Because strength training is often an integrated part of the conditioning programmes for athletes relying on speed, power and aerobic energy utilization, these apparently different responses should be considered in the design of training programmes for these athletes.

Health profile

Anabolic–androgenic steroid free male and female bodybuilders appear to show favourable lipoprotein–lipid profiles. Thus bodybuilders typically possess similar or higher high-density lipoprotein cholesterol (HDL-C) compared to normal and similar or even higher values

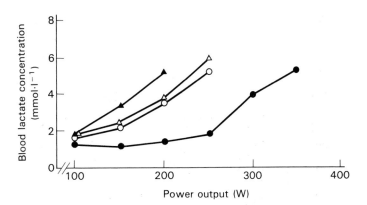

Fig. 17.4 Blood lactate concentration relative to power output during leg cycle ergometry exercise in bodybuilders (○), Olympic weight- and power-lifters (▲), cyclists (●) and controls (△). (Adapted from Tesch, 1987.)

than those reported for endurance runners (Kokkinos & Hurley, 1990). Certainly, the strict diet typical for bodybuilders influences their lipoprotein–lipid profile. Although there are few well-controlled longitudinal studies it is however likely that the specific training has a favourable effect as well. It also appears that strength training is accompanied by a reduced basal plasma insulin concentration and decreased insulin response to a glucose challenge. These responses were demonstrated after a 10-week strength training programme (Miller et al., 1984) and in experienced body-builders (Szczypaczewska et al., 1989). The enhanced glucose tolerance and insulin action in bodybuilders and in response to training appears to be due to the increase in muscle mass and/or the reduced adipose fat tissue content.

There has been some concern whether blood pressure is increased in bodybuilders because of the large increase in arterial blood pressure reported during acute heavy resistance exercise (MacDougall et al., 1985). Thus, intra-arterial pressure increased to 320/250 in strength-trained athletes while performing the leg press. Somewhat in contrast to this view bodybuilders are able to perform resistance exercise with higher absolute and relative weights and yet not show greater increases in systolic or diastolic blood pressure than non-weight-trained individuals (Fleck & Dean, 1987; Chapter 12). Although high resting blood pressures occasionally have

been reported in competitive bodybuilders or power-lifters (Spitler et al., 1980; Staron et al., 1981; Colliander & Tesch, 1988), it is likely that this, at least in part, is attributed to the use of anabolic steroids. In bodybuilders not taking anabolic steroids, systolic and diastolic blood pressures at rest or when performing light to heavy submaximal cycle ergometry exercise were normal or slightly lower than observed in non-athletes (Fig. 17.5; Colliander & Tesch, 1988; Urhausen et al., 1989). Likewise, the bodybuilders showed a much lower rate pressure product (heart rate × systolic blood pressure) than the non-athletes.

The excessive use of drugs and other substances among bodybuilders is not only a serious medical problem and threat. Sometimes it also makes it difficult to interpret results from studies where bodybuilders have been examined, because of the unknown use or the undefined action of the drugs being administered.

Bodybuilding and age

Compared to other athletes competing in physically demanding sports bodybuilders typically reach their peak performance at a relatively high age. Many male and female bodybuilders still show improvements at the age of 30 or even later in their career. In most other sports athletes have retired from high-level competition at that age. For example,

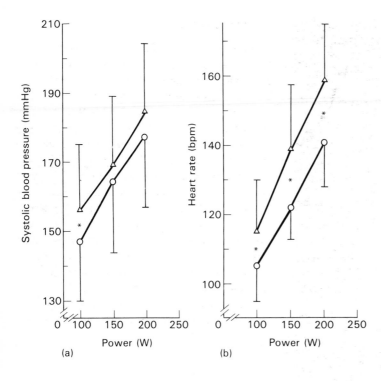

Fig. 17.5 Systolic blood pressure (a) and heart rate (b) during progressive cycle ergometry exercise in bodybuilders (○) and students (△). *, $P < 0.05$.

British bodybuilder Albert Beccles is successfully competing among the very best professionals at the age of 59 (Fig. 17.6). This may be explained by the long time it takes to build overall mass and to sculpture a balanced body. Resistance training can be enjoyed by previously non-strength-trained men at a very high age. There are reports available convincingly demonstrating that 70-year-old men can perform strength-training programmes comprising very intense activities that produce selective fast twitch muscle fibre hypertrophy (Larsson, 1982). Likewise, strength training has been performed by 70–90-year-old individuals (Frontera *et al.*, 1988; Fiatorone *et al.*, 1990). They demonstrated impressive increases in strength that positively impacted on daily functional abilities. The increase in strength was in part explained by increased muscle mass. Hence, this kind of training carried out with reduced intensity seems to be safely performed with beneficial effects in aged populations.

Injuries

There are few data compiled on the incidence of injuries in bodybuilders. Compared to other elite athletes who participate in regular and strenuous physical training programmes, competitive bodybuilders show a low prevalence of injuries. Overuse symptoms located to shoulder and elbow joints appear to be the most common type of injuries (Klein *et al.*, 1979). They seem to be more frequent among beginners or semi-advanced bodybuilders. The cause of the injuries can usually be attributed to erroneous technique or a sudden progression of the load or volume of training. Overuse-induced symptoms from the shoulder, mainly the acromioclavicular joint and muscle or tendon insertions around the shoulder, and inflammation of subacromialis are frequent. According to the report by Klein *et al.* (1979) 14 out of 100 established bodybuilders suffered from these problems at least once during their career. The reason for the high incidence of

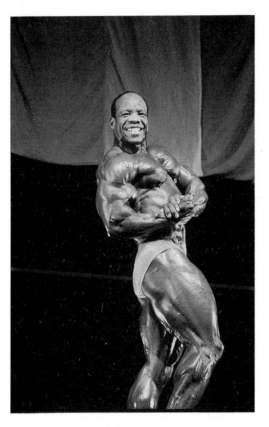

Fig. 17.6 British bodybuilder Albert Beccles. (Couresty of B & K Sports Magazine.)

Training strategies

Although bodybuilders, power-lifters and Olympic weightlifters all display extraordinary muscular strength and mass the training modalities, strategies and goals to be achieved are very different among these athletes. The rationale for these strategies are based mainly on the experiences among the athletes evolved over the years. Whereas strength performance is a major concern for lifters, bodybuilders do not purposely aim at increasing muscular strength. Instead, most of the training carried out by the bodybuilder is devoted to induce muscle hypertrophy. An increase in overall muscle mass is promoted early in the career. Later, the training is focused on maintaining that already achieved and to exercise 'under-developed' body parts in order to achieve perfect symmetry and enhance definition of muscles.

Load

The intensity of heavy resistance or weight training is typically defined as the load that can be raised or lowered for a given number of repetitions. For example the maximum load is the one repetition maximum (1 RM). Bodybuilders use less heavy loads than Olympic weightlifters or power-lifters. Hence they usually exercise with loads that equal 6–12 RM, whereas lifters when aiming at increasing strength output choose heavier loads. There is no scientific proof that the approach taken by the bodybuilder to build muscle mass is more effective. It is not even known if bodybuilders show greater muscle mass than competitive lifters. Thus, no data are at hand to suggest that muscle cross-sectional area for a given muscle group, that is essential in all these categories, is larger in bodybuilders. Neither is it known whether the 'muscle density' or the protein content of muscle is greater in bodybuilders than in untrained individuals or other strength-trained athletes. Very little, if any, data are at hand describing the influences of resistance

shoulder injuries may simply be due to the fact that the shoulders are excessively used and heavily involved in almost all upper-body exercises performed by bodybuilders. The second most prevalent injury was overuse of the triceps insertion at the olecranon, which is highly stressed during many of the elbow extensor exercises. The number of knee injuries reported were very few. Serious injuries among bodybuilders are rare. Because training never uses maximal loads and exercises are typically executed at slow speeds and in a strict and controlled way, accidental injuries are not very common. Infrequently though, more serious injuries such as complete rupture of the pectoralis or biceps muscles may occur in elite bodybuilders.

versus volume of training on the muscle hypertrophic response. Studies that have compared training programmes varying in load and volume have mainly dealt with the effects on muscular strength (Atha, 1981), not muscle mass.

Volume

The volume of training for a given exercise is simply defined as number of sets × repetitions × load. Although the volume of weights lifted, i.e. the amount of work, by bodybuilders is impressive it is not clear if this is a more important feature than maintaining a high resistance.

A recent report showed that increases in 3 RM in the leg press was highly correlated with the progressive increase in resistance, but not volume, during 20 weeks of heavy strength training (Dudley *et al.*, 1991a). Those who showed the largest increases in resistance and 3 RM also displayed the greatest hypertrophic response. This suggests that progression in training should emphasize increases in resistance, not repetitions or number of sets.

Muscle failure

It is a common belief among bodybuilders that muscle failure should terminate each set in order to optimize the beneficial effects of strength training. Statements like 'No pain—no gain' reflects that widespread opinion. In a 36-year-old paper Hellebrandt and Houtz (1956) suggested that 'the rate at which improvement progress depends primarily on the degree to which the person is willing to punish himself'. This may very well be true but there is no proof of this hypothesis. Neither is it clear what mechanism associated with contraction failure would relate to increased protein synthesis, which is the ultimate goal to be achieved by the bodybuilder. The load used in heavy strength exercise influences the acute metabolic and hormonal response. When power output during two 20-min weightlifting sessions was kept constant, but resistance and number of repetitions per set varied, growth hormone secretion was enhanced following high but not low loading (Fig. 17.7; Vanhelder *et al.*, 1984). Similarly, catecholamine levels are markedly enhanced during heavy resistance exercise, but not during cycle ergometry exercise, performed at the same power output (Tesch, 1987). Yet, it should be remembered that there is no evidence to say that the plasma hormonal levels present in response to an acute exercise bout has any influence on the muscle hypertrophic response (see Chapter 11).

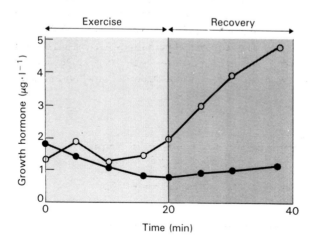

Fig. 17.7 Changes in plasma growth hormone during and after 30 min of heavy-resistance exercise at a given power output executed with high (○) or low (●) loads. (From Vanhelder *et al.*, 1984.)

Table 17.1 Example of '4 days on–1 day off' routine

Day 1	Day 2	Day 3	Day 4	Day 5
Chest	Front thigh	Back	Hamstrings	Rest
Triceps	Calves	Biceps	Shoulders	
		Abdominals		

Frequency

The frequency of training depends on whether a split or an all-round routine is used. For beginners, exercising two or maybe three times a week, it is preferable to exercise all body parts on each day of training. Systems allowing for training on 3 or more consecutive days followed by a day of rest, for example 4 days on and 1 day off, are typical for bodybuilders (see below). It also appears that two workouts per week for most muscle groups is sufficient to induce optimal adaptive responses. There are indications that more frequent all-out training with heavy loads may be too stressful to individual muscle groups and thus produces 'overtraining' symptoms. Since all high-calibre bodybuilders use the split system they typically get more than 48 hours of recovery for each muscle group. It is, however, far from understood what the optimal recovery is, what the individual variation is or how the intensity of training influences the time needed for recovery and optimal adaptive response.

Exercises, sets, repetitions and rest

Using the split system a single workout consists of a series of exercises usually emphasizing two or three major muscle groups or body parts. For example, day 1 may include exercises for chest and biceps. Then, on the following day the back, triceps and abdominals may be exercised. The legs and shoulders are then exercised on day 3. Using this approach the individually designed programme usually includes all muscle groups within a 4-day frame. This is typically followed by 1 day of rest. Examples of '4 on–1 off' and '6 on–1 off' programmes are shown in Tables 17.1 and 17.2. Another alternative is the 'double split' routine where two exercise sessions are performed on each day (Table 17.3). For each muscle group, depending on its complexity, two to five different exercises are usually employed to exhaust and activate all aspects of the muscle or muscle group during a single workout. A typical exercise routine for the shoulders (Table 17.4) may comprise the following sequence of five exercises: seated press behind neck (barbell), military press (barbell), standing side laterals (dumb-bells), seated rear lateral raises (dumb-bells) and standing shoulder shrugs (barbell). Routines for other body parts are designed in a similar manner. Thus one exercise session may comprise 20–25 sets per muscle group or a total of 40–70 sets. The sequence of performing exercises is chosen so that premature fatigue of a single muscle group that has an agonistic function in a sub-

Table 17.2 Example of '6 days on–1 day off' routine

Day 1	Day 2	Day 3	Day 4	Day 5	Day 6	Day 7
Back	Legs	Shoulders	See day 1	See day 2	See day 3	Rest
Chest		Arms				
		Abdominals				

Table 17.3 Example of 'double split' routine

	Day 1	Day 2	Day 3	Day 4
Morning	Shoulders Lower back	Back Aerobics	Chest Aerobics	Rest
Afternoon	Thighs Abdominals	Biceps Calves	Triceps Calves Abdominals	Rest

Table 17.4 Example of a shoulder exercise routine

Exercises	Sets	Repetitions
Seated press behind neck	4–5	10–12
Military press	4–5	10–12
Standing side laterals	4–5	10–12
Seated rear lateral raises	4–5	10–12
Standing shoulder shrugs	4–5	10–12

sequent exercise is avoided. Bodybuilders typically emphasize short (1–2 min) rest periods between sets. One set of exercises usually consists of 6–12 repetitions. In the precontest routine many bodybuilders prefer to reduce the weights and do more sets per muscle group, higher repetitions/set and shorten the rest between sets sometimes to less than 1 min.

Equipment

There is no reason to believe that there are any weight-training devices that are more effective than free weights in producing increases in muscle strength or mass. Exercises with barbells or dumb-bells or simple pulley machines using weight stacks to provide resistance are the brickstones in athletic strength training. Although isokinetic devices, providing accommodated resistance at preselected constant angular velocities, may be effective and safe in clinical settings concerned with rehabilitation of orthopaedic pathologies, there is no scientific proof or indication to say that such dynamometers are more effective. If anything, the available data suggest that isokinetic resistive exercise using concentric or eccentric muscle actions only produce modest muscle hypertrophy compared to training with free weights (Colliander & Tesch, 1990). When exercising with free weights substantial acceleration and deceleration occurs when the trainee starts moving the weight or when bringing it to a stop. This is fundamentally different to what occurs during isokinetic loading. However, how to optimize the adaptive muscle hypertrophic response to resistance exercise remains to be studied.

Circuit weight training

Circuit weight training is a popular form of strength exercise usually performed by individuals who are mainly concerned to maintain or enhance 'overall fitness'. Such programmes consists of series, usually 10–15, of resistance exercises for different body parts. Exercise machines, free weights or body weight bearing exercises are used to produce resistance. For each exercise 12–15 repetitions, using modest weights (approximately 40–60% of 1 RM), are performed. Each exercise is typically completed within 30–40 s. The trainee moves quickly from one exercise to the next with 15–30 s of rest between stations. The circuit is repeated one to three times depending on fitness level. Thus, it takes about 30 min to complete an exercise session. The idea is to enjoy both cardiovascular and strength benefits from the training because circuit weight training is thought to stimulate systems that promote both increases in aerobic capacity and muscle hypertrophic responses.

Unfortunately, the increases in muscular strength and mass or maximal aerobic power in response to circuit weight training are modest (Gettman & Pollock, 1981). It may, however, still be an effective exercise form in enhancing or maintaining overall fitness in healthy individuals or patients undergoing cardiac rehabilitation (Kelemen & Stewart, 1985).

Summary

The intent of training for bodybuilding is mainly to increase muscle mass of all body parts and produce symmetry and harmony and, moreover, to achieve definition so that muscles can be visually separated from each other. This is produced by exercise programmes using 'split' systems, i.e. a few selected muscles or muscle groups are exercised in each exercise session.

Bodybuilders are characterized by large muscle mass and lean body mass relative to stature. The increased muscle size seems to be accompanied by a corresponding increase in muscle strength. They do not, however, show markedly enhanced maximal aerobic power or endurance capacity. It appears that this form of strength training is associated with a low incidence of serious injuries and has some valuable, health promoting effects.

References

Athá, J. (1981) Strengthening muscle. *Exercise and Sport Sciences Reviews*, **9**, 1–73.

Colliander, E.B. & Tesch, P.A. (1988) Blood pressure in resistance-trained athletes. *Canadian Journal of Sport Science*, **13**, 31–4.

Colliander, E.B. & Tesch, P.A. (1990) Effects of eccentric and concentric muscle actions in resistance training. *Acta Physiologica Scandinavica*, **140**, 31–9.

Dudley, G.A., Tesch, P.A., Miller, B.J. & Buchanan, P. (1991a) Importance of eccentric actions in performance adaptations to resistance training. *Aviation Space and Environmental Medicine*, **62**, 543–50.

Dudley, G.A., Tesch, P.A., Harris, R.T., Golden, C.L. & Buchanan, P. (1991b) Influence of eccentric actions on the metabolic cost of resistance exercise. *Aviation Space and Environmental Medicine* (in press).

Fleck, S.J. & Dean, L.S. (1987) Resistance-training experience and the pressor response during resistance exercise. *Journal of Applied Physiology*, **63**, 116–20.

Fiatarone, M.A., Marks, E.C., Ryan, N.D., Meredith, C.N., Lipsitz, L.A. & Evans, W.J. (1990) High-intensity strength training in nonagenarians. Effects on skeletal muscle. *Journal of the American Medical Association*, **263**, 3029–34.

Frontera, W.R., Meredith, C.N., O'Reilly, K.P., Knuttgen, H.G. & Evans, W.J. (1988) Strength conditioning in older men: skeletal muscle hypertrophy and improved function. *Journal of Applied Physiology*, **64**, 1038–44.

Gettman, L.R. & Pollock, M.L. (1981) Circuit weight training: A critical review of the physiological benefits. *Physician and Sportsmedicine*, **9**, 44–60.

Häkkinen, K, Alén, M. & Komi, P.V. (1984) Neuromuscular, anaerobic, and aerobic performance characteristics of elite power athletes. *European Journal of Applied Physiology*, **53**, 97–105.

Hellebrandt, F.A. & Houtz, S.J. (1956) Mechanisms of muscle training in man: Experimental demonstration of the overload principle. *Physical Therapy Review*, **36**, 371–83.

Heyward, V.H., Sandoval, W.M. & Colville, B.C. (1989) Anthropometric, body composition and nutritional profiles of bodybuilders during training. *Journal of Applied Sports Science Research*, **3**, 22–9.

Katch, V.L., Katch, F.I., Moffat, R. & Gittleson, M. (1980) Muscular development and lean body weight in bodybuilders and weight lifters. *Medicine and Science in Sports and Exercise*, **12**, 340–4.

Kelemen, M.H. & Stewart, K.J. (1985) Circuit weight training. A new direction for cardiac rehabilitation. *Sports Medicine*, **2**, 385–8.

Klein, W., Schulitz, K.-P. & Neumann, C. (1979) Orthopädische Probleme beim Bodybuilding. *Deutsche Zeitschrift für Sportmedizin*, **9**, 296–308.

Kokkinos, P.F. & Hurley, B.F. (1990) Strength training and lipoprotein-lipid profiles. A critical analysis and recommendations for further study. *Sports Medicine*, **9**, 266–72.

Larsson, L. (1982) Physical training effects on muscle morphology in sedentary males at different ages. *Medicine and Science in Sports and Exercise*, **14**, 203–6.

MacDougall, J.D., Tuxen, D., Sale, D.G., Moroz, J.R. & Sutton, J.R. (1985) Arterial blood pressure response to heavy resistance exercise. *Journal of Applied Physiology*, **58**, 785–90.

Miller, W.J., Sherman, W.H. & Ivy, J.L. (1984) Effect of strength training on glucose tolerance and post-glucose insulin response. *Medicine and Science in*

Sports and Exercise, **16**, 539–43.

Pipes, T.V. (1979) Physiologic characteristics of elite bodybuilders. *Physician and Sportsmedicine*, **7**, 116–20.

Sale, D.G. & MacDougall, J.D. (1984) Isokinetic strength in weight-trainers. *European Journal of Applied Physiology*, **53**, 128–32.

Spitler, D.L., Diaz, F.J., Horvath, S.M. & Wright, J.E. (1980) Body composition and maximal aerobic capacity of bodybuilders. *Journal of Sports Medicine*, **20**, 181–8.

Staron, R., Hagerman, F. & Hikida, R. (1981) The effects of detraining on an elite power-lifter. *Journal of the Neurological Sciences*, **51**, 247–57.

Szczypaczewska, M., Nazar, K. & Kaciuba-Uscilko, H. (1989) Glucose tolerance and insulin response to glucose load in bodybuilders. *International Journal of Sports Medicine*, **10**, 34–7.

Tesch, P. & Larsson, L. (1982) Muscle hypertrophy in bodybuilders. *European Journal of Applied Physiology*, **49**, 301–6.

Tesch, P.A. & Lindeberg, S. (1984) Blood lactate accumulation during arm exercise in world class kayak paddlers and strength trained athletes. *European Journal of Applied Physiology*, **52**, 441–5.

Tesch, P.A. (1987) Acute and long-term metabolic changes consequent to heavy-resistance exercise. *Medicine and Sport Science*, **26**, 67–89.

Urhausen, A., Hölpes, R. & Kinderman, W. (1989) One- and two-dimensional echocardiography in bodybuilders using anabolic steroids. *European Journal of Applied Physiology*, **58**, 633–40.

Vanhelder, W.P., Radomski, M.V. & Goode, R.C. (1984) Growth hormone responses during intermittent weight lifting exercise in men. *European Journal of Applied Physiology*, **153**, 31–4.

Chapter 18

Training for Power Events

DIETMAR SCHMIDTBLEICHER

Classification of power events

Power refers to the ability of the neuromuscular system to produce the greatest possible impulse in a given time period. The time period depends on the resistance or the load against which the athlete has to work and of the organization of the acceleration. In some sports or disciplines it is necessary to overcome resistance with the greatest possible speed of muscle action at the beginning of the movement (shot put, javelin, etc.). In others, the maximal acceleration should be delayed to reach a maximal velocity for the equipment or the body or parts of the body.

Concentric and isometric actions

A correlation exists between maximal isometric strength (F_{max}) and movement speed. The negative correlation increases from $r = -0.5$ using loads of 2–3 kg up to $r = -0.9$ working against loads close to the individual single repetition maximum (Schmidtbleicher, 1980). This result refers, on the one hand, to the fact that voluntary maximal isometric action is a special case of concentric actions (as can be seen in Fig. 18.1), and on the other hand some other important implications can be demonstrated. If the external loads are low the influence of maximal strength diminishes more and more, and the rate of force development (RFD) increases to be the predominant factor. The maximal rate of force development (MRFD)

is identical with the term 'explosive strength' (Werschoshanskij, 1972; Bührle & Schmidtbleicher, 1981; Bührle, 1985), which describes the ability of the neuromuscular system to develop high action velocities. The MRFD is equal for all loads that are higher than 25% of F_{max} (Müller, 1987). Ballistic movements against resistance lower than 25% of F_{max} are determined from the initial RFD (IRFD), i.e. the beginning of the slope. Werschoshanskij and Tatjan (1975) called the IRFD 'starting strength'. The IRFD is essential in sports where great initial speed is necessary for optimal performance, e.g. boxing, fencing, karate, etc. The RFD depends on the recruitment and firing frequencies of the motor units and the contractile characteristics of the respective muscle fibres. If the load to overcome is light IRFD predominates; if the load is increased (as in the shot put) MRFD is required. In cases where the load is very high (weight-lifting) maximal strength predominates. Beside the load, the movement time also can be chosen as a classification criterion. For movements with a duration of 250 ms or less IRFD and MRFD are the main factors. Movements with a duration of more than 250 ms are dominated by the maximal strength factor (Fig. 18.2).

Stretch–shortening cycle type movements

Beside concentric and isometric actions powerful movements are generated in reactive movements or in a stretch–shortening cycle

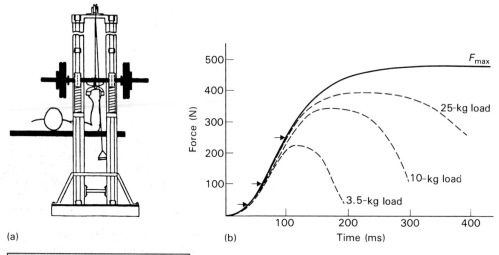

(a)

(b)

Load (kg)	Correlation
25	$r = 0.85$
10	$r = 0.66$
3.5	$r = 0.50$

(c)

Fig. 18.1 (a) Measurement device for the registration of force–time curves. (b) Force–time curves from isometric and concentric actions against different loads of a shot put-like arm movement of one subject. The dashed lines show the concentric phase of the movement. The solid line describes the isometric part of the muscle action. (c) Correlations between strength and movement time of different loads.

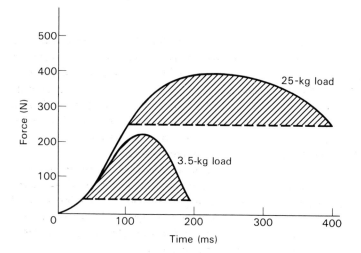

Fig. 18.2 Force–time curves of concentric actions against different loads. The shaded areas describe the acceleration impulse, which is mainly due to the rate of force development (RFD) in lower loads and therefore faster movements. In higher loads the impulse is mainly determined by the maximum strength that can be exerted against this resistance.

(SSC). A stretch–shortening cycle is not only a combination of an eccentric and a concentric movement. Moreover, this type of action is a relatively independent motor quality (Komi & Bosco, 1978; Bosco, 1982; Komi, 1984; Gollhofer, 1987).

Two types of stretch–shortening cycles exist, a long and a short one. A long SSC (e.g. jump

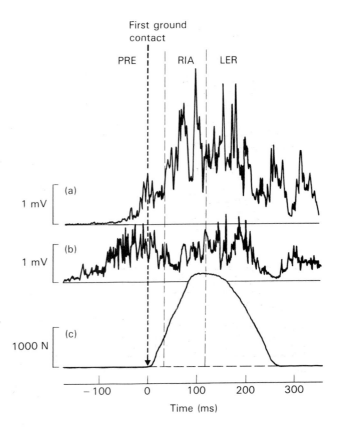

Fig. 18.3 Rectified and averaged EMG pattern of (a) m. vastus and (b) m. gastrocnemius, and (c) angular displacement of the ankle and vertical ground reaction forces from drop jumps ($n = 10$) with a single leg-landing from a dropping height of 16 cm. PRE, pre-innervation phase; RIA, reflex-induced area; LER, late EMG response. (From Gollhofer, 1987.)

to throw in basketball, jump to block in volleyball) is characterized by large angular displacements in the hip, knee and ankle joints and by a duration of more than 250 ms. A short SSC (e.g. ground contact phases in sprinting, high jump or long jump) shows only small angular displacements in the above cited joints and lasts 100–250 ms (Schmidtbleicher, 1986) (Fig. 18.3).

The power production in a short SSC is based on a precise interaction of several mechanisms: before ground contact the extensor muscles are activated as part of the central motor programme (Dietz et al., 1981). The associated cross-bridges are responsible for the short-range elastic stiffness (SRES), which diminishes the lengthening of the muscle during the initial ground contact (Flitney & Hirst 1978a,b; Ford et al., 1981). At the same time, segmental stretch reflex activity serves to enhance the actual

muscle force (Nichols & Houk, 1976) so that the major part of elastic energy can be stored in the tendons of the main extensor muscles of the leg (Gollhofer et al., 1984). This permits a powerful push off of the body, whereas neuronal activation of the leg muscles during the concentric phase of the movement is low (Komi, 1985; Noth, 1985).

The quality of power production in an SSC is essentially dependent on the structure of the innervation pattern and the training state of the tendomuscular system in terms of their contractile and elastic abilities (Komi, 1988; Schmidtbleicher et al. 1988).

We can conclude that maximal strength and power are not distinct entities; they have a hierarchical relationship to one another. Maximal strength is the basic quality that influences power performance. In the case of concentric actions the contribution of maximal strength depends on the magnitude of the resistance. For power performance in a stretch–shortening cycle the correlation between maximal strength and power output are fairly low.

Classification of training methods

Adaptation effects

Traditional designs of strength training methods were originally based on the load used. Other designs were based on the sport, e.g. weightlifting or bodybuilding methods. These designs are still used by athletes, coaches, and scientists, but they raise expectations that stem from the false belief that the 'maximal-strength method' increases maximal strength and that the 'speed-strength method' develops power. In reality, difficulties occur because of confusing the content and the aim of a training method.

In training practice, it is often believed that strength training merely calls for changes in enzymatic quantity or quality within the muscle, which ultimately results in muscle cross-sectional increases. Based on this perceived 'fact', several types of sports (handball, soccer, tennis, boxing, etc.) and even some track and field disciplines, discourage the use of strength training, since the apparently significant increase of body mass arising from muscle cross-sectional hypertrophy negates the desired positive effect of the improvement of power. In this context it has to be pointed out that an increase in maximal strength is always connected with an improvement of relative strength (strength per kg body weight) and therefore with improvement of power abilities. This is proven, aside from the numerous empirical findings, in a very impressive manner by the power performance achieved by heavy athletes in the reach and jump test as well as in the 30 m sprint.

Apart from muscle hypertrophy and perhaps hyperplasia, as a mechanism of hypertrophy (Bischoff, 1979; Mauro, 1979; Ontell, 1979;

Appell, 1983; MacDougall, 1986), there are other means of increasing maximal strength and power. The adaptation of the nervous system to the training stimulus plays an important role here. From the classical cross-innervation studies of Buller *et al.* (1960a,b) and a large number of subsequent studies, we know that the fibre-specific typing of muscle depends on the consistency and utilization or non-utilization of those nerve cells in the spinal column that innervate the corresponding muscle fibres. It could also be shown that the neuromuscular system reacts very sensitively in terms of adaptation to slow or fast contraction stimuli. Longitudinal studies on humans showed clear evidence that following a high intensity strength training session there is an improvement in the ability to quickly mobilize greater innervation activities (Moritani & de Vries, 1979; Schmidtbleicher, 1980; Häkkinen, 1986; Komi, 1986). It was assumed that the cause of this adaptation, in the case of trained athletes, is a rapid recruitment of motor units and an increased firing rate of motoneurones in contrast to untrained people (Schmidtbleicher & Bührle 1987). Besides the ability of the motoneurone pool to tolerate higher activation frequencies there might exist another adaptation phenomenon, i.e. a more synchronized discharge of the motoneurones so that activation bursts discharge a greater number of muscle fibres in a shorter time period (see Fig. 18.4) (Schmidtbleicher, 1984).

The result of this adapted innervation can be seen in a considerable improvement of RFD and therefore in power production.

Another possibility for the improvement of power results from improved intramuscular coordination. The term 'intramuscular coordination' describes, in the author's opinion, the relation between excitatory and inhibitory mechanisms for one muscle for a specific movement. As an example one can observe the muscle activation patterns of human leg extensors and the corresponding force–time curves in jumping exercises under increased stretching loads (see Fig. 18.5). With increasing

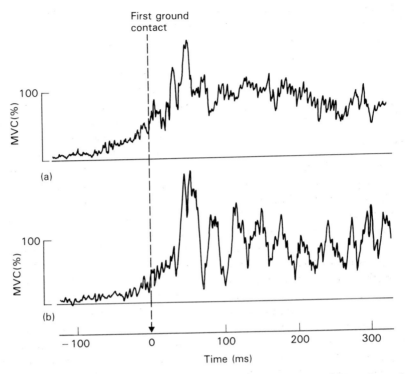

Fig. 18.4 Rectified and averaged EMG pattern ($n = 30$ each) of the m. triceps brachii from a forward fall from vertical position to the ground from one subject, before (a) and after (b) 6 weeks of training. The subjects exercised the forward fall movement four times weekly (3 sets with 5 repetitions and an additional load of 20% of individual body weight). Rhythmic oscillation can be detected after the training process in (b) MVC, maximum voluntary contraction.

stretching loads, the initial impact peak in the vertical ground reaction forces increases and concomitantly with this enhancement a clear reduction in the activation pattern, i.e. the surface electromyogram, occurs. (Schmidtbleicher & Gollhofer, 1982; Gollhofer & Schmidtbleicher, 1988). These inhibitory effects can be interpreted as overload phenomena that serve for the regulation of the stiffness of the tendomuscular system in the initial ground contact. All tested subjects showed this inhibitory effect even though individually beginning from different dropping heights. The higher-trained athletes could resist the impact forces much better, whereas less trained subjects were affected even from the low dropping height of 24–32 cm. After drop jump training these inhibitory effects were reduced.

It was concluded that the inhibitory mechanisms are part of a dynamic performance dependent reaction, functionally serving as a protection system (Schmidtbleicher et al., 1988).

A further way to increase power results from better intermuscular coordination. Intermuscular coordination describes the ability of all muscles involved in a movement, agonists, antagonists, and synergists, to cooperate wholly with respect to the aim of the movement. Improvement of power development of this type is also movement specific, and therefore not transferable to another movement. The specific strength training in training practice strives mainly for the optimization of intermuscular coordination. Therefore, this method is coordination training rather than strength or power training.

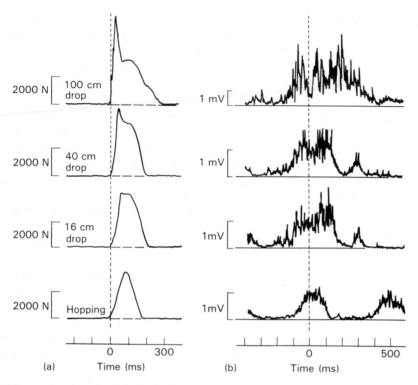

Fig. 18.5 (a) Force–time curves and (b) rectified and averaged EMG pattern of m. gastrocnemius from drop jumps (*n* = 8 each) of different dropping (falling) heights (100 cm, 40 cm, 16 cm) from one subject. The vertical dotted lines mark the first ground contact. Note the increase of initial force peak and the decrease of activation. (From Gollhofer & Schmidtbleicher, 1988.)

As we know from training practice and longitudinal studies, the adaptation of muscle requires considerable time, several months to years, depending on the quality and quantity of the training. On the other hand, measurable adaptation to a training stimulus, directed to muscle hypertrophy, can be detected after a relatively short time span. Biomechanical changes appear in a few hours and lasting improvements in maximal strength and power after 2 weeks. Therefore, short-term increases of performance can be based, on the one hand, on a coordinated learning effect of the inter-muscular type; on the other hand, neuronal changes appear (Sale, 1986) that help the indi-vidual muscle to achieve greater performance capability. This is achieved by shortening the time for the recruitment of motor units and by

increasing the tolerance of the motoneurones to elevated innervation frequencies (Häkkinen & Komi, 1983; Häkkinen, 1986; Schmidtbleicher & Bührle, 1987).

In conclusion, the important long-term factor responsible for muscle hypertrophy is the pro-liferation of contractile material in the muscle (MacDougall, 1986).

The first adaptations are always mainly of an intermuscular coordinative nature and the first stabilization of training effects appears after 2 weeks, by four training units per week. Neuronal adaptations lead after 6–8 weeks (again four training units per week) to far-reaching compensatory modifications, es-pecially in power production. However, only the increase of muscle mass offers considerable improvement possibilities in strength and power behaviour lasting over a period of several years. Experience, as well as investigations from Häkkinen *et al.* (1988) and Häkkinen and Keskinen (1989) indicate that after approximately 9–12 weeks of training, related to the type of training and sex of subjects, the rate of increase drops off dramatically. Based on this knowledge, it is indicated that one should either use another hypertrophy method or emphasize changing to a type of training stress, i.e. geared towards the neuromuscular system. Scientific results, as well as practical experience, allow a rough classification of training methods used in strength and power training based on the above listed results.

Training methods for muscle hypertrophy

The training effects of these methods for periods of maximal duration of 10–12 weeks, with four workouts per week, consist primarily of increases in muscle mass, accompanied by smaller neuronal adaptations and therefore a profitable increase in maximal strength can be detected. These methods are characterized by a large number of sets of repetitions with submaximal loads (60–80%), where 100% is maximal isometric strength. The execution of the movement is rapid to slow and ends with a complete muscular failure. The most widely used methods for training of muscle hypertro-

phy are as follows (see also Table 18.1).

1 Standard method I (constant load): with a load of 80%, 3–5 sets of 8–10 repetitions are performed, with rest intervals of 3 min.

2 Standard method II (progressively increasing load): with the number of sets the number of repetition decreases in the described manner. Frequently, the last repetitions in one set cannot be performed without assistance. In that case a training partner provides slight manual help to allow completion of the prescribed repetitions.

3 Bodybuilding method I (extensive stress): this 'classical' type of training is widely used and aims at bringing about excessive depletion of musculature.

4 Bodybuilding method II (intensive stress): with this method an intensive depletion of the fast twitch fibres is sought.

Both bodybuilding methods aim at the total overloading and depletion of energy stores. The demanded number of sets and repetitions can only be fulfilled with the assistance of a partner. Variations of training strategies, such as forced repetitions, negative repetitions, supersets, burns, cheated repetitions or the use of the pre-exhaustion principle, provide for a long and intensive training stimulus (see also Chapter 17).

5 'Isokinetic' training: this type of training can only be performed with the help of special

Table 18.1 Methods to improve muscle hypertrophy

	Standard method I (constant load)	Standard method II (progressively increasing load)	Bodybuilding method I (extensive)	Bodybuilding method II (intensive)	Isokinetic method
Form of exercise					
Concentric	√	√	√	√	√
Eccentric					√
Intensity load (%)	80	70, 80, 85, 90	60–70	85–95	e.g. 70
Repetitions	8–10	12, 10, 7, 5	15–20	8–5	15
Sets	3–5	1, 2, 3, 4	3–5	3–5	3
Rest interval (min)	3	2	2	3	3

Table 18.2 Methods to improve rate of force development

	Near maximal workouts	Maximal concentric workouts	Maximal eccentric workouts	Concentric–eccentric maximal workouts
Form of exercise				
Concentric	√	√		√
Eccentric			√	√
Intensity load (%)	90, 95, 97, 100	100	c. 150	70–90
Repetitions	3, 1, 1, 1 + 1	1	5	6–8
Sets	1, 2, 3, 4, +5	5	3	3–5
Rest interval (min)	3–5	3–5	3	5

apparatus that provides accommodating resistance for every joint angle, therefore producing a constant external speed of movement. Depending on the type of machine concentric and eccentric exercise can be performed. All 'isokinetic' training methods are characterized by a long duration of stimulation and a slow speed of movement execution. In sports like rowing, canoeing or swimming with 'quasi-isokinetic' movements the exercise machines are integrated into the training process. In other sports, especially power disciplines, 'isokinetic' training should be restricted to the early general preparation phase only.

Training methods for the rate of force development

Training methods of this type produce a neuromuscular adaptation along with only minimal hypertrophy effects. Optimal adaptation occurs after a training period of 6–8 weeks with four training units per week. These methods contribute to an increase in RFD and an improvement in neuronal activation, along with a more effective exploitation of the existing muscle potential with less accompanying muscle mass or body weight increases.

The main characteristics of these methods are short-term extremely fast maximal actions against near maximum loads, or in the case of eccentric actions against supramaximal loads. Difficulties in understanding the demand of the 'extreme fast maximal actions against high loads' occur if one does not differentiate precisely between action and movement velocity, i.e. the action velocity is high, but the movement velocity from the load is very low, because of the high loads. These training methods emphasize neuronal output and therefore should be practised, following an intensive warm-up, in a rested state with each action being executed with maximal voluntary effort as fast as possible. Table 18.2 lists some of the RFD methods. These are explained in more detail below.

1 Near maximal concentric workouts: a 'narrow' pyramid approach is most commonly used. In this case, with the last set, an attempt is undertaken to improve the previous best performance and the principle of progressive resistance is integrated in every training unit. Instead of the pyramid approach some coaches and athletes prefer a programme that contains three sets with three repetitions, each against a load of 90%. Rest intervals in all RFD methods should be at least 5 min for the muscle that is involved in the exercise to avoid fatigue. Other muscle groups can be practised during the pause.

2 Maximal concentric workouts: this method is recommended only for highly trained athletes

and was introduced into the training system by Bulgarian weightlifters. Attempts to improve the performance are made in every new training unit. In the case of weightlifting the principle of coincidence of training and competition movement is easy to fulfil.

3 Maximal eccentric workouts: the load used for eccentric strength development in sport, not in rehabilitation, must be supramaximal, but it should not exceed 150% of the maximal isometric strength. Training partners can be used to overcome the high load with the concentric part of the movement, therefore eliminating the need for special apparatus. In every case the athlete must use the greatest amount of resistance possible. In power sports with hyperextensions (javelin throwing, handball throws, volleyball strokes, etc.) the resistance should be only slightly higher than 100% and the training only practised with assistance to prevent injuries.

4 Concentric–eccentric workouts: this training method combines the superiority of maximal concentric actions in developing RFD with the maximal peak-loading characteristics of maximal eccentric workouts. To perform this technique the almost free falling barbell is decelerated and then accelerated in the shortest possible time. This training form is commonly used in exercises such as the bench press and clean pulls by not allowing pauses while performing a prescribed set of repetitions. German male and female high jumpers have used such training methods, and these have produced good results. This type of training form should not be confounded with a mixed concentric and eccentric training as it was investigated by Kaneko *et al.* (1984).

Mixed methods

All mixed methods deal with the intention to develop maximal strength and power within a unique training programme. Commonly these mixed programmes are performed in a pyramid approach starting with loads at 70% and then set by set with decreasing repetitions up to 100% and vice versa. Experience shows that the mixing of methods has no complications for beginners, children and rehabilitation patients. For top athletes some difficulties occur with this procedure. If an athlete starts with low loads and a lot of repetitions neuronal fatigue will occur before attempting the near maximal contraction that serves for the adaptation in RFD. Working the other way round, and starting with the maximal contractions, leads to high intramuscular lactate concentration during the consecutive sets, with lower loads and high repetitions, therefore reducing the adaptation effects on the nervous system. For a training period of similar length a phase of hypertrophy training followed by RFD training shows better results than a mixed methods training of the classical type over the same period of time.

Training methods for the stretch–shortening cycle

As could be shown empirically there exists basic differences between fast and slow stretch–shortening cycles, not only on the basis of factor analysis but also on learning experiments and training adaptations (Gollhofer, 1987; Schmidtbleicher *et al.*, 1988; Bauersfeld, 1989).

All SSC methods aim primarily at adaptations of the nervous system. Therefore, they should only be performed in a rested state. Easier methods such as single or double-leg hopping or alternate-step hopping are suitable for novices. One should be careful with drop jumps for beginners because the potential for injury is much higher. The use of additional loading even through relatively small weights leads to a reduction of the innervation of the leg extensors and to premature fatigue. Also, orthopaedic considerations validate the concept of not using additional loads.

1 Most common is hopping with both legs (i) at personal rhythm, or (ii) with maximal frequency (maximal number of ground contacts possible), or (iii) with maximal height. In all three methods, 30 repetitions are performed with rest intervals of 5 min between sets. All three methods can be combined in a training unit, since they can be quickly and easily performed and require no apparatus. In single-leg hopping the number of repetitions per set is reduced to 10 jumps.

2 Jump training: alternate step-hopping for 3 sets, with, in each case, 20 repetitions performed with 5 min of rest. Other possibilities are 'triple' or 'pentajumps' for 5 sets of 10 repetitions interspaced by 10-min pause. The distance reached is used as a measure of training adaptation.

3 The most important SSC method is drop jumps. Drop jumps are practised in 3–5 sets of 10 repetitions, along with rest intervals of 10 min between sets. The dropping height (height of the box) is individual and should be set so that the heel of the athlete does not touch the ground in the contact phase. This guarantees an individual loading and progressive load increases. The effect of drop jumps is doubtful if the contact phase with the ground lasts too short or too long a time. The athlete must consciously pretend that he/she will be landing on a hot plate and therefore contract as fast as possible to reach optimal performance. The use of yielding landing surfaces prevents achieving the desired training effect.

Diagnosis of general and sport-specific parameters

Diagnosis

A biomechanical performance diagnosis is based largely on the recording of force–time curves during different types of actions. In order to keep individual lifting ratios, as well as intermuscular coordination, as constant as possible special measuring devices with force transducers (Kistler-Piezo) were constructed for arm extensors (see Fig. 18.1) and leg extensors (see Fig. 18.6). The data are processed on personal computers, whose programs allow the rapid reading of measured values from the AD-converter. All time values are interpolated

linearly and expressed precisely in milliseconds. Differentiation is carried out using a modified central-difference method and the integration according to the trapezius rule (Müller, 1983; Schweizer, 1984; Wörn 1988).

From the resulting force–time curves one can determine isometric maximal strength, IRFD, MRFD and in the case of concentric actions also the movement time and the developed strength level.

The performance diagnosis for SSC consists of a standard programme that includes squat jumps, counter-movement jumps, which are representative for slow SSC, and drop jumps from different dropping heights. The drop jumps were executed with fixed hands at the hip and start from heights of 16 cm, 24 cm, etc. in steps of 8 cm. In all jump conditions the height of the centre of gravity of the body reached in the jump serves as a criterion. Drop jumps were executed until the individual maximum from the corresponding dropping height was reached (Asmussen & Bonde-Peterson, 1974; Kuhlow, 1980; Bosco, 1982; Schmidtbleicher, 1985).

The corresponding force–time curves of the jumps were registered with a force-platform (Kistler) and the data processed on personal computers. The program allows rapid information about maximum ground reaction forces, contact and flight times and height of centre of gravity of the body in the jump (Wörn, 1989).

Prognosis

Only a few components are required to make a valid performance prognosis. For training practice the difference between the measures of maximal isometric strength and maximal eccentric strength provides a raw assessment concerning the voluntary activation capacity of the available muscle mass activated by the test movement. The difference between maximal isometric and eccentric strength varies depending on the momentaneous status of training performance. With better adaptation of the neuronal system the difference diminishes (see

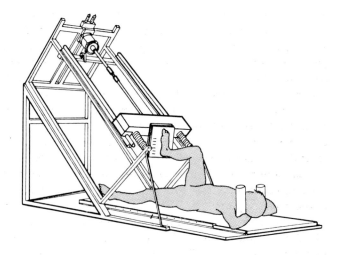

Fig. 18.6 Measurement device for the registration of force–time curves of concentric, isometric and eccentric movements with variable hip, knee and ankle joint angles. The foot is positioned on a force plate, which is fixed on a sledge. Eccentric conditions were produced with a pneumatic system.

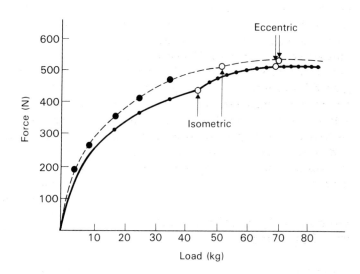

Fig. 18.7 Force–load curves before (——) and after (––––) 6 weeks of strength training using near maximal concentric actions for increasing RFD (rate of force development). Note that the difference between isometric and eccentric maximal strength was reduced.

Fig. 18.7). If a hypertrophy training method is used the difference increases. The value of the difference helps not only to determine which method of training is appropriate at a given time but also delivers information about the momentaneous status of training.

Over a period of about 8 years this diagnostic system has worked very successfully and the individual regulation of the training process was mainly orientated on the described parameters.

Regulation and periodization of training

The regulation and periodization of a training programme requires a detailed knowledge of the athlete's previous training programmes. The same applies for an accurate performance diagnosis of the present training condition. It is also necessary to know how to match the specific methods to the required adaptations of the neuromuscular system. As an example, the

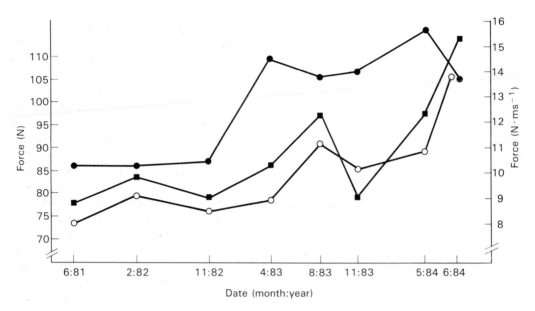

Fig. 18.8 Evolution of maximal rate of force development (MRFD) (■), maximal isometric (○) and eccentric (●) strength and the averaged 10 best results of an athlete in shot-putting competitions within 1 year, over a period of some years. The month and year of the diagnosis are given on the abscissa. Further explanation in the text.

evolution of the power ability of a junior shot-putter is discussed below (see Fig. 18.8).

Based on the knowledge that near maximal concentric workouts performed as fast as possible bring about an adaptation of the nervous system, these workouts were recommended to the athlete in June 1981. It is often mistakenly thought that near maximal or maximal contractions lead primarily to an adaptation of maximal strength. The effects of this training method are a remarkable increase in RFD accompanied by an increase in movement speed, and in a slight increase of maximal isometric strength, whereas maximal eccentric strength stays constant.

The drop in performance observed in November 1982 was a result of the transition phase, when activities were reduced extremely (Bompa, 1983). The return to conditioning orientated training began with a hypertrophy method (standard method II). A subsequent improvement of maximal strength level, especially maximal eccentric strength, was observed in April 1983.

Depending on the training frequency (training injuries aside), the number of strength training units can be increased to four or five per week through the use of microcycles (2 or 3 weeks), during which hypertrophy and RFD methods are alternated. Until the competitive peak was reached in August 1983, this approach produced considerable increases in maximal strength and power. In the subsequent transition phase the values decreased again until November 1983. The preparation period that followed began with an initial phase where the emphasis was placed on increasing muscle mass. Until April 1984 the athlete gradually increased the load intensity while executing the movements as fast as possible. After the preparation phase, the emphasis was placed on the technical component, although the RFD-directed units were never completely eliminated (a minimum of two units per week must be completed).

The excellent results of this training orientation became evident in May 1984. For the short time remaining before the competitive peak of the season (June 1984), microcycling with intensive maximal contractions were added and a slight reduction in body weight was aimed for. This weight reduction was reflected in a slight decrease of maximal eccentric strength. The main training effects were a profitable increase in maximal isometric strength and above all in RFD.

As an example for the regulation and periodization of power training this programme might be sufficient. The same programme as carried out for the arms was done for the legs, but additionally hopping and jump exercises were executed. The SSC programme was undertaken with the procedures described above. At present, simple measuring processes such as touch-sensitive foils and contact mats are used in order to provide less expensive solutions for training environments. An improvement in SSC abilities can be seen in an increase in the height reached by the centre of gravity after a drop jump from a given dropping height. Athletes with good SSC ability show the best jumping heights in the drop jumps. Untrained subjects normally reach the best jumping heights in the counter-movement jumps, whereas the heights reached in the drop jumps often are even worse than the squat jump heights.

Practical recommendations for training purposes

Regardless of the training method practised, the coach as well as the athlete must carefully record the number of training units, the intensity, the number of repetitions, and the rest interval, so that the training goal can be precisely established. To identify only the volume of training in tonnes without identifying other training characteristics is meaningless. For example, a worker who lifts 2 kg, 2000 times a day, would perform 20 t in a week, without any visible training adaptations. Which brings us to the concept of progressive loads. During every training unit or after every training week, the maximal performance capacity must be re-

determined. If this principle is not followed, training progress will soon stagnate. Another principle to be followed is the conformity of the training movement to the competitive movement; the range and direction of movement must be as similar as possible. The difference between the competitive movement and the training movement must be minimal, so that the greatest transfer to the competitive movement can occur. This is valid to an increasing degree in terms of the general goal-oriented preparation and becomes really necessary when doing specific strength training. Another common mistake is made in the elimination of strength training in the competitive phase. This prevents the transfer of the aquired preparatory conditioning to high performance, since most of the peaking is aimed at technical preparation. In the competition phase, one should maintain existing strength and power status by performing two training units per week. To attain absolute high-performance capacity, one should not cease conditioning training more than 5–6 days before the competition. The sophisticated use of macro- and microcycles can bring about relative peaks for 'training competitions'; however, one should realize, that absolute peaking can occur only twice a year. When one increases the number of training units devoted to strength and power training, he/she should elevate the proportion of 'lengthening gymnastics' (stretching, physiotherapeutic procedures, etc.).

Based on the training methods and the specific recommendations given above, the athlete and the coach can develop concrete training procedures and possibly more economic and efficient training.

References

Appell, H. (1983) Mechanismen und Grenzen des Muskelwachstums. *Kölner Beiträge zur Sportwissenschaft*, Jahrbuch der Deutschen Sporthochschule Köln 1983, 7–18.

Asmussen, E. & Bonde-Petersen, F. (1974) Storage of

elastic energy in skeletal muscles in mass. *Acta Physiologica Scandinavica*, **91**, 385–92.

Bauersfeld, M. (1989) Charakteristik der Schnelligkeit und deren Trainierbarkeit im Prozeß der sportlichen Vervollkommnung. *Wissenschaftliche Zeitschrift der Deutschen Hochschule für Körperkultur Leipzig*, **30**, 36–48.

Bischoff, R. (1979) Tissue culture studies on the origin of myogenic cells during muscle regeneration in the rat. In A. Mauro (ed.) *Muscle Regeneration*, pp. 13–30. Raven Press, New York.

Bompa, T. (1983) *Theory and Methodology of Training. The Key to Athletic Performance*. Kendall/Hunt, Dubuque.

Bosco, C. (1982) *Stretch–Shortening Cycle in Skeletal Muscle Function*. Studies in Sport, Physical Education and Health No. 15, University of Jyväskylä, Jyväskylä.

Bührle, M. (ed.) (1985) *Grundlagen des Maximal- und Schnellkraft trainings*. Hofmann, Schorndorf.

Bührle, M. & Schmidtbleicher, D. (1981) Komponenten der Maximal- und Schnellkraft-Versuch einer Neustrukturierung auf der Basis empirischer Ergebnisse. *Sportwissenschaft*, **11**, 11–27.

Buller, A., Eccles, C. & Eccles, R. (1960a) Differentiation of fast and slow muscles in the cat hind limb. *Journal of Physiology*, **150**, 399–416.

Buller, A., Eccles, C. & Eccles, R. (1960b) Interaction between motoneurons and muscles in respect of the characteristic speeds of their responses. *Journal of Physiology*, **150**, 417–39.

Dietz, V., Noth, J. & Schmidtbleicher, D. (1981) Interaction between prectivity and stretch reflex in human triceps brachii during landing from forward falls. *Journal of Physiology*, **311**, 113–25.

Flitney, F. & Hirst, D. (1978a) Cross-bridge detachment and sarcomere 'give' during stretch of active frog's muscle. *Journal of Physiology*, **276**, 449–65.

Flitney, F. & Hirst, D. (1978b) Filament sliding and energy absorbed by the cross-bridges in active muscle subjected to cyclical length changes. *Journal of Physiology*, **276**, 467–79.

Ford, C., Huxley, A. & Simmons, E. (1981) The relation between stiffness and filament overlap in stimulated frog muscle fibres. *Journal of Physiology*, **311**, 219–49.

Gollhofer, A. (1987) *Komponenten der Schnellkraftleistung im Dehnungs-Verkürzungs-Zyklus.* (Components of Power in Stretch–Shortening Cycle.) Sport Fitness Training, Erlensee.

Gollhofer, A. & Schmidtbleicher, D. (1988) Muscle activation patterns of human leg extensors and force-time characteristics in jumping exercises under increased stretching loads. In G. de Groot,

A. Hollander, P. Huijing & G. van Ingen Schenau (eds) *Biomechanics XI A*, pp. 143–7. Free University Press, Amsterdam.

Gollhofer, A., Schmidtbleicher, D. & Dietz, V. (1984) Regulation of muscle stiffness in human locomotion. *International Journal of Sports Medicine*, **5**, 19–22.

Häkkinen, K. (1986) *Training and Detraining Adaptations in Electromyography. Muscle Fibre and Force Production Characteristics of Human Leg Extensor Muscle with Special Reference to Prolonged Heavy Resistance and Explosive Type Strength Training*. Studies in Sport, Physical Education and Health No. 20. University of Jyväskylä, Jyväskylä.

Häkkinen, K. & Keskinen, K. (1989) Muscle cross-sectional area and voluntary force production characteristics in elite strength- and endurance-trained athletes and sprinters. *European Journal of Applied Physiology*, **59**, 215–20.

Häkkinen, K. & Komi, P. (1983) Electromyographic changes during strength training and detraining. *Medicine and Science in Sports and Exercise*, **15**, 455–60.

Häkkinen, K., Pakarinen, A., Alén, M., Kauhanen, H. & Komi, P. (1988) Neuromuscular and hormonal adaptations in athletes to strength training in two years. *Journal of Applied Physiology*, **65**, 2406–12.

Kaneko, M., Komi, P. & Aura, O. (1984), Mechanical efficiency of concentric and eccentric exercises performed with medium to fast contraction rates. *Scandinavian Journal of Sports Sciences*, **6**, 15–20.

Komi, P. (1984) Physiological and biomechanical correlates of muscle function: effects of muscle structure and stretch–shortening cycle on force and speed. *Exercise and Sport Sciences Reviews*, **12**, 81–121.

Komi, P. (1985) Dehnungs-Verkürzungs-Zyklus bei Bewegungen mit sportlicher Leistung. (The stretch–shortening cycle in athletic activities.) In M. Bührle (ed.) *Grundlagen des Maximal- und Schnellkrafttrainings*, pp. 254–70, Hofmann, Schorndorf.

Komi, P. (1986) The stretch–shortening cycle and human power output. In L. Jones, N. McCartney & A. McComas (eds) *Human Muscle Power*, pp. 27–42. Human Kinetics, Champaign, Il.

Komi, P. (1989) The musculoskeletal system. In A. Dirix, H. Knuttgen & K. Tittel (eds) *Olympic Book of Sports Medicine*, pp. 15–39. Blackwell Scientific Publications, Oxford.

Komi, P. & Bosco, C. (1978) Utilization of stored elastic energy in leg extensor muscles by men and women. *Medicine and Science in Sports and Exercise*, **10**, 261–5.

Kuhlow, A. (1980) Hochsprung Frauen-Biomechanische Analyse und Ansteuerung konditioneller Komponenten bei Hochleistungsathleten. In R. Ballreich & A. Kuhlow (eds) *Beiträge zur Biomechanik des Sports*, pp. 37–54. Hofmann, Schorndorf.

MacDougall, J. (1986) Morphological changes in human skeletal muscle following strength training and immobilization. In L. Jones, N. McCartney & A. McComas (eds) *Human Muscle Power*, pp. 269–84. Human Kinetics, Champaign, Illinois.

Mauro, A. (ed.) (1979) *Muscle Regeneration*. Raven Press, New York.

Moritani, T. & deVries, H. (1979) Neural factors versus hypertrophy in the time course of muscle strength gain. *American Journal of Physical Medicine*, **58**, 115–30.

Müller, K. (1983) *Kraftdiagnose*. (Strength diagnosis.) Programmpaket (software package). Universität Freiburg, Freiburg.

Müller, K. (1987) *Statische und dynamische Muskelkraft*. (*Static and Dynamic Strength*.) Deutsch, Frankfurt/M. Thun.

Nichols. T. & Houk, J. (1976) Improvements in linearity and regulation of stiffness that results from action of stretch reflex. *Journal of Neurophysiology*, **39**, 119–42.

Noth, J. (1985) Neurophysiologische Aspekte der Muskelelastizität. (Neurophysiological aspects of elasticity of muscle.) In M. Bührle (ed.) *Grundlagen des Maximal- und Schnellkrafttrainings*, pp. 238–53. Hofmann, Schorndorf.

Ontell, M. (1979) The source of 'new' muscle fibers in neonatal muscle. In A. Mauro (ed.) *Muscle Regeneration*, pp. 137–46. Raven Press, New York.

Sale, D. (1986) Neural adaptation in strength and power training. In L. Jones, N. McCartney & A. McComas (eds) *Human Muscle Power*, pp. 289–304. Human Kinetics, Champaign, Illinois.

Schmidtbleicher, D. (1980) *Maximalkraft und Bewegungsschnelligkeit*. (*Maximal Strength and Speed of Movement*.) Limpert, Bad Homburg.

Schmidtbleicher, D. (1984) Sportliches Krafttraining und motorische Grundlagenforschung. In W. Berger, V. Dietz, A. Hufschmidt, R. Jung, K. Mauritz & D. Schmidtbleicher (eds) *Haltung und Bewegung beim Menschen* (*Posture and Movement in Humans*), pp. 155–88. Springer-Verlag, Berlin.

Schmidtbleicher, D. (1985) Strength training. Parts 1 and 2. *Sports-Science Periodical on Research and Technology in Sport*, Strength W4.

Schmidtbleicher, D. (1986) Neurophysiologische Aspekte des Sprungkrafttrainings. (Neurophysiological aspects of jump-training.) In K. Carl & J. Schiffer (eds) *Zur Praxis des Sprungkrafttrainings*, pp. 56–72. Bundesinstitut für Sportwissenschaft, Köln.

Schmidtbleicher, D. & Bührle, M. (1987) Neuronal adaptation and increase of cross-sectional area studying different strength training methods. In B. Jonsson (ed.) *Biomechanics X B*, pp. 615–20. Human Kinetics, Champaign, Illinois.

Schmidtbleicher, D. & Gollhofer, A. (1982) Neuromuskuläre Untersuchungen zur Bestimmung individueller Belastungsgrößen für ein Tiefsprungtraining. (Neuromuscular investigation to detect the individual loads in drop jump training.) *Leistungssport*, **12**, 298–307.

Schmidtbleicher, D., Gollhofer, A. & Frick, U. (1988) Effects of a stretch–shortening type training on the performance capability and innervation characteristics of leg extensor muscles. In G. de Groot, A. Hollander, P. Huijing & G. van Ingen Schenau (eds) *Biomechanics XI A*, pp. 185–9. Human Kinetics, Champaign, Illinois.

Schweizer, L. (1984) *Programm zur Sprunghöhenbestimmung*. (*Software package to find the centre of gravity in jumpers*.) Universität Freiburg, Freiburg.

Werschoschanskij, J. (1972) Modernes Krafttraining im Sport. In: P. Adam & J. Werschoschanskij (eds) *Trainerbibliothek Bd. 4*, pp, 37–148. Bartels Wernitz, Berlin.

Werschoschanskij, J. & Tatjan, W. (1975) Komponenten und funktionelle Struktur der Explosivkraft des Menschen. *Leistungssport*, **5**, 25–31.

Wörn, K. (1988) *AT kompatibles Programm zur Standardsprungkraftdiagnose*. Universität Frankfurt, Frankfurt/Main.

Wörn, K. (1989) *AT kompatibles Programm zur allgemeinen Kraftdiagnostik*. Universität Frankfurt, Frankfurt/Main.

Index

Reading Economic Geography

Edited by

Trevor J. Barnes, Jamie Peck,
Eric Sheppard, and Adam Tickell

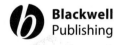

Blackwell
Publishing

Editorial material and organization © 2004 by Blackwell Publishing Ltd

350 Main Street, Malden, MA 02148-5020, USA
108 Cowley Road, Oxford OX4 1JF, UK
550 Swanston Street, Carlton, Victoria 3053, Australia

The right of Trevor J. Barnes, Jamie Peck, Eric Sheppard, and Adam Tickell to be identified as the Authors of the Editorial Material in this Work has been asserted in accordance with the UK Copyright, Designs, and Patents Act 1988.

First published 2004 by Blackwell Publishing Ltd

Library of Congress Cataloging-in-Publication Data

Reading economic geography / edited by Trevor J. Barnes . . . [et al.].
    p.   cm. – (Blackwell readers in geography)
Includes bibliographical references and index.
  ISBN 0-631-23553-1 – ISBN 0-631-23554-X
  1. Economic geography. I. Barnes, Trevor J. II. Series.

  HF1025.R275 2003
  330.9–dc21   2002155058

A catalogue record for this title is available from the British Library.

Set in Sabon 10/12
by SNP Best-set Typesetter Ltd., Hong Kong
Printed and bound in the United Kingdom
by TJ International, Padstow, Cornwall

For further information on
Blackwell Publishing, visit our website:
http://www.blackwellpublishing.com

Dedicated to the memory of
Robert G. Peck
1936–2002

The Editors

Trevor J. Barnes is Professor of Geography at the University of British Columbia. His previous publications include *A Companion to Economic Geography* (co-edited with Eric Sheppard, Blackwell, 2001).

Jamie Peck is Professor of Geography and Sociology at the University of Wisconsin–Madison. He is the author of *Work-place* (1996) and *Workfare States* (2001) and co-editor with Henry Yeung of *Remaking the Global Economy: Economic–Geographical Perspectives* (2003).

Eric Sheppard is Professor of Geography at the University of Minnesota. He is the author of *The Capitalist Space Economy* and *A World of Difference* and the co-editor with Trevor Barnes of *A Companion to Economic Geography* (Blackwell, 2001) and with Robert McMaster of *Scale and Geographic Inquiry* (Blackwell, 2003).

Adam Tickwell is Professor of Human Geography at the University of Bristol. He is editor of *Transactions of the Institute of British Geographers* and review editor of the *Journal of Economic Geography*.

Contents

Acknowledgments

The editors and publisher wish to thank the following for permission to use copyright material:

1. Harvey, D. 2000. "The difference a generation makes." In *Spaces of Hope*, pp. 3–8, 11–18. Edinburgh University Press. Copyright © 2000 David Harvey. Reprinted with permission of Edinburgh University Press. Copyright © Edinburgh University Press.

2. Sayer, A. 1985. "Industry and space: A sympathetic critique." *Environment and Planning D: Society and Space*, 3 (1), 3–7, 9–23. Copyright © 1985 Pion Limited. Reprinted by permission of the publisher.

3. Amin, A. 1999. "An institutionalist perspective on regional economic development." *International Journal of Urban and Regional Research*, 23, 365–78. Copyright © 1999 Joint Editors and Blackwell Publishing Ltd.

4. Thrift, N. and K. Olds. 1996. "Refiguring the economic in economic geography." *Progress in Human Geography*, 20, 311–22, 330–38. Copyright © 1996 Arnold.

5. Gibson-Graham, J. K. 1996. "The economy stupid! Industrial policy discourse and the body economic." In *The End of Capitalism (as we knew it)*, pp. 92–119. Oxford: Blackwell. Copyright © 1996 Julie Graham and Katherine Gibson. Reprinted by permission of the authors.

6. Walker, R. 1985. "Is there a service economy? The changing capitalist division of labor." *Science & Society*, 49, 42–83.

7. Massey, D. 1994. "Uneven development: Social change and spatial divisions of labour." In *Space, Place and Gender*, ed. D. Massey, pp 86–114. Minneapolis, MN: University of Minnesota Press. Copyright © Doreen Massey.

8. Scott, A. J. 1988. "Flexible production systems and regional development: The rise of the new industrial spaces North America and Western Europe." *International Journal of Urban and Regional Research*, 12 (2), 171–83. Copyright © Edward Arnold. Reprinted with permission of Blackwell Publishers.

9. Dicken, P. 1994. "Global–local tensions: Firms and states in the global space-economy." *Economic Geography*, 70 (1), 101–28. Copyright © 1994 Clark University.

10. Wright, M. W. 1999. "The politics of relocation: Gender, nationality, and value in a Mexican maquiladora." *Environment and Planning A*, 31, pp. 1601–17. Copyright © Pion Limited. Reprinted by permission of the publisher.

11. Castree, N. 1997. "Nature, economy and the cultural politics of theory: The 'war against the seals' in the Bering Sea, 1870–1911." *Geoforum*, 28 (1), 1–15, 17–20. Copyright © 1997 Elsevier Science. Reprinted with permission of Elsevier Science.

12. Swyngedouw, E. 1999. "Modernity and hybridity: Nature, *Regeneracionismo*, and the production of the Spanish waterscape, 1890–1930." *Annals of the Association of American Geographers*, 89 (3), 443–54, 456–65. Copyright © 1999 Association of American Geographers. Reprinted with permission of Blackwell Publishers.

13. Watts, M. 1994. "Oil as money: The Devil's excrement and the spectacle of black gold." In *Money Power and Space*, eds. S. Corbridge, R. Martin and N. Thrift, pp. 406–22, 430–35, 438–45. Oxford: Blackwell. Copyright © 1994 Blackwell Publishing.

14. Carney, J. 1993. "Converting the wetlands, engendering the environment: The intersection of gender with agrarian change in The Gambia." *Economic Geography*, 69, 329–48. Copyright © 1993 Clark University.

15. Whatmore, S. and L. Thorne. 1997. "Nourishing Networks: Alternative geographies of food." In *Globalising Food: Agrarian Questions and Global Restructuring,* eds. D. Goodman and M. J. Watts, pp. 287–304. London: Routledge. Copyright © 1997 David Goodman and Michael Watts.

16. O'Neill, P. 1997. "Bringing the qualitative state into economic geography." In *Geographies of Economies,* eds. Roger Lee and Jane Wills, pp. 290–301. London: Arnold. Copyright © 1997 Arnold. Reprinted with permission.

17. Storper, M. 1997. "Territories, flows and hierarchies in the global economy." *Aussenwirtschaft* 50(2), 265–293. Copyright © 1995 *Aussenwirtschaft*. This edited version is reprinted by permission of the publisher.

18. Hudson, R. and D. Sadler. 1986. "Contesting works closures in Western Europe's old industrial regions: Defending place or betraying class?" In *Production, Work Territory – The Geographical Anatomy of Industrial Capitalism*, eds A. J. Scott and M. Storper, pp. 172–93. London: Allen & Unwin. Copyright © 1996 Allen J. Scott, Michael Storper and the Contributors.

19. Fincher, R. 1989. "Class and gender relations in the local labor market and the local state." In *The Power of Geography: How Territory Shapes Social Life*, eds. J. Wolch and M. Dear, pp. 93–117. London: Allen & Unwin. Copyright © 1989 Jennifer Wolch, Michael Dear and Contributors.

20. McDowell, L. 1997. "Thinking through work: Gender, power and space." In *Capital Culture: Money, Sex and Power at Work*, pp. 11–42. Oxford: Blackwell. Copyright © 1997 Linda McDowell. Reprinted with permission of Blackwell Publishers.

21. Graham, S. 1998. "The end of geography or the explosion of place? Conceptualizing space, place and information technology." *Progress in Human Geography*, 22 (2), 165–85. Copyright © 1998 Arnold.

22. Gertler, M. 2001. "Best practice? Geography, learning and institutional limits to strong convergence." *The Journal of Economic Geography* 1 (1), 5–26, by permission of Oxford University Press.

23. Hsing, Y. 1996. "Blood thicker than water: interpersonal relations and Taiwanese investment in southern China." *Environment and Planning A*, 28 (12), 2241–62. Copyright © 1996 Pion Ltd. Reprinted by permission of the publisher.

24. Pratt, G. 1999. "From registered nurse to registered nanny: discursive geographies of Filipina domestic workers in Vancouver, B.C." *Economic Geography*, 75 (3), 215–36. Copyright © 1999 Clark University.

25. Schoenberger, E. 1998. "Discourse and practice in human geography." *Progress in Human Geography*, 22 (1), 1–14. Copyright © 1998 Arnold.

Introduction: Reading Economic Geography

Eric Sheppard, Trevor J. Barnes, Jamie Peck,
and Adam Tickell

The Stuff of Economic Geography

Economic geographers study why, where, and when things are produced: food, shelter, commodities of all kinds, money, cultural meanings, and landscapes. But what do economic geographers produce? Economic geographers, like other natural and human scientists, produce inscriptions – written accounts of the nature of the world, and explanations of it. If writing is the output, reading is one input: The two are utterly interlinked, and co-produced. Economic geographers read the inscriptions of others, and themselves, rearranging and reinterpreting them to produce their own inscriptions, which are in turn read by others, who engage in yet further writing. So turns the world of economic geography. The student of economic geography, then, is first and foremost a reader and a writer – a consumer and producer of inscriptions.

Some may question our claim that economic geography is primarily about reading and writing. While this does describe well how economic geographers (indeed, all scientists) spend much of their time, surely there is more to economic geography? What about data collection and analysis, observation and fieldwork, conversations and debates, interviews and surveys, political interventions and policy work? While at times scientists have sought to give a privileged status to data and facts, it is now widely recognized that they too are a kind of inscription – a description of the world. Secondary databases, such as the census, are produced by particular agencies for particular purposes and represent their accounts of what matters in the world. Even when we go out and collect our own information on our own terms, that information is generally largely a social construct. A landscape, for example, is an inscription of human activities on the earth's surface – either directly, as in the case of an urban neighborhood or an agricultural landscape, or indirectly, as in how even the most remote and seemingly natural landscapes are now being transformed by human-induced global climate change. Biophysical processes are also important in shaping the world we seek to understand – constituting non-human inscriptions – but even these have to be read and interpreted by economic geographers. A fieldtrip is a bit like a trip to the library; we start out with ideas about what we are looking for, sort through the materials deposited there by others, read and interpret them, and then write about them.[1] Of course, economic geographers engage in practices other than reading and writing: operating overhead projectors and Xerox machines, talking with corporate executives and domestic workers, visiting Italian industrial districts and Turkish villages. These would not get us far, however, without reading and writing.

In terms of the inscriptions we produce, surely these are more than "just" writing? Again, practicing scientists often claim that scientific writing is fundamentally different from that of, say, novelists: It provides a definitive analysis of reality, as opposed to story-telling. Yet, again, it is now widely recognized that such claims to the objectivity of scientific accounts are problematic (Longino, 2002). While scientific writing is not the same as that of novelists, scientists also tell stories – about how the world works – that reflect their preexisting beliefs, understandings, and interpretations. By the same token, novelists often seek to provide an account of how the world works through their novels, which, like the scientists' essays, can be more or less compelling, plausible, and insightful. (David Lodge's recent novel *Thinks* . . . provides a humorous narrative of how scientists' and novelists' accounts overlap.)

If reading and writing is the stuff of economic geography, then a Reader should be more than just a collection of economic geography's "greatest hits." Our aim in producing this collection is to help students of economic geography (including ourselves) become better readers and writers. Our strategy is to provide what we think are effective and provocative examples of writing by economic geographers, and some guidance about how to read them critically and place them in context. In doing this, we have faced a series of dilemmas that we have attempted to negotiate. First, there is no canon in economic geography, that is, there is not a common understanding of how to "do" economic geography nor of those articles that are the "classics." Although, as we argue below, this is one of the strengths of economic geography, it made our editorial task difficult. This is compounded by the fact that any selection may well contribute to the canonization of those essays included – and the marginalization and disaffection of those authors excluded. The sheer quantity of writing by economic geographers poses a separate problem. There are, perhaps, a thousand practicing professional economic geographers worldwide. If each of us writes and publishes on average, say, 15,000 words a year, then over a fifteen-year period that would amount to 225,000,000 words. We only had room for less than one-thousandth of that output here.

Rather than providing a definitive selection, then, we offer only a partial collection reflecting our own readings, presuppositions, and opinions. Our choices can only be justified within the context in which it was produced, summarized below. Yet, we hope that even though others inevitably will disagree with our choices, students of economic geography will find our guidance to reading economic geography helpful. Our approach underlines the variegated character of contemporary economic geography in a way that says something about the restlessness and openness of the subdiscipline. Its very dynamism and differentiation is the reason that there is no universally accepted canon, and our selections here have consequently been made in such a way as to highlight some of the diverse ways in which economic geographies have been conceived, practiced, and written. Part of our task has been to illustrate *how* the boundaries of economic geography have been breached, stretched, and remade, but at the same time it is important to hold on to what is *distinctively* economic-geographic. Today, "being an economic geographer" is not just a matter of institutional affiliation, nor is it simply a reflection of substantive empirical concerns; it symbolizes a deeper set of commitments, inclinations, and sensibilities. From our particular historically and geographically situated perspective, the work of economic geographers involves mapping out the geographies of localization and globalization; exploring the geographical foundations of economic structures and restructuring processes; developing accounts for uneven spatial development in the economy; documenting and explaining the spatiality of economic processes; and uncovering the social and institutional bases of economic performance, and the ways in which these vary between places and across scales.

The Broader Context: A Brief History of Economic Geography

The field of economic geography dates back to commercial geography in the nineteenth century – which attempted to compile and give meaning to the geography of economic production, often as a handmaiden to the colonial adventures of European powers (Barnes, 2000). Its current form, direction, and status are largely a result of a remarkable efflorescence of writing in the English-speaking world over the past fifty years (Scott, 2000). Beginning in the early 1960s, economic geography became the primary vehicle through which a new way of doing human geography became popular. The quantitative revolution refashioned geography as a theoretical discipline, whereby geographers sought to explain the spatial organization of human activity rather than just to describe and map it; and as a positivist discipline, developing deductive theories about the world and determining their validity by seeing whether they accurately predict observed spatial patterns. Economic geography proved well suited to this agenda; it could be easily quantified, and there were well-developed deductive theories in economics that some German economists and geographers (notably Johan Heinrich von Thünen, Alfred Weber, August Lösch, and Walter Christaller) had already been adapting to predict the location of economic activities on the basis of rational economic decision-making. It was in the English-speaking world, and to a lesser extent Sweden, that this approach developed particularly rapidly. Initial research adapted statistical methods to test the location theories of von Thünen et al., leading subsequently to new statistical methods and elaborations of these location theories into a rich research program that also gained the attention of urban and regional economists, and even a new interdisciplinary field of study – regional science.[2]

This approach to economic geography has remained an important field of endeavor, but to a significant degree it has been taken up by trained economists rather than trained geographers. The work of Paul Krugman has been particularly influential in recent years, stamping his own personality and engaged writing on this research program (Fujita, Krugman, and Venables, 1999), thereby catalyzing renewed interest from some influential economists under the moniker of the "new" economic geography. Some geographers have protested, with justification, that their contributions within this research program in the 1970s–1990s have been largely ignored, and many have found the program irrelevant to their current preoccupations. But there has been a high-profile attempt to catalyze a conversation between economists and geographers around these issues (Clark, Gertler, and Feldman, 2000), culminating in the establishment of a new journal in 2001, *The Journal of Economic Geography*.

Among trained geographers, the quantitative revolution bequeathed to economic geography an interest in, and commitment to, theory, but neoclassical economic-influenced location theories and positivism have largely been replaced with a succession of different approaches. Beginning in the mid-1970s, political economy became influential. Inspired by the classical economics of Marx, this approach has focused on how the political and economic forces of capitalism shape the space-economy (Harvey, 1982; Swyngedouw, 2000). Economic landscapes are explained as an evolutionary and conflict-laden consequence of contestation among social classes mediated by the state, in contrast to the harmonious equilibrium outcome of rational economic choice favored by location theory. At the same time, with quantitative geography tarred by the brush of positivism, there was a methodological shift away from mathematical models and statistical testing towards a more qualitative, case-study-oriented approach, often grounded in critical realism (Sayer, 1984; Plummer, 2000).

During the 1990s, political economy in turn came under fire, as geographers began to criticize it for over-emphasizing the importance of economic forces relative to culture, for under-playing the importance of human agency in shaping socio-spatial structures, and for its inattention to gender. As a consequence, there is now an unprecedented diversity of approaches to economic geography among geographers, with the creative surge in poststructuralist, feminist, and cultural theoretic approaches (Gibson-Graham, 2000; Oberhauser, 2000; Thrift, 2000), and a related turn to ethnographies and discourse analysis. These approaches emphasize that adequate forms of explanation in economic geography must involve critical reassessments of what we mean by terms like production and consumption, seeking redefinitions that highlight previously neglected aspects of these processes. The boundaries of economic processes do not conveniently coincide with those of firms or labor markets, or those established by censuses or national accounting systems. So, a focus on wage work, for example, can obscure the role of households as places of production, while neglecting the role of women (and other carers) in the process of social reproduction. It is characteristic of much recent work in economic geography to unveil these previously marginalized phenomena, partly in service of the more general argument that economic processes, and the places where production and consumption occur, are shaped by the cultural contexts within which they are embedded. Yet in many senses the research program remains grounded within the broad questions motivating the original forays into political economy: Understanding how the geographical organization of economic activities (now much more broadly defined) is both shaped by, and shapes, the evolution of economic, political, social, and cultural processes; processes that themselves are constituted by the deliberate actions of individuals, and by the social structures and processes of identity formation shaping those actions.

The Immediate Context: The Blackwell *Companion*

This Reader was conceived in parallel with the Blackwell *Companion to Economic Geography* (Sheppard and Barnes, 2000). The *Companion* sought to highlight the predominant focus of geographers working in economic geography, and was organized to reflect the range of theoretical approaches and substantive topics that constitute this diverse research program. It is the richness, breadth, and ambition of this research program that makes economic geography a particularly vibrant area of study at present. Moving beyond the traditional questions of economics, contemporary economic geographers examine what is meant by "economic," and how the economic co-evolves in space with other societal, cultural, political, and environmental processes. One consequence is that what once were considered the "boundaries" of economic geography – say, the interface with environmental issues, gender relations, or the state – are now especially intensive zones of activity. There is no longer a single core or "center" even of Anglo-American economic geography, but a differentiated terrain of debates, emergent questions, fashionable topics, and enduring concerns. Economic geography may defy most attempts at codification and classification: It is not easily bounded, nor can it be easily located within a dominant methodological or theoretical schema; it is fidgety and somewhat unruly, and hardly ever unified or cohesive. But this also means that it is rarely dull.

The original *Companion* was organized into five sections, a basic structure that has been duplicated in this volume. Part I, Worlds of Economic Geography, illustrates the variety of theoretical approaches favored by economic geographers, emphasizing political economy, post-structuralism, feminism, and cultural and institutional approaches. Essays illustrating each of these traditions have been selected here. Part II, Realms of Production, focuses on traditional themes of economics, to examine how they are addressed within geography: Production, labor, firms, competition, growth, and technical change. The essays selected include political economic, post-structural, and feminist approaches to production, firms, regional growth, and work. Part III, Resource Worlds, seeks to bring attention to, and catalyze research on, the relationship between the economy and the biophysical environment – a long-standing area of interest in economic geography that has received less attention within the current research program. Themes emphasized here, as in the *Companion*, include agriculture, resources, and the production of nature, from political economic, cultural theoretic, and feminist perspectives. Part IV, Social Worlds, was designed to emphasize one of economic geography's principal achievements in recent years – recognizing that economic processes cannot be analyzed in isolation from society. Gender relations, class, governance, and the state, and their relationship to space, are the foci of the essays selected here. Finally, Part V, Spaces of Circulation, was developed (like Part III) to refocus attention on some long-standing issues in economic geography that have not had such a high priority in recent research. Beginning with the spatial implications of Sayer's critical realism, and reinforced by more recent interest in territories, local embeddedness, and scale, the nature and implications of the ways in which places are systematically connected together across space have received less attention recently. Connectivity, as expressed through transportation and communications technologies, and the movements of commodities, people, capital, and ideas, is the subject-matter of this section. The essays selected here examine the spatiality of telecommunications, and the connectivity of places through flows of capital and migration.

Selection Strategies

We did not set out to select the best articles ever written in economic geography. Indeed, we do not believe that any such list can be drawn up; its creation would imply the existence of an economic geographical canon that is neither extant nor desirable. It would be possible to compile a list of the most influential papers, based on their measurable influence (say, by the frequency that they are cited), or the ways in which they can be argued to have indirectly influenced subsequent research trajectories, but such approaches are also problematic. For example, the frequency that an article is cited is not a reliable indicator of influence, notwithstanding the popularity of this crude measure among university administrators seeking to quantify research performance. The culture of citation differs across disciplines and research communities within disciplines, and motivations for citation extend beyond formally acknowledging influential ideas to include: marking the intellectual program to which you would like to belong; citing your friends, influential people whose friendship you seek, or what you think potential referees will have expected you to read; citing those whose work you think is poor; and showing off how much you know (Curry, 1991).

Selection is made more difficult by the sheer volume of publication over the past fifteen years, by our own inability to read it all or even recall what we've read, and by language barriers. Despite passing familiarity with a couple of European languages, we are not in a position to survey the relevant non-English literature in any knowledgeable way. To the extent that English has become the *lingua franca* for international scholarship in economic geography, this language barrier might be perceived as less limiting than, say, Japanese. Yet, as noted above, this self-limitation of course also serves to reinforce this English canon, and any broader Eurocentrism that it entails. There is substantial scholarship in economic geography that is not translated into English. The writings by scholars in other languages that are translated are naturally written in such a way as to fit within the English-speaking debates, thus often seeming derivative of the English language literature. It is therefore commonly asserted that the English-speaking realm dominates the research frontiers of economic geography. At the same time, however, we do not wish to underestimate the possibility that very different approaches to the field already exist in the non-English scholarship, or that exposure to these ideas would substantially enrich the English language scholarship. We look forward, therefore, to the development of forums for economic geographers to engage in a multilingual exchange of expertise, from which a very different kind of Reader, relevant for a much broader audience, might emerge.

Our goals are modest: To select articles that reflect our own collective and situated understanding of what is worth reading in the English language. We sought, first, articles that illustrate at least one of the five themes shaping contemporary economic geography as summarized above. In addition, we wanted to include as authors a number of the more influential scholars in the field, people with whose writing we believe any student of economic geography should have some familiarity. Since this volume is conceived of as a complement to the *Companion*, authors whose essays already appear in the *Companion* were not our first choice. Yet, we also selected articles that we find particularly interesting or especially relevant to the thematic structure of the two books, and tried to stay away from conflicts of interest (such as selecting articles by our own students, or ourselves). We sought to provide some balance across the different theoretical perspectives currently shaping geographic work in this field, by gender and location (both of the authors and of the empirical research). Needless to say, this kind of winnowing down and balancing is a very difficult and subjective exercise. In another context, even the same four editors might well have made different choices. Inclusion also entails exclusion, and we can only hope that colleagues who feel left out appreciate the complexity, and understand the contingent nature, of our choices.

Even our choice of just 25 articles from this productive and diverse field transcended limits imposed by the economics of publishing. Constrained to some 200,000 words, we were unable to realize our original aim of publishing the articles in their entirety. While our original goal was to let the readers decide what is important to them, this also abrogates some of our responsibility as editors to provide a representative sample of articles that also is accessible to a student audience, as one referee of the book proposal pointed out. Thus, we decided to include more articles, selectively edited, rather than just three per section in their entirety. In editing the articles, we have again imposed our own particular reading on the writings of others – seeking to make the essays more accessible when necessary, and highlighting those aspects of them that make them relevant to their inclusion in the volume. Some were sufficiently cogent to be included almost in the original length; others had to be cut in half. We cut out all abstracts, acknowledgments, and footnotes from the original papers, and extensive sections that were of limited relevance to their role within this volume. We also engaged in more detailed editing to increase their accessibility, in our view, and to reduce their length. We have not indicated all the places where this more detailed editing occurred, as that would have substantially reduced the legibility of our selections.[3] Our editorial selections, of which parts to include, do not reflect some general and definitive judgment as to which are the "best parts" of an article, but only which parts are most relevant to our context and goals. As always, we urge students of economic geography (or any discipline) to take these readings as only a starting point: Always read the original writings, rather than second-hand accounts or others' abbreviations of the originals; and make your own judgments about which articles are of most use for you, by going beyond edited books and course bibliographies to undertake your own survey of the literature.

Critical Reading

Each section of the Reader is prefaced by a brief introduction, placing the readings in the context of the development of thinking around this theme, and providing some specific questions to ponder with respect to the readings in that section. Here, we offer some tips about reading in a constructively critical manner. This may sound time consuming, but think for a minute about how much effort it took to *write* the article!

- **Gain an overall sense of the argument.** Before reading an article in detail, peruse the introduction and conclusion to get a sense of the research questions driving the scholarship, and the overall argument. A detailed reading will be more meaningful if you can situate it within this overall understanding.
- **Engage in a detailed initial reading.** Take detailed notes, jotting down major arguments advanced, and figuring out how the various parts of the article contribute to constructing the overall argument.
- **Learn the terminology.** Terms mean different things in different contexts, so it is important to know how they are used within economic geography. Make notes of terms you do not understand, and look them up on the Internet or in an encyclopedia or dictionary of human geography (Hanson, 2001; Johnston et al., 2001).
- **Pay attention to writing.** Think about the writing style of the author. What makes it effective, or ineffective? Is the style appropriate for the task at hand? Is the author trying to overwhelm you with fancy words, jargon, and obscure references, thereby undermining your ability to criticize the article, or is he or she adept at making complex ideas accessible and highlighting the most important points?
- **Contextualize the essay.** Determine how authors situate themselves. Which theoretical or philosophical perspective is being adopted? Which kinds of research do the authors engage with, or ignore? How does the article fit within their trajectory of work (visiting authors' web sites often helps)?
- **Take little on faith.** Do not be satisfied with authors' renditions of others' arguments, or their interpretations of empirical material. Wherever possible, go back to the sources, and read critically the various inscriptions that the authors mobilize in support of their argument.
- **Engage in an internalist critique.** An internalist critique pays attention to how well authors achieve the goals they set for themselves. This is essential to any constructive critical reading. Since economic geography is such a diverse field, it is too easy to dismiss an article for taking what you believe to be the wrong general approach, or for asking questions in which you are not interested. This kind of externalist critique (below) is important, but is insufficient. An internalist critique gives due respect to the author and the effort he or she invested. Based on your understanding of the article, how convincing is the overall argument? Is the theoretical argument rigorous, and the use of empirical evidence appropriate and convincing, with respect to the norms of the scholarship within which the article is situated? If not, how could it be improved?
- **Engage in an externalist critique.** What important questions/issues regarding the topic have been omitted in the article? What other approaches to the topic could the author have taken? How would choosing a different approach affect the overall research questions and methodologies? What might be the relative value, in your view, of a different approach?
- **Be reflexive.** Reflect on the critiques you have developed, and how they are shaped by your own personal and intellectual biography (What has interested you? What have you been taught to value? What constitutes your identity and interests?). Use this as an opportunity to reflect on the context from which your critique stems, and to challenge your own preconceptions. To learn from others'

scholarship you have to engage with the research and even change your mind. Finally, ask the ethical question of whether your critical assessment is the kind that you would like to receive from someone reading your essays.

Critical reading is central to the reproduction of economic geography as a vital field of scholarly inquiry. Constructive criticism can contribute to advancing knowledge within a particular research program. It can also lay the foundation for a productive engagement among the different approaches of economic geography (Longino, 2002). At present, different approaches too often seem to be like ships passing in the night; the latest fashions are put on display while last month's styles are scuppered. Effective writing also requires the reflexive application of critical reading skills to our own inscriptions.

Everyone who reads economic geography can, through critical reading, participate in the production of economic geographic knowledge. We thus invite readers to contribute to the vitality of the field by developing and articulating their own critical readings.

NOTES

1. In making this analogy, we do not wish to suggest that fieldtrips can be substituted by trips to the library. To the contrary: arguably economic geography is becoming impoverished because we spend too much time in the library and on the Internet and too little in the field.

2. By "research program" we mean a school of thought that emerges in a discipline, sharing a worldview and a common understanding about what are the most important research questions and how to go about answering them (Lakatos, 1970). Intellectual progress within economic geography, as in any discipline, does not proceed in a steady direction from poor to excellent understandings of the subject matter, but rather proceeds in fits and starts, as older research programs run out of steam, and new ones attempt to replace them.

3. The academic convention when quoting is to indicate every word left out with an "ellipse": . . . We have dispensed with this convention here because space constraints meant that our editing was sometimes extensive and we did not want our editorial presence to be unnecessarily intrusive.

Part I Worlds of Economic Geography

Editors' Introduction:
Paradigms Lost

*Trevor J. Barnes, Adam Tickell, Jamie Peck,
and Eric Sheppard*

David Harvey's essay, which begins this section, is called "The difference a generation makes." It would make an apt title for this editorial introduction. The age span that separates us four editors is less than a generation, but the kind of economic geography into which each of us was first socialized as undergraduates was radically different. Sheppard attended one of the iconic centers of quantitative, model-based geographical training of the late 1960s and early 1970s, Bristol University, and imbibed the purity of those methods. Barnes went to University College London during the mid-1970s, by which time political economic change was in the air, resulting in an incongruous educational mix of Markov chain and Marxian value analysis, sometimes within the same lecture. When Peck finished his BA at Manchester during the early 1980s, there was only one approach to economic geography – political economy, solidified by the publication of Doreen Massey's (1984) watershed book, *Spatial Divisions of Labour*, which for Peck made everything written before seem irrelevant. Finally, when Tickell completed his degree in 1987, again at Manchester, political economy was still central, but there was also the first whiff of a social and cultural sensibility, linked to discussions of gender and local culture (later culminating in the locality project; Cooke, 1989). The difference a generation makes in economic geography, then, is at least three different paradigms.[1]

That term paradigm comes from the work of the historian and philosopher of science, Thomas Kuhn (1962), and is found in his classic, *The Structure of Scientific Revolutions*. There is some debate over what exactly he meant – critics say that there are over twenty separate definitions of paradigm within his slim book – but the gist is clear enough. A paradigm is a way of looking at the world, like Galileo's heliocentric view of the solar system, or David Harvey's class-based (Marxist) view of industrial capitalism. Kuhn was also keen to stress that a paradigm includes an affiliated set of practices that bind practitioners to a common culture and social group. That is, paradigms are not just ethereal abstractions, but are embodied in people, in their relationships and interactions, in institutions, in artifacts, and in a culture's very form of life. This is what made Kuhn's book itself revolutionary: he recognized that academic enquiry, even of the most rarefied form, is never just academic.

For this reason, changing paradigms can be fraught, the stakes and consequence sometimes enormous. Galileo was locked up by the Inquisition for suggesting a change in paradigms from geocentrism to heliocentrism, while Darwin was (and still is) denounced in pulpits, legislatures, and court rooms for favoring an evolutionary paradigm over a creationist one. In economic geography, the consequences of paradigm change have not been quite so dramatic, although it is still likely that some assistant professors and lecturers have been denied tenure or promotion, and certain that some students have done less well in their exams and projects, because of the paradigms that they held. In economic geography there have been some famous paradigm quarrels, such as the mid-1950s Hartshorne–Schaefer debate signaling a move from regional geography to spatial science, or the mid-1970s Berry–Harvey exchange in which the spatial scientist Berry took on Harvey's Marxism on its home turf of *Antipode*, or yet again the early 1990s Harvey–Massey dispute in which Massey castigated Harvey's brand of Marxism for omitting the culture of gender. In line with Kuhn's broader thesis, these various disputes were won or lost partly on rational, intellectual criteria, but also on social and cultural ones. For example, Hartshorne fell to Schaefer not because he lacked good, plausible arguments – Hartshorne wears you down with his inexorable, grinding logic – but because he was fighting against the rising tide of a postwar American culture and society, and the economic geography that emerged from it that valued science and technology, instrumental reasoning, and the young and the new (for more details see Barnes, 2000).

As these examples indicate, and as is clear from our opening story, paradigm change has come thick and fast in economic geography over the past fifty years. It's not quite "if it's Tuesday it must be Marxism," but intellectual change has been the disciplinary name of the game for the past half-century. While this might be viewed as a sign of immaturity, of a juvenile flavor-of-the-month mentality, we believe the opposite. We think it indicates intellectual maturity, and that it is characterized by vibrancy, dynamism, and openness. The contemporary American pragmatist philosopher Richard Rorty argues that there is always hope as long as the conversation continues. From the pieces we have assembled, it is clear that the conversation in economic geography sparkles, and that hope remains vitally alive.

And to prove the point, the first essay by David Harvey (2000) comes from his book, *Spaces of Hope*. Harvey is the foremost Marxist in Anglo-American geography. In his earlier volume *The Limits to Capital*, Harvey (1982) provided a geographical exegesis of Marx's three volumes of *Capital*, and the *Grundisse*, giving economic geographers a body of theory, concepts, and a vocabulary to understand the capitalist space economy. But as Harvey now reflects, the Marxism found in that volume, and in the sometimes-covert seminars and lecture courses he has run on Marx since 1971, is out of fashion, or perhaps even worse, normalized. Marx has become just another dead, white European male we need to know a smattering about in order to pass the exam. For Harvey this is both tragic and comic. Marx's theories, he argues, have never been more relevant to the present generation than they are right now. They are the spitting image of our times. The present generation, including economic geographers, often shuns Marx, however, or provides only ritualistic acknowledgment. They are concerned with carrying out a different paradigm, cultural analysis, rather than political economy, which for them is "much more fun than being absorbed in the dour world and crushing realities of capitalist exploitation." But for Harvey it is on those crushing realities that we must concentrate: it is our political and moral obligation.

Andrew Sayer argues that our obligation as economic geographers is to employ a set of methodological precepts drawn from critical realism. Only by drawing on this paradigm can we ensure that radical (Marxist) theorizing and empirical research of the kind sparked by people like Harvey remains consistent, coherent, and compelling. Originating with the writings of two British philosophers, Roy Bhasker and Rom Harré, during the 1970s, critical realism was introduced into geography by Sayer (1984) in the early 1980s, quickly becoming the unofficial paradigm of economic geography for a decade, especially in the UK.

At its most basic, critical realism is an alternative to positivist science (of the kind that dominated economic geography during the 1960s and 1970s) that sought simple empirical relations of association, taken as equivalent to causes. In contrast, Sayer conceives causation as more complicated. He argues that objects, including social objects, contain within them necessary causal powers and liabilities to make things happen, but which are realized only under specific contingent conditions. To use Sayer's favorite example, a barrel of gunpowder by virtue of its constituent components contains the necessary causal powers to produce an explosion, but whether it does depends upon the contingent fact of someone throwing in a lighted match. Under critical realism, then, we are led to two different but related forms of enquiry. On the one hand, to an abstract examination of the necessary relations that constitute the causative power of an entity (what is it about the abstract chemistry of the various compounds found in gunpowder that makes the combination so volatile?), and, on the other, to a concrete investigation into the multifarious contingent circumstances under which that power is released (Does gunpowder explode when someone accidentally drops a match? Or when a soldier primes the pan of their musket? Or when a miner lights a fuse?).

What does any of this have to do with the project of radical economic geography? Sayer's argument is that it has been methodologically slipshod, undermining the politically important analysis it carries out on such important topics as industrial location and uneven development. The problem is that radical economic geographers foist abstract, necessary relations on to the concrete world without recognizing the effects that contingent, mediating relations produce. For example, a necessary relation within Marx's abstract conception of capitalism is the movement of capital to low-cost, profit-maximizing locations; it is as much a defining feature of an abstract capitalism as is the chemical formula for gunpowder. Some radical geographers have then used this necessary relation to make concrete claims about the world. For example, as in the new international division of labor thesis, the idea that manufacturers in developed countries switch their industrial investment to much cheaper developing countries. The problem, though, as Sayer argues, is that a bevy of contingent, concrete relations interrupt the abstract relation, changing its form and consequence, if not negating it altogether. Note, Sayer is not denying the importance of Harvey's Marxist agenda focusing on a "dour world" and "crushing realities," but he is saying that to achieve the best purchase on them requires use of at least an ancillary paradigm: critical realism.

The paradigm favored by Ash Amin, institutionalism, is quite different. Originally formulated by the maverick American economist Thorstein Veblen, at the turn of the twentieth century, institutionalism is a third way lying between, on the one hand, a more politically driven and often deterministic Marxism, and, on the other, a more abstract and formal orthodox economics with its uncritical belief in the beneficence of the market. In contrast, institutionalism insists on the centrality of contingent and concrete social, cultural, and political institutions, and their interaction, in the constitution and maintenance of the economy. The economy is always embedded in a set of complex institutional relations that shape and animate it. Failure to recognize their importance results in a failure to comprehend both the economy (and its geography), and the means to effect propitious change. It is around this last issue that Amin works out the meaning of an institutionalist paradigm in economic geography by focusing on policies designed to benefit less-favored regions within industrialized countries. During the 1990s, those policies were often predicated on neo-liberalism, the belief that a market-based solution is best. Following institutionalism, Amin convincingly shows the inadequacy of such a policy, and of the wider approach of orthodox economics justifying it. The problem is that market-based solutions appear best only because of the theoretical assumption of an asocial, acultural, maximizing individual, homo economicus. The effect of such an assumption is to make institutions disappear; they are reduced to the sum of the rational maximizing individuals that compose them. For Amin this is nonsense. Institutions are the very stuff of a real economy, and integral to any solution to economic failure such as found in less-favored regions. The answer is not to ignore institutions, but to nurture tighter, broader, and thicker linkages among them, and by doing so unequivocally rejecting fictions such as homo economicus (satirized by Veblen as a "homogenous globule of desire"). Moreover, this is an inherently geographical project. Institutions are not free-floating, waiflike entities, but substantially grounded in particular places. To practice institutionalism is to practice economic geography.

Amin's article begins to push economic geography away from strict political economy as imagined by Harvey and Sayer, allowing through the role of institutions an expanded role for the social and cultural. Such a shift is even more clearly defined in Thrift and Olds' essay that follows. Published in 1996, it has become a manifesto within economic geography for Harvey's dreaded paradigm of "cultural analysis." Thrift and Olds' argument is that there have been sea changes both in the way economies operate, and in the way social sciences represent them, and economic geographers must respond to the new agenda. On the one hand, economy and culture have become "incorrigibly intertwined," which they illustrate using the example of Christmas. Marking the birth of one of the world's greatest cultural religious figures, Christmas in high-income Western countries is now also fundamentally about money: of shopping until you drop, of crowded retail malls and shopping centers, of sales and bargains, of gifting, re-gifting, and de-gifting. Is Christmas a cultural celebration? Or is Christmas a once-a-year economic bonanza for capitalism? It is both. And such hybridity, as Thrift and Olds illustrate, is now pervasive: culture and economy are so blurred that it is difficult to know where one begins and the other ends. On the other hand, if blurring is the new reality, how should economic geography as a social science deal with it? They argue, first, by becoming more polycentric, that is, by "celebrating a qualitative multiplicity of 'economic' times and spaces." And second, by drawing on the panoply of social scientific theorizing available, and not just the one thin slice found in orthodox economics. In doing so, economic geography become "more inclusive and more able to mix in company." More generally, Thrift and Olds recommend a loosening up in how economic geographers theorize; that they move away from the straight and narrow paradigms of orthodox economics and Marxism to more inventive, creative, and experimental theoretical forms. This is what Thrift and Old do at the end of their paper when they offer up a series of topological metaphors to conceive economy and culture. This is not Economics 101, but precisely because it's not, it is so important.

Related arguments about economy and culture, but presented in even starker terms, and expressing perhaps an even more dreaded version of cultural analysis, are continued in Gibson-Graham's essay which appeared in their now classic book, *The End of Capitalism (as we knew it)* (1996). They – Gibson-Graham are two separate authors, Kathy Gibson and Julie Graham – are concerned with metaphor, in this case, metaphors that underpin the very notion of the economy. Metaphors for them are not mere figures of speech, interchangeable, frivolous, and of no consequence. Rather, they produce profound material consequences, determining within the economy, for example, which person does what job, how much they are paid, and whether industries and associated communities are saved or let slip. In particular, they argue that the metaphorical origins of the economy are with the body. But it is not any old body, it is the body of a heterosexual man. In turn, the masculinity of that body shapes the now familiar characteristics of the economy on to which it is transposed: its purity, its sovereignty, its heroicness, and its mastery. These metaphors create, to use Gibson-Graham's vocabulary, a particular discourse about the economy. Discourse is a difficult term, but the general idea is that rather than language reflecting the world, the world comes to reflect language. Furthermore, language is never neutral, and transparent, but reflects all number of social interests, and relations of power. So, in this case, once people begin to use (male) bodily metaphors to represent the economy, and structure their actions and beliefs accordingly, the economy discursively takes on those characteristics, shaping its material form.

Gibson-Graham, however, want to challenge that discourse, which means challenging the dominant cultural metaphor of the male, heterosexual body that underlies it. Only in this way, they suggest, is progressive political change possible. They do so by trying out new metaphors taken from feminist interpretations of the female body, and contra the male body, conceived as porous, non-hierarchical, and partial. Through these alternative metaphors, they argue, it is possible to imagine other discursive possibilities for the economy, and other material prospects than the one promised by capitalism. This too is a space of hope, but the paradigm from which it is envisioned is quite different from Harvey's classical Marxist one.

In reading these essays, we would like you to bear in mind the following questions. As economic geography has moved from Marxism to critical regionalism and now to some form of cultural analysis, has there been any progress? Is economic geography a better discipline now than it was, say, twenty or even thirty years ago? If so, how is it better? What are the criteria? But if we can't claim progress, then how do we interpret the methodological changes represented by the five chapters?

Are we left only with a relativist view that says each approach is as relatively good as any other? But if so, how do we choose among them? Or do we have to choose among them at all? Can we combine different paradigms? Or, again, is it possible to undertake economic geography without using any paradigm at all? What does a paradigm give you that you might need in carrying out economic geography, and what are the grounds for picking one over another?

NOTE

1. Of course, there have been more than just these three. For a fuller discussion see the Introductory essay to this book, and Barnes's (2000) essay which appeared in the *Companion*.

Chapter 1

The Difference a Generation Makes

David Harvey

1 Marx Redux

Every year since 1971 (with the exception of one) I have run either a reading group or a course on Marx's *Capital* (Volume 1). While this may reasonably be taken as the mark of a peculiarly stodgy academic mind, it has allowed me to accumulate a rare time-series of reactions to this particular text. In the early 1970s there was great political enthusiasm for it on the part of at least a radical minority. Participation was understood as a political act. Indeed, the course was set up (in parallel with many others of its sort across American campuses at the time) to try to find a theoretical basis, a way of understanding all of the chaos and political disruption evident in the world (the civil rights movement of the 1960s and the urban uprisings that followed the assassination of Martin Luther King in the United States, the growing opposition to the imperialist war in Vietnam, the massive student movements of 1968 that shook the world from Paris to Mexico City, from Berkeley and Berlin to Bangkok, the Czech "Spring" and its subsequent repression by the Soviets, the "Seven Days' War" in the Middle East, the dramatic events that occurred at the Democratic National Convention in Chicago, just to name a few of the signal events that made it seem as if the world as we knew it was falling apart).

In the midst of all this turmoil there was a crying need for some sort of political and intellectual guidance. Given the way in which Marx's works had effectively been proscribed through the long history of McCarthyite repression in the United States, it seemed only right and proper to turn to Marx. He must have had something important to say, we reasoned, otherwise his works would not have been suppressed for so long. This presumption was given credibility by the icy reception to our efforts on many a campus. I disguised the name of the course, often ran it of an evening, and gave "independent study" credit for those who did not want any mention of it on their transcript (I later learned from someone high up in the administration that since the course was taught in the geography program and was called "Reading Capital" it took them nearly a decade to figure out it was Marx's *Capital* that was being taught).

Capital was not an easy text to decipher, at least for the uninitiated (and there were many of us in that condition and only a few old hands could help us on our way, most of them of European extraction where communist parties had long remained active). But for those of us in universities the intellectual difficulty was, at least, a normal challenge.

In these early years many young faculty members participated, as did many graduate students. Some of them have gone on to be famous (and though some have changed their stripes most will generously acknowledge the formative nature of the whole experience). They came from all manner of disciplines (Philosophy, Math Sciences, Political Theory, History of Science, English, Geography, History, Sociology, Economics . . .). In retrospect I realize what an incredible privilege it was to work through this text with people armed with so many different intellectual skills and political perspectives. This was how I learned my Marx, through a process of mutual self-education that obeyed little or no particular disciplinary logic let alone party political line. I soon found myself teaching the text well beyond the confines of the university, in the community (with activists, teachers, unionists). I even got to teach some of it (not very successfully) in the Maryland penitentiary.

Teaching undergraduates was somewhat more fraught. The dominant tone of undergraduate radicalism in those days was anti-intellectual. For them, the academy seemed the center of ideological repressions; book learning of any sort was inherently suspect as a tool of indoctrination and domination. Many undergraduate student activists (and these were, of course, the only ones who would ever think of taking the course) thought it rather unradical to demand that they read let alone understand and write about such a long and tortuous book. Not many of them lasted the course. They paid no mind to Marx's injunction that "there is no royal road to science" nor did they listen to the warning that many readers "always anxious to come to a conclusion, eager to know the connexion between general principles and the immediate questions that have aroused their passions, may be disheartened because they will be unable to move on at once." No amount of "forewarning and forearming those readers who zealously seek the truth" (Marx, 1967 edition, p. 104) seemed to work with this audience. They were carried forward largely on a cresting wave of intuitions and bruised emotions (not, I hasten to add, necessarily a bad thing).

The situation is radically different now. I teach *Capital* as a respectable regular course. I rarely if ever see any faculty members and the graduate student audience has disappeared (except for those who plan to work with me and who take the course as some kind of "rite of passage" before they go on to more important things). Most of the graduate survey courses in other departments now allot Marx a week or two, sandwiched in between, say, Darwin and Weber. Marx gets attention. But in academia, this is devoted either to putting him in his place as, say, a "minor post-Ricardian" or passing him by as an outmoded "structuralist" or "modernist." Marx is, in short, largely written off as the weaver of an impossibly huge master-narrative of history and an advocate of some totally impossible historical transformation that has in any case been proven by events to be just as fallacious politically and practically as it always was theoretically.

Even before the collapse of the Berlin Wall, in the early 1980s, Marx was definitely moving out of academic and political fashion. In the halcyon years of identity politics and the famous "cultural turn" the Marxian tradition assumed an important negative role. It was ritualistically held up (incorrectly) as a dominant ideology that had to be fought against. Marx and "traditional" Marxism were systematically criticized and denigrated as insufficiently concerned with more important questions of gender, race, sexuality, human desires, religion, ethnicity, colonial dominations, environment, or whatever. Cultural powers and movements were just as important if not more so than those of class, and what was class anyway if not one out of many different and cross-cutting cultural configurations. All of that might have been fair enough (there were plenty of grounds for such criticisms) if it had not also been concluded that Marxism as a mode of thought was inherently antagonistic towards any such alternative formulations and therefore a totally lost cause. In particular, cultural analysis supplanted political economy (the former, in any case, being much more fun than being absorbed in the dour world and crushing realities of capitalist exploitation).

And then came the collapse of the Wall, the last nail in the coffin of any sort of Marxist credibility even if many of a Marxian persuasion had long distanced themselves (some as long ago as the Hungarian uprising of 1956 and still more with the crushing of the Czech Spring in 1968) from actually existing socialism of the Soviet–Chinese sort. To pretend there was anything interesting about Marx after 1989 was to sound more and more like an all-but-extinct dinosaur whimpering its own last rites. Free-market capitalism rode triumphantly across the globe, slaying all such old dinosaurs in its path. "Marx talk" was increasingly confined to what might best be described as an increasingly geriatric "New Left" (I myself passed none too gently into that night known as "senior citizen"). By the early 1990s the intellectual heft of Marxian theory seemed to be terminally in decline.

But some undergraduates still continue to take the *Capital* course. For most of them this is no longer a political act. The fear of communism has largely dissipated. The course has a good reputation. A few students are curious to see what all the fuss with Marxism was about. And a few still have some radical instincts left to which they feel Marx might add an extra insight or two. So, depending on their timetable and their requirements, some undergraduates end up in Marx's *Capital* rather than in Aristotle's *Ethics* or Plato's *Republic*.

This contrast I have drawn between then and now in terms of political and intellectual interest and response to Marx is hardly surprising. Most will recognize the broad outlines of what I have described even if the specific lens I am using exaggerates and distorts here and there.

But there is another tale to be told that makes matters rather more confusing. In the early 1970s it was hard to find the direct relevance of Volume I of *Capital* to the political issues that dominated the day. We needed Lenin to get us from Marx to an understanding of the imperialist war that so unnerved us in Vietnam. We needed a theory of civil society (Gramsci at least) to get us from Marx to civil rights, and a theory of the state (such as Miliband or Poulantzas) to get us to a critique of state repressions and welfare state expenditures manipulated to requirements of capital accumulation. We needed the Frankfurt School to understand questions of legitimacy, technological rationality, the state and bureaucracy, and the environment.

But then consider the historical-geographical conditions. In much of the advanced capitalist world, the trade union movement (often far too reformist for our radical tastes) was still strong, unemployment was broadly contained, everywhere (except in the United States) nationalization and public ownership was still on the agenda and the welfare state had been built up to a point where it seemed unassailable if flawed. Elsewhere in the world movements were afoot that seemed to threaten the existence of capitalism. Mao was a preeminent revolutionary leader in China while many other charismatic revolutionaries from Che Guevara and Castro in the Latin American context to Cabral and Nyerere in Africa actively held out the possibility of a socialist or communist alternative.

Revolution seemed imminent and we have subsequently learned that it was actively feared among many of the rulers of the time (even going beyond what might be expected from the evident paranoia of someone like Richard Nixon). How that revolution might occur and the kind of society to which it might lead were not topics even remotely touched upon in Marx's *Capital* (though there were plenty of other texts of Marx and the Marxists to which we could turn for enlightenment).

In short, we needed a whole host of mediations to get from Marx's *Capital* to the political issues that concerned us. And it frequently entailed an act of faith in the whole history of the Marxist movement (or in some charismatic figure like Mao or Castro) to believe in the inner connection between Marx's *Capital* and all that we were interested in. This is not to say there was nothing in the text to fascinate and delight – the extraordinary insights that came from consideration of the commodity fetish, the wonderful sense of how class struggle had altered the world from the pristine forms of capital accumulation that Marx described. And once one got used to it, the text provided its own peculiar and beguiling pleasures. But the plain fact was that *Capital* did not have that much direct relevance to daily life. It described capitalism in its raw, unmodified, and most barbaric nineteenth-century state.

The situation today is radically different. The text teems with ideas as to how to explain our current state. There is the fetish of the market that caught out that lover of children Kathy Lee Gifford when she was told that the line of clothing she was selling through Wal-Mart was made either by thirteen-year-olds in Honduras paid a mere pittance or by sweated women workers in New York who had not been paid for weeks. There is also the whole savage history of downsizing (prominently reported on in the *New York Times*), the scandals over child labor in Pakistan in the manufacture of carpets and soccer balls (a scandal that was forced upon FIFA's attention), and Michael Jordan's $30 million retainer for Nike, set against press accounts of the appalling conditions of Nike workers in Indonesia and Vietnam. The press is full of complaints as to how technological change is destroying employment opportunities, weakening the institutions of organized labor and increasing rather than lightening the intensity and hours of labor (all central themes of Marx's chapter on "Machinery and Modern Industry"). And then there is the whole question of how an "industrial reserve army" of labor has been produced, sustained, and manipulated in the interests of capital accumulation these last decades, including the public admission by Alan Budd, an erstwhile advisor to Margaret Thatcher, that the fight against inflation in the early 1980s was a cover for raising unemployment and reducing the strength of the working class. "What was engineered," he said, "in Marxist terms was a crisis in capitalism which re-created a reserve army of labour, and has allowed the capitalists to make high profits ever since" (Brooks, 1992).

All of this now makes it all too easy to connect Marx's text to daily life. Students who stray into the course soon feel the heat of what amounts to a devastating critique of a world of free-market neo-liberalism run riot. For their final paper I give them bundles of cuttings from the *New York Times* (a respectable source, after all) and suggest they use them to answer an imaginary letter from a parent/relative/friend from home that says:

> I hear you are taking a course on Marx's *Das Kapital*. I have never read it myself though I hear it is both interesting and difficult. But thank heavens we have put that nineteenth-century nonsense behind us now. Life was hard and terrible in those days, but we have come to our collective senses and made a world that Marx would surely never recognize . . .

They write illuminating and often devastatingly critical letters in reply. Though they dare not send them, few finish the course without having their views disrupted by the sheer power of a text that connects so trenchantly with conditions around us.

Herein, then, lies a paradox. This text of Marx's was much sought after and studied in radical circles at a time when it had little direct relationship to daily life. But now, when the text is so pertinent, scarcely anyone cares to consider it.

2 The Work of Postmodernity

The paradox I have described relates to a massive discursive shift that has occurred over the past three decades. There are all kinds of aspects to this shift and it is easy to get lost in a mass of intricacies and complexities. But what is now striking is the dominance of an almost fairy-tale-like belief, held on all sides alike, that once upon a time there was structuralism, modernism, industrialism, Marxism, or what have you and now there is post-structuralism, postmodernism, postindustrialism, post-Marxism, post-colonialism, and so forth. Like all such tales, this one is rarely spoken of in such a crude or simplistic way. To do so would be particularly embarrassing to those who deny in principle the significance of broad-based "metanarratives." Yet the prevalence of "the post" (and the associated inability to say what it is that we might be "pre") is a dominant characteristic of contemporary debate. It has also become a serious game in academia to hunt the covert modernists (if you are a dedicated postmodernist) or to hunt the decadent postmodernists (if you happen to be in favor of some sort of modernist revival).

One of the consequences of this prevalent fairy tale (and I call it that to capture its beguiling power) is that it is impossible to discuss Marx or Marxism outside of these dominant terms of debate. For example, one quite common reaction to my recent work, particularly *Justice, Nature and the Geography of Difference*, is to express surprise and disbelief at how I seem to merge modernist and postmodernist, structuralist and poststructuralist arguments (see, e.g., Eagleton, 1997). But Marx had not read Saussure or Lévi Strauss and while there are some powerful structuralist readings of Marx (principally by Althusser) the evidence that Marx was a

structuralist or even a modernist *avant la lettre*, as these terms came to be understood in the 1970s, is neither overwhelming nor conclusive. Analyses based on
Marx's work collide with the beguiling power of this fairy-tale reading of our recent
discursive history. Put bluntly, we do not read Marx these days (no matter whether
he is relevant or not) because he is someone whose work lies in a category that we
are supposed to be "post." Or if we do read him, it is solely through the lenses provided by what it is we believe we are "post."

Now it is indeed interesting to look at Marx's *oeuvre* through such lenses. He
was, of course, an avid critic of classical bourgeois political economy and devoted
much of his life to "deconstructing" its dominant principles. He was deeply concerned with language (discourse) and was acutely aware of how discursive shifts (of
the sort he examined in depth in *The Eighteenth Brumaire)* carried their own distinctive political freight. He understood in a deep sense the relationship between
knowledge and "situatedness" ("positionality") though it was, of course, the
"standpoint" of the worker that was the focus of his attention. I could go on and
on in this vein, but my point here is not to try to prove that much of what passes
for innovative in our recent discursive history is already pre-figured in Marx, but
to point to the damage that the fairy-tale reading of the differences between the
"then" and the "now" is doing to our abilities to confront the changes occurring
around us. Cutting ourselves off from Marx is to cut off our investigative noses to
satisfy the superficial face of contemporary intellectual fashion.

Bearing this in mind, let me now focus on two facets of this discursive shift that
have occurred since around 1970: those captured through the terms "globalization"
and "the body." Both terms were little if at all in evidence as analytical tools in the
early 1970s. Both are now powerfully present; they can even be regarded as conceptual dominants. "Globalization," for example, was entirely unknown before the
mid-1970s. Innumerable conferences now study the idea. There is a vast literature
on the subject, coming at it from all angles. It is a frequent topic of commentary in
the media. It is now one of the most hegemonic concepts for understanding the
political economy of international capitalism. And its uses extend far beyond
the business world to embrace questions of politics, culture, national identity, and
the like. So where did this concept come from? Does it describe something essentially new?

"Globalization" seems first to have acquired its prominence as American Express
advertised the global reach of its credit card in the mid-1970s. The term then spread
like wildfire in the financial and business press, mainly as legitimation for the deregulation of financial markets. It then helped make the diminution in state powers to
regulate capital flows seem inevitable and became an extraordinarily powerful political tool in the disempowerment of national and local working-class movements
and trade union power (labor discipline and fiscal austerity – often imposed by the
International Monetary Fund and the World Bank – became essential to achieving
internal stability and international competitiveness). And by the mid-1980s it
helped create a heady atmosphere of entrepreneurial optimism around the theme of
the liberation of markets from state control. It became a central concept, in short,
associated with the brave new world of globalizing neo-liberalism. It helped
make it seem as if we were entering upon a new era (with a touch of teleological
inevitability thrown in) and thereby became part of that package of concepts

that distinguished between then and now in terms of political possibilities. The more
the left adopted this discourse as a description of the state of the world (even if it
was a state to be criticized and rebelled against), the more it circumscribed its own
political possibilities. That so many of us took the concept on board so uncritically
in the 1980s and 1990s, allowing it to displace the far more politically charged concepts of imperialism and neocolonialism, should give us pause. It made us weak
opponents of the politics of globalization particularly as these became more and
more central to everything that US foreign policy was trying to achieve. The only
politics left was a politics of conserving and in some instances downright conservative resistance.

There is, however, one other angle on much of this that may have equally deep
significance. The NASA satellite image entitled "Earth Rise" depicted the earth as
a free-floating globe in space. It quickly assumed the status of an icon of a new kind
of consciousness. But the geometrical properties of a globe are different from those
of a two-dimensional map. It has no natural boundaries save those given by lands
and oceans, cloud covers and vegetation patterns, deserts and well-watered regions.
Nor does it have any particular center. It is perhaps no accident that the awareness
of the artificiality of all those boundaries and centers that had hitherto dominated
thinking about the world became much more acute. It became much easier, with
this icon of the globe hanging in the background, to write of a "borderless world"
(as Miyoshi, 1997, has so persuasively done) and to take a radically decentered
approach to culture (with the massive cultural traditions of China, India, South
America, and Africa suddenly looking as salient and as geographically dominant
across segments of the globe as those of the West). Travel around the world, already
much easier, suddenly had no natural stopping point and the continuity of spatial
relations suddenly becomes both practically and rhetorically a fundamental fact of
life. And it may well be that the focus on the body as the center of all things is itself
a response to this decentering of everything else, promoted by the image of the
globe (rather than the two-dimensional map) as the locus of human activity and
thought.

So what of the body? Here the tale, though analogous, is substantially different.
The extraordinary efflorescence of interest in "the body" as a grounding for all sorts
of theoretical enquiries over the last two decades has a dual origin. In the first place,
the questions raised particularly through what is known as "second-wave feminism"
could not be answered without close attention being paid to the "nature–nurture"
problem and it was inevitable that the status and understanding of "the body"
became central to theoretical debate. Questions of gender, sexuality, the power of
symbolic orders, and the significance of psychoanalysis also repositioned the body
as both subject and object of discussion and debate. And to the degree that all of
this opened up a terrain of enquiry that was well beyond traditional conceptual
apparatuses (such as that contained in Marx), so an extensive and original theorizing of the body became essential to progressive and emancipatory politics (this was
particularly the case with respect to feminist and queer theory). And there is indeed
much that has been both innovative and profoundly progressive within this
movement.

The second impulse to return to the body arose out of the movements of
post-structuralism in general and deconstruction in particular. The effect of these

movements was to generate a loss of confidence in all previous established categories (such as those proposed by Marx) for understanding the world. And it is in this context that the connexion between decentering and the figure of the globe may have done its undermining work. The effect, however, was to provoke a return to the body as the irreducible basis for understanding. Lowe (1995, p. 14) argues that:

> [T]here still remains one referent apart from all the other destabilized referents, whose presence cannot be denied, and that is the body referent, our very own lived body. This body referent is in fact the referent of all referents, in the sense that ultimately all signifieds, values, or meanings refer to the delineation and satisfaction of the needs of the body. Precisely because all other referents are now destabilized, the body referent, our own body, has emerged as a problem.

The convergence of these two broad movements has refocused attention upon the body as the basis for understanding and, in certain circles at least (particularly those animated by writers such as Foucault and Judith Butler), as the privileged site of political resistance and emancipatory politics.

[Let me] comment on the positioning of these two discursive regimes [– "globalization" and "the body" –] in our contemporary constructions. "Globalization" is the most macro of all discourses that we have available to us while that of "the body" is surely the most micro from the standpoint of understanding the workings of society (unless, that is, we succumb to the reductionism of seeing society as merely an expression of DNA codings and genetic evolutions). These two discursive regimes, globalization and the body, operate at opposite ends of the spectrum in the scalar we might use to understand social and political life. But little or no systematic attempt has been made to integrate "body talk" with "globalization talk." The only strong connections to have emerged in recent years concern individual and human rights (e.g., the work of Amnesty International), and, more specifically, the right of women to control their own bodies and reproductive strategies as a means to approach global population problems (dominant themes in the Cairo Conference on Population in 1994 and the Beijing Women's Conference of 1996). Environmentalists often try to forge similar connections, linking personal health and consumption practices with global problems of toxic waste generation, ozone depletion, global warming, and the like. These instances illustrate the potency and the power of linking two seemingly disparate discursive regimes.

The line of argument I shall use is broadly based in a relational conception of dialectics embodied in the approach that I have come to call "historical-geographical materialism." I want, at the outset, to lay out just one fundamental tenet of this approach in order to lay another of the key shibboleths of our time as firmly to rest as I can. And this concerns the tricky question of the relation between "particularity" and "universality" in the construction of knowledge.

I deny that we have a choice between particularity or universality in our mode of thinking and argumentation. Within a relational dialectics one is always internalized and implicated in the other. There is a link between, for example, the particularities of concrete labors occurring in particular places and times (the seamstress in Bangladesh who made my shirt), and the measured value of that labor arrived at through processes of exchange, commodification, monetization, and, of course, the circulation and accumulation of capital. One conception of labor is concrete and particular and the other is abstract and "universal" (in the sense that it is achieved through specific processes of generalization).

Obviously, there could be no abstract labor at all without a million and one concrete labors occurring throughout the world. But what is then interesting is the way in which the qualities of concrete labor respond and internalize the force of abstract labor as achieved through global trade and interaction. Workers engaging in productive concrete labors suddenly find themselves laid off, downsized, rendered technologically obsolete, forced to adapt to new labor processes and conditions of work, simply because of the force of competition (or, put in the terms proposed here, the concrete labor adjusts to abstract conditions at the same time as the qualities of abstract labor depend upon movements and transitions in concrete labor processes in different places and times).

I have used this example to illustrate a general point. The particularity of the body cannot be understood independently of its embeddedness in socio-ecological processes. If, as many now argue, the body is a social construct, then it cannot be understood outside of the forces that swirl around it and construct it. One of those key determinants is the labor process, and globalization describes how that process is being shaped by political-economic and associated cultural forces in distinctive ways. It then follows that the body cannot be understood, theoretically or empirically, outside of an understanding of globalization. But conversely, boiled down to its simplest determinations, globalization is about the sociospatial relations between billions of individuals. Herein lies the foundational connexion that must be made between two discourses that typically remain segregated, to the detriment of both.

Part of the work of postmodernity as a set of discursive practices over the last two decades has been to fragment and sever connexions. In some instances this proved a wise, important, and useful strategy to try to unpack matters (such as those of sexuality or the relation to nature) that would otherwise have remained hidden. But it is now time to reconnect.

There is a final point that I need to make. One important root of the so-called "cultural turn" in recent thinking lies in the work of Raymond Williams and the study of Gramsci's writings (both particularly important to the cultural studies movement that began in Birmingham with Stuart Hall as one of its most articulate members). One of the several strange and unanticipated results of this movement has been the transformation of Gramsci's remark on "pessimism of the intellect and optimism of the will" into a virtual law of human nature. I wish in no way to detract from the extraordinary feats of many on the left who have fought a rearguard action against the wave of neo-liberalism that swept across the advanced capitalist world after 1980. This showed optimism of the will at its noble best. But a powerful inhibitor to action was the inability to come up with an alternative to the Thatcherite doctrine that "there is no alternative" (a phrase that will echo as a recurring refrain throughout this book). The inability to find an "optimism of the intellect" with which to work through alternatives has now become one of the most serious barriers to progressive politics.

Gramsci penned those famous words while sick and close to death in an Italian prison cell under conditions that were appalling. I think we owe it to him to recognize the contingent nature of the comment. We are not in prison cells. Why, then, might we willingly choose a metaphor drawn from incarceration as a guiding light for our own thinking? Did not Gramsci (1978, p. 213) also bitterly complain, before his incarceration, at the pessimism which produced then the same political passivity, intellectual torpor, and skepticism towards the future as it does now in ours? Do we not also owe it to him, out of respect for the kind of fortitude and political passion he exhibited, to transform that phrase in such a way as to seek an optimism of the intellect that, properly coupled with an optimism of the will, might produce a better future? And if I turn towards the end of this book towards the figure of utopia and if I parallel Raymond Williams's title *Resources of Hope* with the title *Spaces of Hope*, then it is because I believe that in this moment in our history we have something of great import to accomplish by exercising an optimism of the intellect in order to open up ways of thinking that have for too long remained foreclosed.

1998 is, it turns out, a fortuitous year to be writing about such matters. It is the thirtieth anniversary (the usual span given to a generation) of that remarkable movement that shook the world from Mexico City to Chicago, Berlin, and Paris. More locally (for me), it is thirty years now since much of central Baltimore burned in the wake of the riots that followed the assassination of Martin Luther King (I moved from Bristol to Baltimore the year after that). If only for these reasons this is, therefore, a good moment to take stock of that generational shift that I began by reflecting upon.

But 1998 is also the 150th anniversary of the publication of that most extraordinary of all documents known as *The Communist Manifesto*. And it happens to be the 50th anniversary of the signing of the *Universal Declaration of Human Rights* at the United Nations. Connecting these events and reflecting on their general meaning appears a worthwhile way to reflect on our contemporary condition. While Marx was deeply suspicious of all talk about rights (sensing it to be a bourgeois trap), what on earth are workers of the world supposed to unite about unless it is some sense of their fundamental rights as human beings? Connecting the sentiments of the *Manifesto* with those expressed in the *Declaration of Human Rights* provides one way to link discourses about globalization with those of the body. The overall effect, I hope, is to redefine in a more subtle way the terms and spaces of political struggle open to us in these extraordinary times.

Chapter 2

Industry and Space: A Sympathetic Critique of Radical Research

Andrew Sayer

1 Introduction

In the last decade there have been major advances in the theory of industrial location and uneven spatial development, both at the international and the subnational
or regional levels. In terms of theory, this research has drawn upon and extended
primarily Marxist concepts, though often in alliance with concepts from institutionalist economics and empirical studies of industry. At both spatial scales many
researchers have recently shifted from theoretical exegesis to empirical application,
with the result that we can now begin to see more clearly how the theories work
in practice. The misgivings voiced here about their adequacy have been developed
in the course of ongoing research on the electronics industry and regional development which I have undertaken with Kevin Morgan. In this paper, I shall outline a
critique and illustrate the points with empirical examples from this concrete
research.

The dissatisfactions cover a variety of particular issues. But beneath almost all
of these lie a few pervasive problems of theory and method whose identification
justifies the use of the term critique rather than criticism. Moreover, it will be
argued that the problems identified in the realm of theory and empirical research
repeatedly carry over into misguided prescriptions about what should be done about
industry and regional development in the realm of practice.

In the second part of the paper these underlying problems are identified in stark
abstract terms. In the third and main section, the particular issues mentioned above
are discussed as instances of these problems and their consequences illustrated in
terms of understanding concrete phenomena by means of examples drawn largely
from our research.

2 Underlying Problems of Theory, Method, and Orientation

These cover the content of theory, method or the way theory is used in concrete
research, and the general orientations or patterns of selection of material in con-

ducting research. Although highly related, I shall separate them into three classes for the purpose of expositional clarity.

Problem A: "Pseudoconcrete analysis"   This concerns the relationship of abstract and concrete research: the problem takes the form either of a reduction of the concrete to the abstract or of a fetishization of certain transient and contingent social forms as the only possible results of capitalist development, with a consequent underestimation of the variety of forms that the latter can take.

My case rests upon a realist interpretation of method (see Sayer, 1982a, 1982b, 1984). On this view, abstract theory isolates one-sided aspects of the objects of interest, particularly those elements of the process or system which are necessarily related; for example, in an abstract analysis of capital accumulation, the necessary conditions for the realization of surplus value. In so doing, it abstracts from the many contingent concrete forms that capital accumulation may take. Concrete forms of development represent combinations of processes and elements, some necessarily related, others contingently related, and each of which may be isolated by abstract theory. These combinations of contingent and necessary relationships can easily mislead. It often happens that, although a particular combination of objects is contingent, when it does happen to occur, certain tendencies follow necessarily; for example, it is contingent whether capital ever uses electric power, but, where it does, its actions are constrained and enabled by the range of inherent (necessary) powers and liabilities of electricity. Moreover, a complicating factor is that the powers and liabilities of people can change as they learn new skills, as they come to understand their situation differently, and as they adopt new forms of organizations with their own powers and liabilities; for example, unions possess powers not wholly reducible to those of the individuals who constitute them.

Despite its extraordinary breadth, Marxism does not monopolize the abstract theory relevant for understanding concrete phenomena. For example, as we shall see, concrete forms of capital accumulation are influenced by technological developments whose explanation lies partly outside Marxism. Whether the combination of abstractions from different sources is successful, or merely eclectic and inconsistent, depends on how it is done. What is certain is that concrete forms of development cannot simply be "read off" from Marxist or neo-Marxist abstract theory, or for that matter, from any other abstract theory. Concrete systems include contingent relations whose form cannot be theorized and hence known in advance, but which must be discovered empirically. Conversely, theories cannot be derived successfully by reading them off from concrete forms: for example, summaries of particular concrete forms of uneven development cannot be turned into theoretical models or ideal types without making a radical underestimation of the range of other possible contingent forms and of their historical specificity. Yet this is precisely what has happened in the study of uneven development. Particular attempts to produce descriptive generalizations about the concrete forms of development have been interpreted – often against the intentions of their authors – as a model or stereotype or way of seeing, such that types of development which do not conform to these local, historically specific generalizations are rendered almost invisible. In some cases, as we shall see, the original descriptive generalizations were not even accurate for their intended objects, let alone others.

Problem B   The second problem concerns space and its identification with process, or more specifically the identification of particular sets of processes with particular spaces, such as a certain kind of economic activity with, say, metropolitan regions. Space and process have to be identified together somehow, because neither can exist independently of the other – but the problem is how? Because the spatial forms in which objects occur are contingent, we abstract from space in abstract theory according to a principal of "spatial indifference." So, for example, Marx's abstract discussion of capital abstracts from the particular spatial contexts in which concrete instances of capital find themselves. However, in a concrete study, we have to take account of how capital (or whatever) is affected by these contingent conditions, and this cannot be understood apart from their spatial and temporal form. So, as Sack (1980) puts it, having been abstracted, space and form must be "recombined." Yet, it is one thing to note that any material process, such as industrial capital, must have spatial extension and hence is not "aspatial," but quite another to recombine space and process by identifying something as heterogeneous as a certain kind of industry (for example, basic production and assembly) with an even more heterogeneous type of region (for example, peripheral regions), so that it appears one can "read off" one from the other. As we shall see, the theoretical grounds for making such identifications are flimsy indeed.

Problem C   The third problem is of a rather different kind, but as will be shown it interacts with problems A and B in a strikingly recurrent manner. It relates to the *theoretical and political priorities of Marxist and other radical research* which govern the relative attention given to different kinds of economic activity and person.

Perhaps the most general of these priorities is now being challenged by feminist research: the priority of paid over unpaid work. Another is the neglect of services, again possibly reinforced by sexist biases with regard to what are considered to be "real" jobs. But even within manufacturing studies, certain biases are clear:

(a)   towards basic standardized mass production and assembly, and away from custom and small batch production, and project production (for example, civil engineering production);
(b)   a slight bias towards consumer industries and away from producer industries, or a tendency to assume that the second are no different from the first;
(c)   towards manual work, away from clerical and administrative work, away from management, research and development, and marketing (consequently, labor-process studies tend to reduce the diverse kinds of labor process going on in a plant to one central stage of manufacture, ignoring prior and subsequent manual work and ignoring administrative labor processes);
(d)   towards the bottom of the status hierarchy;
(e)   towards declining regions and localities and away from relatively prosperous ones;
(f)   towards the more radical kinds of worker and region, and towards combative industrial relations.

Together these biases explain why there is plenty to read on car-workers and the like, and more recently on the female assembly worker, but little on the wages clerk, telephone operator, or technician; also why we know so little about southern non-metropolitan England compared with the assisted areas and inner cities. Even where researchers break out of this system of preferences, it is usually in a very limited way, and within the terms of the remaining priorities; so, for example, recent studies of female workers tend to concentrate on those engaged in manual work such as assembly rather than, say, on canteen staff or office workers (for example, Pollert, 1981; Cavendish, 1982).

In *part,* such biases are perfectly understandable for Left researchers insofar as they prioritize the worse-off (though probably not the worst-off), but they are also influenced by what are little more than prejudices – in particular, leftist intellectuals images of the "ideal" or "real" (either adjective will do) worker. The Left is naturally more interested in workers than in supervisors, managers, and professionals and in radical rather than conservative regions, but *ignoring* the latter does not help our understanding either of economic change or of the political forces supported by the neglected fractions. Insofar as classes (in the Marxist sense) are internally related, one simply cannot expect to understand one class independently of the other. However, some of the biases are also induced by practical considerations of doing research; for example, the greater ease of understanding producers of mass goods relative to producers of highly-differentiated goods and services and the restriction of participant observation to groups with status lower than that of the researcher.

I do not pretend that I have been immune to these biases but I believe that they have supported a distorted and outdated view of existing society and hence one which is unhelpful in guiding our thinking about what an alternative society could be like.

3   Specific Criticisms in Industrial and Regional Studies

Having outlined these three basic problems of theory, method, and orientation, we can now proceed to see how they generate more substantive problems in the study of industry and space. My criticisms of radical research in this area concern both distortions and omissions in the use of theory in interpreting empirical cases, and, as I hope will become clear, many of them overlap and reinforce one another.

3.1   *The neglect of use-values, technology, and product innovation*

As many authors have pointed out (for example, Rosdolsky, 1977; Grossman, 1978; Harvey, 1982), it is wrong to accuse Marx of ignoring use-values. However, as *abstract* theory, *Capital* inevitably has to treat use-values *generically* rather than in terms of their concrete forms and the differences they make. The same could be said of neoclassical economics, even though it conflates value with use-value. As soon as one engages in concrete studies of particular capitalist industries, it becomes apparent that the specific nature of particular use-values and technologies has some crucial effects on capital accumulation and uneven development. Although one cannot (for reasons stated earlier) expect abstract theory to anticipate the actual effects, one might at least expect it to alert us to the problem, so that empirical research does not inadvertently filter these effects out. There are three specific kinds of problems that I will now detail.

3.1.1 Changes in labor processes and deskilling

Many explanations of these changes assume that the range of commodities being produced is fixed or else simply ignore such changes. As a result, excessive explanatory weight is thrown upon capital's attempts to wrest control from labor (Tomlinson, 1982, pp. 23–6; Kelly, 1983). This is not to deny the place of class struggle in the labor process as an ever present condition, but some authors (for example, Aglietta, 1979) erect it into the dominant or sole cause of change, perhaps because such an explanation seems more "radical" than others. Labor processes are often changed because the available process technology and/or nature of the product have changed, rather than as a strategy purely aimed at winning greater control over labor for its own sake. In fact, capital may sometimes replace a labor process over which it has great control by one over which it has *less* control, if the new process is the only existing way of producing a new commodity for which market prospects are better than for its predecessor. Technology is rarely "plastic" in the hands of management; it can create, rather than solve problems of control. Therefore, an increase in labor's control over the labor process may be a "windfall" gain rather than a hard-won victory, and similarly for capital, if its power over labor is increased. In other words, the power of either side can be affected by changes originating *outside* the workplace in terms of changes of markets for products (Kelly, 1983).

Intensification of labor and deskilling are not the only means towards the end of profit maximization, nor the only possible result: product diversification and cheapening of constant capital are alternatives. So new technology may or may not have the effect of weakening labor's control over production, and when that effect does occur it may or may not be the main reason for its introduction. Certainly an explanation of changing work organization which puts all the weight on the historic struggle between capital and labor sounds more radical – until that is, you notice how this gives the impression that labor must lose in the long run as the forces of production develop and capital inexorably deskills labor – but in any case having a radical ring does not make a theory right.

The exaggeration of deskilling owes its influence to Braverman's eloquent but flawed *Labor and Monopoly Capital* (1974); it seems to have become a conventional wisdom that on balance, changes in capitalist labor processes (necessarily) induce a net deskilling effect. If one theorizes or empirically investigates the history of the labor processes used to make a particular product, a long-term deskilling effect seems probable. The problem lies not here but in the assumption that if this is true then it must also be so for the whole economy. As we saw earlier, this is partly an illusion, produced by an abstraction from product innovation and hence from qualitative change in the mix of industries. But it is partly also influenced by a view of early capitalism which ignores its unskilled masses and sees only craft labor, and perhaps by a modern tendency to ignore newer skills whose possessors do not fit stereotypes of real or ideal workers. New technologies, products, and industries may involve reskilling, and, although these are likely to decline too for any product in the long term, there will in turn be successive new products at later dates. Even new process (as opposed to product) technologies need not necessarily involve net deskilling if the new machinery outweighs the higher cost of the more skilled labor needed to run it

In any case, the concept of "deskilling," not to mention "skill" itself, also seems ill defined, insofar as it is sometimes used to refer to individuals and at other times to refer to the content of jobs, often in the same analysis. If large numbers of low skilled are made redundant, as has happened in recent years, the remaining operator jobs may either be deskilled or be reskilled, but overall the proportion of the low skilled jobs will decrease; it seems odd to call this a case of "deskilling." In electronics the proportion of skilled jobs, even allowing for definitional problems, has risen, and at several levels there has been a shift towards "multiskilling" which eludes a simple deskilling–reskilling categorization.

As it is contingent whether deskilling or reskilling is dominant in the economy, it must be treated as an empirical question. Interestingly, I find that those who have done extensive empirical research on skills are far more circumspect about the overall direction of change than those who have merely read Braverman and followers (see EITB, 1981; Kelly, 1983). There is also often some reluctance on the Left to believe that there can ever be serious shortages of technical skills and that such shortages can inhibit development.

3.1.2 Economies of scale

Problems of abstraction from product differentiation also contribute to misinterpretations of the effect of scale on the economies of production. It is easy to get the impression from some theoretical literature that economies of scale are a simple phenomenon or an independent variable, and that optimal scales of production will rise inexorably. Frequently, business or economics literature cites optimal scales which are far beyond that achieved by any firms, for example, in the car industry, the figure of 1 million units per annum for engine plants, even though this has probably never been approached (D. T. Jones, personal communication). Belief in such figures produces puzzlement over how so many firms survive with lower volumes – and not just marginal firms but leading ones too.

There are several reasons for this gap between theoretical expectations and empirical evidence. One is that abstraction from product differentiation conceals the extent to which the market is segmented, thereby limiting scale of output and inducing firms to sacrifice length of production runs for the sake of gaining entry into more sectors of the market. Again, it is not necessarily in the interests of firms to try to homogenize their products excessively because they can also compete more effectively by making themselves different. (Competition is invariably contradictory: sometimes the most effective competitors are those who manage to reduce competition, and product standardization as a means to becoming more competitive may reduce a firm's competitiveness by intensifying competition.) In practice, the stagnation of demand associated with the ending of the postwar long boom has enhanced the attractiveness of product-diversification strategies over maximum-scale strategies.

Further problems arise from the tendency to treat economies of scale as an independent variable when in fact they depend upon a number of conditions internal to the plant, which can be changed: for example, the setup time for machines, the costs of maintaining large inventories and coordinating long production runs of parts needed in different amounts, and more generally particular ways of organizing the production process. Change these conditions, and optimal scale changes, and not necessarily upwards. In fact, the most significant innovations in recent years in process technology and management techniques point to greatly reduced lot sizes in production. On the technical side, computerized numerical control (CNC) and computer-aided design and manufacture (CAD/CAM) have given some respite to smaller producers such as Jaguar in the car industry. More dramatically, on the management side, familiar Western ideas that the secret of profitable production lies in the single-minded pursuit of maximum volumes and line speeds have been turned upside down by the revolutionary Japanese "just-in-time" system of production which unearths and eliminates formerly hidden sources of diseconomies (Ohno, 1982; Schonberger, 1982; Abernathy et al., 1983). This is not to say that firms do not still gain from volume but that volume on its own does not guarantee maximized productivity. Last, a further influence tending to strengthen smaller units of production is the growing consensus in management circles that small plants make for less-adversarial industrial relations.

The spatial consequences of these developments are dealt with later.

3.1.3 The technical and social divisions of labor

Another possibly related problem concerns a common underestimation of nonmarket interactions in exchanges between firms. Frequently, radical distinction is drawn between the technical division of labor within a firm involved in making a particular product and the social division of labor between firms and between different kinds of production. The first is planned *a priori* and carefully controlled by management, whereas the second relies upon the anarchy of the market and is regulated *a posteriori* in response to market signals. However, an important qualification to this contrast, particularly the description of markets as "anarchic," is required to deal with market transactions which are set within a context of buyer–seller interactions which to a certain extent lock the activities of both parties together. These are most obvious in inter-industry transactions where firms do not merely send an order to another firm in return for goods but actually intervene in the management of the subcontracting form in order to guarantee supply and quality. Also, technological interdependencies between the products and components of the firms lock them into a more rigid and controlled relationship than would a simple market exchange. By such means, major firms (for example, oil companies) are able, to a certain degree, to manage labor processes in other firms "at a distance," without the impediment of formal ownership responsibilities. In some cases it might therefore be legitimately argued that the technical division of labor can be extended to embrace a network of firms under separate ownership. Indeed, if as I suspect, this form of industrial organization is becoming more common, a rethinking is required of the concept of industrial concentration, for some of the "largest" companies in revenue terms may do little more than manage production undertaken by other firms.

3.2   Misleading stereotypes of the spatial division of labor

One of the most important sources of progress in understanding the space economy has come from the recognition of the *interdependence* of activities in different areas as parts of a "spatial division of labor." This may take the form of a corporate spatial hierarchy of activities or, at a more aggregate level, a spatially segregated division of labor between different kinds or stages of production undertaken within either a national economy or the international economy. As a result it is now realized that the performance of individual establishments cannot be understood in abstraction from this context and that the nature of national economies, regions, or other localities may be illuminated by examining them in terms of their place within the international division of labor.

But problems start to arise as soon as anyone assumes that these spatial divisions of labor must necessarily take particular forms which are inherent in capital accumulation; indeed such an assumption amounts to what I termed in section 2 a misidentification of space and process. The misleading stereotypes I have in mind can be traced back to the work of individual authors, although what I am attacking is not so much those authors' original positions as the popular views of what they said – views which now seem to constitute part of the "common sense" of the Left. As often happens, there are significant differences between the original arguments and their popularized versions: the latter tend to be shorn of the many and reasonable qualifications made by the original authors.

Three overlapping and similar stereotypes might be distinguished: what I term "Hymer's stereotype"; the product-cycle stereotype; and the new international division of labor (NIDL) thesis.

3.2.1   Hymer's stereotype

The first of these can be traced back to Hymer's ideas about the developing correspondence between global patterns of uneven spatial development and the hierarchical internal structure of multinational firms. Similar ideas – though for different spatial scales – can be found in work by Westaway (1974), Massey (1979), and Lipietz (1980), among others. Hymer's work on multinationals was innovative and extensive, but its limitations are clear in some of his short and more rhetorical articles, and it is probably ideas such as those contained in the following passages which have seeped into radical consciousness:

> a regime of North Atlantic Multinational Corporations would tend to centralize high level decision-making occupations in a few key cities in the advanced countries, surrounded by a number of regional subcapitals, and confine the rest of the world to the lower levels of activity and income, i.e. to the status of towns and village: in a new imperial system, income, status, authority and consumption patterns would radiate out from these centres along a declining curve, and the existing pattern of inequality and dependency would be perpetuated. The pattern would be complex, just as the structure of the corporation is complex, but the basic relation between different countries would be one of the superior–subordinate, head office and branch plant. (1975, p. 38)

The association of space and function is still more clearly stated in the same paper.

Table 2.1: "Hymer's stereotype" (see text), in which the space–process relationship takes the form A–B–C

Level of corporate hierarchy	Type of area		
	Major metropolis (for example, New York)	regional capitals (for example, Brussels)	periphery (for example, South Korea, Ireland)
1 Long-term strategic planning	A		
2 Management of divisions	D	B	
3 Production, routine work	F	E	C

> Since business is usually the core of the city, geographical specialization will come to reflect the hierarchy of corporate decision making, and the occupational distribution of labor in a city or region will depend for its function in the international economic system. (p. 50)

Again it should be stressed that the positive contribution of this work, like that of Murray (1972), was to unite two bodies of theory – on industrial location and regional development – which had formerly been largely separate. But it was the particular *way* in which capital and region, process and form were related that was problematic, particularly if the following relationship between levels of the corporate hierarchy and region were assumed – see Table 2.1.

With certain modifications and adjustments of geographical scale, similar stereotypes could be devised; for example, Lipietz adds a fourth type of region but the principle of his scheme is very similar to that of Table 2.1. According to Hymer's stereotype, the space–process relationship takes the form A-B-C. But of course, D, E, and F are also present. The interpenetration of corporate hierarchies with multinational firms with headquarters in different countries and the influence of preexisting patterns of uneven development make it a poor "model" of the accumulation. At both international and subnational scales and for most sectors, advanced regions dominate levels 2 and 3 in absolute terms, that is, F > E > C.

3.2.2   Product-cycle theory and the new international division of labor thesis

In practice, at least with regard to their spatial implications, these two theories tend to be similar. Although the NIDL thesis has received explicit attention on the Left, for example, through the work of Fröbel et al. (1980), the product-cycle theory is rarely endorsed explicitly by such researchers. However, I believe it to have had a significant unacknowledged influence. In this case too, the errors of the resulting stereotype are compounded by those discussed earlier concerning product differentiation. As with the Hymer stereotype, the target of my criticisms is more the stylized popular version of the spatial implications of the theory than the original work of Vernon (1966).

According to the theory, each product passes through a cycle from innovation to standardization, during which the economics, skill, and gender composition of the workforce and location of production change markedly. After innovation, firms move down the "learning curve," rapidly at first as initial market responses are obtained, then more slowly as the product drops in price and changes from a luxury into a mature product. Innovation and launching the product require close management, research, and technical involvement and also an affluent market which can afford an expensive new product. This suggests a location in a metropolitan region of the home (rich) country. As costs fall, production is moved offshore in search of new markets and cheaper labor so that, by the final stage, the firm imports the product back to the home market.

This theory (or model) certainly has a logic to it, but it is easy therefore to overlook how circumscribed that logic is by (largely hidden) restrictive assumptions about the nature of the firm and industry involved and about its external economic environment. Not surprisingly, very few products resemble the model to any degree or for any length of time. According to Cable and Clarke (1981), hand-held electronic calculators are one of the "better" examples, though even here there are some important divergences, such as the recent tendency to shift straight from innovation to production in a Third World country without the intermediate stage of production in the home country. Second, as with Hymer's "model," the product-cycle model and the NIDL thesis give one the expectation that the general nature of regional or national economies can be "read off" from their place within the corporate divisions of labor. This is an attractive idea, but at the moment it rarely works in practice, as we shall see; although the spatial stereotypes associated with these models and with the "spatial division of labor thesis" are interesting preparations for research, I have not found them very useful for interpreting concrete instances.

The first problem – of an unacknowledged restriction to particular kinds of product – comes out in several ways. One of these is the overestimation of the presence of unskilled labor-intensive production in the later stages of the product cycle, and in *this* respect the model reinforces the biases of the Hymer stereotype towards cheap labor locations. There is no reason why standardization of process technology during the life of a product should not make the production process highly capital-intensive rather than labor-intensive so that the advantages of cheap-labor locations are irrelevant. In fact, given the *persistence* of advanced countries as the most favored locations for direct overseas investment, one suspects that this is usually the case. As has frequently been noted, the "runaway industries" are strictly limited to (certain parts of) a few industries like clothing and electronics. Even within these, changes in the cost structure of production can quickly change the locational strategies of multinationals. For example, many US semiconductor firms have moved assembly stages of production to Third World locations, particularly in Southeast Asia. This appears to support the NIDL thesis that production is being decentralized out of advanced countries. However, more recently, some assembly has been moved back into the advanced countries because increased integration and power of circuitry reduces the relative number of chips to be assembled, and because assembly has become more automated (Rada, 1982). The shift back to the home countries is likely to be slow and uneven as cost balances vary considerably from firm to firm, but some major chip producers, like IBM, have never used offshore manual assembly.

A further limitation concerns the paucity of clear-cut instances of products actually completing the cycle. In particular, it is difficult to identify mature and standardized products: just when they appear to have matured they tend to be modified and/or go through another stage of changing process technology. And in practice it is always difficult to know how big a change in the product must be before it should be treated as a new product. For example, at first sight, cars might appear to be a classic mature product, but significant changes both in process (for example, robots) and in product technology (for example, new wheel designs, ignition, and fuel-efficiency systems) are occurring. They are certainly not cosmetic changes, for success or failure in them can make major differences to sales. In the case of television production, British firms in the early nineteen seventies *did* treat televisions as a mature product (though they failed to decentralize production to the newly industrialized countries), but this was an effect rather than a cause of their lack of expenditure on research and development (R&D); their complacent assumptions were rudely shattered by Japanese producers who proceeded to make major innovations both in process and in product technology which completely changed the nature of the industry (Arnold, 1984). So paradoxically, although in one sense product-cycle theory deals expressly with product innovation, in another it underestimates it by abstracting out changes within the development of a single product, thereby drawing attention away from the connections between the development of one product and the next.

3.2.3   The "branch-plant economy" stereotype

This resulting exaggeration of the importance of standardized production leads to an underestimation of R&D done in production work, especially process engineering, and encourages the belief that all or nearly all "branch plants" are "mere" *"overspill"* plants – simply adding to the production capacity of an already standardized product. We might call this a defining feature of the *"branch-plant economy"* stereotype. However, it hardly makes sense for capital to rest content with existing production methods and products, and to duplicate existing facilities at new locations. Our research on electrical engineering in South Wales and elsewhere shows the stereotype to be inaccurate. Most branch plants we saw make products which are in some ways novel (for example, to meet the characteristics of a national market in which the firm has not previously sold) and they use production methods which are in some ways novel. For example, some new branch plants have been set up in Britain by foreign telecommunications firms, but in most cases they will produce new products. However, it may be that the branch-plant economy stereotype had more validity in the nineteen fifties and nineteen sixties, when mass production of standardized products was more prevalent, but, as we saw earlier, product differentiation, new technologies and management systems require us to rethink our assumption.

Another factor which militates against the duplication of identical overspill plants is the shift in patterns of internationalization of capital towards "complementation." By this is meant the specialization of functions within plants of a multinational and their integration into an international production system, where previously each country might have had its own fairly self-contained plants. This has been widely noted in the car industry with its complex cross-border flows of components between different countries (CIS, undated), but it exists on a possibly larger scale in industries such as electronics and computers. This does not necessarily mean that the *same* model will be sold in all countries. In the car industry it was indeed the intention of the biggest firms to produce a "world car," but diseconomies of scale and resistance to further homogenization of the product has caused a rethink (Jones, 1983).

Coupled with the erroneous view that most branch plants are located in peripheral areas and that most do routine standardized production is the belief that they employ largely "deskilled" "cheap female labor." Many of course do and it is true that feminization serves as a rough index of low skill, given discrimination against women, but the problem is again the treatment of historically specific developments as universal. *Some* decentralization of industry *has* been largely governed by the search for cheap female labor, and this was particularly important in labor-intensive industries prior to the recession, when many firms met rising demand simply by hiring more operators, who would mostly be women. Once again the exaggeration of the relative importance of mass assembly production contributes to the overestimation of the phenomenon.

3.2.4   The stereotypes in practice

At a general methodological level, the basic failing of all these stereotypes is that they freeze, and then present as universal, relationships which are contingent and historically specific. They therefore combine problems A and B in section 2 (pseudo-concrete analysis and misidentification of space and process), but problem C in the shape of the exaggeration of the relative importance of mass standardized production and its workforces is also influential.

When applied in practice, these stereotypes fail to come to terms with the fact that most foreign direct investment is located within the most advanced regions and countries, by exaggerating the significance of labor-intensive production and cheap labor locations and underestimating capital-intensive and high-skill-intensive activity and the consequent need for market locations. This is surely why it seems easier to find literature on electronics in Southeast Asia than it does on electronics in Europe and America, and why the South East is so neglected by researchers in comparison with other British regions!

The stereotypes are also based on a very limited subset of firms, that is, certain kinds of US multinational. In presenting themselves as universally applicable, they encourage a "fallacy of composition" (Elster, 1979) in which it is not realized that what is possible for some individuals (in this case, firms) cannot be possible for all individuals simultaneously.

Now we have seen that the attraction of theories of the internationalization of capital lies in the fact that they suggest the possibility of being able to "read off" the characteristics of regional and national economies from their place in the international order. This would seem to make sense insofar as economies are dominated by international capital. But, as with the Hymer stereotype, whether it is successful depends again on the *way* the corporate structures are portrayed and hence on how process and space are identified.

Obviously there are problems of extrapolating from a few sectors to multisector economies. In our research, we have tried to make more modest inferences about the characteristics of national and regional electronics industries on the basis of their supposed place in the corporate hierarchies.

Attempting to minimize these problems does not mean retreating into a position where any attempt to discover the logic behind behavior is abandoned. Although behavior is more complex than the models suggest, it is not random and it has a rationale. In realist terms, it can be understood by a method which uses abstraction of causal mechanisms and necessary relations coupled with understanding (*verstehen*) of the reasons which cause actors to act as they do, and not by the traditional method of attempting universal generalizations of contingent patterns. In all the examples we have discussed, the logic of capital accumulation is still present, but it constantly adapts to changes in labor, technology, and markets, each of which have their own causal powers and liabilities. Small wonder then that the outcomes continually elude models which freeze and attempt to extrapolate contingent patterns.

Let us consider an illustrative example: we might, on the basis of a rigid and restrictive interpretation of models of corporate structure, conjecture that R&D and marketing functions would be at opposite ends of the corporate hierarchy and so be spatially independent of each other. *If* (contingent fact) the product is a mass one and highly standardized then they probably will be separate. If on the other hand (contingent fact) the product is not standardized but has to be adapted to buyers' needs (for example, business software and custom electronic components) then R&D may be integrated both functionally and spatially with marketing and after-sales service functions. (Actually, a more careful and flexible reading of product-cycle literature would alert one to such a possibility.) Both cases are driven by the dictates of capital accumulation and competition, but the effects are crucially mediated by contingent facts. When one knows what these contingent facts are in a particular situation, the interpretation of the conditional logic of the situation (that is, conditional on whatever contingencies are present) is not difficult. In fact the structure of such explanations is quite ordinary: for example, we know that a bomb has a certain power to explode, but that whether it ever will do so is dependent on the contingent condition of its being detonated; we also know that the effects of its detonation cannot be known if we do not know what the contingent conditions are in which it has been detonated – concrete, glass, or whatever – but when (through empirical investigation), those conditions are discovered, the explanation of the effects is not necessarily difficult. In both cases – capital accumulation or physical events – satisfactory explanation requires care in moving from abstract knowledge about mechanisms through an observation of contingent conditions to the concrete level of events which they codetermine (Sayer, 1984). And such a procedure is our best safeguard against the three basic problems identified in section 2.

As the phenomena we are discussing are social, some of the causes of changes will be reasons held by actors for doing things. Their actions in turn will presuppose certain structures of social relations and other material conditions (for example, buying presupposes relations of exchange, commodity production). But one of the special properties of reasons which is not possessed by physical causes is that they are meaningful and based on some understanding of a situation held by the actor. As such the understanding may be in some way false and yet causally effective nevertheless. It is this relationship of understanding between actors and their situations which makes the realm of contingency seem large in social science relative to natural science. Ironically, understanding and learning – the very things that make knowledge possible – are also the very things that make explanation of social phenomena difficult, because they mean that people's ways of acting are not restricted to a fixed repertoire of responses. Nevertheless, the meaningful character of reasons provides solutions as well as problems: precisely because they can be understood, the explanation of human action, however changeable, need not be particularly difficult, indeed many actions are adequately explained in quite everyday terms. (Students of other cultures in different language communities experience more difficulty in explaining action simply because they lack the advantage of prior acquaintance with the *sense* of actors' reasons; until they acquire this understanding, actions are indeed a mystery. So, far from being a problem, verstehen is a solution.)

Although actors' reasons are never based on perfect understanding of situations (no one's are) their understanding is unlikely to be utterly inadequate if it informs practice. To some degree it is likely to grasp some of the patterns of necessity and contingency in the world, both natural and social, and learning consists largely in refining and extending this grasp. So, for example, the process engineer learns how to improve the manipulations of the inherent (that is, necessary) causal powers and liabilities of machines and materials, and managers learn those of particular organizational forms; indeed, the material process of production is hardly intelligible without an implicit realist ontology (Sayer, 1984).

3.3   Space and proximity

Associated with these stereotypes of spatial divisions of labor are some popular misconceptions about the significance of space, distance, and proximity. The crudest – and fortunately least widely held – of these is the idea that the reduction of transport costs and times has rendered location unimportant and made more firms "footloose." Yet spatial "effects" are invariably double-edged; the removal of the protection of distance and the annihilation of space by time exposes capital to a greater variety of possible operating environments than hitherto and competition forces them to be more selective in their location decisions. In terms of space and distance, the runaway industry phenomenon exemplifies the conquering of space; in terms of spatial *differentiation*, it represents a *heightened* response. The "annihilation of space" for one process allows the significance of proximity for another to increase. Proximity to markets in order to ensure good access is *still* important, especially for the sale of specialized production goods. One of the reasons why large foreign computer firms operating in Britain do better than their British equivalents is that they can afford to set up larger and denser networks of service centers, thereby giving them closer access to customers (Sciberras et al., 1978). Superficially, such instances of the internationalization of production and marketing might be read one-sidedly as evidence of some inexorable annihilation of space, ignoring the complementary localization process.

We have already discussed the possible spatial relationship between R&D and marketing, and the difference between mass marketing standardized products as against highly customized products can be seen as an illustration of the dependence of spatial effects on the processes involved. In the case of R&D and top management, proximity still confers considerable advantages for product innovation.

Boston's Route 128, and Silicon Valley demonstrate the strength of the localization of top scientific and managerial skills and the direct investments by European firms in such areas demonstrate their immobility relative to the mobility of money-capital.

Although there may be "cultural" advantages in separating routine production work and R&D, on account of the different kinds of worker involved, there are also advantages in colocating them, insofar as this allows compatibility between process and product development to be maximized; Japanese consumer electronics firms have exploited such advantages of colocation for some time now and recently IBM have followed suit in combining product development and production of their personal computer at Boca Raton, FL (*Business Week*, 1983). Developments in CAD/CAM also shift the economies of development and production in favor of agglomeration of different spheres of production (Kaplinsky, 1984).

Another development which points to increasing agglomeration is the "just-in-time" method of production, with its need for frequent interplant movements of small lots of goods and close buyer–seller coordination. As these methods begin to diffuse outside Japan we find examples of firms known for their high degree of inter-nationalization, like General Motors, Apple, Motorola, Hewlett Packard, Kawasaki, Sony, and Nissan, setting up *localized* networks of plants and suppliers (*Business Week*, 1984).

This is not to suggest that such firms will "deinternationalize" or that the growth of interest in internationalized production systems has been misplaced – on the contrary. It is merely to point out the double-edged effects of space and the depend-ence of such effects on the nature of the processes involved. Equally, at the same time there are undoubtedly other developments which encourage greater decentral-ization of production, for example computerization of production administration, "modularization" of production processes, not to mention the fear of the power that workers derive from large agglomerations (Murray, 1983).

Again the general thrust behind these points about space takes us back to the three problems identified in section 2: in order of obviousness, first the care needed in identifying space with process (problem B); second the related danger of freezing contingent patterns or reductionist explanations (problem A); and third the neglect of activities such as R&D, marketing and servicing, and customized production relative to less spatially restricted activities such as mass production (problem C).

3.4   The neglect of the nation-state

Capital and labor are not the only economic agents affecting capital accumulation and uneven development – the nation-state also plays a part. Although the capital-ist state always has certain relationships to capital (for example, guarantor of currency, protector of property rights) other aspects of the relationship vary considerably and make a difference to patterns of internationalization of capital. Its variable roles in this respect include: (1) responding to the *net effects* of the myriad of capitals operating within (and outside) its boundaries (for example, responses to balance of payments problems); (2) defensive protectionism, for example, tariffs, regulations on inward investment; (3) aggressive nationalism and corporatism, for example, coordinating and funding R&D, giving investment grants, encouraging restructuring.

In addition to active roles such as these, the particular characteristics of each nation-state form a differentiated context for international capital. There is a continuum of responses to inward investment ranging from "open-door" policies (for example, in the United Kingdom) to aggressively nationalist policies such as those of Japan or France. Defensive protectionist measures such as tariffs may not seem interesting theoretically, but their impact on actual patterns of internationalization of capital – both of foreign and home multinationals – can be significant. Differences in national technical standards can also be important. Defensive protectionism in Europe has been the main reason for Japanese direct investment in Europe, and in the semiconductor industry, as already noted, differences between tariffs governing imports into the USA and Europe partly explain the different locational strategies of their respective multinationals.

Patterns of competition (and collaboration) between states are invariably complex because they work through individual capitals whose interests and spheres of activity bear little correspondence to those of the nation-state. So, for example, the governments of most advanced countries have support programs for microelectronics and, in ESPRIT, the European Economic Community (EEC) has a community-wide program aimed at catching up with the US and Japan in microelectronics and computers. These programs invariably give support to capital in the home country. But this usually includes resident foreign capital; also home multinationals may be technologically dependent on overseas ones. And, although several capitals in one country or the EEC may collaborate to fight off external competition (for example, from Japan), each firm's priority is to defend itself against others whatever their nationality and so they often simultaneously act against such coalitions by entering into deals with foreign competitors. Anarchic though the results of such attempts to regulate competition may be, national differences are still important. For example, the liberalization of British Telecom has been responsible for a major influx of telecommunications firms into Britain in recent years.

Too often such influences have been seen as untheorizable external factors interfering with an otherwise laissez-faire (and more theorizable) international economy. Economic nationalism has also to be explained – and in its concrete forms. Ten years ago there was a lively debate on the relationship of multinational firms to nation-states, but, despite its continuing relevance, interest has fallen off, although Radice has recently reopened the debate (1984). It is also increasingly necessary, both for academic and for political reasons to decide what we mean by the concept of a "national economy" or "the British electronics industry," when most capital is multinationally organized. And in dealing with the relationship between multinationals and host and home governments it is increasingly necessary to take into account intercapitalist competition and interstate rivalries, and these within a context of uneven development and international patterns of technological superiority and dependence.

3.5   The neglect of the social or institutional forms of capital

In any concrete empirical study of capital, contrasts in the social and institutional (or perhaps cultural) forms of capital are striking. Given the internal relation between capital and labor, the same applies to labor. New social forms do not arise automatically out of the particular characteristics of the forces of production, but are born and then succeed or fail in specific cultural contexts, both in the spheres of production and reproduction. Some of these forms fit successfully with emerging technical forces, others do not. At the level of abstract theory the particular nature of these forms can and must be ignored, although as with the effects of use-values, the fact that they can be expected to vary concretely must at least be appreciated at the abstract level. The concrete variations make important differences to workers' experience and political consciousness and therefore need to be understood. Although it is true, at the *abstract* level, as Harvey says, that "Capitalists behave like capitalists wherever they are" (Harvey, 1982, p. 424), at the concrete level this will not do and will only generate false expectations with regard to political consciousness. The concrete variations cannot be dismissed as distractions from the task of developing some essentialist universal theory of capital and labor in general.

In a particular region, the institutional and social forms of capital and labor interact and adapt to one another, and when either side changes it sets up stresses. For example, there is an interdependence between the traditional style of British management and the shop stewards movement. British managers are notoriously status conscious and anxious to distance themselves socially from manual labor. They are generally conservative as regards both technical and social innovations and, although less interventionist on the shop-floor than managers in other countries, they are more prone to aggravate grievances precisely because of their low shop-floor involvement. This is of course a caricature, but nevertheless widely observed on the whole in large plants. The other side of the coin is a ceding of shop-floor control to shop stewards (at least prior to 1979) through whom management's communications with the workforce are channeled. Conversely the growth of the shop stewards movement helped to force management back off the shop-floor – it was not a one-way process. So, although British workers are less radical politically than many of their European counterparts, they are – or perhaps, were – economically stronger within the workplace. Such lines of interdependence can come under attack in a variety of circumstances: through a strengthening of the economic and political leverage of labor; through the effects of a recession in weakening labor and (by intensifying competition) forcing capital to increase its power over labor; through *in situ* development or inward movement of new industries and new institutional and social forms of capital; or through the use of new sources of labor such as women or migrants.

It may be tempting to try to reduce such forms of interdependence to labor process categories such as "Taylorism," "Fordism," and "neo-Fordism," but, although elements of these are common and although they constitute a vaguely discernible periodization of social forms of capital indicative of a learning process, they by no means exhaust the significant differences in social-institutional forms of capital.

There are also contrasts between small and big capital, family-owned and non-family owned capital, and particularly between nationalities of capital. For example, the peculiar nature of Japanese capital has been the subject of much loose speculation in the media, but the inadequacy of the popular accounts does not mean that its peculiarities are of no material significance. The more visible cultural differences (paternalism, workaholism, and obsession with quality) do *make* a difference to

Japanese capital, although few commentators realize how far these "cultural" characteristics are reproduced by very material practices and relationships built into distinctively Japanese forms of management and labor-process organization (Schonberger, 1982). But then significant cultural characteristics always do have a material grounding: exceptionally high productivity is not achieved simply by exhortation or by the influence of a pro-work ethic. And, as Schonberger argues, if Japanese success were attributable purely to a realm of mysterious ethereal cultural characteristics having no material basis, it would hardly be possible for Japanese management methods to be exported and imitated as much as they are.

This implies that, particularly where firms invest overseas, they can act not only as "bearers of market forces" (Murray, 1972) and technologies, and not only as bearers of the social relations of production "writ large," but also as bearers of particular forms of management, work practices, and social organization. Accordingly, capital not only assesses locations as regards labor simply in terms of wage differentials, narrowly defined, but takes into account indicators of existing work "culture" and tradition (for example, rates of absenteeism) in order to evaluate spatial variations in productivity levels. Labor has correspondingly to organize itself to face the challenge of the new social forms of capital, and at the present time it has to do so against the restraining forces of mass unemployment when its resources are at their lowest.

In Britain this is evident not only in the increasing number of non-unionized or anti-union plants (at least in some regions – for example, Central Scotland) but in the shift towards single-union plants in place of traditional multiunion representation and towards corporatist "top-down" forms of unionization. These changes show how labor's own organizations have to restructure too, in this case in a way which destroys the traditional inter-union division of labor and increases inter-union competition. In these ways then, concrete analyses of industry must go beyond seeing uneven development as a simple scarcely mediated expression of the logic of capital-in-general, and grasp the specificities of actual social forms of capital and labor; they are not trivial nuances but an important component of uneven development and political consciousness.

4 Conclusion

I want to conclude by making a few comments about the concern (obsession?) of this paper with *differentiation* and *complexity*. First, I have criticized certain stereotypes not for the sake of scoring pedantic points (which is never difficult where stereotypes are concerned) but because they seemed to be *systematically* misleading both as a way of understanding the world and as a means towards changing it. For the sake of constructing an overview of the state of some system we have to make approximations: the point is not to suggest that all researchers should forsake large scale historical surveys and the like for microstudies – although it would be useful to have a more balanced division of labor on this. Rather, such approximations must be reviewed constantly in the light of more intensive studies, and conversely the latter should always keep in mind the general context. Nor have I been attacking abstract theory: rather I have warned against the dangers of applying it at the concrete level without due regard for contingent mediations.

However, from the point of view of concrete practice, we cannot simply abstract from diversity, distanciation, scale, and complexity, for social and economic organization is itself in part a response to it. Practice always takes place in a highly differentiated context and to engage with it we must understand the local specificities if we are to understand local political responses. If we abstract from these differences and specificities, arriving at generic categories, and then project these back unmediated, onto views of concrete practice, then obviously we will generate a utopian illusion of generic man and woman, living in harmony.

Chapter 3

An Institutionalist Perspective on Regional Economic Development

Ash Amin

Introduction

Until recently, regional policy has been firm-centered, standardized, incentive-based and state-driven. This is certainly true in the case of the Keynesian legacy that dominated regional policy in the majority of advanced economies after the 1960s. It relied on income redistribution and welfare policies to stimulate demand in the less favored regions (LFRs) and the offer of state incentives (from state aid to infrastructural improvements) to individual firms to locate in such regions. Paradoxically, the same principles apply also to pro-market neo-liberal experiments which have come to the fore over the last fifteen years. The neo-liberal approach, placing its faith in the market mechanism, has sought to deregulate markets, notably the cost of labor and capital, and to underpin entrepreneurship in the LFRs through incentives and investment in training, transport and communication infrastructure, and technology. The common assumption in both approaches, despite their fundamental differences over the necessity for state intervention and over the equilibrating powers of the market, has been that top-down policies can be applied universally to all types of region. This agreement seems to draw on the belief that at the heart of economic success lies a set of common factors (e.g., the rational individual, the maximizing entrepreneur, the firm as the basic economic unit, and so on).

The achievements of both strands of such an "imperative" approach (Hausner, 1995) have been modest in terms of stimulating sustained improvements in the economic competitiveness and developmental potential of the LFRs. Keynesian regional policies, without doubt, helped to increase employment and income in the LFRs, but they failed to secure increases in productivity comparable to those in the more prosperous regions and, more importantly, they did not succeed in encouraging self-sustaining growth based on the mobilization of local resources and interdependencies (by privileging non-indigenous sectors and externally-owned firms). The "market therapy" has threatened a far worse outcome, by reducing financial transfers which have proven to be a vital source of income and welfare in the LFRs, by exposing the weak economic base of the LFRs to the chill wind of ever enlarging free market zones or corporate competition, and by failing singularly to reverse the flow of all factor inputs away from the LFRs. In short, the choice has been that between dependent development or no development.

Partly in response to these failings, more innovative policy communities have begun to explore a third alternative, informed by the experience of prosperous regions characterized by strong local economic interdependencies (e.g., Italian industrial districts, certain technopoles, Baden Württemberg). It is an alternative centered on mobilizing the endogenous potential of the LFRs, through efforts to upgrade a broadly defined local supply-base. It seeks to unlock the "wealth of regions" as the prime source of development and renewal. This is not an approach with a coherent economic theory behind it, nor is there a consensus on the necessary policy actions. However, its axioms contrast sharply with those of the policy orthodoxy, in tending to favor bottom-up, region-specific, longer-term, and plural-actor based policy actions. Conceptually, against the individualism of the orthodoxy (e.g., the centrality of homo economicus), it recognizes the collective or social foundations of economic behavior, for which reason it can be described loosely as an institutionalist perspective on regional development.

This chapter seeks to develop the institutionalist perspective by bringing together strands of policy action scattered across the literature, as well as suggesting new strands. It claims that the new perspective opens up novel but challenging opportunities for policy action at the local level. It also claims, however, that the "new regionalism" will amount to very little in the absence of sustained macroeconomic support for the regions, notably a secure financial and income transfer base and expansionary programs to boost overall growth at the national and international level. The first section of the chapter summarizes the axioms of economic action and governance which emerge from a theorization of the economy rooted in institutional economics and socioeconomics. The second section discusses applications of institutionalist thought within regional development studies that seek to explain the importance of territorial proximity for economic competitiveness. Part of the purpose of these two sections is to demonstrate that the new policy orientations, outlined in the third section, are not just ex-post generalizations based on the experience of a small number of regions, but also ex-ante suggestions based on a particular conceptualization/abstraction of the economy and its territoriality.

The Economy and Economic Governance in Institutional Economics

The rise of institutional and evolutionary economics is now well documented (Hodgson, 1988, 1998; Samuels, 1995; Metcalfe, 1998), as is thought in economic sociology which stresses the influence of wider social relations in economic life (Smelser and Swedberg, 1994; Ingham, 1996). Against orthodox assumptions that the economy is equilibrium-oriented and centered on the rational individual or machine-like rules, the stress in these two bodies of thought falls on processes of institutionalization as a means of stabilizing and interpreting an economy that is essentially non-equilibrating, imperfect, and irrational. Three sets of ideas seem to be especially important in this regard.

First, from economic sociology comes the well-known idea that markets are socially constructed (Bagnasco, 1988) and that economic behavior is embedded in networks of interpersonal relations. Crucially, therefore, economic outcomes are influenced by network properties such as mutuality, trust, and cooperation, or their opposite (Dore, 1983; Granovetter, 1985; Grabher, 1993; Fukuyama, 1995; Misztal, 1996). Granovetter, for example, has suggested that networks of weak ties might be more dynamic than those dominated by strong ties (e.g., enforced loyalty) or easy escape (e.g., contract-based ties). While weak ties offer economic agents the benefits of both cooperation and access to a varied selection environment for new learning, strong ties, as in many crime networks, pose the threat of both lock-in and restricted selection, and contractual self-reliance poses very high search costs. In addition, the rising influence of actor-network theory has furthered analysis of the powers of networks by stressing the inseparability of people and things within them, producing distinctive properties that weave together actors, organizational cultures, knowledge environments, machines, texts and scripts (Latour, 1986; Callon, 1991).

Second, and against the rational actor model in standard economics, comes the idea from evolutionary and cognitive psychology (Cosmides and Tooby, 1994; Plotkin, 1994) and the behavioral tradition in economics (Simon, 1959) that different actor-network rationalities produce different forms of economic behavior and decision-making. For example, an instrumentalist or substantive rationality is likely to favor reactive responses to problems, based on a largely rule-following behavior. Reactive responses may prove to be adequate in relatively unchanging and predictable environments but their underlying rationality is not equipped for a varying environment. In contrast, a procedural actor rationality is one which seeks to adapt to the environment, drawing upon perceptive powers and generally more complex cognitive arrangements for solving problems. Finally, while the latter two rationalities tend to assume an invariant environment (therefore largely problem-solving), a recursive rationality is problem-seeking and assumes that the environment can be anticipated and to a degree manipulated through such procedures as strategic monitoring, experimental games, group learning, and so on (Delorme, 1997). It tends to generate creative actor-networks with the ability to shape the environment, owing to the capacity to think and act strategically and multidimensionally (Orillard, 1997). Third, from the recent rediscovery of "old" institutional economics (Hodgson, 1988, 1998; Hodgson et al., 1993) comes the idea that the economy is shaped by enduring collective forces, which make it an instituted process as claimed by Polanyi, not a mechanical system or set of individual preferences. These forces include formal institutions such as rules, laws, and organizations, as well as informal or tacit institutions such as individual habits, group routines, and social norms and values. All of these institutions provide stability in the real economic context of information asymmetry, market uncertainty, and knowledge boundedness, by restricting the field of possibilities available, garnering consensus and common understandings, and guiding individual action. They are also, however, templates for, or constraints upon, future development. It is their endurability and framing influence on action by individuals and actor-networks that forces recognition of the path- and context-dependent nature of economic life, or, from a governance perspective, the wide field of institutions beyond markets, firms, and states which need to be addressed by policies seeking to alter the economic trajectory.

From these strands of institutionalist thought derives an understanding of the economy as something more than a collection of atomized firms and markets driven by rational preferences and a standard set of rules. Instead the economy emerges as a composition of collective influences which shape individual action and as a diversified and path-dependent entity molded by inherited cultural and socio-institutional influences. In turn, the influences on economic behavior are quite different from those privileged by economic orthodoxy (e.g., perfect rationality, hedonism, formal rules, etc.). Explanatory weight is given to the effects of formal and informal institutions, considered to be socially constructed and subject to slow evolutionary change; to values and rationalities of action ensconced in networks and institutions; to the composition of networks of economic association, especially their role in disseminating information, knowledge, and learning for economic adaptability; and to intermediate institutions between market and state which are relatively purposeful and participatory forms of arrangement.

On the basis of these principles, we can begin to derive a number of general axioms of economic governance associated with an institutionalist approach. First, there is a preference for policy actions designed to strengthen networks of association, instead of actions which focus on individual actors alone. Second, part of the purpose of policy action might be to encourage voice, negotiation, and the emergence of procedural and recursive rationalities of behavior, in order to secure strategic vision, learning, and adaptation (Amin and Hausner, 1997). Third, emphasis is given to policy actions which aim to mobilize a plurality of autonomous organizations, since effective economic governance extends beyond the reach of both the state and market institutions (Hirst, 1994). Fourth, the stress on intermediate forms of governance extends to a preference for building up a broad-based local "institutional thickness" that might include enterprise support systems, political institutions, and social citizenship (Amin and Thrift, 1995). Finally, a key institutionalist axiom is that solutions have to be context-specific and sensitive to local path-dependencies.

The Institutional Turn in Regional Development Studies

In recent years, the region has been rediscovered as an important source of competitive advantage in a globalizing political economy (Scott, 1995; Cooke, 1997). In part, this rediscovery is based on studies of the success of highly dynamic regional economies and industrial districts which draw extensively upon local assets for their competitiveness. However, the rediscovery is also based on the insights of institutional economic theory, particularly its explanation of why territorial proximity matters for economic organization. Two conceptual strands stand out.

One strand – perhaps the closest to the economics mainstream – derives from renewed interest in endogenous growth theory, which acknowledges the economic externalities and increasing returns to scale associated with spatial clustering and specialization (Porter, 1994; Krugman, 1995). The contention of Krugman and Porter is that the spatial clustering of interrelated industries, skilled labor, and technological innovations offers some of the key elements of growth and competitiveness. These include increasing returns, reduced transaction costs and economies associated with proximity and interfirm exchange, as well as specialized know-how, skills, and technological advancement.

This "new economic geography" has gained considerable influence and is undoubtedly appealing, as it provides solid economic reasons for local agglomeration in a globalizing economy (reduced transaction costs, economies of specialization, externalities, etc.). It fails, however, to properly investigate the sources of these local advantages, which, according to a second conceptual strand developed largely by economic geographers, lie in the character of local social, cultural, and institutional arrangements. More specifically, insight is drawn from institutional and evolutionary economics concerning ties of proximity and association as a source of knowledge and learning (Amin and Thrift, 1995; Sunley, 1996; Storper, 1997).

A leading exponent is Michael Storper (1997), who has suggested that a distinctive feature of places in which globalization is consistent with the localization of economic activity is the strength of their "relational assets" or "untraded interdependencies." They include tacit knowledge based on face-to-face exchange, embedded routines, habits and norms, local conventions of communication and interaction, reciprocity and trust based on familiarity, and so on.

These relational assets are claimed to have a direct impact on a region's competitive potential insofar as they constitute part of the learning environment for firms. Many of the insights of the literature on the so-called learning regions (Cooke and Morgan, 1998), such as Silicon Valley, Baden Württemberg, and Italian industrial districts, derive from analysis of the learning properties of local, industry-specialist, business networks. These networks of reciprocity, shared know-how, spillover expertise, and strong enterprise support systems, according to Malmberg (1996), are sources of learning, facilitated through such advantages as reduced opportunism and enhanced mutuality within the relationships of interdependence.

Other observers (e.g., Becattini and Rullani, 1993; Asheim, 1997; Maskell et al., 1998; Blanc and Sierra, 1999; Nooteboom, 1999) suggest that geographical proximity plays a unique role in supplying informally-constituted assets. For instance, Maskell et al. argue that tacit forms of information and knowledge are better consolidated through face-to-face contact, not only due to the transactional advantages of proximity, but also because of their dependence upon a high degree of mutual trust and understanding, often constructed around shared values and cultures. Similarly, scholars (Becattini and Rullani, 1993; Asheim, 1997; Nooteboom, 1999) have distinguished between codified knowledge as a feature of trans-local networks (e.g., R&D laboratories or training courses of large corporations) and formally constituted institutions (e.g., business journals and courses, education and training institutions, printed scientific knowledge) and non-codified knowledge (e.g., workplace skills and practical conventions) as aspects locked into the "industrial atmosphere" of individual places. The consensus among these commentators seems to be that in a world in which codified knowledge is becoming increasingly ubiquitously available, uncodified knowledge, rooted in relations of proximity, attains a higher premium in deriving competitive advantage owing to its uniqueness.

Regional Policy Orientations

Both strands of the new regionalism – the "new economic geography" and institutional economic geography – imply practical action which transcends the limits of traditional local economic development initiatives. The focus falls on building the wealth of regions (not the individual firm), with upgrading of the economic, institutional, and social base considered as the prerequisite for entrepreneurial success. In my view there are four novel areas of action which emerge from the "wealth of regions" perspective.

Building clusters and local economies of association

The experience of some of the most dynamic economies in Europe shows that supply-side upgrading of a generic nature (e.g., advanced transport and communications systems or provision of specialized training and skills), though desirable, is not sufficient to secure regional economic competitiveness. Instead, in small nations such as Denmark and successful regional economies such as Emilia-Romagna, Baden Württemberg, and Catalonia, policy action is increasingly centered on supporting clusters of interrelated industries which have long roots in the region's skill- or capabilities-base. This helps not only to secure meaningful international competitive advantage, but also to reap the benefits of local specialization along the supply chain.

In addition, considerable policy attention is paid to building economies of association within clusters. This might include efforts to improve cultures of innovation within firms by encouraging social dialog and learning based on shared knowledge and information exchange. It might include initiatives to encourage interfirm exchange and reciprocity through buyer–supplier linkage programs, incentives for pooling of resources, joint ventures, task specialization, and so on. Finally, in order to maximize the efficiency of collective resources, it might include conscious effort to establish contact between sector-specific organizations (e.g., trade associations, sectorally-based service centers) and other support organizations (e.g., large and small-firm lobbies, function-specific producer services agencies, trade unions, chambers of commerce, local authorities, regional development agencies).

Cluster programs are no longer new to the regional policy community. Indeed, following the spectacular translation of Michael Porter's ideas into policy action through his world-famous consultancy group, Monitor, most regions seem to have a cluster program of some sort. And, ironically, in contradiction to the institutionalist stress on context-specificity and path-dependency, the most common tendency beyond the selection of locally-sensitive industrial clusters has been to copy from the experience of successful regions or from some "expert" manual. Cluster programs are becoming as standardized a mantra as were the incentive packages of preceding regional policy. Very few regions have attempted to develop unique industrial strategies based on deep assessment of local institutional and cultural specificities. To a degree, this failing stems from the inability of the policy community to recognize the centrality of "softer" influences, such as the three considered in turn below.

Learning to learn and adapt

The geographical strand of the new regionalism stresses learning as a key factor in dynamic competitiveness. Indeed, it is claimed that economically successful regions are "learning" or "intelligent" regions (Cooke and Morgan, 1998). It is their capacity to adapt around particular sectors and to anticipate at an early stage new industrial and commercial opportunities that enables them to develop and retain competitive advantage around a range of existing and future possibilities. Their strength lies in "learning to learn" (Hudson, 1999). By contrast, a very large number of less favored regions suffer from the problem of industrial and institutional lock-in and that of reactive adaptation to their economic environment, thus preventing the formation of a learning culture.

Vexing from a policy perspective is that there is no received wisdom on the factors which contribute to regional learning and adaptability. However, some of the contributing factors can be discerned from an observation of the relevant regions. One obvious factor is quite simply the scale and density of "intelligent" people and institutions, as reflected in the skill and professional profile of the labor market, the volume and quality of training and education across different levels, the depth of linkage between schools, universities, and industry, the quality and diversity of the research, science, and technology base, and the availability of intermediate centers of information and intelligence between economic agents and their wider environment (e.g., commercial media, trade fairs, business service agencies). These are vital sources of codified knowledge, grounded in the regional milieu. Many LFRs display a discernible lack of most of these attributes, with policy actions often geared towards the production of low-grade skills and training or towards disembodied ventures such as university expansion, science parks, and training schemes which fail to build the necessary connections.

Less obviously, the quality of ties associated with economies of association is another important source of learning and adaptation, through its impact on the circulation of informal information, innovation, and knowledge. Networks of association in the economy facilitate the spread of information and capabilities and the prospect of economic innovation through social interaction. Of course, there is always the danger that ties which are too strong and long-standing might actually prevent renewal and innovation by encouraging network closure and self-referential behavior (Grabher and Stark, 1997). On the other hand, in contexts where economic agents have the option of participating in many competing networks on the basis of loose ties and reciprocal relations, often through independent intermediaries, the prospect for learning through interaction is enhanced. The policy challenge in this regard for LFRs is to find a way of substituting their traditional ties of hierarchy and dependency (e.g., big firms, state provision, family connections) with links of mutuality between economic agents and institutions.

Third, as mentioned earlier, research has begun to appreciate the connection between rationalities of action and adaptive potential. It would appear that rule-based, substantive rationality, which encourages reactive responses to the external environment, is ill-equipped for learning and adaptation. Procedural rationality, on the other hand, based on cognitive and behavioral interpretation by economic agents of the external environment, favors incremental adjustment and adaptation. In contrast, a reflexive rationality, involving strategic and goal-monitoring behavior (Sabel, 1994), encourages experimental anticipation and actions seeking to shape the external environment. The cognitive frame of regional actors and institutions, in short, is the central source of learning. The culture of command and hierarchy that characterizes so many LFRs has stifled the formation of a reflexive culture among the majority of its economic institutions and, consequently, prevented the encouragement of rationalities geared towards learning and adaptation. Considerable policy attention needs to be paid to the nature of organizational and management cultures and actor rationalities which circulate within a region's dominant institutions. Importantly, but rarely addressed by the policy community, the capacity to change lies centrally in the ability of actor-networks to develop an external gaze and sustain a culture of strategic management and coordination in order to foresee opportunities and secure rapid response. The key factor is the ability to evolve in order to adapt (Amin and Hausner, 1997). The encouragement of this ability requires effort to identify the potential sources of behavioral alternatives – for example the preservation of diverse competencies (e.g., redundant skills and industrial slack – see Grabher and Stark, 1997); the scope for subaltern groups to break the grip of hegemonic interests which gain from preserving the past; the openness of organizations to external and internal influences; the scope for strategic decision-making through agent–environment interaction; and the encouragement of diversity of knowledge, expertise, and capability, so that new tricks are not missed.

Broadening the local institutional base

The last point illustrates the need for wider institutional changes to tackle impediments to economic renewal rooted in institutional dominance and closure. Partly in recognition of this problem, it has become increasingly common to assume that region-building has to be about mobilizing independent political power and capacity. In the European Union this assumption lies at the center of the discourse on "Europe of the regions" and has led to strong endorsement for local fiscal and financial autonomy, together with enlargement of the powers of local government and the establishment of vigorous regional assemblies or parliaments. The linkage made with economic development is that local political power and voice facilitates the formation of a decision-making and decision-implementing community able to develop and sustain an economic agenda of its own.

The institutionalist perspective, however, suggests that region-building cannot stop at simply securing regional political autonomy. Equally – perhaps more important – are matters of who makes decisions and how. Let us recall two institutionalist governance axioms, namely, the desirability of decision-making through independent representative associations and the superiority of participatory decision-making. The added challenge for the regions, therefore, is to find ways of developing a pluralist and interactive public sphere that draws in both the state and a considerably enlarged sphere of non-state institutions. Governance, especially in the institutionally thin regions, has always been in the hands of elite coalitions, and the resulting institutional sclerosis has been a source of economic failure by acting as a block on innovation and the wider distribution of resources and opportunity. In an increasingly global economy, these elites and their charismatic leaders may undoubtedly help regions to jostle for influence with national and international organizations (e.g., the European Commission or transnational corporations), but they will achieve little in terms of mobilizing a regional development path based on unlocking hidden local potential. This is why it is vital that regional actors ask whether their decision-making processes constitute an obstacle to institutional renewal, away from a culture of hierarchy and rule-following, towards one that focuses on informational transparency, consultative and inclusive decision-making, and strategy-building on the basis of reflexive monitoring of goals.

Ultimately, the process of institutional reform has to go beyond the decentralization and democratization of a region's official organizations. Many of the prosperous regions of Europe are also regions of participatory politics, active citizenship, civic pride, and intense institutionalization of collective interests – of society brought back into the art of governance. Within them, associational life is active, politics is contested, public authorities and leaders are scrutinized, public space is considered to be shared and commonly owned, and a strong culture of autonomy and self-governance seeps through local society. They are regions of developed "social capital" (Putnam, 1993), serving to secure many economic benefits, including public-sector efficiency in the provision of services; civic autonomy and initiative in all areas of social and economic life; a culture of reciprocity and trust which facilitates the economics of association; containment of the high costs of social breakdown and conflict; and potential for economic innovation and creativity based on social confidence and capability.

Mobilizing the social economy

The preceding discussion implies that a regional culture of social inclusion and social empowerment is likely to encourage economic creativity by allowing diverse social groups and individuals to realize their potential. This reinforces the view that policies to stimulate regional entrepreneurship should recognize, oblique though it may appear, the centrality of policies to combat social exclusion in this process. This is especially relevant in the context of regions marked by problems of persistent structural unemployment and rudimentary entrepreneurship, both of which act as a severe constraint on economic renewal. In such regions, the depth and scale of unemployment and the trend towards jobless growth in the economy at large, makes a return to full employment highly unlikely through improvements in regional economic competitiveness (via, say, industrial upgrading, clusters and economies of association).

An interesting contemporary policy innovation in the European Union is experimentation with the social economy as a source of local renewal. In countries such as Germany, France, Belgium, the Netherlands, Italy, and Ireland, there is growing public policy support (e.g., subsidies and indirect aids such as training, facilitating legislation, specialized services) for community projects that are run by the third sector and involve excluded groups either as providers or users of socially useful services. This might involve support for a community group that employs school leavers to offer affordable housing to low-income groups or for a cooperative through which the long-term unemployed provide domestic care or transport access to the elderly. In other words, the battle against social exclusion is being combined with reforms to the welfare state, towards building an intermediate economic sphere that serves to meet real local welfare needs. In turn, this intermediate sphere, sustained by both monetary and innovative non-monetary metrics of exchange (e.g., service vouchers or services in kind), is seen as a source of employment and entrepreneurship in "markets" which are of limited interest to state organizations and private-sector firms. In the longer run, it is seen as a vital source for unlocking social confidence and creativity among the excluded.

The policy implication is that regions need to incorporate a social economy program into their efforts to improve regional economic competitiveness. It is important, however, for the reasons given in the preceding section, that support is provided with a light governmental touch, leaving a great deal to local actors. For example, regional, or city-based, "social inclusion commissions" could be established, with an elected chair from a widely-drawn membership of relevant local organizations. The commissions would audit local service needs, propose rules for action, invite and consider applications for funding, work with the local authorities and other economic interest groups, and so on. The local authorities and the central government would play a facilitating role, providing, for example, resources and legislation, but they would not provide a direct steer on local priorities and projects.

Conclusion: Back to the Macro-Economy

The new regionalism offers a solution based on the mobilization of local resources. But it does so on the basis of a very broad definition of what constitutes the economy and economic action. It is an approach that builds outwards from a new industrial policy and effort to strengthen local economies of association to actions to improve institutional reflexivity, learning potential, and social creativity.

To a degree, the focus on endogenous regional solutions has been forced by an uncomfortably pervasive agreement across the policy community around the neo-liberal rejection of macroeconomic actions in favor of LFRs which might hinder market forces. Across the political spectrum, the consensus has grown that national and regional competitiveness is the only pathway to prosperity and that redistributive measures alone will not suffice.

This is a perilous supposition, not least because of the institutionalist axiom that action has to be contextually relevant and medium- to long-term. The policy orientations outlined above are not equally applicable to all types of region, and where they are, they require time to be built up. The orientations are especially appropriate for regions characterized by certain impediments to economic renewal: fragile small-firm entrepreneurship; domination by externally owned or controlled firms with poor levels of local economic integration; restricted diversification, innovation, and learning capacity; and state dependency and institutional closure. These are problems which are rather typical of old industrial regions and their particular institutional legacies. Lagging rural regions face a different set of impediments, and their institutional base might also be less equipped for experimenting with learning-based industrial clusters and reflexive goal-monitoring institutional behavior. Region-building, in short, may not be an option for all regions, owing to the restrictions of context and time.

To a degree, the responsibility for the management of wider connectivity lies in the hands of non-regional actors, notably government. No amount of imaginative region-building will be able to sustain a spiral of endogenous economic growth in the absence of a conducive macroeconomic framework. Interregional competition in a Europe in recession and dominated by restrictive macroeconomic policies will continue to work in favor of the core regions. Therefore, something has to be done to secure the less-favored regions sufficient time and resources to implement boot-strapping reforms.

The reforms suggested here are controversial and need further debate. However, the point of raising them here is that in the absence of a conducive macroeconomic framework, it seems irresponsible to ask the regions to embark upon a long-term and comprehensive overhaul in pursuit of an endogenous pathway to prosperity.

Chapter 4

Refiguring the Economic in Economic Geography

Nigel J. Thrift and Kris Olds

Introduction

> If I had the cash to buy all of my family something to wear I would, but I don't. Last year I did all my shopping on Christmas Eve and spent far too much money on not very nice presents. (Martha in Williams, 1995, p. 5)

> Mum always claims she'd be happy with a kiss, so she's very easy to buy presents for at Christmas. (Milly in Williams, 1995, p. 5)

The full complexity of modern economies only becomes apparent when we move outside of what are often still considered to be the "normal" territories of economic enquiry. Then a whole new world hoves into view.

Take Christmas. Now, at last, the subject of sustained academic enquiry (e.g., Bennett, 1981; Pimlott, 1978; Thrift, 1993; Miller, 1993; Restad, 1995), Christmas is a cultural event of immense economic significance – or an economic event of immense cultural significance. That this is the case can be seen from the case of Great Britain.

In 1993, for example, seasonal factors contributed an extra £5 billion to fourth quarter consumption, compared to the third quarter, and this amount has been increasing steadily since 1960 (A. Scott, 1994). Sectors of the economy that benefited especially included drink, tobacco, and "other goods" like sports equipment, toiletries, jewelry, and greetings cards. To be more specific, in the period leading up to Christmas 1995 various newspapers reported that 1.95 billion Christmas cards were mailed in Great Britain, 14 million turkeys were slaughtered, 5.25 million Christmas trees were harvested (including new varieties like Nordman blue), 5 million poinsettias were sold, and 200,000 children visited Santa Claus' grotto in Selfridges in London.

Nearly all of this seasonal increase in consumption is the result of changing social customs associated with Christmas, and most especially an upward trend in gift-giving (Cheal, 1988; Belk, 1995). Of course, this phenomenon of mass reciprocity is hardly restricted to Great Britain. Since the mid-nineteenth century, Christmas has been a syncretic tradition, which has depended upon symbols drawn from a whole range of different national sources; "the Christmas tree from the German tradition, the filling of stockings from the Dutch tradition, the development of Santa Claus mainly from the United States, the British Christmas card, and many other such elements" (Miller, 1993, p. 4). And this tradition has spread out from Europe and North America to all corners of the world. Thus, as Miller (1993, p. 5) puts it, "by the 1990s we are faced with the extraordinary phenomenon of a global festival which seems to grow in its accumulated rituals and the extravagance of the homage paid to it, even as all other festivals and comparable events have declined."

We could as easily have chosen other examples of practices which until quite recently would have been counted as outside the normal orbit of economic geography, yet which illustrate the extraordinary difficulty of separating out something called "the economic" from "the social" or "the cultural" or "the political" or "the sexual" or what have you – the scent industry, the gambling industry, the "companion animal" industry (all the way from petfood to kennels and catteries), the gardening industry, the music industry, the drugs industry. The list goes on and on. But hopefully the point is made; until quite recently economic geographers would probably have been quite uneasy considering these kinds of industries and, more particularly, the kinds of issues that they raise. This is because economic geography had become stale, when compared with, say, the vibrancy of cultural geography. But now a determined effort is being made to make a space for new kinds of economic geography that can supplement or even replace the older forms of economic geography. That space is meant to be inclusive, critical, and committed. It is a space that cannot help but have roots in the economic geographies of the past – which, after all, produced many good things – but which also represents a determined effort to avoid the bad habits that sometimes (and only sometimes) impoverished them.

The new economic geography will be different, and in three ways. First, it will be polycentric. It will not consist of one narrative (or one narrative and its opposite) but of a set of narrative communities in relation. In turn, this means that it will celebrate a qualitative multiplicity of "economic" times and spaces seen, certainly, as in unequal relation with one another but not thereby giving credence to the composition of an overarching centered, theoretical order, or the fictive telos of a "new world order." Second, it follows that the new economic geography will be much more open to outside influences. It will want to trawl the social sciences and humanities in search of the traces of the economic. But this new emphasis on multiplicity and openness does not mean that the new economic geography needs to be politically quiescent. It will want to generate counter-narratives, it will hunger after critical readings, it will want to disseminate new, alternative economic practices. Third, the new economic geography will necessarily obtain a good part of its impetus from refiguring what is conventionally regarded as "the economic." To use a phrase much favored by Richard Rorty (1989), the assumption of polycentrism, the injection of new perspectives, and the commitment to political action, must produce a shift in the "final vocabulary" that economic geographers fall back on – words like "economy," "market," "industry," and "work" – key words beyond which lies only silence, tautology, or physical force. What seems clear is that attempting to build a unified culture around these key words will become increasingly difficult because the articulations and readings of the economic are proliferating. Indeed, one of the tasks of the new economic geography will be precisely to aid this proliferation by "stretching" its own definition so as to make itself more inclusive and more able to mix in company.

In this paper, we want to address some of these changes in economic geography's final vocabulary through a three-part study. In the first part we want to briefly point to some of the ways in which the practices of the economy have been changing, ways which problematize what we mean by the economic in "economic geography." In turn, in the second part of the paper we want to suggest that these problematizations have produced changing perspectives on how to approach modern space economies which can be encapsulated in four "topological presuppositions." Finally, the last part of the paper presents some brief conclusions about future directions.

1 The Main Changes

There are clearly many important changes taking place in what is conventionally called "economic life." We want to interpret these changes as processes of *problematization*, that is as new practices which set off new accounts which set off new practices . . . on and on in an endless discursive and recursive loop. These new problematizations are only rarely singular and unbending. More often, they are multiple and contested, "dilemmatic" arguments over what the world is like which are, at the same time, constitutive of that world (Billig et al., 1988). Here, we present just our "top ten" of these problematizations. Other writers will no doubt choose other problematizations but most writers would, we are sure, be able to agree on both on a core list and the need to establish the case for change.

1.1 The rise of the social

The first problematization is the rise to prominence of economic concomitants which in previous times might well have been regarded as extra-economic. Recent research has demonstrated perfectly the extraordinary social nature of modern economies and it has done so in four main ways. First, the social basis of economic success has become more and more apparent. Thus, at the national scale, a whole series of writers have pointed to the way in which certain forms of business have proved particularly successful because of the strength of ethnic ties ranging from friendly associations to rotating credit associations. At the international scale, commentators now routinely point to the social differences in national economies as crucial determinants of economic success. For example, Kay (1993) notes how the United States economy is based on a regime of expressive individualism and therefore tends to contractual law and public forms of quality certification like brands. In contrast, Japan's economy is based on a collectivist regime and therefore relies more on building relationships of trust, consensus, and shared knowledge (Hamilton and Biggart, 1992; Orrú, Biggart, and Hamilton, 1991; Whitley, 1991, 1992a). Second, more and more work stresses the importance of the construction of trust in economic interaction, realized through networks of personal contact (e.g., Platteau, 1994a,

1994b; Wong, 1991; Zucker, 1986). This kind of work no longer sees the economic as simply "embedded" in the social – a favorite metaphor of an earlier phase of economic sociology – but instead sees the economic and social as incorrigibly intertwined, unable to be separated off from one another. Third, the rediscovery of the work of Michael Polanyi (1958, 1966) has led to more and more emphasis being placed on the importance of "tacit knowledge," human behavior which habitually escapes verbal formulation or coding but which is seen, in the shape of particular skills, as being at the heart of the economic success of numerous firms, regions, and nations.

Fourth and finally, the honing of social skills, understood as a language of bodily presentation and stance, and conversational skills, is increasingly presented as being determinant of the construction of successful client and customer encounters and, indeed, as being a key component of many modern jobs. That this is the case can be seen in work spanning all manner of economic sectors, from retailing (Crang, 1994) to merchant banking (McDowell and Court, 1994a, 1994b).

1.2   The market

Perhaps the rise of the social is best illustrated by the increasingly explicit problematization of markets (e.g., Swedberg, 1994; White, 1993). Because of events in Eastern Europe, the attempts to form a European Single Market, the increasing use of market regulators, and the rediscovery of the work of Karl Polanyi (1994) on the instituted nature of markets, the inherently social nature of markets has now become much clearer. In turn, this realization of the social nature of markets has changed the idea of the market as a neutral arena in which pure exchange takes place to an arena in which there are complex moral and institutional orders regulating not only the conduct of exchange but also what is defined as exchange in the first place.

The mediated nature of the mediations of markets has been reworked through three main approaches (Swedberg, 1994): the social-structural, the cultural, and the legal-political. In the first approach, the chief focus of attention is social structure, usually identified through networks of affinity. The second approach pays more attention to how actors construct markets through shared meanings. Finally, the third approach emphasizes markets as political arenas within which property rights, governance structures, and transactional rules are primary.

1.3   The rise of the representational

Since the writings of McLuhan and Baudrillard, it has become something of a cliché to point to the image consciousness associated with modern economic formations. Through the action of the media, and technological change, the image becomes a currency in and of itself, one which can be shuttled back and forth between producers and consumers in multiple ways (Wark, 1994). Most particularly, the foregrounding of the image has had important effects in deterritorializing and reterritorializing signs, meanings, and identities around the world (Lash and Urry, 1994). But the process is no longer seen as simply a vehicle of cultural hegemony (driven by, for example, the mass media or Americanism). Rather it now tends to be seen as the fusion of different master narratives (for example, consumerism, enlightenment concepts such as universal rights and citizenship) with local vernaculars (for example, separatism, folklorism, sacred beliefs) (e.g., Appadurai, 1990; Smith, 1994).

1.4 The rise of consumption

The rise of the representational is often associated with consumption. Consumption has, of course, become a major area of problematization in geography and elsewhere (although much of this research has been carried out by cultural rather than economic geographers (Jackson and Thrift, 1995)). Consumption can be seen now as offering four main forms of innovation. First, it has involved major innovations in retailing, from superstores to shopping malls, and more recently, from warehouse clubs to factory outlet villages (Wrigley and Lowe, 1995). Second, it has involved new selling practices (for example, new forms of direct mail and the use of GIS in marketing). Third, it has involved new consumption practices (for example, in Britain, the "consuming Sunday," new forms of gift-giving, and new imported consumption festivals like Father's Day and Halloween). Then, finally, it has involved new forms of material culture based around a process of social and cultural refiguring of both new and old objects (as, for example, in the rise of various forms of heritage culture).

1.5 The rise of new intelligent technologies

Another problematization arises from the new, "intelligent" telecommunicating technologies. No longer seen as a paranoid vision of machines supplanting their builders, these new technologies still problematize the world in several ways. First, they highlight the subject–object relation. The rise of machines that, in a certain fashion, "talk back" has produced reconceptualizations of bodies and selves (new metaphors and figurations now populate the language of self and other which reconstitute the relation between subject and object). Second, the crucial role of information is made much clearer by the machines. It is no surprise that information has become central to the practice of modern economic theory and practice, either as cybernetically inclined systems models or as models of information asymmetry (Stiglitz and Weiss, 1991; Boisot, 1995). Third, intelligent machines suggest many new economic practices by "informating" organizations (Zuboff, 1988).

1.6 Mix 'n' match

A further problematization is the increasing degree of mixing of the functions of the economy which calls all manner of taken-for-granted boundaries into question. What is production and what is consumption? What is supply and what is demand? What is one industrial sector and what is another? What is use and what is exchange? All these and many other categories become increasingly difficult to identify with any clarity. The signs of this recombinant economy are everywhere. Flexible production systems bring production and consumption much closer together and mix and match market and hierarchy in new ways. Ideas of production filières and commodity claims now circulate, including buyer-driven commodity chains. Some authors argue that services now drive production (Lash and Urry, 1994). Software has become more important than hardware. And so on. The ultimate example of this recombinant tendency is probably the biological engineering industry where the "liveware" produced by genetic engineering operates at levels which question the independence of the human subject as a category.

1.7 The gendering of economies

A seventh problematization has been that produced by gender and sexuality. The increasing visibility of women in the waged workforce has been mirrored by their increased visibility as unpaid workers, thus problematizing even further the boundary between the formal economy of work and the informal economy of unwaged and unpaid work for women and this has happened at exactly the same time as many men have become unemployed and had their traditional male roles challenged (Crompton and Sanderson, 1990). In addition, sexuality in the workplace has become a major issue, both because of the issue of sexual harassment and because particular constructions of sexuality have so clearly been a part of the (masculinist) definition of certain kinds of job (McDowell and Court, 1994a, 1994b). Finally, the rise of the gay and lesbian communities has produced a new and relatively distinct source of demand which is now being consciously played to (Edge, 1995; Mort, 1995).

1.8 Informalization

These changes are paralleled by the increasing informalization of work as the world of the mass collective worker is left behind. The informal or shadow economy based on what Smith (1994) calls "idiosyncratic forms of livelihood" spreads. Much of this economy is still, in fact, locked into the institutions of the formal economy, and in some cases, because of the rise of flexible production systems, it is more tightly locked in than ever before. Other parts of it simply represent the survival strategies of the poor and impoverished. Yet other parts represent conscious attempts to buck the prevailing system by building alternative institutions, as in the case of LETS, rotating credit associations, credit unions, community development banks, and the like (Boothroyd and Davis, 1993; Leyshon and Thrift, 1997). It is also worth noting that in this sector of the economy, what we mean by labor becomes increasingly difficult to separate out, because of the highly intersubjective nature of work. What Smith (1994) calls "livelihood practices" often, in one way or another, span the whole day, with no clearly-defined moments of work as opposed to non-work.

1.9 Time and space

It is a *sine qua non* of the current literature that we are witness to sweeping changes in the nature of our practice and understanding of time and space. Epic stories of "time–space compression," "time–space distanciation," "disembedding," "globalization," and new and uncharted "hyperspaces," zones of informational performativity which cannot be tied to one place, circulate (e.g., Castells, 1989; Giddens,

1990; Harvey, 1989). These stories are important constitutive elements of how we problematize the current world, but they are one-sided. They spin a history of detachment without considering the parallel changes in the history of involvement which is only now being written. For, at the same time, it is clear that face-to-face interaction has not died out. Indeed in some senses it has become more important as reflexivity (including an enhanced ability to see ourselves as others see us) has become built into economic conduct (Lash and Urry, 1994). Most particularly, the "core sets" (Collins, 1981) of people in any economic sector still need to build trust: "here it is far from obvious that the world of familiarity, face-to-face interaction, and virtue is indeed lost" (Shapin, 1994, p. 414). These stories also tend to miss, as they make obeisance to new technological developments, how these developments often act as a supplement to face-to-face interaction, rather than as a substitute (Thrift, 1994).

1.10 The rise of new economic discourses

The last problematization has simply been the rise to prominence of new economic discourses in response to all these changes. These discourses have been of three types. First of all, within conventional economics new forms of economic theorizing have been constantly appearing, such as information economics, behavioral economics, and agency theory, which make it much less easy to simply dismiss classical economics out of hand. Second, new discourses have arisen on the borders of conventional economics. For example, the last fifteen years have seen the rise of evolutionary economics (Hodgson, 1988, 1993), ecological economics of various kinds, and so-called rational choice or analytical Marxism (Carling, 1992). Finally, there is a whole area of economics which has appeared quite independently of mainstream economics, arising chiefly out of new economic practices, which is very much the domain of non-economists. This is the area of "new economics," based on "real-world" attempts to institute sustainability, new monetary practices (like revolving credit associations, women's banks, and local economic trading schemes), community economic policies, and ethical investment strategies.

2 Changing Perspectives

There are many other changes that could, no doubt, be pointed to. But already the cumulative effect of the changes we have mentioned is sufficient to suggest that underlying these singular problematizations is a more comprehensive change of perspective on how to approach modern economies; this change of perspective has four main components: the fall of the singular, the disorganization of organization, the multiplication of time, and the erosion of orientalist and occidentalist beliefs.

2.1 The fall of the singular

Of course, economic life has only rarely been characterized by stable accounts of what an economy is or how it proceeds. In retrospect, we can now see that the period from the 1870s to the fall of Bretton Woods was one of these rare periods when relatively stable accounts held sway. It was a period in which grand machines of truth were able to operate with relative impunity, whether in the shape of a number of variants of Marxism or a number of variants of marginalist–neoclassical economics. But now, for all the talk of the triumph of the market, these monumental machines have broken up. They have broken up in theory, partly because of the sheer diversity of approaches that now characterize even mainstream economics, partly because of the challenge from "new" forms of "economics," especially those with their roots in ecology, and partly because of the general acceptance of the importance of instability and change, implicit in the importation of concepts of nonlinearity and chaos (Appadurai, 1990). They have also broken up in practice. The proliferation of the media and telecommunications has produced a war of undecideable narratives which shows no signs of resolution.

There is now, therefore, a vast industry making accounts of economies which we, as academics, have difficulty acknowledging, for three reasons. First, academics do not occupy a privileged place in this industry. There are numerous extra-academic generators of knowledge who now aim to provide guidance, from management gurus to pundits to research analysts to tip sheet editors. In Bauman's (1992) terms, academics are no longer legislators of knowledge, but just one out of many competing groups of interpreters. Second, the economic system is intensely practical. That is, aided by developments like electronic telecommunications, it is based on the needs of the moment and what works. It is therefore ordered, but not in ways which conventional representational theories find easy to come to terms with (Thrift, 1996b). Third, many of the mechanisms through which modern economies cohere are not what have conventionally been regarded as "economic" by academics. They are therefore able to be blanked out.

What seems clear, then, is that the very idea of a singular story of an object denoted "economic" is now lost. It follows that the idea of trying to focus a new economic geography around one concept or theoretical tradition, however broadly defined, cannot hold.

2.2   The disorganization of organization

The second component of the change in perspective on modern economies is in how economic organizations are depicted. Previously, these organizations tended to be enclosed, seen as shells through which transactions with the outside world took place to a greater or lesser degree. Such organizations were also characterized by pre-set goals which they worked towards. But this contained and directed model is now seen to be at odds with what we know of the intensely practical and ad hoc character of most organizations. Four points follow. First, organizations require continual improvisation to maintain, often make mistakes, and can spiral down to collapse at short notice. They will therefore have partial views of the world at best. In other words, organizations are always and everywhere tentative and temporary. Second and consequently, organizations are seen as in *action*, "on the move, if only stumbling or blundering along" (Boden, 1994, p. 192). They are therefore intensely focused on the purposes at hand, on generally local focal points, which will be responded to in part through improvisation and in part through conforming to the organizational field of formal, codified instructions and previous practice. In other words, organizations are talked into being at each moment, by actors who often have to fashion informal solutions to formal goals. Third, organizations are seen as always open to the outside, operating in various kinds of transactional regime. The thrust of modern theory has been to characterize this inevitable process as a problem: there are transaction *costs*. Or, alternatively, attention has focused on a very limited set of successful transactional arrangements, like industrial districts. The result is that we still have only the most limited knowledge of the range of transaction network structures that may exist. Fourth, more attention is now being devoted to new work processes, like teams, and new interactional structures in an acknowledgment that the organizational environment is too complex for an organization to have a fixed strategy, especially as, under the impulse of information technology, response times have had to become faster.

2.3   The multiplication of time

The third component of the change in perspective on modern economies concerns time. In the past, time was seen as a Cartesian bracket around practices, a metric that located them and fixed them in an all-pervasive order. Now time is seen as multidimensional, differential, and produced by participants: "there is no single time, only a multitude of times which interpenetrate and permeate our daily lives" (Adam, 1995, p. 12; Parkes and Thrift, 1980). Thus, the economy is refigured as not one but a series of timelines in which meanings and relevancies are being constantly rekeyed to the moment.

> As social actors look over their shoulders at past actions and decisions, they also look sideways, fitting their current activities with parallel points and agents on their organizational landscape. Simultaneity is a critical contingency of action. Nor are these local relevancies of various aspects and stages of a decision-in-progress simply constructed by temporal contingencies; they are also *constitutive* of them, creating timelines, controlling, to a high degree, the practical enactment of organizational actions and even goals. (Boden, 1994, p. 191)

2.4   The erosion of orientalist and occidentalist beliefs

The fourth component of the change in perspective on modern economies is the erosion of orientalist and occidentalist beliefs. Most particularly, the rise of Japan and the East and Southeast Asia newly industrializing countries has pointed out the limits of the occidental project and not just in theory but also in practice. At the same time, it has undermined the West's sense of itself as *necessarily* different. Nowhere is this clearer than in the economic register. The distinction between the West and the rest was at first drawn in terms of a classical orientalist/occidentalist opposition: the economic success of the countries of East and Southeast Asia was based on a "gift model" which arose from the construction of durable personal relationships which were cemented in place by signs of reciprocity like the gift. These were social procedures that were supposedly in opposition to the West's reliance on a "commodity model" of impersonal transactions, contracts, and the market. But this opposition is now breaking down. For example, Carrier (1995, p. 94) is able to review an impressive amount of evidence which allows him to conclude that:

in different areas of life in industrial capitalist society, identities, relations, and transactions depart from the commodity model and instead resemble what exists in gift
systems in important ways (through this assertion of resemblance is not an assertion
of identity). Impersonal commodity relations and transactions clearly are important in
the modern West. But equally important is the distinction between saying that commodity relations are important in the West on the one hand, and on the other constructing the West as a society in which commodity relations are so essential that we
can ignore the existence of other sorts of relations.

Interestingly, the way in which the new ways of talking about economic practices
is most often summarized is through a spatial description of one kind or another.
We think it is possible to argue that four of these "topological presuppositions" currently coexist, each of them successively more recent, more polymorphous, and less
enveloping (Figure 4.1). We think of each presupposition, following Mol and Law
(1995), as a different cluster of rules for localizing through which the social performs itself, involving different modes of proceeding and different sets of coordinates. The first and most familiar of these presuppositions represents the economy
as a set of *bounded regions* within which different "economic" objects can be identified, constituted, disciplined, by being linked together in various modes of territorial government (e.g., Miller and Rose, 1990). The second topology represents the
economy as a set of interlocking or overlapping *networks*; economic objects are the
result of the interaction between these networks (Grabher, 1993; Hamilton, 1991).
The third topology represents the economy as *flows*; economic objects are continual movements of capital, people, information, commodity, and the like (e.g.,
Castells, 1989; Lash and Urry, 1994). The fourth and final topology represents the
economy as in two places at once: economic objects are *bifocal*, being both point
and wave form (Bohm, 1980, 1994; Virilio, 1993). The economy is always virtual,
never present.

Note that there is no need to take topological sides, since each of these
presuppositions coexists in intricate relation with the others. But clearly these
four presuppositions produce radically different means of framing the world.

3   Conclusions

Dr Ferrari examined 240 mall shoppers, measuring "procrastination scores (on arousal
and avoidance measures), the closeness of the measurement to Christmas, and shoppers' rationales for why they were shopping at that particular time." He reckoned procrastination was "motivated by arousal from working against a deadline and attributed
their lack of diligence to job-related attributes (e.g., work, business commitments) that
compelled them to begin shopping at the last possible opportunity." Or they were motivated by a need to "avoid situations involving threats to self-esteem, attributing their
postponed shopping to personal attributes (e.g., lack of energy, indecisiveness, perceived task aversiveness) reflecting their belief in their own inabilities" (White, 1995,
p. 6).

The outlines of the new economic geography are only just beginning to become
clear. But, already, we think it is possible to see some of the key areas of work that

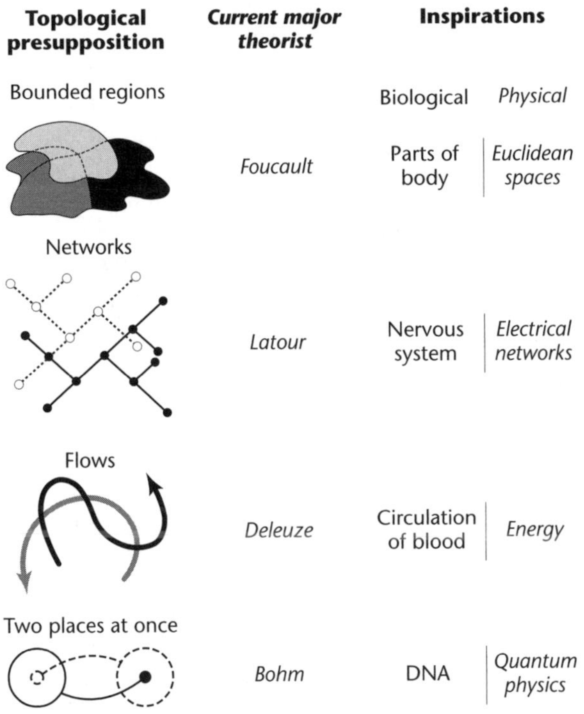

Topological presupposition	Current major theorist	Inspirations	
		Biological	Physical
Bounded regions	Foucault	Parts of body	Euclidean spaces
Networks	Latour	Nervous system	Electrical networks
Flows	Deleuze	Circulation of blood	Energy
Two places at once	Bohm	DNA	Quantum physics

Figure 4.1 Four topological propositions

will occupy its future. For convenience, we have grouped these around the four topological presuppositions set down above.

The first area of work will be based around the topological presupposition of the bounded region. Most especially, it will consist of work that adopts a heterodox but broadly structural approach, which deals in the currency of the nation-state, and multinational corporations, international competitiveness, international regimes, third wave regulation theory, governmentality, and the like, and which increasingly goes under the name of "international political economy." The kinds of concepts gathered under this umbrella title are being leavened by other concerns, for example to do with gender and ethnicity, but they seem likely to remain the most recognizably "economic."

The second area of work will be based around the topological presupposition of the network. It will chiefly be concerned with the social determinants of the economic and will range from the literature on self-organizing networked firms and learning regions, through monetary networks, to ethnic business networks. This area of work will also address the intertwining of different types of networks. In contrast to the chiefly structural approach of the bounded region area of work, this area of work will be founded on pragmatist, constructionist, and ethnographic approaches.

The third area of work will be based on the topological presupposition of flow. It will chiefly be concerned with cultural determinants of the economic and will be most concerned with issues like the body, self, and desire, and with different modes of representation and sensation (moving on from simply the visual) as they relate to different economic processes like money. The kinds of methods deployed will include semiotics, discourse analysis, iconography, and ethnography.

The fourth area of work will be based on the topological presupposition of two places at once. This will be the preserve of a cybergeography. It will consist of work on economies as instantaneous media events (e.g., Wark, 1994) as well as more Nietzschean-inspired work on cyberspace, in the tradition of Plant (1994), Land (1994, 1995), and others, which conjures up a cybernetic world populated by artificial demons and dragons. The kinds of methods employed will include a powered-up poststructuralism and the kinds of approaches to the materiality of communication made popular by Kittler (1990) and Gumbrecht and Pfeiffer (1994).

Yet what will be most interesting, we think, is the kind of work that will be done at the boundaries of these presuppositions, on the borderlines. For example, at the boundaries between international political economy and cultural work is a whole area of work on the transmission of various forms of economic discourse, where discourse is understood in the Foucauldian sense as a transindividual and multi-institutional archive of images and statements providing a common language for representing knowledge about a given theme (e.g., Leyshon and Tickell, 1994).

What all this also shows is the increasing difficulty of stabilizing "the economic" as an entity, in part, because the number of approaches to what we call the economic is multiplying and, in part, because our final vocabulary, to use the Rortyan phrase again, is changing. This last point is worth underlining. What is most striking currently is the degree to which the very borderlines of what we have called "the economic" are now changing. We are moving away from the first round of critiques of economics, such as those offered by McCloskey (1985) or Barnes (1994) or Mirowski (1995a) which pointed to the effects of the different metaphors that can be deployed as descriptions of the economic, towards a second round of reconstruction. This second round, which involves authors like Brennan (1994), Goux (1989, 1990) and Derrida (1992, 1995), questions the whole basis of the occidental model of exchange by drawing on three main sources. The first of these is psychoanalytic models of the ego, most especially drawing on the work of Freud and Lacan. Thus Brennan (1994), for example, argues that proliferation of commodities blocks the mobility of psychical energy and therefore blocks the generation of life and ideas. The second source is the growing body of work on time which challenges prevailing Western "chronotypes" (see, for example, Thrift, 1977; Bender and Wellbery, 1991; Lloyd, 1993). Derrida's (1982) remorseless war on the presence of the present is a case in point. The third and final source is the inspiration provided by Bataille's (1988; Bennington, 1995) theories of expenditure as excess, and equally his appropriation of Mauss's theory of the potlatch as an illustration of the general economy of loss, disequilibrium, and expenditure *without* return, in which exchange does not imply reciprocity. These three sources all challenge the notion of a "restricted" economy of production, equilibrium, and balanced books

– the determined and determinate economy of classical utility – and focus, instead, on loss, excess, chance; an energetics of laughter, excitement, poetry, and all the other activities that are apparently outside "the economic." This challenge, which becomes more concerted day by day, suggests that our final vocabulary is not so final after all. There is no last word.

Chapter 5

The Economy, Stupid!
Industrial Policy Discourse and
the Body Economic

J. K. Gibson-Graham

Once upon a time, people used to talk about ISSUES and HAVE FUN. But then someone invented the economy . . . The economy grew and grew! It took over EVERY-THING and NO-ONE COULD ESCAPE. (Morris, 1992, p. 53, quoting from memory a recent cartoon)

I saw men on television (trade-union stars, Cabinet Ministers, left-wing think-tank advisers) visibly hystericized by talking economics: eyes would glaze, shoulders hunch, lips tremble in a sensual paroxysm of "letting the market decide," "making the hard decisions," "leveling the playing field," "reforming management practices," "improving productivity" . . . those who queried the wisdom of floating the exchange rate, deregulating the banks, or phasing out industry protection were less ignored than washed away in the intoxicating rush of "living in a competitive world" and "joining the global economy." (Morris, 1992, pp. 51–2)

In *Ecstasy and Economics*, Meaghan Morris chronicles the ecstatic submission of white Australian men to "the economy." Humbled before its godlike figure, grown men grovel and shout in fundamentalist rapture, transported in "an ecstasy of Reason" (1992, p. 77). By giving themselves over to a higher power, they have paradoxically gained mastery and authority. They "talk economics" and find themselves speaking the language of pure necessity, unhampered by base specificities of politics and intention. In the face of necessity, and in its despite, they project a willful certainty that their economic "interventions" will yield the outcomes they desire.

During the 1980s and 1990s Australia was one of the few OECD countries governed by a social democratic (albeit right-wing) Labor Party in which interventionist economic and industrial policies were on the national agenda. Recently, though abortively, the Clinton administration promised to concern itself with many of the things that concerned the Hawke and Keating governments from the beginning: deindustrialization, lack of technological innovation, a labor force unsuited to the needs of industry, a weak competitive position in a rapidly changing world. In seeking models of successful intervention that have presumably fostered rather than blocked economic adaptation, American economic strategists looked to Australia for innovative ways of meeting Clinton's mandate to "grow the economy." These American analysts included not merely center and right-wing Democrats but Marxists and other leftists whose pronouncements were suddenly contiguous to debates in the mainstream press.

After 12 years (or maybe a lifetime) in exile, leftists in the US were "talking economics" in a room where just possibly they could be overheard. And the economics they were talking was in some ways very different from what was permissible just a few years before, when "industrial policy" or "managed trade," for example, could not be broached at the national level. Yet despite its release from old strictures and prohibitions, the discussion of economic policy seemed entirely familiar. It moved laboriously in a confined space, as though hobbled by an invisible tether or circumscribed by a jealous and restrictive force – something more potent even than the political realities that also operate to keep debate within narrow and familiar limits.

Despite their divergent positions on every issue, the right and left share a "discourse of economy" that participates in defining what can and cannot be proposed. What from a right-wing perspective may seem like a truly misguided left-wing proposal is nonetheless intelligible and recognizable as a member of the extended family of potential economic initiatives, and vice versa. This is not to say that right- and left-wing policy analysts profess the same economic theories and harbor the same social conceptions. In their positive proposals, their understandings of economy and society are often revealed to be quite different, and indeed they may have been trained in very different schools of thought. Nevertheless, there seems to be a substrate of commonality, detectable in the ubiquitous affective paradoxes of submission and control, arrogance and caution, that structure the range of economic emotions. If the economy of the left is so different in its operations and possibilities from that of the right, why does it produce such similar affective disjunctions? Why is "the economy" at once the scene of abject submission, the social site that constrains activities at all other sites, the supreme being whose dictates must unquestioningly be obeyed and, at the same time, an entity that is subject to our full understanding and consequent manipulation? And how is it, furthermore, that something we can fully understand and thus by implication fully control is susceptible only to the most minimal adjustments, interventions of the most prosaic and subservient sort? What accounts for the twin dispositions of utter submission and confident mastery, and for boldness and arrogance devolving to lackluster economic interventions?

Of course, these questions could be turned upon the questioner, and one might wish to understand how it is that I am positioned to see the left and the right as operating within the same "discourse of economy" despite the cacophony produced by their different starting places, their divergent ends and means, their backgrounds in Marxism or neoclassicism, their heterogeneous present attachments to Keynesianism, post-Keynesianism, and various forms of development economics. In what discursive space am I situated, that left proposals appear strangled and truncated rather than as reasonable or even as exhausting the realm of the possible? If I turned to cultivating that space, to "growing an alternative discourse of the economy," what monstrous novelties might emerge?

The task of cultivation is so daunting that I scarcely know where to begin. But fortunately I do not have to make a beginning, since I too am part of a lineage. Indeed, I can only locate myself outside the "discourse of the economy" by virtue of my association with an alternative economic knowledge, even though the products of that knowledge are few and far between. What follows, then, can be read as the delineation of an existing formation whose magnificent contours can suddenly be seen from the vantage of a new and separate space, itself uncultivated and unformed.

The Body Economic

Ailments in search of a cure

Anorexia, meaning without appetite, is a starvation syndrome that has reached epidemic proportions in wealthy Western social formations. Deindustrialization, defined as the decline of traditional manufacturing, is an economic condition widely perceived as a threat to the industrial capitalist nations. What might be the connection between these two representations of disorder?

A solution to this riddle can be found in the ways in which medical interventions into anorexia, and industrial policy interventions into deindustrialization, are construed as potential "cures" for the ailments of a suffering body. Food is administered intravenously to the anorectic, and investment is lured to declining industrial regions, in order to revitalize an ailing corporeal being. Convincing the anorectic to participate in family therapy and negotiating with the downsized workforce to stem wage growth and introduce a new work culture are both attempts to foster the conditions under which the essential life forces, calories and capital, might restore the body to its natural state of health.

Twenty years of investment policies directed at declining industries and regions have resulted in only marginal success in redressing the deindustrialization disorder. Yet there are few attempts to rethink the economic discourse upon which this "cure" is predicated. By contrast, the human body is currently the focus of a radical rethinking (see, for example, Bordo, 1989; Gatens, 1991; Grosz, 1994; Kirby, 1992). Feminists exploring the social construction of the female body have questioned the centrality of the phallus, or its lack, in governing the actions of the embodied subject. The body is reappearing as a fluid, permeable, and decentered totality in which physiological, erotic, mental, psychological, social, and other processes mutually constitute each other, with no one process or zone being more invested with meaning or effectivity than another.

In part what has motivated this rethinking are the social effects of representing the (female) body as a bounded and structured totality governed by the psyche (or some other locus of dominance) instead of as a "material-semiotic generative node" with boundaries that "materialize in social interaction" (Haraway, 1991, pp. 200–1). The physical and psychological tortures associated with the treatment of anorexia, for example, have prompted a reconceptualization of the body as a complexly overdetermined social site rather than a discrete entity subject to internal governance and medically restorable to self-regulation. Thus psychotherapist Harriet

Fraad sees anorexia as an agonized crystallization of the contradictions "crowding in on [women's] lives" (1994, p. 131) as men, bosses, the media, and women themselves exercise new and demanding expectations of women.

Whereas feminist theorists have scrutinized, and often dispensed with, the understanding of the body as a bounded and hierarchically structured totality, most speakers of "economics" do not problematize the nature of the discursive entity with which they are engaged. Instead, they tend to appropriate unproblematically an object of knowledge and to be constructed thereby as its discursive subjects. In familiar but paradoxical ways, their subjectivity is constituted by the economy which is their object: they must obey it, yet it is subject to their control; they can fully understand it and, indeed, capture its dynamics in theories and models, yet they may adjust it only in minimal ways. These experiential constants of "the economy" delineate our subjective relation to its familiar and unproblematic being.

Constituted in relation to the economy as both submissive and manipulative beings, capable of full knowledge but of limited action, our political effectivity is both undermined and overstated. With the consummate and ultimately crippling arrogance of modernist humanism, we construct ourselves as both the masters and the captives of a world whose truth we fully apprehend. In the face of that world or, more specifically, of the discourse of its economic form, and in the trains of the subjectivity which that discourse posits and promotes, we struggle to mark the existence and possibility of alternate worlds and to liberate the alternative subjectivities they might permit. But in order to re-create or reinform the political subject – a project which is arguably a rallying point for left social theory in the late twentieth century – it is necessary to rethink the economic object. Given the centrality of the economy to modernist social representations, and given its role in defining the capacities and possibilities of the left, it is necessary to defamiliarize the economy as feminists have denaturalized the body, as one step toward generating alternative social conceptions and allowing new political subjectivities to be born.

The birth of the organism: metaphors of totality and economy

Like the anorectic woman constructed as a target of medical intervention, the economy of the economic strategists and planners is depicted as a body, and not just any body. It is a bounded totality made up of hierarchically ordered parts and energized by an immanent life force. In a word, the body economic is an organism, a modern paradigm of totality that is quite ubiquitous and familiar.

The organismic totality emerged, by some accounts, with the birth of "the economy" as a discrete social location. When Adam Smith theorized the social division of labor as the most productive route to social reproduction, he laid the groundwork for a conception of "the economy" as a coherent and self-regulating whole (Callari, 1983, p. 15). By analogy with the individual who labored to produce his own means of subsistence, thereby constituting a unity of production and consumption, Smith saw society as structured by a division of labor among quintessentially "economic" human beings laboring for their own good and achieving the common good in a process of harmonious reproduction.

In the absence of specialization producers are atomized, producing on their own or in small communities the wealth that satisfies their wants and needs; the "economy" is a plurality of practices scattered over a landscape. Increased specialization, however, requires greater social integration, in order for reproduction to take place. The *division of labor*, and the specialization it entails, thus necessitates the *integration of labor*. Over the course of history, then, what was once plural becomes singular. Fragmentation becomes an aspect of unification rather than a state of atomism and dispersal. Scattered economic practices come together as "the economy" – something we all recognize, though may differently define, in economic discourse today.

It is relatively easy to read certain forms of Marxian theory as tracing the lineaments of an economic body. In many versions of Marxism, the capitalist economy or society is represented as a totality governed and propelled by the life force of capital accumulation. The requirements of this life force structure the relationship of parts within the whole, ordaining the extraction of surplus value from labor by capital, for example, which is facilitated by the division of functions among financial, commercial, and industrial capitalist fractions. Social labor is pumped from the industrial heart of the economy and circulates through the veinous circuitry in its commodity, money, and productive forms. As it flows, it nourishes the body and ensures its growth.

As the invisible life force of the capitalist economy, capital accumulation establishes the economy's overarching logic or rationale, its telos of self-maintenance and expanded reproduction. In addition, a regulatory mechanism such as the rate of profit, or competition, or the business cycle, may operate like a thermostat to maintain the economy in a steady state. Ultimately, however, the life "narrative" of the economic organism incorporates not only health and stability but illness and death. Thus a capitalist economy experiences growth punctuated by crises, and may even be susceptible to breakdowns of an ultimate sort. When it eventually fails and dies, it will be succeeded by another organic totality, a socialism that is presumably better adapted to the conditions that brought about capitalism's dissolution.

Some Marxian theories have attempted to dispel or attenuate the economic determinism and functionalism of this story by externalizing the regulatory function and by theorizing reproduction as a contingent rather than a necessary outcome of capitalist existence. French regulation theory and social structures of accumulation (SSA) theory, for example, have invoked the role of political and ideological as well as economic norms, habits, and institutions in the process of economic regulation and have attributed to historical "accident" the maintenance of stability in the relation of production to consumption. Despite these attempts to suppress both the teleological and functionalist aspects of "classical" Marxian theory, these frameworks represent the economy and society as an organic structure that operates as a unity among harmoniously functioning parts. Capitalist history is portrayed as a succession of such structures, each one experiencing maturation and healthy functioning followed by sickness and death. Growth and reproduction are the narrative constants of capitalism's story, revealing the hidden role of accumulation as its life force.

Metaphor and mastery, organism and intervention

Foucault places in a transitional moment at the end of the eighteenth century the first use of organic structure as a "method of characterization" that

> subordinates characters one to another; . . . links them to functions; . . . arranges them in accordance with an architecture that is internal as well as external, and no less invisible than visible. (1973, p. 231)

Man's body, constituted as an organism structured by a life force that produces order from within, became at this time the modern *episteme*, setting unspoken rules of discursive practice that invisibly unified and constrained the multifarious and divergent discourses of the physical, life, and social sciences. Modern economics is grounded in Man's body, finding the essence of economic development in man's essential nature – his labor (the struggle against nature and death), for example, or his needs and desires (Amariglio, 1988, pp. 596–7; Amariglio and Ruccio, 1999). These bodily essences structure a field which is itself the very map of Man, an economy that is organically interconnected, hierarchically organized, and engaged in a process of self-regulated reproduction.

Feminist theorists have argued that it is a gendered body "that was the foundation for representing all things, and thus giving things their hidden meaning" (Amariglio, 1988, p. 586) in the modern age. In the modernist regime of gender, human characteristics and other categories are disaggregated upon a binary discursive template in which one term is dominant and the other subordinate and devalued. Though the two terms exist in and through relation to each other, the regime of gender conveys a license to forget the mutuality of dependence. The dominant term thus becomes independent – in other words, its dependence upon its other for its very existence is forgotten – while the subordinate term is unable to exist without its opposite; it is defined negatively, as all that the dominant term is not.

It is not difficult to see in the story of Man and his body the interplay of an infinite set of gendered oppositions – a brief list might include mind/body, reason/passion, man/nature, subject/object, transcendence/immanence. What is interesting, however, is the way in which the regime of gender is a *colonizing* regime, one that is able to capture other dualities and to partially subsume them. Thus as soon as we produce a dualism incorporating two related terms, gender may operate to sustain meanings of wholeness, positivity, definition, dominance, reason, order, and subjectivity (among others) for the first term and incompleteness, negativity, unboundedness, subordination, irrationality, disorder, and objectification for the second.

In this way it becomes possible to understand the bizarre dance of dominance and submission through which Man addresses the economy. When Man is positioned as the first term in their binary relation, he is the master of the economy and of its processes; but when Man (perhaps in the guise of "society") is positioned as the second term, he bows to the economy as to his god. Each positioning is informed and constituted by an infinity of binary hierarchalizations.

In Man's discursive constitution, dominant (male) human characteristics are represented as universal while subordinate (female) characteristics are externalized or suppressed. They subsist as the Other – woman or nature – to Man, by whose absence or suppression he is defined. Through the operation of the regime of gender, Man becomes a creature who is fundamentally rational and whose fate is mastery and control of nature, of woman, of all non-Man (Sproul, 1993). He is the arrogant knower, whose thoughts replicate and subjugate "reality."

Given its qualities of wholeness, transcendence, and rationality (for which one might read "perfection") the organic economy is sometimes seen as functioning appropriately without intervention. From certain perspectives, the economy is the word to which the flesh is always and necessarily subsumed. From others, however, the existence of reason in the economy signals the possibility of successful intervention but also and simultaneously the limited need and scope for intervention. Thus the economy may need its "pump primed" or its life force "re-ignited"; it may need to be "whipped into shape" or "kick-started" to get it "rolling" again. Someone may need to take the helm, pulling on the "levers" that govern the speed and direction of the machine:

> ("Mr Keating emerges from his bunker"): headlines shouted that he was picking up the reins, handling gears and pulling levers again. (Morris, 1992, p. 24)

> Once Labor was elected, the labour movement made a number of assumptions about taking control of the economic levers of power. (Comment by Chris Lloyd, a left-wing union researcher, from an interview by Curran, 1991, p. 27)

Ultimately, however, these interventions are subservient to the logic and functioning of the economy itself.

Bypass surgery: tinkering with the ticker

The organismic economy calls forth a particular discourse of intervention that establishes the masculinist subject position of intervener/controller. Thus the affective discourse of economy is always to some extent a discourse of mastery: the terrain of the economy is laid out by economic theory, with its entryways and pathways clearly marked and its systems interconnected. Spreading the economy before him as his dominion, economic theory constructs Man as a sovereign/ruler. And the familiar terrain of the body is his domain.

It is not hard to see lurking in the vicinity of economic and industrial policy a body engaged in a battle for survival. Couched in the language of the living body or machine, the economy is portrayed as an organism (machine) whose endemic growth dynamic (or mechanical functioning) is in jeopardy. Diagnoses usually focus upon two key areas of economic physiology, obstructions in the circulation system and/or malfunctioning of the heart. The faltering national economy is often compared to healthier bodies elsewhere, all poised to invade and deprive the ailing, or less fit, organism of its life force. Economic and industry policy is formulated to remove the internal, and create immunity to the external, threats to reproduction.

The analogy of the blood's circulation system and the role of the heart in keeping the volume and rate of flow sufficient to ensure reproduction enables a specific set of interventions and manipulations. In recent years, for example, in most industrialized nations the call for wage restraint has been justified in terms of the presumed negative effect of wage increases upon profitability and economic growth. Wages, it is argued, have been the problem, the obstruction in the system of capital circulation that has prevented growth. In the United States wage cuts have been implemented through such tactics as union decertification, two-tier wage structures, and concession bargaining. In Australia, federally legislated policies of wage restraint have been supported by the unions through the Accord.

Visions of an organized and interconnected economic system in which interventions have predictable (and even necessary) effects have facilitated the acceptance of cuts in real wages in Australia. Wage increases have been portrayed as blocking (via their influence on the rate of profit) the generation of a pool of funds available for investment in the expansion and modernization of Australian industry. The backwardness of national industry has been seen as the major constraint upon the international competitiveness of Australian products. By the straightforward logic of organic reproduction, in which specific and focused interventions have a non-contradictory and presumably restorative effect on the whole, wage cuts have been proposed not only to free up investment capital and increase competitiveness, but to "overcome the problem of a deficit in the current account of the balance of payments" by "curtailing the demand for imports" and "cutting the costs of exporting and import-substituting industries" (Stilwell, 1991, p. 32).

When a totality is centered, internally connected, hierarchically ordered, and governed by laws of motion that can be replicated by reason in the mind of man, the strategist has only to identify the right place to start the treatment (tinkering) and soon the whole will be healthy (working) again. Curtail wages, it is argued, and the flow of investment into the crucial parts of the body economic will take place. At the base of this curative vision is the metaphoric heart of the economy – manufacturing production. It is here that the life blood of the system, capital, is most efficiently created and it is from this site that it is pumped to peripheral sectors and the unproductive extremities.

Given its presumably critical role in economic development and social well-being, it is not surprising that manufacturing investment has long been a concern on the left. In the US in the 1980s, Bluestone and Harrison's influential book *The Deindustrialization of America* (1982) focused attention on disinvestment in the domestic manufacturing sector, identifying foreign investment by multinational corporations and unproductive expenditures on mergers and acquisitions as its principal causes. In Australia, lack of generative investment in manufacturing has variously been attributed to the unwarranted expansionism of the mining sector or the alluring rewards of speculation.

In the context of the prevalent discourse of manufacturing-centrism, it becomes clear that the organicist notion of a hierarchy of functions within the economy – and specifically the essentialist conception that one or several parts are critical while others are peripheral or supportive – has constrained and directed the possibilities of economic intervention. In this, as in other centered formulations, the growth dynamic is perceived as emanating from a single economic location. Manufacturing is viewed as the driver of the economy, and all other parts of the economy (including agriculture, services, government, and households) are seen as ultimately deriving their growth from growth in manufacturing. These other sectors may contribute to the reproduction of capitalist society but they are not the key to its survival – perhaps because they are seen as not generating surplus value, or because they are viewed as low productivity sectors that do not contribute sufficiently to growth, or for some other reason. Growth in these sectors is portrayed as flab, not the hard muscle required for a taut and terrific body economic:

> in order for the shift of employment to services to be developmental and not become a shift to poverty, we (the United States) must maintain mastery and control of manufacturing production. (Cohen and Zysman 1987, p. 16)

Many types of economic activity are thus relegated to secondary status as targets for resources and attention.

Indeed the organicist conception contributes to a very familiar hierarchy of policy priorities. While some types of economic activity are seen as essential to social survival, and as therefore necessitous of intervention, others are viewed as frosting on the social cake. Though it may be widely recognized and lamented that child-care and its low wage providers are in difficult economic straits, policymakers will remind us that unless we take care of manufacturing we are *all* up the creek.

Buttressed by the conception of the organism as a self-maintaining, self-rectifying body, strategists may argue that restoring growth in key or lead sectors will set the entire economy upon a path of growth or recovery. In this view, the principle of efficiency dictates that interventions be targeted at the critical locations. When economic conditions are dire, intervening to improve child-care centers is like offering a bandaid to a patient with a heart attack.

The interconnectedness of the parts, and the accessible logic of their interconnection, enables intervention at some distance from the problem (symptom). It thus becomes perfectly reasonable to argue that if we want decent child-care centers we must start with productivity increases or wage cuts in manufacturing. It is also acceptable to ignore or to postpone dealing with problems in most parts of the economy since these will be rectified by the healthy functioning of the heart.

The truth of all these representations is guaranteed by a rationalist conviction that the reductive logic of economists reflects the orderly and parsimonious logic of the economy itself. These logics dictate that economic interventions will have predictable and noncontradictory outcomes and they define the relation of policymakers to the economy as that of Man to the machine. Thus you may quite easily arrive at the bizarre conclusion that general economic well-being will be enhanced by wage cuts; and by associating this vision with an invincible and deific figure, you may sell this program to an entire nation of wage earners and economic believers.

Matters of life or death

The lawful self-regulation of the economic organism dictates that interventions must ultimately serve or operate within the organism's telos of organized growth. Policy then is affected not only by the essentialism of the organic metaphor, which ascribes generative power and causality to certain aspects of the totality and withholds it from others, but also by the functionalism of this conception. The economy is reduced to a set of functional relations that are coordinated by the rules and require-ments of capitalist reproduction. Thus no matter whether an intervention is well or ill conceived and managed, its effects are necessarily to perpetuate "capitalism" and capitalist class relations. This invisible prescription circumscribes and constrains even the most left-wing economic proposals and analyses.

Organic functionalism subsumes the future to the contours of the present. But it also precludes envisioning diversity and multiplicity in the consequences of eco-nomic intervention. Society as organism is a set of conformable interests in which all benefit from the healthy functioning of the whole:

> Functionalism has been developed on a foundation of organismic metaphors, in which diverse physiological parts or subsystems are coordinated into a harmonious, hierar-chical whole. Conflict is subordinated to a teleology of common interests. (Haraway, 1991, p. 24)

Certainly, in Australia, the interests of business and the organized labor movement have been represented by political and union leaders as effectively harmonious:

> *Australia* needs a sustainable high growth strategy that avoids or minimizes the effects of the boom-bust cycles of the past. Metal workers and *all Australians* simply cannot afford a vision of nation building which leads to low growth and another one or two boom-bust cycles during the 1990s decade. (MEWU, 1992, p. 24, emphasis mine)

In the face of this kind of assertion, which is buttressed by a notion of common "national" interests, it is difficult to maintain a sense that any "growth strategy" – indeed, any intervention in a complex totality – will have uneven and contradictory effects.

That the strategic unionism advocated by leftists has so easily been led into strate-gic functionalism, that is, into advocating policies that help materialize the repro-duction of capitalist practices, has long been a matter of concern to those whose economics focuses less upon reproduction and more upon the potential for eco-nomic dysfunction (MacWilliam, 1989). Bryan (1992) argues, for example, that the Australian left had no business supporting any form of wage restraint, as this only served to shore up the accumulation process and avert, once again, the threat of imminent crisis.

The life/death opposition that lies at the nub of the organic metaphor presents the opportunities for political intervention in the form of a simple duality. If I don't wish to pursue industrial strategies for patching up or resuscitating capitalism, I can upend the analysis and concentrate upon exacerbating the preconditions of death. Though most leftists now abjure the millennial goal of promoting "the revolution" by promoting organic dysfunction, organic functionalism has locked them into the alternative goal of promoting capitalist health. In order to create employment and rebuild communities, they must participate in strategies and programs to foster capitalist development, capitalist reindustrialization, and capitalist growth. Many on the left would like to see an alternative to capitalism, but they face a unitary economy that allows for no such proximate possibility. Their options are to promote the healthy functioning of capitalist economies or to see working people and others marginalized and impoverished. This is not a particularly inspiriting choice, yet its grounding in humanism and organicism is seldom questioned or even brought to light.

Beyond life and death

Donna Haraway argues that if the future is given by the possibility of a past, then an "open future" must rest upon a "new past" (1991, pp. 41–2). This could involve, I would argue, a new conception of totality, one that abandons the organism as we know it. Haraway gives some encouragement that such a discontinuity is possible:

> One is not born a woman, Simone de Beauvoir correctly insisted. It took the political-epistemological terrain of postmodernism to be able to insist on a co-text to de Beauvoir's: one is not born an organism. Organisms are made; they are constructs of a world-changing kind. (1991, p. 208)

In a similar vein, Foucault prepares the way for a rethinking of totality in non-organic and non-anthropomorphic terms. Having shown how the vitalism of organic structure could not have been thought within the discourse of the sixteenth century and thus how Man's body could not have existed as the "ground for discourse" before the nineteenth century (Amariglio, 1988, p. 589), he speculates in the conclusion of *The Order of Things* upon the end of the modern episteme and the fundamental arrangements of knowledge that made it possible for the figure of Man to appear:

> As the archaeology of our thought easily shows, man is an invention of recent date. And one perhaps nearing its end. If those arrangements were to disappear as they appeared, if some event of which we can at the moment do no more than sense the possibility without knowing either what its form will be or what it promises were to cause them to crumble, as the ground of Classical thought did, at the end of the eighteenth century, then one can certainly wager that man would be erased, like a face drawn in sand at the edge of the sea. (1973, p. 387)

In a search for a new social and economic totality, born of the old but perhaps not its semblance, I sometimes turn to discourses of economic change. Certainly, I tell myself at these moments, it is in the discourse of economic restructuring, produced over the last twenty years by Marxist political economists in a variety of social science fields, that I have had the most experience of [re]constructing the organic economy. Perhaps it is also in this context that I might have the greatest chance of perceiving an emergent totality, one that is no longer constrained by essentialism and reproductionism, or inflected with the arrogance of interventionist humanism. Perhaps I might find the ground from which to move beyond the outmoded but still unreplaced "progressive" options of socialist "revolution" or capitalism with a human face.

The Ladder of Evolution

Genealogies of capitalism, metaphors of organic development

The discontinuity which, in Foucault's archaeological terms, marked the beginning of the modern age brought the rise of History as the organizing principle of knowledge. Along with History came an interest in the internal organic relations between elements of a totality, the life and death of organic structures, and the linear sequencing, or succession, of analogous structures (1973, pp. 218–19).

Certainly in the discourse of economic change there has been no shortage of coherent structures succeeding each other in orderly progression. In recent years, for example, one of the distinctive features of Australian left-wing industrial policy has been the promotion of a new "model of industrial development." This model is none other than post-Fordism, an industrial "paradigm" that focuses upon the developmental role of small and medium-sized firms and the reorientation of business and work cultures around flexibility, computerized technology, networking, and strategic alliances both within sectors and between producers and consumers (Mathews, 1990). The aim of industry interventions is to create the conditions under which a fully-fledged post-Fordist economy might be born, unimpeded by obstructionist union regulations or demarcations, business attitudes, or statutory barriers. Underlying the vision of the new industrial model are the familiar metaphor of the economic organism and an associated conception of capitalist development as a succession of organic structures, or "models of development" (this term is taken from Lipietz, 1992), each structurally similar to but qualitatively different from the last.

In his collection of "popular scientific" essays on origins and evolution, Stephen Jay Gould (1991) tells the wonderful story (entitled "Life's Little Joke") of competing depictions of the evolutionary development of the modern-day horse. Until recently, the case of the horse has served as the common illustration of species evolution up a ladder of continuous development from primitive to modern. Each lock step of the ladder is marked by increasing size and height, decreasing number of toes, and an increase in the complexity of the grinding teeth. This standard iconography of evolution has, according to Gould, "initiated an error that captures pictorially the most common of all misconceptions about the shape and pattern of evolutionary change" (p. 171). The metaphor (and illustrative device) of a ladder portrays evolutionary development as an unbroken continuity. It encapsulates the view that horses developed through a series of sequential stages of development, each adapted to the changing environment at hand. In similar fashion, the current penchant for representing the history of twentieth-century capitalist development in terms of a series of progressive steps from pre-Fordism to Fordism to post-Fordism places economic organisms on a ladder of sequential adaptation (see Figure 5.1).

Gould's reading of the fossil evidence, and that now commonly accepted, has caused a radical rethinking of the ladder metaphor and the adaptive functionalism it embodies. He argues that the metaphor of a bush might better suit the evolutionary drama that is partially revealed by the fossil record:

> Evolutionary genealogies are copiously branching bushes and the history of horses is more lush and labyrinthine than most. To be sure, Hyracotherium is the base of the trunk (as now known), and Equus is the surviving twig. We can, therefore, draw a

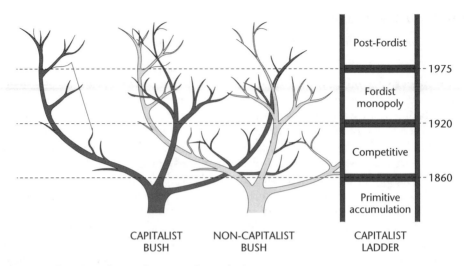

Figure 5.1 Metaphors of economic evolution

> pathway of connection from a common beginning to a lone result. But the lineage of
> modern horses is a twisted and tortuous excursion from one branch to another, . . .
> Most important, the path proceeds not by continuous transformations but by lateral
> stepping. (Gould, 1991, p. 175)

Within economic restructuring discourse some empirical studies likewise question
the hegemony of the ladder of economic development. Salais and Storper (1992),
for example, have produced an interesting discussion of four different models of
technically dynamic industrial development that have coexisted during the twentieth century within different cultural contexts. Only one of these models (found,
not surprisingly, in the United States) is consistent with what we have come to call
Fordism. Piore and Sabel (1984) have highlighted the viability of forms of flexible
specialization within capitalist industry in northern Italy throughout the so-called
Fordist era. The work of economic sociologists and anthropologists suggests a vision
of a diversity of industrial structures, firm types, and models of development interacting in different combinations. The selection of particular models as "universal"
or "dominant" in the accepted narratives of capitalist development reflects, I would
argue, the power of metaphors of organicism and ladders of evolutionary change.

In economic development theory as in biology there has been a tendency to run
"a steamroller over a labyrinthine pathway that hops from branch to branch
through a phylogenetic bush" (Gould, 1991, p. 180) of economic forms (see Figure
5.1). In the process the many capitalist and noncapitalist forms that have coexisted
with the "dominant" form have been obliterated from view. This discursive marginalization functions powerfully to constrain the visions and politics of the future,
prompting, for example, industry interventions designed to facilitate the step into
post-Fordism (seen as currently the most adaptive, advanced, and efficient form of
capitalism) and thereby making it less likely that non-post-Fordist and noncapitalist forms will continue to exist.

As Gould's story shows, the representation of history as a sequential ladder has the effect of reducing economic diversity. By denying the existence of other branches and pathways, the image of development as a ladder of evolution promotes the monolithic capitalism it purports to represent. In its most egregious and easily recognizable manifestation, the development ladder ranges the countries of the world along a unilinear hierarchy of progress, calling forth attempts to eradicate "traditional" economic forms and replace them with capitalist industrialization.

Modern Darwinian evolutionary theory constructs a vision of the "naturalness" of domination. During the early nineteenth century, the representation of the body or population (animal, vegetable, or human) as an organism which is somehow internally motivated by a fight for survival became inextricably linked to concepts of natural dominance (Haraway, 1991, p. 42). In economic terms, dominance came to be understood as the dominance of capitalism and capitalist class processes over all other forms of economy and exploitation. Economic evolution has become a story of the progressive emergence of ever more efficient, more competitive, and therefore dominant forms of capitalist enterprise, technology, and economic organization.

In rethinking the economic totality, perhaps we might begin by abandoning the hegemony of dominance, as some feminist theorists have begun to do. Perhaps we might also abandon the narrative of History as a succession of hegemonic structures, each of which has won a war of survival and adaptation. Finally and most importantly, we might abandon the organic body economic and seek a "new conception of the organism as an intereffective totality of determinations," as Richard Lewontin puts it (quoted in Amariglio, Resnick, and Wolff, 1988, p. 499), or something analogous on the social level.

In an "intereffective social totality" each economic process might be understood as overdetermined by all non-economic processes, and as participating in their overdetermination (Resnick and Wolff, 1987). Privileged economic sites and processes would thereby lose their status as causes that are not simultaneously effects. Lacking its unifying rationale or essential life force, the economy would be deprived of its integrity and its commitment to reproduction. As the desiccated shell of the organism fell away, we might glimpse a region of infinite plurality and ceaseless change, in which economic processes scatter and proliferate, unhampered by a ladder of development or a telos of organized growth.

Here again Gould's story may contribute to a reconceptualization:

> Who ever heard of the evolutionary trend of rodents or of bats or of antelopes? Yet these are the greatest success stories in the history of mammals. Our proudest cases do not become our classic illustrations because we can draw no ladder of progress through a vigorous bush with hundreds of surviving twigs. (1991, p. 180)

My analogous question is "Who ever heard of the development in the contemporary western world of noncapitalist class processes like feudalism or slavery as prevalent forms of exploitation, or of independent commodity production as a locus of self-appropriation?" Yet these are the greatest survival stories in the history of class. Our focus on the development of the different forms of capitalist enterprise (and by implication of capitalist exploitation) has made it difficult to conceptualize the persistence and establishment of many noncapitalist forms of exploitation in households, shops, small factories, farms, and communes (represented in Figure 5.1 as a shadowy bush). Our metaphor of the organism, in its functionalism and holism, has contributed to the portrayal of all noncapitalist class processes as subordinate to and reproductive of "capitalism." It has fostered an understanding of capitalism as a unitary figure coextensive with the geographical space of the nation-state (if not the world) rather than as a disaggregated and diverse set of practices unevenly distributed across a varied economic landscape. On the metaphorical ladder of evolutionary development, noncapitalist forms of exploitation have been denigrated as primitive remnants of a dominance long past, perhaps still existing in Third World countries but not consequential in the social formations of the so-called developed world. Ignored by socialists focused and fixated on capitalist dominance, these noncapitalist forms have been neglected as sites of political activity and class transformation or dismissed as the revolutionary ground of populists and romantics.

No organism, no guarantees

By centering the organic economy on capitalist class processes and on ostensibly dominant economic forms, economic policy discourse curtails and truncates the possible avenues of economic intervention, to the cost of all those interested in the political goal of class transformation (Ruccio, 1992). The ladder of development that places post-Fordism (or some other successful form of capitalism) at the pinnacle of contemporary economic adaptation precludes the possibility that noncapitalist adaptation may be simultaneously taking place and, at the same time, precludes the possibility of successful socialist projects and interventions.

In the face of this restrictive vision and the set of possibilities it allows, some feminist theorists have abandoned the conception of the economy as a unified and singular capitalist entity, emphasizing the role of the household as a major site of noncapitalist production in so-called advanced capitalist social formations (see, for example, Folbre, 1993; Waring, 1988). Eschewing the formulations of what is sometimes known as dual systems theory, in which patriarchy and capitalism are viewed as two forms of exploitation situated respectively in the household and industrial workplace, certain feminist theorists have identified a variety of forms of household class relations (Fraad et al., 1994; Cameron, 1995). They represent the household as a site of difference and change in terms of both the types of production that take place there (including use-values for domestic consumption, like clean rooms and cooked meals) and the ways in which surplus labor is produced and appropriated by household members.

This feminist attempt to retheorize and displace "the economy" has powerful and potentially far-reaching implications. It effectively decenters the discourse of economy from the capitalist sector without at the same time establishing an alternative center for economic theory. At the same time, its emphasis on the diversity of *household* forms of economy and exploitation opens the possibility of theorizing class diversity in the *non-household* sector. Once that possibility exists, we may begin to produce a knowledge of diverse exploitations in "advanced capitalist" social formations. Such a knowledge is one of the conditions of a politics of class diversity, and the absence of such a knowledge is one of the conditions that renders such a politics unthinkable and obscure.

The hegemony of the organism and the ladder within certain types of Marxian (and much non-Marxian) economic theory has prevented a complex, decentered knowledge of an overdetermined economic and social totality from emerging. These metaphors have generated a simple and restrictive vision of "the economy," one that – in ironic counterpoint to the assessed failure of most economic policies and programs – is associated with a discourse of masterful intervention and mechanical eventuation. To the extent that this vision has currency, economic discourse and the economic policy it gives rise to is a drama in which Man aspires to the state of transcendent Reason and mastery. Unfortunately, arrogance and failure are the shadows that play upon the stage.

Though it is not malleable to our manipulations, our totality is what we discursively make it. Perhaps we can make it a site for the envisioning and enactment of a new class future.

Part II Realms of Production

Editors' Introduction:
Problematizing Production

Adam Tickell, Jamie Peck, Trevor J. Barnes,
and Eric Sheppard

For much of its history, economic geography has been preoccupied with various attempts to grasp the geography of production. This was evident in the early descriptive geographies of agricultural and industrial activities. It took on a different form during the quantitative revolution (when economic geographers adopted and developed the classical location models of von Thünen, Weber, Lösch, Christaller, and Palander) by integrating an analysis of raw materials, final manufactured products and distance in the search for systematic explanations of where things were made. An emphasis on production continued with the emergence of Marxist theorizing during the 1970s. In this work, profit and the profit motive were identified as the engines of economic change. It stresses that production was not organized simply for the satisfaction of human needs, nor did it simply respond to consumer demand, but instead, in Marx's words, it represents "accumulation for accumulation's sake." Although Marxist theorizing is no longer *de rigueur* in economic geography (Harvey, Part I), its legacy remains central to the ways in which economic geographers understand the geography of production. To differing degrees, the chapters in Part I explicitly or implicitly embrace, reject, or transform Marxist theorizations. For Marxists, profit-driven production lies at the core of social life in capitalist systems. It is characterized by a fundamental division between capitalists, who own the means of production, and workers, who have to sell their labor in order to survive. (There is also a third group of landlords and resource owners.) There is, thus, an unequal power relationship at the heart of society which produces "systematic conditions of repression, social and ecological exploitation, uneven development, disempowerment, and social exclusion for many, as well as immense wealth, power, and freedom for a few" (Swyngedouw, 2000, p. 44).

Among the following chapters, Richard Walker's paper is the most obviously Marxist. During the 1970s it became clear from a simple reading of the economic statistics of most Western capitalist societies that employment in, and output from, services dwarfed their equivalents in physical production. To some observers such as Daniel Bell (1973), this was indicative of a transformation in the very organization of capitalism itself, with services becoming the motor of growth. Walker's paper is a sustained critique of this argument. In a simple, but erroneous, reading of Marxist thinking, *physical* production lies at the base of capitalism, on which rests the social and legal superstructure that holds society together. A shift to a service-oriented society, therefore, was consequently seen by some to pose a challenge to a political economy apparently rooted in the social relations of material production. Walker shows that this represents a misunderstanding both of the nature of Marxist analysis and of the actual role of services in the organization of the economy. He insists that services should properly be seen as a *continuing* and *integral* part of the production process. For Walker, the key feature of capitalism is that it is dynamic and revolutionary, leading to fundamental changes in both its internal organization and its form of production, but it is also conservative, in that the fundamental class cleavages in society – between those with access to capital and those forced to sell their labor – are enduring. The growth of services, Walker shows, arises precisely because capitalism is sufficiently dynamic to reinvent the way that human needs and desires are satisfied, while remaining sufficiently conservative to leave the fundamental divisions in society unchanged. Consequently, Walker concludes that the prevalent optimism – about living standards and life chances – among theorists of the service society is misplaced and that only a socialist transformation of society can really improve people's lives.

Geographers brought to Marxian analysis the key insight that capitalism *necessarily* leads to "uneven development" because antagonistic relationships between capitalists and workers are organized in real places and over geographical space. In contrast to some of the prevailing liberal explanations, Marxists argued that capitalism produces a necessarily "restless landscape": economic decline in one area does not simply result from bad luck, "suboptimal" decisions, or an "unsuitable" local business climate. Consequently, an adequate analysis requires a focus on the totality of economic relationships and their complex connections with uneven spatial development. In order to maximize their profit rates, firms are constantly adapting (if they don't, they are unable to compete effectively with other firms), making capitalism as a system highly dynamic, characterized by rapid industrial change and considerable locational mobility. Yet capitalism is also unstable, subject to periodic economic cycles of over-production and over-accumulation, where commodities, equipment, money, workers, and the built environment may become under-utilized, leading to "devalorizations" of capital. Inflation, unemployment, stock market crashes, and the destruction of buildings and industrial capacity are among the typical consequences. Marxist geographers emphasize that these devalorizations always take place in specific places, while both capitalists and the state attempt to contain or mitigate crisis through the reorganization of production and geographical relocation, or the transformation of existing built environments (such as the development of dockside housing or retail developments where once industry stood).

In the 1980s in Britain, however, there was growing uneasiness with Marxist analysis. As John Lovering argues, Marxist theorizing in geography

> was pitched at a very general level, throwing little light on specific empirical cases . . . This work was also generally silent on remedies, apart from an implicit or vaguely specified and ultimately millennial revolution. (1989, p. 206)

It is within this context that the reading from Doreen Massey needs to be situated. Massey takes as her starting point the conflictual relationship between capitalists and workers and the centrality of the profit motive, but she goes on to insist that these relationships are manifest in variable forms in geographic space. While the resulting spatial structures may vary considerably, and new ones will develop all the time, axiomatic for Massey is the fact that these geographically constituted relations reflect and reproduce relations of power and control. A common feature of capitalist societies is the emergence of regional economic specialization (for example, into industrial assembly, research and development, or financial services). For Massey, it is not just a matter of productive efficiency or local factor endowments, but, at a deeper level, reflects relations of power. Core regions accumulate power and control by virtue of significant concentrations of financial, managerial, and governmental decision-making functions, whereas others remain in subordinated economic, political, and social positions, often being subject to "external control."

Massey's paper explores the changing economic geography of the United Kingdom between the 1960s and the middle of the 1980s, drawing on empirical evidence to support her argument that the decline of the industrial base of the UK reinscribed existing geographical relations of dominance. Although the southeast of England had always been the favored region, the growing importance of the City of London meant that the southeast was, to an extent, able to dictate its position in the international division of labor, while other parts of the UK were far more dependent on decisions taken elsewhere.

Massey's work on the restructuring of the British economy was produced during a period when the UK appeared to have given up on making things. Within *British* economic geography, the overwhelming emphasis was on grappling with the "geography of deindustrialization" (for example, Martin and Rowthorn, 1986; Marshall, 1987; Massey and Allen, 1988). Claims that capitalism was entering a new period of economic growth, involving new and dynamic forms of production, were consequently met with skepticism. No such reticence is found in Allen Scott's essay. Scott draws upon the theoretical work of the French "regulation school," which is associated with the claims that (a) capitalism is marked by episodes of relatively sustained growth, interspersed with periods of economic instability; and (b) these episodes of growth are in turn sustained by a supportive complex of institutional, cultural, and political conditions (such as patterns of consumption, the behavior of the state, labor relations, business norms, and so on) known as the "mode of social regulation." (This insight, again, owes much to Marxist thinking about the economic "base" and the social and political "superstructure" of capitalist societies.) The paradigmatic case for the regulation school was that of "Fordism," a phase of sustained economic growth between the late 1940s and the early 1970s. During the Fordist period, regulation theorists posit that a virtuous relationship was established between mass production and mass consumption on the one hand and a Keynesian-welfarist mode of regulation on the other. A highly productive factory system, based on assembly-line principles, was variously complemented and underwritten by (a) governments committed to the improvement of standards of living and social welfare (which helped secure incomes) and the sustenance of high employment levels, (b) rising real incomes and a growing financial infrastructure, which provided a material and institutional basis for the extension of mass consumer markets, and

(c) the broad acceptance of various forms of "Keynesian" economic policy, which sought to flatten the economic cycle, making for more stable and predictable market conditions.

By the 1980s, however, it had become clear that this virtuous relationship between production, consumption, and social regulation was no longer working to secure economic growth in Western countries (see Tickell and Peck, 1992). Competition from newly industrializing countries was intensifying, profit rates and labor productivity were falling, and both inflation and unemployment were rising, thereby further undermining the Keynesian-welfarist social settlement. While many economic geographers in northern and western Europe, and in the "rustbelt" regions of North America, were focusing on the readily observable downsides of this process (like deindustrialization and job loss) in their domestic economies, Scott's principal interest is with the upside – the new, flexible economy rising from the ashes of the old. He is particularly concerned with the dynamics of nascent growth sectors and their accompanying forms of social regulation, which he captures in the rubric of "flexible accumulation." Under this emergent regime, a would-be successor to Fordism, companies organize their production flexibly in at least three ways: within the firm, in their relationships with other firms, and in relation to their workers. Furthermore, for Scott, flexible accumulation thrives when it is complemented by supportive social and political structures. For example, firms can only treat labor flexibly if both the local labor laws and the local labor culture allow them to do so. Thus, the economic geography of flexible accumulation is different from its Fordist predecessor: an increased reliance on interfirm transactions is leading to renewed tendencies for spatial agglomeration, the most vivid expressions of which are to be found in the new growth areas, the "new industrial spaces." While Massey, therefore, tends to highlight historical continuities in regional power relationships, Scott emphasizes the potential for fluidity and path-altering change. It is important to note, however, that just as theories of deindustrialization were wrought within a context of economic decline, so were theorizations of flexible accumulation developed within the somewhat atypical context of California's booming industrial economy (Gertler, 1992).

A concern with the changing nature of the capitalist economy is also evident in Peter Dicken's exploration of the relationships between firms and states under conditions of deepening globalization. Dicken was probably the first economic geographer to take seriously the rise of a globally interdependent economy, focusing particularly on the rise of transnational corporations (TNCs). In this reading he attempts to move beyond the dominant rhetorics of globalization, which are sharply polarized between a group of advocates, claiming that globalization is a form of incipient economic homogenization or "market rule," and an opposing group who tend to downplay both the novelty and significance of globalizing processes. Rejecting these polarized views, Dicken argues for a much closer theoretical and empirical examination of the relationship between firms and states. This involves three principal components. First, it is necessary to understand both the nature of TNCs and the relationships between them. TNCs, Dicken argues, do not all behave in the same way. Each has a different structure and strategy, which might be seen as distinctive responses to the same basic dilemma: how to be both globally effective and locally responsive. Second, there is a need carefully to reexamine the role of the nation-state in the international arena (see also Part IV, Social Worlds). Again, Dicken points to a diverse set of behaviors and strategies on the part of states, which must all, to a degree, act as national economic champions. Third, Dicken argues that the relationship between states and TNCs is a multifaceted and dynamic one, subject to significant change over time. Overall, then, Dicken seeks to draw attention to the nuances of the power relationships between TNCs and states. He insists that the consequent economic geography of the world economy is not predetermined. Cautioning against exaggerated accounts of corporations "ruling the world," Dicken nevertheless points out that it is becoming increasingly difficult for nation-states to extract concessions from TNCs. Resurgent local economies, of the kind identified by Scott, are certainly part of the variegated global economy described by Dicken, but his analysis casts some doubt on the claim that networks of "flexible regions" will constitute a new economic paradigm.

Although economic geography has moved a long way from its early productionist ethos, a continuing emphasis on relatively abstract economic categories, such as regions, states, and TNCs, means that, in some respects, many of its accounts remain curiously disembodied. For example, while both Walker and Scott place emphasis on different forms of labor, they have little to say about people. Authors like Melissa Wright, however, tend to be more in agreement with the position of Gibson-Graham (in Part I), asking who fills the "empty spaces" created by these abstract economic categories. In her work on the Mexican *maquiladora*, the belt of intense industrialization on the border with the United States, Wright focuses on the multiplicity of power relationships that are embodied in these apparently simple, if not crude, economic relationships. She draws attention to the complex social constitution of workplace relations, revealing how they are necessarily embodied and socially structured, rather than being mere side-effects of efficient organization. Here, she reports on an empirical exploration of workplace politics in a US factory based in Mexico, demonstrating how gender and nationality complicate class analysis. Like Walker and Massey, Wright is strongly influenced by Marxism, yet she argues that this perspective must be augmented in order to make sense of this empirical case. Consequently, she draws upon feminist theory to convey the multifaceted relations of dominance that are present in the *maquila* workplace (see also McDowell, Part IV; Gibson-Graham, Part I). First, as *women* workers, their labor is regarded as inherently less valuable than that of men. Second, as *Mexican* workers, their labor is likewise seen as inferior to that of US workers (even to the extent that promotion into management positions requires that Mexican workers become US taxpayers). A particular strength of Wright's paper is that it rests upon a critical dialog between empirical and theoretical analysis. The research is based on a combination of in-depth interviews and participant observation over an extended period of time. This allowed Wright both to develop trust relationships with the principal actors and to reflect on the US management's understanding of class, ethnicity, and gender.

While reading the following papers, consider the following questions and issues. All of these readings are influenced by the political economy approach. In what sense do politics and "positionality" – the imprint of the researcher's own class, ethnicity, gender positions, and perspective – shape the research process and the accounts that are presented? Do the accounts simply "report on" the changing economic geographies of production or do they seek to remake our theoretical and political understandings of these economic geographies? Has the production process become "de-centered" in contemporary economic geography, or is it that prevailing analytical treatments of this process have themselves changed? What is the evidence base for the papers? In particular, how do the authors draw upon empirical and theoretical evidence to construct their arguments? Would someone with a different theoretical or political starting point arrive at different conclusions with similar evidence? Finally, and perhaps most challenging, can we distinguish between "real" changes in the economy and shifts in the ways we rationalize, visualize, and understand the economy, and if so how?

Chapter 6

Is There a Service Economy?
The Changing Capitalist Division
of Labor

Richard A. Walker

Introduction

The concepts "services" and "the service economy" have entered the language with little critical examination. The notion is widespread that the advanced economies have entered an era of "post-industrialism" and that the "services sector" has replaced manufacturing as the engine of economic growth (Bell, 1973). These views have begun to come under closer scrutiny (Stanback, 1979; Stanback et al., 1981; Stanback and Noyelle, 1982; Gershuny, 1976; Browning and Singelmann, 1975; Singelmann, 1978; Ginzberg and Vojta, 1981). Nonetheless, the lack of a systematic framework of analysis continues to dog the field. Many disparate phenomena are haphazardly loaded onto a single overburdened concept, "services." Stanback and his colleagues refer to this as "the misconception of homogeneity" (Stanback et al., 1981, p. 2; Singelmann, 1978, p. 24). Marx would have called it a "chaotic conception" (Sayer, 1982a). Our task is to sort out the various aspects of the "service economy" with the help of the Marxian theory of capital.

The service thesis is, first of all, a theory of output. Our analysis must therefore begin with the distinction between services and "goods" as products of labor. The crudest version of the conventional wisdom takes personal consumption, or "consumer services," as its starting point, and argues that consumer tastes now favor services over goods (Fuchs, 1968). More recent approaches focus on "producer services" (Stanback et al., 1981; Stanback and Noyelle, 1982). This still rests on a conception of services as a product – consumed by businesses instead of individuals. Stanback et al. realize, however, that one must not only talk about "what we produce" but "how we produce."

We must, therefore, address the problem of production. To speak of production is to take up the question of labor. The distinction between goods and services turns on the form of labor involved in their production. But this is not enough. One must deal with complex production systems, or what Marx called "the collective laborer." What is needed is a way of handling the division of labor in the modern capitalist economy. Part of this paper is an attempt to dissect the division of labor, focusing on the concrete labor involved in the production and circulation of use-values. It requires a far more complex vocabulary than the impoverished categories of neo-classical economics.

The service thesis is also a theory of economic development. In conventional ter-minology, there has been a shift over time from primary (extractive) to secondary (manufacturing) to tertiary (service) activities (Clark, 1940; Fisher, 1952) or a transformation from an industrial to a post-industrial economy (Bell, 1973). This thesis has two aspects: services have replaced goods as the principal *output* of the economy and service jobs have replaced industrial jobs as the principal *occupation* of workers. Gershuny (1976) has done yeoman work in distinguishing the two inter-pretations, salvaging the first, and directing attention to the changing occupational structure. Nonetheless, he proves unable to break decisively with conventional discourse.

The stalemate arises because the debate never leaves the realm of concrete labor and forms of labor. The issue is not one of outputs versus occupations, but of two kinds of "output" from the actions of labor, use-value and (surplus) value. Gershuny points to the contribution of some occupations to the *productivity* of others. We must therefore consider the kinds of productive labor, in terms of value and surplus value. This is essential to the Marxist case for continuity in the capi-talist character of production and the logic of capital behind economic development and the changing division of labor. But it forces us to reconsider the question of productive and unproductive labor, for which purpose I develop the notion of *indi-rectly* productive labor.

The notion of post-industrialism also carries a sociological and political message: capitalism has been replaced by post-industrial society. Social revolution is unnec-essary because it has already happened. This proposition is not logically distinct from the theory of the post-industrial economy in conventional thinking, which does not distinguish between forces of production (industrialism) and relations of pro-duction (capitalism), nor between class relations and the division of labor (Walker, 1984). The argument that runs throughout this paper is that recent changes in the division of labor can be comprehended within a theory of capitalist development. The products, activities, and types of labor may change over time, but the purpose of labor under capitalism remains the same: the generation and accumulation of surplus value.

What Is a Service? Use-Values and Useful Labor in a Complex Division of Labor

The conventional view sees services everywhere. Apparently, the old-fashioned "good," along with its world of factories, is passing from the scene. In its place has come the "service," a term that implies personalized labor, immateriality, informa-tion, and greater human satisfaction, and fundamentally different modes of pro-duction, movement, and organization than in the industrial age. These presumptions do not hold up to a careful dissection of the forms of useful labor in the modern capitalist economy. The term "services" begs all significant questions about what is done in banks, repair shops, or hotels. Few of these putative "services" are either new or indecipherable in the language of industrialism. This part of the paper is therefore an exercise in disaggregation and analysis of concrete activities, or tasks of labor, in an economy still based on the production, exchange, and consumption of useful products, mostly in the form of commodities and chiefly in the shape of goods.

The product and simple labor

The category "services" is conventionally defined in contrast to goods. Since all goods render a service of some kind, the crux of the distinction must rest with production, not consumption. We therefore begin with the simplest terms regarding concrete labor and its products, or use-values.

The distinction between goods and services lies in the form of labor and its product. A good is a material object produced by human labor for human use. In its simplest form, it is tangible, discrete, and mobile. A labor service, on the other hand, is labor that does not take the intervening form of a material product, such as a play or a lecture. It is thus normally irreproducible by other workers and involves a unique transaction between producer and consumer.

This is not an altogether simple distinction. The crux of the matter is the socio-technical nature of how to produce a desired result, and the consequent ease with which a discrete line can be drawn around the production process and its product. A halfway case is the haircut, which is a tangible product of labor – if it were a toupee it would unquestionably be a good – but adheres to the wearer, making it personal, unique, and irreproducible.

Much confusion is caused by production that joins goods and labor services. Restaurants and other food outlets, for example, are ordinarily considered part of the service sector. Yet the meal is a good produced in the kitchen (notwithstanding some uniqueness in each dish). Waiting table is, however, a separate act of labor, which is often part of the pleasure of dining out. It is a labor service. The restaurant produces a joint product. This is not the case at McDonald's, where the service has been eliminated in the interest of mass production. It is absurd to include fast food outlets in the service economy when they mark the triumph of industrial food preparation.

A good deal of confusion has arisen over the changing physical nature of goods, leading some observers to see services where none exist. This derives in part from increasingly sophisticated manipulations of nature involved in modern production, particularly via electronics. Many people have an antiquated notion of goods derived from the mechanical age. They fail to see that a computer program, which takes the form of electrons on a tape or disk, is every bit as much a material good as a chair. It was produced by labor, it has a continuing existence, and it performs a useful function. It has a discrete and tangible form, unlike a true labor service. The real distinction here is between tactile and non-tactile goods, or things that are easily seen and grasped, and those that are not.

It may be argued that the informational aspect of goods is rising over time, and that it is wrong to emphasize the paper content over the informational content of a written document. My argument is that one should not confuse the use-value (information content) and the materiality of physical objects and, in the process, leap over the tangible acts of labor involved in their production.

Production and the division of labor

Division of labor refers to the differentiation and specialization of labor within complex production processes and diversified production systems. Service theorists have carved the economy into boxes labeled "goods sectors" and "service sectors" in isolation, rather than as parts of an integrated economy.

Too much can be made of the explosion in "producer services." It has long been understood that some commodities serve as means of production for others within complex production processes (Marx, 1967). These are called "intermediate inputs," and may be either goods or labor services. The growth of producer services says nothing about the nature of final output. The term "producer services" implies that all such inputs are labor services when in fact many are goods. But even if there are labor services, they are likely to be intermediate inputs in the production of goods, e.g., engineering consultants hired to help design a factory. The expansion of producer services does not indicate a growth in service outputs; only that the social division of labor in the production of *all* products is steadily expanding. It replicates the stage in 19th century industrialization when capital goods production spun off from consumer goods in separate firms and industries (Marx, 1967).

This expansion cuts both ways. All goods production requires some labor service inputs and all labor services are produced with the use of goods (Gershuny, 1976). Thus an expansion of "health services," for example, requires more pills and x-ray machines, and is, therefore, by no means a triumph of services over manufacturing. The question whether goods or services production predominates leads to a lengthy regress through the input–output matrix of the economy. This task is further clouded by the shifting lines of the social and detail divisions of labor, to which we now turn.

The division of labor is a badly muddled category (Walker, 1984). The social division of labor traditionally means work in different product sectors, e.g., the tin-smith versus the shoemaker. The detail division of labor, on the other hand, refers to the specialization of tasks within the workshop, e.g., between the pattern cutter and sewer in shoe production. The detail division of labor has particularly been associated with the process of breaking production down to discrete steps, either sequential or simultaneous (followed by assembly of parts) (Marx, 1967).

The classic distinction between the two divisions of labor runs into difficulties with intermediate inputs. When is steel-making an industry and when is it a part of automobile manufacture, as it was at Ford's River Rouge plant? The distinction breaks down altogether where single production systems are divided into several smaller factories, as has become more common. We need to redefine the social division of labor in terms of the separation of work groups, normally having a spatial component as work *places*, and confine the term detail division of labor to the task specialization within work groups (Walker and Storper, 1983).

Circulation

The focus has thus far been on the production of use-values. We have said nothing about circulation: the transfer and movement of goods, labor services, money and information between producers and consumers and among units of the social division of labor. Along the way we introduce the notion of *value*, or abstract labor, because certain kinds of concrete labor are applied to the circulation of value.

A commodity is any product of labor sold on the market in exchange for money. Commodities can be either goods or labor services. Commodities are both useful products and embodiments of *value*, a measure of the abstract (socially necessary) labor time involved in their production. Circulation therefore encompasses flows of value as well as of use-values.

Not all goods and labor services circulate as commodities. Markets are not the only mode, or institution, of exchange. This has caused no end of confusion for service theorists, who often confuse the distinction between goods and labor services with that between commodities and non-commodities. There are both market and non-market forms of organizing and integrating the division of labor. Because we take "the market" as a fact of life, we are led to the false conclusion that any other mode of economic integration is an aberration or a complete break with the past.

Markets are socially constructed institutions, built up over centuries (Braudel, 1982). In this century market exchange has been increasingly augmented by the corporate form of business organization. Massive amounts of goods and labor services are transferred within firms, without any price formation, change in property rights, or exchange of money. Whether a company supplies itself via the market or non-market route is strategic for cost and risk, but is often rather arbitrary. The growth of corporate organization is quite separate from the question of the type of output, good or labor service. The mode of exchange does not affect the form of the product.

Corporate organization of the division of labor does not, in my view, annul the law of value, given that the dominant mode of exchange remains the market and large corporations actually replicate the market internally, seeking not to overthrow but to perfect the rules of equalization of (socially necessary) labor time and profit rates among productive activities (Harvey, 1982). Value production and circulation remain the order of the day under internal (non-commodity) as well as external (commodity) exchange. Corporations have as their principal goal organizing industrial production and circulation, not overthrowing it.

Retail and wholesale trade are ordinarily counted among the service sectors. Yet most trade involves goods. Trade activities have grown large wherever commodity exchange has developed, and long before the industrial revolution (Braudel, 1982). Wholesaling dominated the early US economy (Porter and Livesay, 1971; Vance, 1970). Retailing had its greatest growth in the early 20th century, with the spread of mass consumption (Stanback et al., 1981). Today their size is chiefly a measure of industrial productivity, plus the mass of goods in circulation and the competitive sales effort among firms.

The confusion of trade with "services" arises because retail sales often do involve additional labor services, beyond merely handing over the product. The salesperson may provide the buyer with information, instruction, or a package of goods and labor services – as in the case of the holiday tour prepared by a travel agent (Stanback et al., 1981). But in so far as the sales labor merely *transfers* the product from one owner to another, facilitating exchange, or *promotes* the product, as in advertising, nothing has been added to the product or its usefulness – no production has taken place. Such labor is wholly that of circulation, a category apart. Production and the form of the product, good or labor service, is not the issue.

Financial "services," or the circulation of money, are always included among the litany of the service economy. Yet finance is an integral part of the goods-producing, or industrial, system. The development of a money system is part of the construction of the institutions of market exchange. Money serves as the medium of commodity exchange and the measure of exchange value. It everywhere ante-dates capitalism in this role. It also serves as the store of (labor) value accrued through commodity production, which gives the bearer command over a portion of the social product. Finally, it functions as capital to be invested in profit-making activities (Marx, 1967; Harvey, 1982; Braudel, 1982).

In short, the bulk of economic information in circulation parallels the stocks and flows of materials, commodities, money, and capital, and is a basic fiber of market and organizational networks. Of course, information is not just raw data, "mere" reflection of "real" movements; it is also analytic knowledge about the functioning of the economy. In that sense, information production and circulation may grow faster than national product. Nonetheless, in the first instance, the vast bulk of information pertains to the industrial economy itself, and does not form a self-generative "informational economy."

The circulation of information, like that of money, was vital to the merchant of long ago (Braudel, 1982). Improved systems of communications were at the heart of the industrial revolution and the development of the US (Pred, 1973, 1980). AT&T was the largest industrial corporation for much of this century. In short, the information economy is nothing new.

Consumption

Consumption has been a silent partner to the discussion of production and exchange. It merits further comment as to its purposes and modes. Some service theorists believe that as people grow more affluent they tend to satisfy their needs through personal labor services, rather than goods (Bell, 1973). There is no evidence for a trend in this direction. On the contrary, consumer services appear to have declined since a peak earlier in this century (Gershuny, 1976; Stanback et al., 1981). Indeed, the 19th century was a golden age of domestic and personal service, while the 20th century has been characterized by the mass consumption of goods (Gershuny, 1976). The principal objects of mass consumption have been houses, cars and appliances, and their accessories. The chief occupational effect of this con-sumption pattern has been an increase in sales labor, repair labor, and consumer finance.

As Gershuny has pointed out, goods and labor services may be substitutes in the satisfaction of a given need (Gershuny, 1976). One may take concerts or records, a vacuum cleaner or a maid, a French laundry or a home washer and drier, a trip to the doctor or a pill; the results are largely the same, though never precisely so. There are strong reasons of cost for mass-produced goods to replace labor services over time. Yet new needs which can only be satisfied by labor services appear to take their place. The long-run tendency, if any, is difficult to discern.

The growth of "consumer services" is infused with great significance by service theorists, as indicative of the development of human potential. They draw their inspiration from the notion of "a hierarchy of needs," up which people move as they grow more affluent (Ley, 1980; Bell, 1973; Stanback et al., 1981). This theory has no historical or anthropological foundations, other than the trivial notion that as people gain more income they cut back on potatoes and eat more steak. Human needs and the capacity to fulfill them develop in dialectical fashion. There is not a preexisting list of wants to which one turns as one's income goes up. The materially impoverished do not simply fulfill basic needs while the rich attend to all the finer aspirations of humanity. This trivializes human culture and elevates the activities of the wealthy, who are by no means necessarily in the vanguard of civilization (Lebowitz, 1977–8; Walker and Greenberg, 1982).

The growth of consumer products, both goods and labor services, is in part due to the replacement of household labor by commodities purchased in the market. Historically, this transfer from non-capitalist to capitalist production has been a fundamental source of expansion of the home market (Tryon, 1917). The process still goes on with a vengeance, as demonstrated by the growth of fast food outlets. To some extent, no new needs are satisfied; they are just met from a new quarter. Of course, capitalist penetration also ordinarily means the creation of new needs and new products to meet them (Lebowitz, 1977–8). In either case, the expansion of consumer industries in this century is a sign of the triumph of capitalist industrialism.

Organization and management

Conventional service theory commonly includes management among "services," in the form of managerial occupations, headquarters activities, or independent "business services." Because the result of managerial labor is not a "good," it is assumed, by default, to be a "service" to production. But management stands as a category apart in the social division of labor, reducible to the labor of production and circulation it organizes and commands. As such it cuts across all the types of labor considered up to now.

Every workplace requires *some* coordination, oversight and trouble-shooting, whether the product is a symphony or an organic solvent. As the scale and complexity of the labor process increases, an element of technical competence enters into these tasks as well. The labor of "management" may be considered a universal feature of all large-scale and complex production of use-values (Marx, 1967). Its existence bears no relation to the kind of product, good or labor service.

In the modern capitalist economy, work units of diverse kinds are linked to one another by means of corporations as well as by the market. This, too, requires labor of coordination. Corporate management has as its purpose, among other things, reducing the cost and time of circulation, coordinating far-flung production processes, and linking pre- and post-production labor inputs for more effective product development and sale (Chandler, 1977). Corporate administration has grown rapidly with the concentration of capital. Nonetheless, this type of labor is not new (see Chandler, 1977; Porter and Livesay, 1971; Pred, 1980; Braudel, 1982).

Most "business services" are an extension of the division of labor within management. As management has grown, it has commonly become lodged in separate workplaces, known as headquarters. Within these headquarters there are various divisions of management labor, such as the legal unit or accounting unit. Specialized management inputs may also be provided through the market, from outside firms. The growth in "business services" is chiefly due to the emergence as separate industries of work formerly carried on within large corporations (Fuchs, 1968).

This phenomenon seems to raise a contradiction: while management is not itself production, it may utilize inputs that take a simple product/commodity form. There is nothing wonderful in this, however; it parallels the situation in which a consumer service, e.g., medical care, is produced using goods as inputs. Many business services take the form of labor services, but some are provided in the form of goods, such as computer software. In either case, the information content is likely to be high, but this does not alter the form of the product, the mode of circulation, or the managerial purpose of the labor input. As the scale of management operations increases, the provision of managerial inputs can itself become a kind of industrial production, carried out in "back offices" by armies of clerical workers.

So far we have viewed management purely from the point of view of organizing the production and circulation of use-values. Capitalist management encompasses another dimension however: the generation and accumulation of surplus value. The foundation of surplus value production is class power, exploitation and labor control; this function of management permeates all the others previously considered (Braverman, 1974; Edwards, 1979; Marx, 1967; Walker and Storper, 1983). Similarly, the economic calculus of profit is everywhere on the mind of managers. Labor is, indeed, in the service of capital. But this does not make for a service economy.

Development and Productive Labor: The Dynamics of a Changing Division of Labor

The discussion so far has been a static classification of the parts of a modern capitalist economy. It will not do, however, to rest on the ahistorical conclusion that industrialism still reigns (and therefore always will), without addressing the legitimate issues of change raised by the service theorists. What is now needed is an assessment of capitalist development that recognizes the growth of new types and products of labor. This requires a shift in emphasis from the activities of concrete labor (the production and circulation of use-values) to the efforts of abstract labor (the production of surplus value). We have considered only the usefulness of various types of labor, not their productiveness in terms of value and surplus value. To ask *why* the division of labor has changed, we must focus on the capitalist logic of surplus value extraction and accumulation. Marxian value theory must be supple enough to allow for the reallocation of productive labor. It must defend the position that the relations of production, epitomized in the production and accumulation of surplus value, promote the development of the productive forces, rather than vice versa, and remain the heart of the industrial system.

The mass of surplus value: the edifice raised on productive labor

At the outset we may say that capitalist industrialism has not been transcended, but simply extended, deepened and perfected. As has been shown, the great majority of "services" are the classic activities of a goods-producing, industrial economy. To a large degree, therefore, the "service economy" thesis is a fraud. While it is important to study innovation and change, one must not lose sight of an elemental constancy: the growth of so-called "service" activities rests on the productive power of the industrial system. Consumption levels have risen and products proliferated. With the mass production and consumption of goods has come the mass of labor engaged in distribution centers, retail outlets, elaborate sales efforts, and transportation. The value produced along with the goods circulates through a massive financial structure, speeding exchanges, bridging time and space, leveraging capital accumulation. Specialized appendages have sprouted on this financial edifice, from leasing companies to secondary mortgage markets. Information about the economy swirls through communications channels created by that industry. Armies of managers rule over the system, paid out of the surplus of those they supervise; alongside them come the specialists in management inputs.

In short, an enormous superstructure has been erected on the value and wealth generated by modern industry. The superstructure is often called the "service economy" and invoked as a self-generating force, but it would collapse without its industrial foundation.

The image of base and superstructure raises the old question of productive and unproductive labor. This simple distinction has been badly mauled by years of misguided debate. Marx was merely taking a first cut at the distinction between production and circulation labor, in which he wished to maintain consistency with the basic premise of his theory of surplus value: that value must be produced by someone before it can be appropriated by someone else, i.e., it involves class exploitation. In other words, contrary to appearances and bourgeois ideology, money does not breed more money without production and "mere" exchange of commodities does not create value (this is nicely put by Bradby, 1982). Nor, as is commonly held in our own time, does management create its own profits, information give birth to new value, or science create anything without people and practical knowledge being put to work to create new use-values. But the orthodox Marxist view can be equally unsatisfactory when it restricts all productive labor to basic acts of hacking, bending, bolting and hewing, and the like. The problem, then, is how to mesh the distinction between productive and unproductive labor in the value sense with the many varieties of useful labor previously discussed.

The answer lies, I believe, in a structural approach. That is, value relations operate beneath the level of relations of useful labor. They capture certain essential features of the capitalist system, especially the necessity of employing wage-labor to produce value and surplus value somewhere in the economy. But we would not expect to read off tidy distinctions between productive and unproductive labor from everyday occupational categories, any more than we may read off values from everyday prices (Dominic, 1983–4). Therefore, any attempt to carve up a complex, dialectical, and structured division of labor into neat boxes of productive and unproductive labor is bound to be futile.

Thus the simple view of base and superstructure, while a proper antidote to the inverted pyramids of the service thesis, only goes part way toward a correct view of the situation. We need to take a second look at the productive–unproductive labor relation, one which teases out the sources of productivity of the industrial base, many of which lie in the "superstructure" itself. This will not be a fully structural analysis, but a first approach to it which at least recognizes the broad spectrum of productive activities and the shadings across this spectrum from the most directly productive to the most indirectly productive labor.

The rate of surplus value and capital accumulation: the contribution of indirect labor to overall productivity

Capitalist industrialization has been synonymous with raising the productivity of labor, or increasing relative surplus value and lowering the cost and time of circulation. Together these increase the rate of capital accumulation (Marx, 1967; Harvey, 1982). In the press to increase labor productivity and to speed capital accumulation, the emphasis has shifted from direct to indirect labor. As a result, the "hands-on" work of goods production has diminished as a percent of total social labor. This may well indicate a revolution in the organization of production as profound as the 19th century shift from workshop manufacture to factory "machinofacture," or at least as great as that from mechanical to electro-mechanical techniques within the factory in the early 20th century. It is, in any event, the crux of the "service economy" phenomenon.

Primary labor is work expended directly on a product, whether good or labor service. It is "hands-on" labor. The range of direct labor is wider than is often supposed, however, once the complexities of production in space and time are introduced.

Secondary labor embraces those jobs that are a step away from direct labor, the shop floor or the immediate site of primary labor. Two general types may be discerned. The first consists of certain tasks within the immediate workplace; these may be labeled *auxiliary* labor. Such workers do not themselves process, transfer or assemble materials, but their efforts cut down on labor time expended by direct laborers, improve general coordination and intensity, and monitor production data. Another group of secondary workers, *preparatory* labor, opens the way for primary labor. In short, secondary labor releases primary labor from extra tasks, makes production go more smoothly and makes it competitive (conforming to the dictates of socially necessary labor time). The category of secondary labor begins to capture the way in which the division of labor contributes to the productivity of primary workers.

Under the heading of *tertiary* labor are included many types of labor not ordinarily considered productive (of value): trade, management, advertising, banking, leasing, some transport and communication, insurance, etc. These all stand at some distance from direct production, but contribute to the overall integration and coordination of a complex production system, the rate of capital accumulation, and the long-term productivity of the economy.

Most of these activities are circulation labor. The common position that this is "unproductive labor" takes a narrow view of circulation as completion of simple exchanges, a mere property transfer. No new use-value is created, no value added; all that is involved is "realization" of existing value in the form of money. This misses the role of circulation in an ongoing process of production and development of the forces of production. The labor of circulation is an important lever of capitalist growth (Harvey, 1975b).

First, better commodity flows contribute to labor productivity by linking together workplaces, expanding markets, and lowering costs, thereby augmenting the field in which primary, secondary, and complementary labor operate. The same may be said of the flows of money and information that parallel the movement of products. But here we refer only to the simple rate of surplus value. Second, better circulation of *capital*, in terms of fuller realization of value (sales), more rapid turnover, and lower costs of circulation, accelerates the accumulation process. That, in turn, contributes to the successive development of the forces of production by generating larger masses of investible funds, a more rapid rate of investment in new technologies, more funds for R&D, marketing and organizational growth, etc. That is, one must treat the growth of labor productivity and of the rate of surplus value *over time*.

Knowledge production and worker reproduction are the hardest categories to handle: their functional links to capitalist production and circulation were emphasized above. From that perspective, they contribute, from a considerable distance, to the productivity of direct labor. Science and other forms of inquiry contribute to the store of useful knowledge adopted by firms and learned by workers. Education prepares the worker for learning tasks and solving problems. Medical care keeps the worker working. They are all, therefore, preconditions for ordinary labor of all kinds, and add in obvious ways to the growth of labor productivity over time.

Each of the above types of indirect labor is subject to further division in order to raise its productivity. The phenomenon of indirect labor should be clear without spinning out the web any further, however.

Finally, not every contribution to productivity can be captured within the tidy confines of the preceding categories. The whole is greater than the sum of the parts. The development of social labor stimulates the productivity of all the collective human enterprise in unpredictable ways. Some of this rubs off on economic production in the narrow sense and benefits capital.

Use-values and surplus value: shifts in the objects of labor

We have thus far drawn a static picture of the material products of labor, and their use-values. We must now consider the relation between indirect labor, or the shifting base of labor productivity, and product innovation, or the shifting base of commodity production. The production of surplus value requires only that labor be applied to useful products, regardless of their nature. Since product innovation is a fundamental means of gaining competitive advantage and making profit, one should expect capitalists continually to introduce new and unfamiliar goods and labor services.

The industrial revolution transformed the kinds of material inputs handed down from agrarian/handicraft production. That process has continued in this century as wood has given way to fiberglass in boat hulls, steel to concrete in bridges, and copper to plastic in piping. Industrialization has also transformed the kinds of use-values being produced. What I wish to emphasize here is how industrialism creates new needs out of its own development, i.e., serves as its own stimulus to product innovation. Consider again the shift from agriculture to industry – the historical parallel always drawn upon by the service theorists. The agrarian economy was at one time the principal market for manufactured goods, but the industrial economy soon stood on its own feet, becoming its own biggest market (Lindstrom, 1978; Pred, 1966). Today the realm of indirect labor may be the principal locus of industrialism, to which most product development (including means of production) is directed. For example, as US Steel Corporation grows it demands computers for the management of its accounts; computers, in turn, generate demand for microchips, plastic, cathode tubes, etc. – not steel. Similarly, banks generate an enormous demand for money handling, telecommunications and data processing equipment to carry out their financial functions (Hamelink, 1983).

Doesn't this mean a shift from manufacturing to some sort of "service" or "tertiary" economy? The content of output is certainly changing, in three ways. The users of products are increasingly those engaged in indirect labor. The use-value of products increasingly emphasizes "information." And the materials involved in the products have shifted toward such "insubstantial" things as paper and printing, electrical impulses and disk drives. None of these changes is incommensurate with an industrial (manufacturing-based) economy, however.

Furthermore – and this is the point usually missed – the labor involved increasingly takes a commodity form, and goods are substituted for labor services as fast as the latter can appear in new realms of production (Gershuny, 1976). In other words, segments of the "superstructure" continually enter directly into, or generate demands for commodities that are part of the industrial "base." The net effect is a change in the material and use-value content of industrial commodities, but the use of labor to produce marketable products (chiefly goods) and surplus value continues as before. There is nothing sacred about an industrial base of steel and cement used to produce cars and dams. They may go the way of flax and disappear almost completely, or the way of wheat, which while essential and produced in large volume, occupies only a small fraction of the modern labor force. Industry may concentrate increasingly on microprocessors and optical fibers for the use of communications and management. But because of the continual replenishment of the base with new products, there is no discernible tendency for commodity production, or even goods production, *as a whole*, to fade away.

Conclusion

The preceding critique has gone in two directions, both aimed at demolishing the flimsy analytics of conventional service theory. Our first line of attack was to show how much of the purported "new economy" of services could be understood in the classic terms of capitalist industrialism. It argued for the considerable degree of constancy in the basic framework of the economy, even if certain branches of labor have swollen in size in a more productive, more complex, more geographically dispersed, more integrated industrial system. It also repeatedly noted the historical roots of current activities, so as to correct the tendency to confuse the contemporary with the new. A lot of people in the US have been doing something besides basic production for a long time. In fact, employment in manufacturing in the US has never been higher than 27% of the workforce. The United States has long been a "service-intensive" economy relative to other developed capitalist nations (Singelmann, 1978).

On the other hand, there has been continuous upheaval in the shape of industrial capitalism, which I have no wish to deny. The second line of argument therefore spoke to forces for change. That, too, is no surprise given the history of capitalism. We should be prepared for an industrial world that is persistently disorienting. This is the same advice that one would have given our grandparents, but is forever forgotten by generations who consider themselves the embodiment of the modern. Capital is ordinarily far bolder and accepting of the new than most intellectuals. It cares only that people labor to create surplus value; their concrete tasks and products are simply a means to this end.

The revolutionary force of capital has generated dramatic shifts in the division of labor in society. It is this, more than any change in the products or the form of the products, that is at issue in the debate over the "service economy." The locus of competitive advantage – and of capital accumulation in general – has shifted over the last century from simple productive efficiency among direct laborers to the realm of indirect labor, which augments the productivity of social labor and speeds the accumulation of capital. In the process, the "indirect" economy has increasingly become the focus of production, feeding on itself as an engine of growth.

In order to grasp these seemingly contradictory conclusions, we require a supple mode of thinking, capable of seeing change and stasis simultaneously. There is a structural consistency about the last two centuries that is captured by the concept of *capitalism* as a mode of production. It rests on private property, the extraction of surplus value from workers who sell their labor-power, and the production and circulation of commodities bearing the stamp of value. It remains an *industrial* capitalist system, as well, in which such characteristic features of production as the tangible "good," mechanization, and the factory system predominate. It has also long been a *corporate-finance* capitalist system. While these "constants" do, in fact, change through a continual process of restructuring, they nonetheless remain recognizable beneath the flux of everyday life in a way that specific commodities and jobs do not. There may be good reason to add yet another adjective to contemporary capitalism, such as "informational," "electronic," "global," or "indirectly productive." But the case must be made on solid grounds that do not blithely dismiss essential relations and the deep insights of Marxist theory. The concept and theory of "services" are so badly misconceived as to merit rejection in further analytic work.

As for the political debate over the social implications of economic change and the potential for human liberation, that, too, remains open – and little aided by the contribution of the "post-industrial" theorists. The growing technical prowess, changing division of labor, and developing human potential of capitalist civilization *do* create historic possibilities for social change (Block and Hirschborn, 1979). The 20th century revolutionary project is not that of the 19th century, just because wage-labor and factory production can be found in both. The dreams of the post-industrial theorists have some basis in reality. But an idyllic future will not be served to us, as consumers of history, on a silver platter. If there is to be a new age of enlightenment, classlessness, and human service, it will not be born without struggle. And we must all be sobered by the barbaric prospects posed by certain of the weapons, politics, and ideas of capitalist civilization. One sees less liberal optimism about the human prospect in the age of Reagan than when Daniel Bell wrote *The Coming of Post-Industrial Society*. Alas it is not at all clear that civilization can be much further advanced – or even salvaged – as long as it remains tethered to the short leash of capital and its narrow, exploitive motives.

Chapter 7

Uneven Development: Social Change and Spatial Divisions of Labor

Doreen Massey

Uneven Development

The concept of uneven development, if it is to have any purchase on the structure and dynamics of economy and society more widely, must refer to more than the fact that there are more jobs in some places than others, or even that there are better jobs in some places than others. Such measures are interesting, and they are important, but they do not in themselves link that inequality to its causes in the deeper structures of the organization of society. In order to do this, uneven development must be conceptualized in terms of the basic building-blocks of (in this case, capitalist) society. In this paper those are taken to be classes, and the focus will be quite narrowly on the relations within the economy, as these are assumed to be the primary foundation of class structure.

The term "relations" is important, and is actually much more appropriate than "building-blocks." For the classes are not structured as blocks which exist as discrete entities in society, but are precisely constituted in relation to each other. Capitalist is defined in relation to worker, and vice versa. Different classes in society are defined in relation to each other and, in economic terms, to the overall division of labor. It is the overall structure of those sets of relationships which defines the structure of the economic aspect of society. One important element which any concept of uneven development must relate to, therefore, is the spatial structuring of those relationships – the relations of production – which are unequal relationships and which imply positions of dominance and subordination. It is on this that the paper will focus.

The notion of groups/classes being mutually defined by the relationships between them goes beyond the obvious case of capitalist and worker. It is not possible to have work which is predominantly "mental" or "intellectual" (in spite of the frequently applied epithet of "knowledge-based society") without manual work. It is not possible to have supervisory work without there being activity to supervise. It is not possible to have assembly without the manufacture of components. Thus, the different functions in an economy are held together by mutual definition and mutual

1

necessity. They are the basis of the (economic) division of labor in society and of the unequal relations of wealth and power. Those unequal class relations do not, as the saying goes, exist on the head of a pin. They are organized spatially. And it is contended here that this spatial organization must be an important element in any exploration of the nature of uneven development.

One way of approaching this is through the conceptualization of the spatial structuring of the organization of the relations of production. Some spatial structures of the relations of production involve the geographical separation, within one firm, of headquarters and branch plant. Although the precise form will vary (branch plants can, for instance, have varying degrees of autonomy), what is at issue here is the stretching out over space of the relations of economic ownership and of possession (the functions of control over investment, of administration and coordination, and of the hierarchy of supervisory control over labor). Such "managerial hierarchies" have become longer and more complex with the development of capitalist production, and indeed with its increasing geographical spread. Or, again, a spatial structure might involve the geographical separation of the work of strategic conception from that of execution. A classic example here would be the separation of research and development from direct production. Or a production plant may be one in a series within the technical division of labor within a firm, each plant performing only one part of the overall production process. Here the relations between the plants will be planned within the firm rather than determined by the external market. Market relations are also conducted over space and these too may involve systems of unequal power relations, and of domination. Relations between small and large firms come to mind, but unequal power may also exist by virtue of other characteristics which structure the apparently equal relations of market exchange. Highly contrasting degrees of oligopolization between retailing (highly concentrated) and the production of final consumption goods (often very fragmented between firms) in the UK has long meant the dominance by the former over the latter.

Now, the potential variety of actual spatial structures is in principle infinite. Indeed, later sections of this chapter indicate that one of the characteristics of the current structural changes in the economy may well be the spawning of new types. But the point, at least here, is to stress the importance of analyzing the spatial ordering of the relations of production. For these different dimensions (of internal corporate structures, of the relationships of economic ownership and possession, of the technical division of labor) are dimensions along which run relations of power and control, of dominance and subordination. They are also dimensions which develop in systematic ways with the evolution of capitalist society.

So, interregional or inter-area relations, as they are so often called, are actually these relations of production stretched out between areas (at any scale of analysis from the very local to the international). To different degrees they are the relations of class power and control. These relations exist between functions within the overall division of labor. Regions or local areas may be specialized in the performance of a small number of functions and these in turn may be those to which attach power, and strategic control over the operation of the economy, or they may be those which are relatively powerless, subordinated. Most often, there will be a mixture.

But, further, the performance of particular functions within society is part of what defines groups within the class structure. One of the bases of the definition of classes and social strata is their place within the overall relations of production. The location of headquarters in one region/country/local area and of branch plants in another will be reflected in the social compositions of those places. So will the location of the functions of research and development as opposed to shop-floor manufacturing, or of financial functions as opposed to more direct production.

Perhaps more importantly, and to return to the opening theme, to say that one area has all the high-status, white-collar jobs and another all the less well-paid, manual work, while important, is only to capture one element of the full meaning of uneven development. For that distribution of distinct occupational (and social) groups is itself one reflection of a perhaps more fundamental structuring of inequality between those areas – that carried by the organization between them of the relations of production (Massey, 1984).

All this immediately has two further implications. First, if these divisions of labor which are stretched out over space (spatial structures) consist, as we have said they do, of mutually defining elements, then the functional (and social) characteristics of some areas define the functional (and social) characteristics of other areas. If one region has all the control functions, and only control functions (to give an extreme example), then other regions must have all the functions which are controlled, the subordinated functions. This clearly has political and policy implications. Second, it means that as far as the characteristics we are considering here are concerned, any local area (region/country) can only be understood when analyzed in relation to the functions in the wider division of labor which are performed within it, and in the context of its place within the wider system of relations of production. These characteristics of "a local area," in other words, must be conceptualized in terms of the evolution of the wider structures of capitalist economy.

There are, then, certain internal necessities to a spatial structure. The distinct elements within it are held together in a mutually defining tension. There are also likely implications: different spatial structures are likely to have different impacts on local areas. But it is also important to note what is not necessarily implied by a spatial structure. First, the fact that a spatial structure of production implies a particular division into functions within the overall relations of production says nothing about which groups in society will actually perform those functions. That is determined by its own set of causal relations only contingently related (though, indeed, probably related) to the logic of the spatial structure. Second, a division into functions does not necessarily imply the social value which will be accorded to the performers of those functions, their precise social status or, for instance, their monetary reward. All this, again, is contingent although, also again, it is likely to be related to the definitions of the functions themselves and to the nature of the groups performing them. Third, and finally, a spatial structure in itself does not say anything necessarily about its actual geography, in the sense of the particular places in which its constituent parts will be located. Once again, however, and as we shall see in a later section, although there may not be necessity in the form of their interrelation, all the elements above may influence each other.

Finally, the overlapping and interweaving of all these spatial structures is the basis for a spatial division of labor. In the mid-1960s a new spatial division of labor became dominant in the United Kingdom, in which control functions were concentrated, even more than before, in London, scientific and technical functions were clustered in the southeast (with some outliers in other places), and direct production, while present throughout the country, was a higher proportion of economic activity in the regions outside of the south and east. That new spatial division of labor was the outcome of a whole series of changes affecting different parts of the economy in different ways. It was contributed to by shifts in the balance between sectors and the reorganization of, and development of new, spatial structures. It was the combination of spatial structures which produced a new spatial division of labor over the country as a whole. One question which the rest of this chapter will address is how much that scenario has changed in subsequent years.

New Directions

That period of economic and spatial reorganization of which the full establishment of this new spatial division of labor was a part lasted from the mid-1960s to the mid-1970s. Its ending coincided with further shifts both in the economy as a whole (at national and international levels) and in the political climate (see Massey, 1984). It had been a period in which geographical reorganization, and national economic and regional policy, were dedicated to "modernization." Moreover, it was a form of modernization which in turn could be interpreted as an attempt to prolong the life in Britain of what has been called Fordist production, broadly defined, and the social relations which went with it.

The old, basic industries, such as coal and shipbuilding were "rationalized," resulting in major job losses and the creation of additional labor reserves in the "peripheral" regions. Older means-of-production industries in manufacturing saw capacity closure and technical change, resulting in employment declines, especially for male skilled and semi-skilled workers, in the conurbations and nineteenth-century industrial areas. New means-of-production industries, especially in electronics, expanded employment. There was growth of R&D and technical occupations, particularly in the southeast, and also of assembly jobs, mainly for women, in all parts of the country, including some decentralization to "the north." Consumer goods industries grew slowly but did expand, especially those owned by big capital, and continued their longer-established decentralization of employment, including in particular jobs for women, to peripheral regions. Among services it was the public sector which grew most. While employment in the central state exhibited the classic divide, with high-status jobs concentrated in the southeast (mainly London) and some decentralization of lower-status and less well-paid employment to the regions, local authority employment both professional and manual, and that in health and education, was geographically more evenly distributed in its growth. Finally, in private sector services, it was producer services which showed the fastest rate of employment growth overall. Once again, the higher-status professional and higher-technical jobs were concentrated in the southeast.

The decentralization of manufacturing branch plants to the regions was in some sectors associated with technical change, and with an increasingly sharp technical division of labor within production. In other sectors, such as clothing, the move north or west was much more simply a means of cutting labor costs in the face of growing competition in a reorganizing international division of labor. Services, too, began to decentralize, but again it was only the mass-production parts which left the southeast. As an attempt to use spatial reorganization to enable survival in a world where rules were changing, it failed. In those manufacturing sectors where competition was increasingly coming from the Third World, a move to the UK regions was insufficient.

The dominant dynamics reshaping UK economy and geography since the mid-1970s have been different. Not only has the wider economic context changed, so also has the political and ideological prism through which it has been viewed by the prevailing government. Many of the same processes have continued, but in a different tempo or in a different way, and the balance between the processes, and the way they have meshed together, have been distinct from in the earlier period.

At a descriptive level, a number of important changes can be picked out. The decline in manufacturing employment, under way since 1966, sharpened dramatically during the recession of the early 1980s, though easing somewhat again thereafter. Geographically, the impact of this decline was highly differentiated, the bulk of the jobs being lost in the regions outside the southeast, southwest and East Anglia. In part because of the faster decline of manufacturing, the shift from manufacturing to service employment speeded up. But the nature of the growth in service jobs changed too: since the 1970s it has been overwhelmingly private sector services which have dominated employment growth. Not only is the geography of services as a whole different from that of manufacturing, but the geography of the two parts of the service sector is also highly contrasting. Since the late 1970s service-sector employment growth has been overwhelmingly in London and the southeast, as part and parcel of the emergence of London and its region as a world city.

One process which certainly came to an end in the mid-1970s was the decentralization of manufacturing employment. The combination of investment, modernization through cutting labor costs, and geographical shift was abandoned in the face of accelerated decline. Whatever the effect of regional policy in the 1960s and early 1970s, it declined thereafter as the supply of potentially mobile investment dried up. Much of the decentralized employment has itself been subsequently lost.

But if the process of decentralization from the south and east is no longer important, the regions of the north and west are still subject to the arrival of branch plants and to branch-plant status. Now, however, they arrive as part of a different process, more often coming directly from abroad. Most importantly of all, the medium of branch-plant status is shifting from manufacturing to service industries. While services as a whole continued their centralization in the southeast and southwest, the different constituent sectors behaved very differently. There were losses all round in public administration and defense, a continued growth with a (relatively) even distribution across the country in miscellaneous services (which includes education and health), further concentration in distribution (in marginal decline) and professional and scientific services (marginal growth), and evidence of at least some regional decentralization in insurance, banking, finance, and business services. Finally, the last years of the 1980s indicate some new changes on the horizon, in particular a pushing out of growth from its established bases to colonize new areas. There has been a rediscovery by certain service-sector industries, preceded by the property developers, of selected parts of the inner cities, and some reworking of the north–south divide as growth spreads into some of the more southern, and the more rural, areas of "the north."

Spatial Structures

What insight can be gained about these changing patterns by employing the concepts of spatial structure and spatial division of labor?

At the level of occupational structure in the UK as a whole, the changes in direction which took place around the late 1970s seem to have reinforced many of the broad shifts which were already under way. Managerial and professional strata have continued to expand as a proportion of the economically active population; skilled manual workers have continued to decline quite rapidly and semi-skilled and unskilled manual workers together declined more slowly. The geography of the social structure also continued to move broadly in the same direction as previously, although there are some incipient changes, such as the invasion of certain inner-city areas by higher-income groups. But, most obviously, managers, administrators, professionals, and technicians continued to concentrate in the south and east of the country.

In very broad terms, then, the spatial division of labor looks very similar. However, the balance of spatial structures underlying that spatial division of labor has changed somewhat since the late 1970s. There are a number of ways in which this can be illustrated.

First, as far as manufacturing is concerned, the regions of "the north" remain very largely dominated by branch-plant structures. Indeed that subordinate status was reinforced during the eighties. But in some ways the nature of the branch plants has changed: the spatial structure of which they are part is different. A higher proportion of them are responsible to ultimate headquarters outside the UK. Further, although many of these branch plants are clearly part of production, or part-process, hierarchies, dependent on inputs from other plants in the same firm but based elsewhere, the way those hierarchies work may be changing. If it is true that just-in-time systems, for instance, are being adopted by more companies, then these branch plants are less likely to be the classic "cathedrals in the desert" of the 1960s. Increasingly, they may demand that components suppliers locate in their vicinity (Oberhauser, 1987; Schoenberger, 1987).

In other words, the "branch-plant status" of much northern manufacturing remains, yet there is some evidence of two ways in which it may be being transformed – and transformed because of a change in the type of spatial structure into which the branch plants are inserted. The plants are more subject to ultimate control from outside the UK (which may be conceived of as negative) yet they may have rather larger technological multiplier effects locally (usually assumed to be positive). It has to be said, however, that this possibility must be treated highly tentatively.

Almost all the – anyway fragmentary – evidence comes from the car industry (as it also did, of course, for Fordism).

Secondly, and equally still only on the horizon in the late 1980s, is the related possibility that the vertically integrated corporations argued to have been key to the period of Fordism may become rather less important, while more vertically disintegrated, or quasi-integrated, structures may become more important (for example, Christopherson and Storper, 1986). There is, again, little systematic evidence yet of this in the UK, but there are developments which could be seen in this light such as the externalization of certain functions from manufacturing. Thus new parts of the social division of labor, new sectors, are formed out of what were once parts of the technical division of labor within manufacturing-based corporations. What were once planned relations within firms are replaced by market relations between them.

If these things are happening, then some aspects of the spatial structures which underlie the spatial division of labor within the UK are changing. One element of this is a shift in balance towards a sectoral division between north and south, with financial, technical, and professional service firms concentrated in the south, and away from domination of north by south through the part-process hierarchies of the technical division of labor. It is a shift in balance which would also result from the changing relative importance of different sectors in the economy, in particular the continuingly increasing importance of services in relation to manufacturing, and the declining relative importance of electronics.

We shall see later that the picture is actually much more complex than this; but consider the implications of the argument so far. Such a reemergence of an element of sectoral division between north and south would more than anything else be likely to fuel even further the self-feeding cycle of the growth in the southeast. The presence of control functions in London and the southeast is an important reason for the concentration of business services in the same region. It is HQ which deals with those relations. Moreover, the presence of business services is a further condition for the establishment and growth of other firms, especially small ones where buying in such services is necessary. The presence of the City assures a greater availability of venture capital in the southeast than in other regions (Mason, 1987). Even the higher house prices (a product of the concentration of growth, and of the higher incomes of these groups) mean it is easier to raise initial capital. Higher incomes generate further growth through generalized demand. And so on. It was already a virtuous circle which was further strengthened as financial and business services became the key growth sectors of the economy. In electronics, the tendency to cluster already operated both through firms wanting to be "in on the scene" in a technical sense and through their needing to have access to the main pool of highly qualified labor. With vertical disintegration or quasi-integration, however, there is evidence that the tendency for agglomeration of this upper-echelon type of activity may be increased precisely as a result of the increased importance of market relations and thus of the need to be "in on" the important social networks (Christopherson and Storper, 1986).

To the extent that this scenario is correct, it has a further effect, for it reinforces a picture of increasing separation between the economies of the north and the south of the country. North and south are locked in very different ways into international spatial structures and the international division of labor. On the one hand there is the metropolitan region of the southeast of England, with London as one of the three prime world cities at its heart. It has for centuries been true that the financial City of London looked more outward to the world economy than "homeward" to the UK economy. But it is more true today, and increasingly true of the economy of much of the southeast region (Leyshon and Thrift, 1997). The finance and service sectors which are based in the region, and which are a growing part of its economy, are increasingly internationalized. London and the southeast are the first and often only point of entry to the UK for the globalized business service sector (Daniels, 1988). The economy of London and parts of the southeast is in many ways more in competition with and linked to other international metropolitan regions and world cities than it is with the rest of the UK. In contrast, the factories of the north are linked into, and in competition with, similar factories in similar regions in Europe, and also to some extent the Third World. The foreign investment in the north links the region into the world network of branch plants of production, not global financial systems.

And it is not just in terms of spatial structures and systems of competition that north and south are differently linked into the changing international division of labor. The same is true of labor markets. The elite strata of the south and east are increasingly part of international labor markets – indeed "a spell abroad" may be an expected part of the climb up the career ladder.

And yet, of course, north and south are linked. One of those links, however, is much the same as the way in which the economy of London is linked to other parts of the world. It is the location of control. If the south is spawning its own economy relatively unconnected to the north, much of the economy of the north is still subordinate to London. Moreover, there are also increasing signs of an expansion northwards of some of the newer and fast-growing service sectors in the south (Leyshon, Thrift, and Twommey, 1989). This tentative relative decentralization to the regions (or rather, to certain cities within them) can take a number of forms including, in a few sectors, indigenous growth. Important, however, has been the expansion into the regions of large firms based in the southeast, either through the establishment of branch plants or through the acquisition of local companies.

So, it would seem that the new spatial division of labor which was established in the UK in the 1960s in very broad terms continues its dominance. Since the later 1970s, however, there have been some shifts in its constituent spatial structures. As ever, the spatial structures generating a spatial division of labor will be a mixture (Massey, 1984) but since the late seventies that mixture may have changed somewhat in its balance and in its components. Correspondingly some of the effects within local regions may also have changed. If it is possible simply to summarize the evidence examined here, it indicates that the effects in the late eighties are more likely to produce polarization within local labor markets. Finally, there are the effects on relations between regions: the economies of London and the southeast increasingly integrated into the international spatial structures of financial and commercial services, the economies of the north bound into the very different global structures of manufacturing corporations. The southeast embarked on its own process of cumulative growth, the north still tied in, though in ways which are perhaps increasingly complex, to structures of control based in London. It is the ability to grasp these wider relations, that tie local and regional economies in various and changing ways into the evolving structures of capitalist production – the ability to go beyond uneven development as a set of surface distributions – which is provided by an approach through the concept of spatial structures.

The Geography of Social Structures

The concept of spatial structures thus provides a way in to the analysis of the economic relations between regions, the geography of the social relations of production which underlie any particular form of uneven development in capitalist societies. It also provides a basis for examining the geography of social structure, the geography of class.

If class is understood to be importantly (though not solely) defined by place within the relations of production, then the geography of those relations and the places within them, which spatial structures illuminate, begins to define a geography of class. It is not a deterministic relation, but if class is in any way based in production, then this is a way in.

We shall explore just one set of examples here. The fastest-growing occupational groups in the economically active population of the UK are those which fall under the headings managers, administrators, professionals, and technicians. We shall concentrate here on the upper echelons of these groups. What they mainly represent, in descriptive social terms is a relatively high-income, high-status, and non-manual stratum within society. There is a continuing debate about its precise class definition and character, which cannot be addressed here. The question here is what light can be shed on these groups, and on their geography, through an analysis of spatial structures of production.

The first thing to be said is that in fact this broad grouping contains within it a mixture of different groups, each of which has its basis in distinct parts of the division of labor. Managers are distinct from technicians and specialist professional workers (Massey, 1984), public sector employees from those in the private sector. They belong in different parts of the division of labor.

For that reason they also occupy different positions in spatial structures of production. And indeed they have different geographies. All are clustered into the south and east of the country, but managers are more specifically concentrated in London itself, with a very clear hierarchical ordering, the top echelons being in the capital, lower orders forming a larger proportion in the regions. What evidence there is indicates that scientific and technical strata are less focused on the metropolis and more spread through the less urban parts of the southeast region as a whole and its surroundings (Massey, 1984). These, then, are distinct geographies of different types of strategic control over British economy and society.

Moreover, there have been changes in the balance between the different elements of this group and in their class character. The 1960s and the early 1970s were the era of "big is beautiful," of public sector growth and of manufacturing. Lash and Urry (1987), indeed, argue that this was the period of formation of what they call the service class in the UK, and they stress the significance of its public sector base.

It was, precisely, a product of Wilsonian modernization. Today, the emphasis is less on the construction of complex corporate managerial hierarchies, and more on "flexibility" and the promotion of the small firm. This in no way means that real control over society has been dissipated, still less democratized, but none the less the slackening growth of the purely managerial class may be a reflection of the change of emphasis. Similarly, the typical scientist of the 1960s worked in a big corporate R&D lab; the equivalent employee in the late 1980s would be more likely to work in a smaller firm, certainly a smaller unit, and to combine with their scientific and technical functions some elements of management and even of ownership. The class character of the scientific and technical strata appears to be changing, and with it the spatial structures of which they are part. No longer so often are employees buried in corporate structures and, although undoubtedly an elite, with their work subject to "proletarianization," they are now increasingly combining the power which comes from their monopoly over technical knowledge with some of that which derives from ownership and control. The groups which have been growing fastest of all have been the wide range of private sector "professionals" associated with business, and especially financial services (Thrift, Leyshon, and Daniels, 1987). But what all these groups share, simply as a product of their position within the unequal division of labor within society, is participation in and possession of strategic levels of power and control over the economy as a whole.

None of this, however, says anything necessarily about which groups in society fill these different elite positions within the various spatial structures. That is contingent to the division of labor itself; it is not necessarily implied by it. However, to take just one characteristic, even the most cursory of glances at the statistics demonstrates that these positions are filled overwhelmingly by men. The reasons vary, but in no case do they follow simply from class relations or the demands of capital. Cockburn (1985) argues that the design and development of the means of production has always been a peculiarly crucial and powerful function within class societies and she documents the mechanisms by which it has always also been a part of the production system that men, as opposed to simply "capital," have fought to dominate. She looked at three industries, and reported "the significance of the role we have found women playing in all three new technologies is simple: they are *operators*. They press the buttons or the keys . . . What women cannot be seen doing in any of these three kinds of workplaces is managing technology, developing its use or maintaining and servicing it" (p. 142, emphasis in original).

Another characteristic of this group is the degree of autonomy which it has within the workplace, the degree of control over the labor process (Massey, 1984). But this too has implications. One of them is that people work extremely long hours. As Cockburn argues, "Family commitments must come second. Such work is clearly predicated on not having responsibility for childcare, indeed on having no one to look after, and ideally someone to look after you" (1985, p. 181). It is not inherent in the class structure or the technical division of labor that it should not be women who become technologists and have men at home doing the housework. It is, however, in fact men who are the technologists and that fact itself has an impact on the nature of the functions performed, and on how they are performed (Murgatroyd, 1985).

But if one contingent characteristic of these spatial structures (i.e., which social groups actually fill the variety of positions within them) has not changed much in recent decades, other characteristics have been modified. In particular, the relative privilege of these groups within UK society has considerably increased, in both income and status terms.

There is, however, a further contingency to be structured into the discussion. For the actual geography of a spatial structure in terms of where the different elements in the division of labor will actually be located, is not given by the spatial structure itself. It is contingent, that is, dependent on a whole set of other causal systems not necessarily implied by the spatial structure itself. The location in the outer southeast of such a high proportion of these elite, white-collar strata, however, provides a fascinating example of the interaction of all the characteristics summarized above, and one in which spatial form and social form interweave and affect each other. In fact, there is a whole range of factors behind the growth of this area, including nearness to London as a center of control and of international linkages, the presence of Heathrow and good communications generally, and initially for the electronics industry the concentration there of government defense and research establishments. There is also the fact that the structure of these activities at the moment means that, once established, an area is likely to grow through the tendency to clustering. But another element which consistently shows up in research as being important is that the area itself has status.

The question then is, why? The development of the division of labor provides the possibility for these groups to be located separately from direct production. The high status which they have both striven for and been awarded perhaps inclines them to operationalize this possibility, to assert their separateness from the shop-floor and to locate in an area with cachet. But that does not explain why certain areas and not others should be seen in this way, nor indeed why separation from production should be seen as a status asset. The area must be "high amenity" because that is where these people who have choice ("highly-paid, highly-mobile") choose to go. In fact, of course, such preferences are not innate; they have to be constructed.

So what is the attraction of the outer southeast? There is much evidence to suggest that it is mainly about self-assertion and class. It has been argued, for instance, that location in such areas enables self-definition through association with the trappings of some vision of "the gentry" (Thrift, 1988). It is a means of asserting social arrival. Second, however, all this raises the question of whether the "urban–rural shift" was urban–rural at all. Rather, it seems to have been from industrial (meaning manufacturing) to non-industrial. What really does seem to be at issue is distancing from manufacturing production and from the physical and social context that goes with it. The invasion of the Docklands by the private sector middle class is very different from the public sector gentrification of other parts of inner London in the 1960s and 1970s. It involves completely clearing the area or refashioning it. Third, however, the particular groups examined here must be set in a wider context. The southeast is home also to a broad range of other groups, which form part of the basis for the social character of the region, and which in turn forms part of the attraction of the region to the groups being analyzed. They range from employees of the central state to workers in the whole gamut of cultural industries. And in particular they are there because of London, the capital city.

But if spatial structures are geographical systems of mutually defining elements, as argued in the first section of this chapter, then this clustering of certain functions in the overall division of labor has other implications. Most obviously, the existence of clusters in particular functions necessitates the existence also of areas deprived of those functions – in this case, within the UK, the northern regions of the country. Indeed, the evidence is that the concentration of this group in the southeast, and their increased relative incomes, is a prime element in accounting for one of the more obvious descriptive indicators of the north–south divide – that of salaries. While the bottom 10 percent of incomes in the different regions of the country do not vary much, the variation in the top 10 percent of male non-manual earnings is considerable, with the income levels of this decile in the southeast being far higher than those in other regions (Massey, 1988). Further, the fact of this spatial clustering itself has social effects. Most obviously, it has resulted in labor shortages for these groups in the southeast, thereby increasing salary levels still further. Yet at the same time those (far smaller numbers) in regions in the north who have the same skills either remain on lower income levels, or cannot find work and/or cannot afford to move south either to find work or to increase their salaries. In this way, the cumulative dynamics of the initial spatial concentration are reinforcing the income advantages of the already privileged in the south, and even producing geographical inequalities within the group as separate northern and southern circuits develop, those in the former on lower incomes and unable to move in even should they want to, those in the latter in increasingly powerful positions in the labor market, moving increasingly rapidly from job to job, bargaining themselves up the income scale, and seeing their wealth grow still further as house prices continue to rise.

We have then, changing divisions of labor, both technical and social, with a particular social content and consequences, which have enabled – and apparently in some measure been the cause of – new spatial structures, the location of which in turn has further molded the social character of the constituent groups.

Uneven Redevelopment: Reproduction over Time

The structures of uneven development are constantly evolving. While the mid-sixties saw the establishment of a new spatial division of labor, the years since the late seventies have seen some changes in the underlying spatial structures. What seems to be clear, however, is that, although change is continuous, there are also periodic bouts of more thorough-going transformation. There is, in other words, a relationship between the periodization of an economy and its regionalization – its forms of uneven development. And it seems clear that the major shift towards a new spatial division of labor, which began in the mid-sixties, is continuing today. If it began as part of an attempt to install one technocratic, social-democratic view of modernization, it is being perpetuated, probably reinforced, by the economic and political changes since the late seventies.

What the changes we have been discussing produce is a shifting kaleidoscope of local and regional variation. Both the geographical surface and the demands of industry are constantly changing. To give an example of the former, recent evidence would seem to indicate that some regions of the north and west are no longer seen as having reserves of mainly female labor, as they were in the 1960s and 1970s at the height of manufacturing location there. That characterization of the local labor reserves was a result of the women of those regions being seen as "green" labor and hence potentially vulnerable. Now, however, decades of unemployment, and of desperation for jobs, and the existence of a new generation of males without trade union experience, indeed often without experience of paid work at all, have transformed the male labor markets of these regions from being heartlands of trade unionism to ones where it is possible to introduce completely new forms of labor relations. The male labor of those regions may now also be viewed by industry as a vulnerable reserve.

The "geographical surface" and "the demands of industry" always interact. "General processes" only ever exist in the form which they take in particular circumstances. The new spatial structures and their social forms discussed in the last two sections take shape in the context of previously laid down spatial structures and social forms. Each has an impact upon the other. The arrival of vastly increased numbers of white-collar, high-income employees into the outer southeast has transformed the prospects of an older working class already living there. Either they have been able, through employment or through housing, to benefit from the influx or they have been marginalized. Just as the concentration of upper-income groups has had some effect on the character of those strata so also it has affected those on below-average incomes. The experience of living on a fixed (for example, state) income in London or the southeast is very different from that in the north. Apart from the fact that the inequality is more visible, and probably that there are fewer supportive organizations, prices are higher, and housing is very difficult to find at an affordable price; the money goes less far. The southeast is the richest region in average terms, but it is the most unequal.

"Spatial division of labor" is not an explanatory concept in the sense that it embodies an explanation of any particular form of uneven development. In this it is like any other concept of division of labor. A longer perspective on history indicates that the reasons for uneven development taking any particular form will change over time. It is certainly not the case that "labor-force characteristics" are always the dominant consideration. Indeed, patterns of industrial location are not to be explained simply by lists of "factors." There are broad parameters, the maintenance of capitalist accumulation chief among them. But the way in which that operates to produce a particular spatial division of labor will depend on a whole host of things. Of supreme importance in explaining the shifting character, over two centuries, of uneven development in the United Kingdom have been the changing relation of the economy to the international division of labor, the (related) changing sectoral structure of the economy, and the dominant modes of technological and industrial organization. It is the structuring together of all these which will influence the kinds of spatial structures developed, the balance between them, and their overall resultant in a broad spatial division of labor. Further, as we have seen, it is also more than this. As well as the maintenance of capital accumulation, the form of uneven development will also reflect battles over the maintenance of class power and will be refracted also through a wider level of politics, including the political interpretation of what are the requirements of capitalist accumulation. Since the late seventies, for instance, the strategy has been to emphasize and enable a particular dual role for the UK within the international division of labor: a combination of banking center and low-cost production location. It is this, and the ascendancy of particular class strata, which lies behind one of the most important dimensions of uneven development in the UK today.

Chapter 8

Flexible Production Systems and Regional Development: The Rise of New Industrial Spaces in North America and Western Europe

Allen J. Scott

In this paper, I examine some relations between forms of production organization and the dynamics of the space economy in contemporary capitalism. I seek, in particular, to elucidate the locational meaning of certain deeply rooted changes that are currently occurring in the industrial systems of North America and western Europe. These changes consist primarily in a relative decline in the importance of Fordist mass production and an enormous expansion of manufacturing activities based on less rigid and more highly adaptable (i.e., flexible) technological and institutional structures. The same changes are associated with and embedded in a series of wider shifts in what theorists of the French Regulationist School have termed *the regime of capitalist accumulation* (cf. Aglietta, 1979; Lipietz, 1986). We might say, in brief, that the old hegemonic regime of Fordist accumulation has progressively given way to a new regime of *flexible accumulation*. With the steady ascendance of the latter regime a number of new industrial spaces have also started to make their decisive historical appearance on the economic landscape, and these now call urgently for analytical attention.

As it happens, the current situation is one of considerable complexity, for the old regime is far from having disappeared entirely, and the new one by no means yet universally regnant. Moreover, the geographical outcomes proper to each regime intersect with one another in a sometimes disorderly and confusing manner. Despite the intrinsic ambiguities and analytical difficulties raised by this state of affairs, the old industrial spaces of the Fordist regime and the new spaces of flexible accumulation, in their purest and sharpest expression, contrast starkly with one another; and these contrasts are in turn a reflection of the very different patterns of industrialization and regional growth that epitomize each regime.

In the subsequent discussion, I shall attempt to clarify and substantiate the above remarks about the changing regime of accumulation; I shall briefly delineate some of the main features of the new geography of flexible production; and I shall also identify a few guidelines for an appropriately reformulated theory of location and spatial change.

From Fordism to Flexible Accumulation

At the core of all capitalist economic activity lies the institution of commodity production with its overarching logic of accumulation. This institution is at once an
endemic feature of capitalism and yet susceptible to considerable variation in the
concrete shapes it assumes at different historical moments. To exemplify the point,
we need only reflect on the many contrasts between such historical episodes as the
early putting out system, the period of classical factory production towards the
middle of the nineteenth century, the forms of heavy industrialization based on coal,
steel, and chemicals that dominated at the turn of the century, or the era of mass
production that stretched from the early years of the present century down to the
1960s and 1970s. Such episodes constitute more or less specific regimes of accumulation, though they certainly do not exhaust the total set of possibilities that is
observable in practice or imaginable in theory; they are regimes in the sense that
each represents a particular combination of sociotechnical relations through which
commodity outputs are secured, the economic surplus appropriated, and new investments ploughed back into the sphere of production. Relations of this sort are materialized, moreover, within dominant ensembles of industries that help to impress on
each given regime much of its detailed character and dynamics.

No regime of accumulation can function over the long run without encounter-
ing diverse crises and tensions, many of which may threaten its very existence.
Serious threats may spring from such necessary or contingent conditions as class
conflict, overproduction, chronic economic depression, foreign competition, and so
on. Invariably, however, a web of complementary social phenomena comes into
being alongside the regime of accumulation as a means of stabilizing its operation
through time. These phenomena consist of a multiplicity of sociopolitical relations
ranging from established patterns of consumption, through private and public
means of providing education, to governmental legislation on, say, union elections
and norms of business activity. Because of their role in helping the regime of accumulation to adjust to internally and externally generated crisis conditions, relations
of this sort are often referred to in the collective as a *mode of social regulation*. We
can, then, think of specific moments in the historical geography of capitalism as
being analytically representable in terms of the intertwined relations between a
regime of accumulation and a corresponding mode of social regulation. Observe in
passing that I have no intention here of covertly insinuating the functionalist notion
to the effect that a given regime of accumulation calls a corresponding mode of
social regulation into being because that is what it needs in order to survive. But
we may certainly allow ourselves the converse idea that regimes of accumulation
that endure over the long run do so because appropriate regulating mechanisms have been set in place. And as Lipietz (1986) has pointed out, there are in
principle many different possible modes of social regulation for any given regime
of accumulation.

The Fordist regime of accumulation flourished strongly over the period stretching approximately from the 1920s to the 1970s. Over this period of time it was
hegemonic as a type of industrialization, though other types (including, for example,
craft production activities) continued to exist alongside it. The main physical base
of the Fordist regime coincided with an ensemble of mass production sectors such

as cars, capital equipment, and consumer durables. These sectors, in their classical form, are distinguished by a search for massive internal economies of scale based on assembly line methods, technical divisions of labor, and standardization of outputs. The Fordist elements of the system comprise, in their essentials, the deskilling of labor by means of the fragmentation of work while integrating the human operator into the whole machinery of production in such a manner as to reduce to the minimum discretionary control over motions and rhythms of work. Conditions like these were in the past invariably matched by a rigid system of labor relations as manifest in a proliferation of detailed job categories with strong lines of demarcation around each job, and the explicit codification of work rules. As the regime was consolidated in historical terms, so a distinctive and corresponding mode of social regulation was also gradually put into place. In its most fully developed expression, this mode of social regulation comprised both the macroeconomic steering mechanisms of Keynesian economic policy and the socially stabilizing influence of the welfare state. Regulation was further underpinned by a social contract (mediated by the state) in which the labor unions offered concessions to management over shop floor controls and overall production strategies in exchange for guaranteed shares in productivity gains.

At the peak of its development, the regime of Fordist accumulation was geographically associated with a series of great industrial regions in North America and western Europe, as represented by the Manufacturing Belt of the United States and the zone of industrial development in Europe stretching from the Midlands of England through northern France, Belgium, and Holland to the Ruhr of West Germany, with many additional outlying districts at various locations. These regions were the locational foci of propulsive industrial sectors driving forward, through intricate input–output connections, dense systems of upstream producers. The same regions also contained innumerable large urban agglomerations rising out of the industrial base and housing the masses of workers employed in the local area. In the residential districts that emerged within these agglomerations, active processes of collective consumption, community development, and social reproduction – frequently propped up by planning intervention – helped to sustain the viability of the whole socioeconomic system. Also, with steady technological change of the kind described by product cycle models, selected labor processes were periodically resynthesized and deskilled, and as this occurred they were typically reembodied in routinized branch plants and then decentralized to peripheral locations. In this way, core and peripheral regions operated in an interdependent though decidedly unequal relation.

For a time, the entire Fordist regime and its associated mass production system functioned remarkably well. With the ending of the long postwar boom in the late 1960s and early 1970s, however, the system entered into an extended period of crisis, which, even now, has not fully run its course. By the early 1970s, the endemic outflow of capital from core regions was becoming an avalanche, leaving behind large pools of unemployed workers and fiscally crippled municipalities. Competition from Japan and the newly industrializing countries became ever more intense and dealt a serious blow to mass production sectors in core regions throughout North America and western Europe. The crisis was intensified by a rising tide of stagflation, for in a situation of declining industrial productivity and rising unemployment, the public expenditures needed to keep the Keynesian welfare-statist mode in operation could not be maintained without corresponding fiscal distortions. By the late 1970s, the whole regime of Fordist accumulation together with its Keynesian welfare-statist mode of social regulation was beginning to unwind in significant ways. This unwinding manifest in the rise of Thatcherism in Britain and Reaganism in the United States, and it was accelerated by the programs of neo-conservative reform these administrations then began to usher in. In the face of the deepening unworkability of the Fordist regime – in its archetypal form at least – governments in both North America and western Europe started actively to dismantle the Keynesian welfare-statist arrangements that had helped to regulate it but were now only becoming an additional element of the overall crisis.

In the vacuum created by these events, the outlines of an alternative regime of accumulation began to take shape, at first haltingly over the 1960s and early 1970s, and then more assertively in the late 1970s and 1980s. In particular, a number of new flexible forms of productive activity have now appeared (or reappeared) on center stage in all the advanced capitalist societies, and while these often differ markedly from one another in terms of technologies, labor processes, and outputs, they nonetheless share a variety of other basic features in common. Unlike mass production activities which are typically rather rigid in structure, the new forms of production are generally characterized by an ability to change process and product configurations with great rapidity – an ability that is frequently much enhanced by the use of computerized technologies. They are also typically situated in networks of extremely malleable external linkages and labor market relations. By the same token, they tend as far as possible to externalize production processes by buying in services and products that might otherwise be supplied internally, and this sometimes leads in turn to concomitant downsizing of individual establishments. Many sectors that display such attributes are, in addition, the sites of a vigorous revival of entrepreneurial behavior, renewed market competition, and active technological innovation.

Flexible production activities of this general sort are, to be sure, a recurrent phenomenon throughout the history of industrial capitalism (Sabel and Zeitlin, 1985). In their modern guise, however, they possess many unique and novel features, as we shall see. The incipient phases of development of modern flexible production activities coincide with the period immediately following the Second World War, but only of late years have they begun to rival mass production as the dominant core of the advanced capitalist economies. Piore and Sabel (1984) have called this turning point the "second industrial divide" and other commentators such as Cohen and Zysman (1987), Lash and Urry (1987), and Tolliday and Zeitlin (1986) have in their different ways also pointed to the same historical rupture. The forward surge of the new flexible production sectors at the core of the new regime of accumulation has been further underpinned by major changes in the mode of social regulation. There has been a wholesale dismantling of the apparatus of Keynesian welfare-statism and deepening privatization of social life, a marked renewal of the forces of economic competition in industrial production and labor markets, and (in the United States) a sharp rise in governmental allocations for the purchase of military and space equipment. These changes are still in many ways in an experimental stage and no doubt their full extent and form remain yet to be determined. They have nonetheless brought in their train numerous significant mutations in the configuration of urban and regional development over the last decade or so.

Flexible Accumulation and Patterns of Industrialization

The new regime of flexible accumulation is founded preeminently on three major ensembles (or collections) of industrial sectors. These may be enumerated immediately as (a) revivified artisanal and design-intensive industries producing outputs largely but not exclusively for final consumption, (b) various sorts of high technology industries and their associated phalanxes of input suppliers and dependent subcontractors, and (c) service functions, and most especially business services. In what follows, I shall deal for the most part only with the first two of these three ensembles since they are most germane to the issue of new industrial spaces. Obviously, however, service functions are important in their own right and must eventually be accommodated within the overall terms of reference of the analysis. For want of familiarity with recent economic events in other areas (Japan in particular), I shall restrict my remarks to the cases of North America and western Europe.

One of the basic common traits of the flexible production ensembles that have recently made their appearance in modern capitalism is their evident propensity to disintegrate into extended social divisions of labor, thus giving rise to many specialized subsectors. This process is a reflection of the tendency for internal economies to give way before a progressive externalization of the structure of production under conditions of rising flexibility, and it leads at once to a revival of proclivities to locational convergence and reagglomeration. A sort of submerged analytical lineage of key theoretical ideas about these issues can be traced out over two centuries of economic thought. This is a lineage that begins with Smith (1776) in the eighteenth century, passes through Babbage (1835), Marx (1967), and von Bohm-Bawerk (1891) in the nineteenth century, and then reemerges in the twentieth century in the writings of Marshall (1920, 1932), Young (1928), Coase (1937), Stigler (1951), and Williamson (1975, 1985), with an offshoot in the Italian school of industrial economics as represented for example by Becattini (1987) and Brusco (1982). A scrutiny of the works of these authors provides many important insights into the problems of the division of labor, the transactional structure of production, the formation of external economies, and the emergence of Marshallian "industrial districts," i.e., spatially agglomerated production complexes together with their dependent labor markets and intercalated human communities.

I shall not attempt to deal here with all of the innumerable theoretical and analytical questions raised by the authors cited above, and in any case, the interested reader can find extensive treatments of these matters elsewhere (A. J. Scott, 1988a). Instead, I shall broadly summarize a framework of reasoning whose inner intricacies can readily be filled in on a second round of reflection. The foundation stone of this framework reposes on the proposition that when changes in economic conditions bring about intensified uncertainty and instability in production and increased competitiveness in final markets, then internal economies of scale and scope within the firm begin to break down so that the entire production system is liable to display strong symptoms of horizontal and vertical disintegration. Such disintegration enormously enhances flexibility in the deployment of capital and labor for it permits producers to combine and recombine together in loose, rapidly shifting coalitions held together by external transactional linkages. In this way, external economies of scale tend to deepen and widen, and most especially where markets are also expanding so that increasingly specialized service and input suppliers are able to find profitable niches within the total production system. Additionally, new industrial subsectors come one by one into existence thereby giving rise to continual extensions of the social division of labor – a process that may be termed dynamic vertical disintegration. A growing production complex thus makes its historical appearance and becomes steadily more variegated in its internal structure. So long as the pool of external economies is expanding, individual producers can find within the organizational structure of the complex increasingly diverse input options at increasingly lower prices; and the complex thus continues to grow recursively by reason of its own inner momentum of falling production costs.

There is a countervailing disadvantage that accompanies these external benefits, however. As the social division of labor moves forward, inter-establishment transactional structures proliferate, and this immediately encourages certain kinds of costs to rise. These costs comprise the direct expenses of transport, communication, information exchange, search, scanning, and so forth, as well as indirect financial losses caused by the diminished velocity with which circulating capital moves through the whole system. The greater the spatial dispersion of producers, the more onerous these costs will be. The immediate consequence is that selected sets of producers with particularly elevated intragroup interaction costs will tend to converge around their own geographical center of gravity and thus to engender definite nodes of economic activity on the landscape. With the increasing installation in recent years of just-in-time delivery systems, this tendency to agglomeration has been much accentuated (cf. Cusumano, 1985). Hence, via the play of centripetal locational adjustment, external economies of scale (a non-spatial phenomenon) are eventually transmuted into and consumed in the specifically spatial form of agglomeration economies.

The counterpart of rising flexibility in the organization of production is rising flexibility in labor markets. Two main points may be quickly sketched out in this regard. First, vertical disintegration (due primarily to instabilities in production and exchange) is reinforced where employers seek to externalize their consumption of selected labor inputs and thus to head off possible internal upward drift of wages and benefits. This strategy is especially favored among employers with a core of skilled, high-wage workers but who also have a demand for various low-skilled workers. Employers tend frequently to farm such work out to subcontractors ensconced in secondary labor markets. By means of this device, they effectively put bounds around the possible spillovers on remuneration levels that might otherwise occur within the firm from high-wage to low-wage employment segments. One result of this sort of structural response is sharpened dualization of local labor markets. Secondly, where flexible production arrangements are in place, they are frequently accompanied by much fluidity of local labor markets, as manifest, for example, in elevated rates of turnover, extensive part-time and temporary work, and high proportions of politically marginal workers such as immigrants, women, and adolescents in the labor force (Boyer, 1988; Brusco, 1982). In other words, employers attempt to tune their payroll numbers as sensitively as possible to the ups and downs of production, while cultivating fractions of the labor force whose potential for political resistance to this process is likely to be low. All such labor market fluidity is enhanced as the size of the local pool of jobs and workers increases for where this occurs, information and search costs tend to fall and a rising stock of employment alternatives helps to compensate workers for the instability of individual jobs (hence discouraging out-migration of labor). There are therefore strong agglomeration economies in local labor markets and these intersect with and underpin the basic agglomeration economies that arise out of the organizational structure of production.

These different outcomes have an especially intense association with sectors dominated by small and medium-sized firms, though large multiestablishment corporations have also been considerably affected by the recent turn to flexibility in patterns of industrialization. Thus, strategic reductions in make-to-buy ratios and the search for fluid employment practices are apparently becoming an ever more insistent element of the modern corporate world. Even mass production sectors have not escaped these pressures (cf. Abernathy et al., 1983; Cohen and Zysman, 1987). Producers in many of these sectors have been experimenting on a major scale with such aids to flexibility as robotized equipment, workers' quality circles (and other neo-Fordist labor practices), increased subcontracting activity, and just-in-time delivery systems. The managements of mass product industries have also engaged over the last several years in highly successful attacks on the work rule rigidities and entitlements secured in an earlier era by strongly unionized workers. These trends to increased flexibility have been much encouraged by intensified product differentiation and competition in high volume markets and by the importation back into older mass production regions of the regressive labor market norms and practices now being hammered out in the flexible production complexes that form the cores of the new growth centers of the world system.

New Industrial Spaces

We have seen that the emergence and expansion of flexible manufacturing systems has stimulated massive though selective reagglomeration of production. Where, we may ask, has this reagglomeration occurred? How precisely has it come about? And what are its peculiar geographical forms?

A salient feature of the new flexible ensembles of productive activity identified above is that in their incipient phases of development in the 1950s and 1960s there was little to keep them attached locationally to the old centers of Fordist mass production. They had no especial demand for the types of inputs and labor available in such centers, and they were at the outset relatively free to locale in a variety of geographical environments. Moreover, the old centers with their high levels of worker unionization and their relatively politicized working-class populations – leading to stubborn rigidities in both the workplace and the local labor market – constituted hostile milieux in several respects for the new flexible ensembles. It may be said that for a time at least, a window of locational opportunity opened widely as the new regime entered onto the scene of modern capitalism. As a consequence many, *but by no means all*, of the producers in the new ensembles began to seek out alternative kinds of locational environments uncontaminated by previous historical experience of large-scale manufacturing activity and Fordist employment relations (cf. Scott and Angel, 1987; Scott and Storper, 1987). In such environments new and experimental kinds of sociotechnical structures of production can be established with minimum local obstruction. This is doubly important where both avoidance of rigidity and the institutionalization of flexibility are primary goals.

Accordingly, over the last few decades, many new industrial spaces have sprung into existence on the landscape of capitalism. These spaces are the outcome of a twofold process involving a tendency for modern flexible production systems to avoid older centers of accumulation combined with a dynamic of locational implosion resulting from increasing levels of externalization.

For the most part, these spaces comprise either (a) a number of enclaves within older manufacturing regions, or (b) more importantly, a series of areas that have hitherto largely coincided with the extensive geographical margins of capitalist industrialization.

The first of these categories includes many inner-city areas in large metropolitan regions with their revitalized craft industries, such as clothing, furniture, jewelry, leather goods, and, in the case of Los Angeles, the film industry (Storper and Christopherson, 1987). It includes, too, suburban extensions of the same metropolitan regions where high technology industrial complexes may be sometimes found. The outstanding example of the latter phenomenon is the Route 128 industrial complex in Boston's western suburbs (Dorfman, 1983). In all such enclaves, firms usually attempt actively to exclude the traditional male working class from their labor force, and they tend instead to satisfy their demands for unskilled manual labor by preferential employment of recent immigrants and women (cf. Morgan and Sayer, 1985).

In the second category are the diverse sunbelt areas and third development zones of North America and western Europe. These are areas that were formerly peripheral or semi-peripheral zones bordering the old core regions of Fordist industrialization. Their economies have traditionally been based to a large degree on agriculture, trade, and small-scale industry (complemented in some cases by decentralized branch plants), and urban settlement has until fairly recently been comparatively restrained. In many instances (in the US sunbelt above all) these areas possess a sociocultural environment that is relatively free from previous direct contact with big industry and large national unions, and they have thus been especially attractive to industrial sectors that could evade the locational pull of older established industrial centers. These erstwhile peripheral and semi-peripheral areas now constitute many of the new industrial spaces of the regime of flexible accumulation, and numbers of them are presently growing with exceptional vigor as freshly created agglomeration economies begin to build up within them, though there are, to be sure, important differences in patterns of growth between individual cases. To illustrate some of the similarities and differences between these new industrial spaces, let us briefly consider a few empirical examples drawn from Italy, Britain, France, and the United States.

In the so-called "Third Italy" there has been a great expansion of localized production complexes based on highly flexible kinds of artisanal industry over the last two or three decades (Bagnasco, 1977). This part of Italy lies in the northeast and center of the country with its core area focused on the administrative regions of Emilia-Romagna, Marche, Tuscany, and Veneto. In the heyday of Fordist accumu-

lation in the postwar decades, the Third Italy lay conspicuously to one side of a territorial system organized around the large mass production complexes of the north
and the decentralized branch plants of the Mezzogiorno. The industrial base of the
region has traditionally consisted of clusters of craft production activities distributed over a dense network of small and medium-sized towns. Today, this base constitutes one of the most dynamic segments of the modern Italian economy. Its
principal strength resides in its many specialized agglomerations of artisanal firms
producing design-intensive product-differentiated outputs in short production runs,
and with remarkable adaptability of organizational and labor market relations.
Some representative examples of such agglomerations are Arezzo with its gold
jewelry industry, Bologna with its machinery industries and high-performance
car production, Carpi with its knitwear factories, Prato with its woolen textiles,
Sassuolo with its ceramics, and the region of Marche with its furniture and shoe-
producing centers (cf. Russo, 1985; Solinas, 1982). In direct contrast to the US
sunbelt, many municipalities in the Third Italy are politically to the left. In spite of
this circumstance, local administrations have tended to welcome "non-monopolis-
tic" artisanal forms of industry, and the sort of class polarization characteristic of
mass production regions is largely absent. On these foundations, industrial producers in the area have prospered remarkably well in recent years – even over the
crisis period of the 1970s – and in cooperation with specialized marketing organizations they have been able to create and dominate innumerable international
market niches. In many ways, the lessons to be learned from the contemporary
industrialization of the Third Italy are just as important as those of Japan.

In Britain and France, agglomerated high technology industrial complexes are
now thriving at such isolated centers as Cambridge, Grenoble, Montpellier, Sophia
Antipolis, and Toulouse. These complexes, like those of the Third Italy, tend to be
made up of small, interlinked establishments, though in some cases they are also
functionally focused on large propulsive plants. In general, the scale (and hence
internal differentiation) of these complexes is rather modest by comparison with
American standards as final markets for British and French high technology
products are themselves comparatively smaller. That said, two major suburban
technopoles in Britain and France have been developing with great rapidity since
the 1970s, the one aligned along the M4 corridor between London and Reading,
and the other located in the Scientific City in the southernmost portion of the
Greater Paris region. Even though they are adjacent to major metropolitan regions,
these two technopoles are interpenetrated by semirural tracts of land with much
unspoiled open space, and they are in social terms far distant from earlier foci of
accumulation. In this environmental setting, production and local labor market
activity based on sectors such as electronics, computers, biotechnology, software
development, and other sorts of high technology industry is now apparently entering an intensive phase of evolution. Of late years, French regional policy-makers
have started to play a particularly active role in the development of national
technopoles. Much of this role has focused on attempts to stimulate agglomeration
economies in selected areas through publicly funded regional technology innovation
and transfer centers and generous subsidies to innovative firms.

Finally, in the sunbelt of the United States a pattern of agglomeration of high
technology industry can also be observed at isolated urban sites and in suburban

technopoles. The first of these two types of location may be exemplified by centers such as Albuquerque, Austin, Boulder, and Colorado Springs, each representing a particular stage in the process of new high technology industrial growth. The second locational type is strikingly exemplified by Orange County and Silicon Valley, uncontestably two of the world's densest and most dynamic high technology pro- duction complexes (cf. Saxenian, 1983; A. J. Scott, 1988a). These representative cases are all subject to advanced vertical disintegration of production processes combined with extreme labor market instability, not just among secondary workers, but among many kinds of qualified technical and scientific cadres too. In research reported on elsewhere, I have shown how both Orange County and Silicon Valley have grown insistently on the basis of a deepening social division of labor giving rise to dense constellations of interdependent producers and subcontractors situated at the core of burgeoning multifaceted labor markets (A. J. Scott, 1988a; Scott and Angel, 1987). In turn, these industrial complexes have become the functional and spatial hubs of a renewed process of rapid urban growth.

Analogous phenomena of flexible industrialization and reagglomeration have been reported in southern Norway, Denmark, Flanders, Bavaria and Baden Württemberg in West Germany, the Jura region of Switzerland, northeastern Spain, central Portugal, and elsewhere. Some of these areas are growing on the basis of rejuvenated craft production; others have become centers of high technology industrial development. The point must be stressed once more that each of these areas represents a unique configuration of social and political life, which means that each is also caught up in a unique developmental trajectory. That said, a common underlying system of structural dynamics can be detected in virtually every case. These dynamics, as we now know, revolve for the most part around the social divi- sion of labor, the formation of external economies, the dissolution of labor market rigidities, and the reagglomeration of production. Moreover, those places that made an early start down the path of flexible industrialization have tended to forge insis- tently ahead on the basis of their rich and endogenously formed spatial advantages. In this fashion, the window of locational opportunity alluded to above has started in several cases to close again, as firms in flexible production sectors find it increas- ingly difficult to dispense with the intensifying agglomeration economies now avail- able at particular locations in the new industrial spaces of North America and western Europe. Each particular space is the site of an evolving polarized complex of production activities, local labor market phenomena, and social life, in which each element (including educational institutions, residential neighborhoods, the apparatus of local government, and so on) contributes in one way or another to the total process of local territorial reproduction. No doubt, detailed historical ex- egesis of the origins of any given complex are of interest, as in the case, for example, of the standard accounts of the role of Shockley, Terman, and Stanford University in the early development of Silicon Valley; however, such exegesis can never explain subsequent long-run patterns of growth, and in any event, there are likely to be as many different anecdotes about these matters as there are individual cases. What is interesting and significant in theoretical terms are the inner dynamics of each local- ized complex as congeries of interconnected producers and associated local labor markets.

The new industrial spaces that have come to the fore over the last couple of decades are developing at an increasingly fast tempo. Their developmental thrust is all the more forceful given the selective widening of markets for many of their products. Thus, for example, the design-intensive outputs of the Third Italy are now being aggressively exported throughout the world, and in the United States both military and civilian demands for high technology industrial output continue to rise upwards. We must not overlook the circumstance, however, that such conditions are historically reversible. Markets may shrink or give way to outside competition; dramatic resynthesis and routinization of production technologies and work organization may come about; locational decentralization and dispersal may start to undermine the process of agglomeration; and formerly thriving industrial communities may fall into stagnation and decay, just as they have done at previous times over the course of capitalist economic and social development.

Towards a Theoretical Synthesis

Modern capitalist production systems have evidently been evolving over the last couple of decades away from relatively rigid Fordist industrial structures towards more flexible forms of production organization. This evolutionary tendency is enmeshed within concomitant changes in the regime of accumulation and mode of social regulation. The geographical corollary has been a partial but pronounced displacement of the locational foundations of modern capitalism.

As these events were gathering momentum over the crisis years of the 1970s, there seemed to come about a corresponding crisis of urban and regional theory. The old accounts of the forms of spatial development associated with the regime of Fordist accumulation and its cognate mode of Keynesian welfare-statist regulation were patently no longer very satisfactory as descriptions of underlying realities; and an alternative theoretical framework capable of fully assimilating the emerging new contours of capitalist society into its universe of discourse failed signally to make its appearance. Even yet, it can scarcely be claimed that a new theoretical consensus about the current situation has formed. One of the evident responses in human geography to this predicament has been a certain disillusionment with theoretical work in general and a radical return to empirical investigation, the multiplication of case studies, and an insistence on the significance of the local at the expense of the global and universal. This reaction is entirely comprehensible, and it has provided us with many new insights about the detailed workings of contemporary capitalism at both intermediate and micro-scales of analysis. There does, nonetheless, appear to be a burning need to reopen macrotheoretical questions about the logic of capitalist society as a whole. An especially urgent task is to investigate more thoroughly the formation, characteristics, and historical course of flexible accumulation and its attendant mode(s) of social regulation, for only by clarifying these issues can we also effectively explain detailed geographical outcomes currently occurring on the ground (cf. Harvey and Scott, 1988). It is my hope that the arguments deployed above may suggest some potentially fruitful avenues of reconciliation between theoretical and empirical work in human geography as the trend to flexible production organization in modern capitalism deepens and widens.

Meanwhile, we are also faced with the need to provide a meaningful account of the contemporary conjuncture in the space-economies of North America and western Europe, with their conflicting and confusing crosscurrents. These crosscurrents spring in large degree from the copresence of an aging regime of Fordist accumulation alongside an ascending regime of flexible accumulation, giving rise in turn to an intricate pattern of old and new industrial spaces imbricated in a widening international division of labor. Whatever the future evolutionary path of this system may be, it is evident that the landscape of capitalist production is today drastically different from what it was even a couple of decades ago. In this paper I have developed some outlines of a suggested framework for thinking about these changes. There remain innumerable detailed research tasks of conceptual infilling, empirical analysis, and reevaluation.

Chapter 9

Global–Local Tensions: Firms and States in the Global Space-Economy

Peter Dicken

These are exciting and challenging times in economic geography, as we grapple with the problem of understanding the major transformations in the way economic activities are organized and reorganized. Not only does the pace of change pose difficulties, but the complex interplay among processes operating at different, but related, geographic scales has become increasingly intricate as well. I want to frame my argument in the specific context of the "global–local nexus." This is far more than merely a question of the geographic scale at which economic processes occur. More fundamentally, it is a question of where power lies, and it is a central problematic facing both firms and states.

Analysis of these processes is made more difficult by the uncertainty surrounding the interpretation of the current structure of the world economy. Making sense of the present is, of course, always more difficult than making sense of the past, because we do not really know where we are. Throughout history, most observers of the contemporary scene have been tempted to argue for the "specialness" of their own times; the present day is no exception. But, by definition, we cannot know which of the current developments and changes are permanent and which are purely ephemeral. Considerable disagreement exists over the interpretation of current developments in the organization of economic activities at the global scale and their implications for firms and states. The crux of the debate is the extent to which we are moving toward (or already live in) a globalized, rather than an international, economy. Robert Reich's view is that

> We are living through a transformation that will rearrange the politics and economics of the coming century. There will be no national products or technologies, no national corporations, no national industries. There will no longer be national economies, at least as we have come to understand that concept. (1991, pp. 3, 8)

While Reich appears, at least implicitly, to support the view that we are now in a globalizing, if not a globalized, economy, Hirst and Thompson (1992) are more skeptical. On the basis of a comparison between two ideal types of structure – a globalized international economy and a worldwide international economy – and from an analysis of empirical trends in trade, investment, and political restructuring, they conclude, "we do not have a fully globalized economy; we do have an international economy and national policy responses to it" (Hirst and Thompson, 1992, p. 394). Both Reich and Hirst and Thompson agree, in their different ways, that the relationships between firms and states have been drastically changed. Stopford and Strange (1991) express this in terms of mutual dependence, which, they argue, can be explored in terms of a triangular nexus of interactions comprising firm–firm, state–state, and firm–state relationships.

The aim of this paper is to explore some of these complex interactions between transnational corporations (TNCs) and states in the context of the global–local debate through a review of a wide variety of literature drawn from different disciplines. It is important to emphasize that the terms "global" and "local" are not fixed scales; rather, they represent the extreme points of a dialectical continuum of complex mutual interactions.

Firm–Firm Competition: The Changing World of the Transnational Corporation

TNCs today are restructuring their activities in ways that involve (1) reorganizing the coordination of production chain functions in a complex realignment of internalized and externalized network relationships; (2) reorganizing the geography of their production chains internationally and, in some cases, globally; (3) redefining their core activities and repositioning themselves along the production chain, with a particular emphasis on downstream, service functions. These developments reflect the nature of TNCs as highly embedded interacting networks involved in competitive struggles in which a diversity of competitive strategies is used. Such strategies are, themselves, the outcome of contested power relations both inside the firm and, externally, with the constellation of institutions (including the state) with which TNCs interact.

Until relatively recently, much of the business and management literature projected a simplistic sequential path of TNC development. In fact, there is – and always has been – considerable diversity in TNC strategies and in the kinds of organizational coordination and geographic configuration employed to implement them (see, for example, Perlmutter, 1969; Bartlett and Ghoshal, 1989; Martinez and Jarillo, 1989).

Bartlett and Ghoshal (1989) identify three different organizational models, each with distinctive structural, administrative, and management characteristics. Their multinational organization model is characterized by a decentralized federation of activities and simple financial control systems overlain on informal personal coordination. The company's worldwide operations are organized as a portfolio of national businesses. Each of the firm's national units has a considerable degree of autonomy; each has a predominantly "local" orientation. Their international organization model involves far more formal coordination and control by the corporate headquarters over the overseas subsidiaries. Whereas multinational organizations are, in effect, portfolios of quasi-independent businesses, international organizations clearly regard their overseas operations as appendages to the controlling domestic corporation. Thus the international firm's subsidiaries are more dependent on the center for the transfer of knowledge and information, and the parent company makes greater use of formal systems to control their subsidiaries. Their "classic" global organization model is based on a centralization of assets and responsibilities. The role of the local units is to assemble and sell products and to implement plans and policies developed at headquarters. Thus, overseas subsidiaries have far less freedom to create new products or strategies or even to modify existing ones. Although each of these three ideal-type models developed during specific historical periods, there is no suggestion that one was sequentially replaced by another. Each form has tended to persist, to a greater or lesser extent, producing a diverse population of transnational corporations in the contemporary world economy.

Although we can continue to identify these forms of TNC, new forms of transnational organization are also emerging that may – although not inevitably – replace some of the existing forms. Bartlett and Ghoshal argue that each of their three ideal types of organization possesses specific strengths, but each also has severe contradictions and tensions. Thus, the global company capitalizes on the achievement of scale economies in its activities and on centralized knowledge and expertise. But this implies that local market conditions tend to be ignored, and the possibility of local learning is precluded. The more locally oriented multinational organization is able to respond to local needs, but its very fragmentation imposes penalties for efficiency and for the internal flow of knowledge and learning. The international company "is better able to leverage the knowledge and capabilities of the parent company. But its resource configuration and operating systems make it less efficient than the global company, and less responsive than the multinational company" (Bartlett and Ghoshal, 1989, pp. 58–9).

As Bartlett and Ghoshal point out, the dilemma facing firms – especially large firms – in turbulent competitive environments is that to succeed on a global scale they must possess three capabilities simultaneously. They need to be globally efficient, multinationally flexible, and capable of capturing the benefits of worldwide learning all at the same time. A key diagnostic feature of such complex global organizations is their integrated network configuration and their capacity to develop flexible coordinating processes. Such capabilities apply both inside the firm (the network of intrafirm relationships which, it is argued, is displacing hierarchical governance relationships) and outside the firm (the complex network of interfirm relationships).

A central feature of these models of contemporary production organization is that they place particular emphasis on the rich variety of external relationships within production networks. At the international scale, most attention has been devoted to strategic alliances, which, as Kindleberger (1988) has observed, are by no means a new phenomenon.

Such relationships are frequently multilateral rather than bilateral, polygamous rather than monogamous. Collaborative ventures are a long-established form of international business organization that, in the past, involved specific relationships between conventionally organized, hierarchically structured firms as just one element in their competitive strategies. The argument now is rather different: not only have collaborative ventures in the more traditional sense moved to the center of firms' strategies, but also – and more controversially – new forms of collaboration are embedded within a much looser network structure, or *webs of enterprise*

(Reich, 1991). This view, however, is very much a Western perspective. Japanese business organizations have long been embedded in a complex structure of inter-organizational alliances, epitomized by the horizontal and vertical *keiretsu* (Gerlach, 1992; Eli, 1990; Helou, 1991).

Seductive as these various ideas about new forms of international business organization undoubtedly are, we face a major problem in distinguishing what is actually happening (and may happen in the future) from the hype and the rhetoric. When we turn to the hard world of empirical reality we meet up with the intractability – and even total absence – of comprehensive data. The only variable on which we have (reasonably) comprehensive data is that of *foreign direct investment* (FDI), which, unfortunately, exclude coverage of most non-equity relationships and activities, the very ones that are becoming especially important. Within their limitations, however, FDI data provide an important, though partial, indicator of changing levels and patterns of TNC activity at a global scale (Dicken, 1992a; Dunning, 1993).

The recent temporal pattern of FDI growth displays a major upsurge during the 1980s, on a scale exceeding even that of the 1960s. Julius (1990, p. 6) estimates that "whereas in the 1960s FDI grew at twice the rate of GNP, in the 1980s it has grown more than four times as fast as GNP." Not only has FDI been growing faster than GNP, but it also has been growing at a much faster rate than world exports, particularly since 1985 (UNCTC, 1991). This figure alone suggests that FDI has become a more significant integrating force in the global economy than the traditional indicator of such integration, trade (Julius, 1990). Indeed, because TNCs are themselves responsible for a large proportion of international trade (much of this as intrafirm transactions), their global significance becomes even more marked. Another notable trend has been the massive internationalization of services, much of which has been driven by FDI (Dicken, 1992a).

Spatially, a number of important FDI trends can be identified:

(1) Origins have diversified geographically, not only within the industrialized countries, but also from several of the newly industrializing economies (NIEs), notably in East Asia but including some Latin American countries.

(2) Although the United States still accounts for the largest share of the world's stock of FDI, Japan is now the world's leading foreign direct investor on an annual *flow* basis. The collapse of Japan's "bubble economy," however, caused a substantial contraction (and geographic reorientation) of Japanese FDI.

(3) There has been a major intensification of cross-investment between the industrialized economies, an increasingly high level of TNC interpenetration of national economies (Julius, 1990). Overall, the relative importance of TNCs (both foreign and domestic) in each major economy has greatly increased, while the global pattern of FDI has become strongly concentrated in the triad regions.

(4) The intensified concentration of FDI in the industrialized economies means that the share going to developing economies remains low: some 18 percent of the world total compared with more than 60 percent on the eve of World War II. Within the developing countries, the distribution of FDI is extremely uneven: a mere ten countries, primarily the Asian NIEs and "proto-NIEs" and some

Latin American countries (OECD, 1993), account for 75 percent of the FDI inflow.

(5) The recent political developments in the former Soviet Union and in Eastern Europe have unexpectedly opened up investment opportunities for foreign TNCs.

When we turn from FDI to other modes of TNC activity, we face a serious paucity of empirical data and a reliance on case studies and anecdotal evidence. Most strikingly, the majority of strategic alliances are among competitors. Of the 839 agreements analyzed by Morris and Hergert (1987) between 1975 and 1986, no less than 71 percent were between two firms in the same market. In addition, although alliances are certainly not confined to particular sizes or types of firms, they are undoubtedly especially common between large TNCs with extensive international operations. Geographically, most alliances in the Morris and Hergert study were between firms from European Community (EC) countries (31 percent) or between EC and US firms (26 percent). A further 10 percent of the alliances were between EC and Japanese firms and 8 percent between United States and Japanese firms.

Empirical evidence on the existence and nature of the kinds of dynamic network that are becoming especially important in the global economy is even sparser than that on the more conventional collaborative ventures. Here, we are limited to a small number of cases, the most notable being the Italian clothing company, Benetton (Elson, 1989), and the US athletic shoe company, Nike (Donaghu and Barff, 1990).

The clear message is that transnational reality is one of a spectrum of forms of TNC organization, a diversity of developmental trajectories in which consciously planned global operations exist side-by-side with firms that have internationalized in an unplanned, often adventitious, way. Across the spectrum, complex restructuring is occurring at all geographic scales, from the global to the local, as strategic decisions have to be made regarding the organizational coordination and geographic configuration of production chain functions. Decisions to centralize or decentralize decision-making powers, or to cluster or to disperse some or all of the firm's functions in particular ways are, however, contested decisions (Stopford and Strange, 1991), the outcome of power struggles within firms, both within their headquarters and between headquarters and affiliates, and they reflect differences in goals and objectives. How they are resolved depends very much upon the location and nature of the dominant coalition. Such decisions also have to be seen within the context of the fundamental tension facing all firms that operate at a global scale: whether to globalize fully or to respond to local differentiation.

State–State Interaction: The Emergence of the "Competition State"

Having discussed one element of the triangular nexus of interactions identified earlier – firm–firm competition – I now want to address the second element: competition between states. Here, I deliberately avoid discussion of the nature of the state, while accepting that the competitive aspect of state behavior is itself deeply politically, socially, and culturally embedded. My basic approach is that the state in the contemporary global economy may be legitimately regarded as a competition state, whose problem is one of facing "major adjustments to shifts in competitive advantage in the global market place" (Cerny, 1991, p. 183). In this respect, states take on some of the characteristics of firms as they strive to develop strategies to create competitive advantage (Guisinger, 1985). Both are, in effect, locked in competitive struggles to capture global market shares. Specifically, states compete to enhance their international trading position and to capture as large a share as possible of the gains from trade. They compete to attract productive investment to build up their national production base, which, in turn, enhances their competitive position. In particular, states strive to create, capture, and maintain the higher value-adding elements of the production chain.

All states perform a key role in the ways in which their economies operate, although they differ substantially in the specific measures they employ and in the precise ways in which such measures are combined. Although a high level of contingency may be involved (no two states behave in exactly the same way), certain regularities in basic policy stance can be identified. Dahrendorf (1968) distinguished between two ideal types of political economy: the market-rational and the plan-rational. He equated the latter with the state socialist command economies. Johnson (1982), in his seminal work on the growth of the Japanese economy, argued that these command economies were better described as plan-ideological systems, and he applied the term plan-rational to the economies of East Asia, notably Japan and the then-leading NIEs, particularly of South Korea, Taiwan, and Singapore.

Recently, Henderson and Appelbaum (1992) have suggested that a fourth ideal type can be recognized: the market-ideological, which, they suggest, was epitomized by the Reagan and Thatcher "new right" administrations. As always, such simplified typologies require a "health warning," which Henderson and Appelbaum duly provide: "These four constructs (market rational, plan rational, market ideological, and plan ideological) should be regarded as ideal types; actual existing political economies combine them in various historically contingent ways. Still, for any particular society, one will typically dominate, facilitating an overall characterization of its prevailing political economy" (1992, p. 20).

Allowing for these caveats, it is not unreasonable to regard many of the current politico-economic tensions in the global economy as being a reflection of a clash between competition states occupying different positions within the market-rational/plan-rational space. Certainly, the smoldering – occasionally incandescent and inflammatory – disputes between Japan and many Western economies (notably the United States and the European Community) can usefully be set within this context. The various trade disputes between the United States and the European Community and the broader negotiating differences among nations within the Uruguay Round of the GATT can also be interpreted in this way.

The position of states is not necessarily fixed. In this respect, one of the most notable developments of the last few years has been the growing pressure within the most dominant market-ideological state, the United States, for a more overtly strategic policy orientation. The demand in the United States in particular is for a shift away from "free" trade toward "fair" trade – "fairness" being defined by the United States itself. An early sign of this shift in emphasis was apparent in the 1974

US Trade Act; it became quite explicit in the 1988 Omnibus Trade and Competitiveness Act, especially in the so-called "super 301" clause, which aimed to achieve reciprocal access to what the United States defines as unfairly restricted markets. The difference between the 1974 and 1988 Acts is that the clause now applies to entire countries and not, as before, to specific industries. These shifts toward a more strategic policy are particularly evident in high-technology sectors, seen to be at the center of a country's future competitive position. The basic rationale is that, in imperfectly competitive markets, governments must intervene in favor of their domestic firms (Encarnation, 1992; Ostry, 1990). As Ostry (1990) points out, the argument is based upon two issues: "the 'first mover advantage' that a country or firm captures by preempting foreign rivals . . . (which) . . . provides the opportunity for firms and countries to consolidate and extend their competitive advantage" (p. 60), and the issue of externalities or spillovers that enhance the competitiveness of other parts of the domestic economy.

Within market-rational/market-ideological economies like the United States, the pressures for adoption of a more strategic oriented policy emanate from a variety of interest groups (primarily specific industry and labor union lobbies) that may have a particular geographic dimension. Wade and Gates's (1990) analysis of the 1987 vote in the House of Representatives on the Gephardt Amendment to the 1988 Omnibus Trade Act revealed a reordering of the historical regional divisions over trade policy. "Although the old industrial core in the North Atlantic and Great Lakes remains the most protectionist area, the once dependably liberal South now contains much stronger protectionist sentiment than was ever true in the past. And the historically protectionist West, particularly the Northwest, has displaced the South as the regional nucleus of liberal trade opinion in Congress" (Wade and Gates, 1990, p. 297).

One of the diagnostic characteristics of the market-rational (and market-ideological) state is its concern with the regulatory structures in the economy. In such states, a marked feature of the past 10 to 15 years has been the drive toward the deregulation of specific sectors as a competitive weapon. As Cerny (1991) has perceptively observed, however, the process of deregulation is extremely complex; what is propounded as deregulation may actually involve re-regulation in a different form or at a different geographic or political scale.

Each of these measures – from the piecemeal use of trade, industry, and foreign direct investment policies in market-rational/ideological states to their more coherent application in plan-rational states – reflects the diverse attempts by competition states to operate in the volatile environment of the global economy. States, like firms, pursue competitive strategies, although their strategic tool kits are, of course, somewhat different. Another parallel between the competitive behavior of firms and states is that just as firms, especially TNCs, have shown an increasing propensity to enter into collaborative agreements with other firms, so, too, do many nation-states display the same collaborative propensity. As in the case of firms, interstate collaboration can range from the simple bilateral arrangement over a single issue to the complex collaborative network of a supranational economic bloc. Although there are many examples of supranational trading blocs in the global economy, most are relatively ineffectual and some are little more than paper agreements. Such groupings are essentially discriminatory and defensive. They represent an attempt to gain advantages of size in trade and investment by creating large multinational markets for their domestic producers within a framework of protection. As such, they may either create or divert trade, and it is this latter potential that produces apprehension, and possible counteraction, by nonmembers.

One of the major developments in the global economy in recent years has been the strengthening of supranational economic integration in two of the three "global triad" regions and at least the hint of a similar future development in the third. The trend toward increased supranational economic integration is a further aspect of the operation of the competition state. But there are political counterpressures allegedly at work in which increasing emphasis is being placed on the local and regional (i.e., subnational) level. Particularly in Europe, as the momentum toward European integration has increased, the calls for greater degrees of local/regional political and economic autonomy have also grown. The idea of a "Europe of the regions" rather than of nation-states has considerable currency in some quarters. The notion of a shift toward the "local economy," or even the "local state," is embedded in the idea of a transition from Fordism to post-Fordism, the new dynamics of flexible accumulation, and the alleged emergence of new industrial districts (Moulaert and Swyngedouw, 1989; Moulaert, Swyngedouw, and Wilson, 1988; A. J. Scott, 1988b).

Suggestive as these ideas are of, on the one hand, a shift toward supranational integration or, on the other, a move toward greater local economic autonomy, they do not signify the demise of the nation-state as a significant global actor. There is a real need, as Gertler has argued, to "reinstate the nation-state":

> it should be pointed out that, in contrast to the rhetoric of free trade, countries will continue to retain many powers and markets will not be completely and unequivocally "opened up." Although the more subtle powers to harmonize social and economic policies across nations will be strong, the intensified competition expected to prevail will, if anything, enhance the importance of fostering a supportive national system for innovation. Consequently, it is difficult to see how the rise of supranational blocs will undermine these particular powers of the nation-state. (Gertler, 1992, pp. 270–1)

Firm–State Interactions: Dynamic Bargaining Relationships

The third element in the triangular nexus of international interactions is that between firms and states. This is not as straightforward as it may seem, because the actual processes and forms of firm–state interactions at an international scale are deeply intertwined with firm–firm and, especially, state–state interactions. For example, much of the friction between the United States and Japan is actually a dispute between firms, between states, and between states and firms as perceived agents of states. Similar to the situation in the 1960s, when the activities of United States TNCs were seen by many as being a direct extension of United States foreign policy, so today the behavior of Japanese firms is perceived (especially in the United States) as being part of a Japanese strategy of world dominance. The relationships between international firms and nation-states are a complex mixture of conflict and collaboration. The TNC seeks to maximize its freedom to locate its production chain components in the most advantageous locations for the firm as a whole in its pursuit of global profits or global market share. At the same time, the individual state wishes to maximize its share of value-adding activity. As a result, the relationship between firms and states is inevitably an uneasy one (Gordon, 1988; Pitelis, 1991; Stopford and Strange, 1991).

Firm–state interactions tend to differ according to whether the relationship is between a firm and its home country government or a host country government. This does not imply that the former relations are necessarily harmonious and the latter necessarily conflictual. Indeed, many bitter disputes between firms and states have occurred where a state fears that its "domestic" firms are shifting operations overseas or, conversely, where firms allege that their home country government provides inadequate support against external competition. The position, therefore, is extremely complex.

My basic position – contrary to that of Reich (1991) or Ohmae (1990) – is that a TNC's domestic environment remains fundamentally important to how it operates, notwithstanding the global extent of some firms' operations. TNCs are not placeless; all have an identifiable home base, a base that ensures that every TNC is essentially embedded within its domestic environment. Of course, the more extensive a firm's international operations, the more likely it will be to take on additional characteristics. Few, if any, major TNCs have moved their ultimate decision-making operations out of their country (often their community) of origin. The argument that, in effect, there is no longer any real relationship between a firm and its home base is, like many statements in the popular business literature, a considerable exaggeration. Of course, as organizational structures have changed, as hierarchies have "flattened," as network forms have become increasingly significant, things are no longer as simple as they once were. Nevertheless, despite many decades of operation as a TNC, Ford is still essentially a US company, ICI a British company, Siemens a German company. As Stopford and Strange (1991, p. 233) point out, "However great the global reach of their operations, the national firm does, psychologically and sociologically, 'belong' to its home base."

This is not to argue that TNCs necessarily retain a "loyalty" to the states in which they originated. The nature of the embeddedness process is far more complex and national economic welfare is no longer necessarily equated with the performance of national companies (Reich, 1991; Tyson, 1993). But the point I am making is that TNCs are "produced" through a complex historical process of embedding (Dicken and Thrift, 1992), in which the cognitive, cultural, social, political, and economic characteristics of the national home base play a dominant part. TNCs, therefore, are "bearers" of such characteristics, which then interact with the place-specific characteristics of the countries in which they operate to produce a particular outcome. But the point is that the home-base characteristics invariably remain dominant.

This is not to claim that TNCs of a particular national origin are identical; this is self-evidently not the case – but, rather, to argue that there are greater similarities than differences among such firms. Insofar as the nation-state acts as a "container" of distinctive institutions and practices, it remains significant as an influence on the nature of the TNC. Whitley's (1992a, 1992b) work on comparative business systems is especially relevant. Whitley's concern is to counteract the views of the "economic rationalists" that "competitive markets select efficient forms of business organizations and destroy inefficient ones ... that underlying market pressures ensure that the firms which survive by competing successfully in international markets will converge to the same efficient structure, practices and strategic decisions which 'fit' particular technology and market imperatives" (Whitley, 1992a, p. 2). In contrast, Whitley develops the concept of the "business system," which he defines as "particular arrangements of hierarchy market relations which become institutionalized and relatively successful in particular contexts" (1992a, p. 10).

Whitley's analysis, based upon a detailed multidimensional comparison of business systems in East Asia and in Europe, helps to explain international variation in firm structures and behavior, including, for example, the marked differences between Japanese (and other East Asian) business structures on the one hand and those found in the Anglo-Saxon and continental European systems on the other. It adds some depth to the ideal types of political economic system discussed in the previous section. Taken together, these concepts help to clarify our understanding of the complex relationships between firms and their domestic environments, as well as the conflictual economic relationships between firms and states. They illuminate such issues as different state attitudes toward their home firms, including the issue of the "national champion" (Amin, 1992; Reich, 1991) and the bases of such distinctive organizational forms as the Korean chaebol and the Japanese keiretsu. The persistence of distinctive business systems, organized primarily (although not exclusively) within national boundaries, is an important underlying cause for the persistence of distinctive differences between TNCs of different national origins.

The second aspect of firm–state interactions I want to address is the response of firms to state regulatory structures (Dicken, 1992b). For the TNC, the two most critical aspects of state regulatory policy are, first, access to markets and/or resources (including human resources) and, second, rules of operation for firms operating within particular national (or supranational) jurisdictions (Reich, 1989). An obvious assumption would be that TNCs will invariably seek the removal of all regulatory barriers that act as constraints and impede their ability to locate wherever, and to behave however, they wish. The ultimate preference for TNCs would seem to be removal of all barriers to entry; freedom to export capital and profits from local operations; freedom to import materials, components, and operate services; freedom to operate unhindered in local labor markets. Certainly, given the existence of differential regulatory structures in the global economy, TNCs will seek to overcome, circumvent, or subvert them. Regulatory mechanisms are, indeed, constraints on a TNC's strategic and operational behavior.

Yet it is not quite as simple as this. The very existence of regulatory structures may be perceived as an opportunity available to TNCs to take advantage of regulatory differences between states by shifting activities between locations according to differentials in the regulatory surface – that is, to engage in regulatory arbitrage (Leyshon, 1992). One aspect of this is the propensity of TNCs to stimulate competitive bidding for their mobile investments by playing off one state against another as states strive to outbid their rivals to capture or retain a particular TNC activity

(Dicken, 1990; Encarnation and Wells, 1986; Guisinger, 1985; Glickman and Woodward, 1989). More generally, TNCs have a somewhat ambivalent attitude to state regulatory policies (Picciotto, 1991; Rugman and Verbeke, 1992; Yoffie and Milner, 1989). For example, Picciotto (1991) notes that

> TNCs have favoured minimal international coordination while strongly supporting the national state, since they can take advantage of regulatory differences and loopholes ... While TNCs have pressed for an adequate coordination of national regulation, they have generally resisted any strengthening of international state structures. ... Having secured the minimalist principles of national treatment for foreign-owned capital, TNCs have been the staunchest defenders of the national state. It is their ability to exploit national differences, both politically and economically, that gives them their competitive advantage. (1991, pp. 43, 46)

Pitelis (1991) proposes that the relationship between TNCs and nation-states should be analyzed within a rivalry and collusion framework, arguing that "the degree of rivalry and collusion will depend heavily on whether the relationship refers to TNCs' own states or 'host' states as well as whether the states in question are 'strong' or 'weak,' DCs or LDCs" (p. 142). Whether or not a particular situation is one of rivalry or collusion, the essence of the TNC–state relationship is one of overt or covert bargaining (Doz, 1986; Gabriel, 1966; Kobrin, 1987; Poynter, 1985; Stopford and Strange, 1991). As Nixson points out, "it is this process that in large part determines the extent, nature, and distribution between the participating agents of the costs and benefits that arise as a result of direct foreign investment" (1988, p. 318). Little progress has been made, however, in providing either a satisfactory conceptual or empirical basis for understanding these complex relational processes. Stopford and Strange (1991, pp. 134–6) are especially critical of the current literature on bargaining processes in the international relations and international business literature. Part of the problem, of course, is that such bargaining is itself the complex outcome of a myriad of negotiating and bargaining processes within both firms and states as different interest groups and stakeholders themselves attempt to influence the larger-scale bargaining position.

Virtually all the relevant research into TNC–state bargaining relationships has focused on only one set of relationships, those between TNCs and host governments. In such circumstances, the outcome will be a function of the interaction between three elements: (1) the relative demand by each party for resources which the other controls; (2) the constraints on each that affect the translation of potential bargaining power into control over resources; and (3) the negotiating status of the participants involved. It is important to emphasize that the nature of the bargaining process and of the outcome will probably differ according to which part of the production chain is involved. The bargaining stakes on both sides will be much higher for the scarcer, high value-adding functions than for the more ubiquitous functions. Ultimately, however, as Gabriel states so succinctly,

> The price which the receiving country will ultimately pay is a function of (1) the number of foreign firms independently competing for the investment opportunity; (2) the

recognized measure of uniqueness of the foreign contribution (as against its possible provision by local entrepreneurship, public or private); (3) the perceived degree of domestic need for the contribution. The terms the foreign investor will accept, on the other hand, depend on his [sic] general need for an investment outlet; (2) the attractiveness of the specific investment opportunity offered by the host country compared to similar or other opportunities in other countries; (3) the extent of prior commitment to the country concerned (e.g. an established market position). (Gabriel, 1966, p. 114)

The problem, of course, is that the whole process is dynamic; the bargaining relationship changes over time. In most studies of state–TNC bargaining the conventional wisdom is that of the so-called obsolescing bargain, in which, after the initial investment, the balance of bargaining power shifts from the TNC to the host government. This is the situation found most commonly in natural resource-based investments in developing countries. It is less certain, however, that such a relationship will apply in sectors in which technological change is rapid and/or where global integration of operations is the norm (Kobrin, 1987). Even in the case of TNC–host country relationships the current state of research is far from adequate; in the case of bargaining between TNCs and home countries the literature is even sparser.

Conclusion: The Global–Local Debate Revisited

The thread running throughout this paper has been the fact that, within a volatile competitive environment, both firms and states as competitive institutions are subject to fundamental global–local tensions. But precisely what is meant by "global" and "local" is itself problematical and has different meanings for firms, and states. To the firm, the global–local tension is expressed as the question of whether to "globalize" or to "localize" or whether to strive to combine the two in a stance of "global localization." In this case, "local" generally means "national"; the issues are those of the autonomy and responsiveness of national components of the international firm. From the nation-state perspective, the global–local problematic means something rather different. The pressures toward certain kinds of putative supranational organization at one extreme are counterpoised against a pressure toward greater degrees of local political autonomy at the other. The current debates within the European Community around the issue of "subsidiarity" are a reflection of this, as are the growing demands of local states for greater independence. But it is the interaction between international firms and nation-states that gives the global–local problematic a particular twist. To the international firm, the division of the global political map along nation-state boundaries, with the extent of market and factor differentiation this implies, constitutes the major pressure to be sensitive to local differences even while pursuing a global strategy. To the nation-state, the international firm is one of the major channels through which globalizing forces are directed.

The relationship between TNCs and states (at whatever level) is, self-evidently, a power relationship. There is little doubt that, in general terms, the relative power of TNCs and states has shifted, but the position is far less straightforward than has often been supposed. In view of the complexity and degree of contingency of the bargaining process, it is difficult to make broad generalizations about the relative "balance of power" between TNCs and states. There is no doubt that in some areas, most notably that of financial policy, states have become increasingly less able to determine, with impunity, such things as the external value of their currencies. The development of a global financial system, facilitated by electronic trading mechanisms, has vastly increased the exposure of state financial policies to external speculative forces. Some very unwise generalizations have been made over the years, however, which have been used to write the premature obituary of the nation-state. In contrast, Stopford and Strange's view is that

> governments as a group have indeed lost bargaining power to the multinationals. . . . Does it follow that firms as a group have increased their bargaining power over the factors of production? Here, the argument becomes complex, for the power of the individual firm may be regarded as having also fallen as competition has intensified. New entrants have altered the rules and offer governments new bargaining advantage. One needs to separate the power to influence general policy from the power to insist on specific bargains. (Stopford and Strange, 1991, pp. 215–16)

It is this issue of the "specific bargain" that is most relevant to the question of what the processes discussed in this paper mean for the "really seriously local," the local community or region currently being buffeted by the stormy seas of global economic change. The problem facing the local community, in the global scheme of things, is that it is relatively powerless except in very specific circumstances (for example, where it possesses a unique or scarce resource that gives it some leverage). The idea that the transformations that are occurring in the organization of production systems (notably the growth of network organizations and relationships) will automatically lead to a general enhancement of local economic opportunity and well-being is a pipe dream.

The evidence that changes in customer–supplier relations (both inside and outside the firm) will lead to greater local integration is mixed. As McGrath and Hoole (1992) show, global sourcing is far from dead. It is certainly true that customer–supplier relationships do involve a greater emphasis on long-term, closer relationships based upon a high level of mutual trust and that this may be facilitated by geographical proximity. Firms are, however, increasingly operating an upper tier of preferred suppliers that are closely integrated at all stages of the production process, from design to final production. For any one firm, such preferred suppliers are relatively few in number and unevenly distributed geographically. Not every local economy, therefore, can hope to participate in the new integrated networks (Amin, 1992; Amin and Malmberg, 1992).

Ultimately, therefore, it may be that, because of the immense asymmetry of power between TNCs and local institutions, there is little that such institutions can do on their own other than to provide an attractive business environment or to attempt to stimulate the kinds of local businesses that might eventually be embedded in a TNC network. Although much depends on the extent to which a national political system is centralized or decentralized, virtually all effective bargaining power lies not at the local level but at the national level or, in cases like the

European Community, at a supranational level. To that degree, therefore, the prospects of local economies will be influenced as much, if not more, by national policies as by local actions. Within the global–local nexus, the key interactions, in a power sense, remain at the level of the TNC and the nation-state; in that respect, the "seriously local" is a serious problem whose solution requires a broader policy framework.

Chapter 10

The Politics of Relocation: Gender, Nationality, and Value in a Mexican Maquiladora

M. W. Wright

To study changes in corporate decision-making is also to consider the processes for forming social relations and culturally constructed understandings which influence patterns of authority, status, and the meanings of value (Schoenberger, 1997). For example, when emphasis lies on cutting labor costs and enhancing worker productivity, corporate decision-makers often rank the human resources found in different places by correlating certain identities, such as national and gendered ones, with labor skills, innate abilities, and militancy, to name a few features. These methods for comparing the intrinsic traits of one pool of labor against another located in another place reveal how human resources are understood and evaluated through dynamic processes of social construction inside the firm.

In this paper my argument rests on the assumption that corporate managers have, as a group, social power for connecting certain kinds of people with the production of certain kinds of value in the firm. However, their power in the class structure of a capitalist workplace is not independent of the other social relations of power, such as gender and race, that contribute to the formation of hierarchical differences among people within a particular context. In elaborating this assumption, I attempt to illustrate how the managers of a multinational maquiladora establish patterns for correlating the national and sex differences which they identify among their employees with the manufacture of valuable goods. By concentrating on these two social characteristics, I do not intend to imply that others, especially age, race, and wellness, are not of issue in the workplace I explore. Rather, in narrowing my focus to the interplay of nationality, gender, and value, I show that the production of valuable commodities is a social process interwoven with the social construction of differential values in people, and that this process has an impact upon the internal structure of the firm.

This sort of argument emerges from a theoretical dialogue between Marx's critique of the labor theory of value and a poststructuralist feminist emphasis on the productive power behind establishing social identities and their differences (see also Joseph, 1998). Through his critique of capital, Marx reveals a visceral connection linking the manufacture of commodities with the conceptualization of people as embodiments of a specific value which can be transferred to inanimate objects that no longer belong to them. The value of the capitalist good depends upon an ability to imagine people also in terms of value. However, as feminist scholars across disciplines have shown, a strict class analysis limits any inquiry into the complex connections binding the value of things to the people who make them (Kondo, 1990; McDowell, 1997; J. Scott, 1988b). They emphasize how the evaluation of a worker's value to the firm rests upon discourses that regulate the interpretation of the meaning of that worker as a social subject. The performance of work is not independent of one performance, say, as a gendered, sexualized, and raced subject, as the value of one's work emerges through lenses bent on interpreting the value of one's other features.

For this reason, in my study of the politics of relocation within a multinational maquila, I combine a Marxist with a poststructuralist feminist approach to explore how the vicissitudes of value found in people can complicate corporate managers' habits of finding value in their products. A disruption to their historical patterns of recognizing value in people and in the things they make is enough, at least in my estimation of what happened in the case I explore, to justify their costly decision to relocate a critical operation out of Mexico and back to the USA.

The material for my argument originates with a ten-month ethnographic project I conducted between 1993 and 1994 in the maquiladora which I shall refer to as Mexico On the Water (MOTW). This facility represents the Mexican location of a multinational US firm, On the Water (OTW), which manufactures motors, boats, and other water-sporting equipment in operations located in Asia, Europe, South America, and in the USA. MOTW set up shop in Ciudad Juarez in the early years of maquiladora development. It was the first maquila actively to seek male employees at least a decade before it was deemed necessary to compensate for a shortage of female workers in the local labor market. In an interview conducted in 1992, the first General Manager of MOTW had explained that he intentionally excluded women from the labor force: "This is a tool shop, and the girls out here are not the right kind of worker for what we do. Our products are men's products, and I think the men, here or anywhere, understand the work better." In the early, 1990s, however, MOTW expanded its operation to include electronic assembly and began hiring women. This transition raised some harrowing challenges for the MOTW managers.

At MOTW, I studied how managers faced the challenge of producing quality goods with labor which they understood to be lacking in quality. This challenge takes on a particularly gendered and national dimension. These managers need to produce goods for a market which places a premium on American masculinity, a marker of quality in MOTW, and they evaluate their goods in terms of whether they reflect this desired condition. Yet, the MOTW managers attempted to accomplish their goal with laborers who, in their view, represented the opposite of this valuable masculine American condition. In an apparently contradictory move, they had hired Mexican women for a particular new operation specifically because these employees continue to be broadly construed as "dexterous," "patient," and "docile" enough to work under the exigencies of electronic assembly (Salzinger, 1997). At the same time, these women are also widely recognized throughout the industry as "cheap," "unprofessional," and not worth the trouble to train (Wright, 1997). The hiring of such workers signified a shift at MOTW from a factory with a purposely male labor force to one with a sizeable proportion of women. And this transition played havoc with their well-worn customs for recognizing value in MOTW products, peoples, and in the spaces of production that ultimately contributed to decisions about corporate location.

Theoretical Dialogues

In my inquiry into what was at stake when MOTW began hiring women I rely on a Marxist critique of the social construction of value in a capitalist setting. Capital, says Marx, is not concerned with producing just any kinds of things, but of particular things that embody value. This value can only be seen, recognized, and, in effect, valorized under the particular circumstances for evaluating different people as embodiments of a similar kind of value calculated as a condition of their labor.

Marxist scholars have elaborated on Marx's critique of the capitalist labor theory of value to emphasize the importance of understanding that the issue is not only about the construction of value in things, but also about its construction in the people who make those things. As David Harvey has put it:

"The paradox to be understood is how the freedom and transitoriness . . . of living labor as a process is objectified in a fixity of both things and exchange ratios between things." (1982, p. 23)

With this statement, Harvey pushes us to ask how the myriad energies that people express in their activities and in their thoughts can be understood as the conditions of a similar kind of value, which lends itself to quantification and qualification of a trait found in inanimate things. Thus, this is a process for viewing people as well as objects. Feminist scholar Diane Elson emphasizes how this sort of question involves "seeking an understanding of why labour takes the form it does, and [asking] what are the political consequences" (1979, p. 23, my parentheses).

These Marxian concerns are germane to my analysis, as the question that interests me here is not why Mexican women are paid so little for their labor but, instead, why does cheap labor assume a female Mexican form. How does a Mexican woman's labor take on a cheap fixity, and what is at stake in this transformation?

Yet even though I formulate this question with these Marxian critiques in mind, I cannot approach them from a strictly Marxist viewpoint. Feminist scholars have shown that any evaluation of labor as something of value courses through an evaluation of the different kinds of people who embody different properties of labor (Hanson and Pratt, 1988; Pratt, 1990; Rose, 1993). These feminist interventions have forced us to address how the historical constitution of women and racial minorities as laborers of inferior degrees of value have underscored the long-held industrial traditions of paying them less and of not recognizing the skill in what they do.

Taking these feminist interventions as a point of departure, I rely upon a particular kind of feminist scholarship to explore the dilemmas raised by Harvey (1982) and Elson (1979), in relation to certain events at MOTW. Of specific interest to me is Judith Butler's poststructuralist views on materialization: she argues that the social construction of the subject is not an end in itself (1993, 1997). Instead, the constructed subject contributes to a productive continuum, in which the particular identity of the subject is both a product and a producer. The subject is a thing with reverberating productive effects that do not necessarily travel in one particular direction. So, although I look at the social construction of the Mexican woman as the living standard for low-quality production in an American maquila, I do not view this construction of her as a terminus for productive flows. Rather, as the embodiment of low quality, she produces low quality if traces of her are found in the things she makes. In other words, she is not simply marked as a paragon of low value, she marks other things as the bearers of low value. And within the historical MOTW framework for manufacturing quality boat parts, her image as the low-value laborer extends to all products that bear her mark. The trick, therefore, for MOTW managers, is to guarantee that she disappears from the things that she makes. When they fail in this endeavor, they prefer to ship out the product line rather than risk devaluation.

In what follows, I present my material juxtaposing my observations with conversations and interviews conducted over a protracted period of time. The ethnography amplifies the ambiguous details behind the decisions which managers explain as cost-saving or market-enhancing treasures. In the firm I explore here, I had an office located in the administrative area where I was granted unlimited access to meetings, files, and to employees as much as they would tolerate my inquiries. Through conversations and more formal interviews, my informants exposed the politicized negotiations over the meanings of the very categories which are factors in the assessments of corporate efficiency and cost effectiveness, especially with regard to the assessment of people as some kind of valuable resource. Instead, I focus on how managers describe their laborers, with an eye to understanding how their own evaluations of people and the kinds of value they embody and manufacture affect their decisions governing the internal structure of the firm.

Making American

Even though MOTW is a Mexican subsidiary of its parent corporation, the corporate literature reinforces the idea that not only is MOTW an American business, but that all MOTW products are American, no matter where they are produced. The authors of one of the official biographies of the company chronicle "the progress of this American institution" from the patriotic application of OTW technology, motors, and boats in US war efforts, to MOTW's commitment to supporting the US sportsman tradition, and to fighting Japanese "incursions" into the global market. The General Manager of MOTW operations, Steve, explained: "This is an American company to the core." To visualize the Americanness of this Mexican subsidiary, I will begin with the spatial layout of the facility. Within the spatial relations of production, we find determined efforts to buttress the functioning of an American system and the production of unmistakably American things by Mexican laborers.

MOTW consists of two facilities: plants I and II, each with its own production manager, engineering, and American-led supervisory teams who oversee 42 product lines and almost 800 Mexican employees. A Human Resources Manager,

Materials Manager, and Engineering Manager are responsible for the operations of both facilities and answer to the General Manager, who is the primary liaison with clients and other corporate offices. The MOTW administrative area is separated from the production area by a solid wooden door, which is guarded by a security officer who prevents unauthorized individuals from passing into the administrative interior. Inside this protected space, English is the dominant language. As Roger, the Production Manager of the Plant II facility said to me: "This is an American company, so you've got to expect the administration to be English-speaking." The production area, by contrast, is a world of Spanish, where the bulk of MOTW's employees, who are monolingual Spanish speakers, work.

However, managers explain that, even though the vast majority of MOTW's production employees are Mexican, the factory is American by virtue of American control over the labor process. "This is the brains of the operation," the former General Manager told me when describing the administrative area, "we control everything from here." The people in charge are to be American at all times, as is reflected in the corporation's policy which does not allow for any Mexican to hold a position of authority over an American: "You would expect the top people to be American employees here," said Burt, the Manager of Plant I; "We make American products and we need people who understand that."

Corporate policy mandates that all those in management-positions at MOTW be either US citizens or possess a US green card and reside in US territory. Therefore any nonnative US citizen must apply for residency and a green card and pay taxes to the US government in order to qualify for a promotion into management. As a result, a Mexican national promoted into management is, for all intents and purposes, an American employee. Under these rules, it is thus impossible for a Mexican employee to wield corporate authority over an American one. And in those cases where an American and a Mexican employee share the same title, the American employee receives higher wages and supervises the Mexican supervisor. Understanding the national border within the corporation's division of labor is key for individual career strategies in a place where to "Americanize" is to climb and to "Mexicanize" is to descend the social ladder of power and prestige (see Wright, 1998).

When I asked Steve, the General Manager, if he thought the company would ever have Mexican managers – that is managers who were classified as Mexican personnel – he replied: "If we ever try to get into the Mexican market, sure. But as long as we're selling these boats in America, I don't see it happening." Within the logic internal to MOTW, there was a connection linking the national identities of MOTW employees with the marketability of MOTW goods. Even though all labor is technically absorbed in the product, and thereby made invisible according to Marx, the identity of this labor is brought to the surface through marketing strategies that emphasize national content such as "Made in America." MOTW products, in the end, bear the mark "Made in America," the boat and engines undergo final assembly for the US market in the United States. Steve and the other MOTW managers, however, felt a need to guarantee that the internal operations of the factory did not disrupt the identification of MOTW products as American made. The labor itself might be invisible, but its social identity is part and parcel of the process for manufacturing value. For this reason, any identifiable traces of female

Mexican labor within MOTW goods were especially dangerous according to MOTW managers.

The Invisible MOTW Women

Whereas the "Americanization" of the product is assured by the American brains behind its manufacture, the masculinity of the product is protected by the masculinization of the labor process. On my first tour of MOTW in 1992, the then-General Manager, Bob, guided me through the carburetor-assembly area, which he called "the heart" of the operation, which dominates the one large room in Plant I, and then through the "computer numerical control" area that dominates the space in the other part of the building. We observed engineers at their computers and desks, and we walked through the painting section that was soon to be transferred out of the facility. With the exception of the secretarial staff, all of the employees I saw were men. And it was not until the following year, when I began my ethnographic study, that I discovered the women, who then composed about 35% of the production labor force and worked behind the male labor processes. Off in the corners and against the back walls they assembled ignition switches, horns, drive shafts, and fuel systems. They cut and spliced wires and manufactured gauges for dashboards. When I asked the Manager of Plant I, Burt, in 1994, why the former General Manager had not shown me those female work areas, he said, "Bob was proud of our carburetor and tooling operations. We were the first maquila to have those type of operations and to be successful . . . We have the girls in electronic assembly but that's not what we're known for."

The spatial arrangement of male and female workspaces successfully squirreled the women out of view and away from the "heart" of MOTW production. This spatial practice both revealed and embraced a managerial discourse of MOTW as a "man's shop," while the women worked invisibly behind dust-proof doors and against rear walls to fashion the "incidentals" of motor-boat production. The current General Manager, Steve, explained: "We think of ourselves as a tool shop. And across the industry the belief is that men are better at this work than females. It's a macho place. No doubt about it."

Such explanations contributed to a representation pervasive through the maquilas of the Mexican woman as (a) especially suited for unskilled electronic assembly of low-end goods, and (b) particularly unsuited for engineering work, skilled jobs, or any tasks deemed "physical" (Salzinger, 1997). Still, in 1993 women were already putting together many of MOTW products, and by 1997 about half of the 800 production workers were women – a shift having to do with the other pervasive construction of Mexican women as dexterous and innately deft with tedious hair-splitting tasks. Roger, the Manager of Plant II, said, in 1994, "Things are definitely changing here. Plant II is mainly electronic work, and we've just got that going over the last three years. That means we're hiring more female workers because they're good at this work." Steve said, "I think when we decided to put the electronic operations down here it was because we knew that women in Mexico had experience with electrical assembly. And it made more sense to do it here for a lot less money than we were doing it in Europe or in the US." The Human

Resource Manager, Rosalia, explained that MOTW actively pursued female workers for the electrical assembly operations: "Women here are very good with electrical assembly. They have more patience and are better with their hands," she told me.

The hiring of women to work in electrical assembly raised a paradox for the managers of MOTW. Although their labor process had shifted from a purely "man's tool shop" to one including "women's" electrical assembly work, the product, a decidedly man's product, had not changed. When I asked Steve if he thought OTW customers knew that Mexican women were assembling some of their products, he said, "No, and it's my job to make sure they don't find out." The social construction of Mexican women as naturally suited for electronic assembly did not shift their construction as not suited for making MOTW products. If anything, it intensified the managerial conviction that their control over the labor process was even more critical. Now they would not only have to concern themselves with the Americanization of the product, they would also have to supervise its masculinization.

This challenge can be seen in light of the twofold problem raised by the social constructions of MOTW products and of Mexican women as entities of contrasting values. First, the process of social construction is never complete. In order for MOTW products to be seen as "American" and "masculine" they had continually to be seen as the opposite of "Mexican" and "feminine." This process gained backing from managerial efforts to explain that the value in MOTW products was other than the typical value found in electronic feminized maquila production. As the managers reiterated how their products were of a superior caliber compared with an assembly-line television, they repeatedly emphasized how those products associated with female Mexican labor were of inferior quality and value, as opposed to the masculine ones emerging from MOTW.

Second, and related to the first problem, the construction of the Mexican women as incapable of producing masculine value also exercises a productive effect. As Judith Butler (1993) argues, there is no reference to a body that is not, at the same time, a further production of that body. It can then be said, in the case of labor, that there is no reference to someone's labor power (that is, what is exchanged for wages) without further producing a quality of his or her labor. As a result, to view the Mexican woman as naturally adept with electronic assembly and cheap because she has no skills, is at once a construction of her labor as cheap, even as its cheapness generates more wealth for capital. The trick is to take advantage of cheap labor power without jeopardizing the value of the product. At MOTW, this challenge means guaranteeing that no evidence of Mexican women is found in the things that they make. The value of their labor power resides both in its cheapness and in its disappearance from MOTW's quality products.

The complexities underlying this task become clear in the following elaboration of gauge production at MOTW. In this case, we shall see how concerns over the inner workings and outer marking of the Mexican woman's body lead to fears that Mexican women, in electronic assembly, are infiltrating the male spaces of MOTW production and authority and, thereby, threatening the masculine products and the masculine firm with contamination and devaluation.

The Gauges

The events surrounding the short-lived gauge-production operation at MOTW reveal the contradictions inherent to manufacturing a product of high quality with a labor process full of low-quality people. And this transformation absorbed managers from its beginning. Gauge production is a critical operation, with ramifications for client safety and the overall esthetic appeal of the boat. This critical operation had been sent to Mexico from one of the US facilities after Steve, the General Manager, won what he called "a bloody turf battle" with his counterpart in MOTW's China facility. Questions were raised over whether the Mexico facility could handle the task. Steve convinced them that, under his watch, gauges would be up to standard: "My neck is on the line," he told me.

MOTW sought young women for this operation. Rosalia explained: "The younger girls have flexible hands. This area involves a lot of work with fine wires and small pieces." However, expectations for these young women's careers were not high. "I don't think many of them will be here for a long time," Rosalia continued, "Most will come and go. They will start families. These aren't the workers who have the discipline to learn and go through training. That's how it is in the maquilas with electrical assembly. It's not the workers who really want to learn and improve themselves."

MOTW brought in a female American supervisor, Mary, to work with these "unskilled" and nonambitious "girls" to produce the quality-sensitive gauges. MOTW had another woman supervisor in the horn and ignition assembly areas, located against the back wall of Plant I, but Mary was to be the first woman to supervise a "critical" area. Like the other American supervisors, Mary was Mexican-American, bilingual, and had previous experience in manufacturing. When she accepted this position she came out of retirement after a twenty-year career as a supervisor in a clothing maquila. Steve explained why they hired her: "She had experience with sewing operations and had a good reputation. And we knew that this operation would have mainly females because it is electronic assembly." "I always like a challenge," Mary told me as she described why she came out of her brief stint as a "full-time grandmother" helping her daughter with childcare, "My family is a working family." In the summer of 1993, Mary returned to the maquila labor force. "They told me I would be in a sensitive area. That our quality would have to be very good. I knew I was working with young kids. . . . You always do in the maquilas."

Her job was to supervise 35 employees, mostly women in their late teens and early twenties, in the start up of the gauge-production line. The making of gauges entails a painstaking inspection process. Almost half of the workers were inspectors of some sort. They either tested product functions, inspected for paint consistency, or ran durability tests. The production line began when an automatic winder wrapped fine copper wire tightly around a bobbin; this would then be tested for current flow and placed in a housing, after which more wires would be attached, more tests run, and then the painted dial face connected. Only two operators had the delicate task of stamping on the dial face – a process requiring a steady hand and unwavering attention to detail. Two more inspection steps preceded the sealing of the gauge, which was followed by a final test before they would be packaged and shipped to the final assembly plant in Georgia.

Isolated behind the dust-proof doors and in a windowless room, the laborers in gauge production did their work beyond the notice of the rest of the facility. "I guess you could walk around this plant," said Roger, "and never know those girls are back there." And Mary had explicit instructions not to allow the workers to leave their area without permission, and to stagger restroom breaks so that no more than one worker left the area at a time. All of the gauge workers wore gender-distinguished uniforms, and all the women had to cover their hair completely with hair nets – a policy which was only sporadically enforced for the few men in the area. Men wore the nets like caps, over the top of their heads, whereas the women pulled the nets completely down to their necks. Mary explained this preoccupation over women's hair: "Well they're all supposed to wear the nets. But we let the guys just sort of stick them on top 'cause it bothers them more. They don't want the girls' long hair getting in the paint or in the wires. It's the girls we worry about the most."

This heightened attention to evidence of femininity, such as long hair and miniskirts, extended to other body parts as well. Mary described the policies regarding female appearance: "The girls can't wear fingernail polish . . . and we don't want pregnant girls in here. The fumes aren't good for them." Indeed, as in many maquilas, a policy both for refusing to hire pregnant women and for encouraging those who became pregnant to leave their job was tacitly enforced, although such practices violate federal legislation, prohibiting discrimination on the basis of pregnancy. "We all know we're not supposed to hire pregnant girls. It's that way in all the maquilas," said Mary. Roger, Manager of Plant II, echoed the sentiment behind these practices when he said: "We don't want pregnant women here. It's not good for the company and it's not good for them."

Consequently, the young women who worked in MOTW gauge production and who were subject to the practices concentrating on control of their hair, their nails, their clothing choice, and their wombs as they manufactured gauges in the back room of Plant II, also reinforced the traditional gendered pattern for delineating the social hierarchy of the MOTW division of labor. According to the payrolls of MOTW, the women in electronic assembly and gauge production received the lowest wage rates and, over time, had the highest turnover rate. Ramon, a supervisor in carburetors said: "The girls in electronic assembly are important but individually not as important as the guys out here. We need to work with them and try to keep them. The girls come for some experience and then leave when they want a family." Training, in short, is wasted on them. This view of the female employees as not worth training and as likely to leave because of their personal circumstances, rather than because they are not offered wage and training incentives, again reinforces a discourse, pervasive in the maquilas, of the inferior value of the female worker's labor.

Mary had to work with this assumption that training for women in electronic assembly was not warranted. "They put me in with a roomful of girls who didn't have any experience and expected us to do it right the first time," she said. "That's the problem, they want American quality, without the time." Steve explained: "I expected a slower system, but the quality needs to be up to standard. This is an American operation . . . and it's Mary's responsibility to make it work."

Female Contamination

In October 1994, after three months of production, almost two of every three gauges were defective and, making matters worse, demand for gauges was at a high as the company readied for the holiday season. Steve was receiving calls on an almost daily basis from his client – the final production assembly plant in Georgia – to discuss the gauges and predictions for a resolution of the problems. He in turn called meetings with Mary and her immediate boss, Roger. "We're shipping out Mexican product," he said in one such meeting, "And that's got to change."

Mary explained that the problem lay in technological systems and in the lack of training. "It's too much to learn and get good at in two months," she exclaimed in one meeting. In order to "make an American operation out of this," to use Roger's words, they agreed to take the following measures. Roger would tell maintenance that gauges were top priority and Mary would work overtime until things were back on track; within ten days, however, Steve was informed that not only was MOTW still shipping what he would call "Mexican" quality, but that also the lack of acceptable gauges had idled almost 100 workers in the Georgia facility. "I won't be shutting down Georgia!" he announced. By this time, Mary and the operators in her area were putting in 50 to 60 hours in a 6-day, and occasionally 7-day, work week. After a month of overtime in an anxious climate, the operators started to quit. In one week alone, Mary lost more than half of her employees and was spending more time on training new hires than anything else. One operator, an eighteen-year-old woman who had worked at MOTW for about six weeks, said: "We're killing ourselves in here. . . . They're always yelling at us and telling us that we're not doing it right. But they don't even give us time to learn how to do it."

Mary asked Steve for some more time to bring the workers up to speed and to lessen the pressure on everyone: "I've got more new workers than old ones," she said "And it's hard to teach them what to do and get everything out." Steve explained the impossibility of more time. "At this point," he said, "we don't have any time." He and the other managers repeatedly stressed the reasonableness of their expectation that Mexican women ought to be able to pick up this work with little training as this was the kind of work that comes naturally to women. As Burt said, "These girls do electrical assembly all the time."

Mary, exasperated with her bosses' refusal to allow her more training time, decided to take matters into her own hands. She made some *de facto* amendments to the work rules in the gauge area as a way of introducing some flexibility into the labor process while still expecting overtime from the workers. "I had to do something, or everyone would have left," she told me. Without her managers' authority, she immediately relaxed the uniform requirements. Everybody still had to wear the smocks, although she did not object to the women wearing male smocks, which some found more comfortable, and she allowed workers to remove their hairnets as long as their hair was pulled back. "Those things itch," she said, "and after a few hours you're ready to tear them off." She promised coffee and donuts for everyone on Saturdays and announced that anybody working on weekends could work a half day during the week without losing their production or attendance bonuses. They simply had to arrange with her in advance which day they should take. She also took measures to relax the working environment by allowing them to bring in music and by loosening rules governing restroom and water breaks.

Over the next couple of weeks, the turnover rate stabilized and the defect rate improved. Mary was optimistic: "You can't ask these kids to put in six or seven-day weeks without a break . . . Things got better right away."

Although they were not completely out of the woods, the crisis had seemed to pause. The Georgia operation was back in business, and calls had slowed as more gauges were passing the inspection tests of their clients. Mary was not being summoned for daily emergency meetings. And Steve told her: "Whatever you're doing is working." However, he would soon change his mind even though, by Georgia's standards, products were continually improving.

One morning, in a private meeting, the Human Resource Manager, Rosalia, alerted Steve to the fact that things were getting "out of control" in the gauge area. She was concerned that Mary's tampering with the attendance schedules would disrupt the attendance and punctuality policies of the company, introducing Mexican chaos into their professional American system. "This is not a Mexican sweatshop," she said, "She can't just change it around when it's convenient."

Steve decided that he would talk with Mary about the attendance policy on the following Saturday, when she came in for an overtime shift. "I agreed with Rosalia, we have to stick with policy. We need to follow the rules like any American company, but I didn't think it was an emergency." What he encountered, however, when he went to speak with Mary in the gauge area on Saturday morning, shocked him: "I thought I'd walked into a Mexican fiesta," he said, "The only thing missing was a pinata."

According to Steve, after he pushed through the set of dust-proof doors separating the gauge area from the rest of the plant, he saw women talking loudly and walking around the work area with no apparent regard for their work stations. Music, he said, was blaring from a jam box next to the empty donut box located atop a work table. Mary, he said, "looked just like a Mexican grandmother." His American supervisor was beginning to look femininely Mexican in his eyes. Steve described his alarm at the next Tuesday rooming staff meeting: "I don't know what she's doing in there, but there are girls running around everywhere. And they want to bring their children . . . There's no telling how many babies those girls have."

Mary described the scene in this way: "Steve came in ready to jump all over me for not telling Rosalia about our scheduling changes and then he has a heart attack because I told him that one of the girls had asked to bring her baby on Saturdays." She had not let her.

During the staff meeting, concerns over the gauge area shifted from the quality of the product, as it was measured by performance tests, to apparent loss of control by American managers over Mexican females. They agreed that the product was sure to suffer. Burt said that they could not "tolerate" a "Mexican occupation" of the gauge room. Roger raised the issue of fingernail polish. "Some of those girls wear fingernail polish," he said, "Just what we need is a call [from corporate headquarters] asking how purple fingernail polish gets into the gauges." They discussed the dangers of not enforcing the hairnet policy. Roger was sure that hair would slip into the paint and said: "We should just stamp 'Made in Mexico' across the speedometer." They talked about the significance of allowing female operators to wear male uniforms. They voiced doubt over the prudence of allowing the workers to roam the main areas without supervision. And they agreed that, given how things were going, it was only a matter of time before Mary would let someone bring their baby to work. "That's a liability issue," said Steve, "We're not in the day-care business." Burt summed up the meeting by saying: "The thing that bothers me is that we don't know what type of product they're putting together in there. Now that's a problem."

Throughout this meeting, no one mentioned that, as far as their client was concerned, the product was approaching corporate standard. The managers, however, were alarmed over the quality of their gauges, not because of the performance of the gauges in inspection tests, but because they feared that the telltale traces of Mexican women could be identified in them. They made the connection between seeing women roaming the workspaces and relaxing their uniform standards and a loss of managerial control over the labor process. Their lack of control, in turn, meant that the product would not emerge as planned, but instead as a product of undisciplined female and Mexican labor. Steve implied this connection when he said "What I don't want is for someone . . . to walk in this plant and find a bunch of Mexican girls running around . . . I'll hear that we're going Mexican on them and our product going to hell."

The root of the problem, they decided, was that Mary was not "American" enough to "Americanize" the labor process, and was not disciplined enough to keep the feminine influence within its proper bounds. Roger was assigned the task of speaking firmly to Mary about the situation and of advising her that she was being placed on probation. According to Roger, he was trying to be as diplomatic as he could when he told Mary that she needed to "represent the corporation out there" and perform her job to the standards of "American professional behavior." He said, "I told her that we were worried about the product."

Mary was furious. She said, "I told him (Roger), 'I am as American as you are'. I can't believe he said that to me. I know he's saying that I'm not up to their standards. That's what it means when they say something is 'Mexican'." Soon thereafter, the managers decided to demote Mary for being, as Roger recorded on her evaluation form, "unprofessional," "failing in the performance of duties," and not producing quality product. In addition, they demanded that she attend three hours of supervisory-training classes offered by the University of Texas El Paso every week on top of the overtime she was continuing to perform. He also denied her a routine salary inflation compensation. Mary's demotion put her on equal footing with the other Mexican supervisors. She was the only American supervisor who worked under the supervision of another supervisor. Mary begrudgingly attended the supervisor classes. "It's an insult," she said, "they're putting me in there to humiliate me. As far as I can see, they're the ones who aren't being very American. You know they want top quality work without paying for it or even giving enough time for training. And then they turn around say it's because Mexican females don't do good work."

On the heels of her demotion and salary cut, and with mounting evidence that Mary would not mend her attitudes, the managers decided to fire her. When I asked Roger why the managers focused so much on Mary's supervisory style rather than on the obvious improvements, according to performance tests, she made in production he said: "We want a good product. That's what this is about really. It's a long-term issue . . . We're an American operation. We've got an American product . . . Mary doesn't understand." Shortly after Mary's departure, the gauge-production line was returned to a US facility. The politics over Mary's supervisory methods, the uniforms, fingernail polish, hairnets, and whether or not MOTW would turn into a daycare facility had taken its toll on the organization and its budget. The women who could not be placed in other electronic-assembly positions were encouraged to leave. Eventually, the line was out-sourced to an external producer. "This makes us look bad," Burt said, "losing a line means something's gone seriously wrong."

Mary sued the company in court and received some back pay. Steve explained that, despite all of the turmoil, he had no regrets over his actions: "I'd rather lose a line than ship out inferior products," he said.

Conclusion

Clearly, one of the key issues at play in the events surrounding the relocation of the gauge operation is how the production of value at MOTW works out through the processes for identifying nationality and gender. And this calculation revolves around the continual efforts of MOTW managers to resolve the perplexing paradox described, to some degree, by Harvey (1982). How will they turn the vibrant energies of Mexican women into a feature of male, American goods? Another way of putting this question is, how will they manage cheap people in the manufacture of quality goods? We need to recognize the social construction of Mexican women within MOTW as cheap people to understand the difficulty the managers faced when they hired them for their nimble fingers and in the belief that training was not required. The managers knew they were bringing in the worker who had always represented precisely the kind of people MOTW did not employ. If we adjust the Harvey paradox to address Elson's question – how does labor acquire the form that it does – then we can see that the Mexican woman was acquiring a contradictory constitution. On the one hand, she represented the kind of worker whose exclusion reinforced MOTW's superiority among maquiladoras. On the other, she was becoming a member of the MOTW team because of her *natural* ability to assemble electronic components.

The historical social construction of the Mexican woman as a non-MOTW employee had served a useful purpose for the company because it exercised further productive effects. To use Butler's views on this process, we could say that the materialization of the Mexican woman as cheap labor personified was not an isolated event, but rather one interwoven with how value materialized within MOTW goods and within the company itself. The Mexican woman made the recognition of value in MOTW possible by establishing the parameters for recognizing what it was not. She cast the shadow of nonvalue and, against her, value came to light. In MOTW, this relationship of the Mexican woman to the value of company products and people was explained in the designation of the labor process as a masculine one – within an American system for creating American men's goods. Anything that revealed the energies of Mexican women, in their view, such as televisions, was not

a thing of quality in comparison with MOTW goods, which revealed American ingenuity that transformed a Mexican labor process into a top-notch tool shop.

The decision to hire women into the MOTW labor force demonstrates the continuous pattern for protecting the labor process from the influence of cheap Mexican
women. Although MOTW was expanding in the area of electric assembly, managers still described the principal operations as those involving carburetor assembly, tooling, and engineering – all male-dominated occupations in the factory. The
women worked in windowless interior rooms, out of the view of the major production space. Their movements were to be carefully monitored, along with their
clothing, reproductive cycles, and personal hygiene habits. These regulations were
part of the plan for integrating Mexican women into the labor force without con-
taminating the MOTW labor process or its products with evidence of their presence. Perhaps they could protect the value of their products by keeping the women's
contribution to it secret. Steve had guaranteed his executive officers that he could
produce quality gauges at the same time that he was committed to making sure that
customers would never know that Mexican women built parts of their boats. In
this way, the labor of Mexican women could be turned into something that reified
American masculinity.

Problems occurred when Mary subverted the traditional methods for guaranteeing that these vibrant energies of Mexican women could be transformed into the
fixed properties of male American goods. In stressing the need to train the women
with flexible procedures, she appeared to dismantle both the American system that
protected the Americanness of the operation and the masculine domination of
MOTW workspaces and procedures. In so doing, she violated the codes for recognizing quality in this workplace. She declared that these women were worth training if quality was what was expected. In fact, it was the only way that this result
could be achieved. But her bosses, rather than seeing a group of workers learning
and improving over time, encountered the troubling vision of Mexican women
getting out of control while their American supervisor was "Mexicanizing" in front
of them. Their traditional pattern for connecting the value of people to the value
of MOTW goods was unraveling.

The MOTW case also broadly reveals that capitalism is, in the first instance, a
local phenomenon. The ideas behind it may have a global dimension, but the
working out of capitalism occurs when individuals are identified to represent varying
kinds of capitalist subjects, their dimensions being drawn and understood in the
local landscape (see Gibson-Graham, 1996). The evaluation of the quality of the
gauges demonstrates this point. Just as the final-assembly facility in Georgia was
increasingly satisfied with the gauge quality, the MOTW managers were less so.
Both sets of managers equate product quality with product value. However, their
criteria for evaluating these conditions differed and, as a result, that which held
value for one was lacking in value for the other. The value in the gauges depended
upon who was performing the evaluation, and on how they recognized the evidence
for value in people and products.

Finally, the benefits of an ethnographic approach to exploring the dynamics of
corporate behavior ought not to be underestimated. For, had I only conducted interviews with MOTW managers in order to understand why they made particular decisions, I doubt that the kind of story I present with the ethnographic material would

ever have materialized. Likely as not, I would have heard that the decision was made based on the budget and the lack of skills among the Mexican workers. These are the sorts of explanations that abound when a maquila operation fails to function as expected. There is, of course, some validity to both of these contentions, as I think the MOTW case demonstrates, but it is in the conceptualization of the interplay between value, labor, Mexicans, and women that the terms of such explanations come together at MOTW.

Part III Resource Worlds

Editors' Introduction:
Producing Nature

Trevor J. Barnes, Eric Sheppard, Jamie Peck,
and Adam Tickell

The term resources conjures up those sometimes grainy textbook photographs appearing in secondary school geography or social studies texts: drooping bunches of bananas in Caribbean plantations; an oil well gushing black in the Kuwaiti desert; a log boom floating down a Canadian river flanked by forest; a steeply terraced paddy field of rice set among the lush tropical vegetation of Indonesia.

These images of resources, as raw commodities given by nature and ripe for extraction, are also how the first economic geographers conceived them. Indeed, at its institutionalization in the late nineteenth century, economic geography was in effect the geography of resource worlds. The first economic geography textbook in English by the Scottish geographer George Chisholm, *Handbook of Commercial Geography* (1889), provided a meticulous account of the multifarious types of resources found in the world, their geographical distribution, and the natural conditions sustaining them. For Chisholm (1889, p. 1), lying behind resource production is "the great geographical fact...that different parts of the world yield different products, or furnish the same product under unequally favourable conditions." To understand resources, therefore, one must understand differences in *natural* conditions across the globe. It is this "great geographical fact" that creates the mosaic of resource production that Chisholm, and others of his generation, were so keen to claim as economic geography.

With the increased importance of manufacturing during the twentieth century, economic geography shifted emphasis away from resources per se, but they were still present. Even in the late 1930s, well after Henry Ford pioneered his assembly-line techniques, paving the way for mass production more generally (see Sheppard and Barnes, 2000, ch. 1), the American geographer Richard Hartshorne (1939) was still arguing that the fundamental geographical unit was the region, defined principally by its natural resource base. For Hartshorne the world is a patchwork quilt of different economic regions, where each region is a closely delineated complex of interconnected elements that cohere around resource production of which the exemplar is agriculture, and resting on the family farm (it's not surprising that Hartshorne lived all of his working life in the American Midwest).

The emergence of spatial science in late 1950s Anglo-American economic geography, however, pushed Hartshorne's regionalism aside (Barnes, 2000), and in the process marginalized the study of resources. Partly, this was because spatial science upheld general theoretical explanation against the unique description that defined Chisholm's and Hartshorne's approach to resources (all those detailed figures, all those maps, all those lists, facts, and typologies). And partly, it was because the very assumptions under-girding general location theory, especially within the "modeling tradition" (Plummer, 2000), effectively effaced any economic geography of resources. In order to derive simple, tractable mathematical solutions of the kind cherished by spatial science, simplifying assumptions were required. One of the most widespread was the isotropic plain, an infinitely large flat surface undisturbed by resource differentiation. Such an assumption ruled out by default any serious examination of resources, and as a result, they were treated as merely complicating factors, the analysis of which was promised but often indefinitely postponed.

Ironically, perhaps, resources returned to economic geography's agenda in the mid-1970s through Marxism. On the face of it, Marx does not have much to say about resources and nature beyond the philosophical point of dialectical materialism: that human society depends on the material environment. Marx's foci were the Dark Satanic Mills of nineteenth-century industrial capitalism, places where, as in Charles Dickens' description of Coketown, "Nature was bricked out." David Harvey's (1974) influential *Economic Geography* essay, "Population, resources, and the ideology of science," changed that view, however. Closely following Marx, Harvey argued that resources and nature are not asocial givens, but significant only in so far as they are embedded within a particular set of social and economic imperatives such as found under capitalism. As Smith and O'Keefe (1985, p. 80) later put it: "for Marx, nature is related to social activity. He meant that materially as well as ideally; the entire earth bears on its face the stamp of human activity."

Consequently, the earlier interpretation, held by Chisholm and Hartshorne, that resources are given naturally, gave way to one emphasizing their social constitution, and affiliated conflicts, power struggles, and politics. Neil Smith (1984) even spoke of the seemingly oxymoronic "production of nature." Of course, one needs to be careful about that term "production." It doesn't mean that capitalism's social relations defy the Laws of Thermodynamics and create something where nothing existed before. But it does mean that when capitalism emerged on to the scene it transformed preexisting nature (sometimes called "first nature"). Nature still exists, but how it is exploited, used, thought about, and represented is now completely different. Castree (1995, p. 20), following Cronon (1991), provides a useful example: "the 'natural' regions of . . . the Midwestern United States, cannot be understood simply as preexistent natural grasslands, as the traditional notion of 'first nature' would imply. Instead . . . they must be seen as constructed natural environments evolving out of decades of intensive, profit-driven conversion into what they are presently are." Hartshorne's natural economic regions, including those of his native American Midwest – "the corn belt," "the hog belt," "the dairy belt" – were therefore not natural at all, but a consequence of deeply inscribed social relations. The term "second nature" is often used to describe how even the most apparently pristine "natural" ecosystems are now been profoundly shaped by capitalism.

The view that natural resources are social artifacts, rather than simply natural, is the central theme running through the five essays gathered here. This Marxist insight is now ingrained. Debate remains, however, around which kinds of components to include within the social: is it only class relations, the classic Marxist view, or are there other important elements like gender, ethnic allegiance, or environmental discourse? There is no single answer. In large part it depends upon the particular type and context of the resource itself, represented in the essays that follow by: late nineteenth century fur sealing in the Bering Straits; Spanish waterscapes in the first part of the twentieth century; oil exploitation in Venezuela, Iran, and especially Nigeria in the 1970s; rice and vegetable cultivation in postcolonial Gambia; and coffee production in contemporary Peru. The other debate running through the papers turns on the degree to which resources possess a power to assert themselves independently of social relations. One criticism of the orthodox Marxist position is that it gives too much importance to the social; i.e., nature appears malleable, taking any form dictated by capitalism. But doesn't nature resist human wiles, at least sometimes, often responding to human intervention in ways that confound the conceit that we can control the earth's biophysical system? Each author attempts in various ways, and to very different degrees, to give natural resources some agency, an ability to act outside of prevailing social relations.

Noel Castree examines the Bering Straits fur seal industry of the late nineteenth and early twentieth centuries, coming closest to the standard Marxist account of nature and resources. Hunting seals in the North Pacific began systematically around 1870, and by 1911 they were almost extinct. They were saved from eradication only by a treaty signed by the principal sealing nations. Castree asks how we should explain the perilous state of the fur seal hunt. He poses two alternatives. Orthodox economics attributes the crisis to market failure. Because fur seals cost nothing to produce and are not owned by anyone – they are a public good in the language of economics – the normal price mechanism regulating their allocation and use does not apply. Individual capitalists, concerned only with self-interest, will then rationally expropriate the resource as long as revenues exceed costs, eventually wiping it out, and producing what Garrett Hardin (1968) famously called the "tragedy of the commons." In this interpretation, the specific qualities of the good itself, undermining the operation of the market, creates the problem, and not the wider system. Marxism, by contrast, lays the blame entirely at the door of the wider social system, capitalism. Marxists argue that by virtue of its very social constitution capitalism reaps where it sows, destroys what it creates. In particular, Castree traces the destructive impulses of the sealing industry to social class relations, namely, the necessity of capitalists to exploit and to expropriate in the name of profit and accumulation. While following the classical Marxist line, towards the end of the paper Castree adds an interesting wrinkle around what he calls "ideologies of nature." The issue is why didn't the social relations of capitalism, which in so many instances have proved so destructive, carry out the final *coup de grace*, and eliminate the fur seal. For Castree, the existence of a discourse of preservation ("an ideology of nature") blunted the raw, undiluted social relations of capitalism, allowing a less destructive outcome to occur. Note that social relations are still at work here, but they are just not so narrowly defined. It is the broadening of social relations to include "ideologies of nature" that is Castree's special contribution.

Castree provides little autonomy to the seals themselves. In fact, in response to anthropocentric criticisms of Marxism, i.e., that Marxism is too human focused, he says "that it is not possible to 'speak for' 'nature' in any unmediated way." In contrast, Erik Swyngedouw's analysis of the production of the Spanish waterscape, 1890–1930, also written from a Marxist perspective, provides a much greater sense of water having agency, of resisting, and sometimes defeating, the social forces arrayed against it. In part, this is because Swyngedouw adds to the Marxist theoretical canon conceptual arguments taken from researchers in science studies, writers like Donna Haraway and Bruno Latour. Their work is centrally concerned with the relationship between nature and society, which they portray as a hybrid; that is, an inextricable mix of society and nature, interacting and blending, making it very hard to know where society ends and nature begins. Swyngedouw gives hybrids a Marxist gloss through a dialectical interpretation; nature and society are not coherent and separate spheres, but are interrelated through manifold, constantly shifting flows (Harvey, 1996). But less characteristically Marxist is Swyngedouw's willingness to recognize the independent power of water as a resource, whether in the shape of river basins, lakes, aquifers, or the hydrological cycle, as it forms hybrid relations with an emerging social modernity. Modernity is a key term for Swyngedouw, and the moving force behind a political, economic, and cultural movement, "*Regeneracionismo*," that sought to break through conservative, entrenched interests by fundamentally altering the Spanish waterscape from the late nineteenth century onward; through the provision of dams, canals, and irrigation schemes, it pushed traditional Spanish (rural) society into the twentieth century. But it was hard, not only because of resistance from the old political guard, but also because of the engineering task itself, and the very agency of water. Modernity required the conjoining of a myriad of social relations with physical geographical ones, and only then was the reshaping of Spain's hydrological morphology possible. It is not natural resources on the one hand, and society on the other, but both/and, "socionature," hybridity.

Hybridity is there if not in name in Michael Watts' richly drawn and powerfully narrated essay on oil and money, an account of the 1970s oil boom in the "high-absorption" (oil and population rich) developing countries of Venezuela, Iran, and especially Nigeria. Also written from a Marxist sensibility, he joins together, hybrid-like, all manner of different events and entities – the oil itself, mega urban projects, military coups and kidnappings, politics and money, stallions and stereos, Freud and Simmel – in recounting "the spectacle of black gold." What a spectacle! And that's Watts' point. Oil, and the vast sums of money with which it is associated, never stands alone, isolated, but gains meaning from being part of a larger social narrative. The basic lineaments of the story are well known. A cartel, the "Organization of Petroleum Exporting Countries" (OPEC), began flexing its muscles in the early 1970s, resulting in oil prices quadrupling within a year, and increasing the oil-based revenues of OPEC states tenfold within a decade. While this massive infusion of money was supposed to bring development and prosperity, generally it didn't, creating instead dislocation, corruption, massive social inequality, and instability ("social disintegration"). Nigeria is the extreme case, for which Watts relates a hideous downside; oil money becomes "the devil's excrement." As Watts writes, in Nigeria "oil money – as social power, as state corruption and degeneracy, as blind ambition and illusion – has eroded sociability, turning everything it touched into shit: oil money as deodorized faeces that was made to shine." To understand how this happened, Watts turns to Marx and Georg Simmel, an early-twentieth-century Marxist theorist of money. Their story is the same one about resources: money is necessarily embedded within a matrix of social relations, mirroring, mediating, and transforming all at the same time. So, when OPEC states like Venezuela, Iran, or Nigeria were inundated by filthy lucre, inevitably it besmirched and muddied them. More generally, Watts' essay powerfully shows that the natural endowment of rich economic resources such as oil means very little by itself. That's why Chisholm's copious tables of regional resources are in the end also unsatisfactory. Resources take on meaning only when implanted within a set of social relations. Again, natural resources like oil are never simply natural, and sometimes not even a resource. In Nigeria, oil was an anti-resource, creating mal-development, social discord, and political mayhem.

Michael Watts during the early 1980s was a pioneer of political ecology (Watts, 2000). Frequently set within studies of agriculture in developing countries, political ecology argued, in line with the general thesis here, that social relations are key to understanding many ecological problems, particularly stressing inequitable relations of power around land and resource ownership. Watts' later work, such as the essay on oil, retains the general thrust of political ecology, although it is not about ecology per se. Judith Carney's chapter is more typical of the political ecology tradition. Her significant contribution is broadening its remit by incorporating gender – a neglected theme in the other essays. Carney shows that gender is a vital component of the social in her case study of rice and vegetable farming in the Gambia. The gendered nature of social relations forcefully shapes the resources that are produced, the methods by which they are produced, and their degree of success in potentially realizing nation-wide development. In many ways, her story turns on the unintended consequences of aid in the postcolonial period. Under British colonialism, men practiced monoculture in the uplands, farming the cash crop of peanuts, while women worked in the swamplands of the river valley producing rice and vegetables mainly for family subsistence. As a "reward" for contributing to the family household, women were given access to some of the family's land holdings (in a system known as *kamanyango*). Women controlled how that land was used, and could keep financial benefits that accrued. Other land holdings of the family, however, were subject to *maruo*. Here the male head of the household strictly controlled land use and benefits. The end of colonialism was accompanied by a series of aid projects that funded irrigation schemes, especially within the swampland area. They were compromised, however, by gender conflict over the right to control the redeveloped land, and thus income and power within the household. Men claimed the land as *maruo*, while women argued that it is *kamanyango*. The conflict led women to withdraw their labor, reducing land productivity, and undermining the national goal of self-subsistence in rice. Carney's point, then, is that examinations of how social relations make a difference to resource provision must take gender as seriously as other dimensions of social difference and inequality.

Whatmore and Thorne move farthest away from traditional political economy, pursuing instead the writings of Bruno Latour (also discussed by Swygedouw). Latour is especially associated with actor-network theory (ANT). The gist of this complex theory is the assertion that things happen only by "enlisting" or "enrolling" a large number of entities or elements within a larger network, making them work together to produce the desired outcome. That outcome might be the identification of the anthrax bacillus by Louis Pasteur (Latour's favorite example), or it might be the export of Fair Trade coffee from Peruvian farmers to British cafés (Whatmore and Thorne' case study). Persuading entities ("actors") to work together is always difficult, though, and with no guarantee of eventual success. Both Pasteur and Fair Trade coffee repeatedly struggle to maintain their respective networks, fending off rogue "actors" like a contaminated petri dish, or frost in Brazilian coffee fields. Such networks are thus always an achievement, taking a lot of resources, hard work, and dedicated effort; there is nothing natural about them. Also, there is nothing natural, as Whatmore and Thorne argue, about how networks spread. Just because Pasteur identified the anthrax bacillus in a culture flask in his rue d'Ulm Paris lab, it doesn't mean it became instant, universal knowledge, with the technique of pasteurization immediately unfolding. Likewise, because a group of concerned young people gathered in London in 1964 to discuss how to alleviate poverty among developing countries through fair trading practices, there was no necessity for it to become a network that now includes farmers from Latin America to Africa. To effect geographical reach, "action at a distance," requires a whole series of mediating relationships among people and things. Whatmore and Thorne follow Latour in arguing that, rather than making hard and fast geographical distinctions between, say, nature and society, local and global, or cores and peripheries, it is better simply to speak of chains of connections that are more or less long, and more or less strong. More generally, their purpose is to unsettle the political economic privileging of the social over natural resources (and multinational agro-industry over organic smallholders). The social doesn't always get what it wants – networks are precarious and fragile – and there is always more than the social going on. Non-humans also need to be enrolled to achieve results, from machines and tools, to the weather, to the coffee beans themselves. To put it all down to unfettered forces of social relations is both conceited and geographically naive.

The British literary critic Raymond Williams (1976, p. 184) said, "nature is perhaps the most complex word in the language." Consequently, resources must be one of the most complex terms in economic geography, straddling between society *and nature*. Some of the questions the term raises, and which also emerge from the essays, are: What is the role of nature in the definition of a resource? In the social-based definition that was at the core of our review, has nature dropped out, or is it still there, and if so how? In fact, what do we mean when we say a resource is socially defined? What counts as the social? And why should the social be privileged in the first place? Further, how does the work of people in science studies like Donna Haraway and Bruno Latour, who are not economic geographers and are concerned only with science and the material world it studies, bear on how economic geographers should study resources? What are the practical precepts being offered by the mix of theories used in an essay for concrete studies of resources? How, if at all, does adoption of a particular perspective change such studies?

Chapter 11

Nature, Economy, and the Cultural Politics of Theory: The "War Against the Seals" in the Bering Sea, 1870–1911

Noel Castree

Introduction

The last few years have seen the rapid development of a number of approaches to understanding natural resource problems from the perspective of Marxian political-economy. Despite the evident tensions between "red" and "green" thought (well summarized by Eckersley, 1992, ch. 4), several authors have recently sought to fashion a distinctively Marxist approach to environmental questions. More specifically, they have done so by returning to the texts of Marx himself. The work of Elmar Altvater (1993, 1994), Ted Benton (1989, 1991, 1992), Reiner Grundmann (1991, 1992), David Harvey (1993b), and James O'Connor (1989a, b, c) are all attempts to enrich in more ecofriendly ways our understanding of what Neil Smith (1984) provocatively called "the *production* of nature" from within the horizon of classical Marxism. The originality of earlier (and by now well known) exegeses of Marx's understanding of nature were twofold. First, they showed that for Marx nature is not separate from society, but is materially produced by it within a "creatively destructive" capitalist system. The dualism of nature and society is thus dissolved in the labor process, which becomes the flashpoint for social-natural unity centered on capitalist production of "second nature" (Schmidt, 1971; Smith, 1984). Second, they showed that accompanying this process of material transformation, nature was also produced discursively. In particular, Smith's (1984) dissection of what he called "ideologies of nature" illuminated the way in which representations of nature can serve to either conceal or legitimate the often rapacious material production of nature at the hands of capital (see also Fitzsimmons, 1989; Redclift, 1987; Williams, 1980). Overall, this dual focus on the simultaneously material *and* discursive production of nature defines an overarching critical research program in which "the major analytical issue . . . becomes the question of how nature is (re)produced, and who controls this process of (re)production in particular times and places" (Whatmore and Boucher, 1993, p. 167). The more recent ecofriendly commentaries on Marx and nature have enriched this research program by offering a theoretical explanation of the conditions under which capitalism has a specific liability to generate environmental problems, as well as an appreciation of the reciprocal effects these produced problems have upon society (see Castree, 1995). However, these abstract accounts must be supplemented by more detailed historical-geographical investigations. Additionally, with few exceptions (e.g., Harvey, 1993b), the new wave of ecologically-minded Marxist approaches have said little about the discursive production of nature, the hegemonic representations through which nature and environment are understood. There is, in other words, still much to be done.

In this essay I present a Marxian account of the formation and resolution of a major natural resource problem in both its material and its discursive dimensions. That problem was the near total destruction of the north Pacific fur seal (*Callorhinus ursinus*) in the short space of four decades (1870–1911). My overall aim is to suggest the usefulness of Marx's political economy for making critical sense of this episode in the violent life of capitalism in both its material and discursive dimensions. After describing the genesis of the fur seal crisis, I then seek to explain it using neoclassical and ecoMarxist ideas respectively. By exposing the weaknesses of the former I hope to show the perspicacity of the latter, a contrast particularly apposite given the current popularity of market based approaches to environment. Having examined the material destruction of environment, I then consider critically the discursive dimensions of the fur seal conflict. In particular, I focus on the constructions of "nature" proffered by radical American environmentalists which were crucial in saving the Pribilof seals. I seek to show both the effectiveness of those constructions, but *also* their dissimulated ideological dimension: for their success depending on further silencing an already marginalized Pribilof Aleut population sold into what Dorothy Jones (1980) calls a "century of servitude." However, having utilized the Marxian critique to make sense of the fur seal crisis and its resolution, I end by registering the *limits* of that critique. As Donna Haraway (1991) has insisted, theoretical vision is always partial and its privileges are *also* its blind spots, leading to what Sparke (1995, p. 1066, emphasis added) describes as a "usefully dynamic notion of the (im)possibility of *fully adequate* critique."

"The War Against the Seals"

The north Pacific fur seal is triply remarkable. First, in the mid-nineteenth century it was probably the most numerous sea mammal on the planet at around 3.5 million animals. Second, its annual migration pattern from the Bering Sea to the central/north Californian coast is exceeded among mammals only by the great whales. Third, despite its size, the seal herd breeds on only a few small rocks: the Pribilof Islands, which provide some 80% of the total, Russia's Commander Islands, Robben Island off Sakhalin, and the northern Kuriles. The annual cycle begins anew early each summer on just a few miles of rocky Pribilof beaches, the species' principal home. Between April and early June the bulls arrive, mature adult males 7–8 feet long and weighing 400–600 pounds. In June much smaller and lighter pregnant females arrive who are quickly corralled by these "beachmasters" into "harems" of up to 100 seals. The females give birth, nurse their pups, forage far and wide for food at sea, then come into heat and get pregnant again. In July and August the immature males and females arrive for their relatively brief stay, and by October most seals – newly born pups included – have left the rookeries for an elliptical migration 2000 miles and 6–8 months in length during which time landfall is rarely made.

The Pribilof seals were barely touched by humans until Russian fur traders discovered the two main Pribilof Islands (St George and St Paul) in the fog-bound and icy waters of the Bering Sea in 1787. Although not as fine as the pelt of the north Pacific sea otter (which had been hunted virtually to extinction by the late 18th century), it was quickly recognized that the seals' fur, with a density of 300,000 hairs per square inch, could be made into excellent capes and coats. After an early period of unregulated killing, commercial harvesting was eventually consolidated under the control of the Russian-American Company in 1805, whereafter, through a process of trial and error, the management of the seal herd was relatively successful. However, in 1867 Russia ceded the Pribilofs to the United States as part of the $7.2 million sale of Alaska, after which the management of the seals entered a new, dynamic, and dangerous period.

Congress granted the Treasury Department control of the islands on condition that it lease out exclusive rights to harvest seals to a private firm. In 1870, after considering more than a dozen tendered bids, the Treasury granted a twenty-year lease to the recently formed American Commercial Company, an amalgamation of largely San Francisco-based financiers interested in pursuing commercial sealing. The lease stipulated that no more than 100,100 seals could be taken each year, that only non-breeding males be killed, and that killing take place only between June–July and September–October. In return, the Company paid the government a $2.625 royalty on each skin shipped as well as an annual rent of $55,000. The killing and counting were all to be done under the supervision of a Treasury Agent with legal responsibility for the herd, agents serving for a few years at a time. Financially, the ACC lease was a stunning success for both Company and government. Between 1872 and 1889 the Company paid an average dividend of $46.50 per face value $100 share. With an average annual commercial kill over the life of the lease of 92,020, the 1,840,364 skins sold by the Company yielded approximately $27,800,000. From this the US government received just over $6,000,000 (considerably more than the costs it incurred on the islands) which, after deducting sealers' wages, company overheads, and transport costs (approximately $2,000,000), left a net Company profit of $18,102,140 or just under $1,000,000 per year. As Busch Cooper (1985, p. 114) rightly puts it, "even in the age of 'robber barons' this was success to end all successes."

The success is relatively easily explained. From the 1870s onwards, the monied classes of Europe and the US were willing to pay handsomely for fur skin coats and capes, which had become the height of bourgeois fashion. At the London auction of the C. M. Lampson Company (the main destination for Pribilof furs) skins fetched an impressive average of $14.67 each over the lease. With this assured market, monopoly control of the herd, and relatively small costs, it was not hard for the Company to thrive. And yet there was a dark side to this success. In 1889 government agent Charles J. Goff sent a report on seal numbers so alarming that the Treasury sent a special investigator, Henry Elliott. Elliott was considered an authority on the north Pacific fur seal after having first surveyed the Pribilof seals for the Treasury in 1872 when he made an influential, but as it eventually turned out highly spurious, estimate of the herd size, putting it at approximately 4,700,000 animals. Alarmingly, his 1890 estimate was a mere 20% of this earlier calculation, and, warning that the herd was on the brink of extinction, he accused the ACC of over-harvesting males.

When the Pribilof lease expired in 1890, it was awarded to the North American Commercial Company which used its close connections with the Harrison Administration to fend-off a higher bid from the ACC. The new lease was also for twenty years, but the tax raised to $9.25 per skin and the rent increased to $60,000 per annum. The annual quota was reduced and now determined by the Treasury agent yearly. And yet to the frustration of both the NACC and the Treasury seal numbers continued to decline. Over the NACC's lease the average annual commercial kill was just 17,000 seals per annum, a far cry from the ACC average, with the 1910 harvest down to just 13,500 animals (Riley, 1967). Nonetheless, the NACC enjoyed a remarkable profit rate of 45% over the lease, amounting to $4,390,917. Despite the reduced quotas, demand for fur-seal garments in Europe and America exceeded supply, proving once more what a durably lucrative enterprise commercial sealing could be.

But, the herd decline could not be ignored, and by 1890 the real source of the problem had already become apparent: pelagic sealing. Given the phenomenal profitability of commercial sealing the US monopoly could not survive for long, and from the early 1880s onwards a substantial sealing fleet grew up in Victoria, British Columbia and later in Japan. Again figures are imprecise, but Rogers (1976) estimates that approximately 1,311,000 pelagically-taken skins were sold in the London market between 1872 and 1911 (most taken 1885–1905). This vastly exceeds the approximately 360,000 skins taken by the NACC over its twenty-year lease (Riley, 1967).

But even this does not give true measure of the impact of pelagic sealing. Shooting (and spearing) seals at sea was a remarkably inefficient practice: more often than not the seals sank before they could be recovered, or escaped wounded, only to die later. Even a conservative estimate is that for every seal successfully taken at sea, two were lost. On this basis, then, the total pelagic kill was nearer 4,000,000 seals. Consequently, it is not surprising that by 1910 the herd was down to just a few tens of thousands and heading towards extinction unless something was done quickly.

There had been an early attempt to address the seal herd decline, leading to heightened geopolitical tensions, and resulting in the "Bering Sea crisis," as it became known. It would take a multilateral agreement to solve the seal problem: the North Pacific Fur Seal Convention of 1911. The events leading up to the signing of the Convention were complex, as were the negotiations that produced the final document. Apart from the alarmingly low numbers of seals in the rookeries, a new and conciliatory US government under William Taft, the imminent expiration of the NACC lease, and pressure from a new and influential US conservation movement combined fortuitously to encourage the American government to at last resolve the seal problem. Under the aegis of Secretary of Commerce and Labor Charles Nagel, the US, Britain, Canada, Japan, and Russia met in 1911. The resulting treaty has been described as a "historical landmark" (Busch Cooper, 1985, p. 152) and a "splendid bargain" (Gluek, 1982, p. 179), and with good reason. Not only was it the first international and multilateral agreement to conserve a species of marine wildlife; it was also remarkable in satisfying almost all the parties concerned. All pelagic sealing was to be banned (except by aboriginals) and only land-based harvesting permitted. The US, Japan, and Russia thus secured recognition of their island ownership of the seals. But in return for Canada and Japan relinquishing their right to harvest at sea, they would receive 15% of America's Pribilof catch and Russia's Commander catch, with Japan compensating each of the other three nations with 10% of its Robben Island catch. Within a decade seal numbers had recovered and the seals were successfully and profitably harvested more-or-less under the terms of the original agreement for several decades to come (for a history of Pribilof fur seal management see Roppel and Davey, 1965).

Economy and Ecology: Two Paradigms

How, then, are we to make sense of this resource problem and its resolution? Two paradigmatic explanations suggest themselves, orthodox and critical respectively, which have the interesting characteristic of having been formulated at around the same time as the seal crisis developed as well as being, over a century later, very important in the contemporary struggle to explain environmental degradation. In what follows I narrate the seal crisis and its resolution through each paradigm in turn in order to suggest the power of the latter, Marxian political economy, over the former, a free market approach inspired by neoclassical thinking.

A common tragedy?

In the 1870s a theoretical perspective was being developed in a continent far from Alaska – Europe – designed to comprehend a whole spectrum of economic action: namely, neoclassical economics. Over a century later it is that very same perspective, or at least a number of its central precepts, which is currently *de rigueur* within resource management and environmental economics. Seen through this theoretical lens, the near extinction of the north Pacific fur seal is a classic case of what Garrett Hardin (1968) famously called a "commons" problem. And its resolution seems a stunning confirmation of the solution proffered by the environmental embodiment of the neoclassical approach – what Eckersley (1993, p. 1) terms "free market environmentalism" – that creating property rights and markets in natural resources protects them. Let me begin, then, by narrating the seal crisis in terms of this paradigm.

At the heart of the neoclassical approach, of course, is the idea of the maximization of individual satisfaction. Economic activity is seen as a series of voluntary transactions between sovereign individuals who come to market with goods and services to sell or to buy and with particular preference orderings conditioned by resource scarcity. In a "perfect" market, each individual is able to maximize their welfare through rational decision-making. Under these assumptions, free market processes yield an optimum of social welfare, or Pareto optimality, where the latter is defined as the sum of individual welfare maximizations. From this perspective, the fur seal crisis is a case of "suboptimality" or "inefficiency" due to so-called "externalities." Externalities refer to a set of effects of transactions which undermine the capacity of economic actors to freely achieve their desired ends. And in resource management those externalities are, of course, formalized in a model intended to explain a wide range of resource problems: namely, the "commons" model. There is no need to rehearse that model here in any detail (see McCay and Acheson, 1987). Put simply, Hardin's "tragedy" develops under three assumptions (Berkes, 1985, p. 200). First, that resource access is freely open to any user; second, that selfish individualism prevails; and third, that exploitation rates exceed renewal. Under such circumstances, open access ensures that people do not experience fully the costs of their own resource use because they are able to pass a large portion of the costs on to others. This is a case of so-called "market failure." The unintended consequence, or what Elster (1986, p. 24) calls "counterfinal" result, "is said to be a free for all, with users competing with one another for a greater share of the resource to the detriment of themselves, the resource, and society as a whole" (Ciriacy-Wantrup and Bishop, 1975, p. 713).

At first sight the commons model appears to explain the fur seal crisis very well, for two reasons. First, the seals were a "fugitive resource": that is, because they were mobile they did not respect territorial or legal boundaries. Second, for this reason they were effectively a "common" or "open-access" resource which no body owned exclusively. As resource economists like H. Scott Gordon (1954) would later point out, the disjuncture between rights of access to a fishery and responsibility for its overall management created powerful incentives to overharvest. The "tragedy of the commons" develops because each pelagic harvester knows that if they leave a seal in the water someone else will appropriate it and hence the associated profit. As McEvoy (1986, p. 10) puts it, "in a competitive economy no market mechanism ordinarily exists to reward individual forbearance in the use of shared resources." The overall result is the neoclassicist's "externalities" or what R. H. Coase (1960) called "social costs": as *individual* actors try to maximize economic gain the *social* result is resource overexploitation, even exhaustion, and so everyone loses. Seen in this light, the fur seal case is an early, dramatic, and thus classic exemplar of the open-access problem that has bedeviled most twentieth-century commercial fisheries.

However, what makes it of further interest for devotees of the commons approach is its resolution: the 1911 Fur Seal Convention. This brings me to "free market environmentalism," to which the commons model is closely affiliated. The commons tragedy admits of two types of solution. One is governmental intervention through taxes, subsidies, or direct regulation of resource use, an approach with theoretical roots in the work of Pigou (1920). The other, more *laissez-faire*, is to make the resource in question the private property of individual resource users, who via the "invisible hand" will manage the resource in society's best interest. The latter is the distinguishing feature of "free market environmentalism," one important strand of contemporary orthodox approaches to environment which traces its lineage from Coase (1960). Here, as Eckersley (1993, p. 4) puts it, "environmental externalities are seen to arise not from 'market forces' or self-interested behaviour but rather from *an absence of well-defined, universal, exclusive, transferable and enforceable property rights* in respect of common environmental assets." By creating such enforceable (and perhaps tradable) property rights in the commons, and thereby excluding outsiders, externalities are in theory internalized and the market becomes savior not culprit. The consequence of this privatization, again in theory, is that environmental degradation will be averted and Pareto optimality achieved (see Helm and Pearce, 1991; Jacobs, 1994).

As Naughton-Treves and Sanderson (1995) recently pointed out, enforcing property rights in fugitive resources is frequently very difficult: witness the problems of operating Individual Transferable Quotas, especially in international fisheries. For this reason the success of the 1911 Convention seems a striking, if unusual, vindication of the property rights approach in relation to an international resource issue. I say "unusual" for two reasons. First, rather than deploying, say, an ITQ system, the Convention made the seals the sole and exclusive property of the US, a "privatization" made possible by the fact that unlike most commercial fisheries the fur seal spends part of its migration on land. Second, the seals were not – contra the recommendations of free market environmentalism – owned by a private company or individual after 1911, but by a public body, the US government. However, when harvesting resumed in 1916, the US ran sealing as a purely commercial operation and thus effectively acted as a private enterprise. With these caveats in mind, the Convention might thus be claimed as a powerful illustration of the success of the free market approach. Not only did it save the seals. It also – through the ingenious idea of both compensating the Canadian and Japanese seal fleets and sharing the profits of the seal trade equitably between four nations – arguably satisfied the neoclassical precept that social welfare be maximized so far as was possible in what, in this case, was a messy geopolitical resource conflict. Together, finally, these two points seem to support the idea, loudly proclaimed by free market environmentalists, that the "market" corrects itself through a negative feedback mechanism in which, when externalities are felt, action is taken to restore economic optimality. In short, the market knows best.

The political-economy of resource exploitation

So far so good. Except the commons approach and free market environmentalism, with their neoclassical precepts, are not so much "wrong" as, I think, insufficiently penetrating in their assessment of the seal crisis and its resolution. It is, however, possible to draw on an alternative theoretical tradition, also inaugurated in Europe around the time of the Bering Sea controversy, that deriving from political economist Karl Marx. Building on Marx's theoretical legacy, the recent rise of an environmentally focused Marxian political-economy arguably provides a more encompassing and fundamental explanation of the seal case and its consequences (cf. Roberts and Emel, 1991). It is thus to that alternative paradigm that I now turn.

At the heart of an ecologically sensitive Marxism is the idea that "nature" is "produced" within the social relations of capitalism (Smith, 1984). This does not amount to the ludicrous suggestion that society makes the environment, down to the very last atom (Castree, 1995, pp. 19–20): after all, there could have been no sealing without fur seals, which of course preexisted Euro-American exploitation. Rather, it means two things. First, that "natural" resources only become resources through historically and geographically specific social appraisals. Second, it means that those resources are materially appropriated by human labor power. Thus, rather than existing as a pristine "first nature" quite other to society, the environment–society dualism is dissolved through the medium of labor which binds the two into a practical unity. As Smith (1984, p. 18) puts it, "the relation with nature is an historical product, and even to posit nature as external to society . . . is literally absurd since the very act of positing nature requires a certain relation *with* nature." Overall, then, the basic Marxist proposition on environment is that as soon as "first nature" is brought into what Marx called a "metabolic" relation with society through labor then it loses its firstness and originality and becomes a socially produced "second nature."

In economic terms this is all familiar theoretical terrain of course, but it is the ecological dimensions of capitalist growth that have become the subject of recent concern within the Marxian fold. The premise of an ecological Marxism is that economic and ecological transformation are but sides of the same coin. This follows from Marx's well-known argument that labor has the "dual character" of being both concrete and abstract at the same time, just as commodities are simultaneously both specific use-values *and* exchange values capable of general exchange on a world market. As Altvater (1993, p. 188) puts it, this insight "creates the possibility of grasping economic processes at once as *transformations of values* (value formation and valorization) and as *transformations of materials and energy* (labor process, metabolic interaction between man (*sic.*) and nature)." It is here that the negative effects of the "production" or, as Marx put it, the "creative destruction" of nature become particularly important, for the essence of recent theoretical work by eco-Marxists is that capitalist principles of economic organization have *a specific liability to destroy their own resource base*. There have been three notable statements of this argument. The first is James O'Connor's (1989a, b, c) thesis that capitalism underproduces its environmental conditions of production and treats them as if they were available without restriction. The second is Ted Benton's (1989, 1991, 1992) proposition that the value-maximizing intentional structure of capital accumulation leads to what he calls "naturally mediated unintended consequences" of economic activity, or ecological crises like acid deposition, ozone depletion, and the like. The third is Elmar Altvater's (1993) persuasive dual argument that discounting the future routinely leads to resource overexploitation, while the removal and abstraction of individual commodities from their ecosystemic context frequently entails a hidden, because unvalued, cost to those wider ecosystems.

These points weave their way in and out of what follows. Let me thus narrate the fur seal crisis through the Marxian lens, showing that, what from the abstract and clean lines of free market perspective was a property rights problem successfully resolved, is for Marxism a dangerous geopolitical problem that arose from an inherently destructive mode of economic appropriation. The narrative begins with a pre-history to seal exploitation, which the free market approach fails even to register: the sudden intrusion of capitalist social relations into a part of the world that had hitherto been quite peripheral to the major centers of economic power in Europe and the eastern USA. With the purchase of Alaska, the north Pacific quickly entered into the most intimate and transformative relationship with these economic heartlands, as tens of thousands of fur seal skins began to traffick eastwards. This deserves some critical comment, as it can hardly be accepted as a "normal," predestined or inevitable process. Instead, it was the historically contingent result of two forces. First, as Marx argued, capital pushes beyond all previous barriers and batters down "Chinese walls" in its search for profit or what David Harvey (1982) has called a "spatial fix." This was nowhere more true than in the north Pacific, for profit, even in so remote and marginal a location, was still profit. Second, the north Pacific fur trade was wholly dependent on European and eastern American export markets, which highlights how crucial culturally-specific and socially-created effective demand was to making seal skins a valuable "resource." So much for the pre-history. By the time of the "Bering Sea crisis" in the late 1880s, the post-Russian seal trade had been established some 20 years. But the trade, contra neoclassical assumptions, cannot be understood abstractly as the activity of welfare maximizing individuals, all equal and sovereign. Rather, those individuals were situated in specific social relations that placed them in structurally different positions on different sides of the world. In Europe and the eastern USA, as noted, consumers sought finished fur seal garments. But in the north Pacific, producers were not seeking to acquire goods in some generalized pursuit of "preference satisfaction" but to maximize profit: and that has altogether different implications for understanding the development of the fur seal crisis. By 1890, with pelagic sealing well developed, the seal trade depended on specific social relations of production and competition. The former entailed Company shareholders reaping the benefits generated by managers and manual laborers working on the Pribilofs, while most schooner owners were petty bourgeois ex-fishermen, ex-sailors, or tradesmen employing crews seasonally out of Victoria and later several Japanese ports, but also Seattle and San Francisco. There were, then, a complex set of class relations here between workers (themselves divided "vertically" by rank and "horizontally" by nation), petty capitalists, and large capitalists. The competition relation, of course, entailed struggle between pelagic sealers of all nationalities and between them and the commercial companies. When embedded in their geographical and temporal context, these production and competition relations, underpinned by the logic of accumulation for accumulation's sake, reveal commercial sealing to have been a highly conflictual process with serious human, economic, and ecological costs impacting on real people and real environments. Let me elaborate.

Market theory posits an abstract, "pinhead economy" which is spaceless and timeless. Yet in reality the spatial and temporal dimensions of resource over-exploitation become crucial moments in understanding its development. To begin with, for production to take place, capital, as Harvey (1985b, p. 43) has persuasively argued, "must represent itself created in the form of a physical landscape in its own image." In other words, production complexes are necessarily place-specific and geographically localized. The Pribilofs, of course, formed one site of production in the fur seal case, while Victoria, like its American and Japanese equivalents, formed a quite different site as a port whose rapid growth in the 1880s and 1890s was based in large part upon pelagic sealing. It was this differentiated geography of production, in tandem with the national borders between the three nations in question, that provided much of the dynamic for competition in the fur seal case. As fur seal numbers declined throughout the 1890s, then, the cause was not simply preference-maximizing individuals generating externalities which were economically "inefficient," but instead intense competition between place-based class constituencies each seeking to defend their real interests and distribute potential economic surpluses in their favor. Finally, of course, there were the seals themselves. The commons model, betraying its neoclassical basis, is only concerned with environment to the extent that its degradation sets up effects felt as "economic" consequences. The Marxian approach, however, directs attention to the systematicity of that degradation, seeing it as more than just a hiccup in otherwise well-functioning markets. It also, importantly, points to the irrationality of that degradation and thus invites an ecological critique of capitalist principles of resource exploitation. From this perspective, the unregulated slaughter of seals at sea was the horrendous outcome of a mode of economic appropriation whose "normal" functioning would have almost certainly *extinguished* the seal herd unless checked – indeed, at one point, the US government even announced that if pelagic sealing did not cease forthwith then it would slaughter the entire herd on the Pribilofs as a last resort. That such a dreadful course of action was in reality averted was due, of course, to the 1911 Convention. But again, rather than see this landmark agreement as an example of the "self correcting" powers of the market, we might offer a more critical and sober assessment. First, far from being an automatic response to seal herd decline the Convention was the product of years of hard fought diplomacy which persistently broke down as American, British, and Canadian administrations changed and as other international issues were used as bargaining chips in the fur seal negotiations.

Second, it is worth remembering just how unusual the Convention was in successfully conserving the resource: for, arguably, it was successful only because of the ecological peculiarity that unlike most other fugitive resources the seals came ashore and could thus be counted and reliably harvested. In sum, then, an orthodox account of the seal crisis and its resolution is not so much wrong as profoundly inadequate. A "commons" problem based on the absence of well-defined property rights certainly did exist in the north Pacific, but its basis lay in a capitalist mode of resource exploitation whose spatial and temporal dynamics and socio-ecological consequences were more substantial and dangerous than neoclassical precepts or free market concepts can comprehend.

The Discursive Production of Nature

Many greens would broadly concur with this Marxian critique as part of the broader struggle to displace currently popular *laissez-faire* approaches to environment. But they would depart from it insofar as Marxism is frequently seen as being too anthropocentric and so, it is claimed, it fails to respect and defend "nature" *in its own right*. There is, however, a powerful Marxian response to this argument, which is that it is not possible to "speak for" "nature" in any unmediated way. In the Marxian view, representations of "nature" say less about the environment represented and more about the social assumptions of those doing the representing. This is why Smith (1984) talks of "ideologies of nature," to register that representations of nature are both socially produced and invariably geared towards achieving specific social ends. The fur seal case is particularly interesting here, as the formulation of the 1911 Convention, which saved the seals, was crucially influenced by a neophyte preservationist lobby articulating some of the very same concerns as present day greens. Let me, then, now critically examine that preservationist agitation and its effects.

When the Convention was signed in 1911 there was no mention of a moratorium on land-harvesting. Rather, with pelagic sealing banned, Pribilof harvesting would continue, but at levels set by the US Fur Seal Advisory Board. The Board was chaired by eminent biologist and President of Stanford University David Starr Jordan, and consisted of biologists and seal experts. It followed closely the then influential Progressive doctrine that resources should be used efficiently, without wastage, and, if possible, in a renewable way (see Hays, 1959), and enjoyed the support of influential men like George Bird Grinnell (editor of *Field and Stream*). For these reasons Secretary Nagel, whose department was now entirely responsible for the seals, followed closely the Board's advice on harvesting. However, in addition to these establishment conservationists, Nagel also came under pressure from a new and radical preservationist group led by "verbal hit-man," as Dorsey (1991, p. 34) calls him, William T. Hornaday. Hornaday was a wildlife writer who had previously worked in Brooklyn Zoo and was author of such popular titles as *Our Vanishing Wildlife*, written for lay audiences in America and beyond. His "advisor" was none other than Henry Elliott. As Stephen Fox (1981) argues, the rise of preservationism as a complement and rival to conservation was largely a new phenomenon in turn of the century USA, and thus Hornaday's outspoken defense of the seals represented a more radical form of environmental thought and politics than had been seen before in government circles.

This new and strident preservationism quickly proved itself a force to be reckoned with. In alliance with the conservationists, Hornaday and Elliott persuaded Nagel not to issue a new twenty-year lease in 1910 and to buy up the Pribilof operations. However, upon the signing of the Convention, Hornaday was incensed that the US government still intended to continue harvesting on land. As Hornaday asked Nagel in a typically overblown rhetorical outburst, "Did the President . . . or the US Senate, intend for one moment that you go right on in the bloody killing business? No! A thousand times, no! And you know it." His objection was, however, well founded. Fur seal management was still an imprecise science. With margins of error uncertain, continued sealing, as recommended by the Fur Seal Advisory Board, was potentially very risky. Although opposed to any sealing whatsoever, Hornaday recognized that if he could not stop it, he could at least give the herd a breathing space so that it could recover. It was here that the preservationists had their greatest impact. Through intense lobbying of Congressmen in a new Democratic House, Hornaday and his allies managed to secure a five-year closed season on land sealing when the enabling legislation for the Convention was formulated in Congress. This was a daring and dangerous move because it breached the conditions of the Convention and thus gave Canada and Japan a pretext for opting out of it. However, fortunately that eventuality did not materialize and the moratorium, although strongly opposed by Taft, Nagel, and Jordan, was arguably vital in securing the herd's future, since when sealing resumed in 1916 seal numbers were up dramatically.

The discursive production of nature was crucial here. I say this because it was the concatenation of a set of powerful and emotive preservationist *representations* of the seals that swayed the opinions of several Congressmen into supporting a five-year closed season. Moreover, this was, I will suggest, an effective "ideology of nature" whose success depended on a dissimulation of its social constructedness.

Through verbal harrying, numerous letters, and written publications both official and popular, Hornaday and his associates created a battery of images of the Pribilof seals forming what might be called a "discourse of wildest nature." In this discourse, the seals appeared as wild, pristine, and majestic animals, as part of the "natural order" and thus not to be sullied by the grubby machinations of human commerce.

This discourse, rather than innocently reflecting "nature," actively constructed it in interested ways. The preservationist agenda was saving the seals and, accordingly, the animals were "staged" in such a way as to make killing them unthinkable. To say that "nature" is discursively constructed in this way is not, of course, to deny the reality of the seals. But it is to draw attention to what cultural critics call "the materiality of representation." Discourse is proactive and productive, not simply passive, because spoken words and inscriptions on a page can be of world changing consequence. This was particularly so in the seal case, because the preservationists were representing an animal most of them (Elliott excepted) had never personally seen in a part of the world they had never even visited. The preservationists thus deployed what Stephen Greenblatt (1992, p. 23) calls "an immense mimetic machinery" in which representation claimed to "mirror" nature as it was, while dissimulating its construction of that nature. This, then, was a politics of truth masquerading as more-or-less innocent languages of empiricism. But it was no less effective for that because it was precisely the claim *to* truthfulness which allowed the discourse of wildest nature to be so successful. In short, the representation of "nature" was as vital to protecting the seals as had been economic processes in causing seal overexploitation in the first place. Or, as Greenblat (1992, p. 6) aptly puts it, "representations are not only products but *producers*, capable of decisively altering the very forces that brought them into being."

But there was a dark side to this success, and here the Marxian insight that representations of nature are always socially situated and directed becomes particularly useful. EcoMarxists recognize that representations of nature can have a materiality and effectivity that is vital in protecting environments from economic overexploitation, just as it did in the fur seal case. In other words, "ideologies of nature" need not always be directed to exploitative ends. But the Marxian view also recognizes that because those ideologies are aimed at achieving very particular ends, they may conceal as much as they reveal, even when directed to positive goals like environmental protection. In the case of the Pribilof seals this was particularly important: because the preservationist discourse of "wildest nature" largely remained blind to an Aleut population integrally tied to the American seal economy and sold into what historian Dorothy Jones (1980) calls "a century of servitude."

Despite the thousands of words written about the Pribilofs, Hornaday and his associates – like the US government and the other signatories to the 1911 Convention – said remarkably little about the condition of the Pribilof Aleuts. Symptomatic of this was the Pribilofs' alternative name, the "Seal Islands," a title implying that their defining feature was their occupation by wild sea mammals. Yet the Pribilofs were *also* home to a Pribilof Aleut population without whose labor power the American seal trade simply could not have prospered. The Aleuts had been forcibly transported to the Pribilofs from Fox Island by the Russians in the late eighteenth century. Part serfs, part wage laborers, they were retained by the RAC to undertake

much of the annual killing, skinning, and salting of seals. When the Americans purchased Alaska in 1867, serfdom was abolished and the Aleuts were paid for all their
labor by the ACC and NACC respectively. But this shift to an apparently fair and
free system of wage labor concealed a darker side which made the treatment of the
Aleuts one of the scandals of US–native relationships.

True, the Aleuts received wages comparable to those of the average American
worker. But they were paid in credit, not cash, and forced to buy from a limited
range of goods at the Company stores at marked-up prices. It is also true that the
Companies were required to provide schooling and housing for their Aleut workers.
But schooling was based on the white American model and the speaking of the Aleut
language was discouraged. Likewise the provision of "free" housing entailed
destroying traditional Aleut *barabaras* (turf-roofed, half-underground dwellings)
and replacing them with wooden structures which were harder and more costly to
heat. In addition to these relations with the Companies, the Aleuts were overseen
by the Treasury Agent, who exercised enormous power on the islands. Movement
within and between the islands was severely restricted. No unauthorized vessels or
visitors could leave or land there. And modes of work- and public-behavior were
closely regulated through financial penalty, with wages docked or fines levied for
"improper" conduct. In short, even though paid an "acceptable" wage, the Aleuts
were to all intents and purposes a captive population regulated and controlled to a
degree that abrogated all accepted standards of liberty and equality.

Not surprisingly, with little opportunity or power to articulate their claims and
grievances, the condition of the Pribilof Aleuts was little known.

So while the discourse of preservationists helped prevent the seal herd disappearing, it did so at the expense of not improving the condition of those to whom
the seal economy was bound. This, I think, has implications for the present. For
much of modern day North American environmentalism repeats this effacement of
the social habitation of what are constructed as purely "natural" landscapes (see
Willems-Braun, 1997).

Conclusion: The Cultural Politics of Theory

In seeing the "production of nature" as an overarching process, in which material
relationships and discursive representations are both vital and intertwined, an eco-
Marxian approach reveals a complex political economy to seal exploitation that
laissez-faire environmentalism misses and which ecocentrists may only partly grasp.
It also emphasizes the fact that environmental problems emphatically begin and end
in the realms of human practice: there is no representation of "nature" outside social
interests and political agendas. But for all its usefulness, the Marxian approach must
also be vigilant about its own blind spots and aporias. This returns me to the
Pribilof Aleuts. Over the last few years a number of postcolonial critics have drawn
attention to what Shohat and Stam (1994) call the "buried epistemologies" of
Western critical theory, namely the presuppositions they smuggle in to their attempts
to comprehend the world. Marxism, in particular, has come under fire in this regard
because of its Eurocentrism, that is, its imposition of European categories of critical thought onto non-Western settings where they may not be so appropriate
(Serequerbehan, 1990; Slater, 1992). In the case of the Pribilofs, a Marxist optic

usefully directs our attention to the imbrication of Aleuts and seals in an exploitative and ecologically destructive political economy. But in so doing it paradigmati-
cally frames the Aleuts as *class* subjects, whose main defining feature is their place
in social relations of production. As a corollary, it would also have us recover the
class agency of the Aleuts and so reveal a history of exploitation and conflict that
for too long remained hidden. These paradigmatic maneuvers are important and
necessary – for the Aleuts were undoubtedly exploited along rather obvious class
lines and did engage in quotidien acts of resistance – but they are not sufficient. I
say this for two reasons. First, the subjection of the Aleuts *exceeded* class exploitation. The array of exclusionary practices and oppressive restrictions they encountered were very much bound up with their "non-white" status and so equally tied
to an economy of racial and ethnic discrimination. Second, where Marxism would
have us recover the agency and consciousness of the exploited – rather as E. P.
Thompson did for the English working classes – postcolonial critics point out the
problems with such apparently well-intentioned "recovery." As Spivak (1988)
argues in her controversial essay "Can the subaltern speak?," recovering "subaltern" voices is complicated by the fact that those voices are *always already* written
by those in power. In this case, our understanding of Pribilof Aleut agency a century
ago is almost exclusively scripted by the resident Agents and, as such, filtered
through the terms of the dominant culture on the islands. In other words, the historical archive already comes to us infused with the power relations that marginalized Aleuts in the first place. For these two reasons, any critical project to adequately
reconstruct the history of seal exploitation on the Pribilofs in all its dimensions
cannot be based on Marxian precepts alone.

Chapter 12

Modernity and Hybridity: Nature, *Regeneracionismo*, and the Production of the Spanish Waterscape, 1890–1930

Erik Swyngedouw

I am planning something geographical. (Klaus Kinski, the film *Fitzcarraldo*, directed by Werner Herzog)

The Hydraulic ordering of the territory constitutes a structural necessity of Spanish society as an industrial society. (Ortí, 1984, p. 11)

Spain is arguably the European country where the water crisis has become most acute in recent years. Since 1975, demand for water has systematically outstripped supply and, despite major and unsustainable attempts to increase pumping of ground water and to develop a more intensive use of surface water, the problem has intensified significantly. The recent 1991–1995 drought, which affected most of Central and Southern Spain, spearheaded intense political debate, particularly as the cyclical resurgence of diminished water supply from rainwater coincided with the preparation (since, 1985) of the Second National Hydrological Plan (MOPT, 1993; Ruiz, 1993; Gómez Mendoza and del Moral Ituarte, 1995; del Moral Ituarte, 1996).

The political and ecological importance of water is not, however, only a recent development in Spain. Throughout this century, water politics, economics, culture, and engineering have infused and embodied the myriad tensions and conflicts that drove and still drive Spanish society. And although the significance of water on the Iberian peninsula (see Figure 12.1) has attracted considerable scholarly and other attention, the central role of water politics, water culture, and water engineering in shaping Spanish society on the one hand, and the contemporary water geography and ecology of Spain as the product of centuries of socioecological interaction on the other, have remained largely unexplored. Yet very little, if anything, in today's Spanish social, economic, and ecological landscape can be understood without explicit reference to the changing position of water in the unfolding of Spanish society. The hybrid character of the water landscape, or "waterscape," comes to the fore in Spain in a clear and unambiguous manner. Hardly any river basin, hydrological cycle, or water flow has not been subjected to some form of human

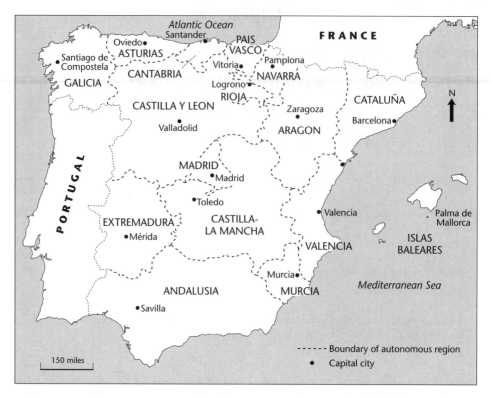

Figure 12.1 The Iberian Peninsula, Spain, and its Autonomous Regions

intervention or use; not a single form of social change can be understood without simultaneously addressing and understanding the transformations of and in the hydrological process. The socionatural production of Spanish society, I maintain, can be illustrated by excavating the central role of water politics and engineering in Spain's modernization process.

I intend to situate the political-ecological processes around water in Spain in the context of what Neil Smith (1984) defined as "the production of nature." In particular, I shall argue that the tumultuous process of modernization in Spain and its contemporary condition, both in environmental and political-economic terms, are wrought from historical spatial-ecological transformations. Modernization in Spain was a decidedly geographical project that became expressed in and through the intense spatial transformation of Spain in this century. This transformation is one in which water and the waterscape play a pivotal role. The contradictions and tensions inherent in the process that is commonly referred to as "modernization" are, I maintain, expressed by and worked through the transformation of nature and society. The "modern" environment and waterscape in Spain is what Latour (1993) would refer to as a "hybrid," a thing-like appearance (a "permanence" as Harvey [1996] would call it) that is part natural and part social, and that embodies a multiplicity of historical-geographical relations and processes.

The main portion of the paper is divided into two parts. In the first, I develop a theoretical and methodological perspective that is explicitly critical of traditional approaches in water-resources studies, which tend to separate various aspects of the hydrological cycle into discrete and independent objects of study. The traditional hydrological, engineering, geographical, political, sociological, economic, and cultural perspectives on water have produced a piecemeal perspective that maintains a particular water ideology, one that is increasingly less able to contribute in creative and innovative ways to the mitigation of growing problems associated with contemporary water practices (Ward, 1997). My perspective, broadly situated within the political ecology tradition, draws critically from recent work by ecological historians, cultural critics, sociologists of science, critical social theorists, and political economists. Although researchers working within mainstream perspectives pay lip service to considering the hydrological cycle as a complex, multifaceted, and global network, one that includes physical as well as human elements, they rarely overcome the dualisms of the nature/society divide, and they continue to isolate parts from the totality (see, for a review, Castree, 1995; Demeritt, 1994; Gerber, 1997). My main objective is to bring together what has been severed for too long by insisting that nature and society are deeply intertwined.

In the second part of the paper, I excavate the origins of Spain's early-twentieth-century modernization process (1890–1930) as expressed in debates and actions around the hydrological condition. The conceptual framework presented in the first part helps structure a narrative that weaves water through the network of socionatural relations in ways that permit the recasting of modernity as a deeply geographical, although by no means coherent, homogeneous, total, or uncontested, project. If the social and the natural cannot be severed, but are intertwined in perpetually changing ways in the production processes of both society and the physical environment, then the rather opaque idea of "the production of nature" may become clearer. In sum, I seek to document how the socionatural is historically produced to generate a particular, but inherently dynamic, geographical configuration.

On Hybrids and Socionature: Flow, Process, and Dialectics

Contemporary scholars increasingly recognize that natural or ecological conditions and processes do not operate separately from social processes, and that the actually existing socionatural conditions are always the result of intricate transformations of preexisting configurations that are themselves inherently natural *and* social. For example, David Harvey (1996) insists that there is nothing particularly unnatural about New York City. Urban areas, regions, or any other outcome of sociospatial processes or conditions exist in a network of interwoven processes that are simultaneously human, natural, material, cultural, mechanical, and organic. The myriad processes that support and maintain social life, such as, for example, water, energy, food, or computers, always combine society and nature in infinite ways; yet simultaneously, these hybrid socionatural "things" are full of contradictions, tensions, and conflicts. They are proliferating objects that Donna Haraway calls "cyborgs" (Haraway, 1991) or that Bruno Latour refers to as "quasi-objects" (Latour, 1993); these hybrid, part social/part natural – yet deeply historical and thus produced – objects/subjects are intermediaries that embody and express nature *and* society and weave networks of infinite liminal spaces. For example, if I were to capture some water in a cup and excavate the networks that brought it there, "I would pass with continuity from the local to the global, from the human to the nonhuman" (Latour, 1993, p. 121). These flows would narrate many interrelated tales, or stories, of social groups and classes and the powerful socioecological processes that produce social spaces of privilege and exclusion, of participation and marginality; chemical, physical, and biological reactions and transformations, the global hydrological cycle, and global warming; capital, machinations, and the strategies and knowledges of dam builders, urban land developers, and engineers; the passage from river to urban reservoir, and the geopolitical struggles between regions and nations. In sum, water embodies multiple tales of socionature as hybrid. The rhizome of underground and surface water flows and the streams, pipes, and canals that come together in water gushing from fountains, taps, and irrigation channels is a powerful metaphor for a deeply interconnected socionature.

The excavation of the production of these hybrid networks and their proliferation with the intensification of the modernization process entails a constructionist view in both a material and discursive sense. In both the *Grundrisse* and *Capital*, Marx insisted on the natural foundations of social development. Any materialist approach necessarily adheres to a perspective that insists that nature is an integral part of the metabolism of social life. Social relations operate in and through metabolizing the natural environment which, in turn, transforms both society and nature and produces altered or new socionatural forms (see Grundmann, 1991; Benton, 1996). While "Nature" (as a historical product) provides the foundation, social relations produce nature's and society's history. Of course, the ambition of classical Marxism was wider than reconstructing the dialectics of historical socionatural transformations and their contradictions. It also insisted on the ideological notion of "nature" in bourgeois science and society, just as it claimed to uncover "Truth" through the excavation of underlying socioecological processes (Schmidt, 1971; Benton, 1989). By concentrating on the labor process per se, however, many Marxist analysts tended to replicate the very problem they meant to criticize. In particular, by rendering nature as the substratum for the unfolding of social relations, especially labor relations, they maintained the material basis for social life, while relegating natural processes to a realm outside of social life and, hence, outside history.

I would argue, with Latour (1993), that the process of separating and purifying things natural and social resides in the conceptual and discursive construction of the world into two separate, but profoundly interrelated realms – nature and society – between which a dialectical relationship unfolds. The debate, then, becomes a dispute about the nature of this dialectical relationship, its implications, and the absence or presence of an ontological foundation from which nature and the social are distinguished and distinguishable. This form of dialectical argumentation runs as follows. Humans encounter nature, with its internal dynamics, principles, and laws, embedded in a society with its own organizing principles. This encounter inflicts consequences on both. The dialectic between nature and society becomes an external one, that is, a recursive relationship between two separate fields, nature and society, which is mediated by material, ideological, and representational practices. The product, then, is the thing (object or subject) that is produced out of this dynamic encounter.

Neil Smith (1984, 1996), in contrast, insists that nature is an integral part of the process of production or, in other words, that society and nature are integral to each other and produce permanencies (or thing-like moments) in their unity. The notion of "the production of nature," borrowed and reinterpreted from Lefebvre (1991), suggests that socionature itself is a historical-geographical process (and therefore time/place-specific). It insists on the inseparability of society and nature and maintains the unity of socionature as a process. In brief, both society and nature are produced, and are hence malleable, transformable, and potentially transgressive. Smith does not suggest that all nonhuman processes are socially produced, although he insists that all nature, including social nature, is a historical-geographical process (see also Levins and Lewontin, 1985; Lewontin, 1993). He argues instead that the idea of some sort of pristine nature ("First Nature" in Lefebvre's account) becomes increasingly problematic as new "nature" (in the sense of different forms of "nature") is produced over space and time. It is this historical-geographical process that led Haraway and Latour to argue that the number of hybrids and quasi-objects proliferates and multiplies. Indeed, from the very beginning of human history, but accelerating as the modernization process intensified, the objects and subjects of daily life became increasingly socionatural.

If we maintain a view of dialectics as internal relations (Olman, 1993; Balibar, 1995; Harvey, 1996) as opposed to external recursive relationships, then we must insist on the need to transcend the binary formations of nature and society and develop a new language that maintains the dialectical unity of the process of change as embodied in the thing itself. "Things" are hybrids or quasi-objects (subjects *and* objects, material *and* discursive, natural *and* social) from the very beginning. By this, I mean that the "world" is a process of perpetual metabolism in which social and natural processes combine in a historical-geographical production process of socionature, whose outcome (historical nature) embodies chemical, physical, social, economic, political, and cultural processes in highly contradictory but inseparable manners. Every body and thing is a mediator, part social, part natural (but without discrete boundaries), which internalizes the multiple contradictory relations that redefine and rework every body and thing.

Figure 12.2 summarizes this argument. None of the component parts is reducible to the other, yet their constitution arises from the multiple dialectical relations that swirl out from the production process itself. Consequently, the parts are always implicated in the constitution of the "thing" and are never outside the process of its making. In sum, then, the above perspective is a process-based episteme in which nothing is ever fixed or, at best, fixity is the transient moment; nothing can be captured in its entirety as the flows perpetually destroy and create, combine and separate. This particular dialectical perspective also insists on the nonneutrality of relations in terms of both their operation and their outcome, thereby politicizing both processes and fluxes. It also sees distinct categories (nature, society, city, species, water, etc.) as the outcome of the infusion of materially discursive practices that are, each time, creatively destroyed in the very production of socionature.

The above perspective will guide my narrative on the production of the modern Spanish waterscape at the turn of the century, when a distinct discourse and rhetoric of modernization emerged. This modernization drive, which permeated the whole of Spanish society, would generate the anchoring framework for key social,

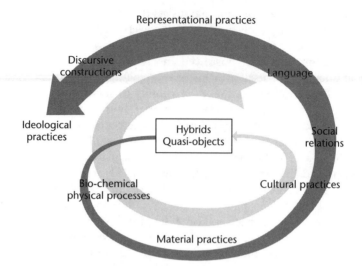

Figure 12.2 Hybridization: the production of socionature

political, cultural, and technical debates and practices until the present day. Multiple narratives that move around the spiral presented in Figure 12.2 will be woven together to reconstruct the relations of power inscribed in the discursive, ideological, cultural, material, and scientific practices through which the Spanish waterscape became constructed and reconstructed as a socionatural space that reflects Spain's contested modernization process and the relations of power inscribed therein.

The Production of Nature: Water and Modernization in Spain

I shall not begin by analyzing the Spanish water map from the available hydrological data and the physical characteristics of the water basins. Such an entrée would surely be important, but prioritizing these things would miss the central tenet of the argument outlined above. Indeed, these very physical conditions and characteristics are not absolute, stable, and God-given characteristics. On the contrary, the history of Spain's modernization has been a history of altering, redefining, and transforming these very physical characteristics. What is more, Spain's hydrological characteristics have been infused with social practices, cultural meanings, political and economic ideologies, and engineering principles for a very long time. It was not until the late nineteenth century that the socionatural production process of contemporary Spain accelerated. From that moment onwards, Spain – belatedly, somewhat reluctantly, and almost desperately – launched itself on a path of accelerating modernization. Of course, modernization through socionatural changes always takes place within already constructed historical socionatural conditions. On occasion, I shall refer to and highlight these conditions. For the present purposes, which are to document and substantiate the notion of the production of nature and to elaborate how Spain's modernization process became, and remains, a deeply geographical project, it will suffice to chart the tumultuous, contradictory, and often

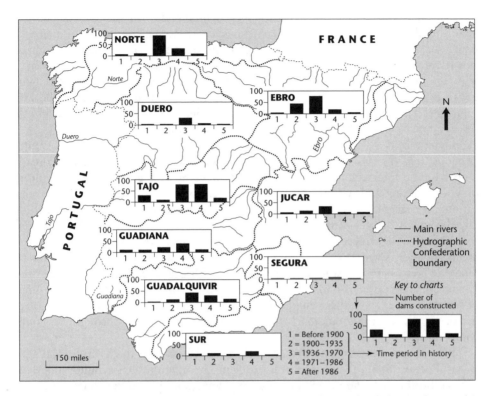

Figure 12.3 Evolution of dam construction in Spain for each of the Hydrographic Confederations (river basin authorities). Data excludes *Islas Canarias* and Pirineo Oriental
Source: Ministerio de Obras Públicas y Urbanismo (1990). *Plan Hidrólogico – Síntesis de la Documentación*. Madrid: Dirección General de Obras Hidraulicas, pp. 32–33.

very complex historical-geography of Spain's modernization through water engineering. Today the country has almost nine hundred dams, more than eight hundred of which have been constructed in this century alone (see Figure 12.3). Not a single river basin has not been altered, managed, engineered, and transformed. Water has been an obsessive theme in Spain's national life during this century, and the quest for water continues unabated (del Moral Ituarte, 1998). From the turn of the century onwards, water rapidly became a prime consideration in national political, socio-economic, and cultural debates.

Modernization as a Geographical Project: The Production of Space/Nature

The dominant form of socioeconomic development in Spain until the late nineteenth century had combined colonial trade with domestic farming. The latter was based on primarily southern large-estate dryland-culture by latifundistas whose economic position depended on a protectionist stance. The effects of increasingly liberalized international trade after 1880 (Carr, 1983), combined with the loss of the last Spanish colonies in 1898, led to disastrous socioeconomic conditions and rapidly rising social conflicts that intensified already sharp social tensions in the countryside (Fontana, 1975; Garrabou, 1975). The traditional agricultural elites were faced with the emergence of modernizing elites, both agricultural and industrial, who began to challenge the political-economic and ideological dominance of the latifundistas. The proletarianization process, combined with sharpening crisis conditions, intensified class struggle in both the city and countryside.

Industrialization, mainly focused in Catalonia and in the Basque Country (Angoustures, 1995), intensified the city/countryside divide, accentuated already long-standing interregional conflicts, and fed demands for greater regional autonomy. Containing and working through these tensions without revolutionary transformation necessitated a vision around which the modernizing social groups could ally through a project of national regeneration. This revitalization, which became formulated as a project of geographical restructuring, combined major environmental change, socioeconomic restructuring, and moral revival, all of which were linked in a regeneracionist ideological discourse. Driever (1998, p. 37) summarizes: "Spain was portrayed as part of a new world order in which Spaniards had to interpenetrate with their natural environment and geographical space in order not to perish as the international marketplace reordered the world through economic competition."

This national geographical project would revolve around the hydrological/agricultural nexus. Spain's "geographical problem" became the axis around which the sociocultural and economic malaise was explained, and where the course of action resided. One of the key protagonists articulating this revival-through-modernization was Joaquín Costa (1846–1911), the most prominent and visible figure of the radical regeneracionism promoted by the intellectuals. Born the son of a poor peasant from Aragon, he was a self-educated intellectual whose influential and prolific writings covered politics, social reform, education, and agricultural and hydraulic policies, among many other themes. His relentless struggle against poverty and the socioeconomic and political disintegration of Spain propelled him to the forefront of the public debates at the time (see Ortega, 1975; Carr, 1983; Pérez, 1999). In 1892, he wrote that state-organized hydraulic politics should be a national objective "capable of reworking the geography of the Fatherland and of solving the complex agricultural and social problems" (Costa, 1892, p. 88). For Costa, fusing the production of a new geography with a revolutionization of the internal operation of the state would help mitigate social tensions and provide the basis for a promodernist and popular petty-production-based development process (Ortí, 1994). The realization of such an ambitious project of mobilizing resources and educating the people demanded thorough geographical knowledge, though of a particular kind. As Gómez Mendoza and Ortega Cantero (1987, p. 80) argue, "the real patriotism is the bedrock of the regeneracionist project and this patriotism flows from the exact knowledge of the geographical reality of the country" (my translation). In 1918, Rafael Altamira (1923, p. 168–69), another leading intellectual, wrote that the description of Spain's geography offers a great lesson in patriotism, while Azorín (José Martínez Ruiz) concluded in 1916 that "the basis of patriotism is geography" (Azorín, 1982, p. 512). In this view, the only means by which to solve the national problem was through the problem of the land – the physical nature of the territory.

This project to remake Spanish geography as a part of modernization combined a decidedly political strategy, a particular ideological vision, a call for a scientific-positivist understanding of the natural world, a scientific-technocratic engineering mission, and a popular base rooted in a traditional peasant rural culture. Plenty of evidence can be found for this in Costa's work and in that of his contemporaries (for a review, see Pérez De La Dehesa, 1966; Tuñon De Lara, 1971; Ortí, 1976). The revolution in the state – but certainly not of the state – was effected through a politics of spatial and environmental transformation that would center around the defense of the small peasant producer-cum-landowner, communal (state) control of water, educational enhancement, technical-scientific knowledge, and the leap to power of an alliance of small holders and the new bourgeoisie that hitherto had been largely marginalized by the aristocratic landowning elite and their associated administrators in the state apparatus. At the same time, the focus on restoring or, in fact, expanding landownership through "internal colonization" fostered growth in and concentrated the efforts of an "organically" organized state that brought reformist intellectuals, some worker movements, and the nascent industrial bourgeoisie together in a more or less coherent vision of reform against the traditionalists (Ortega, 1975). The geographical project became, as such, the glue around which often unlikely partners could coalesce, while excluding both the more radical, left-wing revolutionaries and the "radical" conservatives. Surely, the sublimation of the many tensions and conflicts within this loose alliance of reformists, when accomplished through a focus on reorganizing Spain's hydraulic geography, served the purpose of providing a discursive vehicle to ally hitherto excluded social groups without defining the problem purely in class or other conflictual social terms (see Nadal Reimat, 1981).

Water as the Linchpin to Spain's Modernization Drive

Los Pantanos o la Muerte! [Dams or Death!] (Pérez, 1999, p. 504)

If the "remaking" of Spain's geography became the great modernizing adagio, then water and hydrological engineering were its master tools. Joaquín Costa became one of the prime advocates and potent symbols of this broad social movement for modernization through geographical restructuring. His "hydrological solution" would be the substratum for fostering growth by permitting social and land reforms and encouraging cultural emancipation (Ortega, 1975). His writings would be invoked time and time again by a wide variety of social groups to defend and legitimize national hydraulic programs and the policy of land reform through "internal colonial" settlements. The regeneracionist project became formulated as a "hydrological correction of the national geographical problem" (Gómez Mendoza, 1992, p. 236). For Costa, hydraulic politics sublimated the totality of the nation's economic program, not only for agriculture, but for the whole of Spanish socioeconomic life. Hydraulic constructions for irrigation purposes were regarded as a progressive alternative to the traditional policy of tariffs and import restrictions, which were supported by dryland latifundistas (Torres Campos, 1907). At base, the hydraulic foundation necessitating *el regeneracionismo* resided in the uneven distribution of rainfall and the torrential and intermittent nature of Spain's fluvial system, which was said to make the country "the antechamber of Africa" (de Reparez, 1906). The great modernizing drive of the revivalists therefore demanded not only an imitation and use of nature, but its *creation*: "[increasing] the amount of fertile soil by making a hydraulic artery system cross the whole country – a national network of dams and irrigation channels" (Gómez Mendoza and Ortega Cantero, 1992, p. 174). In "El Problema Nacional," Ricardo Macías Picavea (1899, pp. 318–20), a leading regeneracionist essayist and intellectual, summarizes the hydraulic mission as a necessary strategy for national development:

> There are countries which . . . can solely and exclusively become civilized with such a hydraulic policy, planned and developed by means of designated grand works. Spain is among them . . . And the truth is that Spanish civilized agriculture finds itself strongly subjected to this inexorable dilemma: to have water or to die . . . Therefore, a hydraulic politics imposes itself; this requires changing all the national forces in the direction of this gigantic enterprise. . . . We have to dare to restore great lakes, create real interior seas of sweet water, multiply vast marshes, erect many great dams, and mine, exploit and withhold the drops of water that fall over the peninsula without returning, if possible, a single drop to the sea.

This patriotic mission, requiring the convergence of all national forces, fused around the hydraulic program, which then became the embodiment and representation of a collective myth of national development. This project was sustained and inspired by a *reformist geographical optimism*, which substituted for the social and political pessimism of Spain's turn-of-the-century condition (Ortí, 1984, p. 18). The hydraulic utopia of abundant waters for all would not only produce an "ecological harmony," but also contribute to the formation of a socially harmonious order. The production of a new hydraulic geography would reconcile the ever-growing social tensions in the Spanish countryside, tensions that were taking acute class forms and that resulted from the adverse and conflictual conditions of scarcity and inequality. According to Alfonso Ortí (1984, p. 12), the symbolic power of this material intervention to achieve "hydraulic regeneration" constituted "a mythical power, a collective illusion, and the imagined reconciliation of diverse ideologies." This specific form of regeneration served the productionist logic of the new liberal bourgeoisie that aspired to transform society and space according to the principles of capitalist profitability. It was aimed at facilitating Spain's integration into Europe's modernization process.

The State as Master Socioenvironmental Engineer

"To irrigate is to govern." (Costa, [1892] 1975)

Such an ambitious perspective to regenerate Spain through a geographical project necessitated concerted action and collective control. The regeneracionists welcomed the liberation of international markets and the demise of nineteenth-century protectionism under which the dryland latifundistas of (mainly southern and central) Spain flourished. By 1880, trade liberalization had plunged them into a deep crisis in the aftermath of the expansion of the US wheat export boom. The traditional landed bourgeoisie was economically weakened as a result, but their political commitment to maintain their power at both national and local scales did not abate. This control permitted the continuation, if not the reinforcement, of a strong protectionist economic policy framework.

The central-state intervened nevertheless to produce a nature amenable to the requirements of a modernized, competitive, and irrigated agriculture (Ortega, 1975). This was considered essential to the implementation of hydraulic works that would "remake the geography of the fatherland" (Costa, 1892, cited in del Moral Ituarte, 1998, p. 121), revive the national economy, and "regenerate the people" [la raza] (del Moral Ituarte, 1998, p. 121). The hydraulic politics were, for Costa (1975), a way to place Spain within a European sociospatial framework, after its loss of influence in the Americas, on the basis of a rural development vision that combined a Rousseauan ideal with a small-scaled, independent, and democratic peasant society. The promotion of the rural ideal on the basis of a petty-bourgeois ideology would become the spinal cord of the liberal state and the route to the Europeanization of the nation (Nadal Reimat, 1981, p. 139; Fernández Clemente, 1990).

The growing demand for water and the requirements for a more efficient and equitable distribution of irrigation waters necessitated a fundamental change in the legal status and appropriation rights of water. The liberal revolution in Spain (approximately 1811–1873), which had attempted an institutional (anti)feudal restructuring to promote capitalist forms of ownership and the circulation of goods as commodities, extended also to what Maluquer de Motes (1983, p. 76) called the "depatrimonialization of water." The existence of seignorial rights over water prevented or blocked the development of productive activities that necessitated ever-larger quantities of water. Although the depatrimonialization of land and water reinforced their private character, the growing political and economic crisis of liberalism towards the end of the century prevented the state from embarking on a productivist and privately run program to maximize production "to the last drop of water" (Gómez Mendoza and Ortega Cantero, 1992, p. 174). The regeneracionist vision, then, faced with the failure of privatized and commodified water to operate as an efficient allocative and productive instrument, promoted the emergence of a collective spirit ("illusion" in the words of Alfonso Ortí [1984, p. 14]). The latter implied that the supply of the necessary quantities of water was only possible under a public and socialized form of coordination managed through the state. This collective and state-led but productivist and modernizing vision, would eventually also include the state-led production of "great hydraulic works" (Ortega, 1975; Villaneuva Larraya, 1991). In sum, the regeneracionists turned to the state – after the failure of the Liberal project to defeat the feudal elites – as the agent that could generate a sufficiently large volume of capital to mobilize the nation's natural resources. Moreover, for Costa, the productivist modernization by means of the hydraulic motor would in fact consolidate the liberal state in Spain. In short, a free-market-based, intensive, and productive national economy, whose accumulation process would accelerate on a par with other northern European states, necessitated

a transformation in the state in a double and deeply contradictory sense. Power relations within the state apparatus needed to change in favor of, first, a more modernist alliance of petty-owners, industrialists, and modernizing engineers, and
second, revolutionary social reform supported by the state such that the grand
hydraulic works could lay the foundations for a modernizing Spain. These two tasks
were of course mutually dependent, and yet irreconcilable. Strong traditional forces
fought to maintain control over key state functions and prevented the rise to political power of the nascent petty-owners and middle classes. This firm hold of the
traditional conservative elites blocked most attempts at modernizing the social
economy. The mosaic of contradictory forces and the resistance of the traditionalists would stall state-led modernizing efforts, resulting in more acute and openly
fought social antagonisms throughout the first two decades of the century. These
would eventually pave the way for dictatorial regimes.

Despite the collectivist discourse of much of the regeneracionist literature, it
remained deeply committed to a project of insertion into an international capitalist
market. Although the state needed to take central control over water and forests, it
should do so on the basis of a landownership structure that was essentially private
and market-led (see also Fernández Clemente, 1990). The hydraulic agenda of Costa
and his colleagues was clouded with revolutionary claims but defended as a
reformist route for development against the stronghold of an antireformist, economically and culturally conservative and protectionist elite. In sum, two models of
capitalist accumulation, with evidently different supporting social groups and allies,
crystallized around the hydraulic debates at the time. The social, political, and ecological consequences and implications of these two models would differ fundamentally even while sharing an organicist vision of the world. On the one hand, the
traditionalists defended a protectionist economic stance and the continuation of
existing political and social power relations. On the other, the regeneracionists advocated a more liberal perspective, a rapid modernization of the economy, and a transformation of sociopolitical power relations. The issue of land ownership and the
role of water therein revolved around the question of who would own and control
what part of the land and its waters. For the regeneracionists, for whom petty ownership constituted the way ahead, the hydraulic route was an essential precondition,
while the limited possibilities for accumulation pointed to the state as the only body
that could generate the required investment funds on the one hand and push through
the necessary reforms in the face of strong and sustained opposition from the landed
aristocracy on the other (Ortega, 1975, 1992). At the same time, the very support
of at least some sections of the old elites could be secured via this reformist route,
since it did not threaten their fundamental rights as landowners but defended rural
power against the rising tide of the urban industrial elites and the proletariat. This
was indeed quite central to forging the support of the dominant Catholic groups
that defended a solidaristic and organic model of social cohesion.

Purification and the Transformation of Nature:
Hydraulic Engineers as Producers of Socionature

The hydraulic intervention to create a waterscape supportive of the modernizing
desires of the revivalists, without questioning the social and political foundations

of the existing class structure and social order, was very much based on a respect for "natural" laws and conditions. The latter were assumed to be or thought of as intrinsically stable, balanced, equitable, and harmonious. The hydraulic engineering mission consisted primarily in "restoring" the "perturbed" equilibrium of the erratic hydrological cycles in Spain. This endeavor required a significant scientific and engineering enterprise, first in terms of understanding and analyzing nature's "laws," and, second, in using these insights to work toward a restoration of the "innate" harmonious development of nature. The moral, economic, and cultural "disorder" and "imbalances" of the country at the time paralleled the "disorder" in Spain's erratic hydraulic geography, both of which needed to be restored and rebalanced (as nature's innate laws suggested) to produce a socially harmonious development. Two threads have to be woven together in this context: the pivotal position of a particular group of scientists in the hydraulic arena, the Corps of Engineers (Villaneuva Larraya, 1991), and the changing visions concerning the scientific management of the terrestrial part of the hydrological cycle. Both, in turn, were linked to the rising prominence of hydraulic issues on the sociopolitical agenda at the turn of the century.

The Corps of Engineers, founded in 1799, was (and remains) the professional collective responsible for the development and implementation of public works. It is a highly elitist, intellectualist, "high-cultured," male-dominated, socially homogeneous, and exclusive corporatist organization that has, over the centuries, taken a leading role in Spanish politics and development (Mateu Bellés, 1995). The decision-making structure is hierarchical and all key managerial and institutional bodies, such as the "Junta Consultiva de las Obras Públicas," the hydrological divisions, the provincial headquarters, and various ad hoc study commissions are exclusively "manned" by engineers. In line with the emergent scientific discourse on orography and river-basin structure and dynamics, the engineering community argued for the foundation of engineering and managerial intervention on the basis of the "natural" integrated water flow of a basin, rather than on the basis of historically and socially formed administrative regions (see Figure 12.4). The emergent geographical regionalization overlaid the traditional political-administrative divisions of the country, forcing a reordering of the territory on the basis of the country's orographical structure. The latter, in turn, was portrayed by the engineers as the crucial planning unit for hydraulic interventions. Cano García (1992, p. 312) succinctly summarizes this scientific perspective: "To revert to the great orographical delimitation for organizing the division of the land represents a contribution made from within the strict field of our discipline [engineering] and at the same time, at least initially, it shows the abandoning of traditional political divisions and the importance of other perspectives and concepts."

The history of the delimitation of hydrological divisions is infused with the influence of the regeneracionist discourse on the one hand and the scientific insights gained from hydrology and orography on the other. The attempt to "naturalize" political territorial organization was part and parcel of a strategy of the modernizers to challenge existing social and political power geometries. The construction of and command over a new territorial scale might permit them to implement their vision and bypass more traditional and reactionary power configurations. The complex history of the formation of river-basin authorities and their articulation

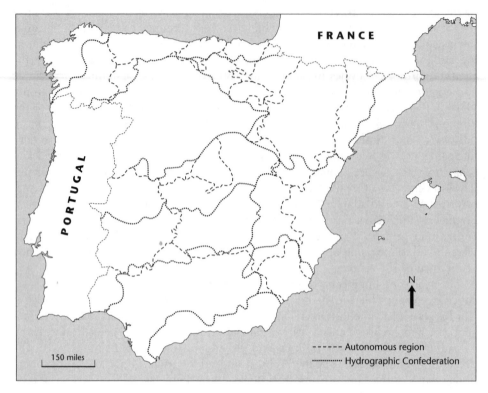

Figure 12.4 Boundaries of the Autonomous Regions and the Hydrographic Confederations

with other political forms of territorial organization, in particular the national state, is a long, complicated, and tortuous one. "Nature" would become inextricably connected to the choreography of power, while the scientific discourse on nature was strategically marshaled to serve power struggles for the control over and management of water. The river basins would become the scale par excellence through which the modernizers tried to undermine or erode the powers of the more traditional provincial or national state bodies. Therefore, the struggle over the territorial organization of intervention expresses the political power struggles between traditionalists and reformers. While the river-basin defenders would become the founding "fathers" of the regeneracionist agenda, the traditional elites held to the existing administrative territorial structure of power. The regeneracionist engineers thereby incorporated the naturalized river basins into their political project. Capturing the scale of the river basin as the geographical basis for exercising control and power over the organization, planning, and reconstruction of the hydraulic landscape was one of the central arenas through which the power of the traditionalists (and the scales over which they exercised hegemonic control) was challenged. In fact, this rescaling of the state and the articulation of different scales of governance became one of the great arenas of struggle for control and power. The modernizers attempted to take hold of the hydrological divisions and develop them as pivotal institutions for instigating the hydrological revolution, while the national scale remained more firmly in the hands of the traditional elites. The bumpy history of the hydrological divisions records this struggle. The instability of their administrative and political organization reflects the relative power of the traditional power brokers. It would await Franco's dictatorship before this issue was resolved, at which time the hydrological dream and its intellectual bearers, the engineers, were aligned with and incorporated into a new fascist-organicist state structure (Gómez Mendoza and Ortega Cantero, 1992).

It was only from 1926 onwards, during the dictatorship of Primo de Rivera, that the current Confederaciones Sindicales Hidrográficas were gradually established as quasi-autonomous organizations in charge of managing water as stipulated by the Water Act of 1879 (Giansante, 1999). The last of these ten Confederaciones was only established in 1961 (see Figure 12.4). What had proven impossible to achieve during the first decades of the century was finally implemented during the dictatorship. It is also from that moment on that their names reflected the river basins for which they were responsible rather than the previous political-territorial naming. In addition, they acquired a certain political status with participation from the state, banks, chambers of commerce, provincial authorities, etc. At each stage, the engineers took the lead roles and became the activists of the regeneracionist project through the combination of their legitimization as the holders of scientific knowledge and their privileged position as a politically elite corps within the state apparatus. The complex and perpetually changing administrative organization and power structures associated with the successive attempts to establish river-basin authorities, and their relative lack of power until the 1930s, reflect the failure of the early modernizers to fundamentally challenge existing power lineages and scales (Mateu Bellés, 1994, 1995). It is only from the later 1920s, and in particular during the Franco era, that the regeneracionist project was gradually implemented.

Conclusions

In sum, the regeneracionist agenda(s) first maintained that the restoration of wealth in Spain should be based on the knowledge of the laws and balances of nature; second, this restoration required the correction of defects imposed by the geography of the country and, particularly, its "imbalances in its climatic and hydraulic regimes" (Gómez Mendoza and Ortega Cantero, 1992, p. 173); and third, this enterprise of geographical rectification could, because of its range and importance, only be carried out by the central public authorities. The hydraulic mission was seen as the solution to the social problems facing Spain at the turn of the century. Failing this, social tensions were bound to intensify, and struggle, if not civil war, would be the likely outcome. Ironically, of course, the voluntarist, powerful, and autocratic hydraulic engineer pursuing a voluntarist program of imposed reform foreshadowed the fascist (falangist) ideology. The latter would gain momentum from the early 1920s onward. Although the debates at the turn of the century indicated a desire to regenerate Spain, conservative forces prevented its actual implementation, and social tension intensified, further destabilizing an already highly fragmented and divisive society. The centralizing fascist regimes that emerged from this turmoil could finally push through the production of a new geography, a new nature, and a new waterscape, something the regeneracionists of the turn of the century had so desperately advocated but failed to accomplish.

This quasi-object and hybrid thing that, until this very day, embodies Spain's modernization process, expresses how modernity is deeply and inevitably a geographical project in which the intertwined transformations of nature and society are both medium and expression of shifting power positions that become materialized in the production of new water flows and the construction of new waterscapes. It is the maelstrom of tensions and contradictions that weave the material, discursive, ideological, and representational, together in often-perplexing, always deeply heterogeneous, collages of changing and shifting positions of power and struggle that decisively shaped the production of the Spanish waterscape over the next century.

I have attempted to reconstruct multiple and often contradictory narratives that span a broad range of apparently separate instances such as engineering, politics, economics, culture, science, nature, ideology, and discourse through which the tumultuous reordering of sociophysical space is shaped and transformed, and out of which a new socioenvironmental landscape emerges; landscapes that are simultaneously physical and social, they reflect historical-geographical struggles and social power geometries, and they interiorize the flux and dynamics of sociospatial change. Geographical conditions, this paper has argued, are reconstructed as the outcome of a process of production in which both nature and society are fused together in a way that renders them inseparable, producing a restless "hybrid" quasi-object in which material, representational, and symbolic practices are welded together. Doing geography then implies the excavation and reconstruction of the contested process of the "production of nature." Of course, this perspective also asks serious questions about who controls, who acts, and who has the power to produce what kind of socionature. The intertwining of nature and society in this production process has indeed profound political implications. As Lewontin (1997, pp. 137–38), a Harvard biologist, maintains:

> The constructionist view of organism and environment is of some consequence to human action. . . . Remaking the world is the universal property of living organisms and is inextricably bound up with their nature. . . . We must decide what kind of world we want to live in and then try to manage the process of change as best as we can approximate it.

Chapter 13

Oil as Money: The Devil's Excrement and the Spectacle of Black Gold

Michael J. Watts

Introduction

Gold which the devil gives his paramours turns into excrement after his departure. (Freud, 1955, p. 174)

I call petroleum "the devil's excrement." It brings trouble.... The [oil money] hasn't brought us any benefits.... We are drowning in the devil's excrement. (Juan Pablo Perez Alfonso, founder of OPEC, 1976, cited in Karl, 1982, p. 316)

After what has been said money is seen to be nothing other than deodorized, dehydrated shit that has been made to shine. (Ferenczi, 1950, p. 327)

This black gold [petroleum], the magical elan vital for ... economic takeoff. (Amuzegar, 1982, p. 814)

Gold by itself is fraught with problems, first of all because of its mysterious origins. It comes from the bowels of the earth.... Gold is instant wealth [yet] it produces corruption ... [it] can signify the loss of the soul ... it scorches fingers and hearts; it is odorless but it is the "devil's dung." (Gille, 1986, pp. 258–9)

In 1975, the founder of OPEC and former Venezuelan oil minister Perez Alfonso wrote a book entitled *Hundiendonos en el excremento de diablo* (We Are Sinking in the Devil's Excrement). Oil, says Perez, is the Third World's black gold. Like gold it brings untold wealth and yet it is a supremely powerful and ultimately uncontrollable force. Like gold in the world of the alchemist, petroleum is a pure fruit of "the subterranean workings of the telluric forces" (Gille, 1986, p. 258), yet it is a brilliant threat. In Perez's powerful and compelling vision, the natural bounty of oil had, in the magical and mysterious process of being transformed into money, become a putrid and toxic waste. It was as if the Venezuelan "body" suffered from bulimia; an excessive, orgiastic appetite was matched by periodic sickness, which contaminated the national metabolism. Indeed, for Perez the digestion of petroleum

– what was referred to in Venezuela as "sowing the oil" – gave birth to a weak and corrupt society, decadent and degenerate under the accumulated weight of waste and excrement (Coronil, 1987; Karl, 1997). "Manna or malediction?" was how one Venezuelan commentator opened his discussion of the legacy of petroleum in Venezuela (Izard, 1986, p. 205). Oil had vastly increased the national appetite and the capacity to consume, yet ingesting petroleum only served to contaminate everything. Black gold, like the devil's counterpart, had turned into excrement. As Coronil puts it in describing Venezuela during the oil boom,

> Venezuela had lost control over itself; intoxicated by oil as waste it had become transformed into waste. . . . The identification of both the nation and individuals with excrement became an ever more common short hand expression for everyday problems . . . "somos una mierda," "es que este es un pais de mierda" ("we are pieces of shit," "it's that this country is made of shit"). (Coronil, 1987, p. 233)

At about the same time that Venezuela's oil wealth was being debated explicitly in terms of waste, corruption, and degeneracy, the Iranian, or more properly the Shah Pahlavi's, petrolic vision of "the Great Civilization" was being derailed by an Islamic revolution made in the name of disciplined Muslim renewal and an autocratic moral order. Several thousand miles away from Caracas, black gold ushered in the collapse of the world's most powerful monarchy and, in its wake, a massive bloodletting.

Oil wealth, the magical elan vital of economic and social transformation, had proven to be a very mixed blessing.

El Dorado: Oil Wealth as Spectacle, Display and Illusion

> The spectacle is not a collection of images, but a social relation among people, mediated by images. (Debord, 1978, para. 4)

> Oil creates the illusion of a completely changed life, life without work, life for free. . . . The concept of oil expresses perfectly the eternal human dream of wealth achieved through lucky accident. . . . In this sense oil is a fairy tale and like every fairy tale a bit of a lie. (Kapuscinski, 1982, p. 35)

For many commentators and critics, the oil bonanza of the 1970s was seen to presage the dawn of prosperity for the privileged few. As the West looked on in horror, oil prices ran out of control, soaring effortlessly, quadrupling in 1973–4 alone, then reaching their zenith during the second boom of 1980. Government revenues of OPEC states mushroomed by over 1,000 percent between 1970 and 1980. Five years after the first boom, nine of the thirteen OPEC members devoted close to 50 percent of their now bloated gross domestic product (GDP) to domestic investment. State treasuries were literally awash with money.

So began the era of blind ambition, "the Great Civilization" in Iran and "La Gran Venezuela." Jahangir Amuzegar describes this sensibility as a "lyrical illusion," an exhilarating state of euphoria in which state planners, blinded by the refulgence of the great God petroleum, came to believe that oil wealth could solve all problems (Amuzegar, 1982, p. 827). El Dorado was finally located, and it was an oil well.

From its inception, the oil boom was a spectacle, with new social relations mediated by images (Debord, 1978). Reza Shah predicted that, in a decade, Iran would have the same living standard as Germany and France (Kapuscinski, 1982, p. 53); in twenty years, he bragged, "we shall be ahead of the United States" (Shah Pahlavi, in Zonis, 1991, p. 65). In the era of the Great Civilization that lay ahead, the Shah saw a world of unbridled material prosperity, thousands of electric buses to shuttle well-endowed workers to and from their workplace, and a three-day work week. The monetary deluge that floated this modern utopia was truly biblical in scale. Hector Hurtado, the Minister of Finance in Venezuela, saw money cascading into the state treasury, money "beyond our wildest dreams" (cited in Karl, 1997, p. 2). Boundless money produced boundless ambition, what was dubbed "Pharaohism" by the popular press. During the 1970s, for example, over three-quarters of the top twenty states classified by scale of public investment (the number of projects exceeding US $100 million) were oil producers. Saudi Arabia and Iran each accounted for over 100 projects costing in excess US $1 billion dollars a shot! (Gelb, 1984, p. 33). To add an extra frisson, the cost overruns on each of these Herculean projects averaged 109 percent!

Anything was possible, even the defeat of nature. Saudi Arabia, for example, aggressively promoted domestically produced wheat, grown in the most inhospitable of desert environments. After massive production subsidies, Saudi wheat could be purchased for US $1050 per ton. US wheat, of vastly superior quality, could be acquired on the world market for less than US $150 per ton (Chaudhry, 1989, p. 128).

Commodity booms are not unusual in themselves, of course. The value of several commodities grew in excess of 20 percent per annum during the 1970s. On a larger historical canvas, the gold and bullion boom in the Americas during the sixteenth century resembles in certain respects the oil windfall four centuries later. Some 450 million pesos of precious metals poured into Spain between 1503 and 1660, stimulating feverish activity in the economy. Seville became a world city for a short while, driven by a manufacturing boom and a cycle of inflationary spending and borrowing (see Braudel, 1973; Wallerstein, 1974; Anderson, 1984; Vilar, 1984). The bullion bonanza lasted a century and a half, producing in its wake inflation, debt, and a crippled Castillian state. Some aspects of the oil boom appear strikingly similar. Both commodities were, after all, central to the mercantilist and capitalist world economies of the time and each, in different ways, contributed to state centralization and state building.

Naturally, there are also radical dissimilarities. These contrasting forms of money were inserted into vastly different political economies and put to quite different uses. The sheer magnitude, duration, and density of the booms also diverge markedly. None the less, these money booms, and the crises they precipitated, if rooted in their historical and cultural specificities, do both provide an opportunity to illuminate the working of societies into which vast fluxes of money are injected, and by extension enable one to outline the social, cultural, and political contours of money. Oil as El Dorado speaks powerfully to what Simmel (1978, p. 175) saw as money's specific role in "reified social functions," as the reified representation of impersonal capitalism. The spectacular manifestations of oil wealth reveal, first, something of the social relations of peripheral capitalisms and, second, how the growth of money in societies often presumed to be partly "traditional" reveals something of how money itself is a "frightful leveler" whose colorlessness and indifference "hollows out the core of things" (Simmel, 1978, p. 414).

Meanings of Oil Money

> Oil *is* almost like money. (Robert O. Anderson, Chairman of ARCO, cited in Yergin, 1991, p. 13)

> Three categories – the imaginary, the symbolic and the real – correspond to the three functions of money: in its capacity as a measure of value money is "imaginary"; as a medium of exchange, money is "symbolic"; and as an instrument of reserve or of hoarding, money is "real." (Goux, 1989, p. 52)

A very great difficulty in talking about money arises from its multiple functions and representations. To simplify such complexity greatly, in this chapter I am going to pursue two broad lines of argument. The first starts from Marx's discussion of the functions of money: as a universal equivalent, as a measure of value, as a medium of exchange, and as social power. But, following Goux (1989), I want to identify these multiple functions as the inseparable symbolic, imaginary, and real aspects of money. Money is both an objectified relation of production (see Marx) and a system of culturally encoded symbols, a sort of transactional order which signifies itself (Smelt, 1980). The specific cultural, social, and historical forms in which these attributes are expressed will vary enormously, giving rise to the multiple meanings of money in capitalist and non-capitalist societies (Zelizer, 1989). Underlying this heterogeneity, however, is a general presumption that money is always in part an abstraction and one that portrays the character, what Simmel (1978, p. 251) called the "modern spirit," of capitalist society. The second line is taken directly from Simmel's *Philosophy of Money* (1978). The central argument here is tripartite in form: first, that the rise of complex and more abstract monetary systems corresponds to a *Gemeinschaft-Gesellschaft* shift; second, that the growing dominance of money represents a progression towards abstraction and convention, which is itself a reflection of impersonal and abstract social relations; third, money promotes increased personal freedom and social exchange at the same time that it subjects human life to growing calculability, bureaucratization, and quantitative regulation (Turner, 1986). For Simmel, money spoke to estrangement under modernity: reification, alienation, and objectification.

I wish to trace these two broad problematics – the symbolic, imaginary, and real unity of money on the one hand, and the simultaneous integrative and disintegrative effects of money *à la* Simmel on the other – as they are played out in oil-based economies awash with money during the 1970s. In this case – and I shall focus primarily on Nigeria – money takes the form of *oil rents*. There are two particular significances to money as rent. First, oil money – as a form of money – must be theorized in terms of specific forms of state landed property (Haussman, 1981). In other words, as owner of the means of production of petroleum, the state mediates the particular social relations by which oil is exploited (royalties, commissions, state-owned enterprises) and converted into money. Changes in the ownership of the state take place through political transformations in the ruling class alliances that govern the state apparatuses.

The second significance of money as rent derives from the dominance of extractive and rentier capitals, which underlie money booms and particular patterns of commodity circulation. In other words, I want to argue that money (or commodity) booms based on extractive and rentier activity rather than on productive capital produce a particular sort of money fetishism. Unlike wealth created through industrial accumulation – in which there is some direct relation between productive labour, investment, work, and money – oil money is effaced and disguised, appearing as it were out of thin air. To put it crudely, the form of capital which corresponds to the proliferation of wealth fundamentally shapes the cultural economy, the particular social and cultural constructions and fetishisms, of money itself.

The Midas Touch: Ingesting Petrodollars and Manufacturing Modernity in Iran and Venezuela

[Your] old socialism is finished. Old, obsolete, finished. . . . I achieve more than the Swedes. Huh! Swedish socialism! It didn't even nationalize forests and water. But I have . . . my White Revolution . . . believe me, in Iran we're far more advanced than you and really have nothing to learn from you. (Shah Pahlavi, interview with Oriana Fallaci, *New Republic*, 1 December 1974, pp. 17–18)

The decision to build a modern industrialized economy was mine. There were others who wanted to move more slowly. But we had to take advantage of this moment given to us, pull Venezuela out of her underdevelopment, and propel her into the twentieth century. (Interview with President Carlos Andres Perez, cited in Karl, 1997, p. 351)

There are about thirty developing countries that are net exporters of oil but they differ markedly in terms of area, size, oil endowment, dependence on petroleum revenues, and economic structure (Watts, 1984). There is a fundamental distinction between the oil-producing city or desert states (Kuwait, Saudi Arabia), which are land and labor poor and in capital surplus, and states such as Iran, Venezuela, and Nigeria, which are large and well-populated, with diversified economies and a substantial domestic economy and home market. In this chapter I shall address oil money in the context of the latter, the so-called "high absorbers" (Gelb, 1984). These petroleum-based economies embarked upon ambitious, and not infrequently disastrous, state-led development programs during the 1970s, ingesting huge quantities of oil revenues. A decade later these same economies were plagued by hyperinflation, economic stagnation, structural balance of payments problems, periodic devaluations, and a massive foreign debt.

What the high absorbers have in common for the purposes of my discussion are the following contradictory traits:

- A dependence on oil as a fully internationalized commodity. All transactions are in dollars (oil *is* money) and the petro-state, as the landlord and entrepreneur, is "internationalized" (i.e., expands its reliance on the world market through a growing monocultural dependence on oil revenues).
- The enclave character of the oil industry within oil producing states, which implies an absence of linkage effects to non-oil sectors. The petroleum industry does not constitute itself as a major determinant of the organization of social life. Hence its impact on the national economy will be determined by the landed property relation (the social relations by which oil is exploited) and the realization of oil rents. What distinguishes an oil country, then, is "not so much the presence of petroleum as the *expenditure of petrodollars*" (Haussman, 1981, p. 75, emphasis added).
- The nationalization of the oil sector such that oil monies flow directly (via taxes, rents, concessions, and sales) to the state treasury, which accordingly acts as a strong centralizing force. Oil accrues to the state as an independent source of revenue, which affords it an unusual degree of political and economic autonomy (i.e., the state is "suspended" from civil society; Katouzian, 1981).
- The centralizing impact of oil revenues confers a central role for the public sector (fiscal linkages) via state investment ("the entire system . . . depends on the size and strategy of state expenditure"; Katouzian, 1981, p. 246), and to this extent the state is "domesticated" (i.e., projected into civil society). The state, in other words, takes on the primary role of "localizing" money capital (oil rents).

Both the Accion Democratic government of Carlos Perez (1974–8) in Venezuela and the Pahlavi regime in Iran saw oil as the ticket to modernity on a grand scale. In Venezuela the centerpiece of "La Gran Venezuela" was the US $52 billion industrial complex in Ciudad Guayana. For the Shah it was the spectacle of modernism; in 1974 he initiated a monumental downtown project in Tehran bearing his name (Shahestan Pahlavi), not simply the largest concentration of service activities in the world but "the equivalent of the Persepolis" (Costello, 1981, p. 170). Grandiosity rested in both instances on extreme political centralization. It took the form of a monarchical clique under an autocratic Shah in Iran, a small power bloc consisting of family, high-ranking state bureaucrats, and a group of industrial and financial bourgeoisies who surrendered political power as a condition of access to oil monies. Under Perez, a bureaucratic oligarchy supported state ownership but actively promoted a domestic capitalist class, "the big manufacturers, large commercial farmers, construction contractors and real estate interests and the large import-exporters who have received the bulk of the investment funds" (Petras and Morley, 1983, p. 26).

The Perez government operationalized a two-prong strategy: sectoral nationalization (iron ore, petrochemicals) and massive investments in upstream sectors (steel); and the redirection of foreign investment into downstream non-oil economic activities (Coronil and Skurski, 1991). The Shah recycled oil money through state development banks which favored large Iranian private capital – in essence a small court clique – particularly in the heavy and capital goods sectors. The small-scale bazaar economy was marginalized and income inequality increased precipitously (Imam-Jomeh, 1985).

In spite of the differences of emphasis there are striking macroeconomic empirical regularities. First, oil money fuels a rapid growth and expansion of state expenditures and parastatal organizations. A huge share of money capital is, in other words, localized by the state to reproduce itself via expenditures on administration and defense/repressive apparatuses. Second, an urban construction boom is stimulated by public investment projects and a vast import boom of both consumer durables and capital goods. Third, there is an increased demand for non-tradables, which promotes an appreciation of the real exchange rate (and hence further stimulates imports). Fourth, a deliberate effort is made to encourage local industrialization through import substitution behind high tariff walls. Fifth, non-oil sectors lag (the so-called Dutch Disease), especially in agriculture. Finally there is a tendency towards "overshooting," that is to say a difficulty in scaling back lumpy state investments, a process compounded by inflation and additional borrowing to cover project completion.

In both Venezuela and Iran, the 1970s witnessed a period of rapid urbanization, industrial growth, and social change. In both cases what emerged was a sort of rentier capitalism in which the state redistributed oil revenues through rents, subsidies, and outright corruption. Huge quantities of public oil monies were privately appropriated and exported; according to Petras and Morley (1983, p. 15) some US $2.3 billion left Venezuela in 1977 for the purchase of property in southern Florida! Sowing oil monies invariably meant seeding foreign bank accounts. Criminality emerged as the normal, and to a degree acceptable, form of sociality and display. For the popular classes, inflation, real estate speculation, administrative chaos, and escalating costs of living (especially food) defined the lived reality of the oil years. The Shah's Great Civilization was, as Kapuscinski (1982) noted, "the Great Injustice." Within several years of the first oil boom, both countries were running substantial balance of payments deficits and were borrowing heavily.

Against this backdrop there are three relevant aspects of the oil boom that provide the vantage point for grasping the form, function, and meaning of petrodollars. The fetishization of money, and the intense activity, much of which was patently and publicly illegal, focused on the acquisition of wealth without apparent effort. Petroleum came to be synonymous with money and the defining force in society. Second, petro-states emerged as rentier and redistributive in form though their social character is locally specific (autocratic and highly centralized personal monarchical rule in Iran, complex political pacts and alliances orchestrated through a powerful oligarchical bureaucracy in Venezuela). The state appears suspended above society – it is represented as *the* source of power since oil *is* power – yet is projected into society as it spends simultaneously to develop and purchase political consent. Finally, the state mediates the contradiction between public petro-wealth and individual appropriation of it. The state distribution of oil monies as rents dominates the investment of money as productive capital. A culture of corruption flourishes in such a way that the state paradoxically becomes *the* major blockage to development (understood as systematic capitalist accumulation) at the same moment that the state is *the* vehicle to promote it.

How, then, can money be traced through the various social, cultural, and political circuits of petrolic capitalism as it is constituted through this trilogy of processes? In the remainder of the chapter I shall focus on another high-absorber oil state, namely Nigeria.

Paradoxes of Prosperity: Oil Money in Nigeria

> Oil is crude or dirty and so are the actions it often inspires. Oil is volatile and so are the expectations that are based on it; oil is a diminishing or vanishing asset, so is the false sense of political power which it could confer. (Festus Marinho, managing director, Nigerian National Petroleum Company, *The African Guardian*, 5 March 1990, p. 19)

She has been called the Texas of Africa: big, brash, and, for a while, oil rich. For a decade oil flowed out and money flowed in. At the peak of production, the mangrove swamps of southeastern Nigeria pumped two million barrels a day and sold them for US $41 a piece. As in Iran and Venezuela, the oil boom created huge windfall profits, a transfer large enough to lay the basis of an economic revolution in Africa's largest nation. The Nigerians chose a capitalist road, an ambitious import-substitution industrialization strategy that required roads, banks, electrification, capital goods, and a developmental state. What they got was a sort of organized chaos: "a massive foreign debt whose size nobody knows, a mountain of expensive equipment that mostly does not work, and a military dictatorship" (*The Economist*, 3 May 1986, p. 3). The oil boom unleashed a spasm of consumption and construction; money and commodities circulated apace and disreputable salesmen from every corner of the globe competed to sell to all manner of Nigerians artifacts they could not possibly make use of. The proliferation of everything from stallions to stereos suggested a sort of African cargo cult.

An independent Nigeria inherited in 1960 an archetypical agrarian export economy dominated by groundnuts, cotton, palm oil, cocoa, and rubber. This economy was starkly regional. Three semi-autonomous regions, each associated with a primary export commodity and a marketing board, tightly circumscribed the power of the federal center. Regional economies were also distinguished by powerful ethnic and religion identifications which produced a fragile and fractured national polity presided over by the Muslim Hausa-speaking north. Behind the facade of political independence during the 1960s lay vicious interregional competition over political office, public contracts, and state resources. Indeed, this delicate federalism exploded into civil war in 1966 and it was into this fragmented political economy, presided over by a military government, that the oil monies of the 1970s were inserted.

The oil revenues flowed directly to the state via the Nigerian National Petroleum Company (NNPC), which both centralized and expanded central (federal) power. Federal revenues grew at 26 percent per annum during the 1970s and expanded state activity unleashed a torrent of imports (capital goods increased from N422 million in 1971 to N3.6 billion in 1979) and urban construction (the construction industry grew at over 20 percent per annum in the mid-1970s). The state invested heavily in industrial development and infrastructure – manufacturing output increased by 13 percent per annum between 1970 and 1982 – but the intense competition for public resources along regional and class lines produced unthinkable corruption and administrative chaos. While serious under the military governments of the 1970s, corruption and state indiscipline radically increased under the civilian government of President Shagari between 1979 and 1983. Cities such as Warri, Port Harcourt, and Lagos doubled (and in some cases tripled) in size during the boom. Consumer prices leapt upward, agriculture collapsed, and the real exchange rate rose steadily, feeding the import boom. Nigeria became ever more a monocultural economy; it simply shifted from one oil (vegetable) to another (petroleum).

The collapse of the boom in 1981 exposed Nigeria to the structural weaknesses of oil-based rentier capitalism. A foreign exchange crisis – the visible trade balance in 1981 was N12 billion – was compounded by mounting external debt obligations. By 1982 the President and his advisors talked of the need for sacrifice and denial: the 1970s, they said, had been a time of illusion. They were promptly ousted in a military coup in 1983. By 1984 the boom was over and the watchword was austerity. By 1986 Nigeria had signed a structural adjustment program (SAP) with the IMF and the World Bank, and the medicine was bitter. The economy contracted, the naira collapsed from US $1.12 to ten cents, and the real wage of industrial workers was savaged. Money was scarce and popular discontent widespread, as the anti-SAP riots in 1988 and 1989 revealed with some clarity.

What began with petro-euphoria and bountiful money in 1973 ended, some fifteen years later, with scarcity, a huge debt, urban looting, and bodies in the streets. Over this period oil money coursed through the Nigerian economy and polity, a sort of a barium meal which charted the decomposing metabolism of Nigerian political economy.

Naira Power: State Degeneracy and the Dikko Affair

Oil is a resource that anesthetizes thought, blurs vision, corrupts. . . . Look at the ministers from oil countries, how high they hold their heads, what a sense of power. (Kapuscinski, 1982, p. 35)

If you haven't got Naira power here, Auntie, you are lost. Money can buy you everything, even justice; and as Auntie replies, "Ah yes, you must be ready to bribe your way openly here, or perish." (Emecheta, 1982, p. 10)

Stansted Airport, 5 July 1984. British customs officers and Scotland Yard's anti-terrorist squad, responding to a reported abduction in central London, intercept two wooden crates addressed to the Ministry of External Affairs, Lagos, that are about to be loaded on board a privately chartered Boeing 707 purportedly containing four tons of catering equipment. In one crate is an Israeli would-be leather manufacturer and a Nigerian employee of the political division of the Nigerian Ministry of External Affairs. In the other, a rather embarrassed Israeli anesthetist by the name of Dr "Lou" Shapiro, and Alhaji Umaru Dikko, former Minister of Transportation and Aviation during the Shagari regime (1979–83), heavily drugged and shackled. Drawn by a "medical smell" that emanated from one of the crates, customs officers forcibly opened the first wooden container to discover Dikko with a tube forced down his throat. As he saw the light of day, Dr Shapiro, a reserve major in the Israeli army, was heard to say: "Well gentleman, what do we do now?" (*Africa Now*, August 1984, pp. 11–15).

Dikko, Nigeria's "most wanted fugitive" (*West Africa*, 16 July 1984, p. 1433), had fled Nigeria early in 1984 in the wake of a military coup, hiding out in Lagos for several days and then driving to the Benin border where he ditched his black Mercedes and casually walked across the border at a rural bush location to avoid capture. Subsequently, having taken up residence in Britain and "living comfortably" in West London according to the *Guardian*, he became an outspoken critic of the new military regime, calling for a jihad to overthrow the Buhari military government. Rumor had it that Dikko had put aside US $300 million to fund an army to overthrow the military government (*Africa Now*, August 1984, p. 14). With other high-ranking politicians and "multi-millionaire exiles" – most conspicuously Joseph Wayas (former President of the Nigerian Senate) and arms dealer Isyaku Ibrahim (*The Observer*, 24 June 1984, p. 12) – Dikko arrived in Britain under a dark cloud of accusation, and quite specifically amid rumor of massive corruption and illicit gain. Dikko himself was estimated to be worth a staggering US $1.4 billion (*Daily Sketch*, 23 January 1984, p. 1).

The Nigerian government denied all knowledge of the kidnapping in spite of the fact that the Israeli abductors claimed to be in the pay of the Nigerian secret police. Extradition orders served by the Nigerian government had placed a good deal of pressure on the Tory Government in Britain to assist in the return of Nigerian exiles to face in camera trials before the Tribunal on the Recovery of Public Property (so-called Decree No. 3). Coupled with the rather dim view of the abduction in the British popular press, the Nigerian generals' aggressive prosecution of ex-President Shagari's National Party of Nigeria (NPN) ruling elite produced an extremely tense diplomatic environment in which the "special relationship" between Britain and Nigeria was severely jeopardized.

What appears on the surface to be the stuff of B-grade movies and pulp spy novels is, I believe, a manifestation of the, in this case political, visage of petrodollars. Umaru Dikko personified Nigerian politics during the euphoric phase of the oil boom and perhaps more than any other personality captured the ethos of a monumentally venal Second Republic (1979–83): the brash and aggressive civil servant-contractor, the corrupt party machine politician, the avaricious rent-seeker for whom public office simply conferred the means to ransack state oil revenues for private gain. The explosion of oil revenues during the 1970s vastly expanded the number and distribution of public offices (there were 850 federal and state parastatals by the late 1970s!) but oil rents were channeled through state apparatuses already cross cut by deeply sedimented regional, ethnic, and religious affiliations and identities. As a consequence, the explosive growth of federal petrodollars had the effect of deepening and intensifying competing claims over highly lucrative state offices and resources. Nigerian political scientist Claude Ake put it well: politics was a ferocious contest to gain access to state monies. The Nigerian public sector became, in this sense, a tool to manufacture a sort of political consent through an unstable and delicate web of pacts and alliances purchased by the distribution of rents (import licenses, contracts) and the seemingly endless extension of federal and state-level employment opportunities. To this extent, the more vast (and myopic) the project – the massive new federal capital project at Abuja, a multi-billion iron and steel program – the greater its political attractiveness as a means to lubricate critical constituencies with petroleum monies. Only in this way can one understand why the costs of irrigation projects or state-funded educational construction throughout the oil boom were obscenely inflated, at least 300–400 percent higher than anywhere else in sub-Saharan Africa.

The intersection of centralized (state) oil monies and a highly segmented, and regionalized, class structure in which northern Muslims maintained, or endeavored to maintain, a precarious hegemony produced a seemingly insatiable source of rents for the privileged, and corruption and fraud of Hobbesian proportions. Chinua Achebe in *The Trouble with Nigeria* put the matter starkly: "Nigeria is without shadow of a doubt one of the most corrupt nations in the world" (Achebe, 1983, p. 42). Not only did Nigerian public servants become "more reckless and blatant" (ibid., p. 43) as oil revenues continued to roll in, but in addition there was a conspicuous failure to apprehend, prosecute, and punish perpetrators.

During the Second Republic, the second oil boom in 1979 unleashed a spasm of fraud and rent-seeking in which the state was mercilessly pillaged. Nigeria "lost" US $16.7 billion in oil income ("Oilgate," so-called) owing to fraudulent activities and smuggling of petroleum between 1979 and 1983 (*New African*, April 1984, p. 11); US $2 billion (over 10 percent of GDP) was "discovered" in a private Swiss bank account; and government ministries regularly went up in flames, the product of arson immediately prior to federal audits. Special military tribunals set up after the December 1983 coup prosecuted governors and high-ranking politicians for spectacular feats of corruption. Governor Lar accumulated N32.6 million in four years; Governor Attah made N2 million through illegal activities associated with a single state security vote in the Kwara state legislature (*West Africa*, 2 July 1984, p. 1373, 23 July, p. 1511). Military officers who raided the home of the governor of Kano state, Bakin Zuwo, discovered millions of naira in cardboard boxes piled up in his bedroom. With money, says Marx, "each individual holds social power in his pocket in the form of a thing" (Marx, 1963, p. 986ff).

Skyrocketing food prices, corruption in high places, hoarding, and speculation were all manifestations of the pillaging of state oil monies, much of which was of course exported. Capital flight not only produced a lack of investment funds, however, but signaled a state fundamentally incapacitated by corruption and rent-seeking. A hugely overvalued exchange rate, in other words, certainly distorted the economy but highlighted how state apparatuses were functionally crippled by a culture of public theft. The bureaucratic inefficiency and administrative anarchy of Nigerian state organizations is, of course, legendary. Electricity and water became the scarcest national resources; the central bank and federal financial institutions were often incapable of providing basic national accounts data; Chase Manhattan was contracted to try and compute the outstanding Nigerian public debt. This is, in other words, the antithesis of the "developmental state"; the public sector is entirely incapable of laying the foundations for systematic capitalist accumulation (as opposed to a flabby and corrupt "pirate" capitalism).

In this regard, the discovery of Umaru Dikko drugged in a wooden crate as part of a pathetic abduction scheme perfectly embodied two features of a Nigerian political economy bloated with oil monies: first, the state as the vehicle for, and obstacle to, capitalist accumulation; second, money as Naira power (to employ the title of Nigerian novelist Buchi Emecheta's popular novel), a general condition that Marx described as the process by which "social power becomes the private power of private persons" (Marx, 1974, p. 133).

The Oil Bust: Scarce Money and the "Great IMF Debate"

> Oil kindles extraordinary emotions and hopes, since oil is above all a great temptation. It is the temptation of ease, wealth, fortune, power. [But] oil, though powerful, has its defects. (Kapuscinski, 1982, pp. 34–5)

On 23 April 1984, the Nigerian Chief of Staff, Tunde Idiagbon, announced via a nationwide broadcast that Nigeria's borders were to be sealed. Simultaneously, all money was to be withdrawn from circulation. Currency exchange was to render worthless the hundreds of millions of naira smuggled out of the country, to force into the open those unscrupulous individuals who accrued untold millions during the civilian binge and who held much of this money outside of the banking system, and not least to squelch large-scale currency counterfeiting. While the Central Bank withdrew N5.3 billion from circulation, it issued only N2.45 billion in new notes, which accordingly generated a huge money scarcity. In the large cities, money was so scarce that the working poor walked to work and pooled food. What was most striking about this disappearance of Nigerian money was that it occurred at a time when the government was rumored to be negotiating a loan from the IMF which involved a substantial currency devaluation. Five years after the second oil boom, Nigeria had a huge external debt and a money that bore no semblance to its value; it was very close to bankruptcy. The oil boom was unequivocally over; 40 percent of the reserves and some US $101 billion in oil revenues had been, to be charitable, "used up."

"One of the effects of the oil boom," said E. C. Edozien, President Shagari's economic advisor, in 1982, "is to make it difficult to engender the necessary spirit of self-sacrifice and self-denial" (*Wall Street Journal*, 2 August 1982, p. 12). The population had simply come to "expect too much from the government." But why should there be a need for self-sacrifice to begin with, and why should there be denial among those, the countless millions of peasants, workers, and informal sector operatives, who had little to show from oil in any case? And how could money, the much touted petro-naira, come and go, how could its value evaporate? How could the expectation and ambition of the boom turn to the disillusionment and austerity of the bust? During the height of the boom, the World Bank classified Nigeria as a middle income country; by the end of the 1980s it was reclassified as "poor." By 1985, talk in Nigeria was of "oil doom" (*West Africa*, 26 August 1985, p. 1735).

The first austerity package had in fact been introduced in September 1981 following a 30 percent fall in oil prices. Further cuts were announced in 1982 but external borrowing increased substantially as the national elections approached. In April 1983 Nigeria initiated negotiations with the IMF to borrow US $2 billion, facing strict conditionalities in the form of devaluation, a tightening of money supply, reductions in current expenditures, and a relaxation in exchange and import controls. Despite progress throughout 1983, three major issues blocked any advance: devaluation, trade liberalization, and petroleum subsidies. By September the parties were stalemated. Three months later the Shagari government was overthrown by a military coup.

The Buhari military government came to power emphasizing discipline, austerity, self-reliance, and populist conservatism. Like Shagari before him, Buhari continued negotiations with the IMF but these stalled over devaluation and subsidies. Nigerian officials feared the destabilizing political consequences of inflation induced by devaluation and the elimination of import licenses (i.e., potential rents for key political constituencies). Trade liberalization would crush the manufacturing sector. As a consequence, Buhari decided to go it alone with a domestically hatched austerity plan wherein 44 percent of the foreign exchange earnings went to debt service. Rather than borrowing from private banks, Nigeria turned to counter-trading oil for current imports. Faced with crashing oil prices (from a high of US $41 per barrel in 1980 to the low teens by 1985) and a severe deflationary budget package, Buhari turned to authoritarian rule in the name of discipline and patriotic self-reliance. In August 1985 he was overthrown in another military coup.

The new Babangida regime immediately confronted the great oil crash; prices slumped below US $10.00 per barrel (in 1986 Nigerian oil earnings were US $6.5 billion compared to US $25.00 billion in 1981) and he declared his intention to break the deadlock with the IMF (Biersteker, 1988). In an extraordinary populist twist, Babangida took the IMF loan to the people: so began, in October 1985, "the Great Debate." It consisted of a flurry of speeches, street demonstrations, and extensive debates in the press and news media (see, for example, Ekpo, 1985; ORC, 1985; Usman, 1986; Phillips, 1987). The articulate middle classes represented the IMF in explicitly nationalist terms; Nigeria would be sold for a mess of pottage. Indeed, in spite of the fact that the Babangida regime mounted a campaign for IMF-type reform, within a short time a broad-based opposition to taking the loan began to form and mobilize. The IMF demands – devaluation, liberalization, anti-inflationary measures – were published and subject to a lively critique by students, organized labor, and academics. To live in debt and bondage or not was the issue.

What began as a thinly disguised effort to build a corporatist alliance around austerity produced a vociferous resistance to cutting petroleum subsidies and devaluation. But what also emerged was a strong popular sentiment against *any* form of borrowing; borrowed money would disappear just as quickly as it had in the past (Lubeck, 1992)! In the wake of popular protest and strikes, the Nigerian government broke off negotiations with the Fund in December 1985. Yet within two weeks the annual budget speech combined nationalist assertion for economic autonomy with savage austerity taken directly from the IMF blueprint: a "realistic exchange rate," an 80 percent reduction in petroleum subsidies, large scale privatization. Six months later came Babangida's new two-year structural adjustment program (SAP): hardship but "Made in Nigeria" as the popular press put it. Within a year, however, the value of the naira had fallen from US $1.12 to 20 cents. By January 1987 an IMF standby loan of SDR650 million had been signed by the Babangida government along with the full battery of SAP cutbacks. The real minimum monthly wage crashed from US $201 to US $16 (Watts and Lubeck, 1989).

Devaluation eroded what Simmel (1978) saw as the precondition for paper money: inter-social trust and social stability. The Great IMF Debate highlights, I would suggest, a long-standing conflict in Western discourse over the possibility of monetary order and in particular the incompatibility of money as a tool of state action and money as a symbol of social trust (Frankel, 1977, p. 86).

Serious Money

> If money is the bond which ties me to human life and society to me, which links me to nature and to man, is money not the bond of all bonds? Can it not bind and loose all bonds? Is it therefore not the universal means of separation? It is the true agent of separation and the true cementing agent, it is the chemical power of society. (Marx, 1975, p. 377)

The dense symbolism and imagery of oil money as the devil's excrement suggests a sort of money fetishism in which extraordinary powers, of a magical and occult variety, are seen to reside in dirty lucre. In this sense it speaks directly to Marx's concern with money fetishism, money's obfuscatory qualities, money endowed with fecundity; in capitalism, money breeds money, he said, "much as it is an attribute of pear trees to bear pears" (Marx, cited in Parry and Bloch, 1989, p. 6).

But there is also a much larger motif here with a very long history in Western thinking (dating at least to Aristotle), in which money has a dark and sinister face, as a source of evil and moral confusion; in short, money as threat.

Marx pursues this line of thinking when he talks of money as the God of commodities, and it is seen in Simmel's vision of money as subversive of "moral polarities," "turning what was formerly black and white into grayness" (Simmel, 1978, p. 72); "honor and conviction, talent and virtue, beauty and salvation of the soul are exchanged against money" (ibid., p. 256). For Chaucer money was filth, for Dickens an awful offal, for Edgar Allen Poe gold was death itself. For Hegel money was a "monstrous system" that required "continual dominance and taming like a beast" (cited in Shell, 1982, p. 154). The particular cultural constructions by which this view of money is articulated across time and space are, as is clear from this chapter, extremely varied. But underlying all these articulations is a strong sense of money as eroding the bases of sociability, as an acid that dissolves social ties, and as a dark almost satanic force that tears asunder the integument of the community, giving rise to greed, avarice, and alienation.

There is, however, a counterweight, another vision of money which stands in a dialectical relation to money as threat (it is also associated with Simmel, and to an extent with Marx), in which money enhances personal freedom, trust, rationality, calculability, and expanded forms of social exchange (Frankel, 1977; Simmel, 1978; Martin, 1986). The community of money tends to be "strongly marked by individualism and certain conceptions of liberty, freedom and equality" (Harvey, 1985, p. 4). Rather than a bland grayness, money produces what Emily Martin (1986, 4) calls "the most intense, clear and passionately directed feelings." Both Marx and Simmel recognized that money can fulfill both these functions – integrative and disintegrative – simultaneously, which produces complex and contradictory tendencies in social, cultural, and political relations. Martin (1986) has brilliantly argued in a comparison of Taiwan and the USA that in the former money works primarily as a form of social integration and in the latter it creates social disintegration.

I have sought to show how the infusion of oil monies in industrializing capitalist states provides a vantage point from which one can show that money contributes to, and reflects, how social integration and disintegration are at work simultaneously. In this light, some of the symbolic, cultural and socio-political expressions of money hold money operations within certain social limits. In other respects, oil money – as social power, as state corruption and degeneracy, as blind ambition and illusion – has eroded sociability, turning everything it touches into shit: oil money as deodorized feces that has been made to shine. Oil money provides a means to pry open the black box of society while the structure of society provides the entry point into understanding the complex ways in which money simultaneously mediates social relations and provides a fundamental means of experiencing them.

Chapter 14

Converting the Wetlands, Engendering the Environment: The Intersection of Gender with Agrarian Change in The Gambia

Judith Carney

The pace of environmental change in the Third World during recent decades has directed increasing attention in regional studies to political ecology, a research framework that focuses on the socioeconomic hierarchies and power relations regulating land use and management (Blaikie and Brookfield, 1987; Bassett, 1988; Zimmerer, 1991; Bryant, 1992). However, the political ecology perspective is most frequently employed in the context of common property regimes in the Third World to refute Hardin's (1968) *free-rider* assertion, which attributes environmental degradation to unchecked use of common property resources. Challenges to Hardin's arguments have, as a consequence, overemphasized analysis of land in political ecological analysis to the exclusion of other important factors. In this paper, I argue that the relationship of common property rights to Third World environmental change may be better understood by adequately conceptualizing labor.

Population growth and consequent pressure on limited land is frequently invoked to explain how common property resources result in environmental change. But the accelerating incorporation of Third World environmental resources into the global economy, particularly evident in recent decades, suggests a different view, in that environmental transformations initiate patterns of income generation by placing new value on land-based resources, which in turn trigger changes in common property resources. The result is often a shift to centralized resource control without a concomitant tendency toward privatization of land (Berry, 1989). Scarcity of land may be artificially created to gain control over labor for accumulation strategies that differentially benefit members within households.

I examine forms of environmental change on the wetlands of The Gambia during the past 25 years. Irrigation schemes play a central role in government policies aimed at diversifying agricultural exports while improving self-sufficiency in food grains. But the intensification of household labor regimes to year-round cultivation is inducing unparalleled gender conflict as communities reorient the common property regime to the new economic emphasis on irrigated production.

An examination of contemporary changes in the Gambian wetlands illuminates the interplay of environmental transformation, accumulation strategies, and women's work to changing common property regimes. In the Gambian system land is managed for individual use but is not individually owned. A number of users enjoy independent rights of usage, which is to say, individual rights to the benefits of his or her labor. Community land access is regulated by households with rights to exclude nonmembers of that collectivity. This political ecological analysis, which examines labor and rights of access to environmental resources, draws attention to the relationship of Gambian women's protests against the changing forms of control exercised over community property systems in the wetlands.

I use multiple case studies of two forms of wetland conversion: irrigated rice schemes and horticultural projects. Both forms of swamp development began in the colonial period when British officials sought to diversify exports from peanuts, the dominant cash crop, and improve domestic rice self-reliance. The projects failed to break down the gender division of labor in rice and vegetables, traditionally cultivated by women. Only in the post-independence period, with successful implementation of irrigation projects, did men labor with their wives in rice cultivation. But male participation also heralded an increasing control over surplus production and, frequently, female land dispossession. Nongovernmental organizations responded to women's declining economic opportunities in rice cultivation schemes by promoting irrigated horticultural projects among village women's groups. Horticultural projects have improved rural women's incomes but, like rice schemes, are rife with gender-based conflicts over access to irrigated land. Tracing the trajectories of the forms of irrigated development consequently reveals a process of land enclosure within the community property system which permits women's land access as laborers but denies full claims to the benefits produced.

In drawing attention to the labor rights that mediate the community property system, this chapter makes two points. First, new patterns of income generation within community property regimes frequently result in a redefinition of rules of access to, and control over, benefits within the household and community. Second, this redefinition is contested by women and given political expression in their growing militancy and nascent social movements. Such "struggles over meaning" in community property regimes may provide a critical perspective for examining Third World women's growing militancy over environmental and economic change.

Building upon previous research in several Gambian wetland communities, the chapter is divided into five sections. The first presents the environmental context of the Gambian wetlands, the extent and significance of wetland farming, as well as women's labor in ensuring its productive use. The next two sections provide a historical overview of the environmental and economic changes that modify women's access to, and use of, wetland resources, as well as recent policy shifts that address the country's environmental and economic crisis. Two case studies then detail the relationship between economic change and the process of land concentration and women's resistance. The chapter concludes by analyzing how wetland commodification has made women's access to resources increasingly tenuous despite income gains.

The Environmental Context of the Gambian Wetlands

The Gambia, a narrow land strip 24–50 kilometers (14–30 miles) wide and nearly 500 kilometers (300 miles) long, encloses a low-lying river basin that grades

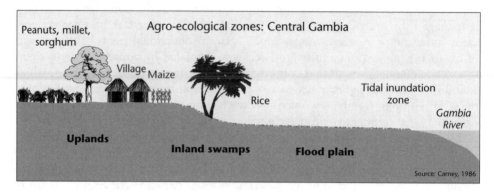

Figure 14.1   Agro-ecological zones: Central Gambia

gradually into a plateau, where the altitude seldom exceeds 100 meters (325 feet). The plateau forms about one-third of the country's land base and depends upon rainfall for farming (Carney, 1986, p. 21). Precipitation during the months of June to October averages 800–1,100 millimeters (31–43 inches) and favors the cultivation of millet, sorghum, maize, and peanuts. As in neighboring Sahelian countries, the Gambian rainfall regime fluctuates considerably between years and within a season. From the 1940s to 1980s, for example, annual rainfall declined by 15 to 20 percent and became increasingly distributed in a bimodal seasonal pattern (Hutchinson, 1983, p. 7). The recurrence of a two-week, midseason dry spell during the month of August increases cropping vulnerability on the uplands and dependence on lowland farming (Carney, 1986, pp. 25–30).

The lowlands are critical for understanding human livelihood and survival in the unstable rainfall setting of the West African Sudano-Sahelian zone. Lowland environments permit a multiple land use cropping strategy that utilizes other forms of water availability, thereby freeing agricultural production from strict dependence on rainfall. Constituting nearly 70 percent of the country's land mass, the Gambian lowlands make available two additional environments for agriculture: (1) the alluvial plain flooded by the river and its tributaries; and (2) a variety of inland swamps that receive water from high water tables, artesian springs, or occasional tidal flooding (Carney, 1986, 20–21) (Fig. 14.1). The lowlands, which enable an extension of crop production into the dry season or even year-round, are planted to rice, although vegetables are frequently grown with residual moisture following the rice harvest (Dunsmore, 1976, pp. 208–11; Carney, 1986, p. 82).

While The Gambia abounds in lowland swamps, not all are suitable for farming. Riverine swamps coming under marine tidal influence are permanently saline within 70 kilometers (42 miles) of the coast, seasonally saline up to 250 kilometers (150 miles), and fresh year-round only in the last 150 kilometers (90 miles) of the Gambia River's course (Carney, 1986, p. 33). The suitability of inland swamps for crop production, moreover, depends on the influence of differing moisture regimes for groundwater reserves. Consequently, although The Gambia contains over 100,000 hectares (247,000 acres) of lowland swamps, only about a third can be reliably planted (ALIC, 1981, p. 19; GGFP, 1988–91; CRED, 1985, p. 127).

Lowland cultivation is thus pivotal to the Gambian farming system, enabling crop diversification over a variety of microenvironments and a reduction in subsistence risk during dry climatic cycles. Wetland farming, however, requires considerable attention to forms of water availability as well as edaphic and topographic conditions. In The Gambia this knowledge is embodied in women, who have specialized in wetland cultivation since at least the early eighteenth century and have adapted hundreds of rice varieties to specific microenvironmental conditions (Jobson, 1623, p. 9; Gamble, 1955, p. 27; Carney, 1991, p. 40). This cumulative in situ knowledge of lowland farming underlies The Gambia's regional importance as a secondary center of domestication of the indigenous West African rice, *Oryza glaberrima*, cultivated in the area for at least three thousand years (Porteres, 1970, p. 47).

Gender, Environment, and Economy: A Historical Overview

Although lowland swamps and production are traditionally women's domain, prior to the mid-nineteenth century men and women were involved in both upland and lowland cropping systems through a division of labor based upon various agricultural tasks. Men assisted in field cleaning for rice cultivation while women weeded upland cereal plots (Weil, 1982, pp. 45–46; Carney, and Watts, 1991, p. 657). The abolition of slavery and the turn to "legitimate commerce" led to Gambia's incorporation into the world economy through commodity production. By the 1830s peanut cultivation was proliferating on the uplands (Carney, 1986, pp. 77–78). The imposition of British colonial rule by the end of the nineteenth century brought taxation and fiscal policies that accelerated reliance on peanuts as a cash crop, resulted in an increasingly specialized use of agricultural space, and led to a more gendered division of labor. These changes became most evident among the rice-growing Mandinka, Gambia's dominant ethnic group and principal wetland farmers.

By the end of the century, Mandinka men's growing emphasis on peanut cultivation resulted in a reduction in millet and sorghum production for household subsistence (Weil, 1973, p. 23; Jeng, 1978, pp. 123–24; Carney, 1986, p. 92). As women compensated for upland cereal shortfalls by augmenting rice production in lowland swamps, the gender division of labor of became increasingly spatially segregated, with the cash crop concentrated on the uplands under male control and women's farm work largely oriented to lowland rice, which emerged as the dietary staple (Carney, 1986, pp. 89–91) (Fig. 14.1). The specialized use of agricultural land and concomitant disruptions in the gender division of labor accompanying nineteenth-century commodity production provide the setting for understanding twentieth-century gender conflicts among the Mandinka over commodification of the Gambian wetlands.

Policy interest in wetland environments began in the early decades of the twentieth century, when colonial officials began documenting farming practices in diverse lowland settings (Carney, 1986, pp. 126–27). The objective was to improve household subsistence security and generate rice surpluses that would feed an expanding pool of migrant laborers, whose seasonal influx accounted for the pace of peanut expansion on the uplands. By the 1960s, swamp development projects had culminated in an expansion of rice planting to some 26,000 hectares (65,000 acres)

(Carney, 1986, p. 178). But limits had been reached on the degree to which women could carry the subsistence burden. The colonial government's inability to persuade Mandinka men to take an active part in rice cultivation brought swamp rice development to a close (Carney, 1986, p. 139; Carney and Watts, 1991, p. 660). In 1949 the colonial government initiated another approach to surplus rice generation by implementing a large-scale irrigation scheme on the site of the present day Jahaly Pacharr project. The Colonial Development Corporation (CDC) scheme departed from the earlier swamp rice improvement project in one important way: land was removed from female rice growers through a 30-year lease program (Carney, 1986, p. 126; Carney and Watts, 1991, p. 666). The project failed due to a poorly designed irrigation system and lack of male or female interest in wage work; yet the CDC scheme is notable for adumbrating the post-independence emphasis on irrigation as well as the gender-based conflicts that would surface in subsequent wetland development projects.

These conflicts center on the invocation of customary tenure "laws" by male household heads and village elites to reduce women's land and labor rights in rice farming or, in Mandinka nomenclature, the conversion of land with individual use rights (*kamanyango*) to land whose product is controlled by the household head (*maruo*). When colonial development policies during the 1940s improved swampland access and productivity, male household heads and village elites called into question women's customary use rights. In one case that reached the colonial authorities, Mandinka men argued that "if women mark the land and divide it, it would become 'women's property' so that when a husband dies or divorces his wife, the wife will still retain the land, which is wrong. Women must not own land" (Rahman, 1949, p. 1). Women's land access was clearly being contested by male claims that female use rights would alienate swampland from the residence unit. A brief review of the meaning of the two Mandinka terms for property access and use of resources illuminates the issues in dispute. Land in rural Gambia is held in communal tenure but carries several forms of property relations. On a general level, the household landholding is termed *maruo* and cannot be alienated from the residence group. But *maruo* additionally refers to a set of labor obligations and crop rights. All able family members are expected by custom to provide labor on household land for family reproduction. Men's *maruo* work responsibility is traditionally met on the uplands through cultivation of millet, sorghum and maize, or groundnuts, which may be traded to purchase cereals. Rice production traditionally fulfills Mandinka women's *maruo* obligations. Because *maruo* crops are produced for household subsistence, they come under control of the male household head, who arranges their distribution.

A second, and important, subset of tenure relations also operates on part of the family landholding. In exchange for providing labor toward household subsistence, junior males and all adult females are given access to some of the family's landholding for their own needs. These land rights and plots are known as *kamanyango*. As long as the farmer remains a member of the household she or he controls the plot's use and benefits from plot output. *Kamanyango* labor rights provide subordinate family members the means to obtain cash from farming, as they control the rights to the crop produced as well as decisions over its use. *Kamanyango* plots are a critical issue in Gambia, where rural society is largely polygynous, male and female budgets are frequently separate, and women traditionally are responsible for purchases of clothing and supplemental foods crucial for the well-being of their children.

The expansion of peanut commodity production during the nineteenth and early twentieth centuries, which shifted food cropping increasingly to wetland environments, resulted in a greater concentration of rain-fed land use into de facto *kamanyango* plots, whether or not it was so termed by male household heads. The reverse process accompanied commodification of lowland environments farmed to rice by women. As colonial rice development projects opened new areas for cultivation, women's *kamanyango* rights were repeatedly contested by male household heads, who placed them instead in the category of *maruo*. By claiming developed rice land as *maruo*, men placed the burden of subsistence responsibility on females, thereby liberating themselves from customary obligations. As women shouldered an ever greater work burden, male responsibility toward subsistence – either through cereal cultivation or purchase from ground nut earnings – diminished (Weil, 1973, p. 23). Women's preexisting labor rights steadily eroded in post-independence irrigation schemes, but with the strikingly different outcome that rural women mobilized to improve their deteriorating situation.

The Environmental and Economic Crisis: Policy Shifts

Since independence, in 1965, The Gambia has experienced rainfall declines and accelerated environmental degradation of its uplands, a massive influx of foreign aid for development assistance (1968–88), policy shifts favoring commodification of the wetlands, and an International Monetary Fund (IMF) structural adjustment program (1985–present). These changes have shaped post-independence accumulation strategies and the gender conflicts among rural households.

Gambia entered independence with a degraded upland resource base and a vulnerable economy. The results of the long-standing monocrop export economy were evident throughout the traditional peanut basin, once mantled with forest cover but substantially deforested during the colonial period (Park, 1983, p. 4; Mann, 1987, p. 85). Reliance on one primary commodity, peanuts, to finance mounting rice imports grew more precarious in the years after independence; peanut export values fluctuated considerably from year to year, but through the 1980s grew less rapidly than the value of food imports (FAO, 1983, p. 4; Carney, 1986, p. 254). Farmers responded to declining peanut revenues through an intensification of land use – namely, by reducing fallow periods in peanut cultivation or by eliminating them altogether. The result was accelerated land degradation, particularly in the North Bank region, which was oriented to Senegalese peanut markets with generally higher producer prices. Subsequent international development assistance brought far-reaching changes to the critical wetland food production zone. Nearly 4,500 hectares (11,115 acres) of riverine swamps were converted to irrigation schemes and another 1,000 hectares (2,470 acres) of inland swamps to horticultural projects (Carney 1992, pp. 77–78). Although affecting less than 10 percent of total swamp land, these conversions in land use have had profound consequences.

By the 1980s, women's mounting economic marginalization from irrigated rice development resulted in nongovernmental organizations (NGOs) targeting them for

horticultural projects developed on inland swamps. The policy emphasis on horticulture intensified with the debt crisis of the 1980s and the implementation of an
IMF-mandated structural adjustment program in 1985 to improve foreign exchange
earnings and debt repayment. Economic restructuring has reaffirmed The Gambia's
comparative advantage in peanuts while favoring the conversion of hydromorphic
swamps to horticulture (UNCTAD, 1986; Government of The Gambia, 1987;
Landell Mills Associates, 1989; Harvey, 1990, p. 3; McPherson and Posner, 1991,
p. 6).

The respective policy emphases of the past 20 years have commodified the wetlands and incurred changes in customary use and access to environmental resources.
As the irrigation schemes provide new avenues for income generation within rural
communities, women's access to improved land for income benefits is increasingly
being contested. The next two sections present an overview of the two post-drought
wetland policy shifts, illustrating how customary laws are being reinterpreted to
reduce women's access to productive resources and the forms of their resistance to
such changes.

"Drought Proofing" the Economy: Irrigated Rice Development

In 1966, one year after independence from Britain, the Gambian government, with
bilateral assistance from Taiwan, initiated a wetland development strategy – the conversion of tidal floodplains to irrigated rice projects. It was to receive increasing
donor emphasis following the 1968–73 Sahelian drought. The rationale for this
development was to promote import substitution by encouraging domestic rice production. Rice imports had reached 9,000 tons per annum, and foreign exchange
reserves had seriously eroded with declining world commodity prices for peanuts.
The 1968–73 Sahelian drought revived the late colonial interest in irrigation and
mobilized foreign aid for investment in river basin development, and irrigated agriculture (UNDP, 1977; CILSS, 1979; Franke and Chasin, 1980, pp. 148–51; Derman,
1984; CRED, 1985, p. 17). Hailed as a way of buffering the agricultural system
from recurrences of a similar disaster, irrigation projects also created a steady
demand for imported technical assistance, machinery, spare parts, and inputs. The
"drought-proofing" strategy embodied in Gambian irrigation schemes targeted rice,
whose import-substitution was prioritized by the post-independence government
(Government of The Gambia, 1966; CRED, 1985, p. 22). From the 1970s to the
mid-1980s the World Bank, the mainland Chinese government, and the International Fund for Agricultural Development (IFAD) continued the Taiwanese development strategy by implementing double-cropped irrigated rice schemes on more
than 4,000 hectares (9,880 acres) of women's tidal swamps (Fig. 14.2).

Despite the contrasting ideological perspectives of the donors involved, all development strategies adhered to a remarkably similar course by introducing the Green
Revolution package for increased production to *male* household heads (Dey, 1981,
p. 109). Developed at a cost of US $10,000 to $25,000 per hectare and inserted
into a preexisting gendered form of agricultural production and land use, these
schemes failed to deliver their technological promise and added to a growing
dependence on imported inputs and spare parts (CRED, 1985, p. 273; Carney, 1986,
p. 275). Donor production targets required double-cropping and thus a shift in

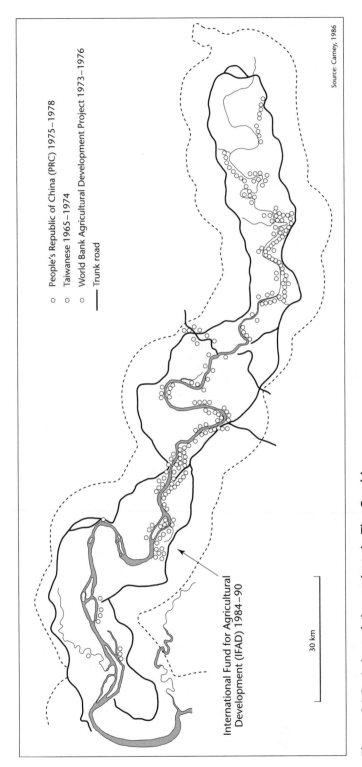

People's Republic of China (PRC) 1975–1978

Taiwanese 1965–1974

World Bank Agricultural Development Project 1973–1976

Trunk road

International Fund for Agricultural Development (IFAD) 1984–90

30 km

Source: Carney, 1986

Figure 14.2 Irrigated rice projects in The Gambia

agricultural production to year-round farming. Although male heads of households were taught this new form of production, cropping calendars could only be followed if women joined their husbands in irrigated rice farming. By placing men in charge of technologically improved rice production, the donors hoped to encourage male participation; instead, they unwittingly legitimized male control over the surpluses gained from double-cropping.

Control over the disposition of marketable surpluses proved pivotal to the gender-based conflicts that erupted within project households over which family members were to assume the increased work load. Male household heads claimed female labor under the customary category, *maruo*, but irrigated rice farming meant that the claim was invoked for year-round labor. As *maruo* labor claims for household subsistence had historically evolved within the confines of a single agricultural season, there was no precedent for women to perform labor obligations during *two* cropping periods when production would yield men a marketable surplus (Carney, 1988, pp. 341–42). Irrigation projects were commodifying rice production, but income gains depended on female labor availability.

Women contested the changing lexicon of plot tenure and the enclosure of traditional *kamanyango* and *maruo* swamp into irrigation schemes. "Development" meant the delivery of female labor for intensified rice farming without concomitant income gains. The reinterpretation of customary tenure by male household heads and village elites aimed to ensure continued female access to rice land, but only as workers on plots whose benefits would flow to men as disposable surpluses. The donors' uninformed view of the Gambian household-based production system was to prove the project's nemesis.

Female rice farmers responded in three principal ways to loss of control over productive swampland and efforts to augment their labor burden: (1) by relocating *kamanyango* production to unimproved swamplands where they could generate small surpluses for sale; (2) when alternative swampland for rice farming was not available, by agreeing to perform *maruo* labor obligations on irrigated rice plots during the dry-season cropping cycle in exchange for using the same plot without irrigation during the rainy season for *kamanyango* production; or (3) by laboring year-round on irrigated schemes but demanding remuneration in rice for their labor during one cropping season (Carney, 1994). All but the first response involved a substantial increase in women's labor. The third pattern represented an even more pronounced departure in female access to resources as *kamanyango* land rights in rice production came to an end and female labor was converted into wage work.

The project's mandate to double-crop as a condition for participation placed intense pressure on household labor, which plot designation as *maruo* could not easily resolve. Previous irrigation schemes had frequently accommodated women's *kamanyango* claims at the cost of year-round pumped production. Because project development had incorporated most of the region's available swampland, preexisting *kamanyango* land access came to an end. Gender-based conflicts exploded throughout the project area as women resisted the erosion of their right to derive benefits from a greatly augmented work burden and sought to reconstitute the rights embraced by *kamanyango* in other ways. While ethnicity, class, and differences among types of irrigated cultivation available within the project shaped the ensuing patterns of conflict resolution, the third response to loss of land access dominated among Mandinka women (Carney, 1994). Nonetheless, many households failed to honor women's demand for access to project land for *kamanyango* cultivation or remuneration in kind for year-round *maruo* labor, resulting in women's outright refusal to work on the family's irrigated plots.

These dispossessed women consequently pursued two complementary economic strategies for income generation: the formation of work groups to carry out the project's labor-demanding tasks of transplanting, weeding, and harvesting; and a shift in *kamanyango* production to upland cultivation. By organizing work groups for hire, women have managed to bid up their daily wage rate within the project and to take advantage of peanut land made available as men intensified their work in the more remunerative rice scheme (Webb, 1989, p. 66). But their efforts to obtain upland *kamanyango* plots were not always successful as they came into direct competition with the claims of junior males for individual land rights. Women have consequently placed considerable effort into gaining the support of nongovernmental organizations to develop village vegetable gardens for income generation (Carney, 1986, p. 311).

In summary, wetland development policy unfolded initially on riverine floodplains. As these areas became technologically improved and commodified, male household heads reinterpreted women's preexisting crop rights and benefits to gain access to their labor for the intensified work burden. Irrigated rice development simultaneously undermined women's customary access to rice land for income generation, while enabling male household heads to capture surplus value. By rupturing the relationship between women's knowledge systems, agronomic expertise, and rice farming, project households are beset with repeated delays in cropping schedules as well as an inability to follow agronomic recommendations. By the 1990s the legacy included poor rates of double-cropping, declining productivities, and failure to achieve rice import substitution.

Notwithstanding repeated state–peasant and male–female conflicts over rice land, irrigated development remains a governmental priority. Gambian political officials and their foreign advisors are currently reviewing ways to more efficiently restructure the irrigation sector. Alternative cropping arrangements in irrigated farming are being explored whereby farmers more "modern" in outlook may be asked to contract irrigated land (Carney, 1994). As policy measures increasingly dictate debt repayment and comparative advantage, the earlier small-scale schemes are being rationalized into larger units for centralized pumping and management (CILSS, 1990). A mounting emphasis is being placed upon crops, like fruits and vegetables, that generate foreign exchange. During the 1980s, the international development assistance community challenged male control over irrigation schemes by funding women's horticultural projects on unimproved inland swamps previously sown to rice. The explicit "women in development" focus of NGOs and multilateral donors aimed to bolster female income earning opportunities by improving seasonally wet swamps, with wells for dry-season planting. As cropping patterns shifted to export production, the process of commodification was brought to inland swamps, with contradictory implications for women.

Comparative Advantage and Horticultural Development

Shortly after the 1968–73 Sahelian drought the Gambian government promoted economic ventures in inland swamps that grew over the years into a major focus of donor assistance and income generation within the country. During the 1970s, the government encouraged onion-growing schemes among village women's groups as a means to increase household incomes in the peri-urban corridor and North Bank district, geographically proximate to the capital (Ceesay, Jammeh, and Mitchell, 1982). During the next decade women's vegetable gardens emerged as a major focus of donor support within the country. By the 1990s over 340 small- (0.5–2 hectares, or 1.1–4.9 acres) and medium-scale (5–15 hectares, or 12.3–37 acres) vegetable gardens were developed by NGOs and multilateral donors (Smith, Jack, and Singh, 1985; Nath, 1985; Sumberg and Okali, 1987; Giffen, 1987; DeCosse and Camara, 1990). The entry of private growers into the burgeoning horticultural sector, along with incipient women vegetable growers' groups (not funded), accounts for an expansion of market gardening that currently exceeds 1,000 hectares (2,470 acres) (Carney, 1992, p. 79).

The boom in market gardening on Gambian wetlands results from the confluence of several policy directions during the past 15 years. Following independence, Gambia began developing its pristine beaches for international tourism; by the 1990s over 100,000 Europeans were taking a six-hour flight to vacation along the Gambian coast between November and April (N'Jang, 1990). The initial onion projects successfully linked local production to the tourist sector and awakened donor agencies to the possibilities of expanding vegetable production for the dry-season tourist demand. These developments, meanwhile, were unfolding against a growing clamor within the international donor community for women in development (WID) projects. The emergent WID focus in The Gambia was pioneered by NGOs that viewed vegetables, traditionally planted by Gambian females, as the solution to women's limited economic opportunities.

Policy support for diversifying wetland agriculture into horticulture received additional impetus in 1985 with an IMF-mandated structural adjustment program. Geographic proximity to Europe encouraged policymakers to exploit The Gambia's comparative advantage as a winter fruit and vegetable supplier, as did favorable tariffs and the removal of export taxes on fresh produce (UNCTAD, 1986; Government of The Gambia, 1987; Jack, 1990). By the 1990s horticultural production had expanded to rain-fed areas in the peri-urban corridor located near the international airport, with boreholes dug to reach underground aquifers. With few exceptions, the projects are operated by the state, senior government officials, and resident Lebanese and Indian landowners and are oriented to European export markets. The same period witnessed the growing involvement of multilateral donors (European Economic Community, Islamic Development Bank, United Nations Development Program, and the World Bank) in women's horticultural production and marketing along the coastal corridor (Ceesay, Jammeh, and Mitchell, 1982; Government of The Gambia, 1987; Barrett and Browne, 1991, p. 244; Carney, 1992, p. 78; World Bank, 1990). Despite this most recent form of donor support, Gambian women's horticultural projects remain concentrated in rural areas, on inland swamps of small areal extent (0.5–2 hectares, or 1.2–4.9 acres), and oriented to local and regional markets.

Although the policy emphasis on converting inland swamps to horticulture dates from the 1970s, Gambian women have long been involved in vegetable production. They were observed marketing vegetables during the dry season as far back as the mid-fifteenth century. Although colonial horticultural programs targeted men, their failure left vegetable growing in women's hands. Females remained the country's principal producers, using residual moisture from inland rice swamps early in the dry season to cultivate traditional crops such as bitter tomatoes, okra, sorrel, and hibiscus for subsistence.

Donor support for well construction from the 1980s has enabled an extension of the vegetable-growing period in inland swamps. Deeply dug, concrete-lined wells have revolutionized Gambian horticultural production by tapping water tables for dry-season cultivation. Vegetable gardening is no longer a seasonal activity, as it was prior to donor involvement. Women's village gardens receiving NGO assistance grow vegetables during the entire dry season and, in some cases, year-round.

The provision of reliable water supplies through well-digging is central to NGO efforts to implement a rural development strategy aimed at improving women's incomes. By promoting village gardens for women's groups interested in commercialized vegetable cultivation, NGOs have launched a development strategy that targets women who were ignored in the previous wetland policy approach. Arrangements to secure female access to improved village gardens, however, vary between communities and depend on the availability of land locally, as well as the swamp's land use history. Consequently, in rural communities with NGO-supported gardens, women are granted either year-round usufruct for cash-cropping vegetables or *kamanyango* dry-season rights, with the plot reverting to subsistence cereal production in the rainy season. Once access to land is accomplished, NGOs provide assistance for constructing concrete-lined wells and barbed wire fences (for protection from livestock damage). When completed, female growers are credited the seeds and tools for vegetable farming.

A labor-intensive process, vegetable gardening during the dry season requires two daily waterings – averaging about two hours per session – weeding, and pest control, as well as transporting the bulky and highly perishable produce to weekly markets. But in a country where rural per capita income averages US $130, efforts are often rewarded (World Bank, 1981). Schroeder (1992, p. 4) records that women vegetable growers in surveyed North Bank villages gross incomes ranging between US $67–265 during the dry season, with more than half of them reporting incomes exceeding their husbands' earnings from peanuts. These income differentials are the new source of contemporary gender conflict in North Bank vegetable gardens.

Vegetable gardening nonetheless remains attractive to women, whose alternative income-earning prospects are limited. While structural adjustment programs have led to a 10 percent reduction in employment within the government sector and have catapulted men into increasing involvement in horticultural production, women have generally maintained usufruct to village land for gardening because donor representatives, located in the capital, are poised to defend them. Proximity to the land border with Senegal and declining peanut production associated with upland environmental degradation underlie the gender conflicts that have emerged in

North Bank horticultural projects. As with peanuts, most vegetable production flows across the border to Senegal, where horticultural import–export distribution networks are of operator antiquity, internal demand for vegetables is more developed, and prices are higher (Mackintosh, 1989, p. 15). NGO improvement of inland swamps with wells has resulted in new avenues for income generation that sharply conflict with the WID objectives of NGOs.

NGO-funded vegetable projects in North Bank communities have transformed the inland swamps and the social relations regulating preexisting cropping and labor patterns. Well construction, in effect, has widened the seasonal window that formerly regulated vegetable cultivation. Crops are no longer confined to the autumnal planting period following the rice harvest; vegetables can be planted throughout the dry season, and frequently year-round, since profits from cross-border sales currently compensate for displaced rice production (Schroeder and Watts, 1991, p. 62).

As North Bank horticultural projects have considerably augmented women's earnings, female rights of disposal over their income and access to vegetable land have come under increasing threat. Schroeder reports men deferring to women the burden for costs formerly met by males and their capture of part of women's earnings through unpaid loans. Additionally, male landholders in numerous communities are contesting women's access rights to vegetable land through the planting of economically valuable trees (e.g., mango and orange) within the vegetable gardens. After five to ten years the canopy closes, blocking the sunlight needed for vegetable growth. Tree planting therefore facilitates the conversion of land use from vegetable gardens to orchards, enabling male landlords to reclaim the improved plots for their own economic strategy based on tree crops within a decade (Schroeder, 1992, p. 9).

By making verbal agreements with NGOs for women's vegetable gardens, landlords are acquiescing to female demands for *kamanyango* land rights. But these rights are honored only for limited number of years – those required to capture women's labor for watering adjacent fruit trees during the initial growth period. The use of economically valuable trees to recapture garden plots as male *kamanyango* over the long run, however, is not lost on women. Schroeder (1992) notes the gender confrontations that have occurred with orchard planting: women cutting back mango and orange trees as they begin shading out vegetables, deliberately setting fires to fatally damage fruit trees, and sending delegations to local officials for legal action.

The inland swamps of the North Bank, formerly used by women for subsistence rice production, are being increasingly commercialized to vegetables. But the process is unfolding within a region of limited economic opportunity and severe environmental degradation. While NGOs attempted to address the gender equity issue ignored in the first wetland development phase, this second development approach indicates that women's gains over the long run are indeed precarious.

Conclusion

The structural dislocation of a monocrop export economy and attendant food shortages brought government attention to the Gambian wetlands during the late colonial period. The pattern of swamp development implemented during colonial rule foreshadowed the large-scale emphasis on the wetlands that materialized with the influx of foreign capital coincident with the Sahelian drought. During the past 25 years, wetland development through irrigation projects has transformed Gambian agriculture from a seasonal to a year-round activity, enabling agricultural diversification, surplus cereal production, and new avenues of income generation among rural households.

The promise of irrigated agriculture, however, depends upon the ability of peasant households to restructure family labor to the dictates of irrigated farming – a labor regime that requires a greater work burden during the entire calendar year. As claims to family labor evolved in the context of a limited wet season, institutional mechanisms within household-based production systems were deformed to mobilize family labor for year-round agriculture. Use of the term *maruo*, for technologically improved swamps, is central to obtaining a female labor reserve for the intensified work burden in irrigated farming. While reaffirming the integrity of the patriarchal family landholding, the naming of developed land, *maruo*, in practice facilitates men's claim to benefits produced by female labor.

Women contest the semantics of *maruo* precisely because this new meaning is a mechanism that deprives them of their customary rights. They are acutely aware that the rules of access to, and control over, environment resources are not a codification of immemorial tradition, but rather the outcome of struggle and negotiation with husbands, male community leaders, state and donor officials (Berry, 1986, p. 5; Okoth-Ogendo, 1989, p. 14). This awareness has sharpened in the past 25 years with irrigation projects that have imbued wetlands with new economic value. Gambian women are not engaging men in mere semantic discussion as they struggle for *kamanyango* rights – their actions reveal growing recognition that commodification of the wetlands is steadily eroding their economic and social status within the household and village community.

The two case studies of irrigated agriculture illustrate the multiple ways in which women contest and renegotiate their access to resources. Struggles in rice schemes have centered on reaffirming claims to a portion of the surplus by requesting seasonal plot use as *kamanyango*; remuneration in the form of paddy rice for year-round labor availability; or, when labor benefits are denied, outright refusal to work on the household's irrigated fields and entry into local wage markets for improved rates of pay. Each outcome of women's struggles, however, has resulted in an intensification of female work burdens without commensurate income gains.

Women's fortunes appear much improved in vegetable projects, where females are granted *kamanyango* cropping rights seasonally or year-round. But female growers find their incomes from garden cultivation being claimed in new ways by their husbands, who, in some cases, refuse to pay back the loans given by their wives or abrogate their contributions toward household expenses (Schroeder, 1992). Moreover, the increasing emphasis on orchards for income generation indicates that women's *kamanyango* gardening rights may only be exercised for a limited number of years – equivalent to the time required for hand-watering of trees until the plot's land use converts to mature orchards (Schroeder, 1992). Despite income gains and growing militancy, women's earnings in vegetable gardening appear precarious over the long run.

These case studies indicate that a process of land concentration is occurring in Gambian wetlands improved with irrigation. Concentration is not the result of absolute land scarcity and overpopulation but rather a response to household labor shortages and new income opportunities with irrigated agriculture. The designation, *maruo*, for irrigated land reveals how land is enclosed to create an artificial scarcity for accessing female labor. This unusual form of enclosure permits women access to irrigated land, while denying them benefits from their work. Land concentration consequently involves the conversion of a developed plot from one with multiple female rights to the surplus product to land with a single claim over the surplus produced by multiple female laborers.

In outlining the social and historical processes of changing land use strategies on the Gambian wetlands, this paper reveals that more than the environment is being transformed. So too are the social relations that mediate access to, and use of, land within rural households. The contemporary pattern of accumulation unfolding in the Gambian wetlands centrally depends on controlling access to irrigated land by "freeing" women from their customary rights and by imposing new work routines that undervalue and intensify their labor contribution. Women, however, are resisting their newly assigned role as cheap labor reserves.

Chapter 15

Nourishing Networks: Alternative Geographies of Food

Sarah Whatmore and Lorraine Thorne

[T]he capitalism of Karl Marx or Fernand Braudel is not the total capitalism of the Marxists. It is a skein of somewhat longer networks that rather inadequately embrace a world on the basis of points that become centers of profit and calculation. In following it step by step, one never crosses the mysterious lines that divide the local from the global. (Latour, 1993, p. 121)

The spatial imagery of a "shrinking world" and a "global village" are the popular hallmarks of an understanding of the limitless compass and totalizing fabric of contemporary capitalism that has become something of a social science orthodoxy, known as *globalization* (Featherstone, 1990; Sklair, 1991). No less heroic than the institutional complexes which it depicts, such an understanding perpetuates a peculiarly modernist geographical imagination that casts globalization as a colonization of surfaces which, like a spreading ink stain, progressively colors every spot on the map. This spatial imagery suffuses the political economy of agro-food through analytical devices like "global commodity systems" (Friedland et al., 1991), "agro-food regimes" (Le Heron, 1994), and "systems of provision" (Fine et al., 1996). In the most cogently argued versions, globalization is animated as a political project of world economic management orchestrated by a regiment of capitalist institutions including transnational corporations (TNCs), financial institutions, and regulatory infrastructures (McMichael, 1996, p. 112). But the most potent agro-food expression of this spatial imagery must surely be George Ritzer's notion of "McDonaldization." He coins the term to describe a process of social rationalization modeled on the fast-food restaurant which he argues has "revolutionized not only the restaurant business, but also American society and, ultimately, the world" (Ritzer, 1996, p. xvii). This is social science at its most triumphant, a rhetorically seductive bestseller which serves up the world on a plate.

That some markets indeed have global reach is not in dispute. What we want to emphasize is that this reach makes the corporations and bureaucracies that fashion such markets both powerful and vulnerable, being woven of the same substances as the more humble everyday forms of social life so often consigned to the "local" and rendered puny in comparison. One of the most serious consequences of orthodox accounts of globalization, whether of the more rigorous or the more populist varieties identified above, has been the eradication of social agency and struggle from the compass of analysis by presenting global reach as a systemic and logical, rather than a partial and contested, process (Amin and Thrift, 1994). TNCs and associated regulatory bureaucracies become magnified into institutional dinosaurs whose scale and mass overwhelms the paltry significance of their social fabric, at the same time as the life practices and milieux of lesser social agents are dwarfed and overshadowed in this colossal landscape. But size, as the dinosaurs discovered, isn't everything.

Our point then, is that there is nothing "global" about such corporations and bureaucracies *in themselves*, either in terms of their being disembedded from particular contexts and places or of their being in some sense comprehensive in scale and scope. Rather, their reach depends upon intricate interweavings of *situated* people, artifacts, codes, and living things and the maintenance of particular tapestries of connection across the world. Such processes and patterns of connection are not reducible to a single logic or determinant interest lying somewhere *outside* or *above* the social fray. This distinction is the difference between systems and networks; a shift in analytical metaphor which takes up critiques of the globalization orthodoxy, notably within geography and anthropology, as a failure of both social and spatial imagination (Strathern, 1995; Thrift, 1996b).

Two complementary influences on the elaboration of these critiques are particularly important for our purposes here, the one concerned with rethinking *political economy* and the other with recognizing *space-time*. In the first case, economic sociology and institutional economics have emphasized the embodied and routinized social practices which constitute markets, corporations, and regulatory bureaucracies against accounts (Marxist and neoclassical) which tend to treat these institutional complexes as abstracted presences, or the product of some historically teleological process (Underhill, 1994; Thrift and Olds, 1996). Economic institutions and practices are conceived of not as some separate, and still less determinant, "sphere" of activity which articulates with other "spheres" of civic society or governance but as socially embedded and contingent at every turn (Smelser and Swedberg, 1994; Murdoch, 1995). In the second case, poststructuralist ideas have informed theoretical efforts to deconstruct the geometric landscapes – what Barnes (1996) has called the "Enlightenment view" – of political economy. By fashioning the modern world as a single grid-like surface, such landscapes make possible the encoding of general theoretical claims as omnipresent, universal rationalities. In contrast, critics point to the *simultaneity* of multiple, partial space-time configurations of social life that are at once "global" and "local," and to the *situatedness* of social institutions, processes, and knowledges as always contextual, tentative, and incomplete (Thrift, 1995).

Such critiques, especially that derived from institutional economics, have been taken up already by those working in agrarian political economy (see Goodman and Watts, 1994; Whatmore, 1994). While it remains "against the grain," such work marks the beginnings of an understanding of globalization as partial, uneven, and unstable; a socially contested rather than logical process in which many spaces of resistance, alterity, and possibility become analytically discernible and politically meaningful. In this paper we want to extend these lines of critique, particularly that concerned with spatial recognition, as a basis for exploring alternative geographies of food that have been eclipsed by mainstream political economy accounts (see Arce and Marsden, 1993; Cook and Crang, 1996, for related forays).

The title phrase "alternative geographies of food" signals an effort on our part to see the world differently in (at least) two senses. We begin by taking up the geographical implications of *actor-network theory* (ANT) which both of us have been exploring in work elsewhere (Thorne, 1997; Whatmore, 1997). As the opening quotation suggests, this involves the elaboration of a *topological* spatial imagination concerned with tracing points of connection and lines of flow, as opposed to reiterating fixed surfaces and boundaries (Thrift, 1996b; Bingham, 1996). In particular, we draw on the work of Bruno Latour (1993, 1994) and John Law (1986, 1991, 1994) to elaborate an understanding of global networks as performative orderings (always in the making), rather than as systemic entities (always already constituted). We then go on to explore some of the analytical and political spaces which such an understanding opens up, by means of a case study of *fair trade coffee networks*. This case study illustrates the fashioning of social and environmental configurations of agro-food production and consumption that coexist with those of industrial food corporations but which in some way counter, or resist, their institutional values and practices.

Global Networks or "Acting at a Distance"

> The two extremes, local and global, are much less interesting than the intermediary arrangements that we are calling networks. (Latour, 1993, p. 122)

The work of Latour and Law, and their respective notions of "hybrid networks" and "modes of ordering," provide ways of reconceptualizing power relations in space from the flat, colonized surfaces of globalization to the frictional lengthening of networks of remote control. In so doing, the key question becomes not that of scale, encoded in a categorical distinction between the "local" and the "global," but of connectivity, marking lines of flow of varying length and which transgress these categories. To put this question in the terms of ANT, what are the conditions and properties of "acting at a distance"? Formulating inquiry in this way refuses the privileged association *a priori* between particular kinds of social institutions (notably TNCs) and global reach and, by implication, the pervasive mapping of the conventional sociological binaries of "macro–micro" and "structure–agency" onto that of the "global–local." Our account builds on the early efforts of geographers to explicate the spatial dimensions of ANT and their import for understanding power as a thoroughly relational process (Murdoch, 1995; Murdoch and Marsden, 1995) and for recognizing the active part of nonhumans in the fabric of social life (Thrift, 1995, 1996b).

Where orthodox accounts of globalization evoke images of an irresistible and unimpeded enclosure of the world by the relentless mass of the capitalist machine, ANT problematizes global reach, conceiving of it as a labored, uncertain, and above all, contested process of "acting at a distance," Law illustrates this conception with the example of Portuguese efforts to expand the reach of European trade in the fifteenth and sixteenth centuries by capturing the spice route to India (1986). This achievement required the Portuguese to refashion contemporary navigational complexes in ways which, as Law puts it, addressed not only the question of social control but also that of

> how to manage long distance control *in all its aspects*. It was how to arrange matters so that a small number of people in Lisbon might influence events half-way round the world and thereby reap a fabulous reward. (Law, 1986, p. 235, original emphasis)

Law's evocative case study of "acting at a distance" centers on the technological metaphor of "remote control" which tends to conjure the dynamics of networking in the rather conventional geographical binary of core (transmitter) and periphery (receiver). Nor are the implications of this metaphor restricted in his work to this particular case study. The imprint of "remote control" marks his elaboration of ANT more widely. Thus, for example,

> heterogeneous socio-technologies open up the possibility of ordering distant events from a center . . . [in which] the center is a place which monitors and represents the periphery and then calculates how to act on the periphery. (Law, 1994, p. 104)

A rather different, and to our mind more promising, exposition of the spatial configuration of actor-networks is that derived from Latour's notion of "network lengthening." Reminiscent of the nomadic cartographies of Deleuze and Guattari (1983), the idea of "lengthening" not only problematizes the process of "acting at a distance" but also disrupts the bi-polarities of "core" and "periphery." These generic spaces, like those of "local" and "global," enshrine a geometric vocabulary concerned with the geography of surfaces. The unilinearity encoded in their relationship makes less sense in a topologic vocabulary concerned with the geography of flows. Here, a network's capacities over space-time represent the simultaneous performance of social practices and competences at different points in the network; a mass of currents rather than a single line of force. In these terms, actor-networks are best understood as "by nature neither local nor global, but [only] more or less long and more or less connected" (Latour, 1993, p. 122).

By implication, the size, or scale, of an actor-network is a product of network lengthening, not of some special properties peculiar to "global" or "core" actors, the "dinosaurs" of our earlier analogy. Furthermore, the power associated with global reach has to be understood as a social composite of the actions and competences of many actants; an attribute not of a single person or organization but of the number of actants involved in its composition (Callon and Latour, 1981; Murdoch and Marsden, 1995). How, then, is this network lengthening achieved? The answer advanced in ANT is that network lengthening requires the mobilization of larger numbers and more intricately interwoven constituents, or *mediators*, to sustain a web of connections over greater distances. In so doing, it focuses analytical attention on describing this process of mediation and its agents in ways which force a challenging, and sometimes disconcerting, shift in the horizons of social research. As Law notes in relation to his Portuguese case study,

if these attempts at long-distance control are to be understood then it is not only necessary to develop a form of analysis capable of handling the social, the technological,
the natural and the rest with equal facility, though this is essential. It is also necessary
that the approach should be capable of making sense of the way in which these are
fitted together. (Law, 1986, p. 235)

At once it becomes essential to talk of network mediators other than people, that
is other than the human actors on whom the whole compass of conventional theories of social agency (including other social network theories) is built. To be sure,
people in particular guises and contexts act as important go-betweens, mobile agents
weaving connections between distant points in the network; for example, the sailors
in Law's Portuguese study, or the managerial elites of corporate business today. But,
insists ANT, there are a wealth of other agents, technological and "natural," mobilized in the performance of social networks whose significance increases the longer
and more intricate the network becomes. Latour calls these agents "immutable
mobiles," such as money, telephones, computers, or gene banks; objects which
encode and stabilize particular socio-technological capacities and sustain patterns
of connection that allow us to pass with continuity not only from the local to the
global, but also from the human to the nonhuman. The more they have proliferated in everyday life the more, it seems, these "objects" have been effaced in social
theory leaving us awed by the subsequently fantastic properties of social entities like
TNCs. By taking such objects into account "one can follow the growth of an organization in its entirety without ever changing levels and without ever discovering
'decontextualized' rationality" (Latour, 1993, p. 122).

It should by now be apparent that a move from "globalization" to global networks as a basis for understanding the conditions and properties of "acting at a
distance" is no small step. It is worth rehearsing three major, mutually reinforcing
elements of the theory as it is advanced by Latour and Law (and Callon): hybridity, collectivity, and durability.

Breaking down the global–local binary through the idea of the lengthening of
networks is intricately tied up with breaking down the nature–society binary
through the idea of *hybridity*. Just as the global–local distinction serves to purify
processes and entities that are not of themselves confined to any particular spatial
scale, so the ontological separation of society and nature purifies the messy heterogeneity of life. Hybrids represent states of being which fall somewhere between the
passive objects of human will and imagination which litter the social sciences, and
the autonomous external forces favored in natural science accounts. Following
Michel Serres (see Serres and Latour, 1995), Latour designates these in-between
states of being as *quasi-objects* which are as "real as nature, narrated as discourse,
collective as society [and] existential as being" (Latour, 1993, p. 89).

Returning to the Portuguese study, Law shows how a composite of agents are
enjoined as emissaries of network lengthening, including documents, devices, and
people fashioned in particular ways. For example, a document called the "Regi-
mento" inscribed a distilled and simplified instruction for navigating by stars which
permitted the navigator to pass beyond the established envelope of North European
travel. Devices included the "carreira," a ship designed for carrying cargo and
avoiding plunder, and "a kind of simplified black box," the astrolabe. Similarly, this

effort to act at a distance mobilized people with very particular kinds of skills or embodied social practices, including navigators, sailors, and merchants.

This example picks up and illustrates a second key step in understanding the process of network lengthening, the fundamentally relational, or *collective* conception of social agency that characterizes ANT. Thus, the significance of the "documents, devices and drilled people" in Law's Portuguese study is the way in which they hold each other in position. "The right documents, the right devices, the right people properly drilled – put together they would create a structured envelope for one another that ensured their durability and fidelity" (Law, 1986, p. 254). Yet the full implications of this conception of social agency are relatively underdeveloped in this early case study. It is in Law's later work and, more particularly, in the notion of the *hybrid collectif* (Callon and Law, 1995) that the importance of the active properties of nonhuman agents in the lengthening of networks is most fully explored. For Latour, these agents are a vital part of a network's collective capacity to act "because they attach us to one another, because they circulate in our hands and define our social bond by their very circulation" (1993, p. 89).

Thus far we have outlined hybridity and collectivity as necessary corollaries of the process of mediation by which networks are sustained over greater distances. Of equal significance is the question of how such networks are strengthened and stabilized over time or, in ANT terms, how they are made *durable*. In Law's book *Organizing Modernity*, he adapts Foucault's notion of "discursive practices" to propose *modes of ordering* as a way of conceptualizing the durability of networks. Modes of ordering are both narrative "ways of telling about the world . . . what used to be, or what ought to happen," and material, "acted out and embodied in a concrete, non-verbal manner in a network" (Law, 1994, p. 20). He shows how organizations perform multiple "modes of ordering," which influence the ways in which agents are enrolled in global networks. While these organizational patternings or habits are invariably plural rather than singular, Law argues that "only a relatively small number of modes of ordering may be instantiated in the networks of the social at a given time and place" (ibid., p. 109). In other words the durability of long-distance networks requires strong fabrics of social organization at all points in the network, making the patterning of social and environmental practices in *particular* times and places integral to the business of network enrolment.

Fair Trade Coffee: An Alternative Net-Working

In this context, alternative geographies of food are located in the political competence and social agency of individuals, institutions, and alliances, enacting a variety of partial knowledges and strategic interests through networks which simultaneously involve a "lengthening" of spatial and institutional reach *and* a "strengthening" of environmental and social embeddedness. Such networks exist alongside the corporate and state networks of orthodox accounts of globalization, sometimes overlapping them in space-time; sometimes occupying separate sites and establishing discrete lines of connection; and sometimes explicitly oriented towards challenging their associated environmental and social practices. In the case of food, the "devices, documents and drilled people" of Law's Portuguese example translate into a broader compass of material concerns than that associated with traditional agrarian political economy. These include the encoding of particular agricultural and dietary knowledges in the form of various technologies; the legal inscription of agro-food practices, from patents to health criteria; and the disciplining of bodies, from obese and skeletal people to industrial animals and plants.

Using this collection of ideas, and working to avoid the bias of scale in structuralist accounts (which inscribe a macro–micro division and then reify the former), we propose that modes of ordering which spin documents, devices, and living creatures (including people) as other than passive agents through multiply sited networks are both possible and extant. In the case study we discuss one such patterning explicitly oriented towards enacting an alternative commodity network, which we have identified as *a mode of ordering of connectivity*. In this mode of ordering, stories are told of partnership, alliance, responsibility, and fairness, but performed in very different ways to the neo-liberal encoding of these terms (Barratt-Brown, 1993). This is a mode of ordering concerned with the empowerment of marginalized, dismissed, and overlooked voices, human or nonhuman. Implicit in this empowering performance is the knowledge that "some network configurations generate effects which, so long as everything else is equal, last longer than others" (Law, 1994, p. 103). The mode of connectivity therefore not only tells and performs but also tries to concretely embody a recursive effect of social, and sometimes environmental, embeddedness.

With roots in nongovernmental organizations dedicated to alleviating poverty in the "Third World," the fair trade "movement" has grown in the UK over the past twenty-five years. The charity Oxfam established a wholly owned trading company in 1964 with other organizations gradually emerging as fully-fledged trading companies from solidarity markets (for example, Equal Exchange Trading Limited), or educational functions (for example, Twin Trading and the Third World Information Network – TWIN). The recently formed British Association of Fair Trade Shops (BAFTS) consists of shops committed to principles of fair trade. Other organizations do not trade at all but provide support in the form of campaigning and lobbying (for example the World Development Movement). The point here is that fair trade organizations in the UK are diverse and numerous, with the physical transactions of trading only one of their component activities. The institutions, transactions, and technologies of fair trade serve to illustrate some of the key concerns highlighted by an analysis of agro-food patterns as hybrid networks. In particular, it shows how the global reach of so-called alternative agro-food networks (or their capacity to "act at a distance") enrols coincident actants and spaces to those of "mainstream" commercial networks. It is the modes of network strengthening (or making durable) that are analytically distinctive between the orderings of fair trade and capitalist commerce and that open up economic and political possibilities for configuring alternative geographies of food.

In this case study we discuss a hybrid network of four UK fair trade organizations and a Peruvian coffee exporting cooperative, although there are many other agents in this network, as becomes clear. In the late 1980s "Oxfam Trading," "Twin Trading," "Traidcraft," and "Equal Exchange Trading Limited" came together to create a consortium called *Cafédirect* which procures, imports, and markets a brand of coffee of the same name, available in ground and freeze-dried forms. The four partners are located in different cities in the UK – Oxford, London, Newcastle-upon-Tyne, and Edinburgh respectively. In the early days, the hybrid network of Cafédirect operated with no central office. Instead, partners had designated responsibilities, for example the buyer working for one organization, the wholesale administration handled by another and so on, with one of the partners, "Twin Trading," acting as the operational focal point. In 1993 the consortium became registered as a private company which has recently appointed a managing director, and the partners are now "shareholders." Cafédirect was the second fairly traded product in the UK to receive the Fair Trademark, which legitimizes the product as fairly traded according to criteria set out by the Fairtrade Foundation, an independent organization recently given charitable status but originally established by several fair trade organizations, including Oxfam and Traidcraft. Thus the product of the Cafédirect network is given institutional legitimacy by a hybridized form of itself.

Cafédirect's southern partners are small-scale farmers whose coffee trees cling to steep mountain slopes in Costa Rica, Peru, and Mexico, in the case of the Arabica component of the brand, while the Robusta component comes from similar producers in Tanzania and Uganda. In this case study we restrict our discussion to some of Cafédirect's partners in Peru, namely the exporting cooperative of CECOOAC-Nor, located in Chiclayo on the northern coast of Peru. CECOOAC-Nor is the central cooperative of nine individual coffee producing cooperatives dotted through the northern Andean mountains. They were all established in the 1970s during a period in which the then military government supported farmers' cooperatives through an Agrarian Bank. But during the 1980s subsequent governments relinquished support and the bank became defunct, leaving farmers vulnerable to commercial bank interest rates and the purchasing strategies of commercial traders (*comerciantes*).

In the 1970s cooperatives were able to provide services to their members, including medical and educational services. Since then, these support services have been eroded, adding to the exposure of the cooperatives to renewed economic pressures. As access to cheap credit dried up the cooperatives have struggled to pay for their members' coffee. The situation worsened in 1989 when the International Coffee Agreement collapsed, leaving prices unregulated. Embedded in a political, economic, and social climate of considerable turmoil, the small-scale coffee producers in the northern Andes were buffeted by the vagaries of the Cocoa, Sugar, and Coffee Exchange in New York (CSCE), which regulates the Arabica futures and spot markets, and the powerful *comerciantes* for whom credit access was not a problem.

In 1990 CECOOAC-Nor made its first sale to a fair trade organization, a key event for its survival. The buyer was a roaster belonging to Max Havelaar, a Dutch-based hybrid network of mainstream coffee roasters who, in exchange for paying a fair price, are able to carry the Max Havelaar trademark on their coffee packaging. Sales to Cafédirect followed, the contracts negotiated with both the Cafédirect buyer and the CECOOAC-Nor export manager paying close attention to the daily market prices in New York. The key difference between fair trade buyers and commercial dealers is that the former pay a guaranteed minimum price (which protects farmers should the market go into free-fall), and a standard number of points above

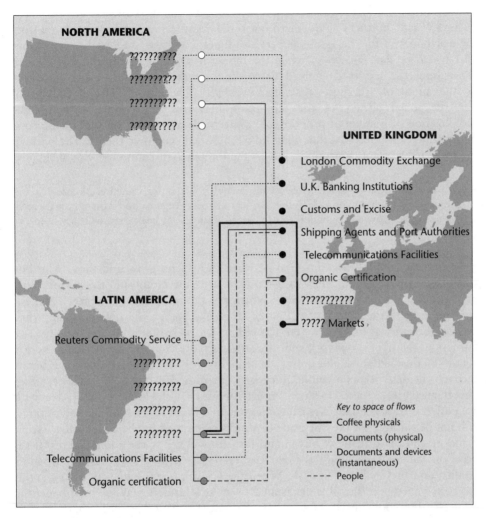

Figure 15.1 Network "lengthening": coincident spaces of a fair trade and commercial coffee network

the CSCE price when the market price exceeds the minimum (in effect, a 10 percent premium). The CSCE is therefore one of many coincident actants and sites in the hybrid network of fairly traded coffee and the commercial coffee networks (see Figure 15.1). Other such coincidences include the export and import authorities for whom documentation must be in order for goods to be granted passage.

Cafédirect pays CECOOAC-Nor using the international financial system (although there may be delays in the release of payments from Peruvian banks for other reasons). The stock exchange, customs officials, and banking clerks are all actants of the hybrid network of fair trade, so too are their computers, telephones, and fax machines. Just as there are coincident actants and spaces between fair trade and commercial coffee networks, so too is there a coincident mode of ordering –

that of *enterprise* – pragmatic, opportunistic, and canny (Law, 1994, p. 1). The "Third World" partners of Northern fair trade organizations are not insulated from the disciplines of the market – delivery deadlines, contracts, and quality conditions all have to be met. However, while the mode of ordering of enterprise is present throughout the fair trade hybrid network, it is mediated and re-articulated by another mode of ordering – that of *connectivity*. The raison d'être of Cafédirect, and the social agency of the fair trade network as a whole, rests on the mobilization of a mode of ordering of connectivity different from that of the cost-minimizing, self-interested individual of neoclassical economic theory. The packaging of Cafédirect coffee products makes the discourse of connectivity explicit.

> This is a fair trade product. More of the money you pay for Cafédirect freeze-dried goes directly to the small-scale coffee farmers in Latin America and Africa. Fair trade means coffee growing communities can afford to invest in healthcare, education and agriculture.

These words establish a connection between those who grow and those who buy Cafédirect coffee. *Connectivity* as a mode of ordering establishes the performance of "fairness," rather than charity, in which the farmer gets a "fair price" and the consumer "gets excellent coffee." In order to strengthen the network, fair trade organizations must make concrete the telling and performing of connectivity and fairness in the hybrid network. But the story is more complicated because another actant in this network, the coffee, is fraught with variabilities that reverberate through the network as a whole. In order to provide consumers of Cafédirect with "excellent coffee," the cooperatives must submit only the highest quality beans. If the coffee is of low quality (reasons may include rainfall, "pests," fermentation) it will not be suitable for the fair trade contracts negotiated by the cooperative export manager and the Cafédirect buyer, and farmers will sell to the *comerciantes*. If the price on the stock exchange is high *comerciantes* will pay well even for this low quality, and they will pay in cash. When the CSCE price is high – if, for example, the coffee harvest in Brazil is devastated by frost – farmers may see little benefit in selling to the cooperative. In such circumstances tensions between the modes of ordering of enterprise and connectivity become immediate and tangible as, for example, the warehouse goes unfilled.

At each point in the hybrid network there is instability and uncertainty, so that strengthening the embeddedness of the cooperatives is as important to the fair trade network as strengthening consumer support for fair trade coffee through marketing strategies and educational campaigns. Network strengthening is a process performed both locally and globally (see Figure 15.2). "Strengthening" social and environmental habits of association amongst producers involves the enhancement of essential services – agricultural, medical, and educational. The second key aspect of the mode of ordering of *connectivity* evidenced in this case study, that of sensitivity to interactions between human and nonhuman actants in the network, is accomplished through organic farming practices. Making the soil fertile by cultivating earthworms (*lombrices*) and mulch, interplanting with shade trees and not burning-off makes coffee growing practices less environmentally destructive. Six of the cooperatives have organic certification granted by the Organic Crop

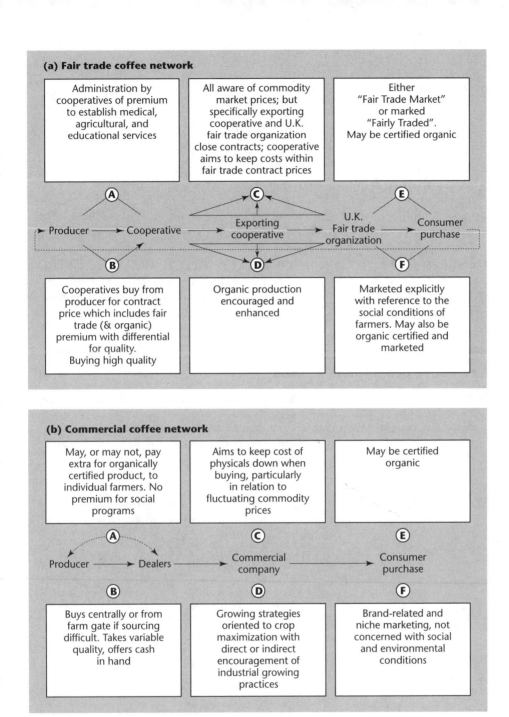

(a) Fair trade coffee network

| Administration by cooperatives of premium to establish medical, agricultural, and educational services | All aware of commodity market prices; but specifically exporting cooperative and U.K. fair trade organization close contracts; cooperative aims to keep costs within fair trade contract prices | Either "Fair Trade Market" or marked "Fairly Traded". May be certified organic |

(A)   (C)   (E)

Producer → Cooperative → Exporting cooperative → U.K. Fair trade organization → Consumer purchase

(B)   (D)   (F)

| Cooperatives buy from producer for contract price which includes fair trade (& organic) premium with differential for quality. Buying high quality | Organic production encouraged and enhanced | Marketed explicitly with reference to the social conditions of farmers. May also be organic certified and marketed |

(b) Commercial coffee network

| May, or may not, pay extra for organically certified product, to individual farmers. No premium for social programs | Aims to keep cost of physicals down when buying, particularly in relation to fluctuating commodity prices | May be certified organic |

(A)   (C)   (E)

Producer → Dealers → Commercial company → Consumer purchase

(B)   (D)   (F)

| Buys centrally or from farm gate if sourcing difficult. Takes variable quality, offers cash in hand | Growing strategies oriented to crop maximization with direct or indirect encouragement of industrial growing practices | Brand-related and niche marketing, not concerned with social and environmental conditions |

Key
A = Premium
B = Buying strategy
C = Relation to commodity market
D - Bean
E = Certification
F = Marketing

Figure 15.2 Network "strengthening": fair trade and commercial coffee networks exhibit distinctive modes of ordering

Improvement Association (OCIA International), drawing into the hybrid network yet other actants and sites across the US, Germany, and the UK. The whole process of organic certification is now regulated in law under European Union legislation (yet another coincident actant and space of fair trade and commercial networks offering organic products). The issue of environmental embeddedness, while a key part of the practices associated with the strengthening of alternative food networks, is no less dynamic than their institutional and technological aspects.

This brief description of a fair trade network is partial not least because there are other coffee growing organizations selling to Cafédirect, creating more heterogeneity than this example is able to convey. Nonetheless, it serves to illustrate how alternative geographies of food lengthen their reach using many of the same actants and spaces as their commercial counterparts. What is analytically distinctive, however, is *how* they strengthen relationships amongst formerly "passive" actants in commercial networks – the producers and consumers – through a mode of ordering of connectivity which works for non-hierarchical relationships framed by "fairness."

Alternative Geographies of Food

> What is to be done, then, with such sleek, filled-in surfaces, with such absolute totalities? Turn them inside out all at once, of course; subvert them, revolutionize them. The moderns have invented at one and the same time the total system, the total revolution to put an end to the system, and the equally total failure to carry out that revolution. (Latour, 1993, p. 126)

The tendency to transform the lengthened networks of modern social life into systematic and global totalities generates heroic accounts of globalization which do not recognize their own partiality (Thrift, 1995, p. 24). For Latour, such accounts of the relentless logic of social rationalization belie "a simple category mistake, the confusion of one branch of mathematics with another" (Latour, 1993, p. 119). Where the concepts "local" and "global" work well for surfaces and geometry, they mean little for networks and topology. While Latour's own style of writing is too supercilious for some – there is nothing simple about this category mistake – it should not detract from the importance of recognizing the power of metaphor and language in shaping economic, as much as scientific, understandings of the world (Mirowski, 1995b; Barnes, 1996); a power that is made flesh in numerous ways. In one sense, such vocabularies become embodied in the performance of individual and collective social identities and practices, both amongst corporate managers and oppositional political movements. In another sense, they become encoded in the authoritative texts and devices of law and science or in the engineered bodies of plants and animals (including humans).

In outlining an alternative understanding of global networks, the main points that we take from actor-network theory are that networks, unlike systems, are not self-sustaining; they rely on hundreds of thousands of people, machines, and codes to make the network. They are *collective*, that is their length and durability are woven between the capacities and practices of actants-in-relation. They are *hybrid*, combining people and devices and other living things in intricate and fallible ways in the performance of social practices. They are *situated*, inhabiting numerous nodes and sites in particular places and involving their own particular frictions (cultural and environmental) to network activity. And, finally, they are *partial* even as they are global, embracing surfaces without covering them, however long their reach.

Our approach shifts concern from a predictable unfolding of social structures in space to the means whereby networks of actors construct space by using certain forms of ordering which mobilize particular rationalities, technological and representational devices, living beings (including people), and physical properties. More than this, unlike the filled-in surfaces of globalization, this approach opens up space-time to the coexistence of multiple cross-cutting networks of varied length and durability, for example in the many coincidences between the institutional spaces and geographical places inhabited by commercial and fair trade coffee networks. TNCs emerge as no longer unique in their substantive capacity for global reach. By exploring the role of the unspoken presences (or immutable mobiles) which hold such connections in place we can begin to talk about "alternative geographies" of food in the same register, not as some pale specter in the colossal landscape of "capital." It is the political competence and social agency expressed through the mode of ordering of connectivity in the fair trade network – including Cafédirect, the exporting cooperative CECOOAC-Nor, and the 3,000 small coffee farmers – which effects the difference.

Part IV   Social Worlds

Editors' Introduction: Bringing in the Social

Jamie Peck, Trevor J. Barnes, Eric Sheppard, and Adam Tickell

One way of looking at the following set of readings is that they each deal with the social *context* in which the economy operates, since they explore issues like the role of the state, the place of gender relations, and the territorial organization of both capital and labor. They move far beyond the narrowly framed view of the market which characterized the economic geographies of the 1960s and 1970s – as a zone of market forces, supply and demand curves, rational responses to price signals – to delve deeply into the economy's social fabric, its institutional texture, and its political constitution. The authors, in their different ways, all reject the notion that "the economic" or "markets" represent a separate and pristine realm of existence in which utilitarian and maximizing actions prevail – the world, if you like, of conventional (neoclassical) textbook economics. But this is merely a point of departure for the following readings, which like so much of contemporary economic geography take it as axiomatic that the notion of a self-regulating market is an abstraction that tells us little or nothing about the operation of actually existing markets. It follows that any adequate understanding of "real world" markets calls for a consideration of the social relations and patterns of behavior that help to make and shape those markets, since economic relations are also social relations, and economic structures and processes are inescapably embedded in social and institutional practices and norms. So, prevailing gender orders and patterns of state regulation, for example, do not merely "distort" otherwise perfectly functioning markets, but are themselves fundamental to the way that markets are constituted and the way that they work. It follows that economic geographies reflect more than the working out of overarching, competitive logics – say, the search for least-cost locations – but in fact are the complex outcomes of a host of intersecting social, political, and institutional processes. As Oscar Wilde might have said, the market is rarely pure, and it is never simple.

What the following readings do is to point to some of the ways in which economic geographies are *socially and politically constituted*. They each draw attention to the various active, enduring, and spatially differentiated forms through which social and political relations shape economic processes, structures, and practices. In the essays that follow, each author pursues a different strategy in excavating and illustrating the role of "the social" in the formation of economic geographies. It is notable that the chapters draw only sparingly on mainstream economic theories of any stripe, drawing inspiration instead from a range of other *social* theories developed by sociologists, anthropologists, state theorists, and management scientists. The influence of Karl Polanyi's (1944) *The Great Transformation* is evident in some of the chapters, while others draw widely on economic sociology, urban social theory, management and organization studies, feminist theory, and political economy. For example, O'Neill's contribution on the role of the state in economic geography engages with the work of political sociologists Claus Offe, Bob Jessop, and Fred Block, while the starting point for Hudson and Sadler is a critical interrogation of Anthony Giddens' theories of social action.

If the economic geography of the 1970s was rather narrowly concerned with the dynamics of manufacturing activity and related questions of regional development, over the course of the past two decades economic geography's field of vision became increasingly global, in every sense of the word. So, research in contemporary economic geography encompasses issues as diverse as service work, consumption, sustainable ecological development, state restructuring, discourses of business, social reproduction, welfare reform, and so on. In the process, prevailing conceptions of the economic have also become substantially enlarged and enriched. Whereas the focus of economic geography was once the search for systematic patterns of "location in space" (Lloyd and Dicken, 1977), now the (conceptually determined) boundaries of the economy have been loosened and the very conception of the space economy has been transformed. The restrictive focus on the market and on manufacturing has been progressively displaced by more complex, integrative, and all-encompassing conceptions of socially embedded, socially regulated, and socially constituted economies (see Lee and Wills, 1997). Increasingly, the task of contemporary economic geography is meaningfully to connect and integrate the economic and the "non-economic", in pursuit of richer and more grounded forms of explanation. For example, this might involve locating the strategies of firms within the context of a supportive milieu of trust relations and institutionalized behavior patterns; it could entail uncovering the gendered nature of local employment practices, or it might mean tracing the dynamic effects of changes in financial, environmental, and labor regulations.

As all the readings that follow point out, but as Fincher, McDowell, and O'Neill argue quite explicitly, this is not simply a matter of "adding on" social, political, or institutional concerns to economic geography's preexisting research agenda. Instead, it implies a radical rethinking of this research agenda. In O'Neill's approach, for example, it involves *beginning* with the understanding that the state and the market are inescapably and necessarily enmeshed, albeit with enormously variable outcomes. "Markets" are not historically and logically prior to the moment of state "intervention," but the relation is one of continual mutual engagement and co-production. The complex and continuous roles performed by the state in making and managing markets – for example, in protecting private property rights, regulating working conditions, or discouraging the formation of monopolies – are crucial both for the operation of markets and the strategies of the state. In practice, the policymaking process cannot be reduced to a "firefighting" role, in which the state acts as a distant "overseer," occasionally moving to attend to market "failures." Instead, state and market are tangled together; their boundaries are not fixed, but porous and mobile. Markets are not self-constituting and self-regulating phenomena, but in an important sense are socially and politically constructed.

Orthodox thinking about market forces and economic processes – particularly in this supposed "era of globalization" – is quite different to the social worldview found in the subsequent essays. The contributions from both Storper and O'Neill make the point that "globalization talk" tends to perpetuate the myth that economic forces, like the weather, are naturally occurring and effectively uncontrollable. In conventional presentations of this argument (for example, Ohmae, 1990), these forces of apparently infinite market extension are also extra-terrestrial in the sense that they are reckoned to overrule and override all other "earthly" forces, such as those associated with government action or local political movements. Behind this caricature, which incidentally serves neo-liberal political interests particularly well, is an infinitely more complex and institutionally cluttered reality. Storper seeks to move beyond the misleading orthodox image of globalization, to parse out conceptually those kinds of economic activities that are "territorialized," in the sense that they depend on resources or relations that are geographically proximate and/or place specific, and those that are not. In carefully probing this flipside of the globalization process, Storper is able to document some of the typical corporate strategies and policy positions associated with different forms of territorialization and deterritorialization. One of his underlying points is that the resultant picture is much more variegated and nuanced than the straightforward stories of globalization-as-homogenous-marketization would suggest. Globalization processes are not as totalizing as many commentaries in the business literature would have us believe, and they do not produce unitary responses such as cutting costs and overheads, getting lean and mobile, and ever staying on the lookout for cheaper locations (see also Dicken, Part II).

Moreover, the heterogeneous organizational terrain described by Storper calls attention to a wide variety of policy options beyond the one-size-fits-all neo-liberal prescription of deregulation, tax-cutting, cost-stripping, and privatization. While some local policymakers may have little room for maneuver in the face of genuine threats of relocation from "footloose" local businesses, others confront situations in which key sectors of the local economy are more or less territorialized, that is, embedded in local networks, relations, and resource linkages. Here, the local policy options and challenges are quite different to those facing classically "globalized" localities, which are pitched into a daily battle to win, or retain, local jobs and businesses. The *reality* of globalization processes is consequently very different from the politically loaded vision of flat-earth market rule.

The way in which the economy is conceived consequently shapes the way in which it is politicized, and the way in which policy "problems" are defined and addressed. In fact, as Hudson and Sadler demonstrate, there are places and moments in which such circumstances of economic vulnerability can create basing points for new forms of political mobilization. Their contribution shows how, in many single-industry communities, threats of plant closure and large-scale job losses were associated with distinctively localized reconfigurations of class politics. Political identities, in this sense, are not "fixed" according to the positions of workers in the production process, but can be remade and re-imagined at the local level, often with far-reaching consequences for the conduct of local politics and the formation of (re)development strategies. And it follows that local economic fortunes are not predetermined by factor endowments or levels of productive efficiency, but are also a function of politics and institutional relations. Again, the emphasis in Hudson and Sadler's contribution is on the socially creative strategies by which communities respond to changing economic circumstances, even in situations where alternative job opportunities may be in limited supply. Through this discussion they also reveal some of the ways in which place complicates class analysis.

Indeed, the contributions here from the 1980s – Hudson and Sadler's paper on responses to plant closures and Fincher's paper on local gender relations – both take as their point of departure the limitations of conventional forms of class analysis. It is important to recall that one of the first means by which the social was brought into economic geography, back in the late 1970s and early 1980s, was in the form of a wave of industrial restructuring studies (see Lovering, 1989; Sayer, Part I), a defining feature of which was the key explanatory role attached to *workplace* social relations. In these studies, capital–labor (or class) relations at the point of production – focused on issues like technical change, job redesign, and industrial relations – provided the privileged point of entry for understanding *distinctively capitalist* forms of industrial restructuring (see Bluestone and Harrison, 1982; Massey and Meegan, 1982). The locational dynamics of industries, it was argued, could not be reduced to an endless search for least-cost production sites, but were also related to the ongoing imperative to control labor, for example, by evading heavily unionized regions and/or seeking out "greener" or more pliable local labor supplies.

By the mid-1980s, those working within this broad framework were beginning to develop less class-centric accounts of economic change, a moment captured in Hudson and Sadler's contribution (see also Massey and Allen, 1984; Gregory and Urry, 1985). Yet the highly influential collection in which Hudson and Sadler's chapter was published, Scott and Storper's (1986b) *Production, Work, Territory*, remained unmistakably production-centric, it being the editors' contention that "the most viable point of departure for an analysis of territorial development in modern capitalism is an investigation of the production system as an articulation of technical, social and political relationships" (Scott and Storper, 1986a, p. 301).

While as *points of departure*, critical studies of production relations continue to provide compelling bases for theories of territorial development – as Storper's contribution to this volume, for example, shows – there is no longer such a broad consensus on where the "explanatory center" lies in economic geography. Indeed, in a companion volume to *Production, Work, Territory*, Dear and Wolch (1989, p. 4, original emphasis) would subsequently argue that there was equal analytical validity in focusing on the linkages between "*reproduction* and territory [encompassing] the wide range of social relations and social practices which derive from, and which serve to protect and maintain, the basic structures of capitalist society." Their collection, which included the contribution by Fincher reprinted here, would explore issues like the production of collective and public services, the gendered nature of labor-market restructuring, the reorganization of welfare systems, the changing form of the voluntary sector, the regulatory activities of the state, and so on. In delving deep into community politics, the state, and the sphere of social reproduction, the

Wolch and Dear collection purposefully stretched prevailing conceptions of "the economic," and in so doing clearly breached the established boundaries of economic geography. Their purpose was not to develop a functionalist rationalization of these apparently extra-economic phenomena – accounting for their existence and their form solely in terms of the narrow requirements of capitalist (re)production – but instead to develop a broader explanation, in which the "formation of territorial outcomes is contingent upon the essentially unpredictable interactions of the spatial with the economic *and* the political and social/cultural spheres" (Dear and Wolch, 1989, p. 4, original emphasis).

The reading from Fincher reflects these broad objectives, since it sets out to explore some of the ways in which the organization of "social reproduction services," like childcare and elderly care, impact on patterns of participation in, and attachments to, the wage labor market. Focusing on the nexus of the local state and the local labor market, her analysis suggests that the geographically uneven nature of service delivery impacts the spatial constitution of job markets. Moreover, the types of jobs that are created in a local economy – what economists understand as "labor demand" – are not just a function of the technical requirements of production, but also reflect prevailing conceptions of "appropriate" work for different groups of men and women. Just as McDowell emphasizes in her reading too, jobs slots are not "out there," waiting to be filled by whomever is available, but the design and functioning of employment systems is instead profoundly gendered (see also Wright, Part II). Again, social relations – on this occasion, gender relations – represent more than a colorful backdrop against which market processes – in this case, labor market processes – operate. Rather, these market processes are themselves understood to be socially structured and socially constituted. So the economy is not a separate sphere with its own logic and dynamics, but its logic and dynamics are inescapably shaped by the social, political, and institutional relations in which all markets are embedded. And the *variable nature* of this embedding process is one of the principal causative factors behind the uneven spatial development of the economy, local differences in the ways in which markets operate having been related to phenomena like the structure of the local state, in Fincher's account, or the institutionalized pattern of "untraded" interdependencies between firms, as Storper emphasizes in his contribution.

Incorporating a deep understanding of the social constitution of economic practices does not simply mean displacing analyses of the "hard economic fundamentals" with a new emphasis on the "fuzzy social context"; it means overcoming this binary distinction altogether. This is one of the reasons why so many contemporary economic geographers draw on economic sociology and institutionalist traditions that emphasize the essential unity of *socioeconomic* processes. "Bringing in the social" is consequently not a one-time event relating to an enlargement of the analytical boundaries and empirical horizons of economic geography, but entails a continuous, recursive process of relating the economic to the extra-economic. The point is not to develop a less materialist and less economistic economic geography for its own sake, but to put this socioeconomic sensibility, and the enlarged field of vision with which it is associated, to work in explanations of the complexity, diversity, and geographical unevenness of economic phenomena. So McDowell observes, for example, that the initial concern in her research on the merchant banking industry was with the everyday practices that constitute gender relations in and around the workplace, not with what some might consider the "harder" economic phenomenon of interest rate-setting or regulatory reform. But she would discover in the course of the project that the gendered employment relations that were the principal focus of her study were in fact decisively implicated in the very structure and practices of this industry. The ways in which business is practiced in merchant banking reflects, remakes, and reproduces gender relations.

In reading the following contributions, therefore, a number of questions can usefully be borne in mind. What are the authors' points of entry into the discussion of the social and the economic – for example, the firm, the global economy, local government, the industry, political events or movements? In what senses does each of the chapters extend the reach of economic geography beyond a narrow concern with market relations? Which institutions, social relations, and political actions are identified as relevant to the formation of economic geographies, and with what *kinds* of economic effects are they associated? Are these relationships quantifiable, for example, and is it appropriate to talk about "degrees" of state involvement in the economy, or "more" or "less" gendered employment systems? In what sense do the different contributions identify a role for explicit social agency – thoughtful and meaningful interventions from social actors like policymakers, corporations, individual workers, or union leaders?

Chapter 16

Bringing the Qualitative State back into Economic Geography

Phillip M. O'Neill

Introduction

It is commonly argued that there has been substantial erosion of state power during the past two decades. This is seen to have occurred as a direct result of changes in the nature of capitalist accumulation which, in turn, are perceived to be driven by enhanced and extended circuits of capital. This chapter will advance three arguments to illustrate how this view of the state is inadequate. First, it is shown that the conception of the state as a totalized entity with centralized structures and purposes is erroneous. It is a conception that fits neatly with periodized views of capitalism (monopoly capitalism, Fordism, post-Fordism, and so on) but which provides little assistance in the analysis of contemporary economic change, at any scale. It is argued in this chapter that a more powerful understanding of contemporary economic change can be derived from depicting the state as a domain where a complex and heterogeneous state apparatus is engaged in constant interplay with non-state institutions and agents, including those from other nations, in an irresolvable contest over accumulation and distributional goals.

Second, the chapter challenges the politically charged discourse that markets are capable of a separate, private existence beyond the actions of the state's apparatus. Rather, a *qualitative* view of the state is preferred. In this view, the state is seen to play an indispensable role in the creation, governance, and conduct of markets, including at the international scale. Consequently, arguments about the *extent* of state intervention are seen as being feeble. Because the state is always involved in the operation of markets, the salient debate should be about the nature, purpose, and consequences of the *form* of state action, rather than about questions of magnitude of intervention.

Third, the chapter shows the depowering outcomes of arguments that the macroeconomic powers of the state are being eroded. At the heart of the neo-liberalist project, for example, is a discourse that promotes a form of capitalism, *laissez-faire*, which thrives under conditions where economic transactions are conducted outside the realm of state action. In this view, it is the very absence of state action that produces the best conditions for the efficient allocation of productive resources and the most desirable distributional outcomes. Similarly, accounts of contemporary economic change such as globalism and certain variations of regulation theory argue that there is a relentless hollowing of nation-state structures and powers. In short, capitalists are seen as being able to accumulate how and where they wish and, thereafter, states intervene to alter distributional outcomes. With the alleged collapse of nationally organized regimes of accumulation, however, opportunities for state-led redistributions are thought to be fading as state effort is redirected into shoring up the conditions for successful accumulation by national capitals in the face of growing international competition. In this contest, extant distributional positions are seen as being bargained away in competition for increasingly mobile investment projects. A *qualitative* construction of the state can avoid this immobilizing view of distributional possibilities. Since capitalism is incapable of operation outside the realm of the state, and since each and every step in the accumulation process involves distributions, then the state is *ever* involved in the distributional processes of capitalism.

These arguments are developed through the four sections of this chapter. The first section reviews the way that the state is perceived in economic geography, referring to three theoretical contexts in which formulations of the state are advanced. These contexts are neo-liberalism, globalization, and regulation theory. The second section of the chapter demonstrates that by decentering the way in which we portray the state and by concentrating on the interactions between the state's apparatus and capitalist processes, the distinction between state and market is broken down and issues of accumulation and distribution become inseparable. The third section of the chapter applies these arguments in an examination of the role of the state at new scales, in the context of rapid growth in international economic transactions. The final section examines distributional implications and new opportunities for intervention to achieve more desirable distributional outcomes.

State–Economy Relations

One of the major difficulties in undertaking an analysis of the role of the state in the construction of economic geographies is finding common answers to the question, What is the state doing? On the one hand, many economic geographers argue that, as a result of liberalized international financial flows over the past two decades, a *global* economic sphere has emerged which is beyond nation-state control (see Martin and Sunley, 1997). On the other, a small number of empirical analyses show how the nation-state plays a major role in both *managing* and *promoting* international financial flows (e.g., Leyshon, 1994; Martin, 1994; Hutton, 1995; O'Neill, 1997). It seems, then, that the major problem with attempts to generalize about the changing role of the modern state on the basis of empirical study is that there is almost always a case study of national economic change available somewhere in the world to match a writer's particular view of the state. Compare, for instance, the Hudson and Williams' (1995) view of an increasingly restricted British state to the active and purposeful state roles depicted by Webber (1994) in the Northeast Asian economies or Enderwick (1997) for the New Zealand state, irrespective of political hue.

Neo-liberalism

Neo-liberalists argue that freely operating private markets are the most capable instrument for maximizing output (technical efficiency), welfare (allocative efficiency), and ease of adjustment (dynamic efficiency). Neo-liberalists see the state as an outsider to the processes of real production and believe that it should constrain private activity to promote public interest only in situations of market failure – where desired goods and services are not supplied at acceptable prices. Yet, even in these circumstances, neo-liberalists point to a dilemma in placing the responsibility for corrective action in the hands of the state apparatus. They argue that the motivation of public regulators is not to maximize public interest but rather they will seek out exclusive benefits (or rents) for themselves and the groups which have secured their patronage. This view is encapsulated in public choice theory (Stigler, 1971) and represents the attempt by neo-liberalists to impugn the principle of public service and the existence of public goods. Neo-liberalist discourse frustrates the development of state distributive actions by arguing, first, that state intervention is best minimized and, second, that it will be corrupted in any event.

It is axiomatic, according to neo-liberalism, that the absence of state intervention *is* the market, that market failures are never failures of the market *per se*, and, therefore, they can only ever be failures of the state (drawing on Hayek, 1948). The political consequence of this view is the drive to deregulate, since modern states are thought to be incapable of managing either the social or the private economies – only through deregulation and privatization can the preconditions of economic growth be reestablished (Francis, 1993). This apparent displacement of a state's distributional functions has meant that not only does the discourse of neo-liberalism drive the accumulation strategies of many nations but, *ipso facto*, it has become the dominant distributional tool. The important point to be made here is that the neo-liberalist vision of "less state" is entirely illusory. Neo-liberalism is a self-contradicting theory of the state. The geographies of product, finance, and labor markets that it seeks to construct require *qualitatively* different, not less, state action. Neo-liberalism is a political discourse which impels rather than reduces state action (Hirsch, 1991; Bonnett et al., 1990; Tickell and Peck, 1995).

Globalism

Internationalization and more recently its descendant, globalism, have been portrayed by economic geographers, and others, as all-powerful tendencies of capitalism which have had major impacts on the role of the state. During the 1970s and 1980s, international capital was commonly seen as controlled by stateless multinational corporations which aimed to penetrate the capital and consumer markets of every country and every region. Analysis drew heavily on the theory of the international division of labor (Fröbel et al., 1980), and privilege was accorded to those events seen to operate at the global scale (e.g., Thrift, 1986; Dicken, 1992a; Chase-Dunn, 1989). In an extreme version of this tale, Ross and Trachte (1990) advise that global capitalism dominates all economic spheres, leading to the crippling of nation-states, whose meager resources shift from the pursuit of legitimation goals (especially social welfare) to the accumulation goals of once-national capitals in their global ventures.

Common to the inexorable-rise-of-global-capitalism accounts of contemporary crisis is the portrayal of the state in classical Marxist form: an organizational unit which serves the dominant classes which, in the contemporary scene, are the controllers of global fractions of capital. Two rebuttals of this position can be made. The first acknowledges that states, acting through autonomous state agents and apparatus, maintain sufficient economic authority and purpose to produce "discontinuous" economic and political spaces (Dicken, 1992a, 1994). The state remains capable of producing "location-specific" supply and demand conditions *within* nations – and these conditions are more than the passive response to globally mobile fractions of capital; they are conditions which *drive* foreign investment itself. Certainly, there is ample evidence that Keynesian macroeconomic management powers are eroded by globalization processes, but one cannot conclude that a powerless nation-state has been left as residue. Inevitably, states are developing new capacities and structures to exert new forms of political and economic power, even across the territories of different states (Dicken et al., 1997).

The second rebuttal of the inexorable-rise-of-global-capitalism-and-decline-of-the-nation-state story is based on distinguishing between globalization as discourse and evidence (or lack of evidence) for the existence of globalization as a general trend (Cox, 1992; Dicken et al., 1997). There is growing understanding that the rise of the vocabularies of globalism has been based on their use for coercive purposes in framing national economic strategies, in reformulating workplace practices, and in garnering community support for national and local economic reforms. These vocabularies necessarily portray the state as a depowered entity – for obvious reasons. Yet there is a difference between a *loss of* state role contained in the globalism story and a *shift in* state role which a qualitative view of the state would assert. However, if indeed the shift in state role is qualitative, then what is changing? What new state capacities and structures have emerged? And what guides their formulation and reformulation? The following section demonstrates the inadequacy of one version of regulation theory in answering these questions.

Regulation theory and the hollowed-out state

One of the major impacts of recent regulation theory on thinking about the state has been the idealization of the postwar Keynesian welfare state and its positioning as a historical yardstick against which subsequent state roles are measured. In particular, regulation theory assigns a nanny role to the postwar state: alleviating crisis in the Fordist economy and nurturing capitalism's drop-outs. Peck and Tickell (1994), for example, argue that the decline of the Keynesian state is a fundamental cause of contemporary economic crisis, a crisis which persists because a stable replacement regulatory order has yet to emerge. In this context, the nation-state is simultaneously coerced by international economic forces and driven by the accumulation needs of its domestic economy (Tickell and Peck, 1995). Similarly, Jessop (1994) argues that the "hollowing-out" of the nation-state is a feature of the contemporary period. Jessop maintains that, at the same time that nation-states have abandoned demand management in favor of supply-side initiatives, supranational state apparatuses have emerged as the new regulators. Activities at the nation-state level are seen to be driven by global economic trends (Jessop, 1994). These include the development of new legal forms to support cross-national cooperation and strategic alliances, the reform of currency and credit systems, rules for technology transfer, trade governance, intellectual property negotiations, and the regulation of international labor migration. At the same time, according to Jessop, investment policies have been devolved to the local state, resulting in new cross-national group-ings of regions. A residual nation-state thereby is left to engage in the development of work practices and other measures to promote international competitiveness, a situation which Jessop labels as the Schumpeterian workfare state.

Jessop's hollowed-out metaphor, then, is an account of *shift in* rather than *diminution of* state role with complex new relationships emerging between state apparatuses at different scales. Yet, irrespective of the original conception, it has become commonplace for the hollowed-out metaphor to be used in the literature to represent a universal condition of state depowerment. The metaphor has come to represent an extreme paralysis of the nation-state, different from the shift process described by Jessop.

Putting aside these misinterpretations of regulation theory, to what extent does regulation theory provide an enduring explanation of state process and behavior? Regulationists Tickell and Peck (1995) are ambivalent. Certainly, they use regula-tion theory effectively to explain the role of the state in the construction of social regulation as a stable form of governance during the Fordist period. Yet they acknowledge that regulation theory offers little explanation for the key processes of transition (Tickell and Peck, 1995), which, surely, have been the key concern of nation-states for at least the past two decades! Regulation theory has insufficient to say about the crucial role of the state in moving societies from one period of stable economic conditions to the next, beyond describing them as intervals of crisis.

Much of this inadequacy stems from regulation theory's attempt to totalize the economy in its form, its history, and its methods of governance. Further, accumu-lation crisis is portrayed by regulation theory as a singular, totalized event. There is no possibility in regulation theory for a multitude of unrelated economic events, in different cycles of growth and prosperity, under different forms of governance. There is no allowance for incremental, strategic, state-driven economic restructur-ing and transition such as has been the hallmark of East Asian economic change since the 1960s; and there is an underlying denial that conflict and tension in the operations of state apparatuses may be normal events.

Further, as a result of presenting an idealized (and nostalgic) view of the social and economic outcomes of Keynesian–Fordist state management, regulation theo-rists have a tendency to conflate successful accumulation with successful distribu-tional outcomes. The theory assumes that the successful management of national accumulation processes is the most important coercive tool in securing state legiti-macy. This view is almost the opposite of the view of many state theorists, such as Claus Offe (see Offe, 1984), and is denied by considerable empirical evidence. Bakshi et al. (1995), for example, point to the racialized and gendered history of the British state in the context of successful national accumulation during the Keynesian–Fordist years. Social compliance was never earned through long periods of economic growth, and fair and reasonable distributions of national income were not automatic for each social group.

It is argued, then, that there is an absence of a theory of the state in regulation theory stemming, first, from the way regulation theory idealizes the *form* and *functions* of the contemporary state and, second, from a heavy reliance on observations of the UK experience – an experience which Hutton (1995) admits is unusual. Regulation theory fails to acknowledge that national economic strategies must be continuously managed and renegotiated since, *per se*, they are continuously involved with both accumulation *and* distribution questions. Better abstractions of state process are needed. These need to draw on a multitude of state experiences and situate the realm of the state *within* accumulation processes. Further, there needs to be greater understanding of the ongoing nature of distributional processes, thereby avoiding the crippling placement of the state in a position where its capacities are limited to *ex post* income transfers through welfare assistance. In summary, what is needed is a theory of the state which says something about (a) the *way* the state functions; (b) how it stabilizes *and* transforms regimes of accumulation; (c) how it operates through geographic scales – not simply how it is constrained by scale; and (d) how it is, and should be, involved with *redistribution*.

The Qualitative State

This chapter advances the paradigm of the *qualitative state* as a way towards a theoretical position which rejects the possibility of a privately constructed realm of freely operating markets and which asserts the indispensable role of the state in providing the means (*inter alia*) for privately performed production and consumption. Block (1994) notes that a qualitative view of the state rejects the assessment or measurement of state role by *degree of intervention*. Wherever, and whenever, commercial transactions occur, the state plays a key role. The new state paradigm begins by rejecting the idea of state intervention in the economy. It insists instead that state action *always* plays a major role in constituting economies, so that it is not useful to posit states as lying outside of economic activity. (Block, 1994, p. 696; emphasis in original)

Qualitative conceptions of the state draw strongly from the historical works of Karl Polanyi (1944). Polanyi demonstrated how, on the one hand, the rise of industrial capitalism could never have been a purely private process and, on the other, that economic institutions are inevitably political creations. He exposed the myth of spontaneous emergence of free-market relationships in post-feudal society. Instead, the emerging modern state is shown to have established crucial conditions for the operation of capitalist relations including exclusive property rights, a legal system based on the inviolability of contracts, the establishment of large national markets (through administrative structures, monetary systems, and common standards such as in food purity, weights and measures), and the means for the penetration of other national markets, especially through imperialism (Block, 1990; Cerny, 1990). The chief message that state theorists have drawn from Polanyi is that markets simply cannot operate in a *laissez-faire* environment.

Block (1994) presents a detailed summary of views of the state which have led to the emergence of the qualitative state paradigm. This is based on four major tenets. First, *economy* is necessarily a combination of three events: markets, state action, and state regulation. A corollary of this constitution is that there is an infinite number of ways in which an economy can be organized. Second, although economic efficiency is dependent on markets, markets are state-constrained and state-regulated and thereby incapable of operating in a *laissez-faire* environment. Third, neither capital nor the state is capable of achieving its goals simultaneously nor independently. Finally, it should be recognized that any coherence that exists about the idea of *economy* derives essentially from our cultural beliefs, which (in Anglo cultures at least) have led to constructions of economy being overlain with the dichotomy of *planned versus market*, which, in turn, has had the effect of denying the existence of multiple forms of economy. This is an extension of the Marxist recognition of the power of economic ideologies to make particular economic arrangements appear as natural and inevitable.

These tenets stand opposed to the basic assumptions of what Block (1994) terms the "old state paradigm." Various forms of the old paradigm construct the state as occupying a position (*a priori*) external to the main economy. The idealized (or normative) *public goods state*, for example, describes the state as having the duty to provide the goods and services, such as blood or policing, which private markets are incapable of supplying efficiently and universally. The *macroeconomic stabilizing* form of the state *intervenes* to adjust market aggregates, especially consumer demand, in order to move equilibrium (or market-clearing) positions of private markets closer to full employment.

Certainly, markets remain the best available device for aggregating individuals' commercial preferences. At the same time, state involvement is inevitable so that markets can be formed and operate efficiently. A common set of roles can be drawn up for all states in all economies. These include the maintenance of a regime of property rights; the management of territorial boundaries; the establishment and administration of legal frameworks to ensure economic cooperation; the provision of basic infrastructure; the creation and governance of financial markets and product markets; ensuring of the production and reproduction of labor; controlling macroeconomic trends; and the conduct of legitimation activities to secure the economic system through time. Table 16.1 details the role of the qualitative state in the construction and maintenance of modern economies and demonstrates the vast and complex operations common to all Western states.

The analysis so far has been concerned with what the qualitative state *does*. Consideration must also be given to the *structures and mechanisms* of the qualitative state which enable the performance of the roles identified. Offe's (1975, 1976, 1984) work provides valuable insights into the *processes* by which the state engages with capitalism. There are two major thrusts in Offe's work. The first is his search for a useful theoretical analysis of economic crisis which incorporates the general questions of state authority and legitimacy as well as the functional problem of how states actually achieve their fiscal and welfare goals. The second is Offe's concern with the question of whether the state is capable of producing the means of overcoming the contradictions of capitalist production. For Offe, state involvement is more than the actions of public institutions *on* various societal groupings. Rather, the state participates directly *in* the domains of other institutions and associations such as political parties, trade unions, and corporations, and in the processes by

Table 16.1:   Roles of the qualitative state in a modern economy

A   Maintenance of a regime of property rights
    i.   maintenance of private property rights
    ii.   recognition of institutional property rights
    iii.   basic rules for the ownership and use of productive assets
    iv.   basic rules for the exploitation of natural resources
    v.   rules for the transfer of property rights (between individuals, households, institutions, and generations)
B   Management of territorial boundaries
    i.   provision of military force
    ii.   economic protection through manipulation of:
- money flows
- goods flows
- services flows
- labor flow
- flows of intangibles

    iii.   quarantine protection
C   Legal frameworks to maximize economic cooperation
    i.   establishment of partnerships and corporations
    ii.   protection of intellectual property rights
    iii.   the governance of recurring economic relations between
- family members
- employers and workers
- landlords and tenants
- buyers and sellers

D   Projects to ensure social cooperation
    i.   maintenance of law and order
    ii.   undertake national image-making processes
    iii.   other coercive strategies
E   Provision of basic infrastructure
    i.   Provision or organization of:
- transportation and communications systems
- energy and water supply
- waste disposal systems

    ii.   assembly and conduct of communications media
    iii.   assembly and dissemination of public information
    iv.   land use planning and regulation

which social and economic interests are represented to government. Not surprisingly, therefore, social turbulence and political resistance – threats to both capital accumulation and state legitimacy – are seen to be continuously internalized within the state apparatus as it seeks to manage and distribute resources in ways that contribute not just to the achievement of economic growth but also to prevailing notions of justice. Offe's point is that the state is neither an arbiter nor a regulator nor an uncritical supporter of capitalism, but is "enmeshed" in its contradictions. Capitalism is anarchic, requiring the state to sustain the processes of accumulation and protect the private appropriation of resources. The social processes necessary for the reproduction of labor, private ownership and commodity exchange, then, are regulated and sustained by *permanent* political intervention. The state is therefore constituted by continuous administrative, legal, bureaucratic, and coercive systems

Table 16.1: *continued*

F   Creation and governance of financial markets
    i.   rules for the establishment and operation of financial institutions
    ii. designation of the means of economic payment
    iii. rules for the use of credit
    iv. maintenance of the lender of last resort
G   Creation and governance of product markets
    i.   regulation of the market power of firms
    ii. the selection and regulation of natural monopolies
    iii. the promotion and maintenance of strategic industries
    iv. the provision of public goods
    v. the provision of goods unlikely to be supplied fairly
H   Production and reproduction of labor
    i.   demographic planning and governance
    ii. provision of universal education and training
    iii. governance of workplace conditions
    iv. governance of returns for work
    v. social wage provision
    vi. supply and governance of childcare
    vii. provision or governance of retirement incomes
I   Control of macroeconomic trends
    i.   fiscal policy
    ii. monetary policy
    iii. external viability
J   Other legitimation activities
    i.   elimination of poverty
    ii. maintenance of public health
    iii. citizenship rights
    iv. income and wealth redistribution
    v. urban and regional development
    vi. cultural development
    vii. socialization
    viii. enhancement of the environment

that not only build relationships *between* the state and other groups in society, but also heavily influence relationships *within and between* these groups. Further, it should not be surprising that different states have different levels of power. The point is that these differences are produced less by extant economic conditions and more by the capacities of states to create or strengthen their organizations, to employ enough appropriate personnel, to co-opt political support, especially through programmes to assist economic enterprises, and to facilitate social programs (Skocpol, 1985). Further, these capacities are in no small part due to historical attitudes to governance and state role. That is, *qualitative* differences in states arise and are sustained by prevailing and historical structures and conditions influencing the state's apparatus.

The National State and the Supranational Scale

This section explores the impact on the state of the growing proportion of market transactions which are international. It is argued that international transactions reinforce the structure and importance of the nation-state, rather than diminish them (see Cerny, 1990). The emergence of global marketplaces has transformed the states' role, and there is ample evidence that global marketplaces themselves are transformed by the involvement of nation-states in the creation and operation of supranational governance regimes and structures. Examples include nation-state involvement in the prudential supervision of international financial transactions through the Bank of International Settlements, the supervision of quality and safety in traded products through the operations of the International Standards Organization, and, of course, the governance of access to domestic product markets by the World Trade Organization. Thus the rise of a more prominent supranational tier of governance has required the *increased* involvement of nation-states, including, in many circumstances, *new* participation by apparatuses of the state at the level of local and regional governments, development agencies, sectoral-industrial and financial instrumentalities, and so on. Paradoxically, then, pressures arising from an increasingly integrated world marketplace reinforce and reconstruct state role rather than usurp it.

The nation-state has also played a key role in the trend towards international regionalism as an avenue for successful international accumulation. Hay (1995) notes that this trend has been accompanied by the emergence of supranational state structures such as the North American Free Trade Agreement, the General Agreement on Tariffs and Trade, and the European Union. In contrast to the Jessop argument that the emergence of supranational state structures is part of the hollowing-out process of the nation-state, Hay argues that tendencies towards strengthening supranational power structures are constrained by "the fact that the inter-state bargaining required . . . is driven by the exigencies of maintaining *national* legitimacy bases" (Hay, 1995, p. 403; emphasis in original). In other words, national state agents pursue national rather than international interests in the global political arena. The irony, according to Hay, is that supranational bodies are incapable of intervening in the circulation of capital unless they are constituted by vibrant national state power. Moreover, global capital circulations *require* state structures in order for accumulation to proceed without persistent chaos.

To assist their supranational operations, nation-states are devising methods which strongly contest both the depowering images of globalism and the growing contestability of domestic markets. Commonly, the nation-state moves to strengthen what its populations see as "national." It is involved increasingly in coercive strategies seeking societal approval of national economic change and to legitimize the adoption or reconstruction of a national accumulation strategy. These strategies build on preexisting national identities which are historical products of myriad state policies dealing with immigration, foreign investment, sport, the arts, school curriculum, telecommunications, and so on. And, not surprisingly, many strategies are erroneous, for they involve the performance of relatively new roles to address new problems in new operational domains. Further, new state actions are not necessarily designed to produce more acceptable distributional outcomes. The argument here is simply that increasingly open and integrated national markets do not so much threaten or undermine the operation and effectiveness of state apparatuses as require that they undergo qualitative change. Critically, this qualitative shift is not optional, for it is fundamental for the continuation of successful accumulation processes and, in the absence of oppression, for the production of distributional outcomes that maintain legitimacy. Along the way, the process of adjustment produces problems which few state managers relish and which require much experimentation in ideas, management structures and cultures, and policies (Cerny, 1990). Some discernible adjustment trends in the current period include a preference for micro- rather than macro-interventions; a shift from the protection of selected industries in specific market segments to the construction of internationally competitive conditions across markets; the adoption of enterprise cultures which promote innovation and competition, including in the public sector; and a shift in state expenditures towards the maximization of economic outcomes rather than the maximization of social welfare. Not surprisingly, there is considerable discontent among progressive groups in all nations with the distributional consequences of these trends.

Two consequences of thinking about the supranational scale in these ways emerge. The first concerns the role of the nation-state in translating activities from the supranational domain to production and consumption activities which take place within national boundaries. Not only does the state create the basic competitive conditions essential for successful accumulation, including trade rules, property rights, and exchange rate stability, it also blends these conditions with emerging apparatuses from the supranational scale. Critically, though, the successful blending of domestic and supranational domains to produce stable national and international circuits of capital with desirable distributional outcomes depends fundamentally on nation-states combining to agree on common objectives and implement common regulations and standards (Hirst and Thompson, 1996).

The second consequence is pointed to by Cerny (1990), who notes that national economic openness in trade, finance, information flows, and communications produces an "overloaded state." This overload consists of problems which arise from the international transmission of recession, the incorporation of both private and public economic goals into an international context, and from struggles to maintain the political legitimacy necessary for national economic management when the traditional tools are found wanting. For example, a common constraint to the maintenance of legitimacy is the persistence of chronic public funding deficits which absorb national savings and exacerbate current-account imbalances. Another constraint is the incompatibility between centralized labor regulation and actions by firms to reduce real unit labor costs through labor shedding, new shift patterns, and outsourcing. A third constraint stems from demands for state assistance in maintaining or restructuring unprofitable economic sectors especially through direct subsidy and microeconomic reforms. Cerny concludes that alongside growing internationalization, "the total amount of state intervention will tend to *increase*, for the state will be enmeshed in the promotion, support, and maintenance of an ever-widening range of social and economic activities" (Cerny, 1990, p. 230; emphasis added). However, Cerny (1990, p. 231) adds that "The domestic redistribution of wealth and power, which is at the heart of the social democratic welfare state, will become more difficult and complex to achieve."

Continued crisis in capitalism, then, maximizes, rather than reduces, the demands for state intervention. Predominantly, however, state intervention seems to favor the types of accumulation practices which involve distributions of incomes in favor of capital – an outcome at the heart of neo-liberalist discourse. The "overloaded state" is faced with addressing distributional problems through targeted welfare assistance from a distressed public budget. In contrast, a reconstructed discourse which takes the view that the state and its apparatus are inherent to the processes of production and consumption, and not lying outside them as detached overseer, regulator, or undesirable intruder, offers opportunities for the identification and manipulation of distributional outcomes at the point of the accumulation process.

Propositions about Distribution

Because capitalism is incapable of an existence outside the realm of state action and because capitalist processes involve distributive processes *per se*, then the state is always involved in redistribution activities. Hence, the argument that the internationalization of the world economy is a natural tendency of modern capitalism resulting in depowerment of the nation-state is simply a restatement of a coercive discourse designed to defer or deny the benefits of restructuring to particular groups. This section of the chapter advances this argument through three propositions about the distributional opportunities of the paradigm of the qualitative state.

The first proposition is that the state and its apparatus constitute an arena for the struggle over distribution (see Offe, 1976, 1984, 1985). Importantly, though, at the same time as being enmeshed in capitalist production and exchange, the state is driven by the need to preserve its own autonomy and power as the arbiter of class conflict and the sustainer of decommodified social production. Accordingly, it is not because of its being a servant of capitalism that makes the state interested in successful accumulation; successful accumulation is critical for the sustenance of the state's own interests, not the least reason being the state's reliance on economic growth for the provision of taxation revenues particularly for redistribution purposes (O'Connor, 1973). A struggle then ensues. The state seeks to fund fiscal actions promised to the electorate. Capital resists regulations which inhibit capacities to secure advantage over competitors, to extract surplus value from labor and to minimize its distribution to consumers. Thus the state's dilemma is the maintenance of the accumulation process (which ideally seeks *minimal* state intervention) while successfully pursuing legitimization goals (which ideally require *maximum* state intervention). In other words, the state has to engage simultaneously in commodification and decommodification.

It can be concluded from this reasoning that, while only the state has the power and apparatus to organize economic spheres of action, the state's redistributive actions inside marketplaces are continuously opposed by agents of capital which claim that economic spheres should be held as "natural and inviolable" (Offe, 1976, p. 395). On the other hand, the state's "natural" domain is seen as being within social systems such as education, health, and welfare which render the "ingredients of a 'decent' life" (Offe, 1975, p. 256). The agents of capital contend that the state's functions should be funded by the state's appropriation of revenue *after* the redistribution processes inherent to accumulation have occurred. Company taxation, for example, is levied on the basis of *net* income flows *following* a financial year of economic activity. Accordingly, when the state accepts a position of *ex post* distributor, it will always suffer fiscal crisis during downturns in the economic cycle when there are increased distributional demands and falling revenues. Hence, the successful simultaneous performance of state functions is impossible for any length of time.

A second proposition that must be inserted into thinking about the qualitative state and its inherent distributive functions is that the state plays a critical role as a coercive instrument during periods of economic restructuring. Globalization presents an attractive image or story to conservative politicians especially in the parts that argue that local labor needs to acquiesce to the demands of international capital and world competitive pressures. This discourse displaces traditional national social democratic strategies and active macroeconomic policies. The point is that the construction of the idea of a market economy that is rational, self-constituting, self-regulating, and independent of the political sphere is a *normative prescription*. This, in turn, is consistent with the view that only a minimalist, non-interventionist, night-watchman state can accompany a maximum performance economy. Thus, the state is at the center of discourses of economic restructuring which, in turn, generate distributional outcomes.

A third proposition picks up from Jessop (1994) and argues that since internationalizing processes involve an expansion of nation-state organization, then internationalization presents greater, not fewer, opportunities for state intervention into distributional outcomes. There is growing evidence that global circulations of capital, goods and services, ideas, and people require supranational state structures and apparatuses. In turn, these depend on the vibrancy of nation-states for legitimacy and power. Only nation-states have territorial authority to deal with the social outcomes, including conflict, which inevitably follow internationalization processes. Obviously, the discourse of internationalization used by nation-states is critical here. Finally, local and regional authorities have little chance of pursuing their international interests unless nation-states "suture" the supranational domain to the national territory. Greater realization of the role of the nation-state in internationalization processes can lead to improved distributional outcomes in regions which have often suffered from the timid explanation that events causing local economic devastation arise from an uncontrollable global capitalism.

Conclusion

Thinking about the qualitative state offers new opportunities for invigorated state action for more desirable distributional outcomes. It involves accepting the autonomy of the state; accepting the crucial role of the state in the governance of private markets; accepting that the state is not a homogeneous unit but exists as a contested domain continuously interacting with society; and accepting that internationalization is not a singular logic of capitalism as investment (allegedly) flees collapsing Keynesian–Fordist national economic spaces. Thinking about the qualitative state also involves rejecting the notion of a hollowed-out state in the sense that internationalization has made the nation-state redundant as a macroeconomic manager; and rejecting the logic that redistribution is an act which follows accumulation processes, the extent of the former being dependent on the success of the latter. Finally, the idea of the qualitative state is not a question of bringing the state back in. Close examination shows that the state never departed. The crucial question concerns the ways in which we have represented the state during the recent decades of economic crisis when commercial transactions have become increasingly internationalized. New discourses about the qualitative state have the potential to enhance opportunities for intervention into economic processes and make them more successful – especially when judged by their distributive outcomes.

Chapter 17

Territories, Flows, and Hierarchies in the Global Economy

Michael Storper

Globalization and the Institutions of Economic Development

In recent years, the flows of goods, services, information, capital, and people across national and regional lines have increased greatly, giving rise to the notion that modern economic activity is somehow becoming "globalized." Do these phenomena mean that contemporary economies are becoming placeless, mere flows of resources via corporate hierarchies, which are themselves not rooted in national or regional territories and therefore not subject to territorially based state institutions? Though many commentators assign territorially based institutions, especially nation-states, a continuing role in the global economy, the balance of power is thought to be tipping in favor of globalized organizations, networks, practices, and flows. Hence, the locus of control over important dimensions of the economic development process – both in the narrow sense of formal decision-making and resource deployment and in the larger sense of influences to which we must respond – is passing from territorialized institutions such as states to deterritorialized institutions such as intrafirm international corporate hierarchies or international markets that know no bounds (Gilpin, 1975; Ohmae, 1990; Reich, 1990). The perfection of hierarchies and markets, as management systems and transactional structures, is said to be gaining on territorial barriers, specificities, and frictions (Julius, 1990).

There is another view, of course, and it comes from the rich literature on different ways that organizations and markets are shaped by political and business institutions. The "Japanese model" and J-firm, the "German model," and the like, are different ways that advanced capitalist activity can be organized (Albert, 1993). There is a competition between such territorially based institutionally organized production systems for world market share in many sectors.

These two views correspond, in many ways, to the two main disciplinary discourses that deal with globalization – economics and political science. Much of the former implies that economic development is becoming deterritorialized, while there is a strong body of research in the latter that indicates continued territorial specificity in development patterns owing to the institutions alluded to previously.

Political economists and political scientists have begun to consider the effects of global capitalism on the margin of maneuver left to nation-states (Carnoy, 1993), but curiously have devoted less attention to scrutinizing how globalized capitalism really is. As a result, the theoretical meaning and practical impact of economic globalization remain obscure.

In this chapter I propose to sketch out what a confrontation between the territorialization of economic development and the emergence of global hierarchies and flows would look like. The reason for this confrontation is the hypothesis that the ability of territorially bounded states and other institutions to bargain with hierarchical global business organizations, and to shape the development process in general, should rise with the territorialization of economic activity. Territorialization thus becomes the analytical key to the debate about the politics and economics of globalization.

Defining territorialization in economic terms

Territorialized economic development may be defined as something quite different from mere location or localization of economic activity. It consists, for our purposes, in economic activity which is dependent on resources that are territorially specific. These "resources" can range from asset specificities available only from a certain place or, more importantly, assets that are available only in the context of certain interorganizational or firm–market relationships that necessarily involve geographical proximity, or where relations of proximity are markedly more efficient than other ways of generating these as set specificities. Geographically proximate relations constitute valuable asset specificities if they are necessary to the generation of spillover effects – positive externalities – in an economic activity system. So territorialization is often tied to specific interdependencies in economic life. Proximity would also be a basis of valuable specific assets insofar as these latter are necessary to the efficient functioning of the firm under normal circumstances, where the firm cannot replace them, either by internalizing functions or by carrying out its external relations in a way that does not involve proximity in them. The assets to which we refer can be hard – labor, technology – or soft – information, conventions of interaction, relation-specific skills. We shall develop this notion of relationally specific assets further as we go along (Asanuma, 1989).

An activity is fully territorialized when its economic viability is rooted in assets (including practices and relations) that are not available in many other places and that cannot easily or rapidly be created or imitated in places that lack them. Locational substitutability is not possible, and feasible locations are small in number, making locational "markets" highly imperfect. This definition of territorialization thus does not cover all cases of agglomeration or localization or urbanization, but a distinctive subset of those cases.

Mainstream Arguments about Globalization and Their Silences

As noted, huge research efforts have been devoted to the behavior of firms in a global economy; to consequences for markets, and to the ways that institutions shape markets and firms. There are major lacunae in these efforts because they do not pose the question of territorialization clearly.

Who is us? Markets versus hierarchies

In the United States, the early 1990s debate over the national economy in a global economy illustrates this conceptual lacuna well. On one side, it was argued that development-inducing investment will flow to those areas that possess appropriate factors of production, which, in the global economy, means high-quality labor ("symbolic analysts"), infrastructure, and so on (Reich, 1990). The argument, then, was implicitly about the importance and mobility of foreign direct investment, and that ownership of assets – the nationality of firms – is unimportant. The role of regions and nations is to develop appropriate factor supplies so as to attract this highly mobile investment. But the argument said nothing about whether those factors are territorialized or not, in the sense defined here. As such, it can be interpreted either as an endorsement of globalization as placelessness or of globalization as the attraction of capital to territorialized economic formations.

On the other side of the debate, it was claimed that ownership – the nationality of firms – is important (Tyson, 1991). It is necessary for political reasons to have firms that produce all technologies essential to national security, and even major multinational firms concentrate their core technology-producing activities in their home territories. Even without security concerns, the existence of technological spillovers means that for an economy to carry out certain innovation and development processes, it must possess a complement of other capacities. Both these claims are probably quite sound, in and of themselves; but they do not say much of anything about globalization. On one hand, the argument does not show why even major multinationals continue to concentrate their principal technology-based activities at home and therefore why the factor/market-attraction argument is not valid (see also Amendola, Guerrieri, and Padoan, 1992; Carnoy, 1993; Patel and Pavitt, 1991). As a result, it could still be claimed that investment is becoming increasingly mobile and that the observed rootedness of major multinationals in their home economies is a transitory, not necessary, condition. On the other hand, while it correctly suggests interdependence-through-spillover as key to many of the most important forms of innovation, it does not say why such spillovers should be localized within a national economy, except for security reasons. There is no economic reasoning about the territorialization of such spillovers, in other words. So the debate over "who is us?" tells us little about who we really are in a global economy.

Commodity trade

The growth of commodity trade figures prominently in claims that the economy is globalizing. Rising intra-industry trade is said to be evidence of globalization as firms create a global functional division of labor. One possibility is that intra-industry trade is accompanied by the advent of global oligopolistic supply structures for many commodities and for knowledge inputs (Ernst, 1990). The big firms who dominate these supply chains benefit from entry barriers due to scale and the firm-specific assets they deploy on a global scale. This argument, however, says nothing about the problem of territorialization *per se*. Global supply structures, even highly oligopolistic ones, could reflect (1) an internalized supply structure of assets, in which case it could be considered deterritorialized (Dicken, 1992a); or (2) an attempt by firms to optimize access to factors of production in order to produce the inputs to their global supply structures (Reich, 1990), another form of deterritorialization, in the sense that regions and nations must simply make themselves attractive to mobile investments; or (3) also an attempt by firms to optimize access to territorialized factors of production (which meet the criteria of our definition). The point is that without a conceptual apparatus specific to the problem, the existing evidence can be made to reveal little about it. Note that the oft-cited rise in foreign direct investment, which is the vehicle of rising intra-industry and intrafirm trade, suffers from the same conceptual void (cf. Julius, 1990). It suggests a rise in activity by major world firms, and the development of a finely grained world division of labor, but little about the meaning of globalization-as-deterritorialization.

The global business hierarchy

Much attention has been devoted to the apparent rise of global business hierarchies, the organizations that manage global supply structures. From theorizing about the "multinational," "transnational," or even "multidomestic" firm in the 1960s and 1970s, concern has shifted to organizations that manage global production and investment systems in "real time," involving simultaneous manipulation and optimization of manufactured inputs, capital, information, and marketing (Ballance, 1987; Dicken, 1992a; Glickman and Woodward, 1989; Ohmae, 1990).

There was considerable optimism about the possibility of such organizations in the late 1970s and early 1980s. Ford Motor Company announced its intention to build a "world car"; General Motors (GM) invested tens of billions of dollars in telecommunications and other infrastructure intended to permit not only worldwide supply and market coordination, but also worldwide concurrent engineering (i.e., innovation and knowledge production). Some analysts label the outcome of such systems the global "hypermobility" of capital, as firms search for ever-better deals from presumably substitutable locations.

The importance of such an approach is the notion of a production system spread across the world, involving intrafirm trade in inputs, between locations lacking specificities (Fröbel, Heinrichs, and Kreye, 1980; Hymer, 1976). Were such a model to become dominant, we would expect intermediate products to account for a very high share of world trade; but this is not the case, as can be seen in Table 17.1. We would also expect international sourcing to be very important, and it is in some industries; the problem is that we cannot know whether such sourcing emanates from substitutable locations or territorialized locations. Further, we would expect that finished product trade, which is high in some industries, would be the result of such locationally substitutable sourcing in intermediates, and not the result of territorialized sourcing, knowledge production, and assets. The statistics shed no light on these issues.

Anecdotally, the results of attempts to build worldwide, locationally substitutable, sourcing systems have been mixed, in that the coordination of such an

Table 17.1: Pattern of globalization of the surveyed industries

Industries included in the survey	Trade				Direct investment				Cooperative agreements		
	Finished prods. (%sales)	Interm prods. (%sales)	Intl. sourcing (%tot.ste)	Intrafirm (%trade)	Flows (%gfcf)	AFFs sales (%gfcf)	M&As (%ops)	Equity parts (%ops)	Devel. purpose (%agrs)	Prod. purpose (%agrs)	Market purpose (%agrs)
Pharmaceuticals	10	8	10–30	70	50–70	40–50	52	48	38–68	13–29	19–41
Computers	26	14	20–60	50–80	30–40	50–60	43	57	50–70	15–28	17–32
Semiconductors	20	n.a.	10–40	70	15–25	20–25	39	61	n.a.	n.a.	n.a.
Motor vehicles	21	13	25–35	50–80	15–25	10–20	33	67	24–48	39–66	9–20
Consumer electronics	55	30	10–40	30–50	20–35	20–30	39	61	24–40	35–62	12–33
Nonferrous metals	21	21a	30–50	30	20–35	15–25	45	55	n.a.	n.a.	n.a.
Steel	27	35–45b	15–25	5–10	5–10	15–25	72	28	n.a.	n.a.	n.a.
Clothing	25–30	25–30c	10–40	5–10	15–20	5–15	n.a.	n.a.	(limited)	n.a.	n.a.

Note: Data from OECD, Industry Division compilation (1993). Elaborated from data sources used for the sector case studies. Please note that gfcf = gross fixed capital formation; ops = overseas partners; agrs = agreements; AFFs = all foreign firms; M&As = mergers and acquisitions; and tot.ste = total subcontracting and exports.
a Unwrought aluminum.
b Iron ore, coking coal, scrap.
c Textiles.

organization has proven to be much more problematic than was initially envisioned. Ford and GM have substantially cut back their earlier ambitions in favor of highly regionalized operations (Morales, 1994). Still, the management literature suggests that it is the ultimate ideal of many firms in both manufacturing and advanced services (Caves, 1982; Dicken, 1992a; Ohmae, 1990; Vernon and Spar, 1989). It would seem that the possibility is limited to a set of special cases, however: certain kinds of assembly and fabrication activities carried out at high scale, involving low levels of firm or industry-specific human and physical capital, and therefore highly substitutable locations for global sourcing. But these operations certainly do not add up to hypermobility-as-deterritorialization of contemporary capitalism as a whole. Indeed, they likely constitute a relatively modest share of the economic process today, by any measure (Carnoy, 1993).

The same is true for discussions of global business hierarchies in the generation of knowledge and technological innovation. It appears that many forms of innovation require investments so great that even the biggest firms, to earn a decent return, attempt to monopolize returns on global markets (Dunning and Norman, 1985; Krugman, 1990). Once such knowledge is developed, it often becomes a global state-of-the-art in product or process. It rests on temporarily non-rival and excludable firm-specific assets which firms use as the basis for earning temporary superprofits (Grossman and Helpman, 1991). The character of these assets encourages firms to internalize them. But does this mean deterritorialization? Not necessarily. The production of firm-specific assets might occur only via use of complementary territorialized resources, that is, the mobilization of territory-specific resources in the firm's core location that permit it to invade world markets by virtue of technological superiority; it could then be made firm-specific via intellectual property rights, and thereby serve as the basis of a global, monopolistic supply structure, deterritorialized from the areas that receive it (Dosi, Pavitt, and Soete, 1990; Patel and Pavitt, 1991). This interpretation is consistent with the fact that intrafirm trade accounts for a high proportion of foreign direct investment in high-technology industries (Table 17.1).

Things are not unambiguous even in these cases, however, for the very same set of risks pushes firms to enter into risk and cost-sharing strategic alliances with other major firms; some such alliances come about because firms want to tap into other firms' expertise in order to avoid the concomitant risk of technological lock-in (by making the wrong, very expensive, firm-specific asset choices) (Mytelka, 1992). Where does such expertise come from? Perhaps from those firms' deterritorialized, fully internalized capabilities, but just as likely from the territorial contexts in which they are inserted. Clearly, the deployment of advanced technology and knowledge, especially if it is firm-specific and where access is subject to significant legal or economic barriers to entry, means major developmental power in today's world, and the global business organization seeks such power of deployment. There are major effects on receiving economies. But the search for this power, again, says little about territorialization or deterritorialization of technology and knowledge generation in the world economy; and much more about corporate supply of such knowledge and technology once developed.

Indeed, in place of the model of the international firm as vertically integrated worldwide business hierarchy, much recent reflection about the organization of global business has turned on the notion of the firm as the central node in a variety of global linkages, ranging from ownership to alliance, and including cross-investment, technology and production partnerships, and research and development (R&D) collaborations (Mowery, 1988; Mytelka, 1992). This may well be a new kind of "nexus" business organization, whose impacts on economic development processes we have barely begun to glimpse; but such a model of the global firm does not so much imply deterritorialization of the economic process as a recasting of the role of territories in complex, intraorganizationally and interorganizationally linked global business flows.

Foreign direct investment

I have left the most obvious category of globalization for consideration until now because, as can be readily seen, it is a chaotic conception. Foreign direct investment is a catchall category that refers to the volume of international investment in subsidiary operations of firms. It leads to intra-industry, inter-industry and intrafirm trade, but, then again, it may reduce commodity trade when it leads to installation of locally serving final output capacity in major markets, so-called "regional" or "Triad" locational patterns. So foreign direct investment may be a vehicle for or substitute for trade. It may reflect firm strategies to control foreign markets via intrafirm trade, but then again it may reflect the need to tap into intermediate inputs produced by firms, through alliances and local trade. It may reflect global supply oligopolies in goods, intellectual property, or technology, but, then again, it may reflect needs to be in contact with territorially rooted foreign contexts of goods or technology development. The statistic reveals little about the territoriality of economic dynamics.

Another argument, which underlies much of the claim that the global economy is deterritorializing in favor of global business organizations, has to do with corporate power. It has been correctly observed that the biggest global firms are getting bigger: there is ongoing concentration of capital. It has also been remarked that there is a certain centralization of capital, in that the shares of the largest 100 or 500 corporations in global output are greater than they were 20 years ago. These large organizations, so it goes, are increasingly powerful across territorial boundaries. Their deployment of investments can shape markets, determine which technologies get developed, and, above all, exercise influence on national and regional governments (Harrison, 1994).

Power, in this sense, probably does have impacts on territorialization as we have defined it. But we need to examine precisely how. One of the paradoxes of globalization, in the sense of interpenetration of markets by companies from different nations, is that many market structures in many industries have actually become less concentrated over the past 30 years; there are more competitors in them than when such markets were composed of national or regional firms, though at a world level the first 10 or 20 companies control high proportions of output in many industries, especially technology-intensive ones. Global firms, while constituting a small club, especially in industries with very high barriers to entry, are therefore locked into competitive battle; they do not rule their world markets in any straightforward sense, as any major automobile, computer, clothing, or chemical company will readily attest.

Still, their power to shift vast quantities of capital, technology, or human capital across territorial borders, into different product markets, into R&D programs, is considerable. These firms can obviously shape the development of markets by shaping supply structures through their decisions. And they can bargain with territorially rooted states in so doing. But the image of nations and regions as Davids facing the global Goliaths cannot be straightforwardly assumed by the mere existence of global firms, for the latter are subject to all the complexities of territorialization described in preceding paragraphs.

The poverty of categories

The traditional categories in which the globalization debate has been framed – foreign direct investment, commodity trade, the global business hierarchy, the global supply structure of commodities, knowledge, and technology – seem instinctively to indicate the steady deterritorialization of economic power. But upon closer observation, these conceptual categories are inadequate to the job of shedding light on the question of territorialization and deterritorialization. It is, indeed, quite curious that a fundamentally geographical process labeled with a geographical term – "globalization"– is analyzed as a set of resource flows largely without considering their interactions with the territoriality of economic development.

Reframing the Question: Territories and Flows

In order to see what the terms territorialized and deterritorialized might mean with respect to the global economy, we can imagine two polar opposite cases, a fully deterritorialized "economy of flows and substitutions" and a fully territorialized "economy of interdependencies and specificities." In constructing these images, we will combine reasoning about organizations (firms), assets, markets, and places.

A pure flow-substitution economy

Imagine the extreme case of a fully realized global supply oligopoly. Resources would flow between parts of a firm, between places, without having any particular dependence on any particular place. Such assets – whether goods or information – would be producible in so many different places as to constitute a true (almost) perfect "market" in locations for their production. This sort of economy could be the result of two possible developmental processes. On one hand, activities that are well developed in a wide variety of places make necessary productive resources available in near ubiquity, but have historically been separated by transport barriers or differentiated tastes. Improvements in transportation, standardization of tastes, or increases in the possible scale of production open up this wide variety of locations to global business organizations, who then profit from a huge potential locational choice and ubiquitous markets, but they are bound by no locational specificities or local interdependencies. On the other hand, such organizations perfect production processes that eliminate the need for locationally scarce specific assets: technological change via product standardization and routinization of production processes does the job.

In both cases, a pure flow form of globalization becomes possible. It matters little whether the flows are via markets or hierarchies: global firms could purchase locally and sell through global commodity trade, for example. It matters little whether the flows concern intermediate or finished products. Those considerations, well analyzed through industrial organization theory, are simply different forms that the global flows of resources and optimization of factor use and capacity may take. The essential condition for a pure flow economy is that locations offer factors of production that could potentially be substituted by a large number of other locations.

This case of nonspecific, locationally substitutable, and perfectly elastic factor supplies is probably not found in pure form anywhere. But in some sectors, notably certain manufacturing industries and consumer services, these conditions are increasingly close to reality. Low-wage, low-skill, low sunk-cost manufacturing processes; certain highly standardized consumer durable manufacturing (where sunk costs are higher, but modular and widely available equipment is used); and certain consumer services where centralized production can be combined with local delivery come to mind.

One could imagine a pure market version of this globalization process, where numerous local economies, characterized by relatively small firms, competed with each other on global markets. Purchasers, armed with perfect information and highly developed and very flexible marketing networks, could switch from one locality's product to another almost instantaneously. Hierarchy is not necessary, then, to the flow economy's definition, in contrast to the image of oligopoly = globalization often implied in the literature. In reality, however, this ability to switch tends to be associated with scale in marketing and an ability to coordinate supplies from different, substitutable sources.

The potential political consequences of flow economies are what bother many of the critics of globalization (e.g., Harrison, 1994). Instead of seeing such flows as the means to resource optimization at a world scale, their point of departure is that economic progress has always depended on political economics, where everything ranging from the distribution of income between labor and capital to the correction of a wide variety of market failures is carried out by territorially rooted institutions such as nation-states. The advent of deterritorialized flow economies would seem to reduce the margin of maneuver of such nation-states dramatically, in favor of that of the private sector and thereby to open up a number of unfavorable consequences in both distributional and efficiency terms.

A pure territorial economy of interdependencies and specificities

A fully territorialized economic activity would satisfy conditions quite opposite to those just described. The essential condition of territorialization is that the activity be dependent on resources with specificities that are strongly territorialized and where the supply of these resources is subject to important inelasticities. The traditional case of scarce natural resources is a pure example but little relevant to most productive activity, where "resources" are mostly produced inputs such as labor and technology. We know that for many labor and technology inputs, there are no functional substitutes at any price, but even though such labor and technology are highly product-specific (heterogeneous is the accepted term), in many cases they are nonetheless widely available or easily produced, at rather different prices. In this case, territorialization is not in evidence. Where they are not widely available at any price, however, that is, where scarcities or inelasticities are in evidence, then not only localization but territorialization exist due to the geographically limited conditions of their production.

It is really with respect to special meanings of the term "labor" and "technology" that territorialization becomes most relevant in today's economy. Certain kinds of labor qualities are different from mere skills. There are many contexts where nonroutine judgments are made and where the success of the judgment depends on how a condition of uncertainty that involves other people is interpreted, or where noncodified traditions and ways of doing things are essential to the job. The former corresponds to demands for creativity or convention, the latter to learned custom. In all these cases, labor qualities are produced in what may be called a relation-specific fashion: they are produced and are exercised via insertion into a system of relations, whether it be interpersonal or bounded by specific, not-fully-codifiable rules of the game (Asanuma, 1989). These skills are not only specific in nature but subject to important supply inelasticities in the medium-run (Amin and Thrift, 1997).

Analogous observations may be made about technology, if what we mean by this is not merely hardware, but know-how, especially know-how that involves an outwardly moving and unknown scientific frontier (as in high technology) or an uncertain movement around such dynamics as product differentiation (for many low-technology or fashion-dependent industries and services). It is likely to involve asset specificities and supply inelasticities (Dosi et al., 1990).

This probably understates the extent of relation and place-specific assets in production. Many production systems turn on an intricate web of external interfirm transactions or internal, intrafirm transactions. In some cases, there are – at one moment or another – various sorts of standard economizing reasons for such transactions to be carried out across limited geographical distances: in these cases, territorialization is the result of necessary *relations of proximity* in the production system, which limit the number of sites at which production can be carried out. Over time, however, such cost barriers tend to be eroded due to transport improvements or to change in the nature of the transactions themselves, which lead to higher scale, greater certainty, and lower costs of covering distance.

But cost barriers are not the only reasons for the existence of relations of proximity in production systems. Many such relationships – buyer–supplier interfirm relations, or R&D–producer relations, or firm–labor market relations – come to be structured in ways that are highly specific to a given, initially geographically bounded, transactional context (usually regions or nation-states). Over time, they become more and more specific as unwritten rules of the game (conventions), formal institutions, and customary forms of knowledge are built up and become indispensable to admission to the producers' community and to efficient interpretation of how to reciprocate via transactions with other agents under conditions of uncertainty. In other words, regional or national production systems become nexuses of interdependencies between organizations and persons which involve relational asset specificities (Amin and Thrift, 1997; Storper, 1997; Storper and Salais, 1997;

Saxenian, 1994). These interdependencies must, of course, be efficient in some sense (e.g., a factor in cost minimization or innovation-improvement).

Territorialization is thus not equivalent to geographical proximity or agglomeration, although such agglomeration may be at some times cause and at others effect territorialization: it is an effect when scarcities and specificities of key resources such as labor and technology draw producers to a place, and when nonsubstitutabilities keep them there; it is a cause when the transactional structure of production draws producers into an agglomeration, and then key dimensions of the production system become relation-specific and key to its ongoing efficiencies.

There are very few industries where pure territorialization, in the sense of a unique possible efficient location for the totality of the industry's output, exists; in this case, there would be a localized global supply monopoly. But the condition of territorialization, in the sense of a few possible locations for significant parts of the industry's output, can be found quite frequently. Certain very high quality goods, those that involve technological innovation or ongoing rapid differentiation, or highly specialized services come to mind as examples. There are two very different versions of this territorialization. One concerns activities that serve such localized tastes that the localized supply structure corresponds to a unique localized demand structure. The more interesting case, of course, is that where the localized supply structure satisfies a national or global demand, and where there is therefore the possibility of entry by competitors in other places. This is likely to show up as a case of commodity trade exports, whether intra- or inter-industry. It is analytically indifferent to ownership (that is, the definition says nothing about whether ownership of territorialized assets must be local). In practice, most such cases of multinational corporations who have core activities in their home country and in a specific region of that country also have national ownership (Patel and Pavitt, 1991; Tyson, 1991), but counterexamples, such as Sony's ownership of Columbia Pictures, are reasonably abundant. Territorialization, therefore, cuts across the standard terms of the globalization debate, such as "who is us?"

The Dynamics of Globalization

What should be clear from the preceding is that global capitalism is being constructed through interactions between flow economies and territorial economies. Internationalization of capitalism has long been measured simply as a function of the increasing intensities of flows, but little was said about territories. Globalization is said to refer to something qualitatively different, in the sense of an economy or its subsystems that operate globally. That is, globalization should involve not merely international flows of resources, but economic systems that operate as international flow economies, as they have been defined here. If globalization is truly gaining on territorial economic organization, then we should find evidence not merely of increasing international flows of resources, but also of decreasing territorialization.

Some of the possible interactions are represented schematically in Figure 17.1. On the horizontal axis is the degree of territorialization of economic activities, and on the vertical axis the level of international flows associated with these activities. The first case (type 1) comprises those activities that are both highly territorialized

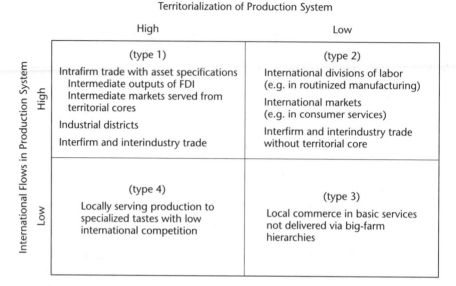

Figure 17.1 Territorialization and internationalization

and highly internationalized, territorially specific, nonsubstitutable assets are involved, but there are relationships that are not bound by such territorialization. Examples include the high-technology production system where the firm has certain important territorialized activities, but engages in intrafirm trade in intermediate inputs, and intrafirm trade for its worldwide marketing network. Intermediate inputs might be sourced for cost reasons alone (in which case this part of the system is effectively deterritorialized) or because the firm is tapping into territorial contexts of expertise elsewhere. Other examples are the now-famous industrial districts, where localized production systems serve world markets. Both interfirm and inter-industry trade, within complex social divisions of labor, can involve highly territo-rialized production for international commodity chains. Foreign direct investment is a means to carry out some of these processes as well.

The second cell (type 2) describes cases of low levels of territorialization and high levels of international flow, and includes territorially dispersed commodity chains where no nonsubstitutable locations are involved (where technological standardi-zation has reached a high level of development, generally) (Fröbel et al., 1980; Hymer, 1976). It also includes dispersed production systems oriented to interna-tional markets, as in many consumer services. Note that this category would lead to interfirm, intrafirm, and inter-industry trade, as well as foreign direct investment.

The third cell (type 3) consists of systems with low territorialization and low levels of international flow, that is, such things as local commerce in basic services that are not provided by far-flung big-firm hierarchies. In this cell we would find the industries of yore, which were localized due to transportation barriers but not truly territorialized; today we might find them there because of very low economies of scale, but less so due to transport barriers.

Finally, in the last cell (type 4), there are highly territorialized systems with few international connections. These are not simply localized due to insurmountable cost barriers to serving other areas from the local production system; they are territorialized because of nonsubstitutable local assets, as in the case of industries producing to specialized regional tastes.

The caricatural version of globalization is based on the notion that advanced capitalism has substituted type 2 production systems for type 3 production systems; and some of this has indeed come about with the progressive reduction of transport barriers, increase in scale of delivery of commodities and services, and changes in trading regimes. Many manufactured goods, including both durables and nondurables, that were formerly produced in isolated regional economies, were first converted to national production systems in the postwar period (most especially in Europe), and then to commodity chains that are now, at least in part, internationalized (Vernon and Spar, 1989).

An even more extreme set of cases is that of type 4 becoming type 2, that is, formerly territorialized and mostly closed production systems now becoming international commodity chains. This is in evidence because as more internationalized, middle-class ways of life and tastes sweep their way across many places, old place-specific tastes disappear and with them the economic reasons for local asset specificity. When needs are redefined, so is demand, which can then be served via other kinds of products, furnished by production systems with assets available at many different locations, and without territorial cores. Crucial to this set of events is *not* changes in transportation, nor even scale, but actual product substitutions – the culture of demand is the key causal mechanism.

Many sophisticated analyses also call attention to a transformation of production systems from type 1 to type 2: this is the movement from "internationalization" of production to its true "globalization." Now it can be seen that the real claim here is not simply that there are high levels of international flow, of whatever sort, involved in the operation of these systems; in and of themselves, they do not transform these production systems into deterritorialized flow economies. The claim is rather that substitutability of locations increases; and territorially specific assets decrease dramatically in their importance to competitive production (Dunning, 1992).

Two other important cases, however, seem to characterize the current era. The first is transformation of type 3 and 4 production systems not to type 2, but to type 1 systems. Formerly highly territorialized but not internationalized systems can become internationalized as they gain the ability to market their products around the world, without losing their locationally specific assets. This requires development of demand for their products beyond local or regional borders. This is precisely what appears to have happened in the cases of many European industrial districts in the postwar period: the product qualities once prized locally have become desired elsewhere, and the relationally specific assets that exist in producer regions now permit those regions to meet broader demands through downstream internationalization, but not through internationalization of production itself (Bianchi, 1993).

Perhaps even more important is the transformation of type 2 production systems into type 1 systems: from highly internationalized but not especially territorialized systems, to ones increasingly territorialized and internationalized. The mass production industries of the postwar period, for example, seemed at one point to be on the road to ever greater standardization and, with it, locational substitutability, but forces such as increased product differentiation, and newly revived product-based technological learning have given a new lease on life to locationally specific relational assets in production.

Indeed, the *principal* trend to which we can call attention today is that in many sectors, there is *simultaneous and ongoing development of the characteristics of both type 1 and type 2 systems*: the latter as ongoing standardization of tastes and techniques occurs, the former as technological learning, product differentiation, and the separating off of new branches of production, materials, and processes occur, all of which are causes of locational specificity, but also precisely outcomes of the interactive processes permitted by the locationally specific relational assets that underlie territorialization. This form of territorialization is qualitatively quite different from that of type 4 systems, in that it is not developed as the result of "tradition via isolation," but via what might be called the ongoing reinvention of relational assets in the context of high levels of geographical openness in trade and communications.

The formation of this *global context* of trade, investment, and communications and organized networks of human relations in production is perhaps the clearest dimension of globalization. The global economy is being constructed as an increasingly widely spread and accepted "grid" of these sorts of transactions, akin to a new global lingua franca of commerce, investment, and organization, based on historical and secular advances in transportation and communication technologies, and the development and diffusion of modern organizational "science," both of these in the context of the increasingly global political order of trade. But the paradox is that it is precisely this global grid or language that leads both to type 2 and to type 1 outcomes. In the former case, it breaks down barriers of taste, transport, and scale. In the latter case, it opens up markets to products based on superior forms of "local knowledge"; it consolidates markets and leads to such fantastic product differentiation possibilities that markets refragment and, with them, new specialized and localized divisions of labor reemerge; and it in some ways heats up the competitive process (albeit among giants), creating new premia on technological learning that require the same firms that become new global supply oligopolists to root themselves in locationally specific relational assets. The point is that globalization and territorialization are not just about the geography of flows and its technological or organizational determinants, but are in some cases dependent on the ways production systems and their products are changed by new patterns of competition unleashed by territorial integration.

To summarize, four principal territorial-organizational dynamics can be isolated from these complex, intersecting forces. In some cases, the opening up of interterritorial relations places previously existing locationally specific assets into a new position of global dominance. In a second set of cases, those assets are devalued via substitution by other products that now penetrate local markets; this is not a straightforward economic process, however; it is culturally intermediated. In a third set of cases, territorial integration permits the fabled attainment of massive economies of scale and organization, devalues locationally specific assets, and leads to deterritorialization and widespread market penetration. In a fourth set of cases, territorial integration is met by differentiation and destandardization of at least some crucial elements of the commodity chain, necessitating the reinvention of territory-specific relational assets.

Hierarchy, Regulation, and Competition: Institutional Dilemmas

State institutions exercise their authority over limited territories. But they do so in fields of forces – whether political or economic – that extend well beyond these borders. At least in matters of economic affairs, for much of the postwar period the economic authority of nation-states and the substantive power to back it up was considerable within the national territory. Globalization of economic processes seems to have weakened that substantive power, if not the formal authority. The global business organizations that control certain important international resource flows seem, in many cases, to be deterritorialized, and thus not directly dependent on processes that states, whether regional or national, can effectively regulate.

Yet, as we have seen, the mere existence of large-scale international flows does not lead directly to a conclusion that a productive activity is deterritorialized. Likewise, we can now see that the mere existence of territorialization does not mean that local or national states can exercise strong regulatory control over the economic development process (Carnoy, 1993; Dunning, 1992). Territorialization is a necessary, but not a sufficient, condition for a strong state role, because territorialization itself may involve hierarchies that are in turn inserted into larger contexts. We now want to sketch out some of the complex interactions between territorial economies and flow economies, and the ways they may mix hierarchical, market, and network forms of governance of production systems. Territorially based state institutions are now forced to confront these sorts of interactions in undertaking economic development strategies.

Figure 17.2 shows different ways of governing production systems, in the context of different levels of territorialization and international flows. Forms of governance where authority is largely internalized within large business organizations are labeled "hierarchies," while those that are carried out via high levels of external relations of large numbers of agents, where no single or small number of agents is dominant, are labeled "networks and markets." These represent two fundamentally different nexuses of decision-making power, centralized and decentralized.

It can be seen from the top half of the Figure 17.2 that for productive activities with high levels of international flow, there is evidence of both territorialization and deterritorialization: high levels of flow do not necessarily imply deterritorialization. Moreover, there is a great diversity of institutional arrangements that govern both the primary dynamic of the production system – that is, investment and technology or knowledge dynamics – and their international flows. For example, many global high technology firms manage extensive intrafirm supply chains, but at the same time are inserted into one or multiple territorialized production systems where network or market relations are dominant. Their power is more absolute with respect to their international flows than it is with respect to the other firms in their industry's territorial core. In certain other industries, global supply oligopolists are highly territorialized and interact locally via hierarchical relations, but then must compete on international markets with other such oligopolists, or they may enter

Territorialization of Production System

	High		Low	
	Hierarchies	Networks/Markets	Hierarchies	Networks/Markets
International Flows in Production System — Low — Networks/Markets	Intrafirm trade, where firm has territorial core	Territorial core systems (especially if high tech industries)	Global supply oligopolists with world division of labor (manufacturing and services)	Isolated captive suppliers to global oligopolists
Hierarchies	Global supply, oligopolists, strategic alliances	Industrial districts	Global supply oligopolists with few intermediaries	Isolated specialist suppliers or contractors
High — Networks/Markets	Local champion firm(s) with little internationalization		Global supply oligopolists via franchising and brand name strategies	
Hierarchies		Locally serving production to specialized tastes		Local commerce in basic services

Figure 17.2   Hierarchies, territories, and flows

into strategic alliances for marketing or for certain input supplies. The paradox is that while such oligopolists may exercise considerable power over those local suppliers and partners, to the extent that they depend on locationally specific relational assets, the state in those places may have considerable potential bargaining power with them.

Industrial districts are frequently characterized by strongly territorialized network relations in the core region, and by networked markets internationally: the institutional construction of international market networks is critical to them. We know from experience that states can play strong roles in supporting the competitiveness of such districts (Bianchi, 1993).

The classical image of globalization is, of course, the global supply oligopolist which has a low level of territorialization and a high degree of hierarchical control over its inputs and markets on a worldwide basis (Hymer, 1976). This can be found as a tendency in certain manufacturing industries and certain consumer service sectors. Isolated captive suppliers to these global oligopolists also have little territorialization and are subject to the strong hierarchy of these firms in their sales relations (semiconductor assemblers in Asia or clothing firms in developing countries are examples). Global supply oligopolists with few intermediate inputs and little territorialization are likely to have little intrafirm trade and foreign direct investment, and instead are likely to internationalize through global sales via markets (Dunning and Norman, 1985). Isolated specialized suppliers or contractors, on the other hand, will interact internationally via networks or markets, as they do with any local suppliers, the terms of their interactions being set by the degree and nature of substitutability of their products by the purchasing firm.

At the bottom half of Figure 17.2 may be found cases of low levels of international flows, and various combinations of both their territorialization and governance. Local champion firms, for example, who dominate a market, will tend to govern their territorialized production systems in a hierarchical way and have little internationalization, whereas other forms of localized production, for localized and specialized tastes, will probably correspond to the nonhierarchical system of traditional local firms. They may export some of their excess output, but this will likely be a small proportion of the total. Global supply oligopolists may not always have high levels of international flow oligopoly can be attained through control of intellectual and intangible assets, such as knowledge and brand names, but carried out through franchising; hence, low flows but hierarchically governed.

These are just a few of the many possible examples of complex configurations of institutions with respect to territoriality and flows in production systems. Small firms can enjoy relatively great market, network, or even hierarchical power, sometimes territorially and other times globally; while big firms can be subject to the forces of other big firms or markets they do not control, whether in their territorialized or their global interactions.

Policy problems

Many dilemmas of aligning the governance of production systems with efficient and desirable patterns of territorialization and flow present themselves in the contemporary world economy; these are problems faced not only by territorially bound state institutions, but also by the private sector.

The most obvious set of problems concerns the cases on the right-hand side of Figure 17.2. Where territorialization is low or declining, that is, where locational substitution becomes more and more possible, there is often a "race to the bottom" for territorially defined states, a competitive bidding war for economic activity that transfers increasing amounts of benefit from the public to the private sector. In the United States, this has been the history of postwar routinized manufacturing, encouraged not only by federalism but by the passage of the Taft–Hartley Act in the late 1940s, which enabled states to make a big institutional concession to employers by making unionization locally more difficult. More recently, such bidding has become a frenetic activity of states and localities. There is evidence that similar trends are developing within the European Union, and we can certainly see them on broader international scales within North America and Southeast Asia.

Moreover, this dynamic is no longer limited to manufacturing. Corporate head-quarters learned that they could demand concessions for remaining in New York, for example, in the 1970s, and since then have generalized these demands. Holly-wood film productions now expect to be wooed to locations in order to shoot films there. Corporations involved in relatively routine administration, such as in the consumer service or retailing sectors, now also regularly demand concessions or threaten to move.

The demands of firms are usually less naked when territorialization of activity is strongly in evidence, precisely because they have less locational substitutability, at least in the short run. Nonetheless, the fact that certain kinds of productive activ-ity are territorialized does not mean that they are wedded permanently to one single territory. Global companies do not just scan the globe for single locations; some interact with multiple territorial economies. To some extent, these territorial economies cannot be substituted by these firms, since the latter are inserted into them in order to tap into the technological or knowledge specificities of such terri-torial systems. The firm thus has a division of labor that involves multiple territo-ries, which are functionally specialized. For the moment global technology firms remain mostly attached to territorialized resources in their nations of origin (Dosi et al., 1990). But one could imagine that for inputs that are not on the cutting edge of technological knowledge, such firms could over time develop parallel territories, in the same way that mass production firms in the 1970s developed parallel assem-bly or fabrication plants. Developmental states in Southeast Asia, for example, have had some successes in helping their firms to build up territory-specific relational assets, and these assets are now enjoyed by firms from elsewhere. The paradox here is that states participate in a kind of *competitive* endogenous development, which creates new forms of capital mobility even in the territorialized parts of the con-temporary economy.

A second concern is that when major hierarchical global business organizations interact with different territorial economies, there may be little harmony between the rules by which such firms intend to relate to these environments and the rela-tional assets already built up in those places. Problems of this nature, however, only become apparent over time, and when they do, multinational firms may not have the commitment required to work them out. And they are problems that are not generally technical, but relational in nature and thus slow to resolve. We might think here of subcontracting policies established by such firms, which are designed to economize for them, but at the medium-term price of the region's subcontracting tissue as a whole (Dunning, 1992).

A third concern has to do with territorialized developmental spillovers. Territo-rial economies exist as such in part because there are knowledge or technology spillovers between activities, and the overall developmental trajectory of a territo-rial economy is strongly influenced by such spillovers. But firms whose primary loy-alties lie outside a particular territorial economy or firms with a highly elaborate interterritorial division of labor may inadvertently make decisions that undercut development of such spillovers, precisely by territorially dividing what might better (from the territory's and technology's standpoint) be kept in proximity. This is not a problem unique to "foreign" firms, but to all multilocational, multiterritorial firms.

A corollary is that when territorialized technological spillovers exist, there is an efficiency rationale for targeted technology policies, even from the standpoint of global output. Where such spillovers do not exist or are not territorialized, however, technology policies tend merely to transfer technological performance from one place to another, usually at a high overall cost (Grossman and Helpman, 1991). The problem is to construct such policies where the community of subjects of the policy is not only local but global; many firms operate in many different institutional and conventional contexts. Such policies therefore have to be "translated" for them, and these global business organizations must find ways to reconcile operations in very different contexts.

Chapter 18

Contesting Works Closures in Western Europe's Old Industrial Regions: Defending Place or Betraying Class?

Ray Hudson and David Sadler

In the 1950s and 1960s, major plant closures in northeast England in most "traditional" industries, but above all coal mining, were largely uncontested by those who were directly or indirectly affected by the accompanying loss of jobs (Hudson, 1986). By contrast, the late 1970s and early 1980s in the same area saw a series of campaigns to contest decisions concerning works closures or major employment losses. By no means all such decisions were challenged, but those that were concentrated in places where the region's "traditional" (and by then often nationalized) industries such as coal mining, iron and steel-making, shipbuilding, and heavy engineering were the major, even sole, source of industrial employment. These anti-closure campaigns were characteristically organized around the threatened works and the community (village or town) reliant upon it for employment and wage income. Furthermore, it was clear that such campaigns were by no means confined to this particular region, as similar ones developed or revived in other "old" industrial regions elsewhere in Great Britain (Scotland, Wales) and in continental Western Europe (Lorraine and the Nord in France, the Ruhr in West Germany, Wallonia in Belgium). In contrast to northeast England, where anti-closure campaigns tended to remain confined to the particular groups of workers, works, villages, or towns directly affected, in several of these other cases protests became generalized within an industry at regional – even national – level, and throughout particular regions across a wide spectrum of social groups. Several of these campaigns, then, were characterized by attachments to place and class becoming contingently conjoined in a variety of often-complex ways, so that these became complementary rather than competitive bases for social organization in defense of place. What was emerging was a series of territorially based campaigns, the aims of which may be summarized in a phrase borrowed from one of the campaign slogans in Longwy (France) in the late 1970s: to defend the right to "live, learn, and work" in particular places, though the ways in which these objectives were pursued and the degree to which they were successfully attained were highly varied. These campaigns were not simply evidence of a deeply felt, and to varying degrees collectively shared, attachment to place that was grounded in the spatially defined routine of everyday life, but also of the active involvement of working people, their families, friends, and neighbors in the restructuring of capital and the changing geography of industrial production as *their* particular places were deemed no longer to be (sufficiently) profitable locations in the context of an increasingly internationalized system of production and trade. How, then, is the emergence of such territorially based protests, at these particular times and in these particular places to be understood? Finding satisfactory answers to this theoretical question took on pressing practical significance as we became actively involved in some of these campaigns in northeast England and sought a better understanding of past practices with a view to informing existing struggles against further closures.

Some preliminary clues were provided by the historical geographic development of this particular set of traditional industries. Frequently they were (a) associated with "one-industry" towns so that the effects of major closure were heavily spatially concentrated (unlike, say, textiles, where aggregate job losses had been very extensive but spatially more diffused); (b) characterized by either public ownership or a high degree of state involvement at national and/or supranational European Community level, so that closure decisions were often transparently "political," while (c) in contrast to the 1960s, by the late 1970s the promises of "alternative jobs" via reindustrialization programs had worn distinctly thin. These provided no more than some general indications, however, and certainly offered no explanation of the rise and variety of territorially based campaigns in defense of place.

Much of the existing literature dealing with attachment to place and capitalism's uneven development provided at best partial insights. For example, much of the debate on nationalism and attachment to the "imagined communities" (Anderson, 1983) of national states is of limited relevance, focusing on issues (such as linguistic distinctiveness) that were of little importance for the defense of particular villages or towns against catastrophic industrial decline. This conclusion holds *a fortiori* for those analyses which pose the issue in terms of territory (nation) versus class (for example, Hobsbawm, 1977), for the precise characteristic of several of the campaigns considered here was their fusion of place and class (at least for a while). While the writings of humanistic geographers (such as Tuan, 1977) on attachment to place and related issues focus more on the spatial scales of village or town, they tend only to describe individuals' experience of place. They do not relate this to the context and structures of the societies in which such people live; to their membership of social groups and classes through which they learn shared meanings, including those relating to the places in which they live and with which they identify. Conversely, the varied contributions within the Marxist tradition on the spatial uneven development of capitalism address themselves to the causally determining powers of unobservable structures (for example, Sayer, 1982b), but tend to neglect the role of people as rational agents affecting change within the limits that these structures impose and reproducing them via their actions. The more sophisticated of these analyses (for example, Harvey, 1982) halt at the point of specifying the structural boundaries to a capitalist society and possible tendencies toward spatial uneven development within them. The cruder versions of such analyses (for example, Carney, 1980) go so far as rather mechanistically to deduce forms of political organization in defense of place from the inner logic of the capitalist mode of production explicitly rather than implicitly reducing people to their ascribed roles of bearers of structures, to the status of "cultural dupes" (Giddens, 1981, pp. 71–2).

A more sophisticated theoretical approach is required in order to begin to grasp the bases for, and character and political potential of, the various campaigns in defense of the right to "live, learn, and work" in particular places. This sophisticated approach is required in order to comprehend more satisfactorily the links between people's knowledge of and feelings about space, their patterns of behavior and social practices, and the spatially uneven development of capitalist societies, and so reveal rather more about the processes of uneven development themselves. This approach views people as active, conscious agents, who are rational in that what they do makes sense to them in terms of their own understanding of their individual and collective interests, while recognizing that the way in which they perceive these interests, and the possibilities that at any time are objectively open to them, will be conditioned by (though not determined by) those deep structural forces that shape the societies in which they live. Seeking to integrate the way in which places and the spatial patterning of (capitalist) societies come to have socially endowed meanings for people presupposes the creation of some significant theoretical space for conscious and meaningful human behavior in the reproduction of uneven development. In so far as it creates this theoretical space it also potentially creates political space within which people can begin to change the societies within which they live.

The Reproduction of Societies as Capitalist

Agency, structure

While in many respects provocative to certain strands of both bourgeois and Marxist thought, Giddens' "theory of structuration" (1981) forms a useful starting point for discussion and is one which accepts the kernel of Marx's arguments about the essential character of capitalist societies. A recognition of the decisive importance of the class structural relation between capital and labor does not imply that the actual development of capitalist societies revolves only around this axis, however. In brief, we must not only recognize the fundamental contradictory relation between capital and labor. We must also recognize the existence of competition between capitals in search of surplus profits. Further, we must acknowledge competition between groups within the (structurally defined) working class, for example on the basis of differences in sector, industry, or occupation.

We must also take account of the possibility of conflict between capital(s) and/or groups within the working class and social groups either located outside of capitalist social relations or located within them, but organized on issues and dimensions other than those of production: gender, race, or an ecological concern for the natural environment, for example. Although the proximate basis of social organization may not be a class issue (in the sense of directly deriving from capital–labor relations of production), it has nevertheless been argued that the capacity of such groups to realize their aims is conditional upon their class location (Wright, 1978). What this suggests is that the relationships between social practice and the reproduction of the class structural relation between capital and labor are complicated and contingent ones.

Central to Giddens' analysis of the links between agency and structure are two related notions: the distinction between system and structure and the duality of structure. He summarizes these points as follows (1981, pp. 26–7):

A distinction is made between *structure* and *system*. Social systems are composed of patterns of relationships between actors or collectivities reproduced across time and space. Social systems are hence constituted of *situated practices*. Structures exist in time-space only as moments recursively involved in the production and reproduction of social systems. Structures have only a "virtual" existence. A fundamental postulate of the theory of structuration is the notion of *duality of structure*, which refers to the essentially recursive nature of social practices. Structure is both the medium and outcome of the practices which constitute social systems. The concept of duality of structure connects the *production* of social interaction, as always and everywhere a contingent accomplishment of knowledgeable social actors, to the *reproduction* of social systems across time-space. (emphases in original)

In this way, Giddens stresses the relations between temporally and spatially situated social interaction and societal reproduction, and emphasizes that the actions of individual agents, pursuing their individually or collectively defined interests, are at once shaped by and reproduce the "basic principles of organization" of societies, above all in capitalist societies that of the fundamental class relationship between capital and labor; and that they do this as a routine, taken-for-granted element in their behavior as rational agents. Whether we are conscious of them or not, and contrary to appearances, structural relationships are not immutably given to us in a manner that renders them unchangeable (or changeable only over time, when the continuing development of the forces of production within the social relations of capitalism attains a critical pitch, after which capitalism somehow mysteriously changes itself into something new and better). The point is that structural relations are routinely socially produced and reproduced in the course of everyday life. This being so, a central task of a critical social theory is to uncover that which is unquestioningly taken for granted, discursively to reveal the real basis of "*practical consciousness* . . . 'knowing how to go on' in a whole diversity of contexts of social life" (Giddens, 1981, p. 27; emphasis in original). For it is in the unquestioning, perhaps even unconscious, acceptance of the legitimacy of the rules governing everyday life that the structural reproduction of capitalist societies is grounded. Of particular importance is the routine acceptance of the legitimacy of wage labor and of going to work in a particular place as a normal feature of such societies, for in this is grounded the reproduction of the class structural capital-labor.

Another important point in Giddens' analysis of the relationships between agency and structure for our purposes is that, while social agents act in a rational manner, it is vital to acknowledge that as a matter of routine they engage in social interaction in circumstances that in part are unknown to them and that, partly because of this, their actions can have outcomes in addition to or other than those that they intended. Furthermore, in pointing out that "the knowledgeability of actors is always *bounded*, by *unacknowledged conditions* and *unintended consequences* of action" (Giddens, 1981, p. 28), Giddens' conclusions highlight the chronic gap between the intentions and outcomes of the policies of capitalist states.

Place, class

Capitalist societies are simultaneously riven with conflict and dissension on several planes. Yet as societies they do hold together with sufficient cohesion and in such ways that capitalist social relations *are* reproduced; precisely how and on what bases such social class groupings form, how the balance of class and other social forces fluctuates, and how capitalist societies are contingently reproduced can only be resolved via theoretically informed empirical investigations. Nevertheless, it is clear that capitalist states, which in practice largely means capitalist national states, play a decisive role in mediating between the claims of competing classes and interest groups (see Jessop, 1982).

Virtually from the outset, capitalist societies have been constituted in the form of competitive *national* states (Anderson, 1983). From the genesis of the capitalist mode of production, there has been a territorial element in the definition of actual class interests. More generally, an important dimension to the historical processes of social class formation in capitalist societies, to divisions between and within the (structurally defined) classes of capital and labor, is the influence of place. This may form a basis for the formation of groups which specify their unifying interests in terms of shared location, either within or cutting across structurally defined class boundaries. Thus space, place, and the organization of social groups, united by a concern with or attachment to a particular locality (be it a factory, neighborhood, or national state), can and in practice persistently and almost without exception do play a key role in the historical processes of social class formation and organization.

Differentiation on the basis of location in space thereby ceases to be something to be appended following the completion of a class analysis, and comes to be regarded as a potentially decisive element in the identification of class interests. It is the recognition of the potentially central role of territorial attachments in actual class formation in Giddens' work that makes it of interest here. While stressing the necessity to ground analysis of capitalist societies in their time-space constitution, Giddens does not focus upon the relationships between spatial uneven development within (as opposed to between) national states, attachment to localities, and the processes of capital accumulation in the way that we seek to do here, however. Location in space must cease to be one way of differentiating between groups within a class once the latter has been formed; rather, the point of departure is a recognition that class interests, organizations, and practices actually (and usually) within capitalism are formulated at least in part with respect to particular localities. This is especially so at a time when capitals' strategies for internationalizing production are accelerating so that the options available to them in fragmenting opposition by playing off workers in an increasing number of areas are growing rapidly.

From this perspective, an important dimension of differentiation (and so a possible basis for competition) between capital and labor, between capitals, or between groups of wage laborers and those linked to them, is location in and attachment to place. Similarly, identification with national territories or supra or subnational territorial units can form the basis or bases for a cross-class identification of interests. It is important to acknowledge, however, that the mechanisms involved in the development of attachment to and identification with territorial units will vary with scale and that even if these all constitute "imagined communities" what is crucial is "the style in which they are imagined" (Anderson, 1983, p. 15).

The way in which such communities are "imagined" is grounded in the daily routine of life in those places, perhaps most vividly in single industry towns (for example, Williamson, 1982; Douglass and Krieger, 1983). It is perhaps not surprising, therefore, that territorially defined competition within the (structurally defined) class of labor can be particularly acute. What is surprising is that much Marxist writing upon issues such as the uneven development of capitalism, while accepting a differentiated view of capital as many competitive capitals, tends to cling (even if only implicitly) to a utopian view of a working class as unified across territorial boundaries by a recognition of its real class interests. While at a deep structural level, this unity of class interests undoubtedly does exist within and across capitalist societies, the real point at issue is to explain why it is not seen in these terms by the relevant agents who perceive their interests in different ways, which then become the basis for particular forms of social organization and practice that become a central element in the uneven development of capitalism.

Defending Places: The Strategies of Capital, Labor, and the State

The necessity for an appropriate theoretical specification of the links between agency, structure, and attachment to place and class is sharply revealed when capitals restructure their activities so as to combat their own crises or to further their own self-expansion. For as Harvey (1982, especially pp. 425–31) has put it, devalorization is and must be place-specific. The validity of this proposition has been sharply brought home to groups of workers throughout the history of capitalism, but it has been particularly accentuated since the transition from a long-period phase of expansion to one of recession in the capitalist world economy in the last decade or so (for example, Mandel, 1980; Frank, 1980). It is this transition, and with it the growing recognition that the option of reindustrialization via state regional policies, which could be presented as having some credibility in the 1960s but is widely seen as having no possibility of success in the "old" industrial regions in the 1980s, that has been important in triggering anti-closure campaigns. Seen from the point of view of workers, their families and dependents in such places, the only feasible solution often appears to be to fight to preserve *their* factory, *their* mine, for their community or region, in the sure knowledge that should their struggle be an unsuccessful one then the jobs lost will not be replaced, while the price of success will be the closure of some other factory or mine, a threat to some other group of workers and *their* community, *their* place. Accepting the competitive ethic of capitalism in this way as a legitimate terrain, and fighting on a territorially defined basis within it, rather than posing broader questions as to why restructuring is regarded as either necessary or justified given its extensive social costs, has the precise (albeit unintended) effect of reproducing the basic structural relations of capitalism. Groups of workers consequently compete with one another, sometimes on the basis of cross-class territorial alliances, for the privilege of being able successfully to sell their labor-power in the marketplace and their places on the place market (Robinson and Sadler, 1985). Put another way, a concern with more general class solidarity, even if this is recognized, is subordinated to a more immediate concern with living and working in a localized, spatially delimited community, in a particular place.

The place-specific campaigns to contest steel closures in the European Community (EC) in recent years illustrate the variety of ways in which this defense of place has been contested, in the course of which identification with place and class have been contingently combined in different times and places, and in which capitals and states have sought to secure their interests in closing steel capacity and restructuring production (Hudson and Sadler, 1983a, 1983b; Morgan, 1983). For in relation to changes in the global pattern of accumulation and the international division of labor in bulk steel production, Western European steel producers have attempted to restore competitiveness and profits, or at least stem hemorrhaging losses, by closing capacity and/or drastically cutting employment in localities which, because of the historical development of the steel industry, depended very heavily upon steel production as a source of wages and employment. The high level of state involvement in the EC – both at the level of national states and the embryonic supranational EC itself – has meant that the locationally concentrated collapse of employment has frequently been perceived, correctly, as a transparently "political" decision rather than simply as the outcome of the logic of "economic" processes and the forces of the market. This deep attachment to such places, built up through generations living, learning, and working in them, was largely taken for granted until such times as the threat of major employment loss with the prospect of no comparable replacement became apparent. For this (and other) reasons such job losses have generally been contested in a variety of ways. These protests have themselves become an active moment in the restructuring process, in shaping *which* steelworks will close as steelworkers have been divided, or more accurately, have divided themselves, on a plant or regional or national basis to fight for the survival of their works at the expense of others.

A particularly stark example of this process was the unsuccessful campaign mounted in 1979 and 1980 to save Consett steelworks in northeast England. This was confined solely to the town of Consett itself and saw steelworkers there isolated both from a wider basis of support within the region and from other steelworks in the northeast and elsewhere, as the "Save Consett" campaign was contested solely on the grounds that it was a profitable steelworks, that its closure was "a grave commercial error" (J. Carney, cited in Hudson and Sadler, 1983a) and, by implication, that it should remain open and some other steelworks within the British Steel Corporation (BSC) should close. At no stage in the campaign was the decisive reason for its proposed closure, BSC's plans to cut overall capacity, and their relation to the political strategies of the UK central government raised or contested. Moreover, even in those cases where there was initially a more marked degree of unity between steelworkers at national level, as in France in the late 1970s where protests against plant closures in Lorraine and the Nord were supported by national strike action, this subsequently crumbled to leave individual plants at best fighting in isolation, at worst competing with one another for survival. In this case, the policies of the French state in terms of differential redundancy payments, differential allocations of resources supposedly to attract new industries and alternative employment in areas affected by steel closures, and so on played an important role in fragmenting steelworkers on a plant and regional basis (see Hudson and Sadler, 1983b). In general, the ways in which steelworkers in these localities identified their interests as place specific and organized to protect them ultimately involved setting themselves in competition with other groups of steelworkers in an attempt to secure some employment. The particular ways in which these campaigns evolved cannot be divorced from the history of trades union organization in the steel industry in France and the UK, with the latter case in particular being characterized by strong tendencies to inter-plant competition and regional chauvinism. Nevertheless, despite the rather specific combination of contemporary and historical circumstances surrounding the steel industry in these two nations in the late 1970s, it would be extremely misleading to leave the impression that territorially based competition between groups of workers is an atypical form of contesting proposed plant closures. Quite the reverse, in fact; it has become increasingly the norm as plant competes with plant, increasingly across not just regional but national boundaries and within a particular transnational corporation.

Furthermore, as the recent history of the steel industry within the EC makes clear, competition between groups of workers in different localities is by no means the only approach to contesting closures. For such closure proposals can also come to form the basis of territorially based alliances, formed for the specific purpose of opposing closures, embracing a broader spectrum of social groups and interests and cutting across (structurally defined) class boundaries. Such alliances can be constructed, for example, because locally based and tied small capitals in retailing and various private service sector activities become aware of the threat to their existence as capitals in those particular places, one that is posed by the imminent precipitous decline of purchasing power that accompanies mass job loss. Once formed, their subsequent development or dissolution becomes integrally involved in the competitive struggles to preserve particular plants as the defense of place, of common territorially defined interests, transcends, at least for a time, (structurally defined) antagonistic class relations. Three examples will be given of this.

The first concerns opposition to steel closures in Lorraine, in France. Partly reflecting a strong sense of regional identity of being Lorrainese, a result of the region's history of being alternately transferred between France and Germany, the regionally based bourgeoisie recognized the threat to their interests posed by steel closures and began to organize against them before the steelworkers and unions did. An organization, the *Avenir du Pays Haut* (APH), was formed with the specific intention of protecting the Lorrainese economy. It played an important role in broadening the social basis of protests against steel closures, at least until February 1979, after which time the onset of violent protests by autonomous groups of steelworkers operating outside the structure and authority of the steel unions challenged the legitimacy of the French state's monopoly of the means of violence. From this point, the APH increasingly distanced itself from the anti-closure protests (Hudson and Sadler, 1983b).

The second example relates to the defense of Ravenscraig steelworks in Scotland. Speculation as to the future of the works grew in the autumn of 1982, against a background of debate about whether BSC could continue to operate its five major integrated production complexes. A broadly based campaign to oppose the threat of closure rapidly developed, embracing not only steelworkers but also groups of workers from other industries in other parts of Scotland. Moreover, drawing on a history of nationalist sentiment in Scotland and an attachment to Scotland as a place with shared, socially endowed meanings that cut across class and other social divisions (for example, Smith and Brown, 1983), the campaign developed to involve a much broader spectrum of class interests and to encompass a wide social basis within Scotland. One important element in it was a powerful cross-party Scottish parliamentary lobby, presented with ammunition by a report of the Parliamentary Committee for Scottish Affairs on the significance of the Ravenscraig plant to the Scottish economy. Such was the breadth and strength of the campaign to preserve Ravenscraig that, despite the fact that it was costing BSC £100 million per annum to keep Ravenscraig open, its future was guaranteed as a steel-making plant until 1985. Even if this turns out to be only temporary, what the success of the 1982–3 campaign demonstrates is that, in certain conditions, territorially based alliances can force a recognition of the fact that, ultimately, closure decisions are political rather than merely narrowly economic (see Sadler, 1984).

The third example is more complicated, also involving individual plant, regionalist, and nationalist dimensions. It relates to Hoesch's decision to end steel-making at Dortmund, in the eastern part of the Ruhr in West Germany. The course of this (unsuccessful) campaign was strongly conditioned by the merger in the 1960s of Hoesch with the Dutch steel company, Hooghoven, and the subsequent breakup of the union of the two companies in the early 1980s. Fears about the ending of steel-making in Dortmund in 1980 led to the formation of a broad cross-class alliance, the *Burgerinitiative Stahlwerk*, in an attempt to guarantee the continuation of steel production in Dortmund rather than its further concentration at Hooghoven's coastal Ijmuidenworks, with Dortmund reduced simply to a steel rolling plant. The broad social base of the protest movement soon dissipated in 1981, however, partly because it had led to the focus of attention being switched to the provision of alternative employment rather than the preservation of steel-making, with the movement to contest the closure proposals becoming much more centered on the Dortmund works and steelworkers. The separation of Hoesch and Hooghoven led to both a revival and a redirection of protest, amid an atmosphere of considerable uncertainty about the proposed restructuring of steel production in West Germany involving the major steel groups (Krupp and Thyssen). Having got rid of the Dutch connection, the way was open to the Dortmund branch of the IG Metall Union to propose, in December 1982, a complete nationalization of West Germany's steel industry as a means of securing Dortmund's future. (Even though the union at national level was opposed to nationalization, a compromise between local and national levels was agreed whereby proposed government financial aid would take the form of it acquiring share capital in the steel companies.) Thus the definition of place altered as the campaign evolved, changing from one that began as a regionally based cross-class protest movement to one with a narrower basis centered on steelworkers in Dortmund itself, and eventually ending up by proposing a national solution as the route to preserving steel-making at Dortmund and, by implication, unity of interests between steelworkers in different plants in West Germany.

There is, then, considerable evidence simply from this review of campaigns against steel closures in the EC of groups within the (structurally defined) working class becoming involved in territorially based cross-class alliances in attempts to pursue what they perceive to be their interests. In fact, there is much more evidence which suggests that historically this process of the formation of such territorially based groupings trying to further the interests of their place has become a persistent one within capitalist societies, a central feature of the reproduction of spatial uneven development within and between them that is deeply embedded in the social practices that are central to their reproduction. Thus groups within the working class become actively involved in the forging of territorially defined alliances, at a variety of spatial scales, unified by their organization around or mediated in a variety of ways through capitalist states. Three examples, at differing spatial scales, will suffice to illustrate the point. At national scale, the formation of cross-class agreements around proposals to nationalize particular branches of industry hinges on a perception of shared interests by some capitals, some elements of labor and the state: for example, in the UK case, the nationalizations of coal, railways, and steel were all seen as satisfying these varying (and ultimately contradicting) interests (Hudson, 1986). It is significant that subsequent decisions to close plants in such nationalized industries have been among the most strongly contested. At a regional scale, the formation of cross-class alliances around a shared perception of the need to modernize old industrial regions by public sector investment programs to build new industrial estates, factories, roads, commercial centers, houses, and so on, providing both fresh opportunities for capitals to reap profits and new employment and better living conditions for some members of the working class, became a recurrent feature of contemporary capitalism, especially in the 1960s. It was a crucial reason why works closures then were generally not contested in the way that they were in the late 1970s and early 1980s. For example, such agreements are discernible in Scotland, Wales, and the peripheral regions of England from the late 1950s (for example, Hudson, 1986) and more generally in Western Europe (Hudson and Lewis, 1982) and the USA (Clavel, 1982), though their roots are often traceable to the interwar years (Carney and Hudson, 1978).

At the same time, in so far as such policies are tied to intraregional settlement policies, as is commonly the case, concentrating new public sector investment in terms of general conditions of production and collective consumption within regions (into selected "growth points," "growth zones," etc.), then their effect is to encourage intraregional divisions on a territorial basis. This arises both because of competition to achieve growth-center designation and because of the divisions engendered between those localities which achieve this and those which do not. Thus the promulgation and implementation of state policies, the formally proclaimed aims of which are to reduce interregional inequalities in employment opportunities and living conditions, presuppose increasing intraregional fragmentation as alliances of interests tied to particular localities form to promote the interests of their particular place. Perhaps the most extreme example of such intraregional growth point policies is that of the UK New Towns. New Town developments in the UK involve the establishment of non-elected development corporations, with a considerable degree of autonomy, cutting across the networks of local political power and control exercised via democratically elected local authorities. In some circumstances, this itself can become a focus for uniting opposition to them within areas (for example, see Robinson, 1983); in others it has served more or less to unite local authorities and local political opinion around coalitions to strive for a New Town in or near their area so as to secure new jobs, better living conditions, and so on.

The final example, to a degree already presaged in the inter and intraregional competition outlined above, refers to the UK in the 1970s. Central government's macroeconomic policies have increasingly been to rely on the market as a steering mechanism, and cut back the scope of regional and urban policy initiatives as part of a more general drive to cut public expenditure and roll back the boundaries of the state itself. As this occurs, cross-class alliances have increasingly formed around the structures of local government (metropolitan, county, and district councils) in defense of the local economy (see Cochrane, 1983). One particularly revealing symptom of competition for jobs between local areas has been the intense lobbying to achieve Enterprise Zone status and so, supposedly, a competitive edge over one's rival areas. Furthermore, as *ad hoc* employment creation agencies such as British Steel (Industry) have proliferated as part of a cosmetic response by national states to place-specific industrial decline, a similar pattern of competition has been set in motion as places strive for the attention of these new organizations.

In summary, then, the "normal" pattern of social organization within capitalist societies is one that chronically involves competition between territorially defined groups attempting to promote the interests of "their place." It is *not* the case that territory replaces class as a basis of social organization and practice but rather that identification with and attachment to place itself becomes integrally involved in the process of class formation. Place and class become contingently related in a complex manner as bases for social organization and thus pivotally involved in the reproduction of spatial uneven development within capitalist societies. Thus the defense of place becomes central to the reproduction of those societies *as* capitalist as an unintended consequence of campaigns to defend or promote the interests of specific places (whether village, town, region, or national state) in competition with other places.

Routinization, Deroutinization, and the Reproduction of Capitalist Societies

A central element in Giddens' theory of structuration is that of the routine, taken-for-granted character of much social interaction within capitalist societies. In this sense, they are routinely, though contingently, reproduced (Giddens, 1981). What is central to the reproduction of capitalist societies as capitalist, then, is the normal routine of "going to work," presupposing as it usually (though by no means always) does the separation of home and workplace in time-space. Put slightly differently, what is central is the normative acceptance by people working for a wage within them of their class position as wage labor (of whatever level of qualification), thereby simultaneously accepting, affirming, and reproducing the decisive central axis of the contradictory structural relationship between capital and labor.

A corollary of this, however, is that when such people become unemployed – when what has been accepted as the normal routine becomes "deroutinized" – then this *might* lead them to question the legitimacy of their class position, particularly given the close links within capitalist societies between being able to earn a wage, and lifestyle and living conditions. The effects of such deroutinization are obviously severe at the individual level, but when they affect comparatively few individuals in a period of full employment it is usually possible for bourgeois accounts to prevail, generally pointing the finger at individual failings or weakness as the cause of unemployment. Where such deroutinization creates mass unemployment in whole localities, with thousands of people losing their jobs as a result of a single and necessarily place-specific devalorization decision by a capital or a national state, then one might reasonably anticipate a challenge to such accounts and a rather different reaction from those adversely affected. Such collectively experienced and simultaneously imposed deroutinization might lead those made redundant to raise questions about the legitimacy of their class position which left them vulnerable, exposed to bearing the costs of decisions over which they could exercise no effective control; or if not to raise this question, then at least to fight for the right to work, albeit as wage labor. Furthermore, one might expect the strength of protests against such imposed deroutinization to be strongest in those communities that substantially depend upon one industry (such as coal or steel) as their source of employment for wage labor, *a fortiori* when the relevant industries are nationalized, formally subject to a logic of politics rather than of the market, so that the normal separation of the economic and political spheres in capitalist societies is broken and these are *seen* to be reconnected.

Giddens (1981) has pointed out that we can learn a good deal about day-to-day life in routine settings from analyzing circumstances in which it is radically disturbed. His point is neatly illustrated by the various examples referred to above of how threats to the everyday lives of members of the working class have frequently been contested, though not necessarily in ways that have raised questions as to the legitimacy of their class position. Rather than question the legitimacy of the class structural relation between capital and labor, and in particular the class position of working people as wage laborers, the struggles by territorially defined groups of workers to fight for *their* jobs transform the contest into one between such groups for a share of those jobs that are offered on the labor market. So, for example, there is conflict between different groups of workers within a factory or mine over differential levels of redundancy payments and therefore over whether to accept or contest proposals for closure. Or there is conflict between plants in different places (regions within a nation-state or different nation-states) for such wage labor employment as capital offers on the market. Furthermore, in particular circumstances this competition for jobs can develop on a broader social basis, from simply the groups of workers directly affected into one based on cross-class alliances. While in general we would accept Giddens' critique of functionalist social theories which presuppose a normative consensus among social agents, in so far as members of the working class fight in various ways to preserve their status as wage labor there is little evidence to support his claim that "those in subordinate positions in a society, particularly those in large-scale societies, may frequently be much less closely caught within the embrace of consensual ideologies than many writers . . . assume" (1981, p. 67). Whether their position as wage labor is willingly accepted is another matter, but in so far as it is accepted, it is central to the reproduction of capitalist societies as capitalist.

Moreover, this territorially defined struggle for employment between groups of workers (and maybe their allies) in particular localities often takes on an additional dimension. Characteristically it can encompass competition for a greater share of state resources for the acquisition of new jobs as well as the defense of "old" ones. Indeed, this has become a persistent feature of contemporary capitalist societies and integrally involves capitalist states in a variety of ways: one diagnostic symptom is the identification of a variety of spatially defined problems (for example, inner city or regional problems, or problems of national economic or industrial development) as various groups press their case for special treatment for their areas. Thus the variety of state spatial policies is to be interpreted not simply in terms of some mechanistic response to the need(s) of capital(s), or as symptomatic of a bad case of false consciousness on the part of members of the (structurally defined) working class, but rather as something fought for by the labor movement, by groups within the working class in such areas, as they rationally engage in forms of social practice intended to further their own interests. Moreover, this is not simply a struggle conducted by such groups within the state as an immutable object, but rather an attempt by them to redefine what are seen as the justified boundaries to the activities of the state in such a way as to protect or further their (territorially specified) interests. It is correct, however, to point out that these spatial policies tend to take their most potent form within capitalist societies when the perception of working-class groups of *their* interests is coincident with the perception of some capitals or the relevant national state of *their* interests. The regional modernization programs in the 1960s in parts of the UK (the northeast of England, Scotland, and Wales, for example), together with what is generally regarded as the strengthening of regional policy by the Labour central government in the UK in the same period and its subsequent dismantling after 1979 by the Conservative government, exemplify this point well.

Nevertheless, the actual outcome of these heightened processes of state involvement has been to reinforce tendencies toward competition for "new" jobs between territorially defined groups within the working class and their party political representatives, sometimes in the context of cross-class alliances. More and more, this competition has been intensified and conducted within the corporate structures of transnational capitals on an increasingly global market for labor power and production sites as part of a new and evolving international division of labor. Increasingly, localities must engage in a bitter and divisive struggle to sell themselves to capitals as the most desirable location for their activities in an attempt to defend the right to live, learn, and work in their place.

Some Concluding Comments

Deep attachments to place in Western Europe's "old" industrial regions (and elsewhere) are grounded in the routine of everyday life there. The emergence from the late 1970s onward of campaigns to defend the right to live, learn, and work in them reflects their heavy reliance on a single industry as a source of jobs and wages, coupled with a perception of the minimal opportunities for the introduction of new sources of employment should the "traditional" industries disappear. Characteristically, these campaigns have conjoined attachment to place and class in complex and shifting ways, and have been conducted on the basis of attempts to promote the interests of one ("our") place at the expense of other ("their") places. Nevertheless, it is important to remember that these sorts of contingent class–place relations as a basis for the defense of the place-defined interests of particular social groups are clearly ones that are associated with the legacy of a territorial division of labor associated with much earlier rounds of capitalist accumulation. It is precisely this material basis for the cultural tradition associated with successive generations living, learning, and working in the one-industry places, thrown up by the historical geography of capitalist development in old industrial regions, that has been and is being removed by the changing intranational and international divisions of labor and the hyper-mobile switching of investment between locations which to their inhabitants are deeply meaningful places but to capitals are merely another piece of space offering possibilities for profitable production.

The net unintended result to date of these various forms of competition to defend particular places between territorially defined groups is doubly to reinforce the hegemonic position of capital as the dominant and decisive social relation. Not only is wage labor legitimated by working-class people competing for the chance to be able to sell their labor power, but to be without the possibility to sell one's labor power (with all that this entails in capitalist societies) is equally recognized as legitimate. To this extent, spatial uneven development is not only an integral part of the development of capitalism, but one that involves working-class people as rational agents, rather than passive cultural dupes, even if the unintended effects of how they engage in social practice in pursuit of their own interests are to reproduce their class position as labor power.

Chapter 19

Class and Gender Relations in the Local Labor Market and the Local State

Ruth Fincher

The local labor market and the local state contribute significantly to the way in which class and gender are experienced by residents and workers in urban communities. They are not independent of one another. The provisions of governments in local areas (part of the local state), in public transport and child day-care, for example, permit people to undertake paid work outside the home. In this sense the spatial scope of local labor markets is defined by virtue of their accessibility to people who must be sustained in paid work by community-based services. Moreover, the hours of operation of paid workplaces and their requirements of workers influence the extent to which existing public services are useful for those workers. It is important to emphasize the obvious point that in people's daily lives the paid work available and the community services that can be used are utterly interrelated. The many analyses that separate production in local labor markets and social reproduction in the use of community services cannot do this.

This chapter aims to indicate some of the characteristics emerging in the local labor markets and local states of Melbourne, and their implications for the formation of class and gender relations. It has the following structure. First, it discusses how the practices of the local state and the nature of the local labor market may structure people's experience of class and gender. In the second section, some of the characteristics of Melbourne's local labor markets are presented, with suggestions for the different and similar class and gender experiences associated with them in different parts of the metropolitan area. Section three documents some of the priorities of local states in Melbourne, and how these priorities are being influenced by changes in federal social policy.

Class and Gender Relations

Theoretical statements usually differentiate class formation – a conscious process of grouping into class collectivities, from class structure – a formal map of class positions in a society, and how many people could be said to hold positions in the capitalist class, the working class, and the middle class (see Wright, 1985). Class

formation is based in varying degrees on class structure, but is never entirely independent of it. Embodied in both the process of class formation and the map of class
structure are class relations; these are the social relationships between people in the
paid workplace, the community, and the home, through which they experience class
(the unequal relationship between capital and labor in a capitalist society), even if
they do not consciously give their experiences that label.

Many of the circumstances affecting the experience of class are institutional features particular to a time and place that differentiate the population along lines not
directly identifiable as class-based. Harvey (1975a) long ago termed these features
of class structuration, and listed them as the division of labor, the consumption
habits and authority relations of a time and place, and the institutional and ideological barriers to mobility there (Harvey, 1975a, p. 362). This chapter seeks to
identify emerging gendered divisions or groupings within Melbourne's working class
that are being produced through class structuration (via the local labor market, and
the local state with its authority over forms of community social reproduction), and
the sorts of class relations they seem to embody.

The changing class relations of the paid workforce in contemporary capitalist
cities have been noted by many authors (Massey, 1984; Massey and Meegan, 1982).
They include the casualization, marginalization, and peripheralization of large
groups within the traditional working class, e.g., male manufacturing workers. New
class relations are appearing as well within groups like part-time women workers,
and between them and other segments of the paid labor force. It is now quite widely
accepted that the reproduction of labor power that occurs in the home and the community, and the fact that household members are often workers in the paid labor
force as well as workers in the household and community, draw class relations into
the household and community as well. Class relations exist in a wide range of daily
activities, then, and through a number of strands of class structuration. Class relations, class formation, and the means of class structuration that affect them both,
are profoundly spatial phenomena; they are restricted or facilitated through use and
reproduction of spatial structures.

Now, gender relations are the socially constructed relationships between men and
women. I suppose analysts committed to the theoretical primacy of class categories
over gender categories would term gender relations one form of class structuration;
others would champion the primacy of socially constructed gender roles over class
as the basis of many everyday experiences. The point is not just to "add on" gender
to class, to adhere feminist concerns to historical materialist ones, but rather to
accept the need for an expanded and reworked concept of a mode of production,
wherein the production of labor power stands on an equally basic footing with the
production of the means of production and subsistence (Livingstone et al., 1982,
p. 9).

This conceptual intermeshing, as well, emphasizes that men's and women's
activities in the paid workforce, in the household or family, and in the community
are not separate spheres but are mutually interrelated. At the simplest level, the
time–space requirements of getting to and being at work restrict people's opportunities to act elsewhere. But less tangible aspects of the social relations of one
"sphere" affect the social relations of another "sphere": for example, a rigid hierarchy in the paid workplace, and strict sex segregation in occupations there, may

have implications for the assumption or allocation of tasks and responsibilities in the household of a worker undertaking paid work in that workplace.

The Local Labor Market

How is the structuring of class and gender relations affected by the (changing) characteristics of local labor markets? First, consider how local labor markets have different characteristics; second, how these may encourage the formation of particular class and gender relations in certain contexts; and third, how changes in economic and other relations may alter all this, and what form some such recently noted changes have taken.

Local labor markets will often have different characteristics, related to the particular industrial and occupational sectors represented in them. Associated with a predominantly manufacturing local economy may be a sexual division of labor and a set of labor processes unlike those of a local economy dominated by personal service provision or tourism. The particular economic base of a local labor market will be important in determining its fate in a time of economic restructuring: traditional manufacturing centers have been hard hit since the 1970s in a number of capitalist countries, as the literature on the deindustrialization of the American northeast and the English north demonstrates. At the same time as traditional manufacturing areas and their predominantly male full-time workforces are experiencing dislocation in the present economic circumstances, other forms of production are emerging and other social groups are finding work, albeit work of different characteristics. Particularly, female participation in the paid labor force is increasing, and is often associated with increasing numbers of part-time jobs.

The dominance of certain employment sectors and forms of work does not determine the class and gender relations of communities, regions, or nations. If this were the case, we would find identical social relations in places with similar economic bases. Rather, continuing economic changes combine with traditions forged out of histories of economic, political, and social interaction in a place, on the part of its long-term residents and indeed on the part of immigrants too. Massey (1984) conceived of layers of past economic and social relationships underlying and influencing the present circumstances of a region. Of importance, too, is the degree to which collective action by local residents and workers can transform local circumstances, despite or in sympathy with exogenous changes.

The challenges to existing class and gender relations in manufacturing communities caused by recent economic upheavals have included: (a) fewer jobs exist in traditional manufacturing. Youth unemployment in places dependent on such jobs is now accompanied increasingly by the unemployment of middle-aged men who had been full-time factory workers. Though the decline of manufacturing in a community does not imply the appearance of a service sector employment base (Murgatroyd et al., 1985, ch. 1), the part-time employment of women, especially in jobs classified as "services," has increased over this period. In some areas, then, one may expect to find a change in the gender characteristics of the workforce in paid employment. (b) This has implications for the characteristics of the unionized labor force, which has traditionally been male-dominated (and often male-centered), and unfavorably disposed towards part-time work. A change in the gender and nature of the workforce and paid work done, then, will see changes in the proportion of the paid labor force that is organized in the traditional manner. (c) Outwork, or homework, is on the increase. A large number of jobs are being performed from the home and there is every indication that this will increase.

Across metropolises, where communities traditionally dependent on manufacturing are juxtaposed with residential suburbs that are also the sites of retail and office development, it appears that women in part-time work in those businesses are also becoming more numerous. And as flexible accumulation grows, a mode of profit-making in which production is disaggregated and spatially decentralized to different communities and households, so suburban residential sites that previously were locations of consumption are the new production sites as well (Nelson, 1986; Harvey, 1987). New social relations will emerge from the placement of these new groups of workers and new forms of employment into any local circumstances, but changes will be especially dramatic where they accompany decline in traditional ways of making a living. Women and men are doing different forms of paid work: their relationships with each other in the workplace and in the home and community will change because of this. New alliances within the working class will emerge from this, and old ones perhaps disappear.

The Local State

The local state is interpreted here as the sphere of political relations associated with the local practice of government (see Fincher, 1987). Studies of the local state therefore include studies of those community conflicts that are associated with the state apparatus and its policies as well as studies of the state apparatus that acts with respect to localities. Clearly, the local state is a sphere of relationships that contains class and gender relations, and can influence their formation or change elsewhere. Consider the following ways the local state (the apparatus and associated political conflicts) influences class and gender relations in paid work and its community support.

First, the local state, through its direct provision (or contract provision, to for-profit firms or charities) of public services to people in paid work who have dependents (children, the elderly), affects the degree to which some people can participate in the paid labor force, quite apart from whether or not employment opportunities are available locally. If suitable child day-care and after-school programs, or domiciliary care for elderly dependents of potential labor force participants, are not available, then those individuals involved in caring will be unable to take up waged work. Second, the local state may, through its direct involvement in employment creation schemes, cause scheme participants to experience work in new ways, and may decrease the incidence of unemployment amongst certain local groups (e.g., women, youth). Third, through its facilitation of different forms of built environment change, the local state can change the nature of work in communities and the demand for public services there, through a change in the nature of the local resident and workforce population. The classic case of this is gentrification, for example the situation in which an alliance of the local state and a major developer locates a luxury waterfront development of offices and expensive, high-density housing in an inner city working-class neighborhood.

A large international literature on the restructuring of the welfare state in advanced capitalist countries since the mid-1970s indicates a ubiquitous reduction in central government financing of, and responsibility for, human services (see Mishrah, 1984; Dear and Wolch, 1987). To the extent that these reductions have locational effects, and are influential in causing local service providers to reduce or change human service provisions, then the local state is involved. Generous provision of child day-care and domiciliary care for elderly dependents would allow more women (especially, as they are the traditional "minders") to participate in paid work, or at least to have more flexibility in doing so. Reductions in human service provisions supporting people in paid work, and the increasing cost of services like child day-care, are most likely to return women to the home by reducing their options to work outside it.

Though the local state is often seen largely as a service provider, as a set of institutions involved in the reproduction of labor power and the provision of collective consumption goods (see Fincher, 1987), local state institutions are becoming involved in employment creation schemes, usually on a fairly small scale. The socialist municipalities of Britain have made their mark here (Boddy and Fudge, 1984). As these and other initiatives show, the activities of the local state have implications for the nature of class and gender relations, as do the activities of employers in the local labor market. Furthermore, the local state influences accessibility to the labor market, and the local labor market creates needs for certain types of public service provision. The local state can be a player in the local labor market through its development of local employment schemes; local businesses can provide community services to support people in paid work, either through employee benefits like work-based day-care, or through being in the business of for-profit human service provision.

Melbourne's Local Labor Markets

This section describes Australian, and then Melbourne's, contemporary labor market characteristics. It goes on to hypothesize the labor market sources of local class and gender relations found in the eastern and western suburbs of Melbourne. Melbourne's local labor markets embody many national trends. These national trends show Australia to be quite like other advanced capitalist countries: its labor market characteristics indicate increasing marginalization in paid work for some employees. The following are Australia's recent labor market features.

(1)   Unemployment has risen drastically in Australia since the mid-1970s. This increase has not been shared equally across different social and economic groups, according to their share of labor force participation. Youth, non-English speaking migrants and women have suffered high relative unemployment, this of course relating to their concentration in particular industries whose labor requirements have decreased.

(2)   There have been different trends since 1966 in full-time and part-time paid labor force participation. Male full-time participation rates have decreased sharply since 1976 and male part-time rates have risen but not offset the full-time rate decreases; female paid labor force participation has increased since

1966, 90 percent of it in part-time work. Married females accounted for all this increase.

(3) Over half the new jobs created since 1973 have been part-time, many of them in community services and retailing. That many of these jobs have gone to women reflects the significant sex segregation of the Australian labor force.

(4) The labor market is further segmented, particularly in Melbourne and Sydney, along another axis relating to the recency of migration of workers, and whether they have non-English speaking backgrounds.

(5) The number of people working at home now forms a significant portion of Australia's paid labor force.

Different parts of Melbourne exhibit these national trends in different degrees: jobs have been growing and declining in number, and changing in type, in different locations within the metropolis. The early 1960s saw "suburbanization" of the considerable job growth in Melbourne. Manufacturing employment was expanding in the east, away from the traditional manufacturing base of the western suburbs. This eastern suburban movement was compounded by commercial job growth between 1966 and 1971, though the inner city also regained some jobs in the early 1980s.

The eastern sector's job growth rates were the highest in the period for each industry category. There was some disparity, too, between the location of jobs and the location of workers' residences. Workers have been moving to the outer suburbs faster than jobs, which are still tending to concentrate in the middle ring suburbs. New offices are locating in the middle eastern suburbs, and more recently in the outer east of the metropolitan area. The disproportionate growth of suburban jobs in the east, compared to the west, is a major difficulty in a large urban area in which regional laborsheds are relatively independent. It is certainly a problem for those without access to a car, and for those whose preferences have been to work locally (traditionally women and blue-collar workers).

What changes in class and gender relations are revealed in the local geographies of the labor market in Melbourne? First, manufacturing workers have in the past been concentrated in western Melbourne. Therefore the decline in manufacturing jobs in the traditional industries and the reappearance of new manufacturing jobs elsewhere (beyond the labor market accessible to western suburbs workers) will be influencing the traditional, male-dominated working class of this region disproportionately. Perhaps marginalization from class practices is increasing with the removal of men from the collective labor processes of the factory floor and the concentration of women in isolating, long homework. Certainly, within households and communities in which males have traditionally held paid positions and women have not, there will be confrontations of class places and gender roles if men are now the unpaid workers.

Second, in the outer eastern region of Melbourne there is a substantial but declining proportion of the labor force in manufacturing jobs, and growth in the proportion of the workforce employed in services, clerical, and professional categories. In the inner east there is a lower and comparatively stable proportion of the population in manufacturing jobs, higher and relatively stable proportions of the workforce in sales, clerical, and services categories, and much larger workforce segments in professional and administrative jobs. Women dominate services and clerical occupations, as elsewhere.

There are higher labor-force participation rates and lower unemployment rates for both men and women in the east than in the west. A higher percentage of women in the workforce works part-time there. And participation rates for women are increasing – probably because of the growing need for households to have two incomes to afford house mortgages. But it is likely that few new part-time service sector or clerical positions are in unionized occupational sectors, and that many jobs are casual or contract-based rather than salaried, permanent, and superannuated. In sum, we find national paid labor force trends exhibited in eastern and western Melbourne in different fashion. Some variations in the class and gender relations associated with these labor force trends have been hypothesized. These, of course, are general expectations. The precise experiences of class and gender in the different locations and workplaces of Melbourne are not indicated adequately by listing trends in occupational and industrial sector data. A range of other factors is relevant, their particular combination to be determined in fieldwork. But one institutional feature that, along with the changing local labor market, differentiates class and gender relations across the city is the local state, and to it we now turn.

Class and Gender Relations in the Local State

A major contributor to the modes of social and economic reproduction in local areas is the local state. Though it does not have complete control over the range of public services available or affordable in an area or investment in jobs there, the apparatus of the local state can influence aspects of economic and social opportunities. For example, local governments may take up or decline federal funds available to set up child day-care centers; they may start local employment creation initiatives or ignore this possibility. As one recent description of local government revenue and expenditure patterns explained: "some councils may decide it is not their role to house needy groups," and "not all municipalities take full advantage of their local entitlements" (City of Camberwell, 1987, pp. 2, 5). The local state is also an arena of local social and political practices that may be channels for changing local class and gender relations – community support networks that help sustain people in paid work are often formed using the resources of local government and local state. Even participation in local community organizing against the local state might weld participants into new groups with new class insights.

There is considerable variation across Melbourne in local government spending on matters that could form better community networks and better prospects for employment. But spatial differentiation in spending is more easily noted between outer and inner municipalities than between east and west. The size and adequacy of amounts spent on education, health, and social welfare depend in part on factors like the age structure of the local population (numbers of elderly, children, needy), income and employment levels.

Since 1983 the federal Labor Government accepted major responsibility for increasing the supply of child day-care places, in contrast to administrations of the previous decade which emphasized that childcare was a family responsibility and which directed most children's services expenditure to pre-schools. A range of strategies enabled the increase in the supply of child day-care places during the mid-1980s. The major federal focus was on expansion of places in local government controlled child-care centers. Family day-care services (where individuals look after others' children in their own homes) were continued, but not emphasized. Government funding of private sector, for-profit centers was avoided altogether, although funding of non-profit, non-government centers was introduced.

In the mid-1980s, the focus of the federal government's role in childcare shifted away from the maintenance of quality standards and the expansion of provision and towards a narrow concern with cost control. Previously, federal subsidies were based on institutionally bargained wages of qualified staff, thus setting staff standards, and center fees were limited by a maximum recommended fee (White, 1986). Together with cuts in funding levels came a new system which established a ceiling of a certain weekly rate above which no federal subsidy will be paid. Service quality, usually regarded as a function of staff experience and training, must now be maintained at the discretion of the centers and the state governments. If centers are to cover their costs, they must either use cheaper (less qualified) staff, or charge higher income parents higher fees than are necessary to cover the cost of the service those parents receive. Subsequently, the federal government indicated that family day-care services (cheaper, but long criticized for their exploitation of care-givers and lack of quality control) would be relied upon for further increase in the supply of child day-care places.

The implication of these changes in federal policy is that the quality of centers will vary according to users' ability to pay for them. Centers will perhaps become the day-care services of higher income users; family day-care providers and informally organized care will perhaps cater to lower income users. Responsibility for enforcing standards will rest more with local and state governments, and will no doubt have to be prompted by continual lobbying: day-care services, their maintenance and extension, have been thrown back into the arena of political competition. It is also, of course, most important to combine this insight with analysis of the workplaces where day-care of children is being done, and their class and gender relations. As family day-care is favored by government funding strategy, with its exploitative, outwork characteristics for women carers, a scenario can be depicted of women working outside the home exploiting women working as child carers within it.

Withdrawals of the federal government from its previously high level of commitment to child day-care are not likely to prompt renewed investment in that service on the part of local government. Should "community management" models of child day-care provision emerge as a way of coping with federal withdrawal, then Mowbray's (1984) comments must be kept in mind. He has argued that community-based and self-help strategies, that place the burden of social service provision on the "community," usually in fact set that burden squarely on the shoulders of women and "the family": they are often very conservative strategies. They do nothing to complement or support increased female participation in the labor force. Government provisions for adults who care for elderly dependents also illustrate this point.

For the last two decades federal government policy in Australia has been to encourage community care of the dependent elderly. Concerns to deinstitutionalize the elderly, however, have been underlain by economic as well as humanitarian motives: some analysts have interpreted the federal government's 1956 Home Nursing Subsidy Act and 1973 Domiciliary Nursing Care Benefit as less an indication of the government's willingness to pay for home-based care than of its desire to encourage more care within the community and the family (Kinnear and Graycar, 1982). The family, they say, is increasingly performing as a "hidden welfare service," especially as community care becomes more favorably viewed in the public eye than institutional care (Kinnear and Graycar, 1983). Its costs to care-givers are hidden, as they are in family day-care provision.

The general implication of a continuing government focus on community care as the most appropriate form of care for elderly dependents, and yet the lack of expanding financial support for this care, is no doubt clear. "The community" will assume the costs and burden of caring for its elderly residents; in practice, this means "the family" will have this responsibility, and in turn this means that women in the family will be care providers. A recent Australian survey of families caring in their homes for elderly relatives echoed the findings of overseas research that family care is usually synonymous with care by women, with little support from spouses, children, and the extended family (Kinnear and Graycar, 1982). A range of changes in carers' lifestyles were observed, with most problems for carers associated with declining leisure activities, and deteriorated work performance, relationships with spouse and siblings, and sleeping patterns. Astoundingly, the survey showed that over 50 percent of the carers interviewed, all women, had given up jobs in the paid labor force in order to provide this care. Clearly "current concepts of community care build on traditional sex roles, and the practice continues a sexual division of labor which makes it a viable and cheap care alternative for the state" (Graycar and Harrison, 1984, p. 6).

Now, there are considerable local spatial variations in access to care for elderly people, and also in access to services for family members caring for dependent relatives. These local variations occur despite the considerable financial involvement of the federal government in service provision which affects the whole of Australia. Howe (1986) shows how the presence of different sorts of providers (public, private, or voluntary sector) in localities dictates the availability of care there, as do the decisions of provider agencies to participate in particular programs. Non-institutional services, that is, community care, are overwhelmingly delivered by local government, and so are potentially universal in their provision. The range and quality of services in a municipality depends on local government's financial capacity and its political will to match funds available from higher levels of government. This is especially true of services giving care to residents outside institutions, which are delivered by local governments.

As with the trend in provision of child day-care services, it appears that the trend in community care for the dependent elderly is one where higher socioeconomic groups will obtain better service levels and where federal government policy will exacerbate this situation. The class and gender implications of this situation, for people working in the paid labor force who have dependent children or elderly relatives, are not entirely clear. For higher incomes and secure jobs do not guarantee that accessible services for dependents will be available to their holders in a locality; this is up to decision-makers in service-providing agencies and organizations. Some local councils accord high priority to provision of these services for their residents, even if those residents are not articulate lobbyists; other councils need to be prodded continually and remain convinced that care of dependents needs council support. However, it does seem very clear that, across all regions of the city and income groups, women bear the major responsibility for dependents. Brennan and O'Donnell (1986) note in the case of child day-care, and Kinnear and Graycar (1982) in the case of care of elderly dependents, that women are the members of the household who most often take on less secure, less well paid and therefore more flexible work in order to meet the need for care of dependents. Federal expenditure on services for adults in the paid labor force, and policy to encourage the "community" basis of care, seems to be reinforcing this reality.

There are groups within the labor force that have particularly low access even to those few services available, however. Non-English speaking immigrants, for example, have been found to make less use of government-sponsored children's services than have families in Australia as a whole (Pankhurst, 1984). This is attributed primarily to the limited information available about centers, to their hours of opening and locations being inappropriate – especially for shiftworkers. Surveys have dispelled the myth that recently immigrated families prefer informal care, and have exposed the anxiety felt by workers whose children have been left alone at home or who have had to make complex child-care arrangements that are constantly breaking down (Pankhurst, 1984). It seems to be the case, even in areas where formal day-care places are relatively numerous, that they are primarily patronized by middle-income, English-speaking Australians. Immigrant women have been less able to use one of the alternatives open to English-speaking women – community-controlled child-care cooperatives. These sorts of centers are only sustained by successful written submissions and frequent meetings, work that requires English language and writing skills (Loh, 1987). The class and gender relations of child day-care provision in the traditionally industrial western suburbs of Melbourne, whose workforce is ethnically very diverse, would reflect this special situation.

Local government provision of services like child day-care and domiciliary care for the dependent elderly, which support adults participating in the paid labor force, is not even in their spatial distribution. The question of how to explain this unevenness is interesting: Why is it that some municipalities have better local government provision than others, some relying more on private or informal provision? Rather than just assuming service levels are set to meet "needs" or depend on the whim of individual bureaucrats, one promising alternative has been suggested by Mark-Lawson et al. (1985) in Britain. They have examined the history of women's involvement in the political arena of the local state, drawing links between this and the provision of community support services. Though local differences may be revealed and explained in Melbourne, federal government changes in social policy threaten everywhere to reduce the accessibility of care for young and old dependents of workers. As these collective consumption goods take on "user pays" characteristics, they will be less affordable. The implications for women, the traditional "carers," may be that they are less able to hold down secure employment: their home, community, and workplace circumstances will combine to alter their experiences of class and gender.

Conclusion

This chapter has suggested ways in which the emerging characteristics of Melbourne's local labor markets and the reactions of local states to the changing priorities of federal social policy may be affecting the class and gender relations experienced in different parts of the metropolitan area. In concentrating on the local labor market and the local state as two institutional features structuring locally experienced class and gender relations, it is easy to think of the labor market as the realm of profit-making firms and the large bureaucracies of the public and private sectors. Equally, it is tempting to regard the local state, especially that part of its apparatus that is local government, as the provider of collective consumption goods for social reproduction. There are two ways in which matters are more complex than this, and I want to raise them as important foci for further research.

First, the local state, far from being only the site of the social reproduction of labor power, has direct effects on the class and gender relations of employment in some localities. British discussions, particularly, illustrate the activity of the state in the formation of urban enterprise zones and freeports, encouraging the relocation of employment opportunities. The involvement of the local state in local employment initiatives, like those of London's Greater London Council, can improve the experience of employment and its availability for people in some localities. To date, these are on such a small scale that they will have little impact on the overall nature of employment-based social relations. But local employment schemes, especially those based around notions of socially useful production, have very interesting implications for the way in which different workplace experiences can facilitate different class and gender relations. There are hints in the Australian initiatives that special efforts may be made by branches of the state apparatus involved to improve the work opportunities and work experiences of women workers there. The involvement of the state in the local labor market, and the degree to which some workplaces can be made the sites of better class and gender relations, is something which should not be overlooked in studies of the local state.

The second point is related to the first. Provision of community services to adults who have dependents and who need those services in order to participate in the paid labor force, is a workplace issue as well as a service delivery use. Services are produced as well as consumed. So the other side of the coin that is marked with declining accessibility of childcare is the side that is marked with the exploitation of women outworkers who are picking up the task of caring for workers' children on an informal basis. That there seems to be a gender bias in both aspects of the situation, that women are often the ones needing the care for their dependents and that women workers are the ones doing the caring under increasingly difficult conditions, has often been remarked and needs to be explained. Class and gender relations are everywhere intertwined, within institutions like the local state as well as in their outcomes.

Chapter 20

Thinking through Work: Gender, Power, and Space

Linda McDowell

Introduction: Organization, Space, and Culture

This chapter counterposes a number of sets of literatures to draw out some questions about the changing organization and distribution of waged work, especially its feminization. As many analyses have made clear, there is an evident, empirically demonstrable, trend towards the "feminization" of work in contemporary Britain. In using this term, I intend to indicate a great deal more than the numerical increase in the numbers of women entering waged employment. I also want to encompass the shift to service sector employment, where the attributes of growing numbers of jobs and occupations are based, in the main, on those purportedly feminine attributes of serving and caring, as well as what organizational theorists and management consultants see as a trend towards the feminization of management structures and practices, with a growing emphasis on less hierarchical, more empathetic and cooperative styles of management. The popular as well as the academic literature in these areas includes praise for nonhierarchical structures, for empathy and caring in the workplace and a range of other essentialized feminine attributes. Indeed, so lyrical has a stream of this literature become about feminized attributes that women have been dubbed "the new Japanese" of organizational theory by one over-enthusiastic advocate (Helgasen, 1990). If these literatures are to be believed, if sheer numbers of women in the labor market are emphasized and the terms and conditions of many women's employment are ignored, it might seem that women are entering a new period of success and empowerment in the late twentieth-century world of work.

The empirical evidence about the purported feminization of organizations has been paralleled by a remarkable expansion in theoretically grounded studies of service-based economies. A particularly noticeable trend in this work has been what we might term a "cultural turn," in which the perception of work and workplaces as active forces in the social construction of workers as embodied beings has become a prominent emphasis. Rather than seeing the workplace as a site which men and women as fixed and finished products enter to become labor power, the ways in which the workplace or the organization plays a key role in the constitution of subjects is becoming clear. It is this work that has been a major influence here, especially studies that have examined the gendering of organizations, the construction of work as emotional labor and the management of feeling, and the significance of embodiment – of men and women as physical beings of different sizes, shapes, skin colors, and sexual proclivities and preferences as well as gendered attributes – in workplace interactions.

To this incisive and significant literature, I want to bring a specifically geographical imagination and suggest that the location and the physical construction of the workplace – its site and layout, the external appearance and the internal layout of its buildings and surrounding environment – also affects, as well as reflects, the social construction of work and workers and the relations of power, control, and dominance that structure relations between them. Here a set of literatures from geography, architecture, and urban sociology are useful. The link between these different literatures, between sociological and geographical imaginations, is the notion of performance, especially the new theoretical work on the body as a site of inscription and cultural analyses of the body. The social constructionist literature has, for several decades from Goffman (1963) onwards, fruitfully used the notion of the stage and performance as a way of understanding everyday behaviors and interactions, and this is mirrored in some of the earliest feminist writing about gender roles. More recently, feminist scholars have developed a psychoanalytically based notion of gender itself as a performance (Butler, 1990). In the work on the built environment, the physical structures of the workplace and the street, Sennett's (1977) classic examination of the decline of the public arena uses the concept of performance as a key to unlock changing attitudes to public and private spaces. A focus on the body as culturally inscribed but also as occupying a range of different spaces in the city, both inside and outside, public and private, is one way of bringing together different theoretical, disciplinary, and methodological approaches.

Men's Jobs, Women's Jobs: Employment Change in the 1980s and 1990s

Like other advanced industrial nations, the last decades of the twentieth century in Britain have been marked by a series of remarkable changes in the nature and location of waged work. So great has been the impact of these changes that Pahl (1988) has suggested that waged work is the dominant but unresolved question at the end of the twentieth century. The postwar certainty about the nature of work, when it was assumed that full-time, waged employment for men was the norm, is now revealed as an exception, dominant only for three brief decades between 1945 and 1975. As in earlier centuries, it seems clear that waged work for growing numbers of people, perhaps even for a majority, was and will be discontinuous, interrupted, and uncertain – in short, a world of employment that has always been familiar to most women.

The remarkable series of changes that was set in motion in Great Britain, and indeed in other advanced industrial economies, from the mid-1960s onwards to their apotheosis in the late 1980s, seems to have finally buried the belief in the permanency of work. In the 1980s, the nature and structure of waged work in these societies, its organization and rewards, the types of tasks undertaken and the people who did them, as well as the places in which they labored, changed irrevocably. The relative certainty of lifetime employment, often for a single employer and frequently in the same place, that had faced men in the postwar decades was swept away in a rhetoric and reality of flexibility, restructuring, casualization, polarization, and feminization. The decline of manufacturing employment in western industrial economies that had been evident for two decades accelerated in the 1980s, and increasing numbers of people found themselves employed in the service economy in a range of occupations from selling haircuts to selling financial advice. These new jobs in the service sector – new only in the sense that they came to dominate these economies – were unevenly distributed across space and between the population. Old manufacturing heartlands suffered serious employment decline, whereas the sunbelt in the south and southwest of the United States, and the golden arc or triangle joined by Bristol, London, and Cambridge in Britain, increased their share of national employment and associated prosperity.

For a time Pahl's thesis about the changing nature of work seemed overly gloomy and, as the 1980s progressed, the huge expansion of employment in the service sector seemed to counter his pessimism. In the southeast of England in particular, economic growth accelerated in the mid-1980s after a period of recession in the early years of that decade, and there was a widespread belief in the buoyant middle years of the decade that the expanding financial services sector heralded a new secure economic future for Britain. New forms of work based on the ownership, control, movement of, and access to money led to the rise of new types of well-paid, middle-class occupations which in combination were dubbed a "new service class" or a new cultural class (Savage et al., 1992; Thrift, 1989). This was the group designated "yuppies" in popular culture. While the term "yuppy" was used, without doubt, to include professional workers in the financial services sector, the label "new service class" tended to be used more restrictively to distinguish a group of workers in what might be referred to as the cultural industries in marketing, advertising, and public relations as well as TV and radio producers and presenters, magazine journalists, fashion writers, and arts administrators and performers. The helping professions – social workers, therapists, etc. – are also often included in this new class fraction.

This group of middle-class workers were identified as being of key significance in the socioeconomic changes that seemed to be sweeping 1980s Britain. Their attitudes to work, it was argued, were different from both the old bourgeoisie and the old manufacturing-based working class. For this new middle class or cultural class, work was fun: indeed, the boundaries between work and leisure were increasingly difficult to define as the social relations of production and consumption merged into each other (Du Gay, 1996). Questions of style and performance, of the ownership and possession of a range of "positional" goods – the Filofax, a Peugeot car, Gucci shoes, a gentrified flat or house in an inner area that was, in estate agents' parlance, "rapidly improving" – all marked out these workers as a distinct class fraction (Thrift, 1989). It is also significant that a spatial referent was attached to the group. Paralleling geographers' arguments about deterritorialization, Featherstone (1991, p. 44) suggested that the new cultural class had a "frequent lack of anchoring in terms of a specific locale or community," although other theorists identified a specifically local impact of the group who were among the key actors in the gentrification of inner area housing markets in the global cities in which they worked (King, 1993; Sassen, 1990).

The remarkably uncritical tone in which the new cultural class is analyzed by some, however, was challenged by the reassertion of the cold world of economics in the celebration of consumption. As Harvey (1989) never ceased to argue, the "postmodern" turn to consumption was little more than "the cultural froth of late capitalism." The mechanisms of class division and exploitation ground on slowly and surely below the surface, and the emphasis on estheticization and lifestyle merely disguised the insecurity of many of those employed in the new service industries. The bubble of service sector expansion burst at the end of the decade. In Britain and the US, between 1990 and 1992, there was recession and a "shakeout" of service sector employment, and Pahl's next examination of work had a pessimistic tide: *After Success* (Pahl, 1995). Financiers, dealers, lawyers, and cultural workers alike were reminded of the harsh world of economic reality as unemployment rose and the housing market suffered an almost unparalleled crisis as real prices fell. Many of those who had bought into the gentrified lifestyle in inner areas or dockland conversions were stranded in negative equity as the value of their property fell below the loan secured to purchase it. A new literature about downsizing and shakeouts and the advantages of a less pressurized lifestyle – an individual's choice to downshift matching enforced corporate downsizing – began to replace the more outrageous of the 1980s texts that had celebrated the "greed is good" ethos.

But even in the boom years, the expansion in service sector employment had not brought prosperity for all. While many of the new jobs were highly paid, demanding increasingly well-qualified employees who were rewarded commensurately, the greatest expansion of employment had been in poorly paid, often casual and temporary work at the bottom end of the service sector – perhaps more accurately called "servicing" rather than service occupations. In the 1980s, the fastest growing jobs in the US economy, for example, included retail assistants, nursing auxiliaries, care attendants in old people's homes, janitors, truck drivers, waitresses and waiters. The list in Great Britain was similar. The net result was a widening pay differential between the well paid and the poorest paid. For those in the bottom decile of the income distribution, for example, the decade brought an absolute as well as a relative decline in their share of the total earnings from employment.

As well as growing income polarization, the 1980s saw the continuation of a shift of employment from men to women which had begun with manufacturing decline in the 1960s. In the ten years after 1966, the net decline in manufacturing output led to significant job losses, of which 73 percent were jobs previously held by men, but only 27 percent by women. Over the same decade, the net increase in private sector services resulted in a 125 percent increase in jobs for women, but a 44 percent decrease in men's service employment (Dex, 1987). In the next 15 years, the loss from the manufacturing sector slowed down but the attrition of men's employment continued. Consequently, by the beginning of the 1990s, there were 3.5 million fewer men in waged employment than at the beginning of the 1960s and almost 3 million more women, although as women were more likely to work part-time, the total number of hours worked had fallen (McDowell, 1991; Walby, 1990). These figures reflect a transformation in the labor market behavior of women in Great Britain in the postwar era. In response to employment restructuring and to social changes from reliable contraception to new patterns of consumption, more and more women entered the workforce. At the beginning of the 1990s, more than half of all women and almost 60 percent of married women were economically active, compared to just over a third of all women and a fifth of married women in 1951.

The feminization of the labor market is not, however, an undifferentiated process. Just as work is becoming increasingly differentiated as a whole in its conditions and rewards, women as waged workers are also becoming increasingly differentiated (McDowell, 1991; Phillips, 1989). Whereas a minority of well-educated women are able to enter and hold on to full-time work in professional occupations, the majority of women in waged work are in part-time jobs at the bottom end of the labor market. Thus, the proportion of women able to return to work after giving birth, for example, differs according to the type of work they do or are willing to accept. In comparison with other occupational groups, women professionals and associate professionals (the latter group includes teachers, health and social workers, and librarians) are more likely to return and most likely to return full-time. Many of these women are in public sector employment where provision for working mothers in the form of flexible working and part-time work is more usual. Women managers and administrators in the private sector, on the other hand, have a lower rate of return, partly reflecting restricted opportunities for part-time employment at this level. Women professionals, as a group, are less likely than either managers and administrators or secretarial and clerical workers to experience downward occupational mobility (Dex, 1987).

These trends reinforce arguments based on the analysis of pay differentials which suggest that women are becoming increasingly differentiated as a workforce. Throughout the 1980s, a growing proportion of women gained educational qualifications and they are beginning to constitute a substantial proportion of those entering professional occupations. Young women improved their performance in school-leaving examinations throughout the 1980s, and as the 1990s began, there was almost no difference between the proportions of men and women aged 20–24 gaining degrees (11 and 10 percent respectively), although considerable differences still exist in the subjects they study. Such is the evident success of women in school, university, and professional examinations, that a crisis of male under-achievement has been recognized as the popular and academic press begins to investigate "boys who fail" and young men with little hope of steady employment (Campbell, 1993).

These trends in the education sector and in the labor market have resulted in a rising number of women gaining access to professional occupations – once the bastions of masculine privilege. In some cases women's representation in the professions has increased dramatically. Examples include law, banking, accountancy, pharmacy, and medicine. In 1991, for example, almost half the new entrants to the legal profession in Great Britain were women, up from 19 percent in 1975. In banking, women accounted for just 2 percent of successful finalists in the Institute of Banking examinations in 1970, but by the early 1990s almost a third of the finalists were women. In 1975 only 7 percent of new chartered accountants and 6 percent of the Chartered Institute of Public Finance Accountants members were women, but a decade later these proportions had risen to 25 percent and 36 percent respectively (Crompton, 1992). Despite their growing presence in higher-level jobs, however, few women make it to the top of the occupational hierarchies in the public or private sector. Although one in four junior managers in Britain was female at the start of the 1990s, at senior management levels the number of women remaining was down to one or two percent.

Explaining Organizational and Workplace Change

Now, I want to shift from an empirical to a theoretical focus and examine the sets of theoretical literatures about work, organizational change and culture, and gender divisions of labor that influenced this study of gendered patterns of recruitment, promotion, and social interaction in the world of investment or merchant banking. I want to outline briefly the ways of thinking that have influenced me in the years in which I have been preoccupied with questions about gender and power. I hope to show that, rather than taking a singular or disciplinary-specific approach, a more complete understanding of why certain types of people are successful merchant bankers can be gained by bringing together a range of different theoretical approaches to occupational segregation and labor market segmentation, the culture of workplaces literatures about the body, about clothes and personal presentation, about success, organizational structures, and the meaning of work, and about the impact that the built environment has on how men and women situate themselves in spaces and places.

In a study of gendered management and employment practices in the insurance industry, Kerfoot and Knights (1994, p. 124) argued that, for them, "financial services are merely a site for empirical research rather than the intrinsic object of investigation." I began this study of merchant banks in the City of London with a somewhat similar belief – my concern was not with the economic niceties of fluc- tuating interest rates, nor with instruments of deregulation and re-regulation, not even with the successive scandals that affected so many City banks in the 1980s and 1990s, but rather with the everyday practices of the men and women who worked in City banks. But, of course, the two cannot be separated. The specificities of finan- cial services as an industry, the particularities of the City in the early 1990s, and the environment, attitudes, and culture of each merchant bank affected the ways in which gender differences in recruitment policies and career opportunities worked out. What economic sociologists term "embeddedness" and geographers "location" cannot be ignored in the investigation of gender segregation at work.

The embeddedness of social and cultural institutions, firms, and individual workplaces is now a key area of study in the new economic sociology (Zukin and DiMaggio, 1990), whereas Bourdieu (1984) used the term "embodiment" to refer to similar processes at the scale of an organization. In the main, however, in analy- ses of the ways in which national and local factors have influenced economic changes, geographers have turned to the revitalized area of economic sociology, rather than to studies of organizational culture, not only to shed light on the loca- tion of industries and their position within national and local systems of political and financial regulation, but also to open up new questions about the cultural meaning of new products, new forms of workplace organization and labor recruit- ment (Schoenberger, 1997; Storper, 1997; Thrift, 1994). Economic sociology focuses on issues of power, the social aspects of markets and business–government links, on social networks and the culture of organizations. It challenges conventional notions of rational economic actors, suggesting rather that economic action is embedded in the social context and the specific institutions within which it takes place. Like all social interactions, economic decisions are as much affected by tradition, historical precedent, class and gender interests, and other social factors as by considerations of efficiency or profit. This is particularly evident in the world of merchant banking, in which networks of familial interests as well as the networks of social elites link directors of banks together and to directors of other British firms and the Conservative Party.

Sets of common social assumptions and cultural understandings shape economic strategies and goals. As Zukin and DiMaggio (1990, p. 17) have argued:

> culture sets limits to economic rationality: it proscribes or limits exchange in sacred objects and relations (e.g. human beings, body organisms or physical intimacy) or between ritually classified groups . . . culture, in the form of beliefs and ideologies, taken for granted assumptions, or formal rule systems also prescribes strategies of self-interested action . . . and defines the actors who may legitimately engage in them (e.g. self-interested individuals, families, classes, formal organizations, ethnic groups). Culture provides scripts for applying different strategies to different classes of exchange. Finally, norms and constitutive understandings regulate market exchange, causing persons to behave with institutionalized and culturally specific definitions of integrity even when they could get away with cheating. On the one hand, it constitutes the structures in which economic self-interest is played out; on the other, it constrains the free play of market forces.

In the 1980s, one of the Conservative government's achievements was to reverse long-standing constraints, creating the circumstances for the spread of a new set of cultural assumptions in the City and in wider society. An ideology of individualism – that people are solely motivated by pecuniary gain – and the associated claims for the efficacy of deregulation in freeing the market from the stranglehold of the state and assuring economic efficiency and success gained the high ground. How these notions progressively infiltrated discourse and practice in a range of economic institutions is a major research challenge for economic sociologists and anthropologists. Merchant banking in particular, within the City as an institution, was one of the prime locations for the successful promulgation and diffusion of these new cultural assumptions. Of all the middle-class occupations in that new service or new cultural class that expanded in the 1980s, it was bankers who were characterized as the personification of the era: the apotheosis of individualistic, profit-oriented "yuppies."

Gender Segregation at Work

Whether in times of economic stability or of marked change, such as those of the 1980s, it seems that women's concentration into a few sectors of the economy and certain types of occupations within them has remained a constant feature of the social division of labor (A. M. Scott, 1994). In the face of this persistence, the unsexed worker, labor power unencumbered by a body or any other social attributes, has almost disappeared from all but the most blinkered of studies, as the lived experience of workers distinguished by, among other characteristics, their gender, ethnicity, age, and family circumstances has become an important focus of research on work and organizations.

In the 1970s and 1980s the dominant perspective was a version of what might be termed the "division of labor" approach (Fröbel et al., 1980; Massey, 1984) in which workers entered the labor market with their gender attributes firmly established. In both the advanced and newly industrializing countries, women were theorized as a reserve of cheap labor, attractive to newly mobile capital in search of higher rates of profit. While the "division of labor" approach implicitly drew on feminist analyses of how women's domestic responsibilities were part of the explanation for their construction as a reserve army, less attention was paid to the reasons for women being drawn into a narrow range of occupations even as the labor market became increasingly feminized. Women's occupational segregation was noted rather than explained. Feminist scholars working within a broad Marxist church, however, explained these patterns through theories of patriarchy, whether conceptualized as a separate system that parallels capitalism, drawing on Marxist notions of exploitation, or as an inseparable part of the capitalist mode of production (Beechey, 1987; Walby, 1990). This stream of explicitly feminist work has the closest links with the divisions of labor school in geography. More recently, Hanson and Pratt's (1995) work has been particularly influential in drawing attention to geographical issues, extending the understanding of the role of residential location and gender differences in job search behavior in the maintenance of occupational sex segregation. They developed a concept of spatial containment, consequent upon women's domestic responsibilities, to explain gender differences.

A second step in the explanation of gender segregation in the labor market came with the recognition that occupations and workers themselves are socially constructed through a variety of practices to conform to a particular set of gender attributes. Occupations are not empty slots to be filled, nor do workers enter the labor market and the workplace with fixed and immoveable gender attributes. Instead these features are negotiated and contested at work. As J. Scott (1988a, p. 47) recognized:

> if we write the history of women's work by gathering data that describe the activities, needs, interests, and culture of "women workers," we leave in place the naturalized contrast and reify a fixed categorical difference between women and men. We start the story, in other words, too late, by uncritically accepting a gendered category (the "woman worker") that itself needs investigation because its meaning is relative to its history.

Jobs are not gender neutral – rather they are created as appropriate for either men or women, and the set of social practices that constitute and maintain them is constructed so as to embody socially sanctioned but *variable* characteristics of masculinity and femininity. This association seems self-evident in the analysis of classically "masculine" occupations; consider, for example, the heroic struggle and camaraderie involved in heavy male manual labor (McDowell and Massey, 1984). The same belief now holds with respect to self-evidently female occupations such as secretarial work, but it is salutary to remember that the latter have changed their gender associations over the century (Bradley, 1989). Less obviously "sexed" jobs and new occupations are struggled over and negotiated to establish their gender coding.

Gendered Organizations: Sexing and Resexing Jobs

An important stimulus to my thinking about the construction and maintenance of gendered occupations in the financial services came from organization theory, especially from recent studies that have drawn attention to the ubiquity of sexuality in organizational processes and the ways in which it is related to the structures of power (Acker, 1990; Hearn and Parkin, 1987; Pringle, 1989). Within this literature, there has been a shift from what might be termed the "gender-in-organization model" – where organizations are seen as settings in which gendered actors behave, as gender-neutral places which affect men and women differently because of their different attributes – to theorizing organizations themselves as embedded with gendered meanings and structured by the social relations of sexuality. In these studies, sexuality is defined as a socially constructed set of processes which includes patterns of desire, fantasy, pleasure, and self-image. Hence, it is not restricted solely, nor indeed mainly, to sexual relations and the associated policy implications around the issue of sexual harassment. Rather the focus is on power and domination and the way in which assumptions about gender-appropriate behavior and sexuality, broadly defined, influence management practices, the organizational logic of job evaluations, promotion procedures and job specifications (Acker, 1990), and the everyday social relations between workers.

The growing recognition of the ways in which male sexuality structures organizational practices counters commonly held views that sexuality at work is a defining characteristic of *women* workers. As Acker (1990, p. 139) has argued:

> their [organization's] gendered nature is partly masked through obscuring the embodied nature of work. Abstract jobs and hierarchies assume a disembodied and universal worker. This worker is actually a man: men's bodies, sexuality and relationships to procreation and waged work are subsumed in the image of the worker. Images of men's bodies and masculinity pervade organizational processes, marginalizing women and contributing to the maintenance of gender segregation in organizations.

The earliest explorations of how organizations are saturated with male power and masculinist values, however, tended to take the social construction of masculinity for granted, instead uncovering in careful detailed work alternative versions of femininity (Kanter, 1977; Marshall, 1984). Although the centrality of a masculine model of employment, based on lifetime, full-time, and continuous employment, and the importance of waged work as a key element in the construction of a masculine identity were clear, the focus was on the ways in which these structures and assumptions exclude women rather than on the different ways in which alternative masculinities are constructed in the workplace. Pringle (1989), for example, in her study of the relationships between secretaries and bosses, noted that the association between masculinity and rationality allowed male sexuality to remain invisible yet dominant, positioning women as the inferior "Other" at work, and yet she interviewed only women.

The realization that male embodiment and masculine sexuality must also be rendered visible and interrogated resulted in a significant shift in feminist analyses of the gendering of occupations. Men began to enter the analyses of feminist work and slowly more organizational sociology where the significance of gender previously had been ignored. Not only the formal structures of institutions, their recruitment, promotion and appraisal mechanisms, and their working hours, but also informal structures of everyday life reinforce women's inferiority. Male power is implicitly reinforced in many of the micro-scale interactions in organizations: in workplace talk and jokes, for example, "men see humour, teasing, camaraderie and strength ... women often perceive crude, specifically masculine aggression, competition, harassment, intimidation and misogyny" (Collinson and Hearn, 1994, p. 3).

The expansion of work about masculinity and organizations, about male power, masculine discourse, and gendered social practices, is part of a wider move in feminist-influenced scholarship to understand the complexity of gendered subjectivities and the ways in which they are constructed in and vary between different sites: the home, the street, and the workplace, for example. It coincided with attempts by feminists, particularly feminists of color, to reveal the assumptions about "woman" that lie behind the early feminist scholarship. Criticized for its implicit focus on a version of white, anglocentric, and middle-class femininity, feminist scholars are increasingly working on the ways in which race, class, and gender are mutually constituted. There has been a parallel rise of queer scholarship. Lesbian feminists, such as Butler (1990), have shown how the "regulatory fiction" of heterosexuality reinforces a naturalized binary distinction between men and women. Similarly, in a remarkable growth of male gay scholarship from the mid-1980s, the construction and dominance of a hegemonic heterosexual masculinity which excludes other forms of masculinity has been revealed (see Kimmel, 1988). In recent work on gender, therefore, in general as well as in the "sociology of organizations" school, the notion of multiple masculinities has been developed to refer to the variety of forms of masculinity across space and time.

Normalizing the Self

The focus on constructing the self at work led to a growing interest in the concept of "normalization" in Foucault's work. The narrow range of socially sanctioned gendered identities and ways of behaving are reinforced and policed through a set of structures that keep in place dominant and subordinate social relations. These structures or mechanisms include not only institutional force and sanctions from above but also self-surveillance and what Foucault termed "capillary power." This interest opened up a way to link analyses of institutional interests and power relations to micro-scale social practices (Foucault, 1979). Here the enormous expansion of interest in subjectivity and in the body by labor analysts and other social scientists is crucial.

New ways of thinking about theory, politics, and the subject have developed in an interesting confrontation between feminism, postmodernism, and poststructuralism. Challenges to the supposed universalism of the rational subject of liberal theory have resulted in a new emphasis in a wide range of different disciplines on the positionality and situatedness of action and knowledge concepts that are not unrelated to the notion of embeddedness in economic sociology. One of the central elements of these arguments is a challenge to the modernist confidence that individuality is grounded in a singular and unique subjectivity that is invariant. In contrast, it is now argued that the self is in a fragile process of construction throughout the life cycle and that a multiplicity of identities are constructed through the symbolic repertoires of everyday actions in institutional contexts (Giddens, 1991). In this sense, the significance of position or location has taken a new precedence in social theory. Here then is a productive coincidence of the notions of embeddedness and embodiment.

The theoretical focus on the body, sexualized performances, and strategies of surveillance parallels material changes in the nature of work in service sector occupations. One of the key features of service sector work, compared with manufacturing jobs, is that the labor power and embodied performance of workers is part of the product in a way that was not the case in the production of manufactured goods. Services that are exchanged, sold, purchased, used up, be they producer or consumer service products – a pedicure, a lecture, or a piece of legal advice – cannot be separated from the workers who are producing and exchanging them. Service occupations revolve around personal relationships or interactions between service providers and consumers, in the main unmediated by a set of exchange professionals as is more usual in the exchange of manufactured goods. In service interactions, the body of the worker be it the "managed heart" of care professionals or flight attendants (Hochschild, 1983), the uniform service of the fast food joint or personalized but scripted service of more upmarket restaurants (Leidner, 1993), the smiling charm of a bank teller or the professional advice of a besuited male manager (Kerfoot and Knights, 1994) – all demand an embodied and visible performance. Special clothing or uniforms may be required for the performance of particular tasks, and prohibitions, for example of facial hair or jewelry, are common in order to produce a specific, usually explicitly heterosexual self-image, both for men and for women. Leidner (1993) has termed these types of service occupations "interactive work," where workers' looks, personalities and emotions, as well as their physical and intellectual capacities, are involved, sometimes forcing them to manipulate their identities more self-consciously than workers in other kinds of jobs.

Bodies at Work

The re-theorizing of work as an embodied performance accords well with the realities of the restructured world of work with which this chapter began. One of the most significant aspects of the 1990s is the ways in which individuals' attachment to the labor force and to a particular job within it has changed. For increasing numbers of workers, there is an expectation of a career that is discontinuous and interrupted, marked by successive contracts rather than the lifetime tenure of a single occupation. Work, once regarded as a (relative) certainty and a central aspect of personal identity, especially for men, has itself become a fluid, multiple, and uncertain performance. Despite these uncertainties, however, and women's greater visibility in the workplace, the most dominant image that continues to structure the world of work in contemporary Britain is that it is a public arena, associated with men and masculinity. As feminist scholars have argued, in western enlightenment societies, embodied social structures, and the physical locations in which they take place, construct acceptable ways of being and "reasonable" behavior on the basis of a set of binaries. As Bourdieu (1984, p. 468) noted:

> The network of oppositions between high (sublime, elevated, pure) and low (vulgar, low, modest), spiritual and material, fine (refined, elegant) and coarse (heavy, fat, crude, brutal), light (subtle, lively, sharp, adroit) and heavy (slow, thick, blunt, laborious, clumsy), free and forced, broad and narrow, or in another dimension, between unique (rare, different, distinguished, exceptional, singular, novel) and common (ordinary, banal, common place, trivial, routine), brilliant (intelligent) and dull (obscure, grey, mediocre) is the matrix of all the commonplaces which find such ready acceptance because behind them lies the whole social order.

And, he continued, they "derive their ideological strength from the fact that they refer back to the most fundamental oppositions between the dominant and the dominated, which is *inscribed in the division of labour*" (1984, p. 469, emphasis added).

In contemporary western societies, therefore, these binaries structure the embodiment of waged labor. They act to define woman as inferior, separating her purportedly natural and private world from the public world of men which, as a public arena, is portrayed as being as distant from the natural world as it is possible to be. Abstract symbols of power, particularly money, are the markers of status and culture. Whereas the natural world is associated with animality, the cultural and cultured world of work is distinguished by its humanity. It is constructed as a rational, objective world in which behavior and decisions are ruled by accepted and conventional norms. In modern industrial societies, the workplace is distinguished by its rational and bureaucratic social order, an arena supposedly unmarked by emotion or by personal characteristics or attributes, one that above all is associated with all that is culturally valued as masculine. Thus, women are literally out of place at work for, as many commentators have pointed out – some approvingly, others critically – woman is to nature as man is to culture. Women, like nature, are viewed as fecund and unreliable, part of the natural order of things, the body rather than the mind, and so unfit for the cool rationality of the public arena. Women are out of place in the embodied social structures of the workplace precisely because they are unable to acquire the cultural markers associated with the attributes valued in the workplace, or perhaps to qualify this, those associated with the rational and bureaucratic workplace. As Young (1990, p. 176) has pointed out, the idealization of a particular notion of (dis)embodiment in the workplace means that "women suffer workplace disadvantage . . . because many men regard women in inappropriate sexual terms and because women's clothes, comportment, voices and so on disrupt the disembodied ideal of masculinist bureaucracy."

The Places and Spaces of Work

Despite the incisiveness of these various sets of literatures about gender, work, power, and organizations, they all seem to have a remarkable blindness to the significance of location. What is happening in the new forms of organizational structures and workplaces has been emphasized to the neglect of where new forms of behavior occur. Yet workplace behavior is both shaped by and shapes the design of the workplace environment at the scale of the city itself, of spaces and localities within it and of individual buildings. The meanings given to different social behaviors, to the characteristics that distinguish femininity and masculinity, are grounded in and accordingly judged more or less appropriate to particular physical spaces.

Lash and Urry (1994) have argued that radical economic changes are paralleled by shifts in the location and structure of industrial spaces. The production and exchange of manufactured products in industrial economies resulted in the production of specialized industrial spaces, the manufacturing heartlands of the industrial nations. Similarly, the production and exchange of commodified signs – the cultural industries and advertising are their example, but financial products such as futures and derivatives are even clearer examples – result in the emergence of post-industrial spaces, even though the goods and services of the late twentieth-century economy are less place-bound in the sense of being reliant on a spatially bound set of raw materials or a local market. As the delivery of services becomes more important and the quality of the interaction between producers and consumers becomes part of the product, the availability both of the right type of labor (often young and personable as well as highly educated for high-status services) and of the *location* of the interaction in an appropriate environment that reinforces the meaning of the commodified signs increases in importance. Indeed, in post-industrial economies, architecture and urban design themselves are a key part of cultural production, both of the products and of performing selves.

Cultural industries are increasingly dominating the economies of large cities (Sassen, 1990; Zukin, 1995). As well as the expansion of financial services in the 1980s and 1990s, global cities became important locations for cultural ventures, from museums and universities to the advertising industry. These industries are part of that "estheticization" of urban life. Zukin (1995) has shown how, in New York at least, the physical reconstruction of urban spaces for workplace and leisure activities for the new middle class is part of the redefinition and reclaiming of inner-city areas. Through the form of the buildings themselves and the nature of interstitial spaces, as well as through mechanisms of physical surveillance and electronic control, undesirable or "dangerous classes" are excluded.

Despite the apparent shift to emphasize representations, the best new work on urban landscapes is distinguished by its determination to link together the material production of the built environment, symbolic meanings and forms of representation, and the sets of material and social practices facilitated or constrained by both physical and symbolic forms. Landscapes are, after all, but the concrete expression of a society, especially its institutions of class and power. Buildings "represent, transmit and transform institutionally embedded power relations" (Zukin, 1991, p. 21). They are not only symbolic representations of discourse, ideologies, and relations of power but also constitute and affect these same attitudes, beliefs, social relations and structures, and so the very distinction between representations and reality falls to the ground. While the relations of power and class have been emphasized in this new "school" of urban scholarship, the way in which the built environment reflects and affects gender relations has been given relatively less attention (Colomina,

1992). Sassen (1996, p. 91) observed that corporate culture is dominated by notions of precision and expertise, imposing its authority on the central area though high-rise, corporate towers: "The vertical grid of the corporate tower is imbued with the same neutrality and rationality attributed to the horizontal grid of American cities." The neutrality and rationality she identified are the same characteristics that construct the female body as out of place in the workplace.

Conclusions

I have argued that the sociology and culture of work literatures, especially those that focus on the gendering of organizational structures and practices, may profitably be brought into juxtaposition with the literatures from urban studies, architecture, geography, cultural studies, and urban sociology, which focus on the built environment not only as a container for the social practices and everyday inter-actions in workplaces that sociologists and anthropologists have documented in increasing and fascinating detail, but also as an active influence on these behaviors. As geographers have claimed for so long and with increasing success, social and spatial processes are mutually constitutive. Where an event or activity takes place shapes its form, and vice versa. The built environment of the City, whether the spatial divisions of the Square Mile and its environs or individual buildings and the layout of workplaces – from the oak-paneled boardrooms and the old open spaces of the trading floors and exchanges to the newer electronic dealing rooms – conveys powerful messages about embodied class and gender attributes.

Part V Spaces of Circulation

Editors' Introduction: From Distance to Connectivity

Eric Sheppard, Adam Tickell, Trevor J. Barnes,
and Jamie Peck

Debates about the importance of space and distance to economic geography are as old as the sub-discipline itself. Their persistence reflects the old geographical idea that what happens in a place depends both on local conditions in that place and on how it is connected to the rest of the world; i.e., on site and situation. In the early "commercial" geographies, such as J. Russell Smith's 1913 foundational text *Industrial and Commercial Geography*, much attention was devoted to trade patterns and the transportation infrastructures that shaped them. They sought to describe how places are connected and how connectivity depends upon ease of travel between them (itself related to distance). The shift to location theory and the search for "scientific laws" in quantitative economic geography in the 1960s made distance into the prime factor in explanations of the geography of economic activities. Location theories generally assumed an isotropic plain, meaning that the only thing varying across the map was distance, whereas uneven distributions of resources or people simply were not considered. Spatial interaction theories sought to predict how the flows of people and goods between places are related to the distance separating them. While spatial analysts devoted much empirical attention to what distance means, distinguishing between economic, social, and Euclidean distance, their theories typically used Euclidean distance as a proxy for relative location.[1] This meant that Euclidean distance became the determinant of location patterns and spatial flows. This causal relationship remains central to the "new economic geography" in economics.

One of the first critiques articulated by Marxian economic geographers against spatial analysts was that this veneration of Euclidean distance is wrong. Marxists argued that economic and social distance are not well approximated by Euclidean distance, because distance is itself a social product. Neil Smith (1984) called this "the production of space." As Marx recognized, in order for capitalists to receive a return on their investment, they must ship their product to distant customers and wait for returning cash payments to be returned to them. The speed and efficiency with which commodities are shipped across space, and money returned, depend on the relative location of linked economic activities and the efficiency of communications technologies. Capitalists and the state thus invest in the built environment and communications infrastructures, in order to accelerate the spatial circulation of commodities and money and thereby enhance profitability. From this perspective, one in which economic distance is produced within the economy, the proposition that Euclidean distance is an externally given determinant of location and spatial interaction amounts to "spatial fetishism" – that is, elevating a social construct (relative location) to the status of a natural feature of the world.

As in discussions about the naturalness of natural resources (cf. Part III Introduction), the conclusion that space is produced by society led Marxist and post-Marxist economic geographers to debate how distance matters in economic geography. If distance is a social product, how can it be isolated as a distinct explanatory factor? After all, if economic activities in a place depend on its connectivity with other places, then connectivity is as much a consequence as it is a cause of socioeconomic processes. Skepticism about the importance of distance has also become more widespread in recent years, as many began to argue that globalization and telecommunications technologies are making Euclidean distance irrelevant anyway – i.e., that we now live in a global village. Frances Cairncross (1997) called this *The Death of Distance*.

Reflecting these debates, Graham examines the role of telecommunications in shaping distance and connectivity, and thereby place and space. He engages in a conceptual comparison of three paradigms: a technological determinist claim that telecommunication is making space and place irrelevant; a co-evolutionary argument that electronic and geographic space are mutually constitutive; and a "recombinant" account, drawing on actor-network theory, that stresses the relational connections between technology, space and place, and social life. Favoring the last approach, and drawing on his own research, he argues that even though space and place are continually reshaped they are not disappearing as material or discursive concepts. Cities remain coherent geographic entities, with communications infrastructures whose geographies are far more coterminous with earlier transportation technologies than technological visionaries suggest. Distance, space, and place thus still matter, despite the space-busting potential of telecommunications.

The next three essays testify to how economic geography over the past two decades has paid more attention to the fortunes of places, and to territoriality, than to the interdependencies connecting places. Yet while their focus is on place, they stress how places are shaped by connectivities with the wider world. Both Gertler and Hsing examine the impact of international flows of foreign direct investment (FDI) on the dynamics of local industrial clusters. FDI connects distant places through intrafirm investments in branch plants as a part of global production or assembly lines (Dicken, this volume). They entail flows of capital, control (over branch plants), influence (over national host governments), and ideas (technologies, labor practices and ideologies). Gertler seeks to extend the research program on industrial districts (Scott, Storper, this volume), arguing that the success of such regions depends on their connectivity to other places, and not just on local conditions. He notes that industrial districts often include branches of multinational firms, whose ability to function effectively in any given industrial district depends on where they originate. He argues that branch plant practices reflect the institutional environment of the home nation, where the parent company is located, and that this environment may differ greatly from that of the host country, where the industrial district is located. His conclusions are grounded in his own research on German-owned branch plants in Ontario, Canada, but his arguments are directed more broadly at the prevailing literature. He is critical of the idea that the prosperity of a region depends on its ability to develop a local culture of learning. Firms gathering there bring cultural norms and practices developed within the institutional context of the nation they come from. The difference (i.e., cultural "distance") between this national context and that of the industrial district may be as important to the success of the cluster as any local learning-based regional development strategies.

Hsing studies industrial cities in southern China. Paying attention to the distinctive geographic and political context of The People's Republic of China, she also concludes that site and situation are important, but in other ways. The willingness of the Chinese central state to devolve responsibility for development to local governments, as it seeks a path to development along the tightrope connecting communism and capitalism in the global periphery, means that local conditions do matter even in this highly centralized society. Yet just as important to her argument is how cultural affinities between Taiwanese owners of local branch plants and local Chinese officials lubricate further investment and growth through traditions of gift exchange. Although she adopts an anthropological account of gift exchange that runs a danger of reducing Chinese culture to a particular trait, she shows, on the basis of extensive interviews, how new investments depend on close connections that have been retained with the overseas Chinese despite mainland China's long-term isolation. In this case, cultural proximity is not shaped by national institutions but by persistent ethnic, familial, and cultural networks spanning space.

Pratt's study of Filipina nannies in Vancouver examines migration, a different but equally important kind of interdependence between places, and takes a different approach to unraveling the cultural dimensions of connectivity. Adopting post-structural discourse analysis, and a feminist methodological strategy of close, situated, and reflexive readings of her interview materials, she seeks both to portray and to disrupt discourses shaping the position that these women occupy as immigrants within Vancouver's labor market. She traces the various geographies of these discourses – situating Filipina domestic workers as somewhere between family members and employees in the households where they work; as housekeepers rather than nannies; and as between visitors and landed immigrants in Canada and Canada's Philippine community. She argues that these discursive geographies stigmatize the nannies' status, but also create a resource for Filipinas and their immigrant organizations to challenge this stigmatization.

These three studies ask how connections across space shape the economic geography of places, but do not seek to conceptualize the processes generating connectivity. Indeed, this question has received limited attention as economic geographers focused on the territoriality of economic activity. Transportation geography has only slowly begun to move beyond traditional location theory, and communications geography was similarly moribund until the recent popularity of telecommunications and the new economy. A number of economic geographers have turned to actor-networks, however, as a way of conceptualizing connectivity. Actor-networks are capable of capturing the complexity and fluidity of the "spaces of flows" and the contingent and negotiable nature of any spatial structures of connectivity (Graham, this volume; Whatmore and Thornes, this volume). Others argue that this focus on fluidity understates the persistence of communications structures. At the opposite extreme, social network analysis conceptualizes networks as relatively fixed relational structures that subdivide the world into self-reproducing cores and peripheries. In this view, sociospatial connectivities are unchanging and determinant of the conditions of possibility of network participants (and of the places they reside in). Reality almost certainly falls somewhere between these extremes, and economic geographers still face the challenge, articulated by Graham, of understanding connectivity in ways that recognize both its fluidity as a social construct and its persistence (Sheppard, 2002).

Beyond theorizing connectivity, a further question is whether attention to connectivity also affects how we can think about and use economic concepts, like competition. Schoenberger seeks to effect such a change; to challenge the now common understanding of competition as an overarching economic logic that determines how firms, regions, and nations should behave, by creating discursive space to consider its social dimension. Her analysis of competition shows well how this seemingly spaceless economic logic can be unpacked to reveal a geographical sensibility that then calls into question the coherence of the original concept. Both of her examples can be interpreted as demonstrating how competitiveness also depends on the interdependencies linking places (Sheppard, 2000). First, drawing on corporate reports, she shows how the profitability (i.e., competitiveness) of Nike reflects the superprofits it makes from underpaying Third World assembly workers. She argues that these wages are not dictated by Nike's struggle to stay competitive, but are a consequence of the ability of Nike to stretch its production chain across space to incorporate national polities with few regulatory structures and low-wage national accumulation strategies. Thus Nike's strategy is one of accumulation, not of achieving competitiveness. Second, drawing from activist research on the living wage campaign in Baltimore MD, she questions the common claim that living wages (successfully negotiated for Baltimore workers in companies with city contracts) undermine local competitiveness.[2] Across the US, firms and the local state have fought against living wage campaigns on the grounds that they make a city unattractive to investors by increasing labor costs. In this view, inter-urban investment flows undermine the economic viability of living wages. By contrast, Schoenberger argues that living wage initiatives may actually attract new money to the city, reducing poverty and thus making the city a more secure place to invest in.

Her argument can be taken one step further. During the 1990s, the US living wage campaign jumped scale, from a few isolated local campaigns to a nationwide grassroots network. The same has happened with the sweatshop campaign that has now put pressure on clothing and shoe corporations, like Nike, to allow inspection of their foreign affiliates and subcontractors. The connectivities created by these activist networks are thus contributing to a shift in how we think about competitiveness, away from bottom-line logic to embrace social considerations. As more localities introduce living wages, it becomes less plausible to argue that when a place introduces living wages it drives investors away. As global clothing manufacturers concede to consumer-led campaigns, allowing inspection of wages and working conditions in assembly plants, social considerations gain more attention. Economic geographers, she argues, must be continually reflexive and self-critical of the concepts and discourses we use. New connectivities on the ground can have the same effect.

In reading these essays, consider the following questions. How does the author conceptualize connectivity and situation? Is connectivity treated as a social construct, a determinant of social processes, or both? What relationships between place and connectivity are highlighted? What theoretical approach does the author adopt (cf. Part I), and how does this affect the questions asked? What kinds of methodologies are used, how are these related to the theoretical approach, and how do they shape the conclusions drawn? How would the adoption of a different theory and/or methodology change the study?

NOTES

1. Euclidean distance is the straight-line distance between two points, measured in miles or kilometers.
2. A living wage is the income necessary to support a family of four at the Federal poverty line, and substantially exceeds the nationally mandated US minimum wage.

Chapter 21

The End of Geography or the Explosion of Place? Conceptualizing Space, Place, and Information Technology

Stephen Graham

It is now widely argued that the "convergence" of computers with digital telecommunications and media technologies is creating "cyberspace" – a multimedia skein of digital networks which is infusing rapidly into social, cultural, and economic life. Cyberspace is variously defined as a "consensual hallucination, a graphic representation of data abstracted from the banks of every computer in the human system" (Gibson, 1984, p. 51); a "parallel universe" (Benedikt, 1991, p. 15); or a "new kind of space, invisible to our direct senses, a space which might become more important than physical space itself [and which is] layered on top of, within and between the fabric of traditional geographical space" (Batty, 1993, pp. 615–16).

Interestingly from the view point of geographers, the recent growth of discourses on "cyberspace" and new communications technologies, even the very word "cyberspace" itself, has been dominated by spatial and territorial metaphors (Stefik, 1996). "Cyberspace," suggests Steve Pile (1994, p. 1817), "is a plurality of clashing, resonating and shocking metaphors." The expanding lexicon of the Internet – the most well-known vehicle of cyberspace – is not only replete with, but actually *constituted* by, the use of geographical metaphors. Debates about the Internet use spatial metaphors to help visualize what are, effectively, no more than abstract flows of electronic signals, coded as information, representation, and exchange. Thus, an Internet point-of-presence becomes a web *site*. The ultimate convergent, broadband descendent of the Internet is labeled the information super*highway*. A satellite node becomes a *teleport*. A bulletin board system becomes a virtual community or an electronic *neighborhood*. Web sites run by municipalities become virtual cities (see Graham and Aurigi, 1997). The whole society-wide process of technological innovation becomes a Wild-West-like electronic *frontier* awaiting colonization. Those "exploring" this frontier become Web *surfers*, virtual *travelers*, or, to Bill Mitchell (1995, p. 7), electronic *flaneurs* who "hang out on the network." The Internet as a whole is variously considered to be an electronic *library*, a medium for electronic *mail*, or a digital market*place* (Stefik, 1996). And Microsoft seductively ask "*Where* do you want to go today?" And so the list goes on and on.

Such spatial metaphors help make tangible the enormously complex and arcane technological systems which underpin the Internet, and other networks, and the growing range of transactions, social and cultural interactions, and exchanges of labor power, data, services, money, and finance that flow over them. While many allege that networks like the Internet tend to "negate geometry," to be "anti-spatial" or to be "incorporeal" (Mitchell, 1995, pp. 8–10), the cumulative effect of spatial metaphors means that they become visualizable and imageably reconstructed as giant, apparently territorial systems. These can, by implication, somehow be imagined similarly to the material and social spaces and places of daily life. In fact, such spatial metaphors are commonly related, usually through simple binary oppositions, to the "real," material spaces and places within which daily life is confined, lived, and constructed.

Some argue that the strategy of developing spatial metaphors is "perhaps the only conceptual tool we have for understanding the development of a new technology" (Sawhney, 1996, p. 293). Metaphor-making "points to the process of learning and discovery – to those analogical leaps from the familiar to the unfamiliar which rally the imagination and emotion as well as the intellect" (Buttimer, 1982, p. 90, quoted in Kirsch, 1995, p. 543). As with the glamorous, futuristic technological visions, or dark, dystopian portraits within which they are so often wrapped, these technological metaphors "always reflect the experience of the moment as well as memories of the past. They are imaginative constructs that have more to say about the times in which they were made than about the real future" (Corn, 1986, p. 219).

Too often, the pervasive reliance on spatial and technological metaphors actually serves to obfuscate the complex relations between new communications and information technologies and space, place, and society. In the simple, binary allegations that new technologies help us to access a new "electronic space" or "place," which somehow parallels the lived material spaces of human territoriality, little conscious thought is put to thinking conceptually about how new information technologies actually relate to the spaces and places bound up with human territorial life. Without a thorough and critical consideration of space and place, and how new information technologies relate to, and are embedded in them, reflections on cyberspace, and the economic, social, and cultural dynamics of the shift to growing "tele-mediation," seem likely to be reductionist, deterministic, oversimplistic, and stale.

In this article I aim to explore some of the emerging conceptual treatments of the relationships between information technology systems and space and place. Building on my recent work with Simon Marvin on the relationships between tele-communications and contemporary cities (Graham and Marvin, 1996), and on conceptualizing telecommunications-based urban change (Graham, 1996), I identify three broad, dominating perspectives and explore them in turn. First, there is the perspective of *substitution* and *transcendence* – the idea that human territoriality, and the space and place-based dynamics of human life, can somehow be replaced using new technologies. Secondly, there is the *co-evolution* perspective which argues that both the electronic "spaces" and territorial spaces are necessarily produced *together*, as part of the ongoing restructuring of the capitalist political-economic system. Finally, there is the *recombination* perspective, which draws on recent work in actor-network theory. Here the argument is that a fully *relational* view of the links between technology, time, space, and social life is necessary. Such a perspective reveals how new technologies become enrolled into complex, contingent, and subtle blendings of human actors and technical artifacts, to form actor-networks (which are sociotechnical "hybrids"). Through these, social and spatial life become subtly and continuously recombined in complex combinations of new sets of spaces and times, which are always contingent and impossible to generalize.

Substitution and Transcendence: Technological Determinism, Generalized Interactivity, and the End of Geography

Both the dominant popular and academic debates about space, place, and information technologies adopt the central metaphor of "impact." In this "mainstream" of social research on technology (Mansell, 1994), and in the bulk of popular and media debates about the Internet and "information superhighway," new telecommunications technologies are assumed directly to cause social and spatial change, in some simple, linear, and deterministic way. Such technological determinism accords with the dominant cultural assumptions of the West, where the pervasive experience of "technology is one of apparent inevitability" (Hill, 1988, p. 23). Here technology is cast as an essential and independent agent of change that is separated from the social world and "impacts" it, through some predictable, universal, revolutionary wave of change.

In terms of the "spatial impacts" of current advances in communications technologies, two broad and related discourses have emerged from the loosely linked group of technological forecasters, cyberspace commentators, and critics who found their commentaries on simple technological determinism (that is, extrapolating the "logic" of the spatial impacts of telecommunications from the intrinsic qualities of the technologies themselves). First, there are widespread predictions that concentrated urban areas will lose their spatial "glue" in some wholesale shift towards reliance on broadband, multimedia communications grids. Advanced capitalist societies are thus liberated from spatial and temporal constraints and are seen to decentralize towards spatial and areal uniformity. Secondly, there are debates about the development of essentially immersive virtual environments, which, effectively, allow the immersive qualities of geographical place to be transmitted remotely.

Areal uniformity, urban dissolution, and generalized interactivity

The geographical effects on space and place of the supposedly wholesale "technological revolution" based on new information and communications technologies become fairly easy to establish, if one follows an essentialist, cause-and-effect, and deterministic logic through. As technologies of media, computing, and telecommunications converge and integrate; as equipment and transmission costs plummet to become virtually distance independent; and as broadband integrated networks start to mediate all forms of entertainment, social interaction, cultural experience, economic transaction, and the labor process, distance effectively *dies* as a constraint on social, economic, and cultural life. Human life becomes "liberated" from the constraints of space and frictional effects of distance. Anything becomes possible anywhere and at any time (see Graham and Marvin, 1996). All information becomes accessible everywhere and anywhere. The "logic" of telecommunications and electronic mediation is therefore interpreted as inevitably supporting geographical dispersal from large metropolitan regions, or even the effective dissolution of the city itself (Gillespie, 1992; Graham, 1997).

Most common here is the assumption that networks of large metropolitan cities will gradually emerge to be some technological anachronism, as propinquity, concentration, place-based relations, and transportation flows are gradually substituted by some universalized, interactive, broadband communications medium (the ultimate "Information Superhighway"). To Baldwin and colleagues (1996), for example, this all-mediating network, this technological Holy Grail of fully converged telephony, TV, media, and data flow, embellished with virtual shopping and interactive video communications, is already in sight, with the trials of so-called full-service networks (FSNs) in cities like Orlando, Florida. "We now have," they write (1996, p. 1),

> a vision of an ideal broadband communication system that would integrate voice, video and data with storage of huge libraries of material available on demand, with the option of interaction as appropriate. The telephone, cable, broadcast, and computer industries, relatively independent in the past, are converging to create these integrated broadband systems.

Such substitutionist arguments, in fact, have a long lineage. Assumptions that advances in telecommunication will "dissolve" the city have a history as long as electronic communication itself. Caroline Marvin (1988), in her book *When old technologies were new*, recounts the many assumptions in the late nineteenth century that the seemingly fantastical technologies of the telegraph, wireless, and telephone would annihilate space constraints through minimizing time constraints. Social, cultural, and geographical differences were to be obliterated in the worldwide shift to ubiquitous, universally accessible telecommunication. According to Edward Bellamy, writing in 1897 (pp. 347–48), "wherever the electric connection is carried . . . it is possible in slippers and dressing gown for the dweller to take his choice of the public entertainment given that day in every city of the earth."

Such technologically determinist predictions also resonate surprisingly strongly with some of the more critical recent perspectives of the relationships between space, place, and technological change. For example, Paul Virilio (1993) recently suggested that a culture of "generalized interactivity" is emerging, based on pervasive, ubiquitous, and multipurpose telematics grids, through which "everything arrives so quickly that departure becomes unnecessary" (Virilio, 1993, p. 8). "The archaic 'tyranny of distances' between people who have been geographically scattered," he writes, increasingly gives way to the "tyranny of real time . . . The city of the past slowly becomes a paradoxical agglomeration in which relations of immediate proximity give way to interrelationships over distance" (Virilio, 1993, p. 10).

"Mirror worlds," the transmission of place and world transcendence

Virilio's predictions of the evaporation of the material, physical dynamics of space and place find support in the more optimistic perspectives of "cyber-gurus" like Nicholas Negroponte (1995) and Bill Gates (1995). Again, the substitution ethos dominates here, with the assumption that sophisticated VR technologies, switched over broadband global grids, will allow immersive, 3D environments to become so life-like that "real" places will easily become substitutable. David Gelerntner (1991) imagined that such technological trends will lead to the construction of "mirror worlds," immersive electronic simulations tied into real-time monitoring apparatus which would allow us to "look into a computer screen and see reality. Some part of your world – the town you live in, the company you work for, your school system, the city hospital – will hang there in a sharp color image" (Gelerntner, 1991, p. 1; see also Graham, 1998).

Such technologically evangelistic debates about "digital living" therefore suggest that we are on the verge of accessing a technological infrastructure which will do little less than provide some single, immersive system to mediate all aspects of human life. The implication is that the very concepts of material space, place and time, and the body, will be rendered problematic, even obsolete. We will shed, as Benedikt (1991) put it, the "ballast of our materiality," escaping the physical, corporeal domains of the body, the territorial earth, and space and time in the process (Slouka, 1995, p. 25). Human societies, cultures, and economies are seen simply to *migrate* into the electronic ether, where identities will be flexibly constructed, any services might be accessed, endless fantasy worlds experienced and any task performed, from any location and at any time, by human agents acting *inside* the limitless domains of constructed electronic environments.

Presumably, as human life becomes more and more dominated by what Thu Nguyen and Alexander (1996, p. 117) call "participation in the illusion of an eternal and immaterial electronic world," the material world of space and place would become gradually eviscerated. Many cyberspace enthusiasts do, indeed, proclaim the need for what Schroeder (1994) has termed "world rejection." Here cyberspace is seen to offer an *alternative* territoriality, an infinitely replenishable and extendible realm of spatial opportunity that counters the finitudes and problems of the increasingly crowded and problematic material spaces on earth.

Of course, the foundations for such technological Utopianism, and determinism, are woven deeply into the very cultural roots of modern capitalist society (Marvin, 1988; Smith and Marx, 1995). Discourses of modernity and "progress" have been widely constituted through technological promises of brave new worlds with universal, beneficent, totalizing shifts and secular technological Utopias variously promulgated by pulp science fiction, comic books, futurists, architects and "city of the future" visionaries, advertisers, and technology firms (Corn and Horrigan, 1984).

Co-evolution: The Parallel Social Production of Geographical Space and Electronic Space

The strong leaning of contemporary technological discourse towards substitution and transcendence perspectives, I would argue, tends to perpetuate little but dangerous myth and fallacy. In proffering new technologies as some complete and simple *substitutes* for the material body, the social world, and for space and place, its proponents do little to advance understanding of the complex *co-evolutionary* processes linking new information technologies and space, place, and human territoriality. Kevin Robins (1995, p. 139) has argued that they say more about their own (usually masculine) "omnipotence fantasies" than about how complex combinations of place-based and telemediated interactions co-evolve. As he suggests, such perspectives rest on a

> common vision of a future that will be different from the present, of a space or a reality that is more desirable than the mundane one that presently surrounds and contains us . . . All this is driven by a feverish belief in transcendence; a faith that, this time around, a new technology will finally and truly deliver us from the limitations and frustrations of this imperfect world (Robins, 1995, p. 135).

Fortunately, however, a much more sophisticated understanding has been developed recently through our second broad perspective which explores how the social production of electronic networks and "spaces" *co-evolves* with the production of material spaces and places, within the same broad societal trends and social processes (see Mosco, 1996, pp. 173–211). Three strands of work have emerged.

Articulations between place-based and telemediated relationships

Rather than assuming some simple substitutional relationship, our second perspective suggests that complex *articulations* are emerging between interactions in geographical space and place, and the electronic realms accessible through new technologies. The argument here is that, because cyber-evangelists are naively obsessed with the abstract *transmissional* capabilities of information technologies, technologically determinist debates usually neglect the richness and embeddedness of human life within space and place. Sawhney (1996, p. 309) criticizes the "very transmission-oriented view of human communication [in cyberspace debates]. The purpose of human communication is reduced to transfer of information and the coordination of human activity. The ritual or the communal aspect of human communication is almost totally neglected."

Technologically determinist commentators are accused of failing to appreciate the social, cultural, and economic dynamics of place and space that cannot be simply telemediated no matter how broadband, 3D, or immersive the substitutes. Quite the reverse, in fact, because the human construction of space and place is seen actually to ground and contextualize applications and uses of new technologies. Kevin Robins (1995, p. 153) believes that "through the development of new technologies, we are, indeed, more and more open to experiences of de-realization and de-localization. But we continue to have physical and localized existences. We must consider our state of suspension between these two conditions."

Telecommunications and the city

This "state of suspension" is especially evident in the contemporary metropolis, which, despite some trends towards the decentralization of routine service functions, shows no sign of simple, wholesale evisceration. Globally, urbanization trends are unmatched in history in their intensity; the global urban system continues to dominate the planet economically, politically, socially, and culturally; transportation flows and demands are spiraling at every scale; and even the large industrial cities in the UK and USA that recently were shedding population are showing some signs of an (albeit patchy) economic and cultural renaissance, and demographic turn round. In short, new communications technologies are not simply substituting for the experience of, or reliance on, metropolitan places. Rather, a complex co-evolution, articulation, and synergy between place-based and telemediated exchange seem to be emerging.

Castells (1996, p. 373) similarly posits that the new, integrated media systems will bring with them what he calls a "culture of real virtuality" drawing diverse participants and fragmented communities into new symbolic environments in which "reality itself (that is, people's material/symbolic existence) is entirely captured, fully immersed in a virtual image setting, in the world of make believe, in which appearances are not just seen on the screen through which experience is communicated, but they become the experience."

Cyberspace is, in fact, a predominantly metropolitan phenomenon which is developing *out of* the old cities. In terms of hard infrastructural investment, demand for services, and rates of innovation, the largest, globally orientated metropolitan areas are clearly maintaining their dominance. Thus, while New York has around 7% of the USA population, 35% of all outgoing USA international calls start there. While London has 17% of the UK population, 30% of all UK mobile phone calls are made there. And while Paris has 16% of the French population, it commands 80% of all investment in telecommunications infrastructure in France (Graham and Marvin, 1996, p. 133).

The work of Jean Gottmann (1982) has clearly demonstrated that the incorporation of computer networks into the economic, administrative, and sociocultural dynamics of the city merely intensifies and adds further capability to the older functions of the post, the telegraph, and the telephone. The maintenance of control over ever-more complex urban and regional systems, straddling ever-larger distances, and spread over larger and larger metropolitan corridors and regions, becomes possible. Rather than simply substituting or revolutionizing the city, and flows of people and material goods, the evidence suggests that new technologies actually diffuse into the older urban fabric offering potential for doing old things in new ways. Urban transportation and infrastructure systems can be managed and controlled more precisely, improving capacity. Telecommunications co-evolve with transportation and physical flows, sometimes replacing (telebanking for branch networks, email for post), sometimes generating (travel TV programs and conference and retail adverts), and sometimes enhancing transport capability (automatic route guidance) (see Graham and Marvin, 1996).

New information technologies, in short, actually resonate with, and are bound up in, the active construction of space and place, rather than making it somehow redundant. William Mitchell's notion of "recombinant architecture" is especially relevant here, because it demonstrates how constructed and produced material spaces are now being infused with cyberspace "entry points" of all kinds (Mitchell, 1995). Material space and electronic space are increasingly being produced together. The power to function economically and link socially increasingly relies on constructed, place-based, material spaces intimately woven into complex telematics infrastructures linking them to other places and spaces. "Today's institutions," argues Mitchell (1995, p. 126), "are supported not only by buildings but by telecommunications and computer software." Thus the articulation between widely stretched telematics systems, and produced material spaces and places, becomes the norm and is a defining feature of contemporary urbanism.

Bookstores, libraries, universities, schools, banks, theaters, museums and galleries, hospitals, manufacturing firms, trading floors, and service providers increasingly become embodied through their presence in both material spaces and electronic spaces. While some substitution is evident – for example, with the closure of banking branches paralleling the growth of telebanking – much of the traditional, nonroutine face-to-face activity within constructed spaces, and the transportation that supports it, seems extremely resilient to simple substitution. In other words, the contemporary city, while housing vast arrays of telematic "entry points" into the burgeoning worlds of electronic spaces, is a cauldron of emotional and personal worlds and attachments, an engine of reflexivity, trust, and reciprocity (Amin and Graham, 1998).

The complex articulations between the local and global dynamics of both material places and electronic spaces have recently been explored by Staple (1993). He believes that the Internet and other communications technologies, far from simply collapsing spatial barriers, actually have a dialectic effect, helping to compress time and space barriers while, concurrently, supporting a localizing, fragmenting logic of "tribalization." Far from unifying all within a single cyberspace, the Internet, he argues, may actually enhance the commitment of different social and cultural interest groups to particular material places and electronic spaces, thus constituting a "geographical explosion of place" (Staple, 1993, p. 52). This "new tribalism," exemplified by the use of the Internet to support complex diasporas across the globe, and to draw together multiple, fragmentary special interest groups on a planetary basis, "folds" localities, cities, and regions into "the new electronic terrain" (Staple, 1993, p. 52).

But it is important to stress that the ways in which places become enmeshed into globally stretched networks like the Internet will be a diverse, contingent process. A wide diversity of relations seems likely to exist between the urban structures and systems, and indeed the particularities of culture, of different spaces and the growth of telemediated interaction.

Telecommunications, "spatial fixes," and the production of space

Theoretical perspectives drawing on critical political economy serve to exemplify further the ways in which new telecommunications systems are materially bound up with the production of complex new social and economic geographies. Reacting against the all-encompassing and overgeneralized concepts of the "global village" and "time–space compression," Scott Kirsch (1995, p. 544, emphasis in original) argues that "by resorting to the rather cartoonish shrinking world metaphor, we lose sight of the complex relations . . . between capital, *technology*, and space, through which space is not 'shrinking' but rather must be perpetually recast."

Perhaps the clearest exploration of how telecommunications become woven in to the production of new geographical landscapes of production, consumption, and distribution at all spatial scales comes from Eric Swyngedouw (1993, p. 305).

Building on the work of Harvey (1985a), he argues that every social and economic activity is necessarily geographical. It is "*inscribed in space and takes place*" (emphasis in original). Human societies "cannot escape place in the structuring of the practices of everyday life" (p. 305). Within an internationalizing economy, capitalist firms and governments must continually struggle to develop new solutions to the tensions and crisis tendencies inherent within capitalism, between what David Harvey calls "fixity" and the need for "motion," mobility and the global circulation of information, money, capital, services, labor, and commodities (Harvey, 1985a). Currently, such tensions and crises arise because increasingly widely dispersed areas of production, consumption, and exchange, befitting of the internationalizing economy, need to be integrated and coordinated into coherent economic systems. Space thus needs to be "commanded" and controlled, on an increasingly international scale.

To do this, relatively immobile and embedded fixed transport and telecommunications infrastructures must be produced, linking production sites, distribution facilities, and consumption spaces that are tied together across space with the transport and communications infrastructure necessary to ensure that a spatial "fix" exists that will maintain and support profitability. Without the elaboration of ever more sophisticated and globally stretched transport and communications infrastructures, Harvey (1993a, p. 7) argues that "the tension between fixity and mobility erupts into generalized crises, when the landscape shaped in relation to a certain phase of development . . . becomes a barrier to further [capital] accumulation." Thus, new telecommunications networks "have to be immobilised in space, in order to facilitate greater movement for the remainder" (Harvey, 1985a, p. 149).

Crucially, then, the political economic perspective underlines that the development of new telecommunications infrastructures is not some value-neutral, technologically pure process, but an asymmetric social struggle to gain and maintain social power, the power to control space and social processes over distance. As any investigation of, say, the growth of global financial centers, or the extending global coverage of corporate telematics networks will soon discover, power over space and power over telecommunications networks go hand in hand. For example, Graham Murdock draws the striking parallel between the "fortress effect" generated by many postmodern office buildings, and the development of vast, private "dataspaces" on corporately controlled networks. He argues (1993, p. 534) that "here, as in territorial space, continuous battle is being waged between claims for public access and use, and corporate efforts to extend property rights to wider and wider areas of information and symbolization."

By demystifying, and unpacking, the social and power relations surrounding telecommunications and the production of space, the political economic perspective does much to debunk the substitutionist myths of technological determinism discussed above. It allows us to reveal the socially contingent effects of new technologies, the way they are enrolled into complex social and spatial power relations and struggles, and the ways in which some groups, areas, and interests may benefit from the effects of new technologies, while others actually lose out. Thus, "the increased liberation and freedom from place as a result of new mobility modes for some may lead to the disempowerment and relative exclusion for others" (Swyngedouw, 1993, p. 322).

Thus, within cities, forms of telematics super-inclusion (Thrift, 1996a) emerge for elite groups, who may help shape cocooned, fortified, urban (often now walled) enclosures, from which their intense access to personal and corporate transport and telematics networks allows them global extensability. Meanwhile, however, a short distance away, in the interstitial urban zones, there are "off-line" spaces (Graham and Aurigi, 1997), or "lag-time places" (Boyer, 1996, p. 20). In these, often-forgotten places, time and space remain profoundly real, perhaps *increasing*, constraints on social life, because of welfare and labor market restructuring and the withdrawal of banking and public transport services. It is easy, in short, to overemphasize the mobility of people and things in simple, all-encompassing assumptions about place-transcendence (Thrift, 1996b, p. 304), which conveniently ignore the splintering and fragmenting reality of urban space.

To Christine Boyer (1996, p. 20), the highly uneven geography of contemporary cities, and the growing severing of the "well designed nodes" of the city from the "blank, in-between places of nobody's concern," allows fortunate groups to "deny their complicity" in the production of these new, highly uneven, material urban landscapes. But perhaps the most extreme example of the complex interweaving of new technologies, power relations, and the production of space and place comes with the small, elite group who run the global financial exchanges in world cities. Here, we find that "the extensible relations of a tiny minority in New York, London, and Tokyo, serve to control vast domains of the world through international networks of information retrieval and command" (Adams, 1995, p. 277).

Recombination: Actor-Network Theory and Relational Time-Spaces

Our third and final perspective takes such *relational* views of the social construction of technology further. Anchored around the actor-network theories of Michel Callon (1986, 1991) and Bruno Latour (1993), and drawing on recent theorizations of Donna Haraway on the emergence of blended human–technological "cyborgs" (or "cybernetic organisms" – see Haraway, 1991), a range of researchers from the sociology of science, science, technology and society, cultural anthropology, and, increasingly, geography have recently been arguing for a highly contingent, relational perspective of the linkage between technology and social worlds. Actor-network theory emphasizes how particular social situations and human actors "enrol" pieces of technology, machines, as well as documents, texts, and money, into "actor-networks."

The perspective is fully relational in that it is "concerned with how all sorts of bits and pieces; bodies, machines, and buildings, as well as texts, are associated together in attempts to build order" (Bingham, 1996, p. 32). Nigel Thrift (1996a, p. 1468) summarizes the approach:

> no technology is ever found working in splendid isolation as though it is the central node in the social universe. It is linked – by the social purposes to which it is put – to humans and other technologies of different kinds. It is linked to a chain of different activities involving other technologies. And it is heavily contextualised. Thus the telephone, say, at someone's place of work had (and has) different meanings from the telephone in, say, their bedroom, and is often used in quite different ways.

This linkage of heterogeneous technological elements and actors, strung across distance, is thus seen as a difficult process requiring continuing efforts to sustain relations which are "necessarily *both* social and technical" (Akrich, 1992, p. 206). The growing *capabilities* of telecommunications, for supporting action at a distance and remote control, do not therefore negate the need for the human actors which use them to struggle to enroll passive technological agents into their efforts to attain real, meaningful remote control. "Stories of remote control tend to tell of the sheer amount of work that needs to be performed before any sort of ordering through space becomes possible" (Bingham, 1996, p. 27). Such "heterogeneous work involving programmers, silicon chips, international transmission protocols, users, telephones, institutions, computer languages, modems, lawyers, fibre-optic cables, and governments to name but a few, has had to be done to create envelopes stable enough to carry [electronic information]" (Bingham, 1996, p. 31).

"Cyberspace" therefore needs to be considered as a fragmented, divided, and contested multiplicity of heterogeneous infrastructures and actor-networks. For example, there are tens of thousands of specialized corporate networks and intranets. The Internet provides the basis for countless Usenet groups, Listservers, corporate advertising sites, specialized Web sites, multi-user dungeons (MUDs), corporate intranets, virtual communities, and increasingly sophisticated flows of media and video. Public switched telephone networks (PSTNs) and the many competing telecoms infrastructures support global systems of private automatic teller machine (ATM) networks, credit card and electronic clearing systems, as well as blossoming applications for CCTV, tele-health, teleshopping and telebanking, global logistics, remote monitoring, back office and telesales flows, electronic data interchange (EDI), electronic financial transactions and stock market flows, as well as data and telephony flows. And specialized systems of satellite, broadband, cable, and broadcasting networks support burgeoning arrays of television flow. Each application has associated with it whole multiplicities of human actors and institutions, who must continually struggle to enroll and maintain the communications technologies, along with other technologies, money, and texts, into producing some form of functioning social order. These, and the hundreds of other actor-networks, are always contingent, always constructed, never spatially universal, and always embedded in the microsocial worlds of individuals, groups, and institutions. Such sociotechnical networks "always represent geographies of enablement and constraint" (Law and Bijker, 1992, p. 301); they always link the local and nonlocal in intimate relational, and reciprocal, connections.

Such a fully relational perspective has important implications for the ways in which we conceptualize place, space, and time. For actor-network theory suggests that, rather than simply being space and time *transcending* technologies, telecommunications systems actually act as technological networks within which new spaces and times, and new forms of human interaction, control, and organization are continually constructed (Latour, 1987).

The merit of the actor-network perspective is the way it articulates human–technological recombinations and relationships through a rich, contextual, mapping which avoids essentializing sociotechnical relations. As an analytic perspective it helps to capture the complex and multiple relational worlds supported by information technologies. Its emphasis on sociotechnical "hybrids" further underlines the growing difficulties of easily separating something called the "social" (or, for that matter, the "spatial") from the "technological." Rather than hypothesizing macrolevel technological "revolutions" it stresses multiple, contingent worlds of social action, underlining the difficulties involved in achieving social ordering "at a distance" through enrolling complex arrays of technological artifacts. In it humans emerge as more than just subjects whose lives are to be "impacted"; as more than bit-players within macrolevel processes of global structural change. Actor-network theory underlines forcefully that "living, breathing, corporeal human beings arrayed in various creatively improvised networks of relation still exist as something more than machine fodder" (Thrift, 1996a, p. 1466).

Work by Thrift (1996a, 1996b) has used actor-network theory to show how highly concentrated urban spaces like the City of London, far from suffering some simple dissolution, have, over the past century, actually been continually recombined with new technological networks: the telegraph, telephone, and, most recently, the telematics trading system. Such new technologies, he writes, do not produce some "abstract and inhuman world, strung out on the wire" (Thrift, 1996a, p. 1480); they are subtly recombined with the spatial and social practices of workers and managers, operating within the complex, material, and social spaces of the City.

Often, the use of faster and faster telematics systems actually *increases* the demands for face-to-face contact so that the interpretive loads surrounding information glut can be dealt with rapidly and competitively. "The major task in the information spaces of telematic cities like the City of London," writes Thrift (1996a, p. 1481), "become interpretation and, moreover, interpretation *in action* under the pressure of real-time events." Thus the production of new material spaces, and the social practices that occur in them, is neither some technological cause-and-effect, nor some simple political-economic machination. Rather, it is

> the hybrid outcome of multiple processes of social configuration processes which are specific to particular differentially-extensive actor-networks (made up of people and things holding each other together) and generate their own space and own times, which will sometimes, and sometimes not, be coincident. There is, in other words, no big picture of the modern City to be had but only a set of constantly evolving sketches (Thrift, 1996a, p. 1485).

Conclusions: Space, Place, and Technologies as Relational Assemblies

Two clear conclusions for how we might address the linkages between space, place, and information technology emerge from our discussion of the three broad substitution, co-evolution, and recombination perspectives.

First, we need to be extremely wary of the dangers of adopting, even implicitly, deterministic technological models and metaphors of technological change. The choice of words here is important. For example, the very notion of a technological "impact," so long a central feature of mainstream technological debates in urban and regional studies (e.g., Brotchie et al., 1987), is problematic, because of its attendant implications of simple, linear, technological cause and societal effect. In their extreme form, deterministic approaches deliver little but the "logic" of apparent technological inevitability, naive assumptions about simple, cause-and-effect, social and spatial "impacts," and even messianic and evangelistic predictions of pure, technological salvation.

The co-evolution perspective teaches us that such perspectives fail to capture the ways in which new technologies are inevitably enrolled into complex social power struggles, within which both new technological systems and new material geographical landscapes are produced. The recombination perspective, on the other hand, teaches us that such broad-brush transition and "impact" models ignore the full, contingent, and relational complexity surrounding the social construction of new technologies, within and between specific places. It argues powerfully that, outside such contingencies, the meaning and effects of new information technologies can never be fully understood or simply generalized.

Secondly, however, we need to be equally wary of the dangers of adopting simplistic concepts of *space* and *place*. Following the arguments of such authors as Giddens (1979), Massey (1993), and Harvey (1993a, 1996) we need to reject the extremely resilient "Euclidean" notions, still implicitly underlying many treatments of the geographies of information technology, that treat spaces and places simply as bounded areas, as definable, Cartesian spatial objects, embedded within some wider, objective framework of time-space. As Doreen Massey (1993, p. 66) suggests, places need to be defined *in relational terms*, too, as "articulated moments in networks of social relations and understandings" rather than as "areas with boundaries around."

The message, then, is clear. Only by maintaining linked, relational conceptions of *both* new information and communications technologies *and* space and place will we ever approach a full understanding of the interrelationships between them. For Latour's "skein of networks" (1993, p. 120) involves *relational assemblies* linking technological networks, space and place, and the space and place-based users (and nonusers) of such networks. Such linkages are so intimate and recombinatory that defining space and place separately from technological networks soon becomes as impossible as defining technological networks separately from space and place.

The example of the contemporary city helps illustrate the point. Here, propinquity in material space has no *necessary* correlation with relational meaning. Complex place and transport-based relational meanings – such as access to physical infrastructure, property, labor markets, an "innovative milieu," social interaction, and the use of cultural facilities – are constantly being recombined with local and nonlocal relational connections, accessed via technological networks (telecommunications, long-distance transport networks, and, increasingly, long-distance energy supplies too).

The "urban" thus can now be seen as a locus for many sociocultural, economic, and institutional networks and practices, spread out over diffuse and extended regions, and mediated by complex combinations of physical "copresence" and technological mediation (see Healey et al., 1995). In some, the interlinkage and superimposition within physical urban space form meaningful nodes and connections – economic, social, cultural, physical. In others, the place-based relations are outweighed by the technologically mediated links to far-off places. Thus, neighbors may or may not know each other's names and have meaningful social relations. Adjacent firms may or may not create meaningful linkages (adjacent back offices are likely to be tied intimately into their own distant corporate telematics networks but poorly linked to each other). Urban public spaces may or may not emerge as common cultural arenas in their articulations with global media flows and exchanges. Complex, subtle, and contingent, combinations of electronic propinquity in the "nonplace urban realm" (Webber, 1964) and place-based relational meanings based on physical propinquity and transport therefore need to be considered in parallel. Such recombinations of "technology" and "place" represent merely the latest processes of urbanism and not some simple post-urban shift (Graham and Marvin, 1996).

While cities are often spreading out to be vast, multicentered urban regions linked into global networks, place-based relational webs that rely on adjacency, propinquity, and physical flows remain central to the experience of human social, economic, and cultural life. The two rely on each other; they recursively interact. For, as Storper (1996) suggests, shifts towards growing reliance on telemediated information, image, electronic transactions, and financial flow, as well as the continuing importance of fashion, art, the media, dance, consumption, leisure, research, play, collective consumption, travel, tourism, education, and governance (Thrift, 1996b), place a premium on reflexivity, interpretation, and innovation – the key assets of urban areas. As he argues, "the worlds of action which make up the [reflexive] city economy and society are hybrids, constrained by the machine-like forces of late modern capitalism, but themselves enabled by the ways that system not only permits, but in certain ways, thrives on social reflexivity" (Storper, 1996, p. 32).

Chapter 22

Best Practice? Geography, Learning, and the Institutional Limits to Strong Convergence

Meric S. Gertler

According to an increasingly accepted view, the sovereignty of national economies has been eroded to the point where nation-states "have become little more than bit actors" (Ohmae, 1995, p. 12). With the development of globalized financial markets, the rising power of multinational corporations (MNCs), and the emergence of a new set of supranational institutions to govern economic processes on a continental or world scale, nation-states are said to have lost the ability to manage their own domestic economic affairs, having ceded control over exchange rates, investment, and even fiscal policy to extranational forces (Strange, 1997). Moreover, with the increasing leverage and reach of MNCs further contributing to the erosion of national economic sovereignty, the once distinctive character of particular national industrial "models" is said to be under imminent threat.

While it may still be possible to identify at least three clearly distinctive national models – an Anglo-American model, a Rhineland (German) model, and a Japanese model – the decline of national institutions, the intensification of competitive forces on a global scale, and the cross-penetration of national markets by MNCs are said to have propelled a process of *convergence* between these different national models. In most representations of this globalization dynamic, convergence is regarded as inexorable and unstoppable.

One of the most important processes underpinning this dynamic is learning. At the global level, large corporate actors are allegedly learning from each other, so that the most successful corporate practices are emulated and diffused crossnationally at an increasingly rapid pace. In the late 1980s and early 1990s, considerable attention was devoted to the diffusion of methods of production and workplace organization perfected by Japanese producers of cars and consumer electronics, in which American, Canadian, and European manufacturers were shown to be learning methods such as just-in-time, kaizen/continuous improvement, and other aspects of lean production techniques from their Japanese competitors (Womack et al., 1990). Since the resurgence of the United States economy beginning in the second half of the 1990s, American practices have apparently become the object of global firms' affections, with large corporations in Europe and Asia adopting the core characteristics of US-style "shareholder capitalism"; especially flexible labor market practices, "reengineering," and the empowerment of shareholders (*The Economist*, 1996a, 1996b).

Closely bound up with this narrative on convergence and learning is the key concept of "best practice," a term which has diffused into the lexicon of business school theory, corporate rhetoric, management consulting, and the popular business press with startling speed. It reflects the idea that there is one universal standard against which firms (anywhere) can and should measure their operational performance. Moreover, best practice is applied to both outcomes (e.g., defect rates per thousand; labor hours per vehicle assembled) and processes (e.g., ISO 9000 and ISO 14000 standards for quality management and environmental practices; as well as specific techniques and modes of production organization). Not surprisingly, an entire industry dedicated to the benchmarking of firms' practices, processes, and achievements has arisen, led by international management consultancies such as McKinsey, Boston Consulting Group, KPMG, PricewaterhouseCoopers, and others.

Despite the compelling nature of this narrative about learning-driven convergence and best practice, at least two major questions remain contentious and unresolved. First, what are the principal mechanisms and channels through which learning-drive convergence is alleged to take place? The absence of detailed analysis of this issue in both the scholarly literature and the business press is troubling. Concepts such as learning and best practice have become, implicitly, both self-evident and unassailable. As a result they have also become deproblematized, in the sense that not only the definition but also their implementation and attainment are accepted as straightforward. The arguments presented in this paper aim to demonstrate the utter folly of this position, while analyzing the principal mechanisms and processes through which learning-driven convergence could conceivably be achieved.

Second, while the evolutionary paradigm in economics (Hodgson, 1988, 1993; Nelson, 1995), as well as the closely associated multidisciplinary field of socioeconomics (Granovetter and Swedberg, 1993), emphasize the central role played by institutions in the structuring of practices inside the firm and in interfirm relations, there remains considerable debate and uncertainty about which institutions matter, how they exert their influence to shape, constrain, limit, or govern firms' practices and ability to learn, and whether or not this is changing at present. In particular, our understanding of the role of these institutions in mediating social learning processes by firms remains rather underdeveloped. These questions also raise the important issue of scale: what is the relative importance of different scales of institutional governance in the regulation of these economic processes? In this paper, the well-known arguments about the declining purchase of the nation-state and the rise of new institutional forms at the regional level to fill the regulatory void will be reconsidered, along with a set of more recent claims about the growing importance of a third source of governance of the firm whose influence allegedly transcends institutional boundaries at both the regional and the national scale.

Mechanisms and Channels of Learning-Driven Convergence

Since "convergence" appears to mean many things to many people, it is best to begin by clarifying the sense in which it is being used in the present context. Simply put, convergence may be said to occur when firms originating in different national institutional spaces implement the same production methods or practices. Here, "methods or practices" must be broadly defined to embrace two different scales. They include practices *internal* to the individual firm, such as the use of particular machinery and process technologies, production systems, and the organization of work flow, the division of labor within individual plants or offices, quality management approaches, inventory management systems, employment relations, and inter-divisional relationships (between, for example, research and development, production, and marketing).

They also include practices *external* to the firm, that is interfirm relationships and transactions of both a vertical and horizontal nature. The former encompass relations with customers and suppliers, the types of relationships established (e.g., contractual/arm's length, collaborative), including what Lundvall (1988) and others refer to as user–producer interaction, as well as the technologies used to support transactions (logistics, information systems). The latter refer to relations between firms in the same or closely related industries (e.g., direct collaboration, other forms of associative action) and firms' relations with institutions (e.g., education and training, research, producers' associations, chambers of commerce).

Two further comments on this definition are warranted. First, this broad definition of "practices" is adopted explicitly to foreground the social context in which they are developed, diffused, and implemented. It also corresponds to broader conceptions of "technology," not dissimilar to classical Marxian definitions which emphasize both forces of production and the social relations in which those forces are applied (Harvey, 1982). Second, notice as well that "convergence" as employed here does *not* refer to the narrow economic definition of diminishing differences in incomes, wages, productivity, or industrial structure between regions over time (for a critical review of this literature, see Martin and Sunley, 1998). While the processes outlined above may ultimately lead to such outcomes, this is by no means a foregone conclusion.

Before considering the actual mechanisms or channels of convergence, it is important to make one further distinction which is frequently overlooked in less-than-systematic accounts of convergence dynamics – that is, the key distinction between weak and strong convergence. When a firm originating in country **A** establishes (or acquires) a branch in a new host country **B**, and adopts the distinctive practices characteristic of the host country (**B**) at its foreign site, this constitutes convergence of a sort. However, when the same firm adopts "country **B**" practices for implementation in its home country (**A**) operations (with or without having first established a foreign branch), arguably a much more profound form of convergence has occurred. One must therefore distinguish between the former (an example of weak convergence) and the latter (strong convergence). This is more than a semantic distinction. While the former case provides evidence of the growing internationalization of production systems, it stops well short of dismantling the characteristic practices that constitute the industrial "model" of either country **A** or country **B**. While some might be tempted to argue that one ultimately leads to the other, that learning and adoption of new practices abroad represent a first step toward their implementation at home, there is no a priori reason why this would be either desirable or easily attainable. We return to these issues below. First, however, we shall consider the precise mechanisms through which such convergence processes might unfold.

Channels of convergence

The issue of how convergence in industrial practices might actually occur has been considered so obvious or self-evident as to require no systematic consideration. Implicitly, the logic runs something like the following. Firms somehow become aware of a best practice (which differs from their own status quo) and, once enlightened, simply implement the new practice in straightforward fashion. Notice the number of hidden assumptions and processes embedded in this simple approach. First, the notion of "the firm": presumably, what is usually meant by this is individual managers within these firms, although the dynamic of competition between individuals or divisions within large firms is not acknowledged (Schoenberger, 1997).

The next step, somehow become aware of a best practice, is equally problematic on two grounds. First, the process by which firms become aware is rarely if ever spelled out; second, the status of best practice is itself assumed to be self-evident. The characteristic of universal superiority is presumed to have been established, as have the criterion/criteria by which this superiority is to be judged. Moreover, there is an implicit presumption above that, once firms have become aware of a new practice which they believe to be superior to their own status quo, they will strive to adopt the new alternative. Clearly, this is somewhat unrealistic since the cost of change may be high and the anticipated benefits must be large enough to justify these costs. It is probably more reasonable to assume that firms depart from the status quo only when they perceive some kind of crisis or major threat to their competitive position. As for the final step, in which firms "simply implement the new practice in straightforward fashion," even a moment's reflection should be sufficient to convince one that this process is nowhere near as simple as it might seem. The annals of technology implementation analysis are replete with case studies in which new process technologies or modes of work organization have encountered serious – sometimes fatal – difficulties (Gertler, 1995). While the origins of these difficulties are often alleged to include insufficient investment in training of managers and workers, poor initial design, and overly enthusiastic sales people who make unsustainable promises concerning the capabilities of new technologies, the real foundations for such problems are usually found at a much deeper, institutional level, as we shall see below.

Although each of the steps outlined above is seriously problematic, the one which has received the least attention in prior research is step two: how firms "become aware of a best practice," and all of the issues implicitly associated with this process. One helpful approach to this question invokes actor-network theory from the sociology of scientific knowledge (Callon, 1991; Blauhof, 1994). This tradition views the diffusion of process innovations as the circulation of conventions which are promoted through three types of channel or media: texts (industry conferences, industry and trade journals); people (actors such as consultants, seconded employees, new hires, other personal contacts, social networks); and artifacts ("hard" technologies, including advanced machinery, information and communication technologies,

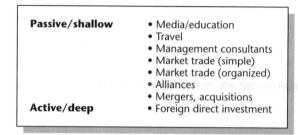

Figure 22.1 Channels of convergence: a continuum of opportunities for learning-through-interaction

database systems). Furthermore, it argues that such innovations are more likely to be adopted when they are perceived by firms to be capable of responding to specific operational problems.

This approach has the virtue of emphasizing the active and social nature of the process by which practices (best and otherwise) migrate between firms, industries, regions, and countries. While it is a helpful beginning, it can be improved upon. Among other things, despite signaling the social nature of the practice-diffusion process, the role accorded to actors (agents) in shaping firms' practices is far too large since it fails to acknowledge a significant enough role for institutions (structures) at a variety of spatial scales. Moreover, the three-way typology of texts, people, and artifacts is not sufficiently specific. By focusing on the *medium* through which interaction occurs rather than the nature of the interaction *process* itself, this scheme is of limited use: a more systematic typology would differentiate between different channels of transmission according to their *degree of activeness* since some forms of interaction are clearly more important while others are more superficial.

[To address the issue of greater differentiation between various channels, Gertler proposes and discusses an eightfold classification of channels, ranging from passive/shallow to active deep (Figure 22.1): Media (print, video, electronic); travel (attending conferences or conducting site visits and tours to witness new practices); hiring management consultants; simple market trade (purchasing commodities "off the shelf"); organized market transactions (significant departures from existing practice requires extended interaction and information sharing between producers and users who ideally are geographically, organizationally, and culturally proximate); alliances (extra-market collaboration for the purpose of sharing and/or jointly developing technology); mergers/acquisitions (where learning occurs through explicit ownership stakes in new practices); and foreign direct investment (acquiring existing assets or establishing new production facilities abroad, a long-term commitment often accompanied by exchange of personnel among branches and the head office).]

Scale and the institutional governance of industrial practices

In this section, I critically assess three sets of arguments concerning institution influences on firm practices which are differentiated primarily on the basis of scale: regional, national, and firm-level.

Regional institutions: "embeddedness" and the learning region thesis

Perhaps no idea has gained currency with more speed and enthusiasm within eco-nomic geography than the notion that place plays a key role in determining the innovative capabilities and performance of individual firms (A. J. Scott, 1988b, 1996; Porter, 1990; Putnam, 1993; Saxenian, 1994; Storper, 1997; Cooke and Morgan, 1998).

The central argument [is] that the geography of economic advantage and innovative capability is highly uneven, owing primarily to spatial variation in the social-institutional character of places. In these lucky places, firms become "embedded" in close vertical and horizontal relationships with other nearby firms, and within a rich, thick local-institutional matrix that supports and facilitates the production (private and socially organized), transmission, and propagation of new technologies (product and process). The ability of firms in such regions to do so is based on shared language, culture, norms and conventions, attitudes, values, and expectations which generate trust and facilitate the all-important flow of tacit and proprietary knowledge between firms (Grabher, 1993; Amin and Thrift, 1994). In other words, a set of characteristic practices emerges and rapidly spreads to many firms within the region, becoming in turn a part of the shared conventions characteristic of the local production cluster (Storper, 1997).

Closely related is the idea that such regions can be characterized as learning regions: that is, places which foster social learning processes amongst firms, between firms and other local organizations, and reflexive learning by local and regional economic development agencies in the public and quasi-public sector (Florida, 1995; Morgan, 1997). Under such conditions, the "region-state" emerges as the scale best suited to the management of economic development and innovation. Especially important institutional entities include research centers and universities, other educational and training institutions, local producers' associations, chambers of commerce, and technology-transfer agencies. Taken together, these elements have been characterized as constituting a *regional innovation system* (Braczyk et al., 1998). It is these institutional forces which are seen as being primarily responsible for producing and reproducing the characteristic firm practices (both internal and interfirm) which are so important to the economic success of such regions.

Underlying these arguments about the rising prominence of the region-state as a source of successful economic governance is the parallel idea that the spread of the global economy has undermined and hollowed out the nation-state. National gov-ernments are viewed as no longer capable of governing the practices of firms within their borders to ensure economic prosperity, having ceded this role to institutions at the subnational (regional) and, to some extent, supranational levels (Ohmae, 1995). Indeed, this view has become so widely accepted as "received wisdom" that it has provided the rationale and guiding framework for economic development policy initiatives at the subnational level in many countries.

However, as we shall see below, there may be good reasons to approach the learn-ing region and region-state hypotheses with a healthy degree of skepticism and caution.

National institutions: innovation systems, business systems, and the nation-state

A growing body of research asserts the following thesis. Notwithstanding the unde-niably increasing influence of supranational institutions such as the European Union, the North American Free Trade Agreement, and the World Trade Organi-zation, and while acknowledging the growing importance of the region-state and other non-state regional initiatives, the nation-state and its institutional legacy still continue to exert a crucial influence over the practices of firms. However, precisely how this influence is exerted remains the subject of some debate, with at least two diverging views evident.

Pauly and Reich (1997) find that multinational corporations forever bear the markings or imprint of their national origins. The path or strategy they choose is most strongly shaped by the national institutional legacy of their *home* country. These findings are consistent with the body of work which has been framed within national systems of innovation perspective. The contributors to Lundvall (1992), Nelson (1993), and Edquist (1997), as well as Pavitt and Patel (1995), assert that distinctive nationally organized constellations of institutions shape firms' innova-tion practices and longer-term trajectories. There is no compelling evidence of con-vergence in national activities for technological accumulation since the 1970s and even some evidence of divergence, implying that national innovation systems have become more (not less) distinctive over time.

Another related literature – on national business systems – offers a complemen-tary perspective which goes well beyond the study of innovation-generating activi-ties alone to argue that virtually *all firm practices* (day-to-day practices as well as long-term strategies) are strongly influenced or governed (though not wholly determined) by national macro-regulatory institutions and "market rules" (Maurice et al., 1986; Christopherson, 1993, 1999; Streeck, 1996; Lane, 1997; Whitley, 1998, 1999; O'Sullivan, 2000). Moreover, firms are quite often not conscious of the influence that this larger institutional matrix exerts on their choice of practices. The argument implicit in this literature is that the contours of the national macro-regulatory framework make certain choices easier or more likely, and others less so.

Other recent work suggests that the framework national institutions of the economies are most influential in shaping the practices and strategies of multi-national firms abroad. Wever (1995) examines the experiences of American firms operating branches in Germany as well as German firms with branches in the United States. In a detailed assessment of these cases, she reports that both sets of firms were frustrated in their attempts to institute the "home" way of doing things in their foreign branch operations. Hence, according to Wever, when MNCs go abroad, the rules of the host country hold sway.

In another study of the transfer of German practices and technology abroad, I conducted interviews with German advanced machinery manufacturers serving the Canadian and American markets (Gertler, 1996), having also interviewed their customers in Canada. The overwhelming conclusion of this work was that the most fundamental sources of difficulty for the North American users (including German-owned user plants) stemmed from the starkly different macro-regulatory environment and institutions regulating labor markets, industrial relations, corporate governance, and capital markets in these two "models" (Gertler, 1999). In other words, the "host rules" prevailed here too, even though they did not provide a very effective framework for the implementation of German manufacturing practices in North America.

Finally, Schoenberger's (1999) recent analysis of US multinationals with Japanese branches lends further support to the argument that rules in the national "host" setting prevail. Her case study of Xerox corporation reveals that the American parent had ample opportunity to learn from the obviously successful practices of its Japanese subsidiary (a joint venture with Fuji), but failed to do so. While Schoenberger attributes this failure to the "cultural crisis of the firm," her analysis raises some important questions about the difficulties or barriers to intrafirm learning across major boundaries between distinct national systems (a theme to which I shall return below).

The work reviewed above offers many important insights in support of the general proposition that the nation-state (whether "home" or "host") is still a primary source of influence over industrial practices. Moreover, this work argues implicitly that all firms are embedded within an institutional matrix whether they realize it or not. This is *not* a process that happens just in those places lucky enough to have abundant trust and local institutional thickness. As a result, according to this view, the success with which firms can transpose a distinctive set of practices from one national space to another (i.e., learn) where the institutional environment is not as conducive or supportive of such practices will be limited at best. Moreover, although there is very little analysis of this issue in the literature, the same limitations ought to apply to *interfirm* as well as *intrafirm* practices. Hence, for example, to what degree and how successfully can German or Japanese firms setting up production operations in North America also re-create the unique set of "network" user–producer (or buyer–supplier) relations that have been so important to the earlier competitive success of their home operations? Moreover, given that the key macro-regulatory features of the German "stakeholder capitalism" model and the Japanese variant are so different from those in North America (Christopherson, 1993, 1999; Wever, 1995; Pauly and Reich, 1997; Lane, 1997; Whitley, 1999; O'Sullivan, 2000), what impact might this have on (i) the ability of these foreign firms to transpose their internal and interfirm practices to North America, or (ii) their ability to transpose lessons learned in their North American operations back to their home plants? After all, in order for us to be able to document strong convergence between national industrial models, we would need to find evidence that North American (or Anglo-American) practices learned abroad were in fact being imported back to Germany or Japan to transform practices there. In order to answer these questions, it is necessary to develop a detailed understanding of the processes by which interfirm learning occurs.

Appealing as this line of argument is, it suffers from limitations. The region remains somewhat underdeveloped in these accounts. Moreover, we should be concerned to avoid the pitfalls of an excessive reliance on "methodological nationalism." Clearly, our explanatory framework must accommodate qualitative variation between firms and the role of management in shaping outcomes.

The firm: capability, absorptive capacity, learning and communities of practice

The large and well-established literature on corporate strategy suggests that there will be important variations from firm to firm in their willingness or ability to implement particular workplace practices or to engage successfully in interfirm and international learning processes (Porter, 1980; Mueller and Loveridge, 1995). Recently, this level of analysis has begun to attract much more attention within economic geography (see, for example, Schoenberger, 1997; Dicken, 1998). Firm-centered approaches privilege the firm as the decisive institution shaping its own practices.

Ever since the publication of Michael Porter's classic *Competitive Strategy* (1980) two decades ago, the fundamental notion – perhaps best thought of as the original conceit of modern management theory – is that firms have the potential to be "masters of their own destiny." In its full-blown form, this idea has even been extended beyond the boundaries of the single firm, suggesting that firms can determine not only their own internal practices and performance, but also actively shape or control the competitive environment around them.

More recent approaches have shown considerably more humility on this matter, in particular the resource-based or capability-based view of the firm. According to this approach, the firm can be thought of as a collection of capabilities. The firm's competitive success is seen to depend especially on its ability to develop and exploit its own distinctive capabilities – that is, those which cannot be easily replicated by competitors (Kay, 1996; Maskell and Malmberg, 1999). In the capability-based approach, most of the assets which constitute a firm's distinctive capabilities must accumulate over time and may include things such as brand identity and reputation, but also knowledge and routines embedded within teams, and relationships between the firm and its customers and suppliers.

Moreover, it is the *tacit knowledge* produced and reproduced in these teams and relationships, based on shared norms and conventions, which is seen to be key. Here, capability and absorptive capacity merge with the closely related competence-based view of the firm, which conceives of the firm as a processor of knowledge (Fransman, 1994). Since the firm's innovative capability is seen to be dependent on its ability to process (generate, maintain, replicate, modify, and, when necessary, forget) knowledge, this approach places key emphasis on cognitive or learning mechanisms and the routines that support them. As in our earlier discussion of learning dynamics at the regional scale, this approach also views learning as fundamentally social in nature. However, the most important scale at which these social learning dynamics unfold is the *community of practice* (Brown and Duguid, 1996; Wenger, 1998). Communities of practice are groups of individuals informally bound together by shared expertise and a common problem. Typically a single large organization will contain multiple communities of practice – leading to a process of "distributed learning" – and the communities may also span the boundary of a single organization to include those in other organizations working on similar issues. These communities serve as the principal ensemble in which "learning-in-working" occurs through a collective, shared process of problem-solving, trial and error, and experimentation which leads to the development of new routines, conventions, and norms. In essence, communities of practice are seen as the principal mechanism through which tacit knowledge relating to new practices is produced and spread.

They are also presented as vehicles through which "best practices" may be spread throughout large (including multilocational) organizations (Ichigo et al., 1998; Brown and Duguid, 2000; Wenger and Snyder, 2000).

Amin (2000) takes this idea one step further by offering a provocative suggestion that the received wisdom within economic geography and related disciplines concerning the centrality of the region as a source of innovation, learning, and tacit knowledge production is perhaps misguided. Instead, he offers up the possibility that *relational organizational proximity* (i.e., that which is achieved through communities of practice) might be more important than *geographical proximity* in constituting "the 'soft' architecture of learning." While relational proximity may depend to some extent on face-to-face interaction, "it can also be achieved at a distance," thanks to modern communications technology and global business travel.

Amin's critique of the learning region hypothesis is salutary, for it reminds us of the importance of nonlocal organizational ties in the production of innovations and the transmission of new practices. It is especially welcome too for emphasizing the existence and importance of diversity and variation within large organizations – a view which dispenses once and for all with the myth of the unitary organization.

Welcome as these insights are, one cannot help but wonder about the accuracy of the assumptions underlying them. The idea that organizational or relational proximity is sufficient to transcend the effects of distance (even when assisted by telecommunications and frequent travel) seems improbable. The contention that communities of practice can serve as the vector through which best practices are disseminated between different locales within the global corporation seems problematic in light of our earlier discussion concerning the limits imposed on the transfer of firm practices by regulatory frameworks at the national level. There is little acknowledgement that systemic institutional influences might play an important role in helping determine which practices will flow between locations most easily and which will not.

This is not to deny the possibility or feasibility of transferring best practices from one national setting to another. Under certain circumstances – that is, when the institutional and regulatory framework in the "sending" and "receiving" country are similar – this kind of "convergence" will be relatively easy to achieve. When they differ, as in the work of Wever (1995) and others discussed above, this will be considerably more difficult even for global firms with deep resources.

Conclusion: Requirements of a New Theory of Firm Practices

Returning to the central question of this paper – how are firm practices determined, and what does this tell us about the likelihood of convergence being achieved – we are now in a better position to evaluate the competing arguments and theoretical perspectives. It seems clear from the foregoing analysis that each of the major contenders does not, on its own, provide an adequate explanatory framework.

If one accepts the central insight of Polanyi (1944) that the market is socially constructed and governed – and *not* a "natural," given, inevitable form – then it makes perfect sense that firms in market economies should also be constructed to some extent by their social-institutional environment. The analysis presented above suggests strongly that firms' choice of practices is constrained by more than the limits of their internal resources (financial, organizational, technological, creative) and strategic vision. However, this view is still not sophisticated enough to help us understand how firm practices arise and change over time.

Among other things, a revised approach must give greater credence to the path-dependent nature of geo-corporate change. For example, when a firm "arrives" in a location inside a new national-institutional space (via FDI), it is not a blank slate – that is, it continues to bear many strong markings and influences from its origins (Doremus et al., 1998). These characteristics are bound to interact with local institutional signals, influences, and characteristics in dialectical ways to produce a new set of practices which conform to neither "original" model – Abo's (1996) "hybrid factories" and the German variant of "lean production" (Streeck, 1996) come to mind here.

Second, it is important to reemphasize the undeniable reality that not all firms or managers are created equal: the agency of these actors does matter. They respond in different ways to the same challenges, based on their own histories, education, experience, temperament, corporate cultures, distinctive capabilities, intangible assets, and so on. Any revised theory of firm practices must make adequate room for individual, collective, and corporate agency within the firm. But at the same time, it is clearly misguided to argue that firms shape their own practices independently of wider, systemic influences.

Third, a revised theory of firm practices should also be supple enough to accommodate a role for regional institutions. For example, in the case of German firms bringing industrial practices to their newly established production operations in the United States, we might expect such influences to be exerted at both ends of the process, especially for small and medium-sized *(Mittelstand)* firms, which typically take on a characteristic set of practices that are strongly shaped by the distinctive institutional contours of many of Germany's *Länder* (states) and substate regions (Sabel, 1989; Herrigel, 1994; Cooke and Morgan, 1998; Braczyk et al., 1998). These analysts stress the dense concentration of institutions at the *Länd* level which shape labor markets, industrial relations, training, investment, and industrial organization, forging important horizontal linkages across firms in the same industry. These institutions include not only government agencies and educational institutions, but also private producers' associations and chambers of commerce. There is also a need to consider the influence of key institutions and characteristics at the regional scale on the "receiving end," as an important intervening force helping to shape the process by which firms transpose industrial practices and strategies from one national space (and continent) to another. How important are regional features such as state- or provincially-regulated industrial relations regimes, education and training systems, research, development, and (more broadly defined) innovation policies? What role does local history play in this process? These questions have received surprisingly little attention thus far.

Coming back to our original question – about the true prevalence of convergence and prospects for future industrial and institutional evolution – it is important to keep in mind that true "strong" convergence requires best practices learned abroad to be transposed (with minimal modification) back home. The arguments presented in this paper suggest that the prospects for strong convergence are limited at best, and will remain so as long as national institutional frameworks retain their distinctive character. They also suggest that the idea of a single, universal, bound-ary-transcending "best practice" is utterly unattainable, even though it may well be in management's interest to perpetuate the myth of a single standard against which all local practices must be measured.

This analysis also reminds us that while *firms'* practices may converge, this does not necessarily translate into convergence of national systems, especially when the firms in question are multinational ones. For example, it will be considerably easier for a German firm to adopt Anglo-American practices by implementing these at pro-duction sites in the US or the UK than in its domestic operations. While there are undeniable pressures for change at home – supported, as Clark et al. (2001, 2002) point out, by the adoption of Anglo-American accounting practices amongst large German firms whose shares are publicly traded – fundamental questions remain. Are these sufficient conditions to bring about *system-wide* change (i.e., strong con-vergence) in a country such as Germany? How do the interests of internationally mobile managers within these large firms interact with those of other stakeholders (labor, consumers, small business, governments) to determine the path of change? Given that the large majority of *Mittelstand* firms remain privately held and con-trolled, how pervasive might such influences actually be?

In addition to advancing the state of our theoretical understanding of how prac-tices are shaped, the accompanying empirical study of how convergence actually works (or doesn't) is also sorely underdeveloped. The multi-channel approach presented in this paper may offer one promising avenue to explore in this regard. It is only through detailed, systematic, historically grounded case studies that we will once and for all be able to distinguish between the rhetoric and the reality of convergence.

Chapter 23

Blood, Thicker than Water: Interpersonal Relations and Taiwanese Investment in Southern China

Y. Hsing

In this paper I explore the question of cultural and institutional conditions that shape the processes of transnational capital flows, by looking at Taiwanese manufacturing investment in southern China. Since the late 1970s, Taiwan, like other Asian newly industrialized economies, has been caught in a squeeze between lower wage Third World competitors and the growing protectionism in the markets of the OECD (Organization for Economic Cooperation and Development). Taiwan's export-oriented manufacturing factories then began to move to Malaysia, Thailand, Indonesia, and the Philippines, where cheap labor was plentiful. However, in the 1980s, the rise in labor costs and the unstable political environment in many of these countries forced Taiwanese manufacturers to look elsewhere. In the meantime, China's Open Door policy caught the attention of Taiwanese manufacturers, who responded quickly to the new opportunity (Hsing, 1997). By 1991 Taiwan had surpassed the USA and Japan to become the second largest investor in China after Hong Kong. Realized direct investment from Taiwan to China totaled US $8–10 billion in 1994, which accounted for 20% of China's total foreign direct investment; and provided more than 5 million jobs, of which 70% were concentrated in the Provinces of Guangdong and Fujian.

Taiwanese manufacturing investment in southern China represents a new pattern of the foreign direct investment found in the rapidly industrializing regions. The new pattern of foreign direct investment is characterized by investors who are not vertically integrated giant transnational corporations. Instead, they are mostly small- and medium-sized, independent manufacturing firms. In addition, in contrast to the common pattern of foreign direct investment, which is based on the interaction between transnational corporations and the national government, the new pattern of investment is shaped by small investors negotiating with low-level local governments in the host country. The investment is made more effective because of two major favorable conditions, namely, the newly gained economic autonomy of local governments in southern China; and the cultural affinity between the Taiwanese investors and their local agents in China.

Beginning from revising the model of a new international division of labor, in which cheap labor is seen as the main driving force of transnational capital flows (Fröbel et al., 1980), in this study of Taiwanese direct investment in southern China I show that although, since the 1980s, capital might have moved freely across national boundaries (see for example Carnoy, 1993; Castells, 1993; Johnston, 1986), it is still confined by institutional and cultural boundaries. Transnational capital has by no means flooded in all directions, as the terms "footloose" or "borderless world" (Ohmae, 1990) might imply. Nor has transnational capital followed a universally applicable set of strategies of accumulation and expansion in different places. Globalization does not produce homogeneity. Such an "unevenness" is generated, on the one hand, from the specificity and diversity of the locality itself. Globalization is conditioned by, and interacts with, local interpretations (Giddens, 1994, p. 5). In their studies of localities in the face of globalization, Bagguley et al. (1990), Ong (1991), and Hall (1991) show that elements such as production organization, power structure, ethnic–racial constitutions, gender and labor relations, the cultural system, historical construction, and the intersections of these elements define the problematic of a locality.

On the other hand, transnational capital is not homogeneous either. Although US, Western European, and Japan-based giant multinationals continue to play a critical role in the global economy, international investments by the newly industrialized countries (NICs), especially investments from Brazil, South Korea, Hong Kong, and Taiwan, have received increased recognition (Agrawal, 1981; Allen and Hamnett, 1995, pp. 88–9; Chang and Thomson, 1994; Jo, 1981; Lall, 1985; Sercovich, 1984; Wells, 1983; White, 1981). In literature on the NIC-based multinationals the focus has been on how they behave differently from the "traditional" multinationals in terms of investment scales, levels of technological input, labor intensity, and the establishment of local production linkages. Though some writers believe that "Third World MNCs" (multinational corporations) have a greater potential to transfer more appropriate technologies to the host country, and are under greater pressure to purchase inputs locally because of their smaller scale (Lall, 1984; Wells, 1983), others argue that, although smaller in scale, the new MNCs are not qualitatively different from the traditional ones (Jenkins, 1987, pp. 159–62). However, given the increasingly diverse organizational characteristics of transnational capitals and their investment strategies (for example, strategic alliance, international subcontracting, etc.), the dichotomy of "traditional" versus "new" multinationals is now less of an aid to understanding the interaction between local societies and transnational capitals. As the production, marketing, and financing arrangements between transnational capitals and local economic systems become increasingly complex, the differences between transnational capitals lie not only between traditional and new multinationals, but also between those of different organizational characteristics (Lim and Fong, 1982). Our inquiry, therefore, should be about the process and impact of specific investment patterns undertaken by specific types of capital in specific places.

Furthermore, corporate strategies and behaviors are not just the results of straightforward economic calculations in a vacuum. Instead, they are shaped by a set of socially and territorially grounded relationships. Economic processes are socially structured by ethnicity, gender, and other social and institutional elements.

In terms of regional production networks, the social and institutional basis for the economic organization is mainly composed of the competitive and cooperative mechanisms among firms, the function of trade associations, the structure of labor markets, the dynamism of the local government, and so on. Some of the institutional elements are less formalized and therefore, more personalized than others. Long term and face-to-face interactions amongst agents also contribute to the establishment and consolidation of interpersonal networks, which in turn generate intellectual ambience, trusting relationships, and information exchanges. The synergy created by interpersonal networks further enhances the flexibility, adaptivity, and competitiveness of firms and regional economies. Interpersonal network building is also a process of culture formation, represented by specific patterns of business practices and social interaction in specific institutional contexts.

If the interpersonal networks are socially embedded and territorially specified, what would happen to the networks when the capitals expand from one territory to another? Under which conditions will investors from outside the region be able to establish effective social networks in the new territory? And again, along which dimensions does the specificity of the capital affect the processes and consequences of such cross-territorial investments? These questions have to be explored in a more specific historical conjuncture. In the case of Taiwanese investment in southern China since the 1980s, one of the most intriguing characteristics of the investment is the historical connection and the cultural affinity between the investors and their local partners. Since the late 1980s Taiwanese investment in China has been a part of the fast growing "Greater China" economic circle (including China, Taiwan, and Hong Kong). In the meantime the formation of the Southeast Asian "growth triangle," composed of Singapore, Malaysia, and Indonesia, has also been conducted mainly by overseas Chinese firms in these regions. These trade and investment alliances seem to suggest that there is some correlation between culture, history, and the direction of transnational capital flows. However, it is still not very clear how such cultural and historical connections affect the establishment of the interpersonal networks in the process of capital expansion, or, what the cultural principles that facilitate the establishment of the interpersonal networks are. If culture is defined as a given set of values and behavior codes of a specific people, and it is assumed that there is such a thing as "Chinese culture," then what are the principles unique to Chinese culture (or, the principles that make Chinese culture different from other cultures) that are shared by Taiwanese investors and their Chinese partners, and have facilitated the interpersonal network building between them? If culture is defined not only as a set of values but also a historically and institutionally situated dynamism (Ong, 1987), how do we understand the interaction between the general cultural principles in Chinese traditions and specific institutional conditions in southern China, which have provided the basis for interpersonal network building between Taiwanese investors and their local Chinese partners?

Most writers agree that the foundation of the Chinese style of business organization is familism (which usually includes nepotism, paternalism, and family ownership in firm organization) and "long-term personalistic ties," or *guanxi* in Chinese, on which a trusting and reciprocal obligatory relationship is built between business partners. The question of interpersonal ties in economic processes has had a long tradition in anthropological studies, especially within the framework of "gift exchange" (Curtin, 1984; Malinowski, 1961; Mauss, 1967; Sahlins, 1972; Yang, 1988, 1989, 1994). Gift exchange is understood as a process of building trusting interpersonal relationships in economic activities. What needs to be explored further is how, if at all, is the gift exchange practiced in the Chinese societies, or in the process of Taiwanese investment in southern China, different from the gift exchange in other societies and cultures.

The historical and institutional contexts in southern China since the economic reform began, especially the increasing fiscal autonomy of local authorities, have shaped the forms and contents of gift exchange and the way Taiwanese investors establish interpersonal relations with local Chinese officials. Decentralized economic policymaking in China provides the basis for local authorities to bypass the central government and to link up with transnational capital directly. The greatly enhanced bureaucratic flexibility at the local level has been particularly crucial for the Taiwanese capital which is characterized by small scales, network form of organization, export orientation, and time sensitivity.

My analysis in this paper is based on my interviews conducted in Taiwan, Hong Kong, Guangdong (the Pearl River Delta), Fujian (Xiaman Special Economic Zone), and Shanghai in 1991, 1992, 1993, and 1994. I conducted interviews with 54 local Chinese officials and 134 Taiwanese and Hong Kong investors, factory managers, and Chinese managers, staff, and workers in the factories. I focused my factory interviews on the export fashion shoe industry, and stayed in two Taiwanese-invested fashion shoe factories in the Pearl River Delta for one month.

Economic Autonomy of China's Local Governments

The decentralization of economic resources from the central government to local governments at the county and municipality levels, and the increasing economic autonomy of local authorities and the active role played by local officials, have been two of the major characteristics of China's recent economic reforms.

The economic autonomy of China's local government is characterized by fiscal sovereignty and responsibility. There have been various revenue-sharing schemes which provide incentives to local governments to collect taxes and to engage directly in profit-making activities. At the same time, the central government permitted provinces to engage in foreign trade through local branches of the national foreign trade corporation (Ho and Huenemann, 1984; Solinger, 1987; Zhang and Zou, 1994).

The county and municipal governments have also enjoyed the authority of approving foreign investment projects. The county government has the full author-ity to grant the permission for those projects under US $3 million; higher rank municipal authorities have as high as US $10 million leeway. The municipal and county governments can also issue import–export licenses, set up independent customs, grant industrial and residential land under a certain size, offer favorable investment conditions for foreign firms, and so on. Many state-owned enterprises have been transformed into collective enterprises which are owned and run by local governments at different levels.

Compared with other regions in China, the provinces of Guangdong and Fujian have enjoyed the greatest economic autonomy. This is because of their geographical position in the periphery and their strong social ties with overseas Chinese funding sources. Guangdong and Fujian could also retain a large portion of the foreign exchange which they earned from exports and tourism as well as a share of the remittances the residents of the two provinces received from abroad.

The increasing fiscal autonomy was accompanied by the gain of financial responsibility by local authorities. Indeed many of the local bureaucrats are highly motivated in exploiting the new opportunities provided by the fiscal reform for their own personal gains. Yet, motivation also came from another source: the greater financial responsibility that the central authority transferred to the local governments. Local governments were required to be self-sufficient financially, and had to search for additional revenues to fund the increasing local shares in the expenditures on infrastructure construction, education, public health, and other items.

The highly motivated local officials with their newly gained economic authority, who were also the only qualified partners for foreign capitals to establish joint ventures in China, have been the most important agents for Taiwanese investment in southern China. Local officials tend to be more flexible than central government officials in their implementation of regulations and are more willing to cooperate with overseas investors. Indeed their practices can be seen as various degrees of corruption. Yet, such a moral judgment can hardly help us to understand the local politics of foreign direct investment in China. Many of the Taiwanese and Hong Kong investors whom I interviewed agreed that it is faster and simpler to deal with the local than the provincial or central authorities. For export-oriented manufacturing, in which most of the overseas Chinese investors were engaged, speedy production and delivery are the most important competitive edges in the world market. Delayed deliveries often result in reduction of payment or cancellation of orders. The need to bypass the formal, bureaucratic procedures and to keep production and delivery moving as quickly as possible is important, particularly for the small- and medium-sized producers with limited operational capital. Lower-level officials at the county and city levels, motivated by the new fiscal schemes, are more willing to accommodate the need of overseas investors to speed up the application process of investment projects and are often willing to make flexible arrangements with individual investors.

The possibility of making "flexible" deals with the low-level Chinese officials has been a major attraction to the small- and medium-sized investors from Taiwan and Hong Kong. Some medium-sized to large-sized investors even split their investment into a number of smaller projects so as to avoid the involvement of higher-level government officials. For instance, one Taiwanese shoe company has built six establishments in different towns in the Pearl River Delta region, hiring more than four thousand workers altogether. Yet each establishment was kept small enough, in terms of the total amount of capital, the number of employees, and the size of land used for factory buildings, in order to qualify as a small project that could be approved by the county government. Investors had to cultivate good relations with local officials of various agencies such as the Public Security Bureau, electricity, water, and telephone companies (which were publicly owned), customs, the Public Health Department, the Tax Bureau, the Committee of Foreign Economic and Trade, the Labor Department, local banks, and so on, in order to ensure a smooth operation of production. The definition of efficiency in this case was the level of cooperativeness of the local officials. It was to the benefit of local officials to attract foreign investors in order to strengthen the economic base of the localities. These officials also gained personal benefits such as a large salary raise as a result of bonuses based on the profits of the joint ventures and collective enterprises. In fact the income levels of government officials in southern China, which vary from town to town, have been an indicator of the success the town has enjoyed in their joint-venture arrangements with overseas investors (interview, China, O-1).

By taking advantage of the linguistic and cultural affinity, Taiwanese investors can successfully cultivate the interpersonal relationship with local Chinese officials and have built social networks with various governmental agencies in the region. It is true that building interpersonal networks between the investors and governmental officials can be corrupt. For example, the owner of a Taiwanese shoe factory, which is located in a fishing village two hours from Shenzhen, told me that he had made a deal with the local party secretary of the county so that if he helped to pay the remittance for the county to the provincial government, the county customs would not inspect the company's exports and imports too closely, nor would the tax bureau audit its accounting books. If I refer to a Chinese idiom, the official would "open one eye, with the other closed" when he visited the factory. Another large shoe factory has managed to maintain good relations with local custom officials. Once every few months this large company reserves an entire Karaoke singing bar to entertain their friends in customs. As a result, the containers of the company's imported materials have never been opened and inspected. The story about smuggling operations is even more stunning. Because of the frequent rotation of custom officers from station to station, a broker might ship the goods to one port this week and to another port the next week in order to follow a particular custom officer who is a "friend" and will help to make sure that the broker's containers go through customs quickly and without being inspected.

It is true that cultural understanding between the investors and local agents does not guarantee the success of the investment projects, and it is very difficult to measure how critical cultural understanding and interpersonal networks are to the formation and operation of the enterprises. However, as they were expressed so frequently in the interviews with Taiwanese investors in China, the cultural factors cannot be ignored. In the following section I will discuss the cultural basis of the interpersonal networks built between Taiwanese investors and local officials in southern China.

Interpersonal Relationship between Taiwanese Investors and Local Chinese Officials

Many Taiwanese investors whom I have interviewed agree that, compared with other overseas production sites, China is more attractive to them because of the cultural and linguistic affinity between Taiwanese and Chinese. Further, Taiwanese investment in China has grown faster than that in the ASEAN (Association of Southeast Asian Nations) countries since the late 1980s. Such cultural affinity has facilitated the establishment of interpersonal relationships between Taiwanese investors and local Chinese officials. Yet, the significance of these interpersonal relationships

is by no means unique to Taiwanese investment in China. The question is, if interpersonal relationships are a key factor in the success of Taiwanese investment
in southern China, and the cultural affinity between the investors and their local
agents is crucial for the establishment of such relationships, what are the culturally
embedded principles of the establishment of such interpersonal relationships?
I adopt Ong's (1987) approach in her analysis of shop-floor gender politics in
the Japanese-funded factories in Malaysia, in which she does not see culture as a
given set of values, but as a historically and institutionally situated dynamism.
She argues that, while culture highlights core social values, there is no direct
relationship between values and behavior that is independent of institutional or
organizational contexts. From this historical and institutional contingent perspective of culture, I will examine the way cultural factors have shaped the processes
and strategies of Taiwanese manufacturing investment in southern China. I focus
on the principles and the practices of interpersonal network building between
Taiwanese investors and local Chinese bureaucrats on the basis of gift exchange in
a specific institutional context in southern China since the reform started in the
late 1970s.

Flexible Interpretation and Implementation of Laws

As suggested before, the increasing local economic authority in China, at the macro
level, has provided the institutional basis for the flexible arrangement between
Taiwanese investors and Chinese officials. At the micro level, one important element
that affects the extent and forms of the networks established between business and
the state is that Chinese bureaucrats are traditionally flexible when they come to
interpreting and implementing the law. It has been a skill of Chinese bureaucrats to
make decisions based on what higher-level officials would not oppose rather than
what they would allow. In Chinese this policy is called "looking for holes" (*zuan
kong-zi*). The philosophy is "if something is not explicitly prohibited, then move
ahead; if something is allowed, then use it to the hilt" (Vogel, 1989, p. 81). The
application of such a philosophy in the local decision-making process is demonstrated by the flexible interpretation and implementation of the regulations that are
imposed by the higher-level governments. A Chinese idiom reflects well such a trend
of superficial compliance of top-down policies and the tension between the high-
and low-level authorities: "policies from the top, counterstrategies at the bottom"
(*shangyou zhengce xiayou duece*).

   The degree of autonomy of local officials and the width of the gap between the
written regulations and the actual practices depend on how well such a culture of
superficial compliance is developed and how fiscally independent the local government in question is. An official in charge of foreign trade and investment in Xiamen,
Fujian Province, explained to me why Guangdong has been one step ahead of Fujian
in economic reform: "leaders in Guangdong have been more willing and daring to
push to the limits of the policies imposed by the central government. They are also
readier to try out new strategies before they receive clear signals from Beijing."
Facing the problems of rapidly declining tax revenue to the central government, in
the early 1990s Beijing began to tighten up the control of loans and project approval
authority. However, in a city district of Guangzhou, an officer of the Land Bureau

told me that since the central government imposed the austerity policies in 1993 and placed a greater restriction on the size of lots that the district government could lend to developers, the district government had adopted the strategy of "small is beautiful," dividing the lot for one project into several smaller lots and granting land-use permission individually in order to avoid the involvement and scrutiny of higher government units. The culture of *shangyou zhengce xiayou duece* thus has blossomed in the institutional context in which opportunities for local accumulation present themselves.

Taiwanese investors obtained favorable investment conditions from local officials on the basis of their understanding of such a flexibility in the interpretation and implementation of regulations. A Taiwanese investor commented that the way he dealt with mainland Chinese officials was very similar to the way he had dealt previously with the Taiwanese officials (interview, China, E-l). Given the loose control of the central government on small business, and the negotiable policy implementation in Taiwan, Taiwanese investors have found little "cultural barrier" to "finding the holes" in southern China. The degree of flexibility tends to increase as the level of government decreases. The tax relief has been one of the most critical favorable investment conditions. The standard enterprise income tax rate of foreign-funded joint ventures was 33%. This tax was totally exempted for the first 2–3 profitable years. For the next 3–4 years half of the tax was exempted. In many cases the tax-free period was extended, or tax rates were kept at 15% after the tax-free period was over.

Other favorable investment conditions that local governments had the authority to grant to foreign ventures entailed the transfer of profit out of China; relaxation of the rules on foreign exchange balance; reduction of power fees, water fees, and land price for factory buildings; exemption of import licenses; provision of cheap loans; relaxation of restrictions on the hiring of nonlocal workers; and exemption of social welfare contributions, etc. There are no upper limits on the size of loans to be granted to enterprises, nor are there any clearly stated policies on the criteria for loan approval. Therefore, local banks have enjoyed a high degree of flexibility in the acquisition and granting of loans. Underneath the guise of stated policies which were supposed to be applicable universally, the actual investment arrangements were mostly tailor-made for individual enterprises and investors, and the profitability of the investment package was mostly dependent upon the relationship between the investor and the local officials. As a Taiwanese investor forthrightly put it, "No favorable investment policies issued by the government can be as favorable as the special deals I made with the local officials."

The increasing economic autonomy of Chinese local governments, combined with the culture of Chinese local bureaucracy in their flexible interpretation and implementation of centrally imposed laws, has provided an institutional framework in which the actual practice of gift exchange is carried out. In Sahlins's (1972) and Malinowski's (1961) works on gift economy, gift exchange differs from market exchange in that it is highly personalized, embedded in ongoing personal relations. The meaning and the effect of the gift depends on who gives it and who receives it and what their relation is and will be. Unlike market exchange, the value of the gift is not always measurable in monetary terms, and gifts have a utility independent of their monetary value. To sustain the exchange relationship it is crucial to meet the expectation of reciprocity and make a fair return. The timescale for returning the gift is not fixed and one is not required to return the gift immediately.

I have identified four cultural–institutional elements that have shaped the practice of gift exchange. These are, measurements of the value of the gift; the sense of time in Chinese culture, which includes the meaning of efficiency, the timelessness of the exchange relationship, and the importance of timing in the giving of gifts; the sense of space in Chinese culture, especially the vague boundaries between the public and the private domain; and last, linguistic commonality as a tool of communication between gift givers and receivers, especially in the understanding of the hidden messages that lie underneath the spoken words, which plays a crucial role in the establishment of personal relations through gift exchanges.

Measurements of the value of the gift

Gift exchange is not always an equal exchange in quantitative terms and the exchanged "gift" is not necessarily of a material form. In fact, the art of gift exchange is to maintain the balance between offering material favors and expressing friendship and loyalty to each other as the basis of mutual trust, which goes beyond immediate material benefits. One needs cultural understanding to perceive where the balance point is and the value of the gift in nonmonetary terms. In many cases the nonmaterial form of gift is even more valuable than the material gifts, especially if the nonmaterial gift can express a greater degree of loyalty. For example, a Chinese official might ask an overseas investor to be the sponsor of his or her child who has planned to attend a US university. The overseas investor might or might not have to take the financial responsibility for the child, but to be a sponsor involves greater risks than simply offering some luxurious gifts or cash. A favor that involves a certain degree of risk is far more effective in winning the trust of the other partner; and it paves a smoother path for future collaboration.

Gifts also have a use-value independent of their monetary value (Sahlins, 1972, p. 12). A rare, but not necessarily expensive gift that cannot be bought "just because one has the money" demonstrates greater sincerity and respect for others. Consequently, a return of the favor of even greater value can be expected.

Sense of time: efficiency, timelessness, and timing

In gift exchange the persons who are engaged in the exchange relationship determine the nature of the exchange. Unlike the market exchange, gift exchange cannot happen between strangers. It only happens between those who have a certain type of preexisting interpersonal relationship, such as classmates, people from the same native place, relatives, colleagues, or those who were sent down to the country villages together during the Sending-Down period in the 1960s and 1970s. When such a preexisting social connection is absent, potential participants can be linked up with the others through a mutual acquaintance and need to establish a basis of familiarity before they can progress in the exchange relationship.

Therefore, although good interpersonal relationships facilitate the investment process and move things along quickly and more efficiently, it takes time to build such relationships. When an investor boasts that he or she could "solve any problem immediately by making a phone call to the governor of the town or the chief officer of the custom," it means that he or she has invested a vast amount of time and energy in advance in order to reach such a level of "efficiency."

The relationship between the participants in a gift exchange does not end immediately after the exchange is completed. It is important to pay back more than one has received, as a Chinese idiom says: "When given a foot, give back a yard." Because gift exchange is not always an equal exchange in quantitative terms, the "favor debts" rarely get cleared in one transaction. As a result, favors are accumulated and interpersonal relationships are strengthened as the exchanges of gifts and favors continue.

According to one Taiwanese investor, the least effective way of making friends with local officials is to shower them with cash or luxurious gifts at the beginning, or to present the gift in a once-and-for-all fashion. Instead, a "constant drizzle" of gifts will facilitate a more stable and lasting relationship. It is also important to present the gift before asking for favors. A joint venture that had a number of trucks frequently delivering materials and finished products had managed to obtain a good relationship with the traffic policemen in town. Three times a year the company would present imported liquor or other gifts to the public security bureau before the three major Chinese festivals of the year – the Dragon Boat Festival, the Mid-Autumn Day, and the Chinese New Year. However, last Chinese New Year (1993) the company did not send the gifts. As a result, immediately after the New Year, their drivers started getting speed tickets. The company soon got the message and brought gifts to the bureau. But the gifts were returned. The policemen told the company that they could not accept the gifts because "it is obvious that you are trying to bribe us."

Sense of space: vague boundaries between the public domain and the private domain

It is often argued that the Chinese do not see the public domain and the private domain as two polar opposites. Instead, the public and the private are considered to be a continuous spectrum or as two concentric circles. The public domain is a congregation of private, individual entities, and there are different levels of publicness. Therefore, the expansion of the private domain is not always considered to be an invasion of the public domain, but an adjustment to the level of publicness (or privateness) in different situations. However, such statements can be overgeneralized. Nevertheless, the way Chinese local officials deal with overseas investors in China qualifies the general observation. As China has been undergoing a transformation from a socialist system in which the public sector is pervasive and because a clear legal framework that redefines the "private" has yet to be built, border crossing between the public and the private domain has been a matter in which legal considerations are mixed with culturally informed interpersonal relations.

The public and the private domain are often intertwined and private and public interests are not always in conflict. A Taiwanese investor commented that the best way to maintain and to enforce the relationship with an official is to offer the opportunity for him or her to gain personal benefits while benefiting his or her institute. For example, if a state-owned factory needs new machinery, it will help the broker to get the contract if he or she can arrange a trip for the decision-makers in the government to visit the foreign equipment supplier. Those who get to represent the customer organization and take the trip gain a direct benefit of a free trip abroad, and therefore owe a favor to the broker, and at the same time the entire organization benefits from getting more information about the new equipment. In fact a US equipment supplier told me that a free trip to visit the suppliers abroad has been part of the deal in his negotiation with his Chinese customers. It has been built into the system as a routine and his company has had a long-term contract with a travel agent who arranged all the trips for his Chinese customers. In the typical 1–2-week visit to the USA, there was a one-day visit to the supplier's factory; the rest of the time usually included trips to Las Vegas, New York, Los Angeles, and so on.

As the benefits are shared by the group, so is the responsibility. One of the most widely used terms in the government is "collective discussion." The official in charge of granting import licenses might tell the applicant, who wishes to have more generous tax breaks on import materials, that the case needs to be discussed collectively with his or her colleagues in the department. This means that the favor expected from the applicant will be shared by a group of officials at different ranks, and so will the risks involved in granting a special tax break to the applicant.

Hidden messages in the language

As mentioned before, when asked about the major advantage of investing in China, compared with other overseas production sites in Southeast Asia, most Taiwanese investors answer that it was the common language they share with local Chinese. The gift receiver is expected to understand what is expected of him or her, without explicit explanations, if he or she is a true friend of the gift giver. To reach such a subtle balance between explicitness and implicitness, it requires effective communication between the participants.

In Xiamen, southern Fujian, Taiwanese speak the same dialect as the southern Fujianese. In Guangdong, the successfully promoted official language in both Taiwan and mainland China, Mandarin, has been an effective tool for communication between the overseas investors and their local agents. Although linguistic commonality is not the only tool to build trusting relationships, it opens doors more quickly.

On many occasions what is spoken is not as important as what is unspoken. Therefore, one of the participants in a gift exchange requires both technical understanding of the spoken words and cultural understanding of the hidden meaning to grasp fully the expectations of the other participant.

For example, when an investor asks for a greater allowance of products to be sold in the local markets, the official in charge might tell the investor, "Let me 'yanjiu', 'yanjiu' about it." Literally "yanjiu" means doing research or looking into the matter carefully. Yet, the conclusion of the research often depends on the favor that the applicant is willing to offer to the official. As the pronunciation of "yanjiu" is close to "cigarettes and liquor" in Mandarin, in the early days of the reform "yanjiu" literally implied the demand of cigarettes and liquor as gifts. The three elements described before – the type (therefore the monetary and the use-value) of the gift, the timing of the offer of the gift, and the occasion on which the gift is presented and received – are all parts of the hidden message. If the cigarettes offered by the applicant are not good enough, the official may reject the gift and at the same time offer one, which is usually of the most expensive brand, to the applicant, as a way to show the applicant the type of cigarettes that is preferred. If the official gives the applicant her or his home address and invites the applicant to have a cup of tea with him or her at home, it usually implies that the gift should be presented and the negotiation made in the official's residence rather than in the office. Furthermore, whether the official accepts the gift or not indicates the chances of whether the favor will be granted to the applicant. If the official feels the favor asked by the applicant is too unrealistic or beyond his or her realm of influence, the official will not accept the gift as a way to tell the applicant that no help can be expected.

Conclusion

Taiwan's economy has been restructuring. After three decades of export-oriented industrialization, the rising production costs in the island and the shrinking world markets have left Taiwanese small-export manufacturers with few choices but to look elsewhere for alternative production sites and markets. Southern China, with its abundant supply of unprotected yet trainable migrant workers, attractive investment packages, and accommodating local officials, fulfills the demand of the Taiwanese small producers. This is an accommodating institutional environment for small investors in southern China, who are matched well with the desperate small Taiwanese export manufacturers, whose competitiveness in the world markets depends heavily on time and low costs. The marriage between Taiwanese capital and mainland Chinese agents is further lubricated by a shared language, the institutional culture of Chinese bureaucracy, and the common cultural tools that facilitate the establishment of interpersonal networks between Taiwanese investors and Chinese local officials.

The dynamism of development comes from the interaction between the national state, the local states, foreign capitals, and the new social forces that are generated from such interactions. Further, as Yang (1994, p. 45) has pointed out, although interpersonal relations are usually regarded as being in line with bureaucratic power, whether as official corruption or as patron–client ties, they are also a force working against state power. To elaborate on this point, the establishment of interpersonal ties between Taiwanese investors and Chinese local officials should be seen as a way that the local states bypass the control of the central state and link up directly with the world market.

"Gift exchange" may be seen as a general principle of the establishment of interpersonal relationships in Chinese societies. It might also be safe to argue that the Chinese tend to rely on gift exchange-based interpersonal relationships more than some other people (Ruan, 1993). Yet, the importance of interpersonal ties is not unique to Chinese societies, nor is gift exchange a principle of establishing inter-personal relations that is adopted only by the Chinese. However, the practice and the form of gift exchange vary, depending on the specific historical and institutional contexts. The culturally available tools that facilitate the practice of gift exchange are unique to the processes of establishing interpersonal networks with local Chinese officials by Taiwanese investors. These tools include the linguistic connection, an understanding of the nonmarket value of gifts, and the sense of time and space in Chinese culture. The principle is applied and the tools are used in an institutional context which is characterized by the increasing autonomy of local Chinese officials and their tradition of flexible interpretation and implementation of the regulations imposed by the central government.

As a preliminary effort to tackle the question of cultural mechanism in develop-ment processes, in this paper I have also brought up several questions to be explored further in the search for "Chinese capitalism." First of all, when I try to identify the cultural elements of the Chinese-style economic activities, I am not looking at atomized cultural factors or the impact of these cultural factors on all the dimen-sions in the process of economic development. Instead I am looking at the *rela-tionship* between certain cultural elements and certain development issues, such as the relationship between familism and firm organizations, the relationship between the definition of partnership and the establishment of business alliances, or the rela-tionship between the definition of public and private sphere and the way the gov-ernment intervenes in the market. This seems to me to be a more promising way to avoid making the sweeping arguments that are often seen in works on the rela-tionship between the Confucian values and East Asian Economic Miracles (see Hamilton and Biggart, 1988, for a very comprehensive critique of this approach). By moving down the ladder of abstraction and reducing the number of definitional attributes of "Chinese capitalism," we might be able to find some measurable vari-ables and therefore a more manageable research project.

Also, the connection between culture and ideology needs to be further developed in the search for Chinese capitalism. For example, the cultural factor in the development of small business, such as familism, is associated with the ideology that being one's own boss is an indicator of success. Therefore it justifies the self-exploitation by the owners of small shops; or, the phenomenon of concentration of investment in property is supported by the cultural association between land, security, and success; and the ideological implication that ownership provides independence.

In the meantime, local government-oriented projects have facilitated a more decentralized process of industrialization and urbanization in China. Overseas investors provide alternative sources of capital and technology transfer for local gov-ernments. A coalition of local governments and foreign capital has also strength-ened the bargaining power of local governments against the national government, creating, in turn, a basis for local governments to take more initiative in regional and urban planning and development. Increasingly, most key planning, manage-ment, and financing issues are decided at the local level. This provides an opportu-nity for local planners to respond to local situations more directly and to shift urban and regional standards of governance away from universal norms set by the central government.

Chapter 24

From Registered Nurse to Registered Nanny: Discursive Geographies of Filipina Domestic Workers in Vancouver, BC

Geraldine Pratt

At the first of a series of workshops with Filipina domestic workers, held at the Philippine Women Centre in Vancouver in 1995, we went around the room and introduced ourselves. With the exception of some of the workshop facilitators, all of the 18 participants were domestic workers, admitted to Canada under the Live-in Caregiver Program. But as we went around that room, there was a surprising (for me) disruption of this uniformity. We heard from women who were trained and certified as midwives or as registered nurses, about the difficulties of finding work in the Philippines as a secondary school science teacher, and about the occupational experiences of a trained social worker. We heard about working in a bank in the Philippines and about the experiences of a bookkeeper. As I listened to these diverse personal histories, I puzzled over a colleague's finding that Filipinas are the most occupationally ghettoized of all women (classified by ethnicity) in the Vancouver labor market (Hiebert, 1999). Analyses of the 1991 census data for Vancouver indicate that Filipinas are especially overrepresented in three occupations: housekeeper, childcare worker (essentially the same occupation labeled in two ways), and medical assistant (e.g., nurses' aid). The Live-in Caregiver Program requires of participants that they work as a live-in caregiver for two full years before applying for an open visa (at which point they are released from the obligation to do live-in domestic work). However, the experience of coming to Canada as a nanny evidently narrows occupational opportunities long after the requirements of the program have been fulfilled. This is a particular, though extreme, case of a familiar immigrant story: deskilling through immigration, followed by ghettoization within marginal occupations.

If the story is familiar, our ability to accommodate it within contemporary labor market theory is less clear. It has become a common, almost clichéd, critique of labor segmentation theory to point to its inadequacy at explaining why and how some groups (women, visible minorities, immigrants) end up in marginal jobs (e.g., Hanson and Pratt, 1995). Recognizing the complexity and specificity of these processes for different groups and in different places has led some (Hanson and Pratt, 1995; Hiebert, 1999; Peck, 1996) to suggest that a lower or middle range of theory and a close attention to empirical detail may be more productive for under-standing these processes. While this position helpfully highlights the contingency and variability of social and economic processes, I now think that it is also poten-tially misleading. This is because it can be interpreted as positing the social and cul-tural processes that lead to the marginalization of certain groups in the labor market as empirical rather than theoretical puzzles. The point is not only that empirical work is never theory free, but that hiving off the empirical from the theoretical might lead us to miss what a substantial body of contemporary cultural theory can offer to our understanding of labor markets.

If much contemporary cultural theory stresses the importance of the everyday and the local, it nonetheless rests on some highly abstract ideas about subjectivity and social and economic life. An emphasis on the local speaks to methodology and not to levels of theoretical abstraction. Foucault (1979), for example, blurred the distinctions between micro/macro, scales of analyses, and levels of abstraction when he observed that even as power relations ultimately become linked to the logic of a great strategy (a logic not conceived as theoretical abstraction), the appropriate *starting point* for analysis lies in everyday local power relations. . . . By analogy, even as labor market segmentation exists and persists as a grand strategy of capitalist imperialist labor control, our point of departure for understanding how individu-als are drawn into this system of class relations lies in a close examination of local power relations and situated practices. It is unhelpful, however, to conceive of local relations and practices as more empirical than systematic strategies. Cultural theo-ries, including theories of subjectivity, are no less abstract when they pertain to individuals and local power relations.

Poststructural theories posit a subject and perspectives on language that are useful for understanding processes of labor market segmentation. Poststructural theorists such as Foucault drew from Althusser's antihumanism to conceive the subject as produced through discourse, rather than as a coherent rational subject who exists prior to language. Language does not simply reflect the world; it is a regulated prac-tice that structures our sense of reality and notions of our own identity. Discourse is material in the sense that it brings into being classifications of objects, bodies, and identities (Butler, 1990; Haraway, 1991) and exists as situated practices, sup-ported by institutions, buildings, and so forth (Mills, 1997). Critics sometimes argue that discourse analysis dissolves the materiality of the world into language, but this misses the messiness of the relations being posited between the material and the dis-cursive (Natter and Jones, 1993). It is not that discourse theorists deny the materi-ality of the world; they argue that how we conceive the world is inextricably bound up with discourse.

Despite the innovative uses to which poststructuralism has been put by political economists (e.g., Gibson-Graham, 1996), suspicion remains that cultural theorists miss the determinate effects of the economy and lose a position from which to cri-tique them (cf. Fraser, 1997; Watts and McCarthy, 1997). Spivak (1988) has argued that discourse analysis can take the form of empiricist reportage, in which the intel-lectual abdicates his or her role as critic. Spivak urges a reconsideration of material interests and the ways in which they come to be represented in discourse; she is par-ticularly concerned with the ways that the international division of labor reflects and structures material interests and how representations veil capitalist, imperialist relations. Without claiming an exhaustiveness for discourse analysis, we can see it as a means of theorizing how subjects come to understand themselves and their capabilities and how material inequalities are produced through everyday situated practices. It is also a powerful tool for disrupting these situated practices.

Poststructural theories of the subject and discourse indicate three possibilities for disruption. First, discourses are productive in the sense that they produce subject positions. These subject positions subjugate individuals but they also function as resources. In the labor market, we can think of how claims of class standing (in solidarity with the working class, for example) work as political resources. A second political possibility comes from the understanding that individuals are "hailed" by multiple, sometimes contradictory, discourses. Managing these contradictions, or bringing one discourse into relation with another, can open points of resistance. Lisa Lowe argues, for example, that the liberal principles of American democracy (including claims to universal rights) are at odds with the various ways that Asian American citizens enter discourse: as "the model minority," or "the invading multitude, the lascivious seductress, the servile yet treacherous domestic, the automaton whose inhuman efficiency will supersede American ingenuity" (1996, p. 18). Placing these discourses in tension creates a space from which to criticize constructions of the American nation and an economic system "that profits from racism" (1996, p. 26). Third, poststructuralists influenced by deconstruction have been attentive to the contradictions *within* any discourse. In Spivak's view (1988), it is by uncovering the disruptions and contradictions between and within discourses that a critical vantage point on discourse is gained. Discourse analysis can lead to an incisive critique of ideology by revealing the "mistakes" that found knowledge, the contradictions within discourses, and the things that are left unsaid or cannot be said, by "*measuring* silences, if necessary – into the *object* of investigation" (Spivak 1988, p. 296; original emphasis).

It is not simply that geographers have much to gain by drawing on poststructural theory; a close reading of geography has much to offer to cultural studies. This is because discourses emerge as situated practices in particular places (they thus are inherently geographic (Pred, 1992)). There are sociospatial circuits through which cultural and personal stories are circulated, legitimated, and given meaning. By mapping these circuits we map types of discursive geography. Moving between places may also be one way in which individuals become aware of contradictions between various discourses. But additionally, geographic terms have important effects within discourse. Feminists have long recognized how constructions of home influence women's work experiences; Moss (1995) and Gregson and Lowe (1994) provide recent examples of how constructions of home affect paid labor performed within that space. We can usefully consider how other discursively embedded geographies work to structure labor markets.

In the following case study, I map discursive constructions that circumscribe subject positions available to Filipina women, delineating for them a limiting space within the labor market. In so doing, I pay special attention to how geographic terms function within discourse. A central discursive struggle surrounds whether domestic workers are interpreted in racial/immigration or class terms. I will examine this struggle, and attempt to get some critical perspective on discursive constructions by attempting to measure some of the silences and contradictions within them.

But I also want to suggest that ruptures between subject positions, as prescribed in different discourses and in different places, open spaces for agency and opportunities for rewriting the meaning of "Filipina" in Vancouver.

My discussion of subject positions is organized by considering paired terms, each defined in relation to the other, reflecting my understanding that identities are relational constructs and that they are defined in relation to what they are not: live-in caregiver is defined in opposition to Canadian citizen; and Filipina domestic workers are constructed in relation to European ones, through the terms "housekeeper" and "nanny," respectively. Within the Filipino community, nanny takes on meaning in relation to the term "immigrant." These categories supplement each other and rigidify Filipina domestic workers' occupational trajectories, such that their entry into the Canadian labor market via the Live-in Caregiver Program narrows their choices thereafter. Complex geographies are woven throughout this trajectory. To fully understand Filipinas' positionings, one would have to consider conditions within the Philippines that drive them to migrate. My analysis is restricted to discursive constructions of Filipinas in Vancouver, but the last discourse considered, one that circulates within the Filipino community in Vancouver, begins to gesture toward important class relations in the Philippines that continue to construct "Filipina" in Vancouver.

Mapping discourse is a vast, open-ended task. I rely on interview material collected between 1994 and 1996. In 1994 I interviewed ten agents operating in the Vancouver area, the only ones who would speak with me and, by their own assessment, the ones who handled the largest volume of placements (see Pratt, 1997 for details of the methodology). In the summer of 1995, I interviewed a randomly selected sample of 52 households in the Vancouver metropolitan area who had advertised for nannies in the previous year in one of two local newspapers. Most were currently employing a nanny when we came to do the interview. Through the summer and fall of 1995 and spring of 1996, I collaborated with the Philippine Women Centre to conduct a series of focus groups with 14 domestic workers. All interviews and focus groups were unstructured, taped, and transcribed, a necessity for a study of discourse in which the framing of meaning is the object of inquiry.

Live-in Caregiver: Noncitizen, Not-Yet-Immigrant

The live-in caregiver is defined in relation and in opposition to the category Canadian citizen, and it is the noncitizen status of job occupants that structures the work conditions of live-in caregivers. Over the years a larger proportion of the mostly women who have come through these programs have come from the Philippines; by 1996 fully 87 percent came from the Philippines. In its informational booklet, the federal government explicitly locates occupants of this job as non-Canadians: "The Live-in Caregiver Program is a special program whose objective is to bring workers to Canada to do live-in work as caregivers when there are not enough Canadians available to fill the available positions. The Live-in Caregiver Program exists only because there is a shortage of Canadians to fill the need for live-in care work. There is no shortage of Canadian workers available for caregiving positions where there is no live-in requirement" (Citizenship and Immigration Canada, 1999). A provincial employee who administers the Live-in Caregiver

Program in one Vancouver employment office stated in a telephone interview in May 1994: "The reason that we have to bring in from abroad is that the occupation is so poorly paid and no one wants to do it. . . . The program is set up for the Canadian employer, to allow them to get on with their lives and get out to work."

This difference between live-in caregivers and Canadian citizens has been encoded in stark terms by provincial employment regulations, which govern the work conditions of live-in caregivers. Regulations vary by province. In British Columbia, until March 1995 live-in domestic workers (along with farm workers and other home-workers) were excluded from regulations governing overtime pay and hours of work. As the West Coast Domestic Workers' Association (1993, p. 2) put it in their brief to the Employment Standards Act Review Committee in March 1993: "by imposing a daily [as opposed to hourly] minimum wage and excluding domestics from hours of work protection, [provincial regulations], in effect, work with the federal immigration program to provide foreign domestic workers as cheap labor."

Why is it that Canadians so readily accept that some categories of people living within Canada are undeserving of protective labor codes available to other citizens? Why are some categories of people assumed to have minimal subsistence requirements? Three geographic concepts are used to negotiate what would seem to be an untenable contradiction between universal rights of Canadian citizens and unequal treatment of workers in different occupational categories. First, the promise of potential citizenship works in a potent way to legitimate labor conditions acknowledged by the Canadian government as unacceptable to Canadians. While, strictly speaking, the Live-in Caregiver Program is a work visa (and not an immigration) program, in practice it entitles the occupant to apply for immigrant status after working two full years as a live-in caregiver. There is a widespread understanding that live-in caregivers endure short-term hardship for the opportunity of applying for landed immigrant status after two years working as a live-in caregiver. As Agent E put it: "Filipinos have a very different motivation [from European nannies]. . . . they are coming to immigrate, to get citizenship, to bring in their families. They will put up with a lot in order to have a clean record, which makes for a whole other set of problems. But it means that they're likely to stay on the job" (interview, May 1994).

Since changes to the Employment Standards Act in 1995, overtime and minimum hourly wage regulations cover all domestic workers in British Columbia. But it is interesting to listen to nanny agents argue against these changes when they were first proposed in 1994. Agents indirectly threatened domestic workers that changes to labor regulations would restrict their opportunities to immigrate.

> Agent D: You're not getting 19 bucks an hour [working as a domestic worker], but the majority of Canadians treat you nicely. And you're getting Canadian citizenship, which is what people are lining up for, dying to come.
> Agent C: And not costing yourself anything. Like I said before, the West Coast Domestic Association [sic] will argue that [domestic workers are exploited]. And they're going to do themselves out of a job.
> Agent D: They'll wreck it for these women, who come in and 99.9 percent of them are happy to be here. And they're not militants. That's just so sad. Because it's just that little few that are banging on.

To me, what is of interest in these passages is the way in which benefits to the Canadian state and Canadian households (which allow Canadian men and women "to get on with their lives and get out to work") are translated into a benefit for domestic workers. A discourse of free and fair exchange (immigration for two years of servitude) is commonplace but it is staged without a careful weighing of the units in exchange; indeed, Agent C cancels out the costs to the domestic worker entirely: "And not costing yourself anything." We need to measure this silence about costs, in part through a more serious analysis of the terms of exchange – that is, whether an opportunity to immigrate can and should be valued against two years of paid servitude. This discussion must be broadened to consider Canada's responsibilities in relation to global patterns of uneven development.

There is a second, fragmented geography that confuses live-in caregivers' rights as employees . . . The federal government has responsibility over the Live-in Caregiver Program, whereas the provincial government regulates employment standards. There is, then, a type of discursive rupture in the way that live-in caregivers are defined in relation to the two levels of the government. For the federal government they are defined as visa holders; for the provincial governments, they are employees. Of particular concern to domestic workers is the federal government's prohibition against educational training for those registered in the Live-in Caregiver Program. In their view, the effect of this prohibition is deskilling:

> *Susan*: It is stated in the work permit that you cannot go to college, you cannot work for others and you cannot work in other provinces.
> After you have not worked for two years in the trade or profession that you have trained for, you begin to doubt if you still have the ability to do your previous work.
> *Jeorgie:* Things are not fresh in your mind anymore.

[The conversation continues and culminates with:]

> *Mhay*: What you know now is only how to clean and polish the bathroom.
> *Elsie*: That's your skills these days. (Focus group discussions, August 1995)

Domestic workers perceive that living within the regulations of the Live-in Caregiver Program makes it difficult to recover a previous occupational identity. Yet it is difficult for them to make a strong case to the federal government because this exceeds the discursive boundaries of the Live-in Caregiver Program, which positions them as noncitizen visa holders.

The governmentally fragmented administration of the Live-in Caregiver Program makes lobbying for change a complicated process. It also lends an air of confusion about entitlements as employees. Among women attending the focus groups, for example, there was a great deal of uncertainty about their entitlement to the federal government's Employment Insurance (EI) program, despite the fact that they paid into the program. This confusion about entitlement is of considerable importance because access to employment insurance benefits could allow a domestic worker to leave an especially exploitative or abusive employment situation.

A third geography is literally written into the Live-in Caregiver Program: regis-trants must live in their employers' homes. The requirement that domestic workers live "in" clearly lowers the costs for employers, because they can deduct $300 a month for room and board from the required minimum wage payment. It thus brings privatized childcare (which costs the employer approximately $900 a month after this deduction) within the reach of middle income families. Problems attend-ing live-in requirements have long been recognized by domestic worker advocacy groups. Living in an employer's home dampens wages, tends to stretch the work day, and can make domestic workers vulnerable to sexual abuse. It also makes it more difficult for the domestic worker to challenge her employer because her work-place is also her home.

Discourses of home and family are woven through these material effects. Aitken (1987) documents how constructions of home as a private space have been used in Ontario to justify minimal state intrusion into the home and thus very weak regu-lation of domestic workers' employment situations (see also Stiell and England, 1997). The domestic worker is sometimes constructed as a family member, who is loved and cherished as such; some have argued that regulation of domestic work within the framework of employer–employee relations penalizes the domestic worker because it degrades her status as a family member.

The West Coast Domestic Workers' Association argues that "Live-in domestic workers can keep time and should be paid for the hours worked" (1993, p. 4). In arguing thus, they were entering a discursive battle, attempting to redefine the domestic worker, not as family member, not as potential immigrant who should be grateful for her temporary lot as a domestic worker, but, quite simply, as an employee. There is much at stake: hours of work and overtime regulations would likely raise wages and shorten hours of work. It is also a struggle to redefine the domestic worker in the language of class so that the politics of class solidarity can be brought into play. Framed in this way, and following Gibson-Graham (1996), we can interpret changes in the Employment Standards Act as a moment of progressive class transformation.

Colonial Geographies: Filipina as Housekeeper

There is another grid of identity formation in which Filipinas are marginalized; they are often unfavorably compared to European women who come to Canada via the same visa program. Filipinas are constructed as housekeepers, while European women are called nannies. The ways that these two groups of women are positioned differently within the same occupational category points to the importance of under-standing the intertwined cultural and social processes of identity formation and labor market segmentation.

Nanny agents who were interviewed in 1994 were very clear on the distinctions between Filipino and European nannies. Many employers absorb the agents' distinction between European nanny and Asian housekeeper, something that came across clearly in interviews with employers who had employed Filipina and European domestic workers. Consider, for example, the comments of a family who first employed a Filipina nanny. She was replaced when their child turned two, an age when the employers became more concerned about the intellectual stimulation of their child. The Filipina nanny was subjected to a covert test, which involved asking her to read to their child during the day and leaving designated books in a marked position on the table. The nanny failed the test – the books were in the same place at the end of the day – and a Slovakian nanny was hired as her replacement. The employers were clearly fond of the Filipina nanny, in part because she did not intrude. They admired their Slovakian nanny for her skills as an early childhood educator, and they spoke in some detail about her other training and skills. They did not, however, like her much, and they were appalled by what they perceived to be her persistent overstepping of social boundaries. I quote from the interview transcript because they express these distinctions in such an open way.

> *Bob*: But I think the big difference between the two was that Rosa [Filipina nanny] never took anything for granted, and when we honored her a privilege, which she thought was a privilege, she would never take advantage of that privilege again unless the honor was there again, whereas with, unfortunately with Brigid [Slovakian nanny] . . .
>
> *Wendy*: She's very good as a caregiver.
>
> *Bob*: Wonderful and stimulating, a good teacher and the whole bit, but as soon as we grant her something . . . Say once she asked if she could use Wendy's skis for the weekend, and we said OK, but after that she used them for the whole season and never asked anymore.
>
> *Wendy*: And she often uses my things. Bob couldn't see my point at first. I mean I had only skied once since Aidan was born. So I said to him, "How would you feel if we hired a gardener and he just used all your golf clubs and stuff?" And that soon put things in perspective!
>
> *Bob*: It was funny, when we would have people over with Rosa we would feel Rosa was part of our family. And a lot of times – not so much on the weekends because she was never here – but on the weekdays, if someone was coming over after work or whatever and we were going out for dinner, we would always invite her to eat with us . . .
>
> *Wendy*: But she would always have eaten before we got home. Whereas with Brigid we feel like we're practically serving her and she's talking back and forth [with our guests].

A little later in the interview, they turned once again to differences between Filipina and Slovakian nannies in terms of intellect and perceptions of entitlement.

> *Bob*: We basically decided in lieu of a Filipino nanny to go with a European nanny, because of the learning skills, the interaction. We were finding that Rosa was really good and loving and hugging and doing everything proper for him and feeding him, but the alphabet, the numbers, the colors, those things weren't happening. . . . I think that's the trade-off. But you've gotta remember that they're educated ladies [Slovakian nannies], and I don't think . . . well I don't know, but I kind of think somewhere down the line it's gonna be: "Well, why am I ironing this man's shirt when I used to be a university scholar?" When we come home at the end of the day, Brigid will have read the paper from front to back. She knows everything in *The Vancouver Sun*. And then she would pull out extracts about taxes going up or the minimum wages going up and she would say to us, "Look, I need a raise, the minimum wage has gone up" . . . Well

you've got to remember that these women [Slovakian nannies] are intellects, and you're not going to have six intellects living in a house at the weekend, sleeping on the floor. Whereas with Filipino nannies, they love to roll all over each other all weekend! [He is referring to the common practice among Filipina nannies of sharing rental accommodations during the weekend.]

Agents themselves play a powerful role in constructing for the prospective employers the idea of Filipina woman as servant/housekeeper. This begins with advice to Filipina women on how they should represent themselves to their prospective employers. Women at the Philippine Women Centre spoke of agents' recommendations to include two pictures of themselves in their files, one showing them caring for children and another displaying them cleaning. Some agents told women not to send a picture that displays them as attractive. Some women were instructed to take off jewelry, wear no makeup, and tie their hair back. An agent in the Philippines cautioned that a picture that displayed a woman as attractive would suggest that "maybe she would go to Canada and seduce her employer." The text that supplements these images of hard-working servants also signals to prospective employers that these women are ripe for exploitation: several domestic workers were told to indicate on their applications forms a willingness to work long hours.

Further, it is often the case that Filipina live-in caregivers have worked previously as domestic workers in Singapore or Hong Kong. Both the agents and employers attempt to bring the highly exploitative conditions for domestic workers from these places to Vancouver. They do this by calling upon personal experiences as domestic workers in Singapore or Hong Kong as they ask Filipina domestic workers to work longer hours and at a wider range of non-childcare-related tasks (such as washing the car) than would be required of European women.

Historical geographies of colonialism and racism continue to define housekeeper and nanny within Vancouver. Filipinas are discursively constructed as housekeepers, with inferior intellects and educations relative to European nannies. Agents encourage Filipina women to represent themselves as exploitable, and they are reminded of their personal and collective histories as domestic workers in Hong Kong and Singapore in the Vancouver context.

Stigmatization within Vancouver's Filipino Community: Filipina Domestic Workers as Husband Stealers

Hegemonic white Canadians have no monopoly on constructions of Filipina domestic workers as inferior. Domestic workers who participated in the focus groups told painful stories about a stigmatization process within the Filipino community, one that revolved around a distinction between immigrant and nanny. The term immigrant was used to refer to individuals who entered Canada through the "regular" immigration system. Some of these would have entered through the family reunification program, some through business class programs, and others through the point system. The point system is complex and the criteria for assembling points periodically readjusted by the federal government, depending on labor requirements. But, among other criteria, points are given for having a sponsor (business sponsorship earns more points than family sponsorship) or specialized training in specifically designated occupations (often technical ones).

Feminized skills are usually undervalued and typically do not score many points. While, strictly speaking, the Live-in Caregiver Program is not an immigration program, in practice it is often the most accessible route for a Filipina woman who wishes to initiate immigration to Canada. Once she has obtained landed immigrant status, she is able to sponsor her family through another immigration program, that of family reunification. The distinction between immigrant and nanny thus carries both class and gender associations; in the former case the lead family member is more likely to be male, with considerable capital and/or educational resources, in the latter a woman. These class and gender dimensions are laden with moral ones: domestic workers who participated in the focus groups saw themselves as being perceived, not only as inferior in class terms, but as promiscuous husband stealers.

> *Mhay*: Because most of us, especially we Filipinos, we go into small groups. One group will say, "Oh, there go the nannies, out on their day off together." It's mostly Filipinos like us who say that. And then there's that other issue about being, since you're a nanny, you're, you know, someone who steals husbands. That's why wives are angry with us. [Mhay is referring to Filipino men and their wives within the Filipino community – not to employers.] (Focus group discussion, September 1995)

This stigmatization may be understandable in the context of what Rafael (1997) has identified as an identity crisis for Filipinos, one that he ties to massive state-encouraged movements of Filipino workers and immigrants over the last 25 years. He argues that middle-class Filipinos are sometimes embarrassed by being mistaken as domestic workers when they travel outside the Philippines: "Embarrassment arises from their inability to keep social lines from blurring (thereby rendering problematic their position as privileged representatives of the nation) and maintaining a distinction between 'Filipino' as the name of a sovereign people and 'Filipino' as the generic term for designating a subservient class dependent on foreign economies" (Rafael, 1997, pp. 276–77).

There are, however, contradictions and silences. In Vancouver, the line between immigrant and nanny may be blurred through a repression of memory and family history. Again, Mhay's remarks are instructive. They follow an incident when she had been insulted by other Filipinos in a public place.

> *Mhay*: It was okay with me, because I really am a nanny, but it was my companion who was hurt. (Laughs) So I asked my friend why he was going into this dark mood, when it was me who was a nanny, not him! [He said,] "No, it's because those people look down on nannies. Where are their roots, anyway?" I said, "Well, from nannies." I was also curious [about his reactions] so I said, "And what about you? If your girl-friend was a nanny, what will you tell your parents about her? Will you say she's a nanny?" "Well, yes" he said. "What if your family looks down on her?" "Well, many people here are like that. If they do that, then they're denying where they came from." It turns out that his family was able to come here because his sister was a nanny. So it was funny that he was reacting like that. But it's really hurting here, that people look down on nannies. (Focus group discussion, September 1995)

Mhay's story shows how the line between nanny and immigrant for many Filipino families in Vancouver is blurry indeed (before this encounter she assumed her friend to be a "regular" immigrant and not an immigrant sponsored by a nanny) and suggests that the distinction is constructed in part through some strategic forgetting within self-identified immigrant families.

There is an interesting geography to these narratives of stigmatization. Moments of stigmatization tend to take place in transit, often quite literally on public transit. The following is typical:

> *Inyang*: I was on the Sky Train and we planned to recruit a person [I saw] to the Centre [Philippine Women Centre]. We had just said, "Oh, you're probably new here, right?" After saying yes, she immediately said, "Wait, but I'm not a nanny, okay?" Look at that! So that time, we never talked to her again. It turns out she was brought over by relatives. (Focus group discussion, September 1995)

These narratives may reflect the fact that contact with other Filipinos is transitory, given that domestic workers live in their employers' homes and work long hours, and that class and other social differences divide the Filipino community. This geography of transition nevertheless stabilizes the construction of Filipina nanny as inferior and immoral because the insults come as incidental, glancing slights, against which she has (literally) no ground for retaliation or renegotiation of discursive categories. She must find other spaces and other grounds for reestablishing self-respect.

Reworking Discourse in Other Spaces and through Boundary Crossings

Although my concern has been to demonstrate how discourses tightly patrol the construction of Filipina in Vancouver, discourses are also productive, open, and polyvalent. In outlining constructions of Filipina, I have tried to mark places where the discursive boundaries might be destabilized by noting silences, contradictions, and patterns of forgetfulness within these constructions. I now turn to other sites where other discourses might be constructed, and then consider how bringing different discourses into tension can be disruptive.

Filipinas undoubtedly construct meanings that disrupt and repair their sense of themselves as supplicant-preimmigrant, inferior nanny, and immoral husband stealer. A number of those who took part in the focus groups spoke of the pressures to earn wages as a dutiful daughter or mother with financial responsibilities in the Philippines. This counterdiscourse of responsibility and duty may reestablish or maintain self-esteem and simultaneously empower women to demand higher wages. It does, however, have mixed effects. Mikita (1994), from her survey of 100 Filipina domestic workers in Vancouver in 1992, estimated the mean monthly remittance to be $245 a month (about 33.4% of gross wages). With such a large proportion of wages going toward family remittances, it is extremely difficult for individual women to contemplate and manage educational upgrading, even when released from the restrictions of the Live-in Caregiver Program. Understanding oneself as a dutiful daughter or sister or mother thus has material effects; in the long run it may lock Filipina women into jobs as domestic workers if the burden of monthly remittances cuts off possibilities for upgrading skills.

Another counterdiscourse may emerge around the identity of consumer, as an individual with the rights and freedoms to consume. Women at the Philippine

Women Centre spoke critically of the many Filipina domestic workers who congregate at the Pacific Center Mall in downtown Vancouver on weekends. One can imagine, however, how consumer consciousness may prepare the ground for resistance if the desire for goods leads domestic workers to challenge employers to comply with new minimum wage and overtime provisions in the Employment Standards Act.

Domestic workers learn another identity at the Philippine Women Centre; they learn to see themselves as exploited Third World women and to understand their situations within a socialist feminist theory of imperialism. We have seen a pedagogic process at work, especially when Cecilia Diocsin, director of the Philippine Women Centre, urges Susan to apply for unemployment insurance for her immediate material benefit and to "learn something about whether there is a different set of rights between you and other Canadians."

A critical potential also emerges from border crossings between sites and discourses, by bringing one discourse into relation with another. The educational process at the Philippine Women Centre, for example, involves not only an exchange of information but a good deal of support and an effort to dislodge the rhetoric of the home as a private, unregulated space, as well as domestic workers' identification with the needs of their employers. The identity of exploited Third World woman that domestic workers learn at the Philippine Women Centre is then introduced to Canadian employers within their homes. In some instances, domestic workers first role play their challenge to their employer with other domestic workers in the safe space of the Centre. As domestic workers attempt to establish their rights as employees rather than family member or supplicant-preimmigrants, they are forcing employers to reconfigure their relations within the terms of labor relations, away from constructions of family or a liberal reading of immigration (which would see individuals entering Canada as lucky, with no appreciation of complicated webs of political economic relations and dependencies between Canada, the International Monetary Fund (IMF), and the Philippines).

Individuals draw strength from transporting meanings from one context to another, even as they recognize the bitterness of their situations in the translation exercise. At the first workshop, I was introduced to a joke among domestic workers in Vancouver when Lisa said: "I was an R.N. in the Philippines and I'm an R.N. in Canada. Only in the Philippines I was a Registered Nurse and in Canada I'm a Registered Nanny" (focus group discussion, August 1995). Their joke points to links between power, discourse, regulation, labor market segmentation, and one geography (transnational migration within neocolonial relations) that mediates them. The joke is political and empowering because it is simultaneously an act of remembering and a recognition of present circumstances. As they remember their professional training in the same term that defines their current situation, memories of the former are reactivated within the latter.

And Back to Labor Market Theory

The challenge of reactivating professional qualifications obtained in the Philippines in the Canadian labor market is clearly going to require more than small instances of decisive wordplay. I have argued that discourses create definitional and social boundaries that contain the horizons of possibilities for individuals and social groups who must live within them. In the case of Filipinas, the discourses of domestic worker seem to constrain them long after they obtain their open visa, given their long-term segregation in the Vancouver labor market. Powerful overlapping of discursive frames of meaning leads to a multiple and polyvalent devaluing of certain categories of people. The word "Filipina" is not only equated with "supplicant-preimmigrant"; the term also connotes "just-a-housekeeper" and "husband stealer."

Contemporary cultural theory also suggests that the overlap of discourses is incomplete, however, and fails to totally envelop individuals caught within them; R.N. is also R.N. In the slippage between discourses and through the contradictions within them, as they are taken up and lived by creative individuals and organized social groups, there is room for agency, and for the creative redirection and redefinition of subject positions.

I am not suggesting that redefining subjective meanings of particular subject positions is sufficient to disrupt labor market segmentation. I do believe that we have to understand how these cultural processes can be put to work as part of this process of disruption. I have attempted to demonstrate how government policy, state regulation, and the informal negotiations that take place between domestic workers, nanny agents, and their employers are all framed within particular discourses that persistently devalue Filipinas. Criticizing these discourses is an important element of disrupting these oppressive institutional practices.

This is a process of critique that sees itself as resistant to, but fully implicated in, the discourses under scrutiny; there is no privileged point from which to claim truth or a vision of nonoppressive social relations. The Philippine Women Centre, for example, is a source of a powerful and productive criticism of neocolonialism, racism, and gender and class oppression in Filipino and Canadian societies. However, their discourse, from a Foucauldian perspective, is no less neutral or "true" than other discourses, although it does produce different subject positions and political possibilities. The task for the critic is not one of uncovering the truth of one discourse but of understanding how subjectivity is produced within these multiple discourses, and to evaluate their effects. Foucault challenges us to generate a critical discourse "whose power effects are limited as much as possible to the subversion of power" (Poster, 1989, p. 30). Like others (Fraser, 1997; Gibson-Graham, 1996; Watts and McCarthy, 1997), I attempt to wed discourse analysis with a critique of exploitation, in my case by assessing how the *effects* of discourse emerge out of and further exploitative north/south international relations through the sedimentation of Filipina immigrants to Canada within a limited range of low-paid occupations.

Whether I have been successful in generating a critique of exploitation that is limited to the subversion of power is an entirely open question. An Immigration Legislative Review, entitled "Not Just Numbers," commissioned by the Ministry of Citizenship and Immigration Canada and released in December 1997, recommended the termination of the Live-in Caregiver Program, in part because of the kinds of criticisms (voiced by academics and activists) leveled in this paper. One assessment (e.g., Philippine Women Centre, 1998) is that the recommended changes would mean that women currently working in Canada as live-in caregivers or admitted through the proposed Foreign Worker Program will no longer be eligible for permanent resident status and possible citizenship. Indeed, current debate among domestic worker advocacy groups in Vancouver turns on how far to criticize the Live-in Caregiver Program, recognizing that one potential effect of this criticism is termination of the program.

Nevertheless, the exposure, politicization, and disruption of conceptual boundaries can be conceived as an important geographic task. My argument has been that geographies are deeply embedded within these boundary projects, in the construction and control of discursive borders. In this sense, geographers have much to bring to cultural theory. Immigration, colonialism, and domestic space are part of the production of borders that define workers as worthy or unworthy, competent or incompetent, skilled or unskilled. These classifications are then intimately tied to the segmentation of labor markets and, in particular, the processes through which particular categories of workers are both allocated to and assume particular occupational niches. Subject positions of "Filipina" are often about, and constructed in relation to, specific places: live-in caregiver is defined through the meanings attributed to the "home"; imagined geographies of "the Philippines" and "Britain" enter into definitions of skills and evaluations of wage requirements. Careful genealogies of place-meanings thus become part of the project of unraveling particular subject positions and releasing certain social categories from particular labor segments.

The case study suggests that geographic strategies of discursive disruption are multiple and complex. When terms from one discourse are used to transform the meanings in another – for example, when a class analysis disrupts the framing of domestic worker as member of the family – we encounter an enabling type of discursive porosity. On the other hand, when the definition of "domestic worker" in Singapore and the definition of the same category of worker in Vancouver leads to more exploitative conditions in Vancouver, we encounter the negative effects of discursive and geographic porosity as poor labor conditions are dragged from one place to another. To point to the particularity and contingency of geographic effects and political strategy is not, however, the same as arguing that low-level theorizing is adequate to the task of conceptualizing these processes. "Big theory" lurks within contemporary claims about subjectivity; this paper is one effort to bring discourse theory into sharper analytical focus in relation to processes of labor market segmentation.

Chapter 25

Discourse and Practice in Human Geography

Erica Schoenberger

What I want to do in this article is to step outside my own work, as much as that can be imagined possible, and try to set up an encounter between my usual analytical style and position and other approaches. There are several reasons for doing this. One is that I think it's a good exercise and good discipline – a way of checking into the rigor of one's own thinking. Another is that I have argued strongly that the inability of corporate strategists to do something like this contributes importantly to the problem of industrial competitiveness, so I thought I ought to try it myself, just as a way of staying honest (Schoenberger, 1997). A third is that it seems a good way of moving out of my comforting little cocoon of thought and engaging productively with other approaches and other concerns. The point is to see if one can critically engage with one's own thought-style (cf. Fleck, 1935).

The alternative terrain on which I want to position myself for this is composed of a couple of themes that crop up in feminist, postimperialist, and/or Foucauldian writings in the history and philosophy of science and social theory. One has to do with the status of the subject and the other with the status of discourse. Given the way I have traditionally worked (spending a lot of time talking with the men who run corporations) you might think that I could hardly have avoided addressing these themes directly, but you would be wrong.

The first issue, then, has to do with what we can say about the knowing subject and the knowledge she produces. Here I wish to follow Harding who provides an intriguing distinction between what she calls weak and strong objectivity in the practice of science. The entire scientific edifice, of course, is built upon and socially legitimated by the claim to objectivity: that the scientist's perception and analysis of "the facts" will not be colored by *a priori* judgments, and that the scientist has no personal stake in the outcome of her research. Objectivity in this sense underwrites the authority of the scientist and her ability to establish widely accepted matters of fact. In the official ideology of science, objectivity, combined with careful adherence to "the scientific method," guarantees the validity of the information produced.

Harding, however, claims that normal scientific practice is only "weakly" objective (Harding, 1991; cf. also Shapin, 1994). Weak objectivity, in this usage, describes the detached and dispassionate stance of the scientist towards the object of research, whether it be a virus or a supernova. It is nothing more than the job of the scientist to analyze rigorously and impartially the data associated with the object or process under study. It is not, however, the normal job of the scientist to subject *herself*, her lab organization, her choice of research questions, and the like to the same careful, dispassionate analysis. For Harding, however, it is precisely this act of locating oneself socially and historically and analyzing how this affects the process of doing science that would constitute "strong" objectivity.

This doesn't amount to a claim that strong objectivity would change what you saw under the microscope or in the particle accelerator. It might make you think twice, though, about why you find certain problems interesting or particularly satisfying, why you ask certain kinds of questions of the data and not others, or how you understand the contributions of different categories of people working with or around you (e.g., lab technicians). And your answers to these new kinds of question might plausibly affect the trajectory of scientific inquiry that you follow.

The second theme I want to draw on has to do with the ways in which discourse enters into the constitution of our social reality and, indeed, of us as social agents. In part here I'm following the lead of McCloskey's (1985) *The rhetoric of economics* which inquires into the nature of the conversation within that discipline, viewing the analysis of rhetoric as an exercise in self-understanding. I am guided also by Poovey's careful investigation of the historical development of epistemological domains such as "the social" and "the economic" in Victorian England (Poovey, 1995). This process involves the establishment of boundaries between domains and the development of discourses and analytical styles appropriate to them. As Poovey shows, the discursive strategies and technologies of representation employed within these domains are involved in the creation of the very social categories they purport to define and analyze. A conceptual apparatus, in this way, takes on the property of materiality: the abstraction becomes a real social entity.

At the same time, academic disciplines, such as sociology or economics, can be seen as nothing more than the study of these epistemological domains and the institutions associated with them. As academics, then, we also have to wrestle with an epistemological and discursive history that not only guides us in the production of knowledge but also tells us in important ways who we are and what we do.

Taking the two themes together, what I'm trying to do is to be strongly objective about how the discursive strategies of others affect my own discursive constructions and how these, in turn, enter into the material work that I do. In other words, what difference does it make that I accept certain ways of talking about the world I'm trying to analyze and what happens if I challenge those rhetorical and discursive conventions?

In what follows, I want to examine the meaning and use of the concept of "competitiveness." The analysis claims, in essence, that the term is not merely an "objective" description of a fact of economic life, but also part of a discursive strategy that constructs a particular understanding of reality and elicits actions and reactions appropriate to that understanding. This is followed by a discussion of why the discourse has the power that it does and how it may influence how we think about and act in the world. I then work through some examples of how an unexamined acceptance of a discursive convention may obscure as much as it reveals.

Competitiveness as an Economic Category and Discursive Strategy

I'm going to make this as simple as possible for myself by reducing the whole problem of discourse to one word: competitiveness. For economic geographers in general and for me in particular, the categories of competition, competitive strategy, and competitiveness have a great deal of importance and might even be thought to pervade our work, even when they are not directly under analysis. All sorts of industrial and spatial economic outcomes are implicitly or explicitly linked to some notion of "competitiveness" (cf. Krugman, 1994). The rise and decline of particular industrial regions have something to do with the competitiveness of the labor force (generally understood in terms of comparative costs and unionization), which (for geographers if for no one else) has something to do with the competitiveness of the region in the first place, understood as its particular mix of resources, infrastructure, location, and cost profile.

More than that, though, "competitiveness" seems to me a term that has become truly hegemonic in the Gramscian sense. It is a culturally and socially sanctioned category that, when invoked, can completely halt public discussion of public or private activities. There is virtually no counterargument available to the simple claim that "doing X will make us uncompetitive," whatever X and whomever "us" might be.

In a capitalist society, of course, it is more than reasonable to be concerned with competition and competitiveness. No matter what your theoretical orientation, mainstream to Marxist, these must be seen as real forces shaping real outcomes in society. They are not just intellectual constructs that lend a false sense of order to a messy world. On the other hand, we can also analyze them as elements of a discursive strategy that shapes our understanding of the world and our possibilities for action in it. In that case, it seems to me the first questions to ask are whose discursive strategy is it, what do they really mean by it, where does its power come from, and what kinds of actions does it tend to open up or foreclose.

Whose discourse?

The discourse on competitiveness comes from two principal sources and in part its power is their power. In the first instance, it is the discourse of the economics profession which doesn't really need to analyze what it is or what it means socially. The market is the impartial and ultimate arbiter of right behavior in the economy and competitiveness simply describes the result of responding correctly to market signals.

The blandness of this "objective" language conceals the underlying harshness of the metaphor. For Adam Smith, the idea of competition plausibly evoked nothing more disturbing than a horse race in which the losers are not summarily executed. Since then, the close identification of marginalist economics with evolutionary theory has unavoidably imbued the concept with the sense of a life or death struggle (cf. Niehans, 1990). In short, on competitiveness hangs life itself. As Krugman (1994, p. 31) defines it: "when we say that a corporation is uncompetitive, we mean that its market position is . . . unsustainable – that unless it improves its performance it will cease to exist."

As with evolutionary theory, our ability to strip the moral and ethical content from the concepts of life and death is not so great as the self-image of modern science suggests. Competitiveness becomes inescapably associated with ideas of fitness and unfitness, and these in turn with the unstated premise of merit, as in "deserving to live" and "deserving to die."

Secondly, competitiveness is the discourse of the business community and represents both an essential value and an essential validation. More generally, it serves as an all purpose and unarguable explanation for any behavior: "We must do X in order to be competitive." Again, the implied "or else" is death.

As hinted, though, the discourse of competitiveness has seeped out beyond these sources and is becoming socially pervasive. University presidents, hospital administrators, and government bureaucrats also discourse quite fluently now about competitiveness and its related accoutrements: customers, total quality, flexibility, and so forth.

It will be objected that competitiveness is a deeply ingrained social category and value in the USA and elsewhere and there is no particular reason to single out economists and business persons as culprits in its dissemination. That objection is true enough, and no doubt contributes to the general power of the discourse since it resonates so well with this broader heritage. But "competitiveness" in the sense of "deserving to live" is not what was commonly meant by this more diffuse social understanding. It is, however, what is meant in economic analysis and business life, and it is increasingly what is meant in other institutional and social settings as well.

The power of the discourse

In my own work, I am constantly engaged in discussions of competitive strategy and competitiveness with the people who run firms. In this context I strive to be a critical and detached interlocutor whose job it is to analyze and interpret – rather than simply report – responses to my questions. When I'm talking with people about what it takes for them to be competitive in a particular market, or whatever, I am not especially shy about debating the substance of their answers. That is to say, I will argue with them about whether or not a given strategy is a good way of being competitive and what you really need to do to implement it. But that there *is* some irreducible category called competitiveness, the fulfilling of which, *in extremis*, overrides all other considerations – that I don't argue about. Or I haven't up to now. I have simply accepted the general idea of competitiveness as the ultimate demonstration of the validity of that behavior.

I don't think I'm alone in this. I think it's characteristic of economic geography to assume the categories of competition and competitiveness in order to answer other questions rather than asking what these categories themselves might be about. I think also that an unexamined notion of competitiveness plays an increasingly strong, if not decisive role in many political and institutional debates with enormous consequences for real people. So it is important to try to understand why the concept is so powerful that it enjoys a kind of social immunity. You can discuss what is more and what is less competitive, but you can't call the category into question.

Within the academy, the power of the discourse of economics has a lot to do with the social power of the discipline. This, in turn, involves some complicated mix of command over material resources, claims of social utility, a certain amount of proselytizing in other disciplines, asserting a family resemblance with other powerful and "hard" disciplines such as physics by virtue of its mathematized and abstract style of reasoning, and so on.

Social power, in turn, can be deployed to set a standard of what constitutes "science" in the social sciences against which other forms of social science (e.g., geography) are implicitly or explicitly valued (cf. Clark, 1998). As McCloskey (1985, p. 82) notes, "The metaphors of economics often carry . . . the authority of Science and . . . its claims to ethical neutrality." One doesn't have to suppose the least degree of cravenness on the part of other social scientists to imagine that the social norms established in this way gradually become part of the general environment and become more generally valued as they are within economics (Foucault, 1995). Certain practices and ways of thinking, as in a Marshallian industrial district, are "in the air" and we are all hard-pressed to avoid inhaling them.

The best evidence of this effect within economic geography that I can think of is actually in the writings of the Marxists within the field, especially in the 1970s and early 1980s. There was a time when none of us could write anything without a lengthy introductory section in which we took great pains to demolish the assumptions and analytical tropes of neoclassical economics. We couldn't leave it alone, and I think it must be the case that the long struggle to valorize an alternative worldview and scientific method has left its mark on all of us. But we're marked in surprisingly subtle ways and it takes real work to see the effects.

But economics also derives some of its power from being able to deploy concepts such as competitiveness which have tremendous ideological weight. Market competition is the guarantor of the fairness of the social system as a whole because markets, by the definition of the discipline, are impartial and competitiveness, though a life or death affair, proceeds on a purely technical basis. That is to say, you are not competitive or uncompetitive because of who you are, but merely as a result of how you respond to market signals that provide the same information to everyone. Further, the idea of economic competitiveness meshes so perfectly with evolutionary theory that it takes on exactly the natural and timeless air that makes it so unarguable. The discipline that owns such a concept – whose discourse this is – is bound to seem inevitable.

In sum, the social power of economics within the academic hierarchy helps anchor the power of its discourse which, in true virtuous circle fashion, reinforces the social power of the discipline. On top of all this, the discourse is shared with another extraordinarily powerful social group: the "business community."

The problems of competition, competitive strategy, and competitiveness are deeply meaningful to people who run businesses. They really see them as authentic life and death issues and, *at the limit*, they are right. But there is arguably a broad range of issues and conditions in which life and death are not at stake, but competitiveness is automatically invoked anyway as the unchallengeable and "natural" explanation for what is about to happen. The degree to which this is accepted and even imitated by people in other spheres entirely is remarkable.

What the discourse produces

What is the relationship, then, between discourse and our material reality and between discourse and our ability to act in the world – at least as it relates to the issue of competitiveness? Here are some thoughts.

The relationship between discourse and material reality/action is mediated by the social power of the discursive agent. The social resources deployed in validating the discourse on competitiveness are really quite impressive. But they can be deployed with great economy or remain entirely latent because of the way the discourse has been successfully naturalized. The beauty of it is that, once the conversation moves on to this terrain, we more or less automatically fall silent of our own accord. This may be a particular instance of Foucault's notion of disciplinary individualism, in which the essence of freedom is voluntary compliance with the rules – in this case, the established order of a particular discipline (Foucault, 1995; cf. Poovey, 1995). Once the word is uttered, its disciplinary force is made manifest.

This isn't meant to imply that we unavoidably end up by simply parroting the economists and business persons. But it does suggest that we may be subtly deflected from certain kinds of questions or challenges to the discourse and the practices associated with it, whether this is in an academic setting or a more general public arena.

This rather simple observation has, I want to stress, real consequences for academics and nonacademics alike. For academics, the substance of our questions and challenges is our stock in trade. We get research funds on the basis of them and write articles which will anchor our careers, allowing us to ask new questions to get more funding and so on. Meanwhile we are contributing to the collective construction of a body of knowledge – an interpretive structure – which shapes a more general understanding of the world. We make and validate ourselves through our discourse.

The silencing and deflecting effect of the discourse on competitiveness can also be seen in various forms of public discourse about any number of issues: the environment, welfare reform, healthcare reform, and, more obviously, the competitiveness of the national economy. Again, when all goes well, no specific exercise of overt power has to be undertaken. The disciplining effect of the discourse has been naturalized and internalized, so it is effective even with people whose interests are plainly not served by it. It also makes it all the more remarkable when some undisciplined groups of people do, in the end, fight back.

The Discourse and Practice of Competitiveness in Everyday Life

In this section, I want to work through a couple of examples of discourse in action on the issue of competitiveness to get a clearer idea of what is at stake. The first example asks to what degree Nike's "competitiveness" depends on having access to low-cost labor in offshore production sites. The second looks at issues of urban competitiveness through an examination of the living wage campaign in Baltimore.

Nike

Nike as a corporation needs no introduction. It is not so much global as omnipresent. It has spread its interests out from athletic shoes to sports equipment and sports clothing, but it is mainly known for transforming athletic shoes into a design and fashion-intensive business, and the company became phenomenally rich in the process (Katz, 1994). According to its 1996 10-K report to the SEC, it is the largest athletic footwear company in the world (Nike, 1996).

Nike also pioneered a shifting international division of labor in athletic shoe production which relies largely on subcontractors in a hierarchically nested set of offshore production locations (cf. Donaghu and Barff, 1990). If local costs become too high, a given location may be either upgraded in its tasks so that costs are not out of line, or abandoned in favor of less expensive locales. This is a production strategy that has been imitated by most of Nike's major competitors.

Shoe assembly remains a highly labor-intensive operation, so wage rates are an obvious location factor. Or we could say that Nike needs access to low-cost labor in order to remain competitive. Unsurprisingly, virtually all the company's athletic shoe output is produced in six Asian countries: Indonesia (38%), the People's Republic of China (34%), South Korea (11%), Taiwan (5%), Thailand (10%), and Vietnam (2%) (Nike, 1996).

Lately the company has come under some fire for the treatment of workers – especially women workers – in these offshore facilities. As well as offering poor wages and working conditions, Nike subcontractors are accused of physical and sexual abuse. In response, Nike has developed a code of conduct for its subcontractors and hired former UN Ambassador and civil rights activist Andrew Young and his consulting firm, Goodworks, to monitor the human rights situation in its offshore operations (ILO, 1996; *The New York Times*, 1997a, 1997b).

Most recently, Nike and several other apparel and footwear companies have reached an agreement with labor and human rights groups to support minimum labor standards in offshore facilities. The standards specify a maximum 60-hour workweek and onsite monitoring for abuses. They ban the employment of children under 15 except where it is permissible to employ 14-year-olds. Companies must pay at least the local minimum wage. Particular points of contention in the negotiations leading up to this agreement reportedly included the independence of the monitors (companies will be allowed to appoint their own) and whether companies should try to pay a local "living wage" – that is, a wage sufficient to live on in the country in question – rather than the local minimum wage. So far, the companies involved have insisted that the legal minimum wage is the appropriate standard (*The New York Times*, 1977c, 1997d).

On another front, Nike has also recently joined a consortium which is working to eliminate pervasive child labor in the soccer ball sewing industry in Pakistan. It was reported that children received 60 cents for sewing a ball that might retail for $30–50. An experienced child can sew two in a day.

Here, then, is the issue. In a labor-intensive industry, we might all agree, low wages have something to do with competitiveness. But how much *exactly* do they have to do with "competitiveness," or the ability to survive economically in a market system, and how much with something else? I was forced to think, in reading about soccer balls in Pakistan, that no company's ability to exist in the world could possibly depend on paying children 60 cents to sew a $50 soccer ball. Why not 90 cents? Why not $3.00? What difference would it make? Similarly, why is it so important to companies that they obligate themselves only to pay the legal minimum wage in places like Vietnam? Would it make such a difference to pay enough to live on there?

I thought I would try to construct a crude numerical analysis of Nike's production costs for its footwear in order to see to what degree the company's competitiveness can be linked to the wages it is actually paying in its low-cost offshore operations – or, at any rate, the wages that its subcontractors are paying on its behalf. In effect, I want to find out what would happen to the company if it 1) simply doubled the prevailing local wage; 2) paid all its offshore workers ten times the prevailing local wage; and 3) paid its offshore workers roughly the USA minimum wage. A first constraint is that it can't pass the cost increase along to its customers so the wage increase presumably won't affect its competitiveness in the market or its revenues. Would it still make money? This can't be calculated with any great precision, but the method is as follows.

Nike acknowledges a total employment figure of 17,200 worldwide. However, this figure almost certainly doesn't include precisely the workers we are interested in, so we simply have to guess. One guess would be that a roughly equivalent number of workers is employed by subcontractors – say 20,000 for ease of calculation. Another guess would be that the number of subcontracted workers is considerably larger – say 50,000.

Average monthly or annual earnings for manufacturing workers in various countries is provided by the ILO's *Yearbook of Labor Statistics* for 1996. Unfortunately, data for Vietnam and Taiwan are unavailable. Because their share of total Nike production in Asia is relatively small (7% total), I took the liberty of simply assimilating them to the nearest Nike country in terms of economic development levels, so that workers in Vietnam are treated as though they earned the same wages as Indonesians in 1990, and workers in Taiwan are treated as though they were Korean women. Korea was the only country on the list for which it was possible to obtain data specifically for women and so all Nike workers in Korea and Taiwan are treated as though they were female. This might tend to understate the actual wage bill for these countries, but on the other hand, using averages for men *and* women in all the other countries probably overstates their actual wage bills.

If there are 20,000 Nike subcontract workers apportioned to each country according to its share in total output, the annual wage bill amounts to some $44 million (see Table 25.1). If there are 50,000 workers, the annual wage bill comes to $111 million.

Table 25.2 shows the results of intervening in the actual wage levels by first doubling them, and then multiplying them by a factor of ten. In both these operations, I have held wages in Korea/Taiwan to current actual levels which happen to be almost exactly equivalent to the annual earnings of a full-time worker in the USA who is paid the current minimum wage of $4.75/hour. In other words, I have granted raises only to workers in Indonesia, the People's Republic of China, Thailand, and Vietnam.

If there are 20,000 workers, doubling low incomes increases the total wage bill by $13.5 million or roughly 31%. Multiplying by ten yields an increase of $122 million or 274%. If there are 50,000 workers, the increases are $34 million and $304 million, respectively (the percentages are the same).

Table 25.1: Estimation of Nike's offshore employment costs

Country	Average annual per capita earnings in manufacturing ($US)	If 20,000 offshore workers		If 50,000 offshore workers	
		Employment	Annual wage bill (US$000s)	Employment	Annual wage bill (US$000s)
Indonesia	573[1,2,3]	7,600	4,354.8	19,000	10,887.0
Vietnam	573[1,2,3]	400	229.2	1,000	573.0
People's Republic of China	739[3,4]	6,800	5,025.2	17,000	12,563.0
South Korea	9,643[5,6]	2,200	21,214.6	5,500	53,036.0
Taiwan	9,643[5,6]	1,000	9,643.0	2,500	24,107.5
Thailand	1,955[3,4]	2,000	3910.0	5,000	9,775.0
Total		20,000	44,376.0	50,000	110,942.0

Notes: 1. Indonesia, 1990; 2. Total labor cost including overheads; 3. Average for men and women; 4. 1994; 5. Korea, 1995; 6. Women only. Figures calculated using exchange rates for March 21, 1997.
Sources: ILO, 1996; Nike, 1996.

Table 25.2: Estimated total annual wage bill under varying conditions, Nike offshore manufacturing

	Employment (20,000)	Increase (US$000s)	Employment (50,000)	Increase (US$000s)
At current earnings	44,377	–	110,942	–
Earnings in low-income countries[1] doubled	57,896	13,519	144,740	33,798
Earnings in low-income countries[1] ×10	166,050	121,673	415,124	304,183
All country earnings at level of Korea	192,860	148,483	482,150	371,208

Note: 1. Indonesia, The People's Republic of China, Thailand, and Vietnam.
Source: Table 25.1.

I then raise everybody to the level of Korea or, roughly, the USA minimum wage. At 20,000 workers, this produces an increase of $148 million or 335%. At 50,000 workers, the wage bill increases by $371 million. This latter figure represents a little under 10% of Nike's total costs in 1996, which were $3.9 billion.

Table 25.3 provides various reference points for judging the impact of these wage increases on Nike's financial results. We can highlight the worst-case scenario to get an overall sense of what is at risk. In the worst case (50,000 workers at Korean wage rates), Nike revenues stay constant at $6.5 billion while costs rise to $4.3 billion. Gross margins accordingly decline from 39.6% to 33.9%. This is

Table 25.3: Financial impact of raising wages, worst case scenario (50,000 workers at Korea-level wages)

	Nike 1996 actual results	Projected results
Revenues (US$000s)	6,470,625	6,470,625
Costs (US$000s)	3,906,756	4,277,964
Income before taxes (US$000s)	899,090	527,822
Net income (US$000s)	553,190	203,235
Net income/common share (US$)	3.77	1.38
Gross margin (US$000s)	2,563,879	2,192,661
Gross margin (%)	39.6	33.9
Return on equity (%)	25.2	9.3
Return on assets (%)	15.6	5.7

Sources: Tables 25.1 and 25.2; Nike, 1996.

significant, given that Nike's gross margins have been at least 38% since 1990, but it is clearly not fatal.

Income before taxes was $899 million in 1996. If we deduct the cost increase entirely from this figure, income before taxes declines to $527.8 million, which is still ahead of the comparable figure for 1994 ($490.6 million). Holding the company's effective income tax rate constant at 38.5%, this yields a net income of $203 million compared with the $553 million actually recorded. Since 1990, Nike's net income has not dropped below $243 million. Net income per common share drops from $3.77 to something like $1.38. Nike's net income per share has not gone lower than $1.61 since 1990.

In 1996, Nike recorded a 25.2% return on equity and a 15.6% return on assets. As near as I can tell (and I know that this is inexact), these ratios drop to 9.3% and 5.7%, respectively. The lowest recorded values for these categories since 1990 are 17.7% and 13.1%.

This worst-case scenario assumes there is zero slack in the system. One might wish to consider, for example, that Nike spent $642.5 million on advertising and promotion in 1996 or roughly 72% of its income before taxes. Now it may be that this is exactly the optimal figure to spend and that any reduction would generate a decline in revenues. On the other hand, it might not be the optimal figure, and it might be possible to lay off some of the increased wage costs against this sum. Or it might be possible to sew the equivalent of a little dolphin on each pair of shoes that has been made under certified humane conditions and charge a little bit more for them.

That doesn't matter, though. What is clear is that if you assume 50,000 offshore workers and you decide to pay them all roughly the USA minimum wage – which is, for most of them, something more than ten times their present earnings – Nike still makes money. The company can absorb 100% of the increased costs and still earn a half billion dollars before taxes. That is to say, the company is still competitive.

Another way of putting this is to say that relying on low-wage offshore workers has nothing to do with Nike's competitiveness. What does it have to do with, then? It may be more accurate to say that, rather than being a necessary part of the firm's competitive strategy, low-wage offshore women workers are a core part of the company's *accumulation* strategy and its *stock market* strategy.

In sum, using ultra-cheap female labor in the Third World allows the company to accelerate the rate at which it accumulates and can redeploy capital, either in expanded and more productive production, or in the kind of global advertising campaigns that simply squash the competition. At the same time, it allows it to boost its financial statistics to more attractive levels. This isn't stupid from a corporate point of view, and companies have the legal right to operate this way. But it is not what we meant by competitive. It is not a life or death situation, and it is not unarguable.

I don't imagine for a minute that anyone really thought that Nike was utterly compelled to pay exactly Indonesian wage levels in order to stay alive. But I do find it possible to imagine that we generally find it plausible that Nike finds it necessary, under the pressures of a competitive market, to pay "low" wages without figuring out what the boundaries of the category of "low" ought to be. I think also that this plausibility reflects the power and pervasiveness of a particular discourse.

Baltimore

Baltimore is, in many ways, a classic case of urban decline. A once robust and diversified manufacturing base has all but collapsed, a thriving port has been downsized and automated, and the white middle class has long since fled to the surrounding counties. Beginning in the 1970s, tremendous state and federal subsidies fed an urban renewal project centered on tourism and services that has redeemed Baltimore's image in the eyes of many without changing the essential fact that an appalling proportion of the city's majority black population lives in poverty. Indeed, the kind of jobs generated by the urban renewal strategy, because they often pay at or near the minimum wage, guarantee that even people working full time will continue to live in poverty. Working full time at a minimum wage of $4.25/hour provides an annual income of just under $9000 a year, assuming no time off. The recent increase to $4.75/hour brings that to $9880. The federal poverty line for a family of four is just under $16,000. Needless to say, these jobs ordinarily do not offer benefits of any sort.

Among the first to decide to take this issue head on was a group of highly respected and influential pastors with long experience in the civil-rights movement. They could hardly avoid noticing that many of the people who were regulars at the soup kitchens run by their churches held full-time jobs and were still a long way from being able to support themselves and their families. The pastors, working through a group called Baltimoreans United in Leadership Development (BUILD), allied themselves with an Industrial Areas Foundation group trying to organize low-income workers. The resulting Solidarity Sponsoring Committee (SSC) is also supported by AFSCME. As a result of their efforts, Baltimore in 1994 became the first city in the USA to pass a "Living Wage" ordinance.

The ordinance requires all providers of services working on contract for the city to pay their employees a living wage – that is to say, an hourly wage sufficient to lift its recipients above the poverty line. That wage is currently pegged at $7.70/hour (compared with the current minimum wage of $4.75) although the ordinance phases in the increase. Thus, at the time of writing the current minimum under the ordinance is $6.60/hour, rising to $7.10 on 1 July 1997 and to $7.70 the following year.

Workers employed directly by the city are already paid at or above this level so the immediate budgetary impacts are restricted to the effects of raising wages on contract costs to the city. The total number of workers involved is thought to be somewhere on the order of 4000, implying that the total direct economic impact on the city will be quite constrained. However, we can suppose that raising the wages of the lowest paid will lead to a certain degree of upward wage drift. And we know that SSC is working hard to organize other low-wage service workers around the living wage. Johns Hopkins University, the largest private employer in Maryland, has so far promised to institute a $6.00 minimum wage on its service contracts in response to this organizing campaign. The ultimate aim in fact is to make the living wage the minimum wage in Baltimore.

Debate about the impacts of the living wage has centered on the costs to the city government and the "competitiveness" of the city. Baltimore's competitiveness or lack thereof is, of course, an extraordinarily touchy subject in the city which has been strenuously fighting to revalorize itself in very particular ways for decades.

The revalorization strategy has essentially had two aspects. The first has been to subsidize publicly the costs to private capital of doing business in the city. The second has been to create geographic enclaves, centering on the Inner Harbor and central business district and including selected outposts such as universities and hospitals, and making these areas "safe" for investment. By safe, of course, we mean (but could never say) free of any threat posed by dangerously poor (black) people. Safest of all is free of their presence entirely.

The living wage appears to be at odds with the first strand of the strategy and essentially irrelevant to the second. The enclave strategy is exclusionary and implies keeping poor people away, not bringing them in and remedying their circumstances. In any case, the second part of the strategy can't be discussed, and so the prevailing discourse, emanating from the traditional centers of power in this city and others where similar proposals are on the table, has been about costs and competitiveness (Weisbrot and Sforza-Roderick, 1996).

And this, indeed, has been the discourse engaged by researchers such as myself. I have been involved in a study designed to assess the impacts of the living wage on Baltimore. This is a follow-up to a 1996 study by the Preamble Foundation which found, actually, that the real cost of city contracts declined slightly and the value of business investments increased in the year following passage of the ordinance. Indeed, positive side-effects of the law appear to be a drastic decrease in turnover and absenteeism and an increase in productivity associated with rising wages (Weisbrot and Sforza-Roderick, 1996).

Now, there's nothing wrong with assessing the costs of this or any other activity. I just went through a whole song and dance about Nike's costs, and I'm very interested to find out what the longer-run cost impacts of the living wage bill are in Baltimore. What if, though, the data had turned out differently in the Preamble Center study, or turn out differently in ours? What if all we can show is that yes, the city's costs increased and at the same time, for whatever reasons, investment in the city declined?

What is disturbing is that the discourse of costs and competitiveness defines the entire terrain of discussion – it constitutes the only valid currency of argument. In part, this is because there is so much going on that can't be said in polite society and in part this is because the "scientifically valid" data that one can find are almost wholly about these categories.

To demonstrate this, I tried to imagine doing an entirely different kind of research project related to the living wage in Baltimore. The hypothesis is that high costs are not a significant deterrent to productive investment in Baltimore; the significant deterrent is poverty, and the insecurity that poverty generates for poor and rich alike. Poverty means no market and poorly prepared workers whose lives are constantly disrupted by small catastrophes which in turn disrupt their ability to work. Poverty also means poor health and a lack of physical security for workers and employers. Poverty means a meager tax base and poor urban infrastructure and services. The cost of doing business could be zero here, and still investment might not be forthcoming. The living wage, in this context, would be *the* leading policy tool to encourage investment and economic growth.

There's another aspect of the kind of place and person that poverty creates that is worth mentioning. Poverty creates scary "others" who, in Baltimore, are predominantly African-American. By the usual social sleight-of-hand, race comes to stand for the general suitability of a person for employment. Or, to put this another way, it is no longer the competitiveness of the *person*, but the competitiveness of the *body* that counts in the first instance in creating a labor supply that is seen to be appropriate for investment (cf. Martin, 1992; Wright, 1996; Harvey, 1998). In a capitalist society, however, the scariness of the Other can be mitigated to the degree that the Other provides a productive basis for accumulation. Again the living wage would seem to be the appropriate policy.

I'm acutely aware that I can't demonstrate any part of this argument in an acceptable scientific fashion. That's the point, really. The discourse, and the real resources that support the discourse, open up a terrain for some kinds of research and make others quite difficult and less valid looking. One is still free to make a moral argument, but that has nothing to do with one's status as a researcher or a scientist in society. Academic freedom or no, it turns out that we're quite constrained in doing our jobs, and as a result, we may end up tacitly supporting the very discourse and practices that constrain us in the first place.

Conclusion

Colonial subjects have long had to struggle with what it means to use the language of the master – even in postcolonial times. In our normal understanding of academic life, we aren't supposed to have anything in common with colonial subjects on this or any other issue. But if we are strongly objective about ourselves and our work as Sandra Harding urges, can we be sure that the desired objectivity of our research is not subtly undermined by our reliance on a language and a discourse that is not entirely of our own choosing and, arguably, is a language and a discourse that represents the interests of particular social groups and not others?

The answer, I think, is that we can't be sure, so we have to check repeatedly and try to figure out what difference it makes. What difference, for example, does it make to conclude that Nike's offshore manufacturing is an accumulation strategy rather than a competitive strategy, or that Baltimore's competitive status is undermined by poverty, not by costs?

I don't think it necessarily means specific, nameable things. I suspect, rather, that over time, if we keep checking back on ourselves and our work in this way, we will contribute to building an alternative ensemble of intellectual and material resources that can be used to pose and answer different kinds of question – our own questions, and questions arising from the discourses and material circumstances of different sorts of people. Among other things, I suspect this would help us to liberate ourselves from the constraining shadows of other disciplines, such as economics, and to re-create geography as a central arena of inquiry and debate within the university and outside it (cf. Clark, 1998).

I don't at all want to argue that, having absorbed the hegemonic discourse, we are all doomed to be Stepford geographers who can only serve that discourse. But I think it must help us to know more clearly why we're doing what we're doing, and why we do it in a particular way. Examining and debating our own discourse and the practices deeply associated with it with some of the same intensity and care with which we examine and debate the world "out there" will help us understand these things better.

Bibliography

Abernathy, W. J., Clark, K. B., and Kantrow, A. M. 1983. *Industrial Renaissance: Producing a Competitive Future for America*. New York: Basic Books.

Abo, T. 1996. The Japanese production system: The process of adaptation to national settings. In R. Boyer and D. Drache (eds). *States Against Markets: The Limits of Globalization*. London: Routledge, 136–54.

Achebe, C. 1983. *The Trouble with Nigeria*. Ibadan: Heinemann.

Acker, J. 1990. Hierarchies, jobs, bodies: A theory of gendered organisations. *Gender and Society*, 4, 139–58.

Adam, B. 1995. *Timewatch*. Cambridge: Polity Press.

Adams, P. 1995. A reconsideration of personal boundaries in space-time. *Annals of the Association of American Geographers*, 85, 267–85.

Aglietta, M. 1979. *A Theory of Capitalist Regulation*. London: New Left Books.

Agrawal, R. G. 1981. Third-World joint ventures: Indian experience. In K. Kumar and M. G. McLeod (eds). *Multinationals from Developing Countries*. Lexington, MA: Lexington Books, 115–31.

Aitken, J. 1987. A stranger in the family: The legal status of domestic workers in Ontario. *University of Toronto Law Review*, 45, 394–415.

Akrich, M. 1992. The description of technological objects. In W. Bijker and J. Law (eds). *Shaping Technology, Building Society: Studies in Sociotechnical Change*. London: MIT Press, 205–24.

Albert, M. 1993. *Capitalism against Capitalism*. New York: Four Walls Eight Windows.

Allen, J. and Hamnett, C. (eds). 1995. *A Shrinking World? Global Unevenness and Inequality*. Oxford: Oxford University Press.

Allen, J. 1988. The geographies of service. In D. Massey and J. Allen (eds). *Uneven Re-Development: Cities and Regions in Transition*. London: Hodder and Stoughton, 124–41.

Altamira, R. 1923. *Ideario Pedagógico*. Madrid: Editorial Reus.

Altvater, E. 1993. *The Future of the Market: An Essay on the Regulation of Money and Nature*. London: Verso.

Altvater, E. 1994. Ecological and economic modalities of time and space. In M. O'Connor (ed.). *Is Capitalism Sustainable?* New York: Guilford, 76–90.

Amariglio, J. 1988. The body, economic discourse and power: An economist's introduction to Foucault. *History of Political Economy*, 20, 583–613.

Amariglio, J. and Ruccio, D. 1994. Postmodernism, Marxism and the critique of modern economic thought. *Rethinking Marxism*, 7, 7–35.

Amariglio, J. and Ruccio, D. 1999. Modern economics and the case of the disappearing body. In M. Woodmansee and M. Osteen (Eds), *The New Economic Criticism: Studies at the Intersection of Literature and Economics*. London: Routledge.

Amariglio, J., Resnick, S., and Wolff, R. 1988. Class, power and culture. In C. Nelson and L. Grossberg (eds). *Marxism and the Interpretation of Culture*. London: Macmillan, 487–502.

Amendola, G., Guerrieri, P., and Padoan, P. C. 1992. International patterns of technological accumulation and trade. *Journal of International and Comparative Economics*, 1, 173–97.

Amin, A. 2000. Organisational learning through communities of practice. *Paper presented at the workshop on "The Firm in Economic Geography,"* University of Portsmouth, 9–11 March.

Amin, A. 1992. Big firms versus the regions in the Single European Market. In M. Dunford and G. Kafkalas (eds). *Cities and Regions in the New Europe: The Global–Local Interplay and Spatial Development Strategies*. London: Belhaven Press, 127–49.

Amin, A. and Graham, S. 1998. The ordinary city. *Transactions of the Institute of British Geographers*, 22, 411–29.

Amin, A. and Hausner, J. (eds). 1997. *Beyond Market and Hierarchy: Interactive Governance and Social Complexity*. Aldershot: Edward Edgar.

Amin, A. and Malmberg, A. 1992. Competing structural and institutional influences on the geography of production in Europe. *Environment and Planning A*, 24, 401–16.

Amin, A. and Thrift, N. J. 1995. Institutional issues for the European regions: From markets and plans to socioeconomics and powers of association. *Economy and Society*, 24, 41–66.

Amin, A. and Thrift, N. J. (eds). 1994. *Globalisation, Institutions and Regional Development in Europe*. Oxford: Oxford University Press.

Amin, A. and Thrift, N. J. 1994. Living in the global. In A. Amin and N. J. Thrift (eds). *Globalisation, Institutions and Regional Development in Europe*. Oxford: Oxford University Press, 1–22.

Amin, A. and Thrift, N. J. 1997. Globalization, socio-economics, territoriality. In R. Lee. and J. Wills (eds). Geographies of Economies. London: Arnold, 147–57.

Amuzegar, J. 1982. Oil wealth: A very mixed blessing. *Foreign Affairs*, 60, 814–35.

Anderson, B. 1983. *Imagined Communities*. London: Verso.

Anderson, P. 1984. *Lineages of the Absolutist State*. London: Verso.

Angoustures, A. 1995. *Historia de España en el Siglo XX*. Barcelona: Editorial Ariel.

Appadurai, A. 1990. Disjuncture and difference in the global cultural economy. *Public Culture*, 2, 1–24.

Arce, A. and Marsden, T. 1993. The social construction of international food: A new research agenda. *Economic Geography*, 69, 291–311.

Arnold, E. 1984. *Competition and Technical Change in the UK Television Industry*. London: Macmillan.

Asanuma, B. 1989. Manufacturer–supplier relationships in Japan and the concept of relation-specific skill. *Journal of the Japanese and International Economies*, 3, 1–30.

Asheim, B. 1997. "Learning regions" in a globalised world economy: Towards a new competitive advantage of industrial districts? In S. Conti and M. Taylor (eds). *Interdependent and Uneven Development: Global–Local Perspectives*. London: Avebury, 143–76.

Azorín. 1982. *Obras Selectas*, 5th edn. Madrid: Editorial Biblioteca Nueva.

Babbage, C. 1835. *On the Economy of Machinery and Manufactures*. New York: A. M. Lelley.

Bagguley, P., Mark-Lawson, J., Shapiro, D., Urry, J., Walby, S., and Warde, A. 1990. *Restructuring: Place, Class and Gender*. London: Sage.

Bagnasco, A. 1977. *Tre Italie: La Problematica Territoriale Dello Sviluppo*. Bologna: Il Mulino.

Bagnasco, A. 1988. *La Costruzione Sociale Del Mercato*. Bologna: Il Mulino.

Bakshi, P., Goodwin, M., Painter, J., and Southern, A. 1995. Gender, race and class in the local welfare state: Moving beyond regulation theory in analysing the transition from Fordism. *Environment and Planning A*, 27, 1539–54.

Block, F. 1990. *Postindustrial Possibilities*. Berkeley, CA: University of California Press.

Baldwin, T., McVoy, D., and Steinfield, C. 1996. *Convergence: Integrating Media, Information and Communication*. London: Sage.

Balibar, E. 1995. *The Philosophy of Marx*. London: Verso.

Ballance, R. H. 1987. *International Industry and Business: Structural Change, Industrial Policy and Industry Strategies*. London: Allen and Unwin.

Barlow, J. and Savage, M. 1986. The politics of growth: Cleavage and conflict in a Tory heartland. *Capital and Class*, 30, 156–82.

Barnes, T. J. 1994. Probable writing: Derrida, deconstruction and the quantitative revolution in human geography. *Environment and Planning A*, 26, 1021–40.

Barnes, T. J. 1996. *Logics of Dislocation: Models, Metaphors and Meanings of Economic Space*. New York: Guilford.

Barnes, T. J. 2000. Inventing Anglo-American economic geography, 1889–1960. In E. S. Sheppard and T. J. Barnes (eds). *A Companion to Economic Geography*. Oxford: Blackwell, 11–26.

Barratt-Brown, M. 1993. *Fair Trade*. London: Zed Books.

Barrett, H. and Browne, A. 1991. Environment and economic sustainability: Women's horticultural production in The Gambia. *Geography*, 776, 241–48.

Bartlett, C. A. and Ghoshal, S. 1989. *Managing Across Borders: The Transnational Solution*. Boston: Harvard Business School Press.

Bassett, T. 1988. The political ecology of peasant–herder conflicts in the northern Ivory Coast. *Annals of the Association of American Geographers*, 78, 453–72.

Bataille, G. 1988. *The Accursed Share*. New York: Zone Books.

Batty, M. 1993. The geography of cyberspace. *Environment and Planning B: Planning and Design*, 20, 615–61.

Bauman, Z. 1992. *Intimations of Postmodernity*. London: Routledge.

Becattini, G. and Rullani, E. 1993. Sistema locale e mercato globale. *Economia e Politica Industriale*, 80, 25–40.

Becattini, G. 1987. L'unita d'indagine. In G. Becattini (ed.). *Mercato e forze f Locali: Il Distretto Industriale*. Bologna: Il Mulino, 35–48.

Beechey, V. 1977. *Unequal Work*. London: Verso.

Belk, R. 1995. *Consuming Societies*. New York: Routledge.

Bell, D. 1973. *The Coming of Post-Industrial Society*. New York: Basic Books.

Bellamy, E. 1897. *Equality*. New York: Appleton.

Bender, J. and Welbery, D. E. (eds). 1991. *Chronotoypes*. Stanford: Stanford University Press.

Benedikt, M. 1991. Introduction. In M. Benedikt (ed.). *Cyberspace: First Steps*. Cambridge, MA: MIT Press, 1–18.

Bennett, T. (ed.). 1981. "Christmas." Popular culture: themes and issues. Milton Keynes: Open University Press (book 1, units 1/2).

Bennington, G. 1995. Introduction to economics. In C. Gill (ed.). *Bataille: Writing the Sacred*. London: Routledge, 63–108.

Benton, T. 1989. Marxism and natural limits: An ecological critique and reconstruction. *New Left Review*, 178, 51–86.

Benton, T. 1991. The Malthusian challenge: Ecology, natural limits and human emancipation. In P. Osborne (ed.). *Socialism and the Limits to Liberalism*. London: Verso, 241–69.

Benton, T. 1992. Ecology, socialism and the mastery of nature: A reply to Reiner Grundmann? *New Left Review*, 194, 55–72.

Benton, T. (ed.). 1996. *The Greening of Marxism*. New York: Guilford.

Berkes, F. 1985. Fishermen and "the tragedy of the commons." *Environmental Conservation*, 12, 199–206.

Berry, S. 1986. Concentration without privatisation: Agrarian consequences of rural land control in Africa. In *Conference on agricultural policy and African food security: Issues, prospects and constraints, toward the year 2000*. Champagne-Urbana, IL: Center for African Studies, University of Illinois.

Berry, S. 1989. Social institutions and access to resources. *Africa*, 59, 41–55.

Bianchi, P. 1993. The promotion of small-firm clusters and industrial districts: European policy perspectives. *Journal of Industry Studies*, 1, 16–29.

Bierstecker, T. 1988. Reaching agreement with the IMF: The Nigerian negotiations 1983–1986. Unpublished manuscript, School of International Relations, University of Southern California, Los Angeles.

Billig, M., Condor, S., Edwards, D., Gare, M., Middleton, D., and Radley, A. 1988. *Ideological Dilemmas*. London: Sage.

Bingham, N. 1996. Objections: From technological determinism towards geographies of relations. *Environment and Planning D: Society and Space*, 14, 635–57.

Blaikie, P. and Brookfield, H. 1987. *Land Degradation and Society*. New York: Methuen.

Blanc, H. and Sierra, C. 1999. The internationalisation of R&D by multinationals: A trade-off between external and internal proximity. *Cambridge Journal of Economics*, 23, 187–206.

Blauhof, G. 1994. Non-equilibria dynamics and the sociology of technology. In L. Leydesdorff and P. van der Desselaar (eds). *Evolutionary Economics and Chaos Theory*. London: Pinter, 152–66.

Block, F. 1994. The roles of the state in the economy. In N. Smelser and R. Smedberg (eds). *The Handbook of Economic Sociology*. Princeton, NJ: Princeton University Press, 691–710.

Block, F. and Hirschborn, L. 1979. New productive forces and the contradictions of contemporary capitalism: A post-industrial perspective. *Theory and Society*, 7/3, 363–96.

Bluestone, B. and Harrison, B. 1982. *The Deindustrialization of America*. New York: Basic Books.

Boddy, M. and Fudge, C. 1984. *Local Socialism*. London: Macmillan.

Boden, D. 1994. *The Business of Talk: Organizations in Action*. Cambridge: Polity.

Bohm, D. 1980. *Wholeness and the Implicate Order*. London: Routledge and Kegan Paul.

Bohm, D. 1994. *Thought as System*. London: Routledge.

Boisot, M. H. 1995. *Information Space*. London: Routledge.

Bonnett, K., Bromley, S., and Jessop, B. 1990. Farewell to Thatcherism? Neo-liberalism and "new times." *New Left Review*, 179, 81–102.

Boothroyd, P. and Davis, C. 1993. Community economic development: Three approaches. *Journal of Planning Education and Research*, 12, 230–40.

Bordo, S. 1989. The body and the reproduction of femininity: The feminist appropriation of Foucault. In A. Jagger and S. Bordo (eds). *Gender, Body, Knowledge*. New Brunswick, NJ: Rutgers University Press, 3–34.

Bourdieu, P. 1984. *Distinction*. London: Routledge.

Boyer, C. 1996. *Cybercities: Visual Perception in an Age of Electronic Communication*. Princeton, NJ: Princeton University Press.

Boyer, R. (ed.). 1988. *The Search for Labour Market Flexibility: The European Economies in Transition*. Oxford: Clarendon.

Braczyk, H.-J., Cooke, P., and Heidenreich, M. 1998. *Regional Innovation Systems*. London: UCL Press.

Bradby, B. 1982. The remystification of value. *Capital and Class*, 17, 114–33.

Bradley, H. 1989. *Men's Work, Women's Work*. Cambridge: Polity.

Braudel, F. 1973. *The Mediterranean and the Mediterranean World in the Age of Philip II*. New York: Harper and Row.

Braudel, F. 1982. *The Wheels of Commerce*. New York: HarperCollins.

Braverman, H. 1974. *Labour and Monopoly Capital*. New York: Monthly Review Press.

Brennan, D. and O'Donnell, C. 1986. *Caring for Australia's Children*. Sydney: Allen and Unwin.

Brennan, T. 1994. *History after Lacan*. London: Routledge.

Brooks, R. 1992. Maggie's man: We were wrong. *The Observer*, June 21, p. 21.

Brotchie, J., Hall, P., and Newton, P. (eds). 1987. *The Spatial Impact of Technological Change*. London: Croom Helm.

Brown, J. S. and Duguid, P. 1996. Organizational learning and communities-of-practice. In M. D. Cohen and L. S. Sproull (eds). *Organizational Learning*. London: Sage.

Brown, J. S. and Duguid, P. 2000. Balancing act: How to capture knowledge without killing it. *Harvard Business Review*, 78, 73–80.

Browning, H. L. and Singelmann, J. 1975. *The Emergence of a Service Society*. Springfield, VA: National Technical Information Service.

Brusco, S. 1982. The Emilian model: Productive decentralisation and social integration. *Cambridge Journal of Economics*, 6, 167–84.

Bryan, D. 1992. Wage policy and the Accord: Comment. *Journal of Australian Political Economy*, 29, 99–110.

Bryant, R. 1992. Political ecology: An emerging research agenda in Third World studies. *Political Geography*, 11, 12–36.

Busch Cooper, B. 1985. *The War Against the Seals*. Montreal: McGill Queen's University Press.

Business Week. 1983. How the PC project changed the way IBM thinks. October 3, pp. 43–4.

Business Week. 1984. Just-in-time inventories: combating foreign rivals. May 14, pp. 44–9.

Butler, J. 1990. *Gender Trouble: Feminism and the Subversion of Identity*. London: Routledge.

Butler, J. 1993. *Bodies That Matter: On the Discursive Limits of Sex*. New York: Routledge.

Butler, J. 1997. *The Psychic Life of Power: Theories of Subjection*. Stanford, CA: Stanford University Press.

Buttimer, A. 1982. Musing on helicon: Root metaphors and geography. *Geografiska Annaler*, 64B, 89–96.

Cable, V. and Clarke, J. 1981. *British Electronics and Competition with Newly Industrialized Countries*. London: Overseas Development Institute.

Cairncross, F. 1997. *The Death of Distance: How the communications revolution will change our lives*. London: Orion Business Books.

Callari, A. 1983. Adam Smith, the theory of value and the history of economic thought. *Association of Economic and Social Analysis Discussion Paper No. 3*, University of Massachusetts-Amherst.

Callon, M. 1991. Techno-economic networks and irreversibility. In J. Law (ed.). *A Sociology of Monsters*. London: Routledge, 132–61.

Callon, M. 1986. Some elements of a sociology of translation: Domestication of the scallops and the fisherman of St Brieuc bay. In J. Law (ed.). *Power, Action and Belief: A New Sociology of Knowledge*. London: Routledge, 196–232.

Callon, M. and Latour, B. 1981. Unscrewing the big leviathan. In K. Knorr-Cetina and A. Cicourel (eds). *Advances in Social Theory and Methodology*. London: Routledge and Kegan Paul, 277–303.

Callon, M. and Law, J. 1995. Agency and the hybrid collectif. *South Atlantic Quarterly*, 94, 481–507.

Cameron, J. 1995. Ironing out the family: Class, gender and power in the household. Mimeo, Department of Geography and Environmental Sciences, Monash University, Clayton VIC, Australia.

Campbell, B. 1993. *Goliath*. London: Methuen.

Cano García, G. 1992. Confederaciones Hidrográficas. In A. Gil Olcina and A. Morales Gil (eds). *Hitos Históricos de los Regadíos Españoles*. Madrid: Ministerio de Agricultura/Pesca y Alimentación, 309–34.

Carling, A. 1986. Rational choice Marxism. *New Left Review*, 160, 24–62.

Carling, A. 1992. *Analytical Marxism*. London: Verso.

Carney, J. 1980. Regions in crisis: Accumulation, regional problems and crisis formation. In J. Carney, R. Hudson, and R. Lewis (eds). *Regions in Crisis*. London: Croom Helm, 28–59.

Carney, J. 1986. The social history of Gambian rice production: An analysis of food security strategies. Unpublished Ph.D. dissertation, University of California, Berkeley.

Carney, J. 1988. Struggles over crop rights within contract farming households in a Gambian irrigated rice project. *Journal of Peasant Studies*, 15, 334–49.

Carney, J. 1991. Indigenous soil and water management in Senegambian rice farming systems. *Agriculture and Human Values*, 8, 37–58.

Carney, J. 1992. Peasant women and economic transformation in The Gambia. *Development and Change*, 23, 67–90.

Carney, J. 1994. Contracting a food staple in The Gambia. In P. Little and M. Watts (eds). *Peasants under Contract: Contract Farming and Agrarian Transformation in Sub-Saharan Africa*. Madison, WI: University of Wisconsin, 167–87.

Carney, J. and Hudson, R. 1978. Capital, politics and ideology: The North East of England, 1870–1946. *Antipode*, 10, 64–78.

Carney, J. and Watts, M. 1991. Disciplining women? Rice, mechanization, and the evolution of Mandinka gender relations in Senegambia. *Signs*, 16, 651–81.

Carnoy, M. 1993. Multinationals in a changing world economy: Whither the nation-state? In M. Carnoy, M. Castells, S. Cohen, and F. H. Cardoso (eds). *The New Global Economy in the Information Age*. University Park, PA: Pennsylvania State University Press, 45–96.

Carr, R. 1983. *Espana: de la Restauración a la Democracia, 1875–1980*. Barcelona: Editorial Ariel.

Carrier, J. G. 1995. Maussian occidentalism: Gift and commodity systems. In J. G. Carrier (ed.). *Occidentalism: Images of the West*. Oxford: Oxford University Press, 85–108.

Castells, M. 1989. *The Informational City*. Oxford: Blackwell.

Castells, M. 1983. The informational economy and the new international division of labor. In M. Carnoy, M. Castells, S. Cohen, and F. H. Cardoso (eds), *The New Global Economy in the Information Age*. University Park, PA: The Pennsylvania State University Press, 15–44.

Castells, M. 1996. *The Rise of the Network Society*. Oxford: Blackwell.

Castree, N. 1995. The nature of produced nature: Materiality and knowledge construction in Marxism. *Antipode*, 27, 12–48.

Cavendish, R. 1982. *Women on the Line*. London: Routledge and Kegan Paul.

Caves, R. 1982. *Multinational Enterprise and Economic Analysis*. Cambridge: Cambridge University Press.

Ceesay, M., Jammeh, O., and Mitchell, I. 1982. *Study of Vegetable and Fruit Marketing in The Gambia*. Banjul, The Gambia: Ministry of Economic Planning and Industrial Development and the World Bank.

Center for Research on Economic Development [CRED]. 1985. *Rural Development in the Gambian River Basin*. Ann Arbor, MI: CRED.

Cerny, P. G. 1990. *The Changing Architecture of Politics*. London: Sage.

Cerny, P. G. 1991. The limits of deregulation: Transnational interpenetrations and policy change. *European Journal of Political Research*, 19, 173–96.

Chandler, D. A. 1977. *The Visible Hand*. Cambridge, MA: Harvard Belknap.

Chang, K.-T. and Thomson, C. N. 1994. Taiwanese foreign direct investment and trade with Thailand. *Singapore Journal of Tropical Geography*, 15, 112–27.

Chase-Dunn, C. 1989. *Global Formation*. Cambridge, MA: Blackwell.

Chaudhry, K. 1989. The price of wealth: Business and state in labor remittance and oil economies. *International Organization*, 43, 101–45.

Cheal, D. J. 1988. *The Gift Economy*. London: Routledge.

Chisholm, G. G. 1889. *Handbook of Commercial Geography*. London and New York: Longman, Green, and Co.

Christopherson, S. 1993. Market rules and territorial outcomes: The case of the United States. *International Journal of Urban and Regional Research*, 17, 274–88.

Christopherson, S. 1999. Rules as resources: How market governance regimes influence firm networks. In T. J. Barnes and M. S. Gertler (eds). *The New Industrial Geography: Regions, Regulation and Institutions*. London: Routledge, 155–75.

Christopherson, S. and Storper, M. 1986. The city as studio; the world as back lot: The impact of vertical disintegration on the location of the motion picture industry. *Environment and Planning D: Society and Space*, 4, 305–20.

CILSS [Permanent Interstate Committee for Drought Control in the Sahel]. 1979. *Development of Irrigated Agriculture in Gambia: General Overview and Prospects. Proposal for a second program 1980–1985*. Paris: Club du Sahel.

CILSS. 1990. *Study on Improvement Irrigated Farming in The Gambia*. Paris: Club du Sahel.

Ciriacy Wantrup, S. V. and Bishop, R. C. 1975. Common property as a concept in natural resource property. *Natural Resources Journal*, 15, 713–26.

CIS [Counter Information Services] n.d. *Anti-Report on Ford*. London: Counter Information Services.

Citizenship and Immigration Canada. 1999. *The Live-in Caregiver Program: Information for Employers and Live-In Caregivers from Abroad*. Ottawa: Minister of Public Works and Government Services.

City of Camberwell. 1987. *Melbourne Inter-Council Comparison*. 3rd edn. Melbourne: City of Camberwell.

Clark, G. L., Gertler, M., and Feldman, M. (eds). 2000. *The Oxford Handbook of Economic Geography*. Oxford: Oxford University Press.

Clark, G. L., Mansfield, D., and Tickell, A. 2001. Emergent frameworks in global finance: Accounting standards and German supplementary pensions. *Economic Geography*, 77, 250–71.

Clark, G. L., Mansfield, D., and Tickell, A. 2002. Global finance and the German model: German corporations, market incentives, and the management of employer-sponsored pension institutions. *Transactions of the Institute of British Geographers*, 27, 91–110.

Clark, C. 1940. *The Conditions of Economic Progress*. London: Macmillan.

Clark, G. 1998. Stylized facts and close dialogue: Methodology in economic geography. *Annals of the Association of American Geographers*, 88, 73–87.

Clavel, P. 1982. *Opposition planning in Wales and Appalachia*. Philadelphia: Temple University Press.

Coase, R. H. 1937. The nature of the firm. *Economica*, 4, 386–405.

Coase, R. H. 1960. The problem of social cost. *Journal of Law and Economics*, 3, 1–44.

Cochrane, A. 1983. Local economic policies: Trying to drain an ocean with a teaspoon. In J. Anderson, S. Duncan, and R. Hudson (eds). *Redundant Spaces in Cities and Regions?* London: Academic Press, 285–312.

Cockburn, C. 1985. *Machinery of Dominance: Women, Men and Technical Know-How.* London: Pluto Press.

Cohen, S. S. and Zysman, J. 1987. *Manufacturing Matters: The Myth of the Post-Industrial Economy.* New York: Basic Books.

Collins, H. M. 1981. The role of the core set in modern science. *History of Science*, 19, 6–19.

Collinson, D. and Hearn, G. 1994. Naming men as men: Implications for work, organisation and management. *Gender, Work and Organisation*, 1, 2–22.

Colomina, B. (ed.). 1992. *Sexuality and Space.* New York: Princeton Architectural Press.

Cook, I. and Crang, P. 1996. The world on a plate: Culinary culture, displacement and geographical knowledges. *Journal of Material Culture*, 1, 131–53.

Cooke, P. (ed.). 1989. *Localities.* London: Hyman.

Cooke, P. 1997. Regions in a global market: The experiences of Wales and Baden-Wurttemberg. *Review of International Political Economy*, 4, 349–81.

Cooke, P. and Morgan, K. 1998. *The Associational Economy.* Oxford: Oxford University Press.

Corn, J. 1986. Epilogue. In J. Corn (ed.). *Imagining Tomorrow: History, Technology and the American Future.* Cambridge, MA: MIT Press, 219–29.

Corn, J. and Horrigan, B. 1984. *Yesterday's Tomorrows: Past Visions of the American Future.* Baltimore, MD: Johns Hopkins University Press.

Coronil, F. 1987. The black El Dorado: Money fetishism, democracy and capitalism in Venezuela. Unpublished Ph.D. dissertation, University of Chicago.

Coronil, F. and Skurski, J. 1991. Dismembering and remembering the nation: The semantics of political violence in Venezuela. *Comparative Studies in Society and History*, 26, 288–337.

Cosmides, L. and Tooby, J. 1994. Better than rational: Evolutionary psychology and the invisible hand. *American Economic Review*, 84, 327–32.

Costa, J. 1892. *Política Hidráulica y Misión Social de los Riegos en España.* Madrid: Edición de la Gaya Ciencia.

Costello, V. 1981. Tehran. In M. Pacione (ed.). *Problems and Planning in Third World Cities.* New York: St. Martin's, 137–56.

Cox, K. R. 1992. The politics of globalization: A sceptic's view. *Political Geography*, 11, 427–9.

Crang, P. 1994. It's showtime: On the workplace geographies of display in a restaurant in Southeast England. *Environment and Planning D: Society and Space*, 12, 675–704.

Crompton, R. 1992. Where did all the bright girls go? Women's higher education and employment since 1964. In N. Abercrombie and A. Warde (eds). *Social Change in Britain.* Cambridge: Polity Press.

Crompton, R. and Sanderson, K. 1990. *Gendered Jobs and Social Change.* London: Unwin Hyman.

Cronon, W. 1991. *Nature's Metropolis: Chicago and the Great West.* New York: A. A. Norton.

Curran, C. 1991. Change of heart: Interview with Meg Smith, Peter Ewer, Chris Lloyd and John Rainford, four of the authors of "Surviving the Accord: From Restraint to Renewal." *Australian Left Review*, 134, 24–9.

Curry, M. 1991. On the possibility of ethics in geography: Writing, citing, and the construction of intellectual property. *Progress in Human Geography*, 15, 125–48.

Curtin, P. 1984. *Cross-Cultural Trade in World History*. New York: Cambridge University Press.

Cusumano, M. A. 1985. *The Japanese Automobile Industry*. Cambridge, MA: Harvard University Press.

Dahrendorf, R. 1968. Market and plan: Two types of rationality. In R. Dahrendorf (ed.). *Essays in the Theory of Society*. London: Routledge and Kegan Paul, 215–31.

Daniels, P. 1988. Producer services and the post-industrial space-economy. In D. Massey and J. Allen (eds). *Uneven Re-development: Cities and Regions in Transition*. London, Hodder and Stoughton, 107–23.

de Reparez, G. 1906. Hidráulica y Dasonomiá. *Diario de Barcelona*, July 21.

Dear, M. and Wolch, J. 1987. *Landscapes of Despair*. Princeton NJ: Princeton University Press.

Dear, M. J. and Wolch, J. R. 1989. How territory shapes social life. In J. R. Wolch and M. J. Dear (eds). *The Power of Geography*. Boston: Allen and Unwin, 1–18.

Debord, G. 1978. *Society of the Spectacle*. Detroit: Black and Red Books.

DeCosse, P. and Camara, E. 1990. *A Profile of the Horticultural Production Sector in Gambia*. Banjul, The Gambia: Department of Planning and Ministry of Agriculture.

del Moral Ituarte, L. 1996. Sequía y Crisis de Sostenibilidad del Modelo de Gestión Hidráulica. In M. V. Marzol, P. Dorta, and P. Valladares (eds). *Clima y Agua: La Gestión de un Recurso Climático*. Madrid: La Laguna, 179–87.

del Moral Ituarte, L. 1998. L'état de la Politique Hydraulique en Espagne. *Hérodote*, 91, 118–38.

Deleuze, G. and Guattari, F. 1983. *Anti-Oedipus*. Minneapolis: University of Minnesota Press.

Delorme, R. 1997. The foundational bearing of complexity. In A. Amin and J. Hausner (eds). *Beyond Market and Hierarchy: Interactive Governance and Social Complexity*. Aldershot: Edward Elgar.

Demeritt, D. 1994. The nature of metaphors in cultural geography and environmental history. *Progress in Human Geography*, 18, 163–85.

Derman, W. 1984. USAID in the Sahel. In J. Barker (ed.). *The Politics of Agriculture in Tropical Africa*. Beverly Hills: Sage, 77–97.

Derrida, J. 1982. *Given Time: Counterfeit Money*. Chicago: Chicago University Press.

Derrida, J. 1992. *Given Time*. Chicago: Chicago University Press.

Derrida, J. 1995. *The Gift of Death*. Chicago: Chicago University Press.

Dex, S. 1987. *Women's Occupational Mobility*. London: Macmillan.

Dey, J. 1981. Gambian women: Unequal partners in rice development projects? *Journal of Development Studies*, 17, 109–22.

Dicken, P. 1990. Seducing foreign investors: The competitive bidding strategies of local and regional agencies in the United Kingdom. In M. Hebbert and J.-C. Hansen (eds). *Unfamiliar Territory: The Reshaping of European Geography*. Aldershot: Avebury, 162–86.

Dicken, P. 1992a. *Global Shift*. 2nd edn. London: Chapman.

Dicken, P. 1992b. International production in a volatile regulatory environment: The influence of national regulatory policies on the spatial strategies of transnational corporations. *Geoforum*, 23, 303–16.

Dicken, P. 1994. Global–local tensions: Firms and states in the global space-economy. *Economic Geography*, 70, 101–28.

Dicken, P. 1998. *Global Shift*. 3rd edn. New York: Guilford.

Dicken, P., Peck, J., and Tickell, A. 1997. Unpacking the global. In R. Lee and J. Wills (eds). *Geographies of Economies*. London: Arnold, 158–66.

Dicken, P. and Thrift, N. J. 1992. The organization of production and the production of organization: Why business enterprises matter in the study of geographical industrialization. *Transactions of the Institute of British Geographers*, 17, 279–91.

Dominic, G. 1983/84. Beyond the transformation riddle: A labor theory of value. *Science and Society*, 47, 427–50.

Donaghu, M. and Barff, R. 1990. Nike just did it: International subcontracting and flexibility in athletic footwear production. *Regional Studies*, 24, 537–52.

Dore, R. 1983. Goodwill and the spirit of market capitalism. *British Journal of Sociology*, 34, 459–82.

Doremus, P., Keller, W., Pauly, L., and Reich, S. 1998. *The Myth of the Global Corporation*. Princeton, NJ: Princeton University Press.

Dorfman, N. S. 1983. Route 128: The development of a regional high technology economy. *Research Policy*, 12, 299–316.

Dorsey, K. 1991. Putting a ceiling on sealing: Conservation and cooperation in the international arena, 1909–11. *Environmental History Review*, 15, 27–46.

Dosi, G., Pavitt, K., and Soete, L. 1990. *The Economics of Technical Change and International Trade*. London: Harvester.

Douglass, D. and Krieger, J. 1983. *A Miner's Life*. Henley: Routledge and Kegan Paul.

Doz, Y. 1986. *Strategic Management in Multinational Companies*. Oxford: Pergamon.

Driever, S. L. 1998. "And since Heaven has filled Spain with goods and gifts": Lucas Mallada, the Regeneracionist Movement, and the Spanish Environment, 1881–90. *Journal of Historical Geography*, 24, 36–52.

DuGay, P. 1996. *Consumption and Identity at Work*. London: Sage.

Dunning, J. H. 1992. The global economy, domestic governance strategies and transnational corporations: Interactions and policy implications. *Transnational Corporations*, 1, 7–45.

Dunning, J. H. 1993. *Multinational Enterprises and the Global Economy*. Reading, MA: Addison-Wesley.

Dunning, J. H. and Norman, G. 1985. Intra industry production as a form of international economic involvement: An exploratory analysis. In A. Erdilek (ed.). *Multinationals as Mutual Invaders: Intra Industry Foreign Direct Investment*. New York: St. Martin's, 9–28.

Dunsmore, J. R. 1976. *The Agricultural Development of The Gambia: An Agricultural, Environmental and Socio-Economic Analysis*. Land Resource Study No. 22. Surrey: Land Resources Division, Ministry of Overseas Development.

Eagleton, T. 1997. Spaced out. *London Review of Books*, April 27, pp. 22–3.

Eckersley, R. 1992. *Environmentalism and Political Theory: Toward an Ecocentric Approach*. London: University College Press.

Eckersley, R. 1993. Free market environmentalism: Friend or foe? *Environmental Politics*, 2, 1–19.

Edge, S. 1995. Consuming in the face of hatred. *Soundings*, 1, 163–74.

Edquist, C. (ed.). 1997. *Systems of Innovation: Technologies, Institutions and Organizations*. London: Pinter.

Edwards, R. 1979. *Contested Terrain*. New York: Basic Books.

EITB [Engineering Industry Training Board]. 1981. *Maintenance Skills in the Engineering Industry*. Stockport, Cheshire: Engineering Industry Training Board.

Ekpo, E. 1985. *IMF Loan Comes to Nigeria*. Apapa: Nigerian Problems and Issues.

Eli, M. 1990. *Japan Inc.: Global strategies of Japanese Trading Corporations*. London: McGraw-Hill.

Elson, D. (ed.). 1979. *Value: The Representation of Labour in Capitalism*. London: CSE Books.

Elson, D. 1989. The cutting edge: Multinationals in the EEC textiles and clothing industry. In D. Elson and R. Pearson (eds). *Women's Employment and Multinationals in Europe*. London: Macmillan, 80–110.

Elster, J. 1979. *Logic and Society*. Chichester: John Wiley.

Elster, J. 1986. *Making Sense of Marx*. Cambridge: Cambridge University Press.

Emecheta, B. 1982. *Naira Power*. London: Macmillan.

Encarnation, D. J. 1992. *Rivals Beyond Trade: America versus Japan in Global Competition*. Ithaca, NY: Cornell University Press.

Encarnation, D. J. and Wells, L. T. 1986. Competitive strategies in global industries. In M. E. Porter (ed.). *Competition in Global Industries*. Boston, MA: Harvard Business School, 267–90.

Enderwick, P. (ed.). 1997. *Foreign Investment: The New Zealand Experience*. Palmerston North: Dunmore Press.

Ernst, D. 1990. *Global Competition, New Information Technologies and International Technology Diffusion: Implications for Industrial Latecomers*. Paris: OECD Development Centre.

Featherstone, M. 1991. *Consumer Culture and Postmodernism*. London: Sage.

Featherstone, M. (ed.). 1990. *Global Culture: Nationalism, Globalisation, and Modernity*. London: Sage.

Ferenczi, S. 1950. *Sex in Psychoanalysis*. New York: Holmes.

Fernández Clemente, E. 1990. La Política Hidráulica de Joaquín Costa. In T. Pérez Picazo and G. Lemeunier (eds). *Agua y Modo de Producción*. Barcelona: Editorial Crítica, 69–97.

Fincher, R. 1987. Space, class and political processes: The social relations of the local state. *Progress in Human Geography*, 11, 496–515.

Fine B., Heasman, M., and Wright, J. 1996. *Consumption in the Age of Affluence: The World of Food*. London: Routledge.

Fisher, G. B. A. 1952. A note on tertiary production. *Economic Journal*, 62, 820–34.

Fitzsimmons, M. 1989. Reconstructing nature. *Environment and Planning D: Society and Space*, 7, 1–3.

Fleck, L. 1935. *Genesis and Development of a Scientific Fact*. Chicago: University of Chicago Press.

Florida, R. 1995. Toward the learning region. *Futures*, 27, 527–35.

Folbre, N. 1993. *Who Pays for the Kids? Gender and the Construction of Constraint*. New York: Routledge.

Fontana, J. 1975. *Cambio Económico y Actitudes Políticas en la España del Siglo XIX*. Barcelona: Editorial Ariel.

Food and Agriculture Organization. 1983. *Rice Mission Report to The Gambia*. Rome: Food and Agriculture Organization.

Foucault, M. 1973. *The Order of Things: An Archaeology of the Human Sciences*. New York: Vintage Books.

Foucault, M. 1979. *History of Sexuality*. Vol. 1. London: Allen Lane.

Foucault, M. 1995. *Discipline and Punish*. 2nd edn. New York: Pantheon.

Fox, S. 1981. *John Muir and his Legacy: The American Conservation Movement*. Boston, MA: Little Brown.

Fraad, H., Resnick, S., and Wolff, R. 1994. *Bringing it all Back Home: Class, Gender, and Power in the Modern Household*. London: Pluto.

Francis, J. 1993. *The Politics of Regulation*. Cambridge, MA: Blackwell.

Frank, A. G. 1980. *Crisis in the World Economy*. London: Heinemann.

Franke, R. and Chasin, B. 1980. *Seeds of Famine*. Montclair, NJ: Allanheld.

Frankel, H. 1977. *Money: Two Philosophies*. Oxford: Blackwell.

Fransman, M. 1994. Information, knowledge, vision and theories of the firm. *Industrial and Corporate Change*, 3, 1–45.

Fraser, N. 1997. *Justice Interruptus: Critical Reflections of the "Postsocialist" Condition*. London: Routledge.

Freud, S. 1955. *Standard Edition of the Complete Psychological Works*. London: Hogarth Press.

Friedland, W., Busch, L., Buttel, F., and Rudy, A. 1991. *Towards a New Political Economy of Agriculture*. Boulder, CO: Westview Press.

Fröbel, F., Heinrichs, J., and Kreye, O. 1980. *The New International Division of Labor*. New York: Cambridge University Press.

Fuchs, V. 1968. *The Services Economy*. New York: Columbia University Press.

Fujita, M., Krugman, P., and Venables, A. J. 1999: *The Spatial Economy: Cities, Regions and International Trade*. Cambridge, MA: MIT Press.

Fukuyama, F. 1995. *Trust*. New York: Free Press.

Gabriel, P. 1966. The investment in the LDC: Asset with a fixed maturity. *Columbia Journal of World Business*, 111, 3–20.

Gamble, D. 1955. *Economic Conditions in Two Mandinka Villages: Kerewan and Keneba*. London: Colonial Office.

Garrabou, R. 1975. La Crisi Agrária Espanyola de Finals del Segle XIX: Una Etapa del Desenvolupament del Capitalisme. *Recerques*, 5, 163–216.

Gatens, M. 1991. Representations in/and the body politic. In R. Diprose and R. Ferrel (eds). *Cartographies: The Mappings of Bodies and Spaces*. Sydney: Allen & Unwin, 79–87.

Gates, W. 1995. *The Road Ahead*. London: Viking.

Gelb, A. 1984. *Adjustment to Windfall Gains: A Comparative Analysis of Oil Exporting Countries*. Washington, DC: World Bank.

Gelerntner, D. 1991. *Mirror Worlds*. New York: Oxford University Press.

Gerber, J. 1997. Beyond dualism: The social construction of nature and the natural and social construction of human beings. *Progress in Human Geography*, 21, 1–17.

Gerlach, M. L. 1992. *Alliance Capitalism: The Social Organization of Japanese Business*. Berkeley, CA: University of California Press.

Gershuny, J. 1976. *After Industrial Society*. London: Macmillan.

Gertler, M. S. 1992. Flexibility revisited: Districts, nation-states and the forces of production. *Transactions of the Institute of British Geographers*, 17, 259–78.

Gertler, M. S. 1995. "Being there": Proximity, organization, and culture in the development and adoption of advanced manufacturing technologies. *Economic Geography*, 71, 1–26.

Gertler, M. S. 1996. Worlds apart: The changing market geography of the German machinery industry. *Small Business Economics*, 8, 87–106.

Gertler, M. S. 1999. The production of industrial processes. In T. J. Barnes and M. S. Gertler (eds). *The New Industrial Geography: Regions, Regulation and Institutions*. London: Routledge, 225–37.

Giansante, C. 1999. *In-Depth Analysis of Relevant Stakeholders: Guadalquivir River Basin Authority*. Mimeo, Department of Geography, University of Seville.

Gibson, W. 1984. *Neuromancer*. London: Harper and Collins.

Gibson-Graham, J.-K. 1996. *The End of Capitalism (As We Knew It): A Feminist Critique of Political Economy*. Oxford: Blackwell.

Gibson-Graham, J.-K. 2000. Poststructural interventions. In E. Sheppard and T. Barnes (eds). *Companion to Economic Geography*. Oxford: Blackwell, 95–110.

Giddens, A. 1979. *Central Problems in Social Theory*. London: Macmillan.

Giddens, A. 1981. *A Contemporary Critique of Historical Materialism*. London: Macmillan.

Giddens, A. 1990. *The Consequences of Modernity*. Stanford, CA: Stanford University Press.

Giddens, A. 1991. *Modernity and Self-Identity*. Cambridge: Polity.

Giddens, A. 1994. *Beyond Left and Right*. Cambridge: Polity.

Giffen, J. 1987. *An Evaluation of Women's Vegetable Gardens*. Banjul: Oxfam.

Gille, D. 1986. Maceration and purification. In *ZONE ½*. New York: Urzone, 226–83.

Gillespie, A. 1992. Communications technologies and the future of the city. In M. Breheny (ed.). *Sustainable Development and Urban Form*. London: Pion, 67–77.

Gilpin, R. 1975. *US Power and the Multinational Corporation: The Political Economy of Foreign Direct Investment*. New York: Basic Books.

Ginzberg, E. and Vojta, G. 1981. The service sector of the US Economy. *Scientific American*, 244/3, 48–65.

Glickman, N. J. and Woodward, D. P. 1989. *The New Competitors*. New York: Basic Books.

Gluek, A. C. 1982. Canada's splendid bargain: The North Pacific Fur Seal Convention of 1911. *Canadian Historical Review*, LXIII, 179–200.

Goffman, E. 1963. *Behavior in Public Places*. Glencoe, IL: Free Press.

Gómez Mendoza, J. 1992. Regeneracionismo y Regadíos. In A. Gil Olcina and A. Morales Gil (eds). *Hitos Históricos de los Regadíos Españoles*. Madrid: Ministerio de Agricultura. Pesca y Alimentación, 231–62.

Gómez Mendoza, J. and del Moral Ituarte, L. 1995. El Plan Hidrológico Nacional: Criterios y Directrices. In A. Gil Olicna and A. Morales Gil (eds). *Planificación Hidráulica en España*. Murcia: Fundación Caja del Mediterráneo, 331–98.

Gómez Mendoza, J. and Ortega Cantero, N. 1987. Geografía y Regeneracionismo en España. *Sistema*, 77, 77–89.

Gómez Mendoza, J. and Ortega Cantero, N. 1992. Interplay of state and local concern in the management of natural resources: Hydraulics and forestry in Spain 1855–1936. *Geo-Journal*, 26, 173–79.

Goodman, D. and Watts, M. 1994. Reconfiguring the rural or fording the divide? Capitalist restructuring and the agro-food system. *Journal of Peasant Studies*, 22, 1–49.

Gordon, D. M. 1988. The global economy: New edifice or crumbling foundations? *New Left Review*, 16, 824–64.

Gordon, H. S. 1954. The economic theory of a common property resource: The fishery. *Journal of Political Economy*, 62, 124–42.

Gottmann, J. 1982. Urban settlements and telecommunications. *Ekistics*, 302, 411–16.

Gould, S. J. 1991. *Bully for Brontosaurus: Reflections on Natural History*. New York: Norton.

Goux, J.-J. 1989. *Symbolic Economies after Marx and Freud*. Ithaca, NY: Cornell University Press.

Goux, J.-J. 1990. General economies and postmodern capitalism. *Yale French Studies*, 78, 206–24.

Government of The Gambia. 1966. *Five Year Plan for Economic and Social Development*. Banjul: Ministry of Economic Planning and Industrial Development.

Government of The Gambia. 1987. *Donors' Conference on the Agricultural Sector in The Gambia*. Banjul: Ministry of Agriculture.

Grabher, G. and Stark, D. (eds). 1997. *Restructuring networks in postsocialism: Linkages and localities*. Oxford: Oxford University Press.

Grabher, G. (ed.). 1993. *The Embedded Firm*. London: Routledge.

Graham, S. 1996. Imagining the real-time city: Telecommunications, urban paradigms, and the future of cities. In S. Westwood and J. Williams (eds). *Imagining Cities: Scripts, Signs and Memories*. London: Routledge, 31–49.

Graham, S. 1997. Liberalized utilities, new technologies, and urban social polarization: The UK case. *European Urban and Regional Studies*, 4, 135–50.

Graham, S. 1998. Spaces of surveillant-simulation: New technologies, digital representations, and material geographies. *Environment and Planning D: Society and Space*, 16, 483–504.

Graham, S. and Aurigi, A. 1997. Virtual cities, social polarisation and the crisis in urban public space. *Journal of Urban Technology*, 4, 19–52.

Graham, S. and Marvin, S. 1996. *Telecommunications and the City: Electronic Spaces, Urban Places*. London: Routledge.

Gramsci, A. 1978. *Selections from Political Writings, 1921–26*. London: Verso.

Granovetter, M. 1985. Economic action and social structure: The problem of embeddedness. *American Journal of Sociology*, 91, 481–510.

Granovetter, M. and Swedberg, R. (eds). 1993. *The Sociology of Economic Life*. Boulder, CO: Westview Press.

Graycar, A. and Harrison, J. 1984. Ageing populations and social care: Policy issues. *Australian Journal on Ageing*, 3, 3–9.

Greenblatt, S. 1992. *Marvellous Possessions: The Wonder of the New World*. Chicago: Chicago University Press.

Gregory, D. and Urry, J. (eds). 1985. *Social Relations and Spatial Structures*. London: Macmillan.

Gregson, N. and Lowe, M. 1994. *Servicing the Middle Classes*. London: Routledge.

Grossman, H. 1978. Marx, classical political economy and the problem of dynamics. *Capital and Class*, 2, 67–99.

Grossman, G. and Helpman, E. 1991. *Innovation and Growth in the Global Economy*. Cambridge, MA: MIT Press.

Grosz, E. 1994. *Volatile Bodies: Towards a Corporeal Feminism*. Bloomington, IN: Indiana University Press.

Grundmann, R. 1991. *Marxism and Ecology*. Oxford: Clarendon Press.

Grundmann, R. 1992. The ecological challenge to Marxism. *New Left Review*, 187, 103–120.

Guisinger, S. 1985. *Investment Incentives and Performance Requirements*. New York: Praeger.

Gumbrecht, H. U. and Pfeiffer, K. L. (eds). 1994. *Materialities of Communication*. Stanford, CA: Stanford University Press.

Hall, S. 1991. The local and the global: Globalization and ethnicity. In A. King (ed.). *Culture, Globalization, and the World-system: Contemporary Conditions for the Representation of Identity*. Binghamton, NY: State University of New York Press, 21–40.

Hamelink, C. (ed.). 1983. *Finance and Information*. Norwood, NY: Greenwood Publishing Group.

Hamilton, G. and Biggart, N. W. 1988. Market culture, and authority: A comparative analysis of management and organization in the Far East. *American Journal of Sociology*, 94, S52–S94.

Hamilton, G. 1991. The organizational foundations of Western and Chinese commerce: A historical and comparative analysis. In G. Hamilton (ed.). *Business Networks and Economic Development in East and Southeast Asia*. Hong Kong: Centre of Asian Studies, University of Hong Kong, 48–65.

Hamilton, G. and Biggart, N. W. 1992. Market, culture, and authority: A comparative analysis of management and organization in the Far East. In M. Granovetter and R. Swedberg (eds). *The Sociology of Economic Life*. Oxford: Westview Press, 81–221.

Hanson, S. and Pratt, G. 1988. Reconceptualizing the links between home and work in human geography. *Economic Geography*, 64, 299–321.

Hanson, S. and Pratt, G. 1995. *Gender, Work and Space*. London: Routledge.

Haraway, D. 1991. *Simians, Cyborgs, and Women: The Reinvention of Nature*. New York: Routledge.

Hardin, G. 1968. The tragedy of the commons. *Science*, 162, 1243–8.

Harding, S. 1991. *Whose Science? Whose Knowledge?* Ithaca, NY: Cornell University Press.

Harrison, B. 1994. *Lean and Mean: The Resurrection of Corporate Power in an Age of Flexibility*. New York: Basic Books.

Hartshorne, R. 1939. *The Nature of Geography: A Critical Survey of Current Thought in Light of the Past*. Lancaster, PA: Association of American Geographers.

Harvey, C. 1990. *Improvements in Farmer Welfare in The Gambia: Groundnut Price Subsidies And Alternatives*. Institute of Development Studies Discussion Paper No. 277. Sussex: Institute of Development Studies.

Harvey, D. 1974. Population, resources and the ideology of science. *Economic Geography* 50, 256–277.

Harvey, D. 1975a. Class structure in a capitalist society and the theory of residential differentiation. In R. Peel, M. Chisholm, and P. Haggett (eds). *Process in Physical and Human Geography: Bristol Essays*. London: Heinemann, 354–69.

Harvey, D. 1975b. The geography of accumulation: A reconstruction of the Marxian theory. *Antipode*, 7, 9–21.

Harvey, D. 1982. *The Limits to Capital*. Oxford: Blackwell.

Harvey, D. 1985a. *Consciousness and the Urban Experience*. Oxford: Blackwell.

Harvey, D. 1985b. *The Urbanization of Capital*. Oxford: Blackwell.

Harvey, D. 1987. Flexible accumulation through urbanization: Reflections on postmodernism in the American city. *Antipode*, 19, 260–86.

Harvey, D. 1989. *The Condition of Postmodernity*. Oxford: Blackwell.

Harvey, D. 1993a: From space to place and back again: Reflections on the condition of postmodernity. In J. Bird, B. Curtis, T. Putnam, G. Robertson, and L. Tickner (eds). *Mapping the Futures: Local Cultures, Global Change*, London: Routledge, 3–29.

Harvey, D. 1993b. The nature of environment: The dialectics of social and environmental change. *Socialist Register*, 29, 1–51.

Harvey, D. 1996. *Justice, Nature and the Geography of Difference*. Oxford: Blackwell.

Harvey, D. 1998. The body as an accumulation strategy. *Environment and Planning D: Society and Space*, 16, 401–21.

Harvey, D. 2000. *Spaces of Hope*. Berkeley, CA: University of California Press.

Harvey, D. and Scott, A. J. 1988. The practice of human geography: Theory and empirical specificity in the transition from Fordism to flexible accumulation. In W. D. Macmillan (ed.). *Remodelling Geography*. Oxford: Blackwell, 217–29.

Hausner, J. 1995. Imperative vs. interactive strategy of systematic change in central and eastern Europe. *Review of International Political Economy*, 2, 249–66.

Haussman, R. 1981. State landed property, oil rent and accumulation in Venezuela. Unpublished Ph.D. dissertation, Cornell University, Ithaca, New York.

Hay, C. 1995. Re-stating the problem of regulation and re-regulating the local state. *Economy and Society*, 24, 387–407.

Hayek, F. A. 1948. *Individualism and the Economic Order*. Chicago: University of Chicago Press.

Hays, S. 1959. *Conservation and the Gospel of Efficiency*. Cambridge, MA: Harvard University Press.

Healey, P., Cameron, S., Davoudi, S., Graham, S., and Madani Pour, A. (eds). 1995. *Managing Cities: The New Urban Context*. London: Wiley.

Hearn, G. and Parkin, P. W. 1987. *Sex at Work*. Brighton: Wheatsheaf.

Helgasen, P. 1990. *The Female Advantage*. London: Sage.

Helm, D. and Pearce, D. 1991. Economic policy towards the environment: An overview. In D. Helm (ed.). *Economic Policy Towards the Environment*. Oxford: Blackwell, 1–25.

Helou, A. 1991. The nature and competitiveness of Japan's *keiretsu*. *Journal of World Trade*, 25, 99–131.

Henderson, J. and Appelbaum, R. P. 1992. Situating the state in the East Asian development process. In J. Henderson and R. P. Appelbaum (eds). *States and Development in the Asian Pacific Rim*. Newbury Park, CA: Sage, 1–26.

Herrigel, G. 1994. Industry as a form of order: A comparison of the historical development of the machine tool industries in the United States and Germany. In J. R. Hollingsworth, P. C. Schmitter, and W. Streeck (eds). *Governing Capitalist Economies: Performance and Control of Economic Sectors*. New York: Oxford University Press, 97–128.

Hiebert, D. 1999. Local geographies of labor market segmentation: Montreal, Toronto, and Vancouver, 1991. *Economic Geography*, 75, 339–69.

Hill, S. 1988. *The Tragedy of Technology*. London: Pluto.

Hirsch, J. 1991. From the Fordist to the post-Fordist state. In B. Jessop, H. Kastendiek, K. Nielson, and O. K. Pederson (eds). *The Politics of Flexibility*. Aldershot: Edward Elgar, 67–81.

Hirst, P. 1994. *Associative Democracy*. Cambridge: Polity.

Hirst, P. and Thompson, G. 1992. The problem of "globalization": International economic relations, national economic management and the formation of trading blocs. *Economy and Society*, 21, 357–96.

Hirst, P. and Thompson, G. 1996. *Globalization in Question*. Cambridge: Polity.

Ho, S. P. S. and Huenemann, R. W. 1984. *China's Open Door Policy: The Quest for Foreign Technology and Capital*. Vancouver: University of British Columbia Press.

Hobsbawm, E. 1977. Some reflections on "the break-up of Britain." *New Left Review*, 105, 3–24.

Hochschild, A. 1983. *The Managed Heart*. Berkeley, CA: University of California Press.

Hodgson, G. M. 1988. *Economics and Institutions*. Cambridge: Polity.

Hodgson, G. M. 1993. *Economics and Evolution: Bringing Life Back Into Economics*. Cambridge: Polity.

Hogdson, G. M. 1998. The approach of institutional economics. *Journal of Economic Literature*, 36, 162–92.

Hogdson, G. M., Samuels, W. J., and Tool, M. R. (eds). 1993. *The Elgar Companion to Institutional and Evolutionary Economics*. Aldershot: Edward Elgar.

Howe, A. 1986. Aged care services: An analysis of provider roles and provision outcomes. *Urban Policy and Research*, 4, 2–20.

Hsing, Y.-T. 1997. *Making Capitalism in China: The Taiwan Connection*. New York: Oxford University Press.

Hudson, R. 1999. The learning economy, the learning firm and the learning region: A sympathetic critique of the limits to learning. *European Urban and Regional Studies*, 6, 59–72.

Hudson, R. 1986. Producing an industrial wasteland: Capital, labour and the state in North East England. In R. L. Martin and B. Rowthorne (eds). *The Geography of Deindustrialisation*. London: Macmillan, 169–213.

Hudson, R. and Lewis, J. (eds). 1982. *Regional Planning in Europe*. London: Pion.

Hudson, R. and Sadler, D. 1983a. The closure of Consett steelworks: Anatomy of a disaster. *Northern Economic Review*, 6, 2–17.

Hudson, R. and Sadler, D. 1983b. Region, class and the politics of steel closures in the European Community. *Environment and Planning D: Society and Space*, 1, 405–28.

Hudson, R. and Williams, A. M. 1995. *Divided Britain*. Chichester: Wiley.

Hutchinson, P. 1983. *The Climate of The Gambia*. Banjul: Ministry of Water Resources and the Environment.

Hutton, W. 1995. *The State We're In*. London: Jonathan Cape.

Hymer, S. H. 1975. The multinational corporation and the law of uneven development. In H. Radice (ed.). *International Firms and Modem Imperialism*. Harmondsworth: Penguin, 37–62.

Hymer, S. 1976. *The International Operations of National Firms: A Study of Direct Foreign Investment*. Cambridge, MA: MIT Press.

Ichigo, K., von Krogh, G., and Nonaka, I. 1998. Knowledge enablers. In G. von Krogh, J. Roos, and D. Kleine (eds). *Knowing in Firms: Understanding, Managing and Measuring Knowledge*. London: Sage, 173–203.

Imam-Jomeh, I. 1985. Petroleum-based accumulation and the state in Iran: Aspects of social and geographical differentiation, 1953–1979. Unpublished Ph.D. dissertation, University of California, Los Angeles.

Ingham, G. 1996. Some recent changes in the relationship between economics and sociology. *Cambridge Journal of Economics*, 20, 243–75.

Izard, M. 1986. *Tierra Firme: Historia de Venezuela Contemporanea*. Madrid: Alianza America.

Jack, I. 1990. *Export Constraints and Potentialities for Gambian Horticultural Produce*. Banjul: Ministry of Agriculture.

Jackson, P. and Thrift, N. J. 1995. Geographies of consumption. In D. Miller (ed.). *Acknowledging Consumption*. London: Routledge, 204–37.

Jacobs, M. 1994. The limits to neo-classicism: Towards an institutional environmental economics. In M. Redclift and T. Benton (eds). *Social Theory and the Global Environment*. Routledge, London, 67–91.

Jeng, A. A. O. 1978. An economic history of The Gambian groundnut industry 1830–1924: The evolution of an export economy. Unpublished Ph.D. dissertation, University of Birmingham.

Jenkins, R. 1987. *Transnational Corporations and Uneven Development: The Internationalization of Capital and the Third World*. London: Methuen.

Jessop, B. 1982. *The Capitalist State*. Oxford: Martin Robertson.

Jessop, B. 1994. Post-Fordism and the state. In A. Amin (ed.). *Post-Fordism: A reader*. Oxford: Blackwell, 251–79.

Jo, S.-H. 1981. Overseas direct investment by South Korean firms: Direction and pattern. In K. Kumar and M. G. McLeod (eds). *Multinationals from Developing Countries*. Lexington, MA: Lexington Books, 53–77.

Jobson, R. 1623. *The Golden Trade*. Devonshire: Speight and Walpole.

Johnson, C. 1982. *MITI and the Japanese Economic Miracle: The Growth of Industry Policy, 1925–1975*. Stanford, CA: Stanford University Press.

Johnston, R. J. 1986. The state, the region, and the division of labor. In A. J. Scott and M. Storper (eds). *Production, Work, and Territory: The Geographical Anatomy of Industrial Capitalism*. Boston, MA: Allen and Unwin, 265–78.

Johnston, R., Gregory, D., Pratt, G. et al. (eds). 2001: *The Dictionary of Human Geography*. Oxford: Blackwell.

Johnston, R., Gregory, D., and Smith, D. M. (eds). 1994: *The Dictionary of Human Geography*. Oxford: Blackwell.

Jones, D. T. 1983. Technology and the UK automobile industry. *Lloyds Bank Review*, 148, 14–27.

Jones, D. K. 1980. *A Century of Servitude*. Washington, DC: University Press of America.

Joseph, M. 1998. The performance of production and consumption. *Social Text*, 16, 25–62.

Julius, DeAnne. 1990. *Global Companies and Public Policy*. London: Pinter.

Kanter, R. 1977. *Men and Women of the Organization*. New York: Basic Books.

Kaplinsky, R. 1984. *Automation*. Harlow: Longman.

Kapuscinski, R. 1982. *Shah of Shahs*. New York: Harcourt Brace Jovanovich.

Karl, T. 1982. The political economy of petro-dollars: Oil and democracy in Venezuela. Unpublished Ph.D. dissertation, Stanford University, California.

Karl, T. 1997. *The Paradox of Plenty: Oil Booms and Petro-States*. Berkeley, CA: University of California Press.

Katouzian, H. 1981. *The Political Economy of Modern Iran 1926–1979*. New York: New York University Press.

Katz, D. 1994. *Just do it: The Nike Spirit in the Corporate World*. New York: Random House.

Kay, J. 1993. *Foundations of Corporate Success*. Oxford: Oxford University Press.

Kay, J. 1996. *The Business of Economics*. Oxford: Oxford University Press.

Kelly, J. 1983. *Scientific Management, Job Redesign and Work Performance*. London: Academic Press.

Kerfoot, D. and Knights, D. 1994. The gendered terrains of paternalism. In S. Wright (ed.). *Anthropology of Organisations*. London: Routledge.

Kimmel, M. 1988. *Changing Men*. London: Sage.

Kindleberger, C. P. 1988. The "new" multinationaliation of business. *ASEAN Economic Bulletin*, 5, 113–24.

King, A. 1993. Identity and difference: The internationalization of capital and the globalization of culture. In P. Knox (ed.). *The Restless Urban Landscape*. Englewood Cliffs, NJ: Prentice Hall.

Kinnear, D. and Graycar, A. 1982. Family care of elderly people: Australian perspectives. *Social Welfare Research Centre Research Paper 23*, University of New South Wales, Kensington NSW, Australia.

Kinnear, D. and Graycar, A. 1983. Non-institutional care of elderly people. In A. Graycar (ed.). *Retreat from the Welfare State: Australian Social Policy in the 1980s*. Sydney: Allen and Unwin.

Kirby, V. 1992. Addressing essentialism – thought on the corporeal. *Women's Studies Occasional Paper Series # 5*, University of Waikato, New Zealand.

Kirsch, S. 1995. The incredible shrinking world? Technology and the production of space. *Environment and Planning D: Society and Space*, 13, 529–55.

Kittler, F. A. 1990. *Discourse Networks 1800/1900*. Stanford: Stanford University Press.

Kobrin, S. J. 1987. Testing the bargaining hypothesis in the manufacturing sector in developing countries. *International Organization*, 41, 609–38.

Kondo, D. K. 1990. *Crafting Selves: Power Gender and Discourses of Identity in a Japanese Workplace*. Chicago: University of Chicago Press.

Krugman, P. 1990. *Rethinking International Trade*. Cambridge, MA: MIT Press.

Krugman, P. 1994. Competitiveness: A dangerous obsession. *Foreign Policy*, 73, 28–44.

Krugman, P. 1995. *Development, Geography and Economic Theory*. London: MIT Press.

Kuhn, T. S. 1962. *The Structure of Scientific Revolutions*. 2nd edn. Chicago: University of Chicago Press.

Lakatos, I. 1970. Falsification and the methodology of scientific research programmes. In I. Lakatos and A. Musgrave (eds). *Criticism and the Growth of Knowledge*. Cambridge: Cambridge University Press, 91–195.

Lall, S. 1985. *Multinationals, Technology and Exports: Selected Papers, A Study of Multinational and Local Firm Linkages in India*. New York: St Martin's.

Land, N. 1994. Machinic desire. *Textual Practice*, 7, 471–82.

Land, N. 1995. Machines and technocultural complexity. *Theory, Culture and Society*, 12, 131–40.

Landell Mills Associates. 1989. *A Market Survey for Gambian Horticultural Crops in the UK, Sweden, The Netherlands and The Federal Republic of Germany*. London: Commonwealth Secretariat.

Lane, C. 1997. The social regulation of inter-firm relations in Britain and Germany: Market rules, legal norms and technical standards. *Cambridge Journal of Economics*, 21, 197–215.

Lash, S. and Urry, J. 1994. *Economies of Signs and Space*. London: Sage.

Lash, S. and Urry, J. 1987. *The End of Organized Capitalism*. Cambridge: Polity.

Latour, B. 1986. The powers of association. In J. Law (ed.). *Power, Action and Belief*. London: Routledge and Kegan Paul, 264–80.

Latour, B. 1987. *Science in Action*. Oxford: Oxford University Press.

Latour, B. 1993. *We Have Never Been Modern*. Brighton: Harvester Wheatsheaf.

Law, J. 1986. On the methods of long-distance control: Vessels, navigation and the Portuguese route to India. *Sociological Review Monograph*, 32, 234–63.

Law, J. (ed.). 1991. *A Sociology of Monsters*. London: Routledge.

Law, J. 1994. *Organising Modernity*. Oxford: Blackwell.

Law, J. and Bijker, W. 1992. Postscript: Technology, stability and social theory. In W. Bijker and J. Law (eds). *Shaping Technology, Building Society: Studies in Sociotechnical Change*. London: MIT Press, 290–308.

Le Heron, R. 1994. *Globalized Agriculture*. Oxford: Pergamon.

Lebergott, S. 1966. Labor force and employment, 1800–1960. In National Bureau of Economic Research. *Output, Employment and Productivity after 1800*. New York: National Bureau of Economic Research, 117–210.

Lebowitz, M. 1977–8. Capital and the production of needs. *Science and Society*, 41, 430–48.

Lee, R. and Wills, J. (eds). 1997. *Geographies of Economies*. London: Arnold.

Lefebvre, H. 1991. *The Production of Space*. Oxford: Blackwell.

Leidner, R. 1991. *Fast Food, Fast Talk*. Berkeley, CA: University of California Press.

Levins, R. and Lewontin, R. 1985. *The Dialectical Biologist*. Cambridge, MA: Harvard University Press.

Lewontin, R. 1997. Genes, environment, and organisms. In R. B. Silvers (ed.). *Hidden Histories of Science*. London: Granta Books, 115–39.

Lewontin, R. 1993. *The Doctrine of DNA: Biology as Ideology*. Harmondsworth: Penguin.

Ley, D. 1980. Liberal ideology and the post-industrial city. *Annals of the Association of American Geographers*, 70, 238–58.

Leyshon, A. 1992. The transformation of regulatory order: Regulating the global economy and environment. *Geoforum*, 23, 249–67.

Leyshon, A. 1994. Under pressure: Finance, geo-economic competition and the rise and fall of Japan's postwar growth economy. In S. Corbridge, N. J. Thrift, and R. L. Martin (eds). *Money, Power and Space*. Oxford: Blackwell, 116–46.

Leyshon, A., Thrift, N. J., and Twommey, C. 1989. The rise of the British provincial financial centre. *Progress in Planning*, 31, 151–229.

Leyshon, A., Thrift, N., and Daniels, P. 1987. The urban and regional consequences of the restructuring of world financial markets: The case of the City of London. *Working Papers on Producer Services No. 4*, Department of Geography, University of Liverpool.

Leyshon, A. and Thrift, N. J. 1997. *Money/Space*. London: Routledge.

Leyshon, A. and Tickell, A. 1994. Money order? The discursive construction of Bretton Woods and the making and breaking of regulatory space. *Environment and Planning A*, 26, 1861–90.

Li, T. K. 1992. Why we invest in Canada. *Dialogue*, 6 (1), 8.

Lim, L. and Fong, P. E. 1982. Vertical linkages and multinational enterprises in developing countries. *World Development*, 10, 585–95.

Lindstrom, D. 1978. *Economic Development of the Philadelphia Region, 1810–50*. New York: Columbia University Press.

Lipietz, A. 1980. Inter-regional polarisation and the tertiarisation of space. *Papers of the Regional Science Association*, 44, 3–17.

Lipietz, A. 1986. New tendencies in the international division of labor: Regimes of accumulation and modes of social regulating. In A. J. Scott and M. Storper (eds). *Production, Work, Territory: The Geographical Anatomy of Industrial Capitalism*. Boston, MA: Allen and Unwin, 16–40.

Lipietz, A. 1992. *Towards a New Economic Order: Post-Fordism, Ecology and Democracy*. New York: Oxford University Press.

Livingstone, D., Luxton, M., and Seccombe, W. 1982. *Steelworker Families: Workplace, Household and Community in Hamilton, Ontario*. Ottawa: Social Sciences and Humanities Research Council of Canada.

Lloyd, G. 1993. *Being in Time*. London: Routledge.

Lloyd, P. E. and Dicken, P. 1977. *Location in Space*. London: Harper and Row.

Lodge, D. 2001. *Thinks*. New York: Viking Press.

Loh, M. 1987. On-the-job child care. *Australian Society*, April, 38.

Longino, H. 2002. *The Fate of Knowledge*. Princeton, NJ: Princeton University Press.

Lovering, J. 1989. The restructuring debate. In R. Peet and N. J. Thrift (eds). *New Models in Geography*. Vol. 1. London: Unwin Hyman, 198–223.

Lowe, D. 1995. *The Body in Late Capitalist USA*. Durham, NC: Duke University Press.

Lowe, L. 1996. *Immigrant Acts*. Durham, NC: Duke University Press.

Lubeck, P. 1993. Restructuring Nigeria's urban-industrial sector within the West African region: The interplay of crisis, linkages, and popular resistance. *International Journal of Urban and Regional Research*, 16, 7–23.

Lundvall, B. A. 1988. Innovation as an interactive process: From user–producer relations to the national system of innovation. In G. Dosi, C. Freeman, G. Silverberg, and L. Soete (eds). *Technical Change and Economic Theory*. London: Pinter, 349–69.

Lundvall, B. A. (ed.). 1992. *National Systems of Innovation: Towards a Theory of Innovation and Interactive Learning*. London: Pinter.

Lupton, D. 1986. *Food, the Body and the Self*. London: Sage.

Macías Picavea, R. 1899. *El Problema Nacional*. Madrid: Instituto de Estudios de Administración Local.

Mackintosh, M. 1989. *Gender, Class and Rural Transition*. Atlantic Highlands, NJ: Zed.

MacWilliam, S. 1990. Manufacturing, nationalism and democracy: A review essay. *Journal of Australian Political Economy*, 24, 100–20.

Malinowski, B. 1961. *Argonauts of the Western Pacific*. New York: E. P. Dutton.

Malmberg, A. 1996. Industrial geography: Agglomeration and local milieu. *Progress in Human Geography*, 20, 392–403.

Maluquer de Motes, J. 1983. La Despatrimonialización del Agua: Movilización de un Recurso Natural Fundamental. *Revista de Historia Económica*, 1, 76–96.

Mandel, E. 1980. *Long Waves of Capitalist Development: The Marxist Interpretation*. Cambridge: Cambridge University Press.

Mann, R. 1987. Development and the Sahel disaster: The case of The Gambia. *The Ecologist*, 17, 84–90.

Mansell, R. 1994. Introductory overview. In R. Mansell (ed.). *Management of Information and Communication Technologies*. London: ASLIB, 1–7.

Mark-Lawson, J., Savage, M., and Warde, A. 1985. Gender and local politics: Struggles over welfare policies, 1918–1939. In L. M. Murgatroyd, M. Savage, D. Shapiro, J. Urry, S. Walby, and A. Warde with J. Mark-Lawson (eds). *Localities, Class and Gender*. London: Pion, 195–215.

Marshall, A. 1920. *Principles of Economics*. London: Macmillan.

Marshall, A. 1932. *Industry and Trade*. 3rd edn. London: Macmillan.

Marshall, J. 1984. *Women Managers*. London: John Wiley.

Marshall, M. 1987. *Long Waves of Regional Development*. London: Macmillan.

Martin, E. 1986. The meaning of money in China and the United States. Mimeo, University of Rochester, New York.

Martin, E. 1992. *Flexible Bodies*. Boston, MA: Beacon Press.

Martin, R. L. 1994. Stateless monies, global financial integration and national autonomy: The end of geography? In S. Corbridge, N. J. Thrift, and R. L. Martin (eds). *Money, Power and Space*. Oxford: Blackwell, 253–78.

Martin, R. L. and Rowthorn, B. (eds). 1986. *The Geography of Deindustrialisation*. London: Macmillan.

Martin, R. and Sunley, P. 1997. The post-Keynesian state and the space economy. In R. Lee and J. Wills (eds), *Geographies of Economies*. London: Arnold, 278–89.

Martinez, J. I. and Jarillo, J. C. 1989. The evolution of research on coordination mechanisms in multinational corporations. *Journal of International Business Studies*, 20, 489–514.

Marvin, C. 1988. *When Old Technologies were New: Thinking about Electric Communication in the Late Nineteenth Century*. Oxford: Oxford University Press.

Marx, K. 1963. *Early Writings* (ed. T. Bottomore). Harmondsworth: Penguin.

Marx, K. 1967. *Capital*. Vol. 1. New York: International Publishers.

Marx, K. 1973. *Grundrisse*. New York: Vintage.

Marx, K. 1974. *Capital: Volume 1* (trans. B. Fowkes). New York: Vintage.

Marx, K. 1975. *Early Writings*. New York: Vintage.

Maskell, P., Eskelinen, H., Hannibalsson, I., Malmberg, A., and Vatne, E. 1998. *Competitiveness, Localised Learning and Regional Development*. London: Routledge.

Maskell, P. and Malmberg, A. 1999. Localised learning and industrial competitiveness. *Cambridge Journal of Economics*, 23, 167–85.

Mason, C. 1987. Venture capital in the United Kingdom: A geographical perspective. *National Westminster Bank Quarterly Review*, May, 47–59.

Massey, D. 1979. In what sense a regional problem? *Regional Studies*, 13, 233–43.

Massey, D. 1984. *Spatial Divisions of Labor*. New York: Methuen.

Massey, D. 1988. A new class of geography. *Marxism Today*, May, 12–17.

Massey, D. 1993. Power-geometry and a progressive sense of place. In J. Bird, B. Curtis, T. Putnam, G. Robertson, and L. Tickner (eds). *Mapping the Futures: Local Cultures, Global Change*. London: Routledge, 59–69.

Massey, D. and Allen, J. (eds). 1984. *Geography Matters!* Cambridge: Cambridge University Press.

Massey, D. and Allen, J. (eds). 1988. *Uneven Re-Development: Cities and Regions in Transition*. London: Hodder and Stoughton.

Massey, D. and Meegan, R. 1982. *The Anatomy of Job Loss*. London: Methuen.

Mateu Bellés, J. F. 1994. Planificación Hidráulica de las Divisiones Hidrológicas 1865–1899. Mimeo, Department of Geography, University of Valencia.

Mateu Bellés, J. F. 1995. Planificación Hidráulica de las Divisiones Hidrológicas. In A. Gil Olicna and A. Morales Gil (eds). *Planificaion Hidráulica en España*. Murcia: Fundación Caja del Mediterráneo, 69–106.

Matthews, J. 1990. Towards a new model of industrial development in Australia. *Industrial Relations Working Paper Series 78*, School of Industrial Relations and Organizational Behaviour, University of New South Wales, Kensington NSW, Australia, 1–21.

Maurice, M., Sellier, F., and Silvestre, J.-J. 1986. *The Social Foundations of Industrial Power: A Comparison of France and Germany*. Cambridge, MA: MIT Press.

Mauss, M. 1967. *The Gift*. New York: W. W. Norton.

McCay, B. and Acheson, D. (eds). 1987. *The Question of the Commons: The Culture and Ecology of Communal Resources*. Phoenix, AZ: Arizona University Press.

McCloskey, D. 1985. *The Rhetoric of Economics*. Madison, WI: University of Wisconsin Press.

McDowell, L. 1991. Life without father and Ford: A new gender order of post-Fordism. *Transactions of the Institute of British Geographers*, 16, 400–19.

McDowell, L. and Massey, D. 1984. A woman's place. In D. Massey and J. Allen (eds). *Geography Matters!* Cambridge: Cambridge University Press, 128–47.

McDowell, L. 1997. *Capital Culture: Gender at Work in the City*. Oxford: Blackwell.

McDowell, L. and Court, G. 1994a. Gender divisions of labour in the post-Fordist economy: The maintenance of occupational sex segregation in the financial services sector. *Environment and Planning A*, 26, 1397–418.

McDowell, L. and Court, G. 1994b. Missing subjects: Gender, power, and sexuality in merchant banking. *Economic Geography*, 70, 229–51.

McEvoy. A. F. 1986. *The Fisherman's Problem: Ecology and Law in the California Fisheries, 1850–1980*. Cambridge: Cambridge University Press.

McGrath, M. E. and Hoole, R. W. 1992. Manufacturing's new economies of scale. *Harvard Business Review*, May–June, 94–102.

McMichael, P. 1996. *Development and Social Change: A Global Perspective*. Thousand Oaks, CA: Pine Forge Press.

McPherson, M. and Posner, J. 1991. Structural adjustment in sub-Saharan Africa: Lessons from The Gambia. *Paper presented at the 11th annual symposium of the Association for Farming Systems Research Extension*, Michigan State University.

Metcalfe, J. S. 1998. *Evolutionary Economics and Creative Destruction*. London: Routledge.

MEWU [Metal and Engineering Workers' Union]. 1992. *The Australian Economy and Industry Development: Issues and Challenges for Metal Works in the 1990s*. Sydney: Metal and Engineering Workers' Union.

Mikita, J. 1994. The influence of the Canadian state on the migration of foreign domestic workers to Canada: A case study of the migration of Filipina nannies to Vancouver, British Columbia. Unpublished M.A. thesis, Department of Geography, Simon Fraser University.

Miller, D. 1993. *Unwrapping Christmas*. Oxford: Clarendon Press.

Miller, P. and Rose, N. 1990. Governing economic life. *Economy and Society*, 19, 1–31.

Mills, S. 1997. *Discourse*. London: Routledge.

Ministerio de Obras Públicas y Urbanismo. 1990. *Plan Hidrólogico – Síntesis de la Documentación Básica*. Madrid: Dirección General de Obras Hidraulicas.

Ministerio de Obras Públicas y Transportes 1993. *Plan Hidrólogico Nacional – Memoria*. Madrid: Dirección General de Obras Hidraulicas.

Mirowski, P. 1995. *More Heat than Light*. Cambridge: Cambridge University Press.

Mirowski, P. 1995. *Natural Images in Economic Thought*. Cambridge: Cambridge University Press.

Mishrah, R. 1984. *The Welfare State in Crisis*. Brighton: Harvester Press.

Misztal, B. 1996. *Trust in Modern Societies*. Cambridge: Polity.

Mitchell, W. 1995. *City of Bits: Space, Place and the Infobahn*. Cambridge, MA: MIT Press.

Miyoshi, M. 1997. A borderless world. In C. David and J. F. Chevrier (eds). *Politics-Poetics Documenta X*. Munich: Kassel, 102–202.

Mol, A. and Law, J. 1994. Regions, networks and fluids: Anaemia and social topology. *Social Studies of Science*, 24, 641–71.

Morales, R. 1994. *Flexible Production: Restructuring of the International Automobile Industry*. Cambridge: Polity.

Morgan, K. 1983. Restructuring steel: The crises of labour and locality in Britain. *International Journal of Urban and Regional Research*, 7, 175–201.

Morgan, K. 1997. The learning region: Institutions, innovation and regional renewal. *Regional Studies*, 31, 491–503.

Morgan, K. and Sayer, A. 1985. A modern industry in a mature region: The restructuring of labour–management relations. *International Journal of Urban and Regional Research*, 9, 383–404.

Morris, D. and Hergert, M. 1987. Trends in international collaborative agreements. *Columbia Journal of World Business*, 22, 15–21.

Morris, M. 1992. *Ecstasy and Economics*. Sydney: EMPress.

Mort, F. 1995. Archaeologies of city life: Commercial culture, masculinity and spatial relations in the 1980s. *Environment and Planning D: Society and Space*, 13, 505–630.

Mosco, V. 1996. *The Political Economy of Communication*. London: Sage.

Moss, P. 1995. Inscribing workplaces: The spatiality of the production process. *Growth and Change*, 26, 23–57.

Moulaert, F. and Swyngedouw, E. 1989. A regulation approach to the geography of flexible production systems. *Environment and Planning D: Society and Space*, 73, 27–45.

Moulaert, F., Swyngedouw, E., and Wilson, P. 1988. Spatial responses to Fordist and post-Fordist accumulation and regulation. *Papers of the Regional Science Association*, 64, 11–23.

Mowbray, M. 1984. Localism and austerity: The community can do it. *Journal of Australian Political Economy*, 16, 3–14.

Mowery, D. (ed.). 1988. *International Collaborative Ventures in US Manufacturing*. Cambridge, MA: Ballinger.

Mueller, F. and Loveridge, R. 1995. The "Second Industrial Divide"? The role of the large firm in the Baden-Wurttemberg Model. *Industrial and Corporate Change*, 4, 555–82.

Murdoch, J. 1995. Actor-networks and the evolution of economic forms: Combining description and explanation in theories of regulation, flexible specialisation and networks. *Environment and Planning A*, 27, 731–57.

Murdoch, J. and Marsden, T. 1995. The spatialization of politics: Local and national actor-spaces in environmental conflict. *Transactions of the Institute of British Geographers*, 20, 368–80.

Murdock, G. 1993. Communications and the constitution of modernity. *Media, Culture and Society*, 15, 521–39.

Murgatroyd, L. 1985. Occupational stratification and gender. In The Lancaster Regional Group. *Localities, Class and Gender*. London: Pion.

Murray, F. 1983. The decentralization of production – the decline of the mass-collective worker. *Capital and Class*, 19, 74–99.

Murray, R. 1972. Underdevelopment, the international firm and the international division of labour. In European Conference of the Society for International Development. *Towards a New World Economy*. Rotterdam: Rotterdam University Press, 159–247.

Mytelka, L. (ed.). 1992. *Strategic Partnerships: States, Firms, and International Competition*. Rutherford, NJ: Farleigh Dickinson University Press.

Nadal Reimat, E. 1981. El Regadío Durante la Restauración. *Revista Agricultura y Sociedad*, 19, 129–63.

Nath, K. 1985. Women and vegetable gardens in The Gambia: Action aid and rural development. *African Studies Center Working Paper No. 100*. Boston, MA: Boston University.

Natter, W. and Jones, J. P. 1993. Signposts toward a poststructuralist geography. In J. P. Jones, W. Natter, and T. R. Schatzki (eds). *Postmodern Contentions: Epochs, Politics, Space*. New York: Guilford,165–203.

Naughton-Treves, L. and Sundcrson, S. 1995. Property, politics and wildlife conservation. *World Development*, 23, 1265–75.

Negroponte, N. 1995. *Being Digital*. London: Hodder & Stoughton.

Nelson, K. 1986. Labor demand, labor supply and the suburbanization of low-wage office work. In A. J. Scott and M. Storper (eds). *Production, Work, Territory: The Geographical Anatomy of Industrial Capitalism*. Boston, MA: Allen and Unwin, 149–71.

Nelson, R. R. 1995. Recent evolutionary theorizing about economic change. *Journal of Economic Literature*, 33, 48–90.

Nelson, R. R. (ed.). 1993. *National Innovation Systems: A Comparative Analysis*. New York: Oxford University Press.

New York Times. 1997a. Peering into the shadows of corporate dealings. March 25, p. D1.

New York Times. 1997b. Nike's boot camps. March 31, p. A21.

New York Times. 1997c. Apparel industry group moves to end sweatshops. April 9, p. A14.

New York Times. 1997d. Accord to combat sweatshop labor faces obstacles. April 13, p. A1.

Niehans, J. 1990. *A History of Economic Theory*. Baltimore, MD: Johns Hopkins University Press.

Nike. 1996. 10-K statement of US Securities and Exchange Commission. SEC File 001-10635. Washington, DC: Securities and Exchange Commission.

Nixson, F. 1988. The political economy of bargaining with transnational corporations: Some preliminary observations. *Manchester Papers on Development*, 4, 377–90.

N'Jang, A. 1990. *Characteristics of Tourism in The Gambia*. Banjul: Ministry of Information and Tourism.

Nooteboom, B. 1999. Innovation, learning and industrial organisation. *Cambridge Journal of Economics*, 23, 127–50.

O'Connor, J. 1973. *The Fiscal Crisis of the State*. New York: St. Martin's.

O'Connor, J. 1989a. Capitalism, nature, socialism: A theoretical introduction. *Capitalism, Nature, Socialism*, 1, 11–38.

O'Connor, J. 1989b. Political economy and ecology of socialism and capitalism. *Capitalism, Nature, Socialism*, 1, 93–106.

O'Connor, J. 1989c. Uneven and combined development and ecological crisis: A theoretical introduction. *Race and Class*, 30, 1–11.

O'Neill, P. M. 1997. So what is internationalisation? Lessons from restructuring at Australia's "Mother Plant". In S. Conti and M. Taylor (eds). *Interdependent and Uneven Development: Global–Local Perspectives*. Aldershot: Ashgate, 283–308.

Oberhauser, A. 1987. Labour, production and the state: Decentralization of the French automobile industry. *Regional Studies*, 21, 445–58.

Oberhauser, A. 2000. Feminism and economic geography: Gendering work and working gender. In E. Sheppard and T. J. Barnes (eds). *Companion to Economic Geography*, Oxford: Blackwell, 60–76.

Offe, C. 1975. The theory of the capitalist state and the problem of policy formation. In L. N. Lindberg, R. Alford, C. Crouch, and C. Offe (eds). *Stress and Contradiction in Modern Capitalism*. Lexington, MA: Lexington Books, 125–44.

Offe, C. 1976. Political authority and class structures. In P. Connerton (ed.). *Critical Sociology*. London: Penguin, 388–421.

Offe, C. 1984. *Contradictions of the Welfare State*. London: Hutchinson.

Offe, C. 1985. *Disorganized Capitalism*. Cambridge: Polity.

Ohmae, K. 1990. *The Borderless World: Power and Strategy in the Interlinked Economy*. London: Collins.

Ohmae, K. 1995. *The End of the Nation State: The Rise of Regional Economies*. New York: Free Press.

Ohno, T. 1982. How the Toyota production system was created. *Japanese Economic Studies*, 10, 83–103.

Okoth-Ogendo, H. 1989. Some issues of theory in the study of tenure relations in Africa agriculture. *Africa*, 59, 56–72.

Olman, B. 1993. *Dialectical Investigations*. London: Routledge.

Ong, A. 1987. *Spirits of Resistance and Capitalist Development: Factory Women in Malaysia*. Albany, NY: State University of New York Press.

Ong, A. 1991. The gender and labor politics of postmodernity. *Annual Review of Anthropology*, 20, 279–309.

ORC [Opinion Research and Communications]. 1985. *The Great Debate: What Is IMF?* Owerri: Gunson Headway Press.

Organization for Economic Cooperation and Development. 1993. *International Direct Investment-Policies and Trends in the 1980s*. Paris: OECD.

Orillard, M. 1997. Cognitive networks and self-organisation in a complex socio-economic environment. In A. Amin and J. Hausner (eds). *Beyond Market and Hierarchy: Interactive Governance and Social Complexity*. Aldershot: Edward Elgar.

Orrù, M., Biggart N. W., and Hamilton, G. 1991. Organizational isomorphism in East Asia. In W. Powell and P. DiMaggio (eds). *The New Institutionalism in Organizational Analysis*. London: University of Chicago Press, 361–89.

Ortega, N. 1975. *Política Agraria y Dominación del Espacio*. Madrid: Editorial Ayuso.

Ortega, N. 1992. El Plan Nacionál de Obras Hidráulicas. In A. Gil Olcina and A. Morales Gil (eds). *Hitos Históricos de los Regadíos Españoles*. Madrid: Ministerio de Agricultura. Pesca y Alimentación, 335–64.

Ortí, A. 1976. Infortunio de Costa y Ambigüedad del Costismo: Una Reedición Acrítica de "Política Hidráulica." *Agricultura y Sociedad*, 1, 179–90.

Ortí, A. 1984. Política Hidráulica y Cuestión Social: Orígenes, Etapas y Significados del Regeneracionismo Hidráulica de Joaquín Costa. *Revista Agricultura y Sociedad*, 32, 11–107.

Ortí, A. 1994. Política Hidráulica y Emancipación Campesina en el Discurso Político del Populismo Rural Español entre las dos Repúblicas contemporáneas. In J. Romero and C. Giménez (eds). *Regadíos y Estructuras de Poder*. Alicante: Instituto de Cultura "Juan Gil-Albert," Diputación de Alicante, 241–67.

Ostry, S. 1990. *Governments and Corporations in a Shrinking World*. New York: Council on Foreign Relations.

O'Sullivan, M. 2000. *Contests for Corporate Control: Corporate Governance in the United States and Germany*. Oxford: Oxford University Press.

Pahl, R. 1988. *On Work*, Oxford: Blackwell.

Pahl, R. 1995. *After Success*. Cambridge: Polity.

Pankhurst, F. 1984. *Workplace Child Care and Migrant Parents*. Canberra: National Women's Advisory Council/AGPS.

Park, M. 1983. *Travels into the Interior of Africa*. London: Eland.

Parkes, D. and Thrift, N. J. 1980. *Times, Spaces, Places*. Chichester: John Wiley.

Parry, J. and Bloch, M. (eds). 1989. *Money and the Morality of Exchange*. Cambridge: Cambridge University Press.

Patel, P. and Pavitt, K. 1991. Large firms in the production of the world's technology: An important case of non-globalization. *Journal of International Business Studies*, 22, 1–21.

Pauly, L. W. and Reich, S. 1997. National structures and multinational corporate behavior: Enduring differences in the age of globalization. *International Organization*, 51, 1–30.

Pavitt, K. and Patel, P. 1995. Corporate technology strategies and national systems of innovation. In J. Allouche and G. Pogorel (eds). *Technology Management and Corporate Strategies: A Tricontinental Perspective*. Amsterdam: Elsevier Science, 313–40.

Peck, J. 1996. *Work-place: The Social Regulation of Labor Markets*. New York: Guilford.

Peck, J. and Tickell, A. 1994. Searching for a new institutional fix: The after-Fordist crisis and global–local disorder. In A. Amin (ed.). *Post-Fordism: A Reader*. Oxford: Blackwell, 280–316.

Pérez De La Dehesa, R. 1966. *El Pensamiento de Costa y su Influncia en el 98*. Madrid: Editorial Sociedad de Estudios y Publicaciones.

Pérez, J. 1999. *Historia de España*. Barcelona: Editorial Crítica.

Perlmutter, H. V. 1969. The tortuous evolution of the multinational corporation. *Columbia Journal of World Business*, January–February, 24–31.

Petras, J. and Morley, M. 1983. Petrodollars and the state: The failure of state capitalist development in Venezuela. *Third World Quarterly*, 5, 8–27.

Philippine Women Centre. 1998. Commentary on "Not just numbers." Brief to the Honourable Lucienne Robillard, Minister of Citizenship and Immigration, March 9, 1998.

Philips, D. 1987. *Structural Adjustment of What, by Whom, for Whom?* Lagos: Centre for Management Development.

Phillips, A. 1989. *Divided Loyalties*. London: Virago.

Picciotto, S. 1991. The internationalization of the state. *Capital and Class*, 43, 43–63.

Pigou, A. 1920. *The Economics of Welfare*. London: Macmillan.

Pile, S. 1994. Cybergeography: 50 years of *Environment and Planning A*. *Environment and Planning A*, 26, 1815–23.

Pimlott, B. 1978. *The Englishman's Christmas*. Hassocks: Harvester Press.

Piore, M. and Sabel, C. 1984. *The Second Industrial Divide: Possibilities for Prosperity*. New York: Basic Books.

Pitelis, C. 1991. Beyond the nation-state? The transnational firm and the nation-state. *Capital and Class*, 43, 131–52.

Plant, S. 1994. Beyond the screens: Film, cyberpunk and cyberfeminism. *Variant*, 16, 12–17.

Platteau, J.-P. 1994a. Behind the market stage where real societies exist – Part I: The role of public and private order institutions. *Journal of Development Studies*, 30, 533–77.

Platteau, J.-P. 1994b. Behind the market stage where real societies exist – Part II: The role of moral norms. *Journal of Development Studies*, 30, 753–817.

Plotkin, H. C. 1994. *Darwin, Machines and the Nature of Knowledge*. Harmondsworth: Penguin.

Plummer, P. 2000. The modeling tradition. In E. S. Sheppard and T. J. Barnes (eds). *A Companion to Economic Geography*. Oxford: Blackwell, 27–40.

Polanyi, K. 1944. *The Great Transformation*. New York: Rinehart.

Polanyi, M. 1958. *Personal knowledge: Towards a Post-Critical Philosophy*. London: Routledge and Kegan Paul.

Polanyi, M. 1966. *The Tacit Dimension*. London: Routledge and Kegan Paul.

Pollert, A. 1981. *Girls, Wives, Factory Lives*. London: Macmillan.

Poovey, M. 1995. *Making a Social Body*. Chicago: University of Chicago Press.

Porter, G. and Livesay, H. 1971. *Merchants and Manufacturers*. Baltimore: Johns Hopkins University Press.

Porter, M. E. 1980. *Competitive Strategy*. New York: Free Press.

Porter, M. E. 1990. *The Competitive Advantage of Nations*. New York: Free Press.

Porter, M. E. 1994. The role of location in competition. *Journal of the Economics of Business*, 1, 35–9.

Porteres, R. 1970. Primary cradles of agriculture in the African continent. In J. Fage and R. Oliver (eds). *Papers in African Prehistory*. Cambridge: Cambridge University Press, 43–58.

Poster, M. 1989. *Critical Theory and Poststructuralism: In Search of a Context*. Ithaca, NY: Cornell University Press.

Poynter, T. A. 1985. *Multinational Enterprises and Government Intervention*. London: Croom Helm.

Pratt, G. 1990. Feminist analyses of the restructuring of urban life. *Urban Geography*, 11, 594–605.

Pratt, G. 1997. Stereotypes and ambivalence: Nanny agents' stereotypes of domestic workers in Vancouver, B.C. *Gender, Place and Culture*, 4, 159–77.

Pred, A. 1966. *The Spatial Dynamics of Urban Growth in the United States, 1800–1914*. Cambridge, MA: Harvard University Press.

Pred, A. 1973. *Urban Growth and the Circulation of Information, 1790–1840*. Cambridge, MA: Harvard University Press.

Pred, A. 1980. *Urban Growth and City Systems in the United States, 1840–60*. Cambridge, MA: Harvard University Press.

Pred, A. 1992. Languages of everyday practice and resistance: Stockholm at the end of the nineteenth century. In A. Pred and M. Watts (eds). *Reworking Modernity: Capitalisms and Symbolic Discontents*. New Brunswick, NJ: Rutgers University Press, 118–54.

Pringle, R. 1989. *Secretaries Talk*. London: Verso.

Putnam, R. 1993. *Making Democracy Work*. Princeton, NJ: Princeton University Press.

Rada, J. 1982. Structure and behaviour of the semiconductor industry. Mimeo, United Nations Center on Transnational Corporations, New York.

Radice, H. 1984. The national economy – a Keynesian myth? *Capital and Class*, 22, 111–40.

Rafael, V. 1997. "Your grief is our gossip": Overseas Filipinos and other spectral presences. *Public Culture*, 9, 267–91.

Rahman, A. K. 1949. Unpublished notes on land tenure in Genieri, courtesy of David Gamble.

Redclift, M. 1987. The reproduction of nature and the reproduction of the species. *Antipode*, 19, 222–30.

Reich, R. 1990. Who is us? *Harvard Business Review*, January–February, 53–64.

Reich, R. 1991. *The Work of Nations: Preparing Ourselves for 21st Century Capitalism*. New York: Vintage Books.

Reich, S. 1989. Roads to follow: Regulating direct foreign investment. *International Organization*, 43, 543–84.

Resnick, S. and Wolff, R. 1987. *Knowledge and Class: A Marxian Critique of Political Economy*. Chicago: Chicago University Press.

Restad, P. L. 1995. *Christmas in America. A History*. New York: Oxford University Press.

Riley, F. 1967. Fur Seal Industry of the Pribil of Islands, 1786–1965. *Bureau of Commercial Fisheries Circular No. 275*, U.S. Department of Interior, Fisheries and Wildlife Service, Washington, DC.

Ritzer, G. 1996. *The McDonaldization of Society*. Thousand Oaks, CA: Pine Forge Press.

Roberts, R. and Emel, J. 1991. Uneven development and the tragedy of the commons: Competing images for nature-society analysis. *Economic Geography*, 67, 247–71.

Robins, K. 1995. Cyberspace and the world we live in. In M. Featherstone and R. Burrows (eds). *Cyberpunk/Cyberspace/Cyberbodies*. London: Sage, 135–56.

Robinson, J. F. F. 1983. State planning of spatial change: Compromise and contradiction in Peterlee New Town. In J. Anderson, S. Duncan, and R. Hudson (eds). *Redundant Spaces in Cities and Regions?* London: Academic Press, 263–84.

Robinson, J. F. F. and Sadler, D. 1985. Routine action, reproduction of social relations and the place market: Consett after the closure. *Environment and Planning D: Society and Space*, 3, 109–20.

Rogers, G. 1976. An economic analysis of the Pribil of Islands. 1870–1946. *U.S. Department of Justice, Indian Claims Commission Dockets 352 and 369*, Institute of Social, Economic and Government Research, University of Alaska, Fairbanks AL.

Roppel, A. Y. and Davey, S. P. 1965. Evolution of fur seal management on the Pribilof Islands. *Journal of Wildlife Management*, 29, 448–63.

Rorty, R. 1989. *Contingency, Irony and Solidarity*. Cambridge: Cambridge University Press.

Rosdolsky, R. 1977. The *Making of Marx's* Capital. London: Pluto Press.

Rose, G. 1993. *Feminism and Geography: The Limits of Geographical Knowledge*. Minneapolis: University of Minnesota Press.

Ross, R. J. S. and Trachte, K. C. 1990. *Global Capitalism*. Albany, NY: State University of New York Press.

Ruan, D. 1993, Interpersonal networks and workplace controls in urban China. *Australian Journal of Chinese Affairs*, 20, 89–105.

Ruccio, D. 1992. Failure of socialism, failure of socialists? *Rethinking Marxism*, 5, 7–22.

Rugman, A. M. and Verbeke, A. 1992. Multinational enterprise and national economic policy. In P. J. Buckely and M. Casson (eds). *Multinational Enterprises in the World Economy: Essays in honor of John Dunning*. Aldershot: Edward Elgar, 194–211.

Ruiz, J. M. 1993. La Situación de los Recursos Hídricos en España, 1992. In L. R. Brown (ed.). *La Situación en el Mundo – 1993*. Madrid: Ediciones Apóstrofe S.L., 385–450.

Russell Smith, J. 1913. *Industrial and Commercial Geography*. New York: Henry Holt & Co.

Russo, M. 1985. Technical change and the industrial district: The role of interfirm relations in the growth and transformation of ceramic tile production in Italy. *Research Policy*, 14, 329–43.

Sabel, C. 1989. Flexible specialization and the re-emergence of regional economies. In P. Hirst and J. Zeitlin (eds). *Reversing Industrial Decline?* Oxford: Berg, 17–70.

Sabel, C. 1994. Learning by monitoring: The institutions of economic development. In N. Smelser and R. Swedberg (eds). *Handbook of Economic Sociology*. Princeton, NJ: Princeton University Press, 137–65.

Sabel, C. and Zeitlin, J. 1985. Historical alternatives to mass production: Politics, markets and technology in nineteenth-century industrialization. *Past and Present*, 108, 133–76.

Sack, R. D. 1980. *Conceptions of Space in Social Thought*. London: Macmillan.

Sadler, D. 1984. Works closure at British Steel and the nature of the state. *Political Geography Quarterly*, 3, 297–311.

Sahlins, M. 1972. *Stone Age Economics*. New York: Aldine.

Salais, R. and Storper, M. 1992. The four "worlds" of contemporary industry. *Cambridge Journal of Economics*, 16, 169–93.

Salzinger, L. 1997. From high heels to swathed bodies: Gendered meanings under production in Mexico's export-processing industry. *Feminist Studies*, 43, 549–74.

Samuels, W. 1995. The present state of institutional economics. *Cambridge Journal of Economics*, 19, 569–90.

Sassen, S. 1990. *The Global City*. Princeton, NJ: Princeton University Press.

Sassen, S. 1996. Analytic borderlands: Race, gender and representation in the new city. In A. King (ed.). *Re-Presenting the City*. London: Macmillan.

Savage, M., Barlow, J., Dickens, P., and Fielding, T. 1992. *Property, Bureaucracy and Culture*. London: Routledge.

Sawhney, H. 1996. Information superhighway: Metaphors as midwives. *Media, Culture and Society*, 18, 291–314.

Saxenian, A. 1983. The urban contradictions of Silicon Valley. *International Journal of Urban and Regional Research*, 17, 237–61.

Saxenian, A. 1994. *Regional Advantage: Culture and Competition in Silicon Valley and Route 128*. Cambridge, MA: Harvard University Press.

Sayer, A. 1982a. Abstraction: A realist approach. *Radical Philosophy*, 28, 6–15.

Sayer, A. 1982b. Explanation in economic geography. *Progress in Human Geography*, 6, 68–88.

Sayer, A. 1984. *Method in Social Science: A Realist Approach*. London: Hutchinson.

Schmidt, A. 1971. *The Concept of Nature in Marx*. London: New Left Books.

Schoenberger, E. 1987. Technological and organizational change in automobile production: Spatial implications. *Regional Studies*, 21, 199–214.

Schoenberger, E. 1997. *The Cultural Crisis of the Firm*. Oxford: Blackwell.

Schoenberger, E. 1999. The firm in the region and the region in the firm. In T. J. Barnes and M. S. Gertler (eds). *The New Industrial Geography: Regions, Regulation and Institutions*. London: Routledge, 205–24.

Schonberger, R. J. 1982. *Japanese Management Techniques: Nine Hidden Lessons in Simplicity*. New York: Free Press.

Schroeder, R. 1992. *Shady Practice: Gendered Tenure in The Gambia's Garden/Orchards*. Yundum: Department of Agriculture Horticultural Unit and Oxfam America.

Schroeder, R. 1994. Cyberculture, cyborg postmodernism and the sociology of virtual reality technologies. *Futures*, 26, 519–28.

Schroeder, R. and Watts, M. 1991. Struggling over strategies, fighting over food: Adjusting to food commercialization among Mandinka peasants. *Research in Rural Sociology and Development*, 5, 45–72.

Sciberras, E., Swords-Isherwood, N., and Senker, P. 1978. Competition, technical change and manpower in electronic capital equipment: A study of the UK minicomputer industry. *Occasional Paper No. 8*, Science Policy Research Unit, University of Sussex, Brighton, Sussex.

Scott, A. M. (ed.). 1994. *Gender Segregation and Social Change*. Oxford: Oxford University Press.

Scott, A. 1994. Hark, the herald cash tills ring . . . *Financial Times*, December 24, p. 7.

Scott, A. J. 1988a. *Metropolis: From the Division of Labor to Urban Form*. Berkeley and Los Angeles: University of California Press.

Scott, A. J. 1988b. *New Industrial Spaces*. London: Pion.

Scott, A. J. 1995. The geographic foundations of industrial performance. *Competition and Change*, 1, 51–66.

Scott, A. J. 1996. Regional motors of the global economy. *Futures*, 28, 391–411.

Scott, A. J. 2000. Economic geography: the great half century. *Cambridge Journal of Economics*, 24(4), 483–504.

Scott, A. J. and Angel, D. 1987. The US semiconductor industry: A locational analysis. *Environment and Planning A*, 19, 875–912.

Scott, A. J. and Storper, M. 1987. High technology industry and regional development: A theoretical critique and reconstruction. *International Social Science Journal*, 112, 215–32.

Scott, A. J. and Storper, M. 1986a. Industrial change and territorial organization: A summing up. In A. J. Scott and M. Storper (eds). *Production, Work, Territory*. Boston, MA: Allen and Unwin, 301–11.

Scott, A. J. and Storper, M. (eds). 1986b. *Production, Work, Territory*. Boston, MA: Allen and Unwin.

Scott, J. 1988a. Deconstructing equality versus difference; or, the uses of post-structuralist theory for feminism. *Feminist Studies*, 14, 33–50.

Scott, J. 1988b. *Gender and the Politics of History*. New York: Columbia University Press.

Sennett, R. 1977. *The Fall of Public Man*. New York: Knopf.

Sercovich, F. C. 1984. The case study of Brazil. *World Development*, 12, 575–600.

Serequerberhan, T. 1990. Karl Marx and African emancipatory thought: A critique of Marx's Eurocentric metaphysics. *Praxis International*, 10, 161–81.

Serres, M. and Latour, B. 1995. *Conversations on Science, Culture, and Time*. Ann Arbor, MI: University of Michigan Press.

Shapin, S. 1994. *A Social History of Truth*. Chicago: Chicago University Press.

Shell, M. 1982. *Money, Language and Thought: Literary and Philosophic Economies from the Medieval to the Modern Era.* Los Angeles: University of California Press.

Sheppard, E. S. 2000. Competition in space and between places. In E. S. Sheppard and T. J. Barnes (eds). *A Companion to Economic Geography.* Oxford: Blackwell, 169–86.

Sheppard, E. S. 2002. The spaces and times of globalization: Place, scale, networks, and positionality. *Economic Geography*, 78, 307–30.

Sheppard, E. S. and Barnes, T. J. (eds). 2000. *A Companion to Economic Geography.* Oxford: Blackwell.

Shohat, E. and Stam, R. 1994. *Unthinking Eurocentrism: Multiculturalism and the Media.* New York: Routledge.

Simmel, G. 1978. *The Philosophy of Money.* London: Routledge.

Simon, H. A. 1959. Theories of decision-making in economic and behavioral sciences. *American Economic Review*, 49, 253–83.

Singelmann, J. 1978. *From Agriculture to Services.* Beverly Hills: Sage.

Sklair, L. 1991. *Sociology of the Global System.* Baltimore: Johns Hopkins University Press.

Skocpol, T. 1995. Bringing the state back in: Strategies of analysis in current research. In P. B. Evans, D. Rueschemeyer, and T. Skocpol (eds). *Bringing the State Back In.* Cambridge: Cambridge University Press, 1–43.

Slater, D. 1992. On the borders of social theory: Learning from other regions. *Society and Space*, 10, 307–28.

Slouka, M. 1995. *War of the Worlds: The Assault on Reality.* London: Abacus.

Smelser, N. and Baltes, P (eds). 2001. *International Encyclopedia of the Social & Behavioral Sciences.* Oxford: Pergamon, 26 vols.

Smelser, N. and Swedberg. R. (eds). 1994. *The Handbook of Economic Sociology.* Princeton: Princeton University Press.

Smelt, S. 1980. Money's place in society. *British Journal of Society*, 31, 204–23.

Smith, A. 1776. *The Wealth of Nations.* Harmondsworth: Penguin.

Smith, F., Jack, I., and Singh, R. 1985. *The Survey of Rural Women's Vegetable Growing and Marketing Programme.* Banjul: Action Aid.

Smith, G. 1994. Toward an ethnography of idiosyncratic forms of livelihood. *International Journal of Urban and Regional Research*, 18, 71–87.

Smith, M. and Marx, L. 1995. *Does Technology Drive History? The Dilemma of Technological Determination.* Cambridge, MA: MIT Press.

Smith, N. 1984. *Uneven Development: Nature, Capital, and the Production of Space.* Oxford: Blackwell.

Smith, N. 1996. The production of nature. In G. Robertson, M. Mash, L. Tickner, J. Bird, B. Curtis, and T. Putnam (eds). *Future-Natural: Nature/Science/Culture.* London: Routledge, 35–54.

Smith, N. and O'Keefe, P. 1985. Geography, Marx and concept of nature. *Antipode* 17, 79–88.

Smith, P. and Brown, P. 1983. Industrial change and Scottish nationalism since 1945. In J. Anderson, S. Duncan, and R. Hudson (eds). *Redundant Spaces in Cities and Regions?* London: Academic Press, 241–62.

Solinas, G. 1982. Labour market segmentation and workers careers: The case of the Italian knitwear industry. *Cambridge Journal of Economics*, 6, 331–52.

Solinger, D. J. 1987. Uncertain paternalism: Tensions in recent regional restructuring in China. *International Regional Science Review*, 11, 23–42.

Sparke, M. 1995. Writing on patriarchal missiles: The chauvinism of the "Gulf War" and the limits of critique. *Environment and Planning A*, 27, 1061–89.

Spivak, G. C. 1988. Can the subaltern speak? In C. Nelson and L. Grossberg (eds). *Marxism and the Interpretation of Culture.* Urbana, IL: University of Illinois Press, 271–313.

Sproul, C. 1993. Mastering the other: an ecofeminist analysis of neoclassical economics. PhD dissertation. Department of Economics, University of Massachusetts-Amherst.

Stanback, T. 1979. *Understanding the Service Economy*. Baltimore: Johns Hopkins University Press.

Stanback, T. and Noyelle, T. 1982. *Cities in Transition*. Totowa, NJ: Allenhheld.

Stanback, T., Bearse, P., Noyelle, T., and Karasek, R. 1981. *Services: The New Economy*. Totowa, NJ: Allenheld.

Staple, G. 1993. Telegeography and the explosion of place: Why the network which is bringing the world together is also pulling it apart. *CITI Working Papers No. 656*, Columbia University, New York.

Stefik, M. 1996. *Internet Dreams: Archetypes, Myths and Metaphors*. Cambridge, MA: MIT Press.

Stiell, B. and England, K. 1997. Domestic distinctions: Constructing difference among paid domestic workers in Toronto. *Gender, Place and Culture*, 4, 339–59.

Stigler, G. J. 1951. The division of labor is limited by the extent of the market. *Journal of Political Economy*, 59, 185–93.

Stigler, G. 1971. The theory of economic regulation. *Bell Journal of Economics and Management*, 2, 3–21.

Stiglitz, J. E. and Weiss, A. 1991. Credit rationing in markets with imperfect information. In G. Mankiw and D. Romer (eds). *New Keynesian Economics*. Cambridge, MA: MIT Press, 247–76.

Stilwell, F. 1991. Wages policy and the Accord. *Journal of Australian Political Economy*, 28, 27–53.

Stopford, J. M. and Strange, S. 1991. *Rival States, Rival Firms: Competition for World Market Shares*. Cambridge: Cambridge University Press.

Storper, M. 1996. The world of the city: Local relations in a global economy. Mimeo, School of Public Policy and Social Research, University of California, Los Angeles.

Storper, M. 1997. *The Regional World*. New York: Guilford.

Storper, M. and Christopherson, S. 1987. Flexible specialization and regional industrial agglomeration: The case of the US motion picture industry. *Annals of the Association of American Geographers*, 77, 104–17.

Storper, M. and Salais, R. 1997. *Worlds of Production: The Action Frameworks of the Economy*. Cambridge, MA: Harvard University Press.

Strange, S. 1997. *The Retreat of the State*. Cambridge: Cambridge University Press.

Strathern, M. (ed.). 1995. *Shifting Contexts*, London: Routledge.

Streeck, W. 1996. Lean production in the German automobile industry: A test case for convergence theory. In S. Berger and R. Dore (eds). *National Diversity and Global Capitalism*. Ithaca, NY: Cornell University Press, 138–70.

Sumberg, J. and Okali, C. 1987. *Workshop on NGO-sponsored Vegetable Gardening Projects in The Gambia*. Yundum: Department of Agriculture Horticultural Unit and Oxfam America.

Sunley, P. 1996. Context in economic geography: The relevance of pragmatism. *Progress in Human Geography*, 20, 338–55.

Swedberg, R. 1994. Markets as social structures. In N. J. Smelser and R. Swedberg (eds). *The Handbook of Economic Sociology*. Princeton and New York: Princeton University Press and Russell Sage Foundation, 255–82.

Swyngedouw, E. 1993. Communication, mobility and the struggle for power over space. In G. Giannopoulos and A. Gillespie (eds). *Transport and Communications in the New Europe*. London: Belhaven, 305–25.

Swyngedouw, E. 2000: The Marxian alternative: Historical-geographical materialism and the political economy of capitalism. In E. Sheppard and T. J. Barnes (eds). *Companion to Economic Geography*. Oxford: Blackwell, 41–60.

The Economist. 1996a. Past masters: Present pupils. November 23, p. 16.

The Economist. 1996b. Showing Europe's firms the way. July 13, p. 15.

Thorne, L. 1997. Towards ethical trading space? Unpublished Ph.D. dissertation, Department of Geographical Sciences, University of Bristol.

Thrift, N. J. 1977. Time and theory in human geography: Part 1. *Progress in Human Geography*, 1, 65–103.

Thrift, N. J. 1986. The geography of international economic disorder. In N. J. Thrift and P. Williams (eds). *Class and Space*. London: Pion, 207–53.

Thrift, N. J. 1989. Images of social change. In C. Hammnett. L. McDowell, and P. Sarre (eds). *The Changing Social Structure*. London: Sage, 12–42.

Thrift, N. J. 1993. The light fantastic: Culture, postmodernism and the image. In G. L. Clark, D. K. Forbes, and R. Francis (eds). *Multiculturalism, Difference and Postmodernism*. Melbourne: Longman Cheshire, 1–21.

Thrift, N. J. 1994. On the social and cultural determinants of international financial centres. In S. Corbridge, N. J. Thrift, and R. L. Martin (eds). *Money, Power and Space*. Oxford: Blackwell, 327–55.

Thrift, N. J. 1995. A hyperactive world. In R. Johnston, P. Taylor, and M. Watts (eds). *Geographies of Global Change*. Oxford: Basil Blackwell, 18–35.

Thrift, N. J. 1996a. New urban eras and old technological fears: Reconfiguring the goodwill of electronic things. *Urban Studies*, 33, 1463–93.

Thrift, N. J. 1996b. *Spatial Formations*. London: Sage.

Thrift, N. J. 2000. Pandora's box? Cultural geographies of economics. In G. Clark, M. Gertler, and M. Feldman (eds). *The Oxford Handbook of Economic Geography*. Oxford: Oxford University Press, 689–704.

Thrift, N. and Olds, K. 1996. Refiguring the economic in economic geography. *Progress in Human Geography*, 20, 311–37.

Thu Nguyen, D. and Alexander, J. 1996. The coming of cyber space-time and the end of polity. In R. Shields (ed.). *Cultures of Internet: Virtual Spaces, Real Histories, Living Bodies*. London: Sage, 125–32.

Tickell, A. and Peck, J. 1992. Accumulation, regulation and the geographies of post-Fordism: Missing links in regulationist research. *Progress in Human Geography*, 16, 190–218.

Tickell, A. and Peck, J. 1995. Social regulation after Fordism: Regulation theory, neoliberalism and the global–local nexus. *Economy and Society*, 24, 357–86.

Tolliday, S. and Zeitlin, J. 1986. Introduction: Between Fordism and flexibility. In S. Tolliday and J. Zeitlin (eds). *The Automobile Industry and its Workers: Between Fordism and Flexibility*. Cambridge: Polity, 1–26.

Tomlinson, J. 1982. *The Unequal struggle: British Socialism and the Capitalist Enterprise*. Andover: Methuen.

Torres Campos, R. 1907. Nuestros Ríos. *Boletín de la Sociedad Geográfica de Madrid*, 37, 7–32.

Tryon, R. 1917. *Household Manufacturers in the United States, 1640–1860*. Chicago: University of Chicago Press.

Tuan, Y.-F. 1977. *Space and Place: The Perspective of Experience*. London: Arnold.

Tuñón De Lara, M. 1971. *Medio Siglo de Cultura Española 1885–1936*. 2nd edn. Madrid: Editorial Tecnos.

Turner, B. 1986. Simmel, rationalisation and the sociology of money. *Sociological Review*, 34, 93–114.

Tyson, L. D. 1991. They are not us. *The American Prospect*, Winter, 49–54.

Tyson, L. D. 1993. *Who's Bashing Whom? Trade Conflict in High-Technology Industries*. Washington, DC: Institute for International Economics.

Underhill, G. 1994. Conceptualising the changing global order. In R. Stubbs and G. Underhill (eds). *Political Economy and the Changing Global Order*. London: Macmillan.

United Nations Center on Transnational Corporations. 1991. *World Investment Report 1991: The Triad in Foreign Direct Investment*. New York: United Nations.

United Nations Commission on Trade and Development. 1986. *Post-Harvest Handling and Quality Control for Export Development of Fresh Horticultural Produce*. Geneva: United Nations Commission on Trade and Development.

United Nations Development Program. 1977. *Development of the Gambia River Basin: Multi-disciplinary Mission and Multidonor Mission. Programme of action*. New York: United Nations Development Program.

Usman, B. 1986. *Nigeria Against the IMF*. Kaduna: Vanguard Printers.

Vance, J. 1970. *The Merchant's World*. Englewood Cliffs, NJ: Prentice-Hall.

Vernon, R. 1966. International investment and international trade in the product life cycle. *Quarterly Journal of Economics*, 80, 190–207.

Vernon, R. and Spar, D. L. 1989. *Beyond Globalism: Remaking American Foreign Economic Policy*. New York: Free Press.

Vilar, P. 1984. *A History of Gold and Money*. London: Verso.

Villanueva Larraya, G. 1991. *La "Politica Hidráulica" durante la Restauración 1874–1923*. Madrid: Universidad Nacional de Educación a Distancia.

Virilio, P. 1993. The third interval: A critical transition. In V. Andermatt-Conley (ed.). *Rethinking Technologies*. Minneapolis: University of Minnesota Press, 3–10.

Vogel, E. 1989. *One Step Ahead in China: Guangdong Under Reform*. Cambridge, MA: Harvard University Press.

Von Bohm-Bawerk, E. 1891. *The Positive Theory of Capital*. New York: G. E. Stechert.

Wade, L. L. and Gates, J. B. 1990. A new tariff map of the United States (House of Representatives). *Political Geography Quarterly*, 9, 284–304.

Walby, S. 1990. *Theorizing Patriarchy*. Oxford: Blackwell.

Walker, R. 1984. Class, division of labor and employment in space. In D. Gregory and J. Urry (eds). *Social Relations and Spatial Structures*. London: Macmillan: 164–89.

Walker R. and Greenberg, D. 1982. Post-industrialism and political reform in the city: A critique. *Antipode*, 14, 17–32.

Walker, R. and Storper, M. 1983. The theory of labor and the theory of location. *International Journal of Urban and Regional Research*, 7, 1–44.

Wallerstein, I. 1974. *The Modern World System*. New York: Academic Press.

Ward, C. 1997. *Reflected in Water – A Crisis of Social Responsibility*. London: Cassell.

Waring, M. 1988. *Counting for Nothing: What Men Value and What Women are Worth*. Sydney: Allen and Unwin.

Wark, M. 1994. *Virtual Geography*. Bloomington, IN: Indiana University Press.

Watts, M. 1984. State, oil and accumulation: From boom to crisis. *Environment and Planning D: Society and Space*, 2, 403–28.

Watts, M. 1992. The shock of modernity. In A. Pred and M. Watts (eds). *Reworking Modernity*. New York: Rutgers University Press, 21–64.

Watts, M. 2000. Political ecology. In E. S. Sheppard and T. J. Barnes (eds). *A Companion to Economic Geography*. Oxford: Blackwell, 257–74.

Watts, M. and Lubeck, P. 1989. Structural adjustment, academic freedom and human rights in Nigeria. *Bulletin of Concerned Africanist Scholars*, 28.

Watts, M. and McCarthy, J. 1997. Nature as artifice, nature as artefact: Development, environment and modernity in the late twentieth century. In R. Lee and J. Wills (eds). *Geographies of Economies*. London: Arnold, 71–86.

Webb, P. 1989. *Intrahousehold Decisionmaking and Resource Control: The Effects of Rice Commercialization in West Africa*. Washington, DC: International Food Policy Research Institute.

Webber, M. 1964. The urban place and the nonplace urban realm. In M. Webber, J. Dyckman, D. Foley, A. Guttenberg, W. Wheaton, and C. Whurster (eds). *Explorations into Urban Structure*. Philadelphia, PA: University of Pennsylvania Press, 79–153.

Webber, M. 1994. Enter the dragon: Lessons for Australia from Northeast Asia. *Environment and Planning A*, 26, 71–94.

Weil, P. 1973. Wet rice, women, and adaptation in The Gambia. *Rural Africana*, 19, 20–29.

Weil, P. 1982. Agrarian production, intensification and underdevelopment: Mandinka women of The Gambia in time perspective. In *Proceedings of the Title XII conference on women in development*, University of Delaware, Newark, DE.

Weisbrot, M. and Sforza-Roderick, M. 1996. *Baltimore's Living Wage Law*. Washington, DC: Preamble Center for Public Policy.

Wells, L. T. 1983. *Third World Multinationals: The Rise of Foreign Investment from Developing Countries*. Cambridge, MA: MIT Press.

Wenger, E. C. 1998. *Communities of Practice: Learning, Meaning and Identity*. Cambridge: Cambridge University Press.

Wenger, E. C. and Snyder, W. M. 2000. Communities of practice: The organizational frontier. *Harvard Business Review*, 78, 139–45.

West Coast Domestic Workers' Association. 1993. Brief to Employment Standards Act Review Committee, West Coast Domestic Workers' Association, #302, 119 West Pender Street, Vancouver, BC.

Westaway, J. 1974. The spatial hierarchy of business organizations. *Regional Studies*, 8, 145–55.

Wever, K. 1995. *Negotiating Competitiveness: Employment Relations and Organizational Innovation in Germany and the United States*. Cambridge, MA: Harvard Business School Press.

Whatmore, S. 1994. Global agro-food complexes and the refashioning of rural Europe. In A. Amin and N. J. Thrift (eds). *Globalization, Institutions and Regional Development in Europe*. Oxford: Oxford University Press, 46–67.

Whatmore, S. 1997. Dissecting the autonomous self: Hybrid cartographies for a relational ethics. *Environment and Planning D: Society and Space*, 15, 37–53.

Whatmore, S. and Boucher, S. 1993. Bargaining with nature: The discourse and practice of environmental planning gain. *Transactions of the Institute of British Geographers*, 18, 166–78.

White, E. 1981. The international projection of firms from Latin American countries. In K. Kumar and M. G. McLeod (eds). *Multinationals from Developing Countries*. Lexington, MA: Lexington Books, 155–86.

White, G. 1993. Towards a political analysis of markets. *IDS Bulletin*, 24, 4–11.

White, J. 1995. Two days to go. *The Independent*, December 23, p. 6.

White, M. 1986. Child care funding: A change of direction. *Australian Journal of Early Childhood*, 11, 38–41.

Whitley, R. 1991. The social construction of business systems in East Asia. *Organization Studies*, 12, 1–28.

Whitley, R. 1992a. *Business Systems in East Asia: Firms, Markets and Societies*. London: Sage.

Whitley, R. (ed.). 1992b. *European Business Systems: Firms and Markets in their National Contexts*. London: Sage.

Whitley, R. 1998. Internationalization and varieties of capitalism: The limited effects of cross national coordination of economic activities on the nature of business systems. *Review of International Political Economy*, 5, 445–81.

Whitley, R. 1999. *Divergent Capitalisms: The Social Structuring and Change of Business Systems*. Oxford: Oxford University Press.

Willems-Braun, B. 1997. Buried epistemologies: The politics of nature in (post)colonial British Columbia. *Annals of the Association of American Geographers*, 87, 3–32.

Williams, R. 1976. *Keywords: A vocabulary of society and nature*. London: Fontana.

Williams, R. 1980. *Problems in Materialism and Culture*. London: Verso.

Williams, S. 1995. All I want for Christmas . . . *The Independent*, December 16, p. 5.

Williamson, B. 1982. *Class, Culture and Community*. Henley: Routledge and Kegan Paul.

Williamson, O. 1975. *Markets and Hierarchies: Analysis and Antitrust Implications*. New York: Free Press.

Williamson, O. 1985. *The Economic Institutions of Capitalism*. New York: Free Press.

Womack, J., Jones, D., and Roos, D. 1990. *The Machine that Changed the World*. New York: Macmillan.

Wong, S.-L. 1991. Chinese entrepreneurs and business trust. In G. Hamilton (ed.). *Business Networks and Economic Development in East and Southeast Asia*. Hong Kong: Centre of Asian Studies, University of Hong Kong, 13–29.

World Bank. 1981. *The Gambia: Basic needs in The Gambia*. Washington, DC: World Bank.

World Bank. 1990. *Women in Development project: Staff appraisal report*. Washington, DC: World Bank.

Wright, M. W. 1996. Third world women and the geography of skill. Unpublished Ph.D. dissertation, Department of Geography and Environmental Engineering, The Johns Hopkins University, Baltimore, MD.

Wright, M. W. 1997. Crossing the factory frontier: Gender, place and power in a Mexican *maquiladorda*. *Antipode*, 29, 278–302.

Wright, M. W. 1998. The maquiladora mestiza and a feminist border politics: Revisiting Anzaldua. *Hypatia: A Journal of Feminist Philosophy*, 13, 114–31.

Wright, E. O. 1978. *Class, Crisis and the State*. London: New Left Books.

Wright, E. O. 1985. *Classes*. London: Verso.

Wrigley, N. and Lowe, M. (eds). 1995. *Retailing, Consumption and Capital: Towards the New Retail Geography*. Harlow: Longman.

Yang, M. M-h. 1988. The modernity of power in the Chinese socialist order. *Cultural Anthropology*, 3, 408–427.

Yang, M. M-h. 1989. The gift economy and state power in China. *Comparative Studies in Society and History*, 31, 25–54.

Yang, M. M-h. 1994. *Gifts, Favors and Banquets: The Art of Social Relationships in China*. Ithaca, NY: Cornell University Press.

Yergin, D. 1991. *The Prize: The Epic Quest for Oil, Money and Power*. New York: Simon and Schuster.

Yoffie, D. B. and Milner, H. V. 1989. An alternative to free trade or protectionism: Why corporations seek strategic trade policy. *California Management Review*, 31, 111– 31.

Young, A. 1928. Increasing returns and economic progress. *Economic Journal*, 38, 527–42.

Young, I. M. 1990. *Justice and the Politics of Difference*. Princeton, NJ: Princeton University Press.

Zelizer, V. 1989. The social meaning of money: Special monies. *American Journal of Sociology*, 95, 342–77.

Zhang, A. and Zou, G. 1994. Foreign trade decentralization and its impact on central–local relations. In J. Hao and L. Zhimin (eds). *Changing Central– Local Relations in China: Reform and State Capacity*. Boulder, CO: Westview Press, 153–80.

Zimmerer, K. 1991. Wetland production and smallholder persistence: Agricultural change in a highland Peruvian region. *Annals of the Association of American Geographers*, 81, 443–63.

Zonis, M. 1991. *Majestic Failure: The Fall of the Shah*. Chicago: University of Chicago Press.

Zuboff, S. 1988. *In the Age of the Smart Machine*. London: Heinemann.

Zucker, L. 1986. Production of trust: Institutional sources of economic structure, 1840–1920. *Research in Organizational Behaviour*, 8, 53–111.

Zukin, S. 1991. *Landscapes of Power*. Berkeley, CA: University of California Press.

Zukin, S. 1995. *The Cultures of Cities*. Oxford: Blackwell.

Zukin, S. and DiMaggio, P. (eds). 1990. *Structures of Capital*. Cambridge: Cambridge University Press.

Index

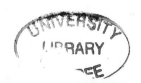